# A CHRONOLOGY OF MEDICINE AND RELATED SCIENCES

# A CHRONOLOGY OF MEDICINE AND RELATED SCIENCES

## Leslie T. Morton
### FLA

FORMERLY
LIBRARIAN, NATIONAL INSTITUTE FOR MEDICAL RESEARCH, LONDON

and

## Robert J. Moore
### BA, ALA, MIInfSc, MIBiol

LIBRARIAN
NATIONAL INSTITUTE FOR MEDICAL RESEARCH, LONDON

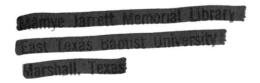
SCOLAR
PRESS

Published by
SCOLAR PRESS
Gower House
Croft Road
Aldershot
Hants GU11 3HR
England

Ashgate Publishing Company
Old Post Road
Brookfield
Vermont 05036-9704
USA


British Library Cataloguing-in-Publication Data

Morton, Leslie T. (Leslie Thomas)
A chronology of medicine and related sciences
1.Medicine – History – Chronology
I.Title II.Moore, Robert J.
610.9

Library of Congress Cataloging-in-Publication Data
Morton, Leslie T. (Leslie Thomas)
A chronology of medicine and related sciences / Leslie T. Morton and Robert J. Moore.
Includes indexes.
ISBN 1-85928-215-6
1. Medicine—History—Chronology. 2. Medical sciences—History—Chronology.
3. Medicine—Bibliography. 4. Medical sciences—Bibliography. I. Moore, Robert
J. II. Title. (DNLM: 1. History of Medicine—chronology. 2. Science—History—
chronology. WZ 30 M889c 1997)
R133.M717 1997    96-42257
610'.9—dc20    CIP

ISBN 1-85928-215-6

Printed in Great Britain at the University Press, Cambridge

# Contents

# Introduction

When we first considered the possible value of a chronology of medicine and related sciences – which would give, year-by-year, significant events in medicine and the supporting sciences, together with information about the participants – we surveyed existing sources of this type. These seemed to fall into various categories, i.e. specialized chronologies such as D'Arcy Power and Thompson's *Chronologia Medica* (1923), Darmstaedter's *Handbuch der Geschichte der Naturwissenschaften und der Technik* (1902) (neither of which gives bibliographical references), general chronologies which included medicine and science, and bibliographical sources which covered the field using a subject arrangement, such as *Morton's Medical Bibliography* (5th edition, 1991).

After some thought we came to the conclusion that such a work would be worth while and, on consulting potential users, we were encouraged to proceed. The responses we received confirmed that a strictly chronological approach had an important role to play. The general feeling was that such a work would be of considerable use in giving a good indication of the overall development of the field, showing the relationship of advances in specific areas to those in others, revealing historical coincidences, providing information on individuals, given in the year of their birth, and would supplement the standard historical texts and bibliographies. We hope that this work will be of value to those interested in the history of medicine, to those needing a broad outline of the development of medicine and details of particular fields or individuals, and to those requiring information on anniversaries.

It should be borne in mind that this work does not claim to be exhaustive but aims to portray the broad development of a wide field over a long period – and that the need to maintain an historical perspective means that the advances of more recent decades are probably better identified from contemporary medical/scientific review publications. One difficulty in adequately covering the period since the Second World War is that before that time 'breakthroughs' are more easily identified and in most cases can be related to a specific publication. In many fields knowledge was relatively shallow, fewer people were working in specific areas, competition was present but there was a freer and easier exchange of information. In recent decades, discoveries are to a far greater extent 'incremental'; this could be explained by research areas being much narrower, more and larger groups working on them, the increased speed and sophistication of the methodology of research, and faster and more frequent publication of results influenced by intense competition. Despite these obstacles we consider our attempt broadly to chart the progress of medicine to be worth while.

**Arrangement**

Each year's entries are divided into three groups:

a) *Events*: Nobel Prizes, the establishment of institutions, hospitals, societies, journals, etc., significant publications in periodicals or monographs.

b) *Births*: entries for individuals whose work appears in the chronology, which include a description, actual day of birth (where known), year of death, and details of all contributions recorded in the *Chronology*.

c) *Deaths*: entries giving name, year of birth (where the full entry for the individual appears), and subject keywords to assist users in anniversaries of individuals active in related fields.

Both a) and b) include a brief annotation and a bibliographical reference. We also include, when available, the citation number of *Morton's Medical Bibliography*, 5th edition, edited by Jeremy M. Norman, 1991; we feel it will be useful for readers to be able to refer readily to *MMB* (which is arranged by subject and contains far more bibliographical entries than the *Chronology*) and thus readily obtain further information on the development of a particular subject.

A *Journal code list* is also included, as are an *Index of personal names*, normally referring to the birth entry, and *Subject index*, referring to subjects or corporate/institutional names.

We should like to record our appreciation of the kind cooperation of Mr Norman in allowing us to make use of material appearing in many annotations in *MMB*. We have benefited from his interest and encouragement throughout the preparation of the *Chronology* and hope that it will, through its different arrangement and scope, be seen as complementary to his work.

We should like also to record our indebtedness to the Librarian and his staff at the Wellcome Institute for the History of Medicine for invaluable assistance, and our gratitude to Dr E.M. Tansey, also of the Wellcome Institute, for her firm encouragement at times when our efforts and spirits flagged.

We are particularly grateful to Rachel Lynch and her colleagues at Scolar Press for the technical advice and help throughout the preparation of this book.

As compilers we are aware that our work will inevitably be imperfect, but are not prepared to blame our errors on the computer or on others. We shall be grateful to learn of any sins of commission or omission that our readers may discover.

L.T.M.
R.J.M.

# Chronology of medicine and related sciences

**3000 BC:**

(*c*) **Edwin Smith Papyrus**. A papyrus acquired by Edwin Smith at Luxor, Egypt, in 1862. Facsimile and hieroglyphic transliteration, with translation and commentary, 1930. Consists of **Egyptian surgical** case reports. *5547*

**2700 BC:**

(*c*) **Emperor Shen Nung** (2727 BC), putative father and founder of **Chinese medicine**, is said to have originated the Chinese materia medica; the *Pentsao* (Great herbal) is attributed to him and the *Nei-ching* (Canon of medicine) to **Emperor Huang-ti** (2697 BC). Paul Unschuld's *Medicine in China*, 1985, a comprehensive analytical history of therapeutic concepts and practices, includes a number of primary texts in translation. The *History of Chinese medicine*, by K. Chimin Wong and Wu Lien-Tei, 2nd edn, 1936, is the first important contribution to the subject. *6495.4, 6493*

**1792–1750 BC:**

**Hammurabi**, *King of Babylon* (*fl*); he laid down a legal code, discovered in the library of Ashurbanipal in 1902. Clauses 215–223 relate to medicine and lay down the fees payable to **Babylonian physicians** following successful treatment, and the punishment for an unsuccessful outcome. R.E. Harper, *The code of Hammurabi, King of Babylon, about 2000 BC*, 1904. *1*

**1550 BC:**

(*c*) **Ebers Papyrus**. Purchased by Georg Ebers, 1873. The most complete record of ancient **Egyptian medicine**. Written in hieratic script. Facsimile published, with partial translation, 1875. Translation by B. Ebbell, 1875. *2*

**1400–1200 BC:**

(*c*) **Ayurveda**. The Ayurvedic system is the most ancient system of **Hindu medicine**. Published, 3 vols, 1901–7 (reprinted 1984). *8*

**800 BC–AD 78:**

**Charaka** is said to have lived at dates varying between 800 BC and AD 78. The Charaka Samhita is one of the most ancient and complete systems of **Hindu medicine**. Published in Sanskrit, 1877; published with translations in English, Hindi and Gujerati, 6 vols, 1949. *9, 10*

**500–400 BC:**

(*c*) **Susruta**. The system of medicine taught by Dhanwantari and compiled by Susruta. The Susruta Samhita and the Charaka Samhita formed the groundwork of all subsequent **Hindu medical and surgical systems**. First published in the West in Latin translation, 5 vols, 1844–55. English translation, 2nd ed., 1963. *11*

**460–*c*375 BC:**

**Hippocrates**; Greek physician, taught at Cos. The major figure in **Greek medicine**. Although he contributed to a significant body of writing, it is difficult to determine which are his and which are by his contemporaries at Cos and Cnidus. They are the earliest extant source of

Western medical thought and practice. He gave the earliest known description of **puerperal fever** (*Works* ... transl. by W.H.S. Jones, 1923, **2**, 127). Credited with the first mention of **epilepsy** in children (*Works*, 1923, **1**, 193). *13, 14, 15, 16, 16.1, 4807, 6267*

### 430–425 BC:
**Plague of Athens**

### 384–322 BC:
**Aristotle**; Greek physicist, **biologist** and **comparative anatomist**. His *Works* were published in English (12 vols, 1908–1952); the Loeb Classical Library has published them in 23 vols (Greek and Latin text), 1926–70. *See also* W.D. Ross, *Aristotle*, revised ed., 1964. *17, 18*

### 360 BC:
**Diocles** *of Carystus fl.*, Greek physician. Author of numerous works of which only fragments remain. First physician to use a collection of the Hippocratic writings. Wrote the first book on **anatomy**, and used that term in the title. First to complete a **herbal** and thus has claim to be the founder of **pharmacy**. His *Fragments* were published in 1901. *16.2*

### 350 BC:
**Herophilus**, Greek anatomist, physiologist and physician *fl.* He laid the foundations of the scientific study of **anatomy** and **physiology**. Existing texts of his works, with English translations, in *Herophilus*, by H. von Staden, 1989. *18.1*

### 340 BC:
**Praxagoras** *of Cos*, Greek physician, born. Wrote several books on **Greek medicine and science**. *Fragments* of his works were published in 1958. *16.3*

### 304 BC:
(*c*) **Erasistratus**, Greek anatomist and physiologist, born. He wrote many works on **anatomy** and **physiology** of which none have survived. With his teacher, **Herophilus**, he laid the foundations for the scientific study of these subjects, providing a basis and stimulus for the investigations of **Galen**. He studied the **brain**, stressed the importance of **hygiene**, and pioneered the study of **pathological anatomy**.

### 130–40 BC:
(*c*) **Asclepiades**, Greek physician in Rome, where he did much to overcome the Roman prejudice against **Greek medicine**. Fragments of his works were published, 1955. *19, 1984*

### AD

### 30
30:1 The *De medicina* of **Aulus Aurelius Cornelius Celsus** (25 BC to AD 50), oldest medical document after the Hippocratic writings, one of the first medical works to be printed, and the first Western **history of medicine**. Written around AD 30 and first published in 1478. Latin and English text in Loeb Classical Library, 3 vols, 1935–38. *20, 21, 6375*

### 50
50:1 **Athenaeus** *fl.* Greek physician, founded the Pneumatic School of **Greek medicine**. Selections from his writings were published in *Corpus Medicorum Graecorum*, **VI**, 1–3, 1926–31 (reprinted 1964).

**54**

54:1 The *De materia medica* of **Dioscorides** (*fl.* AD 54–68), Greek physician, is the authoritative source on the **materia medica** of antiquity. It first appeared in print in 1499. *1786*

**81**

81:1 **Aretaeus** *of Cappadocia* (81–?138) Greek physician. He left a number of excellent descriptions of disease. He is considered to have given the first accurate description of **diabetes mellitus** (recorded in his *Extant works*, [Adams] p. 338, 485) and the first unmistakable description of **diphtheria** (*Extant works*, p. 253, The *Extant works* were first published in Latin, 1552, and in Greek, 1554. A Greek text with Latin translation, ed. F. Adams, appeared in 1856 (reprinted 1972). *22, 3925, 5046*

**100**

100:1 **Rufus** *of Ephesus fl.* Greek surgeon. Particularly remembered for his work on **haemostasis**; he wrote much, including a treatise on **gout**, and he added much to the **materia medica**. A Greek-French edition of his works appeared in 1879. *23, 24*

**129**

129:1 **Galen** (129–199) Greek physician born in Pergamum. He is second only to Hippocrates in ancient **Greek medicine** but his **anatomy** and **physiology** suffered from his lack of opportunity to examine human cadavers. His extensive writings dominated medicine until the time of Vesalius, Harvey and Boerhaave. His *Opera Omnia* appeared in the *Corpus Medicorum Graecorum* (20 vols, 1914–, so far published). *27, 28, 29*

**250**

250:1 **Antyllus** *fl.* Greek surgeon, notable for his work on the surgical management of **aneurysm**. A compilation of his works by Oribasius was published, in German, in *Janus*, 1847, **2**, 298–329, 744–71; 1848, **3**, 166–84. *30*

**369**

369:1 **Hospital of St Basil** erected at **Caesarea** by **Justinian**

**400**

400:1 (*c.*) First **hospital in Western Europe** (Rome) founded by **Fabiola**, a wealthy Roman lady, who became a nurse

**500**

500:1 **Caelius Aurelianus** *fl.*, Roman physician, gave one of the best early descriptions of **epilepsy** and a humane treatment of **insanity**; in his *Tardarum passionum libri V*, first printed in 1529, English translation, 1950. *4808.1, 4915.1*

**502**

502:1 **Aetius** *of Amida* (502–575), Byzantine physician. His *Tetrabiblion* collected together the works of others which might otherwise have been forgotten. The standard Greek edition of his works (books 1–8) is in the *Corpus Medicorum Graecorum*, **VIII**, 1–2, 1935–50. *33*

**542**

542:1 **Hospitals** founded at **Lyons** by Childebert I, and at **Arles** by Caesarius

**580**

580:1 **Hospital** at **Merida** founded by Bishop Masona

**583**

583:1 **Council of Lyons** interdicts migration of **lepers**

**610**

610:1 **Hospital** of **St John the Almsgiver** at **Ephesus**

**625**

625:1 **Paul** *of Aegina* (625–690), Greek physician and surgeon in Alexandria. He wrote an epitome of **medicine** in seven books, which transmitted the whole range of classical **Greek medical** thought to the Islamic world. *The Seven Books of Paulus Aegineta* were translated from the Greek by F. Adams and published, 3 vols, 1844–47. *36, 37*

**651**

651:1 **Hospital**: **Hôtel Dieu** founded by St Landry, Bishop of **Paris**

**738**

738:1 **School of Montpellier** founded

**776**

776:1 **Rabanus Maurus** (776–856), Archbishop of Mainz. His *De sermonum proprietate sive Opus de universo*, ?1467, is the earliest known printed book to include a section on medicine. *2190*

**794**

794:1 **Leprosarium** at **St Albans**, England

**830**

830:1 **Monastic infirmary** at St Gall

**848**

848:1 **School of Salerno** first mentioned. At Salerno, not far from Naples there arose something resembling a medical school. From it came the *Regimen sanitatis*, a poem on the laws of health, which went through hundreds of editions. An English version by John Harington (1560–1612) with a history of the school was published by F.R. Packard, 1920. It reached its peak in the 12th–13th centuries, then declined and was formally suppressed by Napoleon in 1811. *49–51*

**854**

854:1 **Rhazes** [Abu Bakr Muhammad ibn Zakariya al-Razi] (854–925(*c*)), Persian physician born; ranks with Hippocrates and Galen as one of the founders of **clinical medicine**. Wrote popular textbook, the *Almansor* (first printed 1476) and the *Al-Hawi* or *Continens*, 1486 (which may however have been written posthumously by his students. First to devote an entire treatise, *De curis puerorum in prima aetate*, to **diseases of children** (first printed in his *Opuscula mediolani*, 1481. First to differentiate between **measles** and **smallpox** and to give the first medical account of smallpox, *c*910, the first Arabic and Latin account of which, *De variolis et morbillis commentarius*, was published in 1766; see *A treatise on the smallpox and measles*, transl. by A. Greenhill, 1848. Died 925 or 935. *39, 40, 923, 6313, 5441, 5404*

**930**

930:1 **Haly Abbas** [Ali-ibn-al-'Abbas al Majusi] (930–994), Persian physician. Author of the *Almaleki*, the leading medical treatise for 100 years, until displaced by Avicenna. It was first printed in 1492. *42*

**936**

936:1 **Abulcasis** [Abul Quasim] (936–1013), Arabian physician, born Cordova, Spain. Wrote the *Al-Tasrif*, a medical and surgical encyclopaedia. A Latin translation of the medical section, *Liber theoricae nec non practicae Alsaharavii*, printed 1519, includes his, probably first, description of **haemophilia** (fol.145). The surgical section was a complete and illustrated treatise, with illustrations of surgical (including dental) instruments (first printed in Latin, 1497; definitive edition of Arabic text with English translation, 1973). *3048, 5550*

936:2 **Hospital of St Peter and St Leonard** established in **York**, England

**962**

962:1 **Hospice of St Bernard**, Great St Bernard Pass

**980**

980:1 **Avicenna** [Abu-'Ali al-Husain ibn Abdallah ibn-Sina] (980–1037), Persian physician. His *Liber canonis*, first printed 1473, is a complete exposition of Galenism, 'the final codification of all Graeco-Arabic medicine' (Neuberger). A translation of Book 1 of the *Canon* appeared in 1930. *43, 44, 45*

**1070**

1070:1 **Knights Hospitallers (Order of St John of Jerusalem)** founded

**1080**

1080:1 **Leper hospital** at Harbledown, near **Canterbury**, England (rebuilt 1276)

**1088**

1088:1 **University of Bologna** founded

**1092**

1092:1 **Avenzoar** [Abumeron] (1092?–1162), born in Spain; considered the greatest of the **Moslem physicians** in the Western Caliphate; possibly a Jew. Wrote *Liber Teisir*, first printed 1490. *47*

**1107**

1107:1 **St Thomas' Hospital, London**, founded (as part of the Priory of St Mary Overie); rebuilt 1215

**1110**

1110:1 **University of Paris** founded 1110–13: (granted Papal licence 1215)

**1123**

1123:1 **St Bartholomew's Hospital, London**, founded

**1126**

1126:1 **Averroes** (1126–1198), born in Cordova, Spain. Wrote the *Kitab-al-Kullyat* or *Colliget*, 'an attempt to found a system of medicine upon the neo-Platonic modification of Aristotle's philosophy' (Garrison); printed 1482. *48*

## 1135

1135:1 **Maimonides** [Moses ben Maimon] (1135–1204), Jewish physician born in Cordova, Spain; settled in Cairo (1166) where he became Court Physician to Saladin and head of the Jewish community. His medical writings include a treatise on **poisons**, another on personal **hygiene** and a collection of aphorisms derived from Galen. *53*

## 1136

1136:1 **St Cross Hospital, Winchester**, founded

1136:2 **Leper hospital** at Ilford, near **London**

## 1180

1180:1 **University of Montpellier** founded, declared a free **school of medicine**, 1181

## 1193

1193:1 **Albertus Magnus** [Albert von Bollstadt] (1193–1280), Dominican monk, the most eminent naturalist of the 13th century. Works include *De animalibus*, printed 1478, and *De vegetabilibus, libri vii*, printed 1867, which includes some therapeutic information. *276, 1792*

## 1201

1201:1 Community of scholars at **Oxford** first termed a **university**; chartered 1244 (oldest university in Britain

## 1210

1210:1 Guglielmo da **Salicetti** (1210 (*c*)–1277), Italian surgeon, professor at Bologna. His book on **surgery**, written around 1275 and first printed in 1474 is the first medical book printed in Italian and the most important on the subject during the 13th century. *5552*

1210:2 **Ibn-al Nafis** (1210:2 (*c*)–1288), Syrian physician; in a commentary on Avicenna's *Canon* he described the **lesser circulation** in 1268 (1933, *QSGM* **4**:37). *753*

## 1222

1222:1 **University of Padua** formed by migration of students from Bologna

## 1223

1223:1 Community of scholars at **Cambridge** first called a **university**

## 1224

1224:1 **University of Naples** founded

## 1231

1231:1 **Salerno** constituted a **medical school** by Frederick II, Holy Roman Emperor; suppressed by Napoleon I, 1811

## 1235

1235:1 **Arnold of Villanova** (1235–1312), Catalan Arabist, associated with the medical school at **Montpellier**

**1240**

1240: 1 **University of Siena** founded

**1247**

1247: 1 **Hospital of St Mary of Bethlehem** founded in **London**; by 1377 used as a **lunatic asylum** ('**Bedlam**'); removed from London in 1930

**1250**

1250: 1 **Petrus de Abano** (1250–1315), Italian physician and philosopher; compiled first printed book on **toxicology**, *Tractatus de venenis*, printed in 1472. *2070*

**1256**

1256: 1 **Chateau Bicêtre** built by Bishop of Winchester at **Chantilly**; became hospital, almshouse and prison, 1657

**1257**

1257: 1 **Sorbonne** founded in **Paris**

**1260**

1260: 1 Henri de **Mondeville** (1260–1320 ?), French anatomist and surgeon. Lectured on anatomy at Montpellier. Regarded as a key link between Italian and French surgery. His *Anatomie* (1304) was first printed under the editorship of Julius Pagel, Berlin, 1889. His *Chirurgie*, also edited by Pagel, was first printed in 1892. *362, 5554*

**1266**

1266: 1 **University of Perugia** founded

**1270**

1270: 1 **Spectacles** produced by Venetian glassmakers, 1270–1280

1270: 2 Simone **Cordo** [Simon Januensis] (1270–1303), Italian physician; compiled the first printed **medical dictionary**, *Synonyma medicinae, seu clavis sanationis*, 1473. *6788*

**1275**

1275: 1 **Mondino de'Luzzi** [Mundinus] (1275(?)–1326), Italian anatomist; author of *Anothomia*, first modern book devoted solely to **anatomy**, written in 1316 and published in 1478. *361*

**1280**

1280: 1 **John** *of Gaddesden* (1280(?)–1361), English physician; his *Rosa anglica* is the first printed medical book compiled by an Englishman, *c*1314, published 1492. *2191*

**1290**

1290: 1 **Lanfrancho** *of Milan* [Lanfranc] (*fl.* 1290–1296), Italian surgeon, regarded as the founder of French **surgery**; his *Chirurgia magna*, completed in 1296 was first published in 1490, with French (1490) and English (1565) translations. *5553*

**1298**

1298: 1 Guy de **Chauliac** (?1298–1368), French surgeon. The most eminent surgeon of his time; wrote *La pratique en chirurgie* in 1363 (the first French medical book printed, 1478). *5556*

**1305**

1305:1 **City hospital** established at **Siena**

**1307**

1307:1 **John** *of Arderne* English surgeon (1307–?1380); his operation for **anal fissure** was his most important contribution to **surgery**, *c*1376; in his *Treatise of the fistulae in the fundament* (printed 1588). Also wrote *De arte phisicale et de cirurgia*, 1370. *3416*

**1321**

1321:1 **Medical school** established at **Perugia**

**1341**

1341:1 Public **dissection** at **Padua** by Gentile da **Foligno**

**1345**

1345:1 **Apothecary shop** in **London**

1345:2 **School of Medicine** established at **Valencia**, 1345–1350

**1346**

1346:1 **Edward III** issues ordinance driving **lepers** from **London**

**1348**

1348:1 A **Board of Health** and **quarantine regulations** established at **Venice**

1348:2 **University of Prague** established

1348:3 **Black death** introduced into **Europe** from Africa and Asia, 1348–1350

**1349**

1349:1 **University of Florence** founded

**1350**

1350:1 **Joannes Actuarius** *fl.*, Byzantine physician, wrote the most complete medieval treatise on **urinoscopy**, *De urinis libri vii*, first published in Latin, 1529. *2666*

**1357**

1357:1 **Public hygiene**: a royal order in **London** against throwing filth into River Thames

**1361**

1361:1 **University of Pavia** founded

**1364**

1364:1 **Jagiellonian University**, with medical faculty, created at **Krakow**

**1365**

1365:1 **University of Vienna** founded

**1383**

1383:1 **Quarantine** established at **Marseilles** harbour

**1386**

1386:1 **Heidelberg University** founded

**1388**

1388:1 First **English Sanitary Act** (17. Richard II)

**1400**

1400:1 (*c*) **Ortolff von Bayrlant**, German physician, born; compiled first German pharmacopoeia, *Artzneibuch*, 1477. *1794*

**1403**

1403:1 **Quarantine** lazaretto established at **Venice**

**1404**

1404:1 First public **dissection** at **Vienna**

**1411**

1411:1 **University of St Andrews** (Scotland) founded

1411:2 **Leprosarium** at **St Jørgen's Hospital, Bergen**, first mentioned

**1422**

1422:1 **University of Parma** founded

**1425**

1425:1 **University of Louvain** founded

**1429**

1429:1 **Syphilis** mentioned in Italian and Swiss archives, 1429–1431

**1440**

1440:1 Ulrich **Ellenbog**, German physician, born; his tract on the diseases of miners, *Von den gifftigen besen Tempffen und Reuchen*, written in 1473 and published in 1524, was the first known work on occupational medicine and toxicology. Died 1499. *2118*

**1445**

1445:1 Gabriele **Zerbi**, Italian anatomist, born; published *Gerontocomia*, first printed work on geriatrics, 1489. Died 1505. *1589.1*

**1450**

1450:1 (*c*) Hieronymus **Brunschwig** [Braunschweig], Alsatian surgeon, born; wrote the first printed treatise on surgery in German; *Dis ist das buch der Cirurgia Hantwirckung der wundartzny*, 1497. Died *c*1512. *5559*

**1451**

1451:1 **University of Glasgow** founded

**1452**

1452:1 **Barber surgeons** of **Hamburg** incorporated

---

1452:2 **Leonardo da Vinci**, Italian artist and scientist, born 15 Apr. 'Founder of iconographic and physiologic anatomy' (Garrison). *Leonardo da Vinci on the human body. The anatomical, physiological and embryological drawings. With translations, emendations, and biographical introduction*, by C.D. O'Malley and J.B. de C.M. Saunders, 1952. *Corpus of the anatomical studies in the collection ... at Windsor Castle.* Edited by K.D. Keele and C. Pedretti, 3 vols, 1980. Died 1519. *364–366.1*

**1456**
1456:1 **Ospedale Maggiore, Milan,** founded

**1460**
1460:1 **University of Basel** opened

---

1460:2 (*c*) Giacomo **Berengario da Carpi**, German anatomist and surgeon, born; gave the first authentic report of vaginal hysterectomy for prolapse; in his *Commentaria cum amplissimus additionibus super anatomia Mundini*, 1521, fol.ccxxv. Died ?1530. *6010*

---

1460:3 Giovanni **Arcolani** died; the first documentation of the use of gold fillings for teeth is in his *Chirurgia practica*, 1493. *3666.84*

**1462**
1462:1 Rodrigo Ruiz **Diaz de Isla**, Spanish surgeon, born; in his *Tractado cótra el mal serpentino*, 1539, he was among the first to propose the West Indian (Haitian) origin of syphilis. Died 1542. *2367*

**1467**
1467:1 ? Earliest known printed book to include a section on medicine is *De sermonum proprietate sive Opus de universo*, of Rabanus Maurus (776–856). *2190*

**1472**
1472:1 First printed book on **toxicology**, *Tractatus de venenis*, was compiled by Petrus de Abano (1250–1315) and printed in 1472. *2070*

1472:2 The *De infantium aegritudinibus et remediis* of Paolo Bagellardo (d.1494), was the first printed book dealing exclusively with **paediatrics** and the first treatise to make its first appearance in book form rather than having prior circulation in manuscript. *6315*

---

1472:3 Symphorien **Champier**, French physician, born; his *Libelli duo* includes *De medicine claris scriptoribus*, ?1506, the first history of medicine of any importance. This biographical study of famous medical writers also includes an attempt at a medical bibliography. Died 1539. *6376*

**1473**
1473:1 The first printed **medical dictionary** was *Synonyma medicinae, seu clavis sanationis*, compiled by Simone Cordo [Simon Januensis] (1270–1303). *6788*

**1474**
1474:1 The earliest printed book on **ophthalmology** was *De oculis eorumque egritudinibus et curis*, by Benevenuto Grassi (*fl.* 12th century). *5816*

**1477**

1477:1 **University of Tübingen** founded

1477:2 **University of Uppsala** founded

1477:3 First German **pharmacopoeia**, *Artzneibuch*, compiled by Ortolff von Bayrlant (b.*c*1400). *1794*

1477:4 Earliest printed **herbal**, *Macer floridus: De virtutibus herbarum*, published. It is ascribed to various authors. *1791*

**1478**

1478:1 *Anothomia* written in 1316 by Mondino de'Luzzi (?1275–1326) published; first modern book devoted to **anatomy**. *361*

---

1478:2 Girolamo **Fracastoro** [Fracastorius], Italian physician, born; wrote *Syphilis sive morbus gallicus*, 1530, the most famous of all medical poems; in it he recognized a venereal cause of the disease. In his *De sympathia et antipathia rerum liber unus: De contagione et contagiosis morbis et curatione*, 1546, he was first to state a germ theory of infection, and gave one of the first accounts of typhus (p. 43). The book also marks an epoch in the history of medicine: in it Fracastoro enunciated the modern doctrine of the specific character and infectious nature of fevers. Died 1553. *2364, 2528, 5371*

**1479**

1479:1 **University of Copenhagen** founded

**1480**

1480:1 A Latin text of the *Regimen sanitatis* (*Salerno*) printed

**1485**

1485:1 Johann **Lange**, German physician, born; gave first definite description of chlorosis; in his *Medicinalium epistolarum miscellanea*, xxi, p. 74, 1554. Died 1565. *3109*

**1486**

1486:1 Jason **Pratensis**, Dutch physician, born; wrote the first work devoted entirely to brain disorders, *De cerebri morbis*, 1549. Died 1558. *4511.02*

1486:2 Euricius **Cordus**, German physician, born; provided an early account of sweating sickness; in his *Ein Regiment: wie man sich vor der newen Plage der Englische Schwaisz gennant, bewaren*, etc., 1529. Died 1535. *5520*

**1488**

1488:1 Mariano **Santo di Barletta** [Marianus Sanctus Barolitanus], Italian surgeon, born; popularized the operation of median lithotomy, introduced by his father; it became known as the 'Marian operation'; in his *De lapide renum curiosum opusculum nuperrime in lucem aeditum*, 1535. Died 1577. *4278*

**1489**

1489:1 **[Hospital for Insane]** opened at **Valladolid**, Spain

1489:2 *Gerontocomia*, first printed work on **geriatrics**, published by Gabriele Zerbi (1445–1505). *1589.1*

1489:3 Nicola **Massa**, Italian anatomist and syphilologist, born; in his *Liber de morbo gallico*, 1527, he includes a description of the neurological manifestations of syphilis. Died 1569. *2365*

## 1490
1490:1 (?) Andrew **Boorde** [Borde], English physician, born; his *Breviary of helthe*, 1547, is considered the earliest 'modern' work on hygiene. Died 1549. *1591*

## 1492
1492:1 **[Hospital for Insane]** founded at **Granada** by Ferdinand and Isabella of Spain

1492:2 The **first printed medical book** by an English author is the *Rosa anglica*, compiled *c*1314, by John of Gaddesden (?1280–1361). *2191*

## 1493
1493:1 The use of **gold fillings** for **teeth** first documented by Giovanni Arcolani (d.1460 or 1484); in his *Chirurgia practica*. *3666.84*

1493:2 **Paracelsus** [Theophrastus Philippus Aureolus Bombastus von Hohenheim], Swiss physician, surgeon and alchemist, born 17 Dec; initiated chemotherapy, 1526. In his *Von der frantzösischen kranckheit drey Bücher*, 1553, he confused syphilis with gonorrhoea, and suggested hereditary transmission. His book on miners' diseases, *Von der Bergsucht oder Bergkranckheiten drey Bücher*, 1567, was the first work concerning the diseases of an occupational group. Was first to note the coincidence of cretinism and endemic goitre; in his *Opera*, **2**, 174–82, 1603. Died 1541. *2118.1, 2369, 3805*

1493:3 Nicolás **Monardes**, Spanish physician, born; wrote first work on Central American materia medica, 1565, *Dos Libros. El uno trata de todas las cosas que traen nuestras Indias Occidentales* etc. Died 1588. *1817*

## 1494
1494:1 **Syphilis** in south of **France**

1494:2 Paolo **Bagellardo**, Italian paediatrician, died; his *De infantium aegritudinibus et remediis*, 1472, was the first printed book dealing exclusively with paediatrics and the first treatise to make its first appearance in book form rather than having prior circulation in manuscript. *6315*

## 1495
1495:1 **University of Aberdeen** founded

1495:2 (*c*) The first book on **obstetrics** printed in the vernacular was *Büchlein der schwangeren Frauen* by Ortolff von Bayrlant (b.*c*1400). *6137.1*

## 1496
1496:1 Four salaried medical chairs created at **Montpellier** by Charles VIII

1496:2 Beginning of spread of **syphilis** in **Europe**

**1497**

1497:1 **Scurvy** on voyage to **India** by **Vasco da Gama**

1497:2 The first printed treatise on **surgery** in German was *Dis ist das buch der Cirurgia Hantwirckung der wundartzny* by Hieronymus Brunschwig (*c*1450–*c*1512). *5559*

1497:3 Jean **Fernel**, French physiologist and physician, born; published first systematic treatise on pathology; *Medicina, pt. 2, Pathologia,* 1554. Died 1558. *2271*

**1498**

1498:1 First official **pharmacopoeia** (*Ricettario*) of **Florence** issued

1498:2 **Syphilis** noticed in **England and Scotland**

**1499**

1499:1 The *De materia medica* of Dioscorides (*fl.* AD 54–68) is the authoritative source on the **materia medica** of antiquity. It first appeared in print in 1499. *1786*

1499:2 Andrés **Laguna**, Spanish anatomist and physician, born; among the first to suggest a method of excising **vesical caruncles**; in his *Methodus cognoscendi, extirpandique excrescentes in vesicae collo carunculas,* 1551. Died 1560. *4159*

1499: Ulrich **Ellenbog** died, **born** 1440. *occupational medicine, toxicology*

**1500**

1500:1 Hans von **Gersdorff**, German military surgeon, *fl.*; illustrations of early surgical procedures appear in his *Feldtbuch der wundartzney,* 1517. He carried out some 200 amputations and opposed Paré's abandonment of boiling oil for cauterization of wounds. *5560*

1500:2 Pietro Andrea **Mattioli**, Italian physician, born; in his *Morbo gallici novum ac utilissimum opusculum ...,* 1533, he considered mercury a specific in the treatment of syphilis; he worked particularly on neonatal syphilis. Died 1577. *2366*

1500:3 Pierre **Franco**, French surgeon, born; considered to be the best lithotomist of the 16th century. Gave the first recorded description of herniotomy for strangulated hernia, used the perineal route, and introduced suprapubic cystotomy in operating for stone; in his *Petit traité contenant une des parties principalles de chirurgie,* 1556; also wrote *Traité des hernies,* 1561. Died 1561. *3573, 3574, 4279*

1500:4 Jacob **Rueff**, Swiss obstetrician, born; published an improved version of Rösslin's *Swangern frawen ...* under the title *Ein schön lustig Trostbüchle von dem Empfengknussen und Geburten der Menschen,* 1554. It contains the first true anatomical pictures in a book on obstetrics. Died 1558. *6141, 6138*

**1501**

1501:1 Leonhart **Fuchs** born 17 Jan; he published in 1542 *De historia stirpium commentarii,* most important herbal of the 16th century. Died 1566. *1808*

1501:2 Girolamo **Cardano** [Hieronymus Cardanus], Italian physician, born 24 Sep; gave an early account of typhus; in his *De malo recentiorum medicorum medendi usu libellus,* cap.xxxvi, 1536. Died 1576. *5370*

16

1501:3 **Garcia d'Orta**, Portuguese physician, born; his *Coloquios dos simples, e drogas he causas mediçinais da India*, 1563, besides being the first textbook on tropical diseases written by a European, gives the first accounts of Indian materia medica and Asiatic cholera. Died 1568. *1815, 5104*

## 1505

1505:1 **Craft of Barbers and Surgeons** founded in **Edinburgh**; became **Royal College of Surgeons of Edinburgh** in 1788

1505: Gabriele **Zerbi** died, **born** 1445. *geriatrics*

## 1506

1506:1 (?) The first **history of medicine** of any importance is *De medicine claris scriptoribus*, in the *Libelli duo* of Symphorien Champier (1472–1539). This biographical study of famous medical writers also includes an attempt at a **medical bibliography**. *6376*

1506:2 **Savoy Palace, London**, rebuilt as a **hospital** (by order of Henry VIII); dissolved 1702

## 1507

1507:1 Thomas **Gale**, English military surgeon, born; his *Certaine works of chirurgerie*, 1563, includes the first mention of syphilis in the English literature and support for the views of Paré concerning treatment of gunshot wounds. Died 1587. *2140, 2371*

## 1510

1510:1 John **Caius**, English anatomist and surgeon, born 6 Oct; published first book in English on the sweating sickness, *A boke, or conseill against the disease commonly called the sweate, or sweatyng sicknesse*, 1552. Died 1573. *5522*

1510:2 (c) Bartolomeo **Eustachi** [Eustachius], Italian anatomist, born; his *Tabulae anatomicae*, completed in 1552 but remained forgotten in the Vatican Library until published in 1714. Had they been published when originally completed he would have been ranked with Vesalius as one of the founders of modern anatomy. In his *Opuscula anatomica*, 1564, he described the thoracic ducts, the adrenal glands and the 'Eustachian tube', but was not the first to do so. However, he was first to describe the chorda tympani as a nerve in his *De auditus organis* and published the first detailed study of the teeth in his *Libellus de dentibus* (both in his *Opuscula anatomica*). Died 1574. *391, 1093, 1139, 1538, 3668*

1510:3 Thomas **Phaer** [Phayer, Phayr], English physician, born. The first work on diseases of children by an Englishman was written by him and published as an addendum to a translation of a work by J. Goeurot; *The regiment of life, whereunto is added A treatise of the pestilence, with the Boke of Children*, 1545. Died 1560. *6317*

1510:4 Ambroise **Paré**, French army surgeon, born; the greatest army surgeon before Larrey. Published a treatise on gunshot wounds, *Méthode de traicter les playes par hacquebutes*, 1545. Repopularized podalic version (described by Soranus of Ephesus), in his *Briefve collection de l'administration anatomique ... avec la manière ... d'extraire les enfans tant mors que vivans du ventre de la mere*, 1549. He had a large dental practice and his books (such as *Dix livres de la chirurgerie*, 1564) contain much information on dentistry. His *Oeuvres* were first published in 1575; among other things he abandoned boiling oil and the cautery in the treatment of wounds and distinguished syphilis from smallpox. Died 1590. *2139, 6140, 3668.1, 5564, 5565*

1510: 5 (?) Giovanni Filippo **Ingrassia**, Italian physician, born; gave the first known description of an epidemic disease resembling scarlet fever, and was first to differentiate it from chickenpox (varicella); in his *De tumoribus praeter naturam*, 1553, p. 194, He is by some accredited with the discovery of the stapes (in his posthumous *In Galeni librum de ossibus*, 1603). Died 1580. *5073, 5437, 1541*

## 1511

1511: 1 Michael **Servetus**, Spanish physician and theologian, born 29 Sep; in his *Christianismi restituto*, 1553, he described the lesser circulation. He was burned at the stake as a heretic, 27 Oct 1553. *754*

1511: 2 **Amatus Lusitanus** (João de Castello Branco Rodrigues), Portuguese physician and surgeon, born; gave first description of purpura as a separate entity, not associated with fever; in his *Curationum medicinalium centuriae quatuor*, 1556. Died 1568. *3050*

## 1512

1512: 1 (*c*) Hieronymus **Brunschwig** died, **born** *c*1450. *surgery*

## 1513

1513: 1 The earliest textbook for **midwives** was *Der swangern frawen und hebammen roszgarten*, by Eucharius Rösslin (d.1526); it survived 40 editions and was in use as late as 1730. *6138*

## 1514

1514: 1 Andreas **Vesalius**, Flemish anatomist, born 31 Dec; a founder of modern anatomy; his *De humani corporis fabrica* (1543) revolutionized the science and teaching of anatomy. Made first diagnosis of aortic aneurysm in living, and confirmation at autopsy, 1555; reported in G.H. Welsch: *Sylloge curationum et observationum medicinalium*, pt.4, 46, 1667. Advocated surgical treatment of empyema, 1562, in P. Ingrassia, *Quaestio der purgatione*, 1568. Died 1564. *375, 376, 2972, 3164*

## 1515

1515: 1 Valerius **Cordus**, German botanist and pharmacist, born 18 Feb. Author of the first real pharmacopoeia to be published, the *Pharmacorum omnium ... vulgo vocant dispensatorium*, 1546, official pharmacopoeia of Nuremberg. Died 1544. *1810*

## 1516

1516: 1 Conrad **Gesner**, Swiss botanist and zoologist, born 26 Mar; his *Historia animalium*, 5 vols, 1551–1587, was the starting-point of modern zoology. Died 1563. *280*

1516: 2 Johann **Weyer** [Wier], Dutch physician and psychiatrist, born; the first European physician to take a scientific approach to psychiatric conditions; his *De prestigiis daemonum*, 1567, 'reduced the clinical problems of psychopathology to simple terms of everyday life and everyday, human, inner experiences' (Zilborg). Died 1588. *4916*

## 1517

1517: 1 Illustrations of early **surgical** procedures appear in *Feldtbuch der wundartzney* by Hans von Gersdorff (*fl*.1500). He carried out some 200 **amputations** and opposed Paré's abandonment of boiling oil for **cauterization** of wounds. *5560*

## 1518

1518:1 **(Royal) College of Physicians of London** founded, 23 Sep

1518:2 **Bibliothèque Nationale** founded in **Paris**

1518:3 **Public hygiene**: ordinance issued at **Nuremberg** regulating sale of food

1518:4 Felix **Würtz**, Swiss surgeon, born; wrote *Practica der wundartzney*, 1563. Died 1574. *5563*

## 1519

1519:1 **Haemophilia** probably first described by Albucasis (936–1013); in his *Liber theoricae necnon practicae Alsaharavii*, first published in 1519. *3048*

1519:2 The first 'clinical' manual on diseases of the **ear** was *De compositione medicamentum; De orbis oculorum et aurium* by Girolamo Mercuriali (1530–1606). *3343*

1519:3 Andrea **Cesalpino**, Italian physician and botanist, born 6 Jun; studied circulation and recognized heart as centre, but did not discover the main blood circulation; in his *Peripateticarum quaestionum libri quinque*, 1571. Died 1603. *755*

1519:4 (c) Leonardo **Botallo**, Italian physician, born; first described hay fever in his *De catarrho commentarius*, 1564. Died 1587/8. *2581.99*

1519: **Leonardo da Vinci** died, **born** 1452. *anatomy, physiology, embryology*

## 1521

1521:1 **Gaol fever** at **Cambridge Assizes** (Black Assizes)

1521:2 The first authentic report of **vaginal hysterectomy** for **prolapse** given by Giacomo Berengario da Carpi (c1460–?1530); in his *Commentaria cum amplissimus additionibus super anatomia Mundini*, fol.ccxxv. *6010*

## 1523

1523:1 Gabriele **Falloppio** [Fallopius], Italian anatomist, born; in his *Observationes anatomicae* (1561) he gave first descriptions of numerous anatomical structures which he had discovered, including the Fallopian tubes, the chorda and membrana tympani, and the semicircular canals. Died 1562. *378.2, 1208, 1537*

1523:2 Girolamo **Capivaccio** born; demonstrated hearing by bone conduction of some who cannot hear by air conduction; in his *Opera omnia quinque*, cap.1, pp. 587–91, 1603. Died 1589. *3343.1*

## 1524

1524:1 Thomas **Linacre** (1460–1524) founded **medical lectures** at **Oxford** and **Cambridge**

1524:2 First **hospital** in city of **México** erected by **Cortes**

1524:3 **Occupational medicine**; Ulrich Ellenbog's (1440–1499), tract on the diseases of miners, *Von den gifftigen besen Tempffen und Reuchen*, written in 1473 and published in 1524, was the first known work on **occupational medicine** and **toxicology**. *2118*

## 1525

1525:1 Earliest English printed **herbal**. It was published anonymously and printed by Rycharde Banckes and is known as *Banckes' herbal. 1799*

---

1525:2 Boudewijn **Ronsse**, Belgian physician, born; gave one of the earliest medical accounts of scurvy, and its cure by eating citrus fruits; in his *De Hippocratis magnis lienibus, Pliniique stomacace seu, ac sceletyrbe [i.e. scelotyrbe]*, 1559. Died 1597. *3710*

## 1526

1526:1 **Chemotherapy** initiated by **Paracelsus** (1493–1541)

1526:2 First illustrated English **herbal**, *The grete herball. 1802*

---

1526:3 Eucharius **Rösslin**, German physician, died; wrote the earliest textbook for **midwives**, *Der swangern frawen und hebammen roszgarten*, 1513; it survived 40 editions and was in use as late as 1730. *6138*

## 1527

1527:1 First **Protestant university** founded at **Marburg**

1527:2 **Neurosyphilis** was probably first described by Nicola Massa (1489–1569); *Liber de morbo gallico. 2365*

## 1529

1529:1 The most complete medieval treatise on **urinoscopy**, *De urinis libri vii*, was written by Joannes Actuarius (*fl.* 1350) and first published in Latin, 1529. *2666*

1529:2 An early account of **sweating sickness** provided by Euricius Cordus (1486–1535); in his *Ein Regiment: wie man sich vor der newen Plage der Englische Schwaisz gennant, bewaren*, etc. *5520*

---

1529:3 Walter **Bayley** [Bailey, Baley], English physician, born; wrote the first separate work on ophthalmology printed in England, *A briefe treatise touching the preseruation of the eie sight*, 1586. Died 1592. *5819*

## 1530

1530:1 **Collège de France** founded

1530:2 **Syphilis:** *Syphilis sive morbus gallicus*, by Girolamo Fracastoro (1478–1553), is the most famous of all medical poems; in it Fracastoro recognized a venereal cause of the disease. *2364*

1530:3 The first book on **dentistry** is the anonymous *Artzney Buchlein* .... *3667*

---

1530:4 Girolamo **Mercuriali**, Italian physician, born; his *De compositione medicamentum; De orbis oculorum et aurium*, 1519, was the first 'clinical' manual on diseases of the ear. Published one of the earliest books on the therapeutic value of gymnastics, *Artis gymnasticae*, 1569. His *De morbis cutaneis*, 1572, was the first systematic textbook on dermatology. Died 1606. *3343, 1986.1, 3980*

1530: 5 (c) Francisco **Bravo**, Mexican physician, born; gave the original description of Spanish or Mexican typhus (tabardillo); in his *Opera medicinalia*, Mexico, ff.1–90, 1570, the first medical book published in the New World. Died 1594. *5372*

1530: (?) Giacomo **Berengario da Carpi** died, **born** c1460. *vaginal hysterectomy*

## 1531
1531: 1 **University of Granada** founded

## 1532
1532: 1 **Commissions of Sewers** in **England** instituted by Act of Parliament (23. Henry VIII, cap.5)

1532: 2 Parish **Bills of Mortality** in **England**

## 1533
1533: 1 Chair of **materia medica** at **Padua**

1533: 2 **Mercury** considered a specific in the treatment of **syphilis** by Pietro Andrea Mattioli (1500–1577); in his *Morbo gallici novum ac utilissimum opusculum* .... *2366*

1533: 3 Girolamo **Fabrizio** [Fabricius ab Aquapendente], Italian anatomist, embryologist and surgeon, born 20 May. Described the valves of the veins (in his *De venarum ostiolis*, 1603). Wrote at length on embryology, which he elevated to a science (*De formato foetu*, 1604, and *De formatione ovi et pulli*, 1621). Died 1619. *757, 465, 466*

1533: (c) Girolamo **Fracastoro** [Fracastorius] died, **born** 1478. *syphilis, typhus, fevers*

## 1534
1534: 1 The first-known medical monograph on **gout** was *Ob das Podagra möglich zu generen oder nit*, by Dominicus Burgauer *fl*.1534. *4484.1*

1534: 2 Volcher **Coiter**, Dutch anatomist, physiologist and embryologist, born; published first monograph on the ear, his *De auditus instrumento* in his *Externarum et internarum principalium humani corporis partium tabulae*, 1572. Died 1576. *1539*

## 1535
1535: 1 Spread of **epidemic pneumonia** from **Venice**, 1535–1598.

1535: 2 The operation of median **lithotomy**, introduced by his father, was popularized by Mariano Santo di Barletta (Marianus Sanctus Barolitanus) (1488–1577) ; it became known as the '**Marian operation**'; in his *De lapide renum curiosum opusculum nuperrime in lucem aeditum*. *4278*

1535: 3 Georg **Bartisch**, German ophthalmic surgeon, born; wrote *Οφθαλμοδονλεια das ist Augendienst*, 1583, the first extensively illustrated treatise on eye surgery, and one of the first to use movable flaps to illustrate a medical book. Died 1606. *5817*

1535: 4 François **Rousset**, French gynaecologist, born; recorded 15 successful caesarean sections carried out by various people during the previous 80 years; in his *Traitte nouveau de l'hysterotomotokie, ou enfant caesarien*, 1581. Died ?1590. *6236*

1535: Euricius **Cordus** died, **born** 1486. *sweating sickness*

**1536**

1536:1 **Dissolution of monasteries** in England

1536:2 An early account of **typhus** given by Girolamo Cardano [Hieronymus Cardanus] (1501–1576); in his *De malo recentiorum medicorum medendi usu libellus*, cap.xxxvi. *5370*

1536:3 Giovanni Battista **Carcano Leone**, Italian anatomist, born; described lacrimal duct, in his *Anatomici libri II*, 1574. Died 1606. *1479*

1536:4 Felix **Platter**, Swiss physician, born; made the first attempt at classification of diseases according to symptoms; *Praxeos seu de cognoscendis ... homini incommodantibus*, 1602. Described a meningioma and gave first description of flexion contracture deformity of the fingers ('Dupuytren's contracture'); in his *Observationum in hominis affectibus*, 1614. Died 1614. *2195, 4511.1, 4297.9*

**1537**

1537:1 Simon de **Vallambert**, French paediatrician, *fl.* 1537–1565; published the first French work on paediatrics, *Cinque livres, de la maniere de nourrir et gouverner les enfants dans leur naissance*, 1565. *6318*

**1538**

1538:1 Recording of **baptisms**, **marriages** and **deaths** in English parish churches ordered by Henry VIII

1538:2 Marcello **Donati**, Italian physician, born; in his *De medica historia mirabili*, 1586, first to record a case of gastric ulcer, lib.IV, cap.iii, p. 196, and first to describe angioneurotic oedema, lib.VI, cap.iii. Died 1602. *3417, 4011.2*

1538:3 Guillaume de **Baillou** [Ballonius], French physician, born; gave the first description of whooping cough, 1578; recorded in his *Epidemiorum et ephemeridum libi duo*, 1640, p. 237, Wrote the first book on rheumatism, a term he introduced, *Liber de rheumatismo et pleuritide dorsali*, 1642. Died 1616. *5085, 4485*

**1539**

1539:1 **Syphilis**: West Indian origin first proposed by Rodrigo Ruiz Diaz de Isla (1462–1542); *Tractado cótra el mal serpentino. 2367*

1539:2 José de **Acosta**, Spanish naturalist, born; first described mountain sickness – altitude sickness, 'Acosta's disease'; in his *Historia natural y moral de las Indias*, 1590. Died 1600. *2244*

1539: Symphorien **Champier** died, **born** 1472. *history of medicine*

**1540**

1540:1 **Guild of Barbers and Surgeons** formed in **England**

1540:2 Four **dissections** annually in **England** permitted by statute of Henry VIII

1540:3 William **Clowes**, English surgeon, born; published the first original English treatise on syphilis, *A short and profitable treatise touching the cure of the morbus gallicus by unctions*, 1579. Died 1604. *2373*

## 1541
1541:1 Rodrigo de **Castro**, Portuguese physician, born; published first 'modern' work on medical ethics, *Medicus-politicus*, 1614. Died 1627. *1759*

1541: **Paracelsus** died, **born** 1493. *occupational medicine, syphilis, gonorrhoea, cretinism, goitre*

## 1542
1542:1 *De historia stirpium commentarii*, most important **herbal** of the 16th century, published by Leonhart Fuchs (1501–1566). *1808*

1542: Rodrigo Ruiz **Diaz de Isla** died, **born** 1462. *syphilis*

## 1543
1543:1 **Apothecaries** in **England** legalized by Act of Parliament

1543:2 **Botanic garden** established at **University of Pisa**

1543:3 *De humani corporis fabrica* and its *Epitome* published by Andreas Vesalius (1514–1564); a founder of modern **anatomy**. *375, 376*

1543:5 Costanzo **Varoli**, Italian anatomist, born; described the 'pons varolii' in his *De nervis opticis*, 1573. Died 1575. *1377.2*

## 1544
1544:1 **St Bartholomew's Hospital, London**, refounded

1544:2 **Botanic garden** established at **University of Padua**

1544:3 George **Whetstone**, English poet, soldier and traveller, born; the author of *Cures of the diseased, in remote regions*, 1598, the first English work on tropical disease. Died ?1587. *2262*

1544: Valerius **Cordus** died, **born** 1515. *pharmacopoeia*

## 1545
1545:1 The first work on **diseases of children** by an Englishman, written by Thomas Phaer [Phayer, Phayr] (1510–1560), and published as an addendum to a translation of a work by J. Goeurot *The regiment of life, whereunto is added A treatise of the pestilence, with the Boke of children. 6317*

1545:2 Treatise on **gunshot wounds**, *Méthode de traicter les playes par hacquebutes*, published by Ambroise Paré (1510–1590). *2139*

1545:3 John **Gerard**, English surgeon and herbalist, born; published *The herball or generall historie of plantes*, 1597; one of the best remembered of all English herbalists. Died 1612. *1820*

## 1546

1546:1 **Regius Professorship of Physic** established at **University of Cambridge**

1546:2 Valerius Cordus (1515–1544) was author of the first real **pharmacopoeia** to be published, the *Pharmacorum ominium ... vulgo vocant dispensatorium*, official pharmacopoeia of Nuremberg. *1810*

1546:3 *De sympathia et antipathia rerum liber unus. De contagione et contagiosis morbis et curatione* by Girolamo Fracastoro [Fracastorius] (1478–1533) contains one of the first accounts of **typhus** (p. 43) and his statement of the **germ theory of infection**. It also marks an epoch in the history of medicine in that he enunciated the modern doctrine of the specific character and infectious nature of **fevers**. *5371, 2528*

1546:4 Gaspare **Tagliacozzi**, Italian surgeon, born; a pioneer in plastic surgery, famous for his work on rhinoplasty; he wrote *De curtorum chirurgia per insitionem*, 1597. Died 1599. *5734*

## 1547

1547:1 **Bethlehem Royal Hospital**, **London**, closed at the Dissolution (1536), reopened as a **lunatic asylum** ('Bedlam')

1547:2 *Breviary of helthe* published by Andrew Boorde [Borde] (?1490–1549); considered the earliest 'modern' work on **hygiene**. *1591*

1547:3 Giovanni Battista **Codronchi**, Italian physician, born; wrote first important treatise on diseases of the larynx, *De vitiis vocis*, 1597; and first important work on forensic medicine, *Methodus testificandi*, etc., pp. 148–232 of *De vitiis vocis*, 1597. Died 1628. *1718, 3244*

## 1548

1548:1 (*c*) The first monograph on **dentistry** for the layman included in the health guide, *Nützlicher bericht ... Wie man den Mundt, die Zän und Biller ... etc.*, by Walther Hermann Ryff, Strassburg physician and surgeon (died 1548). *3667.1*

## 1549

1549:1 **Anatomical theatre** opened at **Padua**

1549:2 The first work devoted entirely to **brain disorders**, *De cerebri morbis*, written by Jason Pratensis (1486–1558). *4511.02*

1549:3 **Podalic version**, described by Soranus of Ephesus, repopularized by Ambroise Paré (1510–1590); in his *Briefve collection de l'administration anatomique ... avec la manière ... d'extraire les enfans tant mors que vivans du ventre de la mere. 6140*

1549: Andrew **Boorde** [Borde] died, **born** ?1490. *hygiene*

## 1550

1550:1 Geronimo Scipione **Mercurio**, Italian obstetrician, born; he published the first Italian book on obstetrics, *La commare o riccoglitrice*, 1596. In it he advocated caesarean section in cases of contracted pelvis. Died 1616. *6144*

24

1550:2 Nicholas **Habicot**, French surgeon born; reported four successful laryngotomies in his *Question chirurgicale* ..., 1620. Died 1624. *3244.1*

1550:3 Jacques **Guillemeau**, French surgeon, born; produced the first French work on ophthalmology, *Traité des maladies de l'oeil*, 1585, an epitome of existing knowledge. His *La chirurgerie françois* ..., 1594, contains a good deal of information on dentistry, including the first description of pyorrhoea alveolaris. Wrote *De l'heureux accouchement des femmes*, 1609. He was actually responsible for the so-called 'Mauriceau manoeuvre' for delivery of the after-coming head and was also the first to employ podalic version in placenta previa. Died 1613. *5818, 3669, 6145.1, 6147*

**1551**
1551:1 **Anatomical theatres** opened at **Paris** and **Montpellier**

1551:2 Among the first to suggest a method of excising **vesical caruncles** was Andrés Laguna (1499–1560); in his *Methodus cognoscendi, extirpandique excrescentes in vesicae collo carunculas*. *4159*

1551:3 *Historia animalium* by Conrad Gesner (1516–1563) was the starting-point of modern **zoology**. *280*

1551:4 Ercole **Sassonia**, Italian physician, born; gave early description of heart block; in his *De pulsibus*, 1604. Died 1604. *2726*

1551:5 (?) Timothy **Bright**, English physician, born; gave the first comprehensive description of depression in English; in his *Treatise of melancholie*, 1586. Died 1616. *4918*

**1552**
1552:1 *Tabulae anatomicae* of Bartolomeo Eustachi [Eustachius] (*c*1510/20–1574) completed in 1552 but not published until 1714; if published, on completion Eustachi would have ranked with Vesalius as one of the founders of modern **anatomy**. *391*

1552:2 The first English book on the **sweating sickness**, *A boke, or conseill against the disease commonly called the sweate, or sweatyng sicknesse*, published by John Caius (1510–1573). *5522*

**1553**
1553:1 The first known description of an epidemic disease resembling **scarlet fever**, and first differentiation from **chickenpox** (**varicella**) by Giovanni Filippo Ingrassia (?1510–1580); in his *De tumoribus praeter naturam*, p. 194. *5073, 5437*

1553:2 Lesser **circulation** described by Michael Servetus (1511–1553) in his *Christianismi restitutio*. *754*

1553:3 **Syphilis**: confused with **gonorrhoea**, and hereditary transmission suggested, by Paracelsus (1493–1541) in his *Von der frantzösischen kranckheit drey Bücher*. *2369*

1553: Michael **Servetus** died (burned at the stake 27 Oct), **born** 1511. *lesser circulation*

1553: Girolamo **Fracastoro** died, **born** 1478. *germ theory of infection, syphilis*

**1554**

1554:1 **Pathology**; first systematic treatise published by Jean Fernel (1497–1558); *Medicina, pt. 2, Pathologia. 2271*

1554:2 First definition of **chlorosis** given by Johann Lange (1485–1565); in his *Medicinalium epistolarum miscellanea*, xxi, p. 74. *3109*

1554:3 **Aortic aneurysm** first described by Antoine Saporta (d.1573); in his *De tumoribus praeter naturam libri V.*, published 1624. *2971*

1554:4 An improved version of Rösslin's *Swangern frawen* ... was published by Jacob Rueff (1500–1558) under the title *Ein schön lustig Trostbüchle von dem Empfengknussen und Geburten der Menschen.* It contains the first true **anatomical** pictures in a book on **obstetrics**. *6141, 6138*

**1555**

1555:1 First diagnosis of **aortic aneurysm** in living, and confirmation at autopsy, by Andreas Vesalius (1514–1564); reported in G.H. Welsch: *Sylloge curationum et observationum medicinalium*, pt.4, 46, 1667. *2972*

1555:2 Federico **Bonaventura**, Italian physician, born; wrote *De natura partus octomestris adversus vulgatam opinionem*, 1600, an encyclopaedic work on ancient and contemporary medical, scientific and juridical opinion on premature birth and the period of gestation. Died 1602. *6144.1*

**1556**

1556:1 **Purpura** first recorded as a separate entity, not associated with fever, by Amatus Lusitanus (João de Castello Branco Rodrigues) (1511–1568); in his *Curationum medicinalium centuriae quatuor. 3050*

1556:2 The first recorded description of **herniotomy** for strangulated **hernia** given by Pierre Franco (1500–1561), considered the best **lithotomist** of the 16th century, in his *Petit traité contenant une des parties principalles de chirurgie* (in which he also introduced suprapubic **cystotomy** in operating for stone). He also wrote *Traité des hernies*, 1561. *3573, 4279, 3574*

**1558**

1558:1 **University of Jena** opened

1558:2 Giovanni **Colle**, Italian physician, born; gave first definite description of a blood transfusion; *Methodus facile parandi iucunda tuta et nova medicamenta*, 1628. Died 1631. *2011*

1558:3 André **Du Laurens** [Laurentius], French physician, born; maintained that goitre was contagious; in his *De mirabili strumas sanandi*, 1609. Died 1609. *3806*

1558: Jean **Fernel** died, **born** 1497. *pathology, physiology*

1558: Jason **Pratensis** died, **born** 1486. *brain disorders*

1558: Jacob **Rueff** died, **born** 1500. *obstetrics*

## 1559

1559:1 **University of Geneva** founded

1559:2 Boudewijn Ronsse (1525–1597) gave one of the earliest medical accounts of **scurvy**, and its cure by eating citrus fruits; in his *De Hippocratis magnis lienibus, Pliniique stomacace seu, ac sceletyrbe [i.e. scelotyrbe]*, 1559. *3710*

## 1560

1560:1 **Syphilis** distinguished from **smallpox** by Ambroise Paré (1510–1590); in his *Oeuvres*. *5565*

_____

1560:2 Wilhelm **Fabry** [Fabricius Hildanus], German surgeon – 'the Father of German surgery', born; published first book to describe and classify burns, *De combustionibus*, 1607. His excellent collection of case records, *Observationum et curationum chirurgicarum*, 6 vols, 1606–41, records that he removed a gallstone from a living patient (1618) and at his wife's suggestion extracted an iron splinter from the eye with the use of a magnet. Died 1634. *2245, 5570*

1560:3 Peter **Lowe**, Scottish surgeon, born; wrote the first systematic work on surgery in England, *A discourse on the whole art of chyrurgerie*, 1596. Died 1610. *5567*

1560:4 John **Harington**, English courtier and writer, born; invented a water-closet in which the disposal of excreta was mechanically controlled; in his *The metamorphosis of Ajax*, 1596. Died 1612. *1594*

_____

1560: Andrés **Laguna** died, **born** 1499. *vesical caruncles*

1560: Thomas **Phaer** [Phayer, Phayr] died, **born** 1510. *diseases of children, hygiene*

## 1561

1561:1 **St Thomas' Hospital** (London) re-founded

1561:2 **Fallopian tubes**, other **female genitalia**, and other **anatomical structures**, including the **chorda tympani, membrana tympani,** and **semicircular canals**, described by Gabriele Fallopio (1523–1562) in his *Observationes anatomicae*. *1208, 1537, 378.2*

_____

1561:3 Santorio **Santorio** [Sanctorius], Italian physician, born. Invented several instruments, including a pulse-clock ('pulsilogium'), a hygrometer, a thermometer, a chair scales, a syringe for extracting bladder stones. His first book, *Methodi vitandorum errorum omnium qui in arte medica contingunt* (1603) was a study on how to avoid errors in healing, and included the first mention of his pulse-clock. The first printed mention of the air thermometer appeared in his *Commentaria in artem medicinalium Galeni*, 1612. Introduced quantitative experimentation into biological science, and was the founder of the physiology of metabolism (*Ars de statica medicina*, 1614). The principles of construction of his instruments are revealed in his *Commentaria in primam fen primi libri canonis Avicennae* (1625). Died 1636. *572.1, 572.2, 573, 2668*

_____

1561: Pierre **Franco** died, **born** 1500. *hernia, herniotomy, lithotomy*

## 1562

1562:1 **University of Lille** founded

1562:2 **University of Douai** founded

1562:3 **Poor Laws** in England enacted under Elizabeth I, 1562–1601

1562:4 Surgical treatment of **empyema** recommended by Andreas Vesalius (1516–1564); in P. Ingrassia, *Quaestio de purgatione*, 1568. *3164*

---

1562: Gabriele **Fallopio** [Fallopius] died, **born** 1523. *anatomy, Fallopian tubes, membrana tympani, chorda tympani, semicircular canals*

## 1563

1563:1 **Gunshot wounds**; in his *Treatise of wounds made with gonneshot*, Thomas Gale (1507–1687) supported the views of Paré concerning treatment. *2140*

1563:2 **Syphilis** first mentioned in the English literature by Thomas Gale (1507–1587); *Certaine works of chirurgerie. 2371*

1563:3 The first account of Asiatic **cholera** was that of Garcia d'Orta (1501–1568); in his *Colloquios dos simples, e drogas he causas mediçinais da India*, which was the first textbook on **tropical medicine** by a European and includes the first account of **Indian materia medica**. *1815, 5104*

1563:4 Felix Würtz (1518–1574), an important **surgeon** of the 16th century, wrote *Practica der wundartzney. 5563*

---

1563:5 Louise **Bourgeois**, French midwife, born; published *Observations diverses sur la sterilite, perte de fruict, foecondite, accouchements*, etc., 1609, the first book on obstetrics published by a midwife. Died 1636. *6145*

---

1563: Conrad **Gesner** died, **born** 1516. *zoology*

## 1564

1564:1 The **thoracic ducts** and **adrenal glands** first described by Bartolomeo Eustachi (*c*1510/20–1574) in his *Opuscula anatomica*. He also described, although not first to do so, the **Eustachian tube**, and was first to describe the **chorda tympani** as a nerve, in his *De auditu organis* (a section of his *Opuscula*). He published the first detailed study of the **teeth** in *Libellus de dentibus*, also a section of the *Opuscula*. The *Libellus* has a special title page, dated 1563. *1093, 1139, 1538, 3668*

1564:2 **Hay fever** first described by Leonardo Botallo (*c.*1519–1587/88); in his *De catarrho commentarius. 2581.99*

1564:3 Ambroise Paré (1510–1590) had a large dental practice and his books (such as *Dix livres de la chirurgie*) contain much information on **dentistry**. *3668.1*

---

1564: Andreas **Vesalius** died, **born** 1514. *empyema, anatomy, aortic aneurysm*

## 1565

1565:1 **Dissection** of executed **criminals** permitted in **England** by statute of Elizabeth I

1565:2 First work on Central American **materia medica** published by Nicolás Monardes (1493–1588), *Dos libros. El uno trata de todas las cosas que traen nuestras Indias Occidentales*, etc. *1817*

1565:3 The first French work on **paediatrics** was *Cinque livres, de la maniere de nourrir et gouverner les enfants dans leur naissance* by Simon de Vallambert (*fl.* 1537–1565). *6318*

1565: Johann **Lange** died, **born** 1485. *chlorosis*

## 1566
1566: Leonhart **Fuchs** died, **born** 1501. *herbal, materia medica*

## 1567
1567:1 **Occupational medicine**; Paracelsus' (1493–1541) book on **miners'** diseases, *Von der Bergsucht oder Bergkranckheiten drey Bücher*, is the first book on the diseases of an occupational group. *2118.1*

1567:2 The first European physician to take a scientific approach to **psychiatric conditions** was Johann Weyer [Wier] (1516–1588), whose *De prestigiis daemonum* 'reduced the clinical problems of **psychopathology** to simple terms of everyday life and everyday, human, inner experiences' (Zilborg). *4916*

1567:3 Pascal **Lecoq**, French medical bibliographer, born; produced the first systematic medical bibliography, *Bibliotheca medica*, 1590. It includes an annotated list of 1224 authors. Died 1632. *6743.1*

1567:4 John **Parkinson**, English apothecary, born; published *Paradisi in sole*, 1629, and a larger herbal, *Theatrum botanicum*, 1640. Died 1650. *1823*

## 1568
1568:1 Alexo de **Abreu**, Portuguese physician, born; published the first important work on tropical medicine, *Tratado de las siete enfermedades*, 1623. It include an early account of yellow fever (fol.193v) and one of the first precise descriptions of scurvy – he used fresh milk and rose syrup in treatment (fol.150v–193). Died 1630. *2262.1, 5449.5, 3712*

1568: **Amatus Lusitanus** (João de Castello Branco Rodrigues) died, **born** 1511. *purpura*

1568: Garcia **d'Orta** died, **born** 1501. *materia medica, cholera*

## 1569
1569:1 *Artis gymnasticae*, by Girolamo Mercuriali (1530–1606), one of the earliest books on the **therapeutic value of gymnastics**, published. *1986.1*

1569: Nicola **Massa** died, **born** 1489. *neurosyphilis*

## 1570
1570:1 The original description of Spanish or Mexican **typhus (tabardillo)** given by Francisco Bravo (c.1530–1594); in his *Opera medicinalia*, Mexico, ff.1–90, the first medical book published in the New World. *5372*

1570:2 John **Woodall**, English military surgeon, born; published the first textbook on naval medicine and surgery, *The surgions mate*, 1617. Among other things he advocated limes and lemons as a preventive against scurvy. Died 1643. *2144, 3711*

## 1571

1571:1 **Barber-surgeons Board** constituted at **Stockholm**

1571:2 Andrea Cesalpino (1519–1603) studied the **circulation** and recognized the **heart** as the centre, but did not discover the main blood circulation; in his *Peripateticarum quaestionum libri quinque*. *755*

## 1572

1572:1 The *De morbis cutaneis* of Girolamo Mercuriali (1530–1606) was the first systematic textbook on **dermatology**. *3980*

1572:2 First monograph on the **ear** by Volcher Coiter (1534–1576), his *De auditus instrumento* in his *Externarum et internarum principalium humani corporis partium tabulae*. *1539*

1572:3 Daniel **Sennert**, German physician, born 25 Nov; gave the first scientific description of scarlet fever; in his *De febribus*, libri IV, 1641. Died 1637. *5074*

1572:4 François **Citois**, French physician, born; his description of 'Poitou colic' (lead poisoning) led to its recognition as a definite syndrome, 1616, in his *De novo et populari Pictones dolore colico bilioso diatriba*. Died 1652. *2092*

## 1573

1573:1 The '**pons varolii**' described by Costanzo Varoli (1543–1575); in his *De nervis opticis*. *1377.2*

1573:2 Antoine **Saporta**, French surgeon, died; first described aortic aneurysm; in his *De tumoribus praeter naturam libri V.*, published 1624. *2971*

1573: John **Caius** died, **born** 1510. *sweating sickness*

## 1574

1574:1 **Lacrimal duct** described by Giovanni Battista Carcano Leone (1536–1606), in his *Anatomici libri II*. *1479*

1574: Bartolomeo **Eustachi** [Eustachius] died, **born** 1510/20. *anatomy, adrenal gland, chorda tympani, teeth*

1574: Felix **Würtz** died, **born** 1518. *surgery*

## 1575

1575:1 **University of Leiden** founded

1575: Costanzo **Varoli** died, **born** 1543. *pons varolii*

## 1576

1576: Volcher **Coiter** died, **born** 1534. *hearing*

1576: Girolamo **Cardano** [Hieronymus Cardanus] died, **born** 1501. *typhus*

## 1577
1577:1 **Botanic garden** opened at **Leiden**

1577:2 **Gaol fever** at **Oxford** (Black Assizes) (510 deaths from **typhus**)

---

1577:3 Robert **Burton**, English humanist and writer, born 8 Feb; wrote the first encyclopaedia of psychiatry, quoting nearly 500 medical authors, is his *Anatomy of melancholy*, 1621. Died 1640. *4981.1*

---

1577: Pietro Andrea **Mattioli** died, **born** 1500. *syphilis, mercury*

1577: Mariano **Santo di Barletta** (Marianus Sanctus Barolitanus) died, **born** 1488. *lithotomy*

## 1578
1578:1 **Chair of Medicine** established at **University of Mexico**

1578:2 The first description of **whooping cough** given by Guillaume de Baillou [Ballonius] (1538–1616); recorded in his *Epidemiorum et ephemeridum libi duo*, 1640, p. 237, *5085*

---

1578:3 William **Harvey**, English physiologist and physician, born 1 Apr; in *De motu cordis*, 1628, one of the most important books in the history of medicine, he described the circulation of the blood through the heart. Published *Exercitationes de generatione animalium*, 1651, an early work on embryology; the chapter on labour (De partu) is the first original work on obstetrics to be published by an English author. Died 1657. *759, 467*

---

1578:4 Adriaan van den **Spieghel** [Spigelius], Belgian anatomist, born; his *De semitertiana libri quatuor*, 1624, was the first extensive account of malaria. Died 1625. *5229*

## 1579
1579:1 **Syphilis**: the first original English treatise, *A short and profitable treatise touching the cure of the morbus gallicus by unctions*, published by William Clowes (1540–1604). *2373*

---

1579:2 Johannes Baptista van **Helmont**, Flemish chemist and physician, born 12 Jan. A founder of biochemistry who did important work on the role of acids in digestion, and was first to recognize the physiological importance of ferments and gases. Writings collected in his *Ortus Medicinae*, 1648. Died 1644. *665*

---

1579:3 Juan Pablo **Bonet**, Spanish physician, born; used a 'combined' system of teaching the deaf to speak and the dumb to communicate with others; in his *Reduction de las letras, y arte para enseñar a ablar los mudos*, 1620. Died 1633. *3345*

## 1580
1580:1 Francisco **Diaz**, Spanish urologist, *fl.*; wrote the first treatise on diseases of the urinary tract, *Tratado de todas las enfermedades de los riñones, vexiga, y carnosidades de la verga, y urina*, 1588; sometimes called the 'Father of urology'. *4160*

---

1580:2 Marco Aurelio **Severino**, Italian anatomist and pathologist, born; published first textbook on surgical pathology, *De recondita abscessuum natura*, 1632. Died 1656. *2273*

---

1580: Giovanni Filippo **Ingrassias** died, **born** 1510. *varicella, scarlet fever, stapes*

## 1581
1581:1 Ordinance against **plague** in **London (Bills of Mortality)**

1581:2 Fifteen successful **caesarean sections** carried out by various people during the previous 80 years recorded by François Rousset (1535–?1590); in his *Traitte nouveau de l'hysterotomotokie, ou enfant caesarien. 6236*

1581:3 Gaspare **Aselli**, Italian anatomist, born; discovered the lacteal vessels; in his *De lactibus*, 1627. Died 1626. *1094*

## 1582
1582:1 **University of Edinburgh** chartered by James VI of Scotland

1582:2 Measures taken against **overcrowding** and overbuilding in **London**

## 1583
1583:1 Οφθαλμοδονλεια *das ist Augendienst*, was the first extensively illustrated treatise on **eye surgery**, and one of the first to use movable flaps to illustrate a medical book. It was written by Georg Bartisch (1535–1606). *5817*

## 1584
1584:1 Walter **Raleigh** brings **curare** from **Guiana**

1584:2 Paolo **Zacchias**, Italian physician, born; contributed significantly to medical jurisprudence; his 9–volume treatise, *Quaestiones medico-legales*, appeared in 1621–61. Died 1659. *1720*

## 1585
1585:1 The first French work on **ophthalmology**, *Traité des maladies de l'oeil*, an epitome of existing knowledge, produced by Jacques Guillemeau (1550–1612). *5818*

## 1586
1586:1 **University of Graz** chartered

1586:2 **Gastric ulcer** first recorded by Marcello Donati (1538–1602); in his *De medica historia mirabili* lib.IV, cap.iii, p. 196, *3417*

1586:3 **Angioneurotic oedema** first described by Marcello Donati (1538–1602); in his *De medica historia mirabili*, lib.vi, cap.iii. *4011.2*

1586:4 The first comprehensive description of **depression** in English is the *Treatise of melancholie*, by Timothy Bright (?1551–1616). *4918*

1586:5 The first separate work on **ophthalmology** printed in England, *A briefe treatise touching the preseruation of the eie sight*, written by Walter Bayley [Bailey, Baley] (1529–1592). *5819*

## 1587
1587: (?) George **Whetstone** died, **born** ?1544. *tropical disease*

1587: Leonardo **Botallo** died, **born** *c*.1519. *hay fever*

1587: Thomas **Gale** died, **born** 1507. *syphilis, gunshot wounds*

## 1588
1588:1 **Anatomical theatre** at Basel opened

1588:2 The first treatise on diseases of the **urinary tract**, *Tratado de todas las enfermedades de los riñones, vexiga, y carnosidades de la verga, y urina* published by Francisco Diaz (*fl.* 1580), sometimes called the 'Father of urology'. *4160*

1588: Nicolás **Monardes** died, **born** 1493. *materia medica*

1588: Johann **Weyer** [Wier] died, **born** 1516. *psychiatry*

## 1589
1589:1 Lazare **Rivière** [Riverius], French physician, born; first to note aortic stenosis ; in his *Opera medica universa*, 1674. Died 1655. *2727*

1589: Girolamo **Capivaccio** died, born 1523. *hearing*

## 1590
1590:1 The first systematic **medical bibliography** published, the *Bibliotheca medica* of Pascal Lecoq (1567–1632); includes an annotated list of 1224 authors. *6743.1*

1590:2 The first clinical manual on **diseases of the ear** was *De compositione medicamentum; De orbis oculorum et aurium* by Girolamo Mercuriali (1530–1606). *3343*

1590:3 **Altitude sickness** described by José de Acosta (1539–1600); in his *Historia natural y moral de las Indias*. *2244*

1590: Ambroise **Paré** died, **born** 1510. *surgery, gunshot wounds, dentistry, podalic version, syphilis, smallpox*

1590: (?) François **Rousset** died, **born** 1535. *caesarean section*

## 1591
1591:1 **Trinity College Dublin** founded

## 1592
1592:1 Jacob de **Bondt** [Bontius], Danish physician and naturalist, born; gave the first modern scientific description of beriberi; in his *De medicina Indorum*, pp. 115–20, 1642. Died 1631. *3736*

1592: Walter **Bayley** [Bailey, Baley] died, **born** 1529. *ophthalmology*

## 1593
1593:1 **Dublin University** founded

1593:2 **Marischal College, Aberdeen** founded

1593:3 Nicholas **Tulp**, Dutch physician, born 11 Oct; gave one of the earliest accounts of **beriberi**; in his *Observationes medicae*, 1652, p. 300. Died 1674. *3737*

**1594**

1594:1 **Pyorrhoea alveolaris** first described by Jacques Guillemeau (1550–1613); in his *La chirurgerie françois ...*, which contains a good deal of information on **dentistry**. *3669*

1594:2 Stephen **Bradwell**, English physician, born; wrote the first book on first aid, *Help for suddain accidents endangering life*, 1633. Died 1636. *5569*

1594: Francisco **Bravo** died, **born** c.1530. *typhus*

**1596**

1596:1 The first Italian book on **obstetrics** is *La commare o riccoglitrice* by Geronimo Scipione Mercurio (1550–1616), who advocated **caesarean section** in cases of contracted pelvis. *6144*

1596:2 *The metamorphosis of Ajax* describes a **water-closet** invented by John Harington (1560–1612). *1594*

1596:3 The first systematic work on **surgery** written in England was *A discourse on the whole art of chyrurgerie* by Peter Lowe (1560–1610). *5567*

1596:4 René **Descartes**, French philosopher and mathematician, born 31 Mar; his first experiment in reflex action (1644) recorded in his *Des passions de l'âme*, 1649. Died 1650. *4965*

**1597**

1597:1 **Guild of Surgeons** organized in **Bergen**

1597:2 **Jardin des Plantes, Paris**, founded

1597:3 *The herball or generall historie of plantes* published by John Gerard (1545–1612), one of the best-known English herbalists. *1820*

1597:4 First important treatise on diseases of the **larynx**, *De vitiis vocis*, published by Giovanni Battista Codronchi (1547–1628), included the first important work on **forensic medicine**, *Methodus testificandi*, etc., on pp. 148-232. *3244, 1718*

1597:5 A pioneer in **plastic surgery** was Gaspare Tagliacozzi (1546–1599), famous for his work on **rhinoplasty**; he wrote *De curtorum chirurgia per insitionem. 5734*

1597:6 Francis **Glisson**, English physician, born; his *De rachitide*, 1650, contained the fullest account of rickets that had appeared up to that time, it also (chap. 22) gave the first description of infantile scurvy. Described the capsule of the liver, 'Glisson's capsule', in his *Anatomia hepatis*, 1654. Died 1677. *3729, 972*

1597: Boudewijn **Ronsse** died, **born** 1525. *scurvy*

**1598**

1598:1 **Tropical disease**; first English work, *Cures of the diseased, in remote regions*, published by George Whetstone (?1544–?1587). *2262*

## 1599

1599:1 **Royal Faculty of Physicians and Surgeons of Glasgow** founded by Peter Lowe; became Royal College in 1962

---

1599:2 Guerner **Rolfinck**, German physician, anatomist and chemist, born; first to demonstrate the location of cataract in the lens; in his *Dissertationes anatomicae methodo synthetica exaratae*, 1656. Died 1673. *5821.1*

---

1599: Gaspare **Tagliacozzi** died, **born** 1546. *rhinoplasty*

## 1600

1600:1 *De natura partus octomestris adversus vulgatam opinionem*, by Frederico Bonaventura (1555–1602), is an encyclopaedic work on ancient and contemporary medical, scientific and juridical opinion on **premature birth** and the period of **gestation**. *6144.1*

---

1600: José de **Acosta** died, **born** 1539. *altitude sickness*

## 1602

1602:1 **Bodleian Library, Oxford** founded

---

1602:2 The **classification of diseases** according to symptoms was attempted by Felix Platter (1536–1614); *Praxeos seu de cognoscendis ... homini incommodantibus*. *2195*

---

1602:3 Athanasius **Kircher**, German physician, microscopist and priest, born 2 May; was probably the first to use the microscope to study the cause of disease. In his *Scrutinium physico-medicum contagiosae luis, quae pestis dicitur*, 1658, he remarked that the blood of plague patients was filled with a 'countless brood of worms not perceptible to the naked eye'; he was the first to state explicitly the theory of contagion by animalculae as the cause of infectious diseases. Died 1680. *5118*

---

1602: Marcello **Donati** died, **born** 1538. *gastric ulcer, angioneurotic oedema*

---

1602: Federico **Bonaventura** died, **born** 1555. *premature birth, gestation*

## 1603

1603:1 **Venous valves** described by Girolamo Fabrizio [Fabricius ab Aquapendente] (1533–1619); in his *De venarum ostiolis*. *757*

---

1603:2 Santorio Santorio [Sanctorius] (1561–1636) invented many **scientific instruments**. His first book, *Methodi vitandorum errorum omnium qui in arte medica contingunt* was a study on how to avoid errors in healing; it included the first mention of his **pulse-clock**. *572.1*

---

1603:3 Giovanni Filippo Ingrassia (?1510–1580) is by some accredited with the discovery of the **stapes** (in his posthumous *In Galeni librum de ossibus*, 1603). *1541*

---

1603:4 **Hearing** by bone conduction of some who cannot hear by air conduction demonstrated by Girolamo Capivaccio (1523–1589); in his *Opera omnia quinque*, cap.1, pp. 587–91. *3343.1*

---

1603:5 Paracelsus (1493–1541) was first (1517) to note the coincidence of **cretinism** and endemic **goitre**; in his *Opera*, **2**, 174–82. *3805*

---

1603: Andrea Cesalpino died, **born** 1519. *heart, circulation*

## 1604

1604:1 Girolamo Fabrizio [Fabricius ab Aquapendente] (1533–1619) wrote at length on **embryology**, which he elevated to a science; *De formato foetu. 465*

1604:2 Early description of **heart block** given by Ercole Sassonia (1551–1607); in his *De pulsibus. 2726*

---

1604: William **Clowes** died, **born** 1540. *syphilis*

## 1605

1605:1 Thomas **Browne**, English physician, born 19 Oct; wrote *Religio medici*, 1642, one of the best works in English literature written by a physician; an attempt to reconcile scientific scepticism with faith. Died 1682. *6612.90*

## 1606

1606:1 Wilhelm Fabry's (1560–1634) excellent collection of case records, *Observationum et curationum chirurgicarum*, 6 vols, 1606–41, records that he removed a **gallstone** from a living patient (1618) and at his wife's suggestion extracted an **iron splinter** from the **eye** with the use of a **magnet**. Died 1634. *5570*

1606: Giovanni Battista **Carcano Leone** died, **born** 1536. *lacrimal duct*

1606: Girolamo **Mercuriali** died, **born** 1530. *therapeutic gymnastics, dermatology, diseases of ear*

1606: Georg **Bartisch** died, **born** 1535. *eye surgery*

## 1607

1607:1 **University of Giessen** chartered by Rudolph II

1607:2 **Burns**; first book to describe and classify them published by Wilhelm Fabry [Fabricius *Hildanus*] (1560–1634), *De combustionibus. 2245*

---

1607: Ercole **Sassonia** died, **born** 1551. *heart block*

## 1609

1609:1 **Jalap**, a **purgative** drug, brought from **Mexico**

1609:2 André Du Laurens [Laurentius] (1558–1609) maintained that **goitre** was contagious; in his *De mirabili strumas sanandi. 3806*

1609:3 *Observations diverses sur la sterilite, perte de fruict, foecondite, accouchements*, etc. by Louise Bourgeois (1563–1636) was the first book on **obstetrics** published by a midwife. *6145*

1609:4 Jacques Guillemeau (1550–1613), who wrote *De l'heureux accouchement des femmes*, was actually responsible for the so-called '**Mauriceau manoeuvre**' for delivery of the after-coming head and was also the first to employ **podalic version** in **placenta previa**. *6145.1, 6147*

---

1609: 5 Ysbrand van **Diemerbroeck**, Dutch physician, born; gave an important early account of plague; in his *De peste libri quatuor*, 1646. Died 1674. *5117*

---

1609: André **Du Laurens** [Laurentius] died, **born** 1558. *goitre*

## 1610
1610: 1 **Galileo** devises a **microscope**

---

1610: 2 Johannes Michael **Fehr**, German physician, born; with Elias Schmidt, first to report a case of trigeminal neuralgia, 1671, *MCMP* 2. Died 1688. *4512*

---

1610: Peter **Lowe** died, **born** 1560. *surgery*

## 1611
1611: 1 **University of Santo Tomas, Manila** founded

---

1611: 2 Willem **Piso**, Dutch physician and botanist, born 9 May; first to differentiate yaws from syphilis; in *Historia naturalis Brasiliae* (De medica Brasiliensi p. 35, 1648. Died 1678. *5303*

1611: 3 Job Janszoon van **Meekeren**, Dutch surgeon, born; first to record a bone graft (Chap. 1 of *Heel- en geneeskonstige aanmerkkingen*, 1668). Unfortunately the Church ordered the removal of the graft. Died 1666. *5735*

## 1612
1612: 1 The first printed mention of the **air thermometer** appeared in *Commentaria in artem medicinalium Galeni* by Santorio Santorio (1561–1636). *572.2*

---

1612: John **Harington** died, **born** 1560. *water-closet*

1612: John **Gerard** died, **born** 1545. *herbal*

## 1613
1613: 1 **University of Córdoba, Argentina** founded

---

1613: Jacques **Guillemeau** died, **born** 1550. *ophthalmology, dentistry, pyorrhoea alveolaris, obstetrics*

## 1614
1614: 1 **University of Groningen** founded

1614: 2 In his *Observationum in hominis affectibus* Felix Platter (1536–1614) gave the first known report of a case of fatal hypertrophy of the **thymus** and described a **meningioma**. *3789, 4511.1*

1614: 3 Santorio Santorio [Sanctorius] (1561–1636) invented several **scientific instruments**, introduced **quantitative experimentation** into biological science, and was the founder of the **physiology of metabolism**. His ideas are presented in his collection of aphorisms, *Ars de statica medicina aphorismorum ... . 573*

1614:4 **Medical ethics**; first 'modern' work, *Medicus-politicus*, published by Rodrigo de Castro (1541–1627). *1759*

1614:5 **Flexion contracture deformity of the fingers** ('**Dupuytren's contracture**') first described by Felix Platter (1536–1614); in his *Observationum in hominis affectibus*, Lib. 1, 140. *4297.9*

1614:6 Thomas **Wharton**, English anatomist and endocrinologist, born 31 Aug; his *Adenographia*, 1656, included a description of the submaxillary salivary gland ('Wharton's duct'). Died 1673. *1116*

1614:7 Franciscus de le **Boë** [Sylvius], German/Dutch physician born. First to describe tubercles in tuberculosis, asserting that they are often found in the lung and that they softened and suppurated to form cavities; *Opera omnia*, 1679. Died 1672. *2321*

1614:8 Conrad Victor **Schneider**, German physician, born; showed that nasal mucus originates in the nasal mucous membrane ('Schneider's membrane'); in his *Liber ... de catarrhis*, 1660. Died 1680. *3245*

1614: Felix **Platter** died, **born** 1536. *thymus, meningioma, flexion contracture deformity of fingers, classification of disease*

## 1615
1615:1 William Harvey (1578–1657) commences lectures on the **circulation of the blood**

1615:2 Jean Claude de **la Courvée**, French physician, born; reported a case of successful symphysiotomy, in his *De nutritione foetus in utero paradoxa*, 1655, p. 245. Died 1664. *6146.1*

## 1616
1616:1 **Poitou colic** (due to **lead poisoning**) described by François Citois (1572–1652), in his *De novo et populari Pictones dolore colico bilioso diatriba*. *2092*

1616:2 **Sign-language** for **deaf-mutes**, using almost every part of the body, introduced by Giovanni Bonifacio; in his *L'arte di cenni* .... *3344*

1616:3 Nicholas **Culpeper**, English herbalist, born 16 Oct; his *Pharmacopoeia Londinensis*, Boston, 1720, is the first herbal and the first full-length medical book printed in North America. Died 1654. *1828.2*

1616:4 Thomas **Bartholin**, Danish anatomist and physiologist, born 20 Oct; discovered human thoracic duct, published in his *De lactis thoracicis in homine brutisque*, 1652; his claim, in his *Vasa lymphatica*, 1653, of priority in the discovery of the lymphatics was disputed by Rudbeck and Joyliffe. Died 1680. *1096, 1097, 1098.1*

1616:5 John **Wallis**, English mathematician, born 23 Nov; a prominent teacher of deaf-mutes, a professor of mathematics at Oxford, classified the various sounds of the human voice; in his *Grammatica linguae Anglicae*, 1653. Died 1703. *3348*

1616:6 William **Holder**, English priest, born; described paracusis; in his *Elements of speech* ..., Appendix, p. 166, 1669. Died 1698. *3349*

38

1616: Timothy **Bright** died, **born** ?1551. *depression*

1616: Guillaume de **Baillou** [Ballonius] died, **born** 1538. *whooping cough, rheumatism*

1616: Geronimo Scipione **Mercurio** died, **born** 1550. *obstetrics*

**1617**
1617:1 **Society of Apothecaries of the City of London** chartered

1617:2 The first textbook on **naval medicine and surgery** is John Woodall's (1570–1643) *The surgions mate.* Among other things he advocated limes and lemons as a preventive against **scurvy**. *2144, 3711*

**1618**
1618:1 *Pharmacopoeia Londinensis,* first London **pharmacopoeia** published by the (Royal) College of Physicians of London. *1821*

1618:2 A **gallstone** removed from a living patient by Wilhelm Fabry (1560–1634); recorded in his excellent collection of case records, *Observationum et curationum chirurgicarum,* 6 vols, 1606–41. Died 1634. *5570*

**1619**
1619: **Fabricius ab Aquapendente** [Girolamo Fabrizio] died, **born** 1533. *venous valves, embryology*

**1620**
1620:1 Four successful **laryngotomy** operations were carried out by Nicholas Habicot (1550–1624); in his *Question chirurgicale .... 3244.1*

1620:2 A 'combined' system of teaching the **deaf** to speak and the **dumb** to communicate with others was used by Juan Pablo Bonet (1579–1633); in his *Reduction de las letras, y arte para enseñar a ablar los mudos. 3345*

1620:3 Theophile **Bonet** Swiss pathologist born, 6 Mar; published first systematized collection of pathological descriptions, *Sepulchretum,* 1679. Died 1689. *2274*

1620:4 John **Graunt**, English statistician and demographer, born 24 Apr; published first book on vital statistics, *Natural and political observations ... upon the Bills of Mortality of London,* 1662; some authorities attribute the work to his friend Sir William Petty. Died 1674. *1686*

1620:5 Johann Jacob **Wepfer**, Swiss physician, born 20 Dec; showed apoplexy to be a result of a haemorrhage into the brain; in his *Observationes anatomicae, ex cadaveribus eorum, quos sustulit apoplexia,* 1658. Died 1695. *2703, 4511.2*

**1621**
1621:1 **University of Strasbourg** founded

1621:2 Girolamo Fabrizio [Fabricius ab Aquapendente] wrote at length on **embryology**, which he elevated to a science, *De formatione ovi et pulli. 466*

1621:3 Paolo Zacchias (1584–1659) began publication of his treatise on **medical jurisprudence**, *Quaestiones medico-legales*, 1621–61. *1720*

1621:4 The first encyclopaedia of **psychiatry**, quoting nearly 500 medical authors, is Robert Burton's (1577–1640) *Anatomy of melancholy*. *4981.1*

1621:5 Thomas **Willis**, English physician and anatomist, born 27 Jan. His writings include *Diatribae duae*, etc., 1659, in which he gave the first description of epidemic typhoid (De febribus, cap.X, xiv); *Cerebri anatome*, 1664, in which he gave the most complete and accurate account of the nervous system that had hitherto appeared and (cap.I and plates 1, 2) a description (but not the first) of the 'circle of Willis'; *Pathologia cerebri*, 1667, where he gave the first account of cerebral syphilis – without recognizing cause; *Affectionum quae dicuntur hystericae*, etc., 1670, where he showed hysteria to be a nervous disease and not a uterine disorder; *De anima brutorum*, 1672, where he gave a probable description of myasthenia gravis (pars. 2, cap.IX); a description of the 'paracusis of Willis' (cap.XIV, 73), general paralysis (4to edn, p. 392, 8vo edn, p. 278), and lethargy (pars 2, cap.III); *Pharmaceutice rationalis*, 1675, in which he gave a clear account of whooping cough (pars.2, 99) and noted the sweetness of urine in diabetes mellitus, differentiating the condition from diabetes insipidus (2, IV, cap.3); and *Practice of physick*, 1684, where he gave what is probably the first report of cerebrospinal meningitis (VII, 46). Died 1675. *5020, 1378, 4839, 4730, 1544, 4793, 4819, 3926, 5086, 4673*

## 1622
1622:1 Hendrik van **Roonhuyze**, Dutch gynaecologist, born; wrote the first modern work on operative gynaecology, *Heel-konstige aanmerkkingen betreffende de gebreeken der vrouwen*, 1663. Died 1672. *6015*

## 1623
1623:1 First important work on **tropical disease** published by Alexo de Abreu (1568–1630); *Tratado de las siete enfermedades* ... etc. It includes one of the first precise descriptions of **scurvy** and its treatment using fresh milk and rose syrup, together with an early account of **yellow fever**. *2262.1, 3712, 5449.5*

1623:2 The earliest scientific work dealing with **spectacles**, was *Uso de los antojos para todo genero de vistas*, etc., by Benito Daza de Valdes (fl. 17c); it included sight-testing tables. *5821*

## 1624
1624:1 The first extensive account of **malaria** provided by Adriaan van den Spieghel [Spigelius] (1578–1625); in his *De semitertiana libri quatuor*. *5229*

1624:2 Thomas **Sydenham**, English physician – 'the English Hippocrates', born (or baptized) 10 Sep. His efforts to base treatment on observable phenomena and his concern for epidemic variations encouraged more bedside observation of disease. He gave many excellent accounts of diseases including (*Observationes medicae*, 1676) scarlet fever (p. 387) and a most minute and careful description of measles (pp. 272–80). He clearly differentiated gout from rheumatism (*Tractatus de podagra et hydrope*, 1683). His important account of smallpox was published in *Observationes medicae* Ed. quart, Book 3, cap.2; Book 5, cap.4), 1685; and Sydenham's chorea (chorea minor) was described in his *Schedula monitoria de novae febris ingressus*, 1686, p. 25. Died 1689. *5075, 5441.1, 4486, 5407, 4514*

1624:3 Georg Hieronymous **Welsch**, Austrian physician, born 24 Oct; gave an exhaustive survey of dracontiasis; in his *Exercitatio de vena Medinensis*, 1674. Died 1677. *5336.1*

1624: Nicholas **Habicot** died, **born** 1550. *laryngotomy*

## 1625

1625: 1 Santorio Santorio [Sanctorius] (1561–1636) invented several **instruments**, including a **pulse-clock** ('**pulsilogium**'), a **hygrometer**, a **thermometer**, a **chair scale**, a **syringe for extracting bladder stones**. The principles of construction of his instruments are revealed in his *Commentaria in primam fen primi libri canonis Avicennae*. *2668*

1625: Adriaan van den **Spieghel** [Spigelius] died, **born** 1578. *malaria*

## 1626

1626: 1 Francesco **Redi**, Italian physician, born 19 Feb; published the first methodical account of snake poison, *Osservazione intorno alle vipere*, 1664. Died 1697. *2102*

1626:2 Gerard **Blaes** [Blasius], Dutch anatomist, born; published first work solely on the spinal cord, *Anatome medullae spinalis, et nervorum*, 1666. Died 1682. *1354.9*

1626:3 (?)George **Dalgarno**, English schoolmaster, born; invented an alphabet for the use of deaf-mutes; in his *Didascalocophus or the deaf and dumb mans tutor ...*, 1680. Died 1687. *3350*

1626: Gaspare **Aselli** died, **born** 1581. *lacteal vessels*

## 1627

1627: 1 The **lacteal vessels** were discovered by Gaspare Aselli (1581–1626), as recorded in his *De lactibus sive lacteis venis*, 1627. *1094*

1627:2 Robert **Boyle**, English chemist, born 25 Jan; Boyle's Law contained in his *A defence of the doctrine touching the spring and weight of the air*, 1662; first analysis of blood in *Memoirs for the natural history of humane blood*, 1684, regarded as his most important medical work. Died 1691. *666, 861*

1627: Rodrigo de **Castro** died, **born** 1541. *medical ethics*

## 1628

1628: 1 **Circulation** of the **blood** described by William Harvey (1578–1657) in *De motu cordis*. *759*

1628:2 First definite description of a **blood transfusion** given by Giovanni Colle (1558–1631); *Methodus facile parandi iucunda tuta et nova medicamenta*. *2011*

1628:3 Marcello **Malpighi**, Italian physician and biologist, born 10 Mar; in *De pulmonibus ...*, 1661, he described the capillary circulation; in *De viscerum structura ...*, 1666, gave an excellent description of the 'Malpighian bodies' and the uriniferous tubules of the kidney; published *De ovo incubato* and *De formatione pulli in ovo*, 1673, these works placed the study of embryology on a sound basis; gave the first description of leontiasis ossea; in his *Opera posthuma*, 1700, p. 68. Died 1694. *468, 469, 760, 1230, 4299*

1628: Giovanni Battista **Codronchi** died, **born** 1547. *medical jurisprudence, larynx*

## 1629
1629:1 **London Bills of Mortality** begin to include causes of death

---

1629:2 Valentine **Greatrakes**, English faith healer, born; wrote the earliest scientific account by a practitioner of psychotherapy by the 'laying on of hands'; in his *A brief account of Mr Valentine Greatrakes, and divers of the strange cures lately performed by him*, 1666. Died 1683. *4992*

## 1630
1630:1 Treatment of **malaria** with **cinchona** bark known in Peru

---

1630:2 Alexo de **Abreu** died, **born** 1568. *tropical disease, scurvy, yellow fever*

## 1631
1631:1 Richard **Lower**, English physician, born; transfused blood from one live animal into another (dogs), 1665, *PT* **1**:353. In *Tractatus de corde*, 1669, he noted the scroll-like structure of cardiac muscle. Died 1691. *2012, 761*

1631:2 William **Boghurst**, English apothecary, born; differentiated plague from typhus; in his *Loimographia*, written in 1666 but not published until 1894. Died 1685. *5120*

---

1631:3 Peter **Chamberlen** (the elder) died. He was probably the first to use the **Chamberlen (midwifery) forceps**, a secret of the family, including Peter (the younger, 1572–1626), his son Peter (1601–1683), Hugh (the elder, b.?1632), his brother Paul (1635–1717), and Hugh (the younger, 1664–1728), a London obstetrician

1631: Giovanni **Colle** died, **born** 1558. *blood transfusion*

1631: Jacob de **Bondt** [Bontius] died, **born** 1592. *beriberi*

## 1632
1632:1 **University of Dorpat** founded

1632:2 **Botanic garden** established at **Oxford** (oldest in Britain)

1632:3 **Surgical pathology**; first textbook, *De recondita abscessuum natura*, published by Marco Aurelio Severino (1580–1656). *2273*

---

1632:4 Antoni van **Leeuwenhoek**, Dutch pioneer microscopist, born 24 Oct. Described and illustrated spermatozoa (originally pointed out to him by his student, Hamen, in 1674), studied structure of muscle, discovered protozoa, introduced histological staining; in his *Ontledingen en ontdekkingen*, 1693–1718. Gave the first accurate description of the red blood corpuscles (previously noted by Swammerdam in 1658), 1674, *PT* **9**: 121; described and illustrated bacteria, 1684, *PT* **14**:568. Died 1723. *67, 860, 2464.1*

---

1632: Pascal **Lecoq** died, **born** 1567. *medical bibliography*

## 1633

1633:1 The first book on **first aid**, *Help for suddain accidents endangering life*, written by Stephen Bradwell (1594–1636). *5569*

---

1633:2 Bernardino **Ramazzini**, Italian physician, born 5 Nov; his *De morbis artificum diatriba*, 1700, was the first comprehensive and systematic work on occupational diseases. Died 1714. *2121*

---

1633: Juan Pablo **Bonet** died, **born** 1579. *communication by deaf and dumb*

## 1634

1634:1 **University of Utrecht** founded

---

1634:2 Johann Daniel **Major**, German physician, born; made successful intravenous injections of drugs; *Chirurgia infusoria*, 1667. Died 1693. *1963*

1634:3 Pierre de **La Martinière**, French physician, born; first to describe gonococcal arthritis, in his *Traité de la maladie vénérienne*, 1664. Died 1690. *4485.1*

1634:4 Heinrich **Vollgnad**, German physician, born; gave the first authentic account of variolation (inoculation against smallpox); in his *Globus vitulinus*, 1671. Died 1682. *5405*

---

1634: Wilhelm **Fabry** [Fabricius *Hildanus*] died, **born** 1560. *surgery, burns, gallstone, eye splinter removal with magnet*

## 1635

1635:1 **Académie Française** founded by **Richelieu**

---

1635:2 Robert **Hooke**, English natural philosopher, born 17 Jul; published earliest work devoted entirely to an account of microscopical observations, 1665. Died 1703. *262*

## 1636

1636:1 **Harvard College (University)** founded; oldest such in USA

---

1636: Santorio **Santorio** [Sanctorius] died, **born** 1561. *medical and scientific instruments, quantitative experimentation, physiology of metabolism, air thermometer*

1636: Stephen **Bradwell** died, **born** 1594. *first aid*

1636: Louise **Bourgeois** died, **born** 1563. *obstetrics*

## 1637

1637:1 Jan **Swammerdam**, Dutch biologist and physician, born 12 Feb. Discovered that the lungs of newborn infants will float on water if respiration has taken place (an important medico-legal point); in his *De respiratione usuque pulmonum*, 1667. Disputed priority of de Graaf in his demonstration of ovulation; in his *Miraculum naturae, sive uteri muliebris fabrica*, 1672. Died 1680. *1724, 1211*

---

1637:2 Richard **Morton**, English phthisiologist, born 30 Jul; first important pathological study of pulmonary tuberculosis, and first account of anorexia nervosa; in his *Phthisiologia*, 1689. Died 1698. *3216*

---

1637:3 Giacinto **Cestoni**, Italian naturalist, born; with Giovanni Cosimo Bonomo, observed the scabies mite, *Sarcoptes scabiei*, the first proof of infection by a microparasite; in *Osservazioni intorno a' pellicelli del corpo umano*, 1687. Died 1718. *2529.1, 4012*

1637:4 François **Mauriceau** born; leading French obstetrician of his day, wrote *Des maladies des femmes grosses et accouchées*, 1668, the outstanding textbook on obstetrics of the time. Died 1709. *6147*

---

1637: Daniel **Sennert** died, **born** 1572. *scarlet fever*

## 1638

1638:1 **University of Lima**, Peru, founded 1553, acquires a Medical Faculty

---

1638:2 Niels **Stensen** [Nicolaus Steno], Danish anatomist and priest, born 10 Jan. His *Observationes anatomicae*, 1662, includes the first description of the excretory duct of the parotid gland ('Stensen's duct') and the ceruminous glands; he studied the structure and function of muscle (*De musculis et glandulis observationum specimen*, 1664; *Elementorum myologiae specimen*, 1667); he first described 'Fallot's tetralogy' in his *Embryo monstro affinis Parisiis dissectus*, 1671. Died 1686. *973, 1543; 576–7; 2726.1*

1638:3 Heinrich **Meibom**, German physician and anatomist, born 29 Jun; described Meibomian (conjunctival) glands, already known to Galen, in his *De vasis palpebrarum novis epistola*, 1666. Died 1700. *1481*

---

1638:4 Frederik **Ruysch**, Dutch anatomist, born; first to describe the valves of the lymphatics, in his *Dilucidatio valvularum in vasis lymphaticis et lacteis*, 1665. In his *Thesaurus anatomicus i–x*, 1701–16, described his method for injecting blood vessels, was first to describe the bronchial blood vessels and made other important anatomical discoveries. Died 1731. *1099, 389*

## 1639

1639:1 First **hospital** in **Canada** founded

1639:2 **Law regulating medical practice** in Virginia passed

1639:3 *Codex medicamentarius seu pharmacopoeia Parisiensis*, first Paris **pharmacopoeia**, published. *1824*

1639:4 **Cinchona** introduced into Spain and Portugal by **Juan del Vigo**

## 1640

1640:1 **University of Åbo (Turku)**, **Finland**, founded

1640:2 *Theatrum botanicum*, largest English-language **herbal**, published by John Parkinson (1567–1650). *1823*

---

1640:3 Sebastiano **Bado** [Baldi], Italian physician, *fl.* 1640–1676; defended the virtues of 'Peruvian bark' (cinchona) in malaria; in his *Anastasis corticis Peruviae, seu chinae defensio*, 1663. He also includes evidence that '**fever bark**' was introduced into Spain in 1632. *5230.1*

1640:4 Jean **Denis** [Denys] born; performed first blood transfusion into a human; *Lettre ... touchant deux expériences de la transfusion ...*, 1667. Died 1704. *2013*

---

44

1640: Robert **Burton** died, **born** 1577. *psychiatry*

## 1641

1641:1 The first scientific description of **scarlet fever** given by Daniel Sennert (1572–1637); in his *De febribus*, libri IV. *5074*

1641:2 John **Mayow**, British physician and chemist, born 24 May. In his *Tractatus duo*, 1668, his first tract covers respiration and he describes the role of oxygen in respiration and combustion; the second tract deals with rickets. An improved exposition is contained in his *Tractatus quinque medico-physici* (a revision of *Tractatus duo*), 1674, which also records a probable case of mitral stenosis. Died 1679. *578, 2726.2*

1641:3 Regnier de **Graaf**, Dutch physician and physiologist, born 30 Jul; in his *De virorum organis generationi inservientibus*, 1668, he gave an exact and detailed account of the male reproductive system, and in his *De mulierum organis generationi inservientibus*, 1672, demonstrated ovulation and included the first account of the 'Graafian follicle'. Died 1673. *1210, 1209*

1641:4 Raymond **Vieussens**, French physician, born; in his *Nevrographia universalis*, 1684, described the centrum ovale for the first time, and threw new light on the structure of the brain and nerves; gave an important account of various heart disorders, including mitral stenosis; in his *Novum vasorum corporis humani systema*, 1695. Died 1715. *1379, 2729*

## 1642

1642:1 The first modern scientific description of **beriberi** was given by Jacob de Bondt [Bontius] (1592–1631); in his *De medicina Indorum*, pp. 115–20. *3736*

1642:2 The first book on **rheumatism**, a term introduced by its author, was *Liber de rheumatismo et pleuritide dorsali*, by Guillaume Baillou (1538–1616). *4485*

1642:3 Thomas Browne (1605–1682) wrote ***Religio medici***, one of the best works in English literature written by a physician; an attempt to reconcile scientific scepticism with faith. *6612.90*

1642:4 John **Browne**, English physician, born; gave first description of cirrhosis of the liver, 1685, *PT* **15**:1266. Died 1700? *3613*

1642:5 William **Briggs**, English physician and oculist, born; gave the first known description of nyctalopia, 1684, *PT* **14**:561. Died 1704. *5822*

## 1643

1643:1 Lorenzo **Bellini**, Italian physician and anatomist, born 3 Sep. His *Exercitatio anatomica de structura et usu renum*, 1662, an important description of the kidney, includes the first description of the renal excretory ducts ('Bellini's ducts' or 'tubules'). Demonstrated the importance of urine in diagnosis; in his *De urinis et pulsibus*, 1683. Died 1704. *1229, 4162*

1643: John **Woodall** died, **born** 1570. *scurvy, naval medicine*

## 1644

1644:1 **Hôtel Dieu, Montreal**, founded

1644:2 The first works by an Englishman on teaching of **deaf-mutes**, *Chironomia* and *Chirologia*, published by John Bulwer (*fl.*1654). *3346, 3347*

1644:3 An experiment in **reflex action** performed by René Descartes (1596–1650); recorded in his *Des passions de l'âme*, 1649. *4965*

_____

1644: Johannes Baptista van **Helmont** died, **born** 1579. *biochemistry, digestion, physiology*

## 1645
1645:1 Precursor of **Royal Society** founded in **London**; formally established in 1660

## 1646
1646:1 **Syphilis** appears in **Boston, Massachusetts**

1646:2 An important early account of **plague** given by Ysbrand van Diemerbroeck (1609–1674); in his *De peste libri quatuor*. *5117*

_____

1646:3 James **Yonge**, English surgeon, born; recorded an account of the first flap amputation in his *Currus triumphalis ...*, 1679. Died 1721. *4436*

## 1647
1647:1 Walter **Harris**, English paediatrician, born; his *De morbis acutis infantum*, 1689, served for nearly a century as the standard English work on diseases of children. Died 1732. *6321*

## 1648
1648:1 Johannes Baptista van Helmont (1579–1644) was a founder of **biochemistry**, who did important work on the role of acids in **digestion**, and first to recognize the physiological importance of ferments and gases. Writings collected in his *Ortus Medicinae*. *665*

1648:2 First differentiation of **yaws** from **syphilis** by Willem Piso (1611–1678); in *Historia naturalis Brasiliae* (De medica Brasiliensi p. 35). *5303*

_____

1648:3 Joseph Guichard **Duverney**, French anatomist and physician, born 5 Aug; published first scientific account of the ear, its structure, function and diseases, *Traité de l'organe de l'ouie*, 1683. Died 1730. *1545*

_____

1648:4 Frederik **Dekkers**, Dutch physician, born; first described albuminuria; in his *Exercitationes medicae practicae*, cap. V., 1672; gave the first clear account of proteinuria; in his *Exercitationes medicae practicae circa medendi methodum*, 1673. Died 1720. *4161, 4204.1*

## 1649
1649:1 **Act regulating the practice of medicine in Massachusetts** passed

1649:2 **[Royal Academy of Medical Sciences]**, **Palermo**, established

_____

1649:3 Govert **Bidloo**, Dutch physician, professor, University of Leiden, born 12 Mar. His *Anatomica humani corporis*, 1685, is remarkable for its 105 fine copperplate engravings by Pieter van Gunst, afterwards plagiarized by William Cowper (1698). Died 1713. *385*

_____

1649:4 John **Floyer**, English physician, born; first clearly described bronchial asthma, in his *Treatise on the asthma*, 1698; invented a pulse-watch, as recorded in *The physician's pulse-watch*, 1707; his *Medicina gerocomica*, 1724, is the first English work devoted to geriatrics. Died 1734. *3166, 2670, 1595*

## 1650

1650:1 Francis Glisson's (1597–1677) *De rachitide* contained the fullest account of **rickets** that had appeared up to that time, it also (chap.22) gave the first description of infantile **scurvy**. *3729*

1650:2 Edward **Tyson**, English anatomist and physician, born; gave early anatomical description of *Ascaris lumbricoides*, 1683, *PT* **13**:133. Died 1697. *2448*

1650:3 Antoine **Maître-Jan** born; the 'Father of French ophthalmology'. He wrote *Traité des maladies de l'oeil*, 1707, and supported Brisseau's views on the nature of **cataract**. Died 1730. *5824*

1650: John **Parkinson** died, **born** 1567. *herbal*

1650: René **Descartes** died, **born** 1596. *philosophy, mathematics, reflex action*

## 1651

1651:1 **La Salpêtrière, Paris**, founded; opened 1657

1651:2 *Exercitationes de generatione animalium* published by William Harvey (1578–1657); an important early work on **embryology**. The chapter on **labour** (De partu) is the first original work on **obstetrics** to be published by an English author. *467, 6146*

1651:3 Hendrik van **Deventer**, Dutch obstetrician and orthopaedist, born 16 Mar; gave the first accurate description of the female pelvis and its deformities, and the effect of the latter in complicating labour, in his *Manuale operatien, I. deel zijnde een neiuw ligt voor vroed-meesters en vroed-vrouen*, 1701. Died 1724. *6253*

## 1652

1652:1 **Academia Naturae Curiosorum** founded in **Germany**

1652:2 Nicholas Tulp (1593–1674) gave one of the earliest accounts of **beriberi**; in his *Observationes medicae*, 1652, p. 300. Died 1674. *3737*

1652:3 Human **thoracic duct** discovered by Thomas Bartholin (1616–1680); published in his *De lactis thoracicis in homine brutisque. 1096*

1652:4 **Haemolytic jaundice of newborn** described by Domenico Panaroli (d.1657); in his *Iatrologismorum seu medicinalium observationum …. 3050*

1652:5 Daniel **Le Clerc**, Swiss physician, born 4 Feb; he wrote the first large history of medicine, *Histoire de la médecine*, 1729; he is sometimes termed the 'Father of the history of medicine'. Died 1728. *6379*

1652:6 John **Radcliffe**, British physician to William III, Queen Mary and Queen Anne, born; Radcliffe Infirmary, Oxford, erected from the residue of his estate, 1770. Died 1714.

1652: François **Citois** died, **born** 1572. *lead poisoning*

## 1653

1653:1 *Vasa lymphatica* published by Thomas Bartholin (1616–1680), in which he claimed priority in the discovery of the **lymphatics**; this was disputed by Rudbeck and Joyliffe. *1096, 1097, 1098.1*

1653:2 A prominent teacher of **deaf-mutes**, John Wallis (1616–1703), a professor of mathematics at Oxford, classified the various sounds of the human **voice**; in his *Grammatica linguae Anglicae. 3348*

1653:3 Johann Conrad à **Brunner**, Swiss anatomist, born 16 Jan; performed pioneer experiments on the pancreas and recorded extreme thirst and polyuria after its excision in the dog, which almost led him to the discovery of diabetes mellitus; in his *Experimenta nova circa pancreas*, 1683. Died 1727. 3927

## 1654

1654:1 **Fraternity of Physicians** formed in **Ireland** (College in 1667; **Royal College of Physicians of Ireland**, 1890)

1654:2 '**Glisson's capsule**', the capsule of the liver, described by Francis Glisson (1597–1677) in his *Anatomia hepatis. 972*

1654:3 Giovanni Maria **Lancisi**, Italian physician, born 26 Oct; gave an important account and classification of the heart diseases then recognized; in his *De subitaneis mortibus*, 1707. Suggested that malaria was a poison emanating from marshes and possibly transmitted by mosquitoes; in his *De noxiis paludum effluviis, eorumque remediis*, 1717. Died 1720. *2731, 5232*

1654:4 John **Bulwer** *fl*; published the first works by an Englishman on teaching of deaf-mutes, *Chironomia* and *Chirologia* (1644). *3346, 3347*

1654: Nicholas **Culpeper** died, **born** 1616. *herbal*

## 1655

1655:1 **University of Duisberg** founded

1655:2 A report on successful **symphysiotomy** is contained in *De nutritione foetus in utero paradoxa*, p. 245, by Jean Claude de la Courvée (1615–1664). *6146.1*

1655:3 Caspar **Bartholin**, Danish anatomist and physician, born 10 Sep; described the sublingual salivary gland and ducts, later named after him, in his *De ductu salivati hactenus non descriptio*, 1684. Died 1738. *974.2*

1655:4 (*c*) Clopton **Havers**, English physician, born. His *Osteologia nova, or some new observations of the bones*, 1691, was the first complete account of the microscopic structure of bone. The 'Haversian canals' are named after him. Died 1702. *387*

1655: Lazare **Rivière** [Riverius] died, **born** 1589. *aortic stenosis*

**1656**

1656:1 **Lazar houses** abolished in **France**

1656:2 The location of **cataract** in the lens first demonstrated by Guerner Rolfinck (1599–1673); in his *Dissertationes anatomicae methodo synthetica exaratae. 5821.1*

1656:3 Thomas Wharton's (1614–1673) *Adenographia* included a description of the **submaxillary salivary gland** ('**Wharton's duct**'). *1116*

1656:4 Edmund **Halley**, British astronomer and mathematician, born 8 Nov; compiled the so-called 'Breslau tables' of mortality rates and other vital statistics, 1693, *PT* **17**:596. Died 1742. *1687*

1656: Marco Aurelio **Severino** died, **born** 1580. *surgical pathology*

**1657**

1657:1 **Chateau Bicêtre** built by Bishop of Winchester at **Chantilly**, 1256; became **hospital, almshouse and prison**, 1657

1657:2 **La Salpêtrière, Paris**, opened; founded 1651

1657:3 **Accademia del Cimento, Florence**, founded 16 June by Ferdinand II, de Medici

1657:4 Domenico **Panaroli** died; described haemolytic jaundice of newborn ; in his *Iatrologismorum seu medicinalium observationum ...*, 1652. *3050*

1657: William **Harvey** died, **born** 1578. *blood circulation, embryology, labour*

**1658**

1658:1 Athanasius Kircher (1602–1680) was probably the first to use the **microscope** to study the cause of disease. In his *Scrutinium physico-medicum contagiosae luis, quae pestis dicitur*, he remarked that the blood of **plague** patients was filled with a 'countless brood of worms not perceptible to the naked eye'; he was the first to state explicitly the theory of **contagion** by **animalculae** as the cause of **infectious diseases**. *5118*

1658:2 **Apoplexy** shown by Johann Jacob Wepfer (1620–1695) to be a result of a cerebral haemorrhage into the brain; in his *Observationes anatomicae, ex cadaveribus eorum, quos sustulit apoplexia. 2703, 4511.2*

1658:3 Alexis **Littré**, French surgeon, born 21 Jul; described diverticulum hernia ('Littré's hernia') and Littré's glands, 1700, *HARS Mém*:300, 311 (1719); first to suggest colostomy in intestinal obstruction, 1710, *HARS*, Mém:36 (1732). Died 1726. *3575, 1215, 3418*

1658:4 Marko **Gerbec** [Gerbezius] born; first to note Stokes-Adams syndrome, 1692, *MCT* **10**:115. Died 1718. *2728*

1658:5 Francesco **Torti**, Italian physician and pharmacologist, born; established the specific effectiveness of cinchona in malaria; in his *Therapeuticae specialis ad febres quasdam perniciosas, inopinato, ac repente lethales, una vera china china*, etc., 1712. He is also credited with the introduction of the term **malaria**. Died 1741. *5231*

1658:6 Nicolas **Andry**, French physician, born; published first medical textbook on human parasitology, *De la géneration des vers dans le corps de l'homme*, 1700. Wrote the first book on orthopaedics, *L'orthopédie*, 1741; he introduced the term. Died 1742. *2448.2, 4301*

## 1659
1659:1 **[Royal Library]** founded in **Berlin**

1659:2 The first description of **epidemic typhoid** given by Thomas Willis (1621–1675); in his *Diatribae duae*, etc. (De febribus, cap.X, xiv.). *5020*

---

1659:3 Giacomo **Pylarino** [Pilarini], Italian physician, born; he is accredited with the 'medical' discovery of variolation; in his *Nova et tuta variolas excitandi per transplantionem methodus*, 1715, he described its practice in Constantinople. Died 1718. *5409.1*

---

1659: Paolo **Zacchias** died, **born** 1584. *medical jurisprudence*

## 1660
1660:1 **Royal Society of London** formally constituted

1660:2 **Nasal mucus** shown to originate in the nasal mucous membrane ('**Schneider's membrane**') by Conrad Victor Schneider (1614–1680); in his *Liber ... de catarrhis*. *3245*

---

1660:3 Friedrich **Hoffmann**, German physician, born 19 Feb; gave classic description of chlorosis; in his *De genuina chlorosis indole, origine et curatione*, 1731. Died 1742. *3110*

1660:4 Georg Ernst **Stahl**, chemist and physician, born 21 Oct. The first to treat lacrimal fistula, on the basis of correct anatomical understanding; he described it in an addendum, *De fistula lacrimali*, 1702, to the thesis of his student E.C. Lange, *De affectibus oculorum*. His *De motus haemorrhoidalis et fluxus haemorrhoidum* was a classical work on the subject, 1730. Died 1734. *5823, 3421*

---

1660:5 (?) Patrick **Blair**, surgeon and botanist, born; first to describe congenital hypertrophic pyloric stenosis, 1717. Died 1728. *3419*

## 1661
1661:1 **University of Lemberg (Lwow)** founded

1661:2 Capillary **circulation** described by Marcello Malpighi (1628–1694) in *De pulmonibus* .... *760*

---

1661:3 François **Poupart**, French surgeon and naturalist, born; described the inguinal ligament ('Poupart's ligament'), 1730, *HARS* 51. Died 1708. *977*

## 1662
1662:1 **Charles II** grants charter to **Royal Society of London**, 15 July

1662:2 **Anatomical theatre** built in **Uppsala** by Olof **Rudbeck** (1630–1702)

1662:3 Lorenzo Bellini's (1643–1704) *Exercitatio anatomica de structura et usu renum*, an important description of the **kidney**, includes the first description of the **renal excretory ducts** ('**Bellini's ducts**' or 'tubules'). *1229*

1662:4 **Ceruminous glands** and excretory duct of **parotid gland** ('Stensen's duct') described by Niels Stensen [Nicolaus Steno] (1638–1686), in his *Observationes anatomicae*. *973, 1543*

1662:5 **Boyle's law**, Robert Boyle (1627–1691), contained in his *A defence of the doctrine touching the spring and weight of the air*. *666*

1662:6 First book on **vital statistics**, *Natural and political observations ... upon the Bills of Mortality of London*, published by John Graunt (1620–1674). *1686*

1662:7 Thomas **Dover**, English physician and privateer, born; his *Ancient physician's legacy to his country*, 1732, contains the original prescription for Dover's powder: equal quantities of opium, ipecacuanha, liquorice, saltpetre and tartar vitreolus (ipecacuanha and opium powder BP, 1958), a former favourite for the relief of pain, coughs, etc. In 1708 he embarked on a privateering voyage, and in the following February, on the island of Juan Fernandez, discovered the castaway Andrew Selkirk, who inspired Defoe's *Robinson Crusoe*. Died 1742

## 1663

1663:1 First **hospital** established in **American colonies** (Long Island, NY)

1663:2 **Collegium Medicorum** established in **Stockholm**

1663:3 The virtues of '**Peruvian bark**' (**cinchona**) in **malaria** defended by Sebastiano Bado [Baldi] (*fl.*1640–1676); in his *Anastasis corticis Peruviae, seu chinae defensio*. He also includes evidence that '**fever bark**' was introduced into Spain in 1632. *5230.1*

1663:4 The first modern work on **operative gynaecology**, *Heel-konstige aanmerkkingen betreffende de gebreeken der vrouwen*, written by Hendrik van Roonhuyze (1622–1672). *6015*

1663:5 Johann Konrad **Amman** born; a successful teacher of deaf-mutes, published his method in *Surdus loquens*, 1692. Died 1730. *3352*

## 1664

1664:1 The structure and function of **muscle** studied by Niels Stensen [Nicolaus Steno] (1638–1686); in his *De musculis et glandulis observationum specimen*, 1664; *Elementorum myologiae specimen*, 1667. *576, 577*

1664:2 **Nervous system** accurately and completely described by Thomas Willis (1621–1675) in his *Cerebri anatome*. *1378*

1664:3 First methodical work on **snake poison**, published by Francesco Redi (1626–1697); in his *Osservazione intorno alle vipere*. *2102*

1664:4 **Gonococcal arthritis** first described by Pierre Martin de La Martinière (1634–1690); in his *Traité de la maladie vénérienne*. *4485.1*

1664:5 François **Pourfour du Petit**, French physiologist and surgeon, born; discovered the vasomotor nerves, 1727, *HARS*:1. Died 1741. *764*

**1665**

1665:1 *Journal des Sçavans*, **first independent scientific journal**, commences publication (5 January)

1665:2 **Royal Society of London** commences publication of *Philosophical Transactions* (6 March)

1665:3 **Great Plague of London**

1665:4 **University of Kiel** founded

1665:5 **[Royal Library, Copenhagen]** founded

1665:6 **University of Lund** founded

1665:7 *Micrographia*, earliest work devoted entirely to account of **microscopical** observations, published by Robert Hooke (1635–1703). *262*

1665:8 **Blood transfusion** from one live animal into another (dogs) by Richard Lower (1631–1691), *PT* **1**:353. *2012*

1665:9 **Sunstroke** described by Georg Horst (d.1688); in his *De siriasi. 2246*

1665:10 Frederik Ruysch (1638–1731) was first to describe the **valves of the lymphatics**, in his *Dilucidatio valvularum in vasis lymphaticis et lacteis. 1099*

—————

1665:11 Giuseppe **Zambeccari**, Italian anatomist and surgeon, born; showed that the spleen is not essential to life; in his *Esperienze ... intorno a diverse viscere tagliate a diversi animali viventi*, 1680. Died 1728. *3761*

**1666**

1666:1 **Académie des Sciences** founded in **Paris**

1666:2 **Great Fire of London**

1666:3 First work solely on the **spinal cord** published by Gerard Blaes [Blasius] (1626–1682); in his *Anatome medullae spinalis, et nervorum. 1354.9*

1666:4 **Plague** differentiated from **typhus** by William Boghurst (1631–1685); in his *Loimographia*, written in 1666 but not published until 1894. *5120*

1666:5 The earliest scientific account by a practitioner of **psychotherapy** by the 'laying on of hands' was that of Valentine Greatrakes (1629–1683); in his *A brief account of Mr Valentine Greatrakes, and divers of the strange cures lately performed by him. 4992*

1666:6 **Meibomian (conjunctival) glands** described by Heinrich Meibom (1638–1700); in his *De vasis palpebrarum novis epistola. 1481*

1666:7 **Malpighian bodies** and **uriniferous tubules** described by Marcello Malpighi (1628–1694); in his *De viscerum structura .... 1230*

—————

1666:8 Antonio Mario **Valsalva**, Italian anatomist, born 15 Feb; described Valsalva's manoeuvre in his *De aure humana tractatus*, 1704. Died 1723. *1546*

1666:9 William **Cowper**, English anatomist and surgeon, born 8 Mar; described Cowper's glands, 1699, *PT* **21**:364; they had earlier been noted by Jean Méry, 1684. First described aortic insufficiency, 1706, *PT* **24**:1970. Pioneered the surgical treatment of diseases of the maxillary sinus; he wrote on this in James Drake's *Anthropologia nova*, **2**, 526–49, 1707. Died 1709. *1214, 2730, 3670.1*

1666:10 Bernard **Connor** (or O'Connor), Irish physician, born; gave the first description of ankylosing spondylitis; in his *Lettre écrite à Monsieur le Chevalier Guillaume de Waldegrave*, 1693? Died 1698. *4298*

1666:11 Giovanni Cosimo **Bonomo** born; with Giacinto Cestoni gave first clinical and experimental proof of infection by a microparasite (*Sarcoptes scabiei*); in *Osservationi intorno a' pellicelli del corporo umano*, 1687. Died 1696. *2529.1, 4012*

1666: Job Janszoon van **Meekeren** died, **born** 1611. *bone grafts*

**1667**
1667:1 **College of Physicians, Ireland** (formerly Fraternity, 1654)

1667:2 Jan Swammerdam (1637–1680) discovered that the **lungs** of newborn infants will float on water if **respiration** has taken place (an important medico-legal point); in his *De respiratione usuque pulmonum*. Died 1680. *1724*

1667:3 **Intravenous injections of drugs** reported by Johann Daniel Major (1634–1693); in his *Chirurgia infusoria*. *1963*

1667:4 **Blood transfusion** into a human first performed by Jean Denis [Denys] (1640–1704); *Lettre ... touchant deux expériences de la transfusion ...*. *2013*

1667:5 The structure and function of **muscle** studied by Niels Stensen [Nicolaus Steno] (1638–1686); in his *Elementorum myologiae specimen*, 1667. *577*

1667:6 Thomas Willis (1621–1675) gave the first account of **cerebral syphilis**, without recognizing the cause, in his *Pathologia cerebri*.

1667:7 Charles de **Saint-Yves**, French ophthalmologist, born 10 Nov; reported the removal *en masse* of a cataract from a living subject; in his *Nouveau traité des maladies des yeux*, 1722. Died 1736. *5827*

1667:8 Daniel **Turner**, English physician, born; his *De morbis cutaneis. A treatise of diseases incident to the skin*, 1714, is the first English text on dermatology; he may be regarded as the founder of English dermatology. Died 1741. *3981*

**1668**
1668:1 **University of Agram (Zagreb)** founded

1668:2 An exact and detailed account of the male **reproductive system** published by Regnier de Graaf (1641–1673); in his *De virorum organis generationi inservientibus*. *1210*

1668:3 First recorded **bone graft** by Job Janszoon van Meekeren (1611–1666) (Chap. 1 of *Heel- en geneeskonstige aanmerkkingen*). Unfortunately the Church ordered the removal of the graft. *5735*

1668:4 In John Mayow's (1641–1679) *Tractatus duo*, his first tract covers respiration and describes the role of **oxygen** in respiration and combustion, the second tract deals with **rickets**. *578*

1668:5 François Mauriceau (1637–1709), leading French obstetrician of his day, wrote *Des maladies des femmes grosses et accouchées*, the outstanding textbook on **obstetrics** of the time. *6147*

1668:6 Herman **Boerhaave**, Dutch physician and chemist and eminent teacher at Leiden (1701–1729), born 31 Dec. The modern medical curriculum owes much to him. The *Institutiones medicae*, 1708, one of the earliest textbooks of physiology, was used in every medical school. His *Aphorismi de cognoscendis et curandis morbis*, 1709, enshrines much of his ripe clinical wisdom. First to separate out urea from urine (*Elementa chemiae*, 1732). Died 1738. *581, 2199, 666.1*

## 1669
1669:1 Leopold I founds **University of Innsbruck** (as **Academia Leopoldina**)

1669:2 Richard Lower (1631–1691), in *Tractatus de corde*, noted the scroll-like structure of **cardiac muscle**. *2012, 761*

1669:3 **Paracusis** described by William Holder (1616–1698); in his *Elements of speech …*, Appendix, p. 166. *3349*

1669:4 Pedro **Virgili**, Spanish surgeon and anatomist, born; successfully performed tracheotomy for quinsy, 1743, *MARC* 1 (3):141. Died 1776. *3248*

## 1670
1670:1 **Physic Garden** (later **Royal Botanic Garden**) established at **Edinburgh**

1670:2 *Miscellanea Curiosa Medico-Physica*, **first scientific journal in Germany**, commences publication

1670:3 In his *Affectionum quae dicuntur hystericae*, etc., Thomas Willis (1621–1675) showed **hysteria** to be a nervous disease and not a uterine disorder, as had been traditionally believed. *4839*

1670:4 Francis **Fuller** born; published *Medicina gymnastica*, first English text on therapeutic value of gymnastics, 1705. Died 1706. *1986.3*

## 1671
1671:1 'Fallot's tetralogy' first described by Niels Stensen (1638–1686); in his *Embryo monstro affinis Parisiis dissectus*. *2726.1*

1671:2 The first authentic report of **trigeminal neuralgia** given by Johannes Michael Fehr (1610–1688) and Elias Schmidt, *MCMP* 2. *4512*

1671:3 The first authentic account of **variolation** (inoculation against **smallpox**) given by Heinrich Vollgnad (1634–1682); in his *Globus vitulinus*. *5405*

1671:4 Jan Swammerdam (1637–1680) disputed priority of de Graaf in his demonstration of **ovulation**; in his *Miraculum naturae, sive uteri muliebris fabrica*. Died 1680. *1211*

1671:5 George **Cheyne**, Scottish physician, born; attributed hypochondria to the moisture of the air and the variability of the weather in the British Isles; in his *The English malady*, 1733. Died 1743. *4840*

**1672**
1672:1 Isaac **Newton**'s (1642–1727) theory of **light** and **colours** announced

1672:2 **Graafian follicle** and **ovulation** described by Regnier de Graaf (1641–1673) in his *De mulierum organis generationi inservientibus*. *1209*

1672:3 Thomas Willis (1621–1675) described, in his *De anima brutorum*, **general paralysis** (4to edn, p. 392, 8vo edn, p. 278), **myasthenia gravis** (pars 2, Cap.ix), **lethargy** (pars 2, cap.III) and **paracusis of Willis**. *4793, 4730, 4919, 1544*

1672: Hendrik van **Roonhuyze** died, **born** 1622. *gynaecology*

1672: Franciscus de le **Boë** [Sylvius] died, **born** 1614. *tuberculosis, tubercles*

**1673**
1673:1 *De ovo incubato* and *De formatione pulli in ovo* published by Marcello Malpighi (1628–1694); these works placed the study of **embryology** on a sound basis. *468, 469*

1673:2 The first clear descriptions of **proteinuria** and **albuminuria medendi** given by Frederik Dekkers (1648–1720); in his *Exercitationes medicae practicae circa medendi methodum*. *4161, 4204.1*

1673:3 Richard **Mead**, English physician, born 11 Aug; a popular and wealthy physician, his advice about the plague, *A short discourse concerning pestilential contagion*, 1720, was later expanded to become almost a prophecy of the English public health system. He advocated inoculation against smallpox, *De variolis et morbillis liber*, 1747, and he persuaded Thomas Guy to establish Guy's Hospital, London. Died 1754. *5123, 5417*

1673: Thomas **Wharton** died, **born** 1614. *salivary gland*

1673: Regnier de **Graaf** died, **born** 1641. *Graaffian follicle*

1673: Guerner **Rolfinck** died, **born** 1599. *cataract*

**1674**
1674:1 First **Medical Act** of **Norway** and **Denmark**

1674:2 The first accurate description of the **red blood corpuscles** (previously noted by Swammerdam in 1658) given by Antoni van Leeuwenhoek (1632–1723), *PT*, **9**: 121. *860*

1674:3 **Aortic stenosis** described by Lazare Rivière [Riverius] (1589–1655); in his *Opera medica universa. 2727*

1674:4 An improved account of the role of **oxygen** in respiration and combustion described by John Mayow (1641–1679) in his *Tractatus quinque medico-physici*, 1674 (a revision of his *Tractatus duo*, 1668) which also records a probable case of **mitral stenosis**. *2726.2*

1674:5 An exhaustive survey of **dracontiasis** given by Georg Hieronymous Welsch (1624–1677); in his *Exercitatio de vena Medinensis. 5336.1*

1674:6 Jean Louis **Petit**, French surgeon, born 13 Mar; he is particularly remembered for his work on bone diseases, *L'art de guérir les maladies des os*, 1705; he gave the first account of **osteomalacia**. In his *Traité des maladies chirurgicales*, 1774, recorded his successful treatment of mastoiditis (**1**,153, 160) and described 'Petit's hernia' and 'Petit's triangle' (**2**, 256). Died 1750. *4300, 3357, 3577*

1674: Ysbrand van **Diemerbroeck** died, **born** 1609. *plague*

1674: John **Graunt** died, **born** 1620. *vital statistics*

1674: Nicolaas **Tulp** died, **born** 1593. *beriberi*

## 1675

1675:1 Thomas Willis (1621–1675) noted the sweetness of urine in **diabetes mellitus** and differentiated this condition from **diabetes insipidus**; in his *Pharmaceutice rationalis ...*, **2**, IV, cap.3. He also gave a clear account of **whooping cough**, **2**, p. 99. *3926, 5086*

1675:2 James **Douglas**, Scottish physician, born; described the 'pouch', 'line', and 'fold of Douglas'; in his *A description of the peritonaeum ...*, 1730. Died 1742. *1217*

1675:3 John **Freind**, English chemist and physician, born; the first English historian of medicine, wrote *The history of physick, from the time of Galen to the beginning of the sixteenth century*, 2 vols, 1725–6. Died 1728. *6378*

1675: Thomas **Willis** died, **born** 1621. *nervous system, paracusis of Willis, diabetes, cerebral meningitis, hysteria, myasthenia gravis, general paralysis, typhoid, whooping cough, lethargy, syphilis*

## 1676

1676:1 **Chelsea Physic Garden (Society of Apothecaries)** founded

1676:2 **Hôpital des Enfants Malades** founded in **Paris**

1676:3 Thomas Sydenham (1624–1689) gave many excellent accounts of diseases including, in his *Observationes medicae circa morborum acutorum historiam et curationem*, 1676, his description of **scarlet fever** (p. 387) and the most minute and careful description of **measles** that had so far appeared (pp. 272–80). *5075, 5441.1*

1676:4 Michel **Brisseau** born; first demonstrated the true nature and location of cataract; in his *Traité de la cataract et du glaucoma*, 1709. Died 1743. *5825*

**1677**

1677:1 **Kaiserliche Leopoldinische Akademie der Naturforscher** founded

1677:2 Stephen **Hales** born 17 Sep; inventor of artificial ventilation; in his *A description of ventilators*, 1743. His invention of the manometer, 1733, enabled him to measure blood pressure; published in his *Statical essays*. Died 1761. *1596, 765*

1677: Francis **Glisson** died, **born** 1597. *liver capsule, rickets, scurvy*

1677: Georg Hieronymous **Welsch** died, **born** 1624. *dracontiasis*

**1678**

1678:1 **University of Modena** founded (chartered 1683)

1678:2 Robert **Houstoun** born; first to treat ovarian dropsy by tapping the cyst, 1701, reported in 1724, *PT* **33**:8. Died 1743. *6017*

1678:3 Pierre **Fauchard** born; considered the 'Father of dentistry', published *Le chirurgien dentiste*, 1728. Died 1761. *3671*

1678:4 François de **La Peyronie**, French surgeon, born 15 Jan; first described plastic induration of the penis ('Peyronie's disease'), 1743, *MARC* 1:425. Died 1747. *4163*

1678: Willem **Piso** died, **born** 1611. *yaws, syphilis*

**1679**

1679:1 **First independent medical periodical** (*Nouvelles Découvertes sur toutes les Parties de la Médecine*) published by Nicolas de Blegny

1679:2 **Botanic garden** at **Amsterdam**

1679:3 **Pathological anatomy**; first systematized collection of cases, *Sepulchretum*, by Theophile Bonet (1620–1689). *2274*

1679:4 Franciscus de le Boë [Sylvius] (1614–1672) was first to describe **tubercles** in **tuberculosis**, asserting that they are often found in the lung and that they softened and suppurated to form cavities; *Opera omnia*, 1679. *2321*

1679:5 An account of the first **flap amputation** recorded by James Yonge (1646–1721); in his *Currus triumphalis* .... *4436*

1679:6 Zabdiel **Boylston**, American physician, born 9 Mar. First in America to introduce smallpox inoculation (Boston 26 June 1721); *An historical account of the small-pox inoculated in New England*, 1726. Died 1766. *5415*

1679:7 Gaspar **Casal y Julian**, Spanish physician, born; wrote the first recognizable description of pellagra (*mal de la rosa*) but published posthumously; *Historia natural, y medica de el Principado de Asturias*, 1762. Died 1759. *3750*

1679:8 Dominique **Anel**, French surgeon, born; first to catheterize the lacrimal duct; in his *Observation singulière sur la fistule lacrimale*, etc., 1713. Died 1730. *5826*

1679: John **Mayow** died, **born** 1641. *oxygen, respiration, rickets, mitral stenosis*

## 1680
1680:1 The fact that the **spleen** is not essential to life proved by Guiseppe Zambeccari (1665–1728); in his *Esperienze ... intorno a diverse viscere tagliate a diversi animali viventi. 3761*

1680:2 An alphabet for the use of **deaf-mutes** invented by George Dalgarno (?1626–1687); in his *Didascalocophus or the deaf and dumb mans tutor .... 3350*

1680:3 (?) Claudius **Amyand**, English surgeon, born; performed the first recorded successful appendicectomy, 1736, *PT* **39**:329. Died 1740. *3559*

1680: Thomas **Bartholin** died, **born** 1616. *thoracic duct, lymphatics*

1680: Conrad Victor **Schneider** died, **born** 1614. *nasal mucus*

1680: Athanasius **Kircher** died, **born** 1602. *microscopy, plague, infectious disease*

1680: Jan **Swammerdam** died, **born** 1637. *lungs, respiration, ovulation*

## 1681
1681:1 **Royal College of Physicians of Edinburgh** founded

1681:2 **[Hospital for Insane]** opened at **Avignon**, France, 11 Feb

## 1682
1682:1 Giovanni Battista **Morgagni**, Italian anatomist and pathologist, born 25 Feb; his *De sedibus et causis morborum per anatomen indagatis*, 1761, is a foundation stone of pathological anatomy; it includes his account of a case of angina pectoris observed in 1707. Died 1771. *2276, 2885*

1682: Heinrich **Vollgnad** died, **born** 1634. *smallpox, variolation*

1682: Gerard **Blaes** [Blasius] died, **born** 1626. *spinal cord*

1682: Thomas **Browne** died, **born** 1605. *Religio medici*

## 1683
1683:1 First scientific account of the **ear** and its structure, function and diseases, by Joseph Guichard Duverney (1648–1730); in his Traité *de l'organe de l'ouie. 1545*

1683:2 *Ascaris lumbricoides*; early anatomical description by Edward Tyson (1626–1697), *PT* **13**:133. *2448*

1683:3 **Diabetes mellitus** almost discovered by Johann Conrad à Brunner (1653–1727) who performed pioneer experiments on the **pancreas** and recorded extreme thirst and polyuria after its excision in the dog; in his *Experimenta nova circa pancreas. 3927*

1683:4 Importance of **urine** in **diagnosis** demonstrated by Lorenzo Bellini (1643–1704); in his *De urinis et pulsibus. 4162*

1683:5 Thomas Sydenham (1624–1689) clearly differentiated **gout** from **rheumatism** in his *Tractatus de podagra et hydrope. 4486*

---

1683:6 Lorenz **Heister**, German surgeon, born 19 Sep; founder of scientific surgery in Germany, wrote *Chirurgie in welcher alles was zur Wund-Artzney gehoret*, 1718, most popular surgical text of the 18th century. Died 1758. *5576*

---

1683: Valentine **Greatrakes** died, **born** 1629. *psychotherapy*

## 1684

1684:1 **First English medical journal** (*Medicina Curiosa*) published

1684:2 **Bartholin's duct** and **gland**, the sublingual salivary gland and ducts described by Caspar Bartholin (1655–1738), in his *De ductu salivati hactenus non descriptio. 974.2*

1684:3 **Blood analysis** carried out by Robert Boyle (1627–1691); in his *Memoirs for the natural history of the blood. 861*

1684:4 **Bacteria** in the **mouth** discovered by Antoni van Leeuwenhoek (1632–1723), *PT* **14**:568. *2464.1, 3669.4*

1684:5 Raymond Vieussens (1684–1715) in his *Nevrographia universalis* described the **centrum ovale** for the first time, and threw new light on the structure of the **brain** and **nerves**. *1379*

1684:6 The first to report **cerebrospinal meningitis** was probably Thomas Willis (1621–1675); in his *Practice of physick*, VIII, 46. *4673*

1684:7 The first known description of **nyctalopia** given by William Briggs (1642–1704), *PT* **14**:561. *5822*

---

1684:8 Jean **Astruc**, French anatomist and physician, born 19 Mar; considering the period in which it was written, his *De morbis veneris libri sex*, 1736, provides an admirable and comprehensive account of venereal disease. Died 1766. *5195*

## 1685

1685:1 **Medical faculty** established at **University of Edinburgh**

1685:2 **Barber-Surgeons' School, Stockholm**, reorganized as **Societas Chirurgica**

1685:3 **Prussian ordinance** regulating **medical fees**

1685:4 An important account of **smallpox** published by Thomas Sydenham (1624–1689); in his *Observationes medicae*, Ed. quarta, Book 3, cap.2, Book 5, cap.4. *5407*

1685:5 Govert Bidloo's (1649–1713) *Anatomica humani corporis* is remarkable for its 105 fine copperplate engravings by Pieter van Gunst, afterwards plagiarized by William Cowper (1698). *385*

1685:6 **Liver cirrhosis** first described by John Browne (1642–170?), *PT* **15**:1266. *3613*

1685:7 Charles Allen's (*fl.* 1685) *The operator for the teeth* was the first British book on **dentistry**. *3670*

---

1685:8 Henri François **Le Dran**, French surgeon, born; improved the operation of lithotomy; in his *Parallèle des différentes manières de tirer la pierre hors de la vessie*, 1730; he was by some accredited with originating the lateral operation usually attributed to Cheselden. Died 1770. *4283*

---

1685:9 John **Atkins**, English naval surgeon, born; gave the first description in English of African trypanosomiasis (sleeping sickness); in his *The navy surgeon*, 1734, p. 364. Died 1757. *2148, 5265*

---

1685: William **Boghurst** died, **born** 1631. *plague, typhus*

## 1686

1686:1 **Chorea minor** ('**Sydenham's chorea**') reported by Thomas Sydenham (1624–1689); in his *Schedula monitoria de novae febris ingressus*, p. 25. *4514*

---

1686: Niels **Stensen** [Nicolaus Steno] died, **born** 1638. *parotid glands, ceruminous glands, Fallot's tetralogy, muscle*

## 1687

1687:1 Course of **anatomical lectures** at **Collegiium** in **Zürich**

---

1687:2 Giovanni Cosimo Bonomo (1666–1696) and Giacinto Cestoni (1637–1718) observed the **scabies mite**, *Sarcoptes scabiei*, the first proof of infection by a **microparasite**; in *Osservazioni intorno a' pellicelli del corpo umano. 2529.1, 4012*

---

1687: George **Dalgarno** died, **born** ?1626. *alphabet for deaf-mutes*

## 1688

1688:1 William **Cheselden**, British anatomist and surgeon, born 19 Oct; better known for his surgical accomplishments, he wrote *Anatomy of the humane body* (1713), for many years a textbook of the English medical schools. He described his method of suprapubic lithotomy in his *Treatise on the high operation for the stone*, 1723; he abandoned it in favour of the lateral operation in 1727, as recorded by Alexander Reid in 1746. His *Osteographia*, a fine atlas of human and animal bones, appeared in 1733. Carried out iridotomy and the construction of an artificial pupil on a patient whose natural pupil had been damaged by inflammation, 1729, *PT* **35**:447 Died 1752. *390, 395, 4282,4284, 5828*

---

1688:2 John **Freke**, English physician, born; gave what is probably the first description of myositis ossificans progressiva, 1740, *PT* **41**:369. Died 1756. *4731*

---

1688:3 Georg **Horst** died; described sunstroke: in his *De siriasi*, 1665. *2246*

---

1688: Johannes Michael **Fehr** died, **born** 1610. *trigeminal neuralgia*

## 1689

1689:1 First account of **anorexia nervosa** by Richard Morton (1637–1698); in his *Phthisiologia. 3216*

1689:2 First important pathological study of **pulmonary tuberculosis** by Richard Morton (1637–1698); in his *Phthisiologia*. *3216*

1689:3 The *De morbis acutis infantum* of Walter Harris (1647–1732) served for nearly a century as the standard English work on **diseases of children**. *6321*

1689: Theophile **Bonet** died, **born** 1620. *pathology*

1689: Thomas **Sydenham** died, **born** 1624. *chorea minor, rheumatism, gout, scarlet fever, measles, smallpox*

**1690**
1690: Pierre de **La Martinière** died, **born** 1634. *gonococcal arthritis*

**1691**
1691:1 **University of Dôle** (1422) moved to **Besançon**

1691:2 **Regia Accademia dei Fisiocritici** established in **Siena**

1691:3 Clopton Havers' (*c*1655–1702) *Osteologia nova, or some new observations of the bones*, was the first complete account of the microscopic structure of **bone**. The 'Haversian canals' are named after him. *387*

1691:4 (?) William **Douglass** born; gave the first adequate clinical description of scarlet fever; in his *Practical history of a new epidemical eruptive miliary fever, with an angina ulcusculosa*, etc., 1736. Died 1752. *5076*

1691: Robert **Boyle** died, **born** 1627. *Boyle's law, blood analysis*

1691: Richard **Lower** died, **born** 1631. *blood transfusion, cardiac muscle structure*

**1692**
1692:1 **Stokes-Adams syndrome** first recorded by Marko Gerbec [Gerbezius] (1658–1718), *MCT* 10:115. *2728*

1692:2 Successful teacher of **deaf-mutes**, Johann Konrad Amman (1663–1730), published his method in *Surdus loquens*. *3352*

1692:3 John **Huxham**, English physician, born; his best work was his *Essay on fevers*, 1750. Studied relationship between atmospheric conditions and disease, 1752; in his *Observationes de äere et morbis epidemicis*. In his *Dissertation on the malignant, ulcerous sore-throat*, 1757, gave an excellent account of diphtheria and was first to observe the paralysis of the soft palate, although not differentiating the disease from scarlatinal angina. Died 1768. *2201, 1675, 5050*

**1693**
1693:1 **College of William and Mary** founded at **Williamsburg**, Virginia

1693:2 Antoni van Leeuwenhoek's studies on **spermatozoa**, **muscle**, **bacteria**, **protozoa**, **blood corpuscles**, **histological staining** are recorded in his *Ontledingen en ontdekkingen*, 1693–1718. Died 1723. *67, 860, 2464.1*

1693:3 'Breslau tables', showing mortality rates and other vital statistics, published by Edmund Halley (1656–1742), *PT* **17**:596. *1687*

1693:4 (?) The first description of ankylosing spondylitis given by Bernard Connor (or O'Connor) (1666–1698); in his *Lettre écrite à Monsieur le Chevalier Guillaume de Waldegrave. 4298*

1693:5 Jacques **Daviel**, French ophthalmologist, born 11 Aug; introduced the modern method of treatment of cataract by extraction of the lens, 1753, *MARC* **2**:337. Died 1762. *5829*

1693: Johann Daniel **Major** died, born 1634. *intravenous injection of drugs*

## 1694
1694:1 Zacharias **Platner**, German surgeon, born 16 Aug; he affirmed the tuberculous nature of kyphosis; in his *De iis, qui ex tuberculis gibberosi fiunt*, 1744. Died 1747. *4302*

1694: Marcello **Malpighi** died, born 1628. *capillary circulation, embryology, kidney tubules, Malpighian bodies, leontiasis ossea*

## 1695
1695:1 Raymond Vieussens (1641–1715) gave an important account of various heart disorders, including mitral stenosis; in his *Novum vasorum corporis humani systema. 2729*

1695: Johann Jacob **Wepfer** died, born 1620. *apoplexy*

## 1696
1696: Giovanni Cosimo **Bonomo** died, born 1666. *Sarcoptes scabiei, scabies mite*

## 1697
1697:1 **Anatomical theatre** installed in **Surgeons' Hall, Edinburgh**

1697:2 Bernhard Siegfried **Albinus**, German anatomist, professor at Leiden, born 22 Feb. His *Tabulae sceleti et musculorum corporis humani*, [1737]–1747, with its 40 large copperplate engravings established a new standard in anatomical illustration. Died 1770. *399*

1697.3 Sauveur-François **Morand**, French surgeon, born 2 Apr; gave the first description of cleidocranial dysostosis, 1760, *HARS* (1766), p. 47. Recorded a successful operation for temporo-sphenoidal abscess; in his *Opuscules de chirurgie*, Pt. 1, p. 161, 1768. Died 1773. *4302.2, 4851*

1697:4 Georg Erhard **Hamburger**, German physician, born 21 Dec; gave first description of duodenal ulcer; in his *De ruptura intestini duodeni*, 1746. Died 1755. *3424*

1697:5 John **Burton**, British obstetrician, born; first to suggest the contagious nature of puerperal fever; in his *An essay towards a complete new system of midwifery*, 1751. Died 1771. *6268*

1697:6 William **Smellie**, British obstetrician, born; contributed more to the fundamentals of obstetrics than virtually any other individual. Wrote *A treatise on the theory and practice of midwifery*, 1752. He accurately described the mechanism of parturition, stressing the importance of exact pelvic measurements; laid down safe rules regarding the use of forceps, of which he himself introduced several types; introduced the 'Smellie manoeuvre' and published the first illustration of a rachitic pelvis. Published *A sett* [sic] *of anatomical tables, with explanations, and an abridgement of the practice of midwifery*, 1754, the celebrated atlas for his *A treatise on the theory and practice of midwifery* (1752). Died 1783. *6154, 6154.1*

1697: Francesco **Redi** died, **born** 1626. *snake poison*

## 1698
1698:1 Statute at **Montpellier** requiring visits of **medical students** to hospital and city patients

1698:2 **Bronchial asthma** was first clearly described by John Floyer (1649–1734); in his *Treatise on the asthma. 3166*

1698:3 John **Rutty**, Irish physician, born; gave the first clear description of relapsing fever; in his *A chronological history of the weather and seasons and of prevailing diseases in Dublin*, 1770, p. 75. Died 1775. *5309*

1698: Richard **Morton** died, **born** 1637. *pulmonary tuberculosis, anorexia nervosa*

1698: William **Holder** died, **born** 1616. *paracusis*

1698: Bernard **Connor** (or O'Connor) died, **born** 1666. *ankylosing spondylitis*

## 1699
1699:1 **Cowper's glands** described by William Cowper (1666–1709), *PT* **21**:364; they had previously been noted by Jean Méry in 1684. *1214*

1699:2 Paul Gottlieb **Werlhof**, German physician, born 24 May; gave classical account of purpura haemorrhagica ('Werlhof's disease'); in his *Epistologica de variolis et anthracibus*, 1735. Died 1767. *3052*

1699:3 Frank **Nicholls** born; gave first description of dissecting aneurysm of the aorta, 1761, *PT* **52**:265. Died 1778. *2734.1*

## 1700
1700:1 **Königliche Preussische Akademie der Wissenschaften** founded in **Berlin**

1700:2 **Real Academia de Medicina y Cirugía, Seville**, founded

1700:3 **Quarantine Act, Pennsylvania**

1700:4 **Littré's hernia (diverticulum hernia)** and **Littré's glands** described by Alexis Littré (1658–1726), *HARS Mém* 300, 311 (1719). *3575, 1215*

1700:5 **Occupational medicine**; the first comprehensive and systematic work was Bernardino Ramazzini's (1633–1714) *De morbis artificum diatriba. 2121*

1700:6 Human **parasitology**; first medical textbook, *De la géneration des vers dans le corps de l'homme*, published by Nicolas Andry (1658–1742). *2448.2*

1700:7 First description of **leontiasis ossea** given by Marcello Malpighi (1628–1694); in his *Opera posthuma*, p. 68. *4299*

---

1700: (?) John **Browne** died, **born** 1642. *liver cirrhosis*

1700: Heinrich **Meibom** died, **born** 1638. *conjunctival glands*

## 1701
1701:1 **Variolation** against **smallpox** practised in Constantinople

1701:2 **Smallpox Prevention Act, Massachusetts,** authorizing the impressment of houses for the isolation of patients

1701:3 **Yale College** (so named 1718), **New Haven** founded, became **Yale University**

1701:4 Treatment of **ovarian dropsy** by tapping the cyst first carried out by Robert Houstoun (1678–1743), reported in 1724, *PT* **33**:8. *6017*

1701:5 The first accurate description of the female **pelvis** and its deformities, and the effect of the latter in complicating **labour,** is given in *Manuale operatien, I. deel zijnde een neiuw ligt voor vroed-meesters en vroed-vrouen,* by Hendrik van Deventer (1651–1724). *6253*

1701:6 Frederik Ruysch (1638–1731) described in his *Thesaurus anatomicus i–x,* his method for injecting **blood vessels** and was first to describe the **bronchial blood vessels** and made other important anatomical discoveries. *389*

## 1702
1702:1 **University of Breslau** founded

1702:2 The first to treat **lacrimal fistula,** on the basis of correct anatomical understanding, was Georg Ernst Stahl (1660–1734). He described it in an addendum, *De fistula lacrimali,* to the thesis of his student E.C. Lange, *De affectibus oculorum. 5823*

---

1702:3 Robert **Bunon,** French surgeon, born 1 May; published the first book incorporating specialized odontological research, *Essai sur les maladies des dents,* 1743. Died 1748. *3672.1*

1702:4 George **Martine,** *the younger,* Scottish physician, born; first to perform tracheotomy for diphtheria, 1730, *PT* **36**:448. The first important work on clinical thermometry was included in his *Essays medical and philosophical,* 1740. Died 1741. *5048, 2671*

---

1702: Clopton **Havers** died, **born** *c*1655. *bone*

## 1703
1703:1 **Apothecaries** in **England** authorized by Parliament to prescribe as well as to dispense drugs

---

1703:2 Jean **Baseilhac** (*Frère Côme*), French physician and surgeon, born Apr; invented several new instruments for use in suprapubic lithotomy; described in his *Nouvelle méthode d'extraire la pierre de la vessie urinaire,* 1779. Died 1781. *4285*

1703:3 André **Levret**, French obstetrician, born; introduced a curved obstetric forceps; in his *Observations sur les causes et les accidents de plusiers accouchemens laborieux*, 1747; invented several obstetric instruments and made fundamental observations on pelvic anomalies; in his *L'art des accouchemens.* Died 1780. *6152, 6153*

1703: Robert **Hooke** died, **born** 1635. *microscopy*

1703: John **Wallis** died, **born** 1616. *deaf-mutes, classification of human voice*

## 1704
1704:1 **Valsalva's manoeuvre** described by Antonio Mario Valsalva (1666–1723), in his *De aure humana tractatus. 1546*

1704:2 William **Battie**, British physician, born; was the first to teach psychiatry at the bedside; his *Treatise on madness*, 1758, was the first textbook in English on the subject. Died 1776. *4919.1*

1704: Jean **Denis** [Denys] died, **born** *c*1640. *blood transfusion*

1704: Lorenzo **Bellini** died, **born** 1643. *diagnosis, urine, kidney*

1704: William **Briggs** died, **born** 1642. *nyctalopia*

## 1705
1705:1 First professorship of **anatomy** in **Edinburgh** (Robert Eliot)

1705:2 *Medicina gymnastica*, first English text on **therapeutic value of gymnastics**, published by Francis Fuller (1670–1706). *1986.3*

1705:3 Jean Louis Petit (1674–1750) is particularly remembered for his work on **bone diseases**, *L'art de guérir les maladies des os*; he gave the first account of **osteomalacia**. *4300*

1705:4 Robert **James**, British physician, born; compiled *A medicinal dictionary*, 2 vols, 1743–45. It was the largest and most learned medical dictionary written in English prior to the early 19th century. Samuel Johnson contributed to it. Died 1776. *6799*

## 1706
1706:1 **Académie des Sciences, Montpellier**, founded

1706:2 **Moscow Court Hospital** founded

1706:3 **Aortic insufficiency** first described by William Cowper (1666–1709), *PT* **24**:1970. *2730*

1706:4 Carl Friedrich **Kaltschmied**, German physician and surgeon, born 21 May; gave first description of a parotid tumour; in his *De tumore scirrhoso trium cum quadrante librarum glandulae parotidis*, 1752. Died 1769. *3424.1*

1706:5 Edmé Gilles **Guyot**, postmaster at Versailles, born; first to attempt catheterization of the Eustachian tube; this was done by way of the mouth, 1724, *HARS*, p. 37. Died 1786. *3354*

1706:6 Nils **Rosén von Rosenstein**, Swedish physician, born; his *Underrättelser om barn-sjukdomar och deras botemedel*, 1764, was considered by Still 'the most progressive work which has yet been written' on paediatrics. It gave an impetus to research influencing the future course of paediatrics. English translation 1776. Died 1773. *6323*

1706: Francis **Fuller** died, **born** 1670. *therapeutic gymnastics*

## 1707
1707:1 [**Senckenburg Foundation for the Advancement of Science**], **Frankfurt am Main**, founded

1707:2 Antoine Maître-Jan (1650–1730), the 'Father of French **ophthalmology**', wrote *Traité des maladies de l'oeil* and supported Brisseau's views on the nature of **cataract**. *5824*

1707:3 **Angina pectoris** observed by Giovanni Battista Morgagni (1682–1771); recorded in his *De sedibus, et causis morborum*, 1761, 1, 282. *2885*

1707:4 A **pulse-watch** was invented by John Floyer (1649–1734), as recorded in *The physician's pulse-watch*. *2670*

1707:5 The surgical treatment of diseases of the **maxillary sinus** was pioneered by William Cowper (1666–1709); he wrote on this in James Drake's *Anthropologia nova*, 2, 526–49. *3670.1*

1707:6 *De subitaneis mortibus*, by Giovanni Maria Lancisi (1654–1720), includes an important account and classification of the **heart diseases** then recognized. *2731*

1707:7 John **Pringle**, British physician, born 10 Apr; showed typhus to be identical to 'hospital fever'; in his *Observations on the nature and cure of the hospital and jayl fevers*, 1750 – he advocated better ventilation in hospitals and prisons as a preventive measure. Regarded as the founder of modern military medicine, he stated the principles in his *Diseases of the army*, 1752. Died 1782. *5374, 2150*

1707:8 Carl von **Linné** [Linnaeus], Swedish botanist and taxonomist, born 23 May; in 1735 published *Systema naturae*, first modern and logical classification of plants, animals and minerals. First described aphasia, 1745, *SAH* 6:116. Died 1778. *99, 4616*

## 1708
1708:1 The *Institutiones medicae*, by Herman Boerhaave (1668–1738) was one of the earliest textbooks of **physiology** and used in every medical school. *581*

1708:2 Albrecht von **Haller**, Swiss physician, anatomist, physiologist, botanist and bibliographer, born 16 Oct. Haller, one of the most imposing figures in medicine, was professor of anatomy, surgery and medicine at Göttingen. His *Primae lineae physiologiae*, 1747, was the first textbook of physiology; he completed four great bibliographies of botany, anatomy, surgery and medicine, forming the most complete reference works of the time. They are respectively *Bibliotheca botanica*, 2 vols, 1771–72, *Bibliotheca anatomica*, 2 vols, 1774–77; *Bibliotheca chirurgica*, 2 vols, 1774–75; *Bibliotheca medicinae practicae*, 4 vols, 1777–88. Died 1777. *1833, 438, 5789, 6747*

1708: Edward **Tyson** died, **born** 1650. *Ascaris lumbricoides*

1708: François **Poupart** died, **born** 1661. *inguinal ligament*

## 1709
1709:1 *Aphorismi de cognoscendis et curandis morbis*, by Herman Boerhaave (1668–1738) enshrines much of his ripe clinical wisdom. *2199*

1709:2 The true nature and location of **cataract** first demonstrated by Michel Brisseau (1676–1743); in his *Traité de la cataract et du glaucoma*. *5825*

1709: William **Cowper** died, **born** 1666. *Cowper's glands, aortic insufficiency, maxillary sinus*

1709: François **Mauriceau** died, **born** 1637. *obstetrics*

## 1710
1710:1 **Hospital** at **York, England**

1710:2 **Charité Krankenhaus** opened in **Berlin**

1710:3 **Quarantine Act** in **Britain**

1710:4 **Konglige Vetenskaps-Societeten i Uppsala** founded

1710:5 **School of Physic** established at **Trinity College, Dublin**

1710:6 First suggestion of **colostomy** for **intestinal obstruction** made by Alexis Littré (1658–1726), *HARS Mém* 36 (1734). *3418*

1710:7 William **Heberden** Sr, English physician, born Aug; gave classic description of angina pectoris, and introduced the term, 1768; lecture published in 1772, *MTr* **2**:59. First definitely differentiated varicella from smallpox, 1768, *MTr* **1**:427. In his *Commentarii de morborum historia*, p. 130, 1802, he described the form of rheumatic gout in which nodules ('Heberden's nodes') appear in the interphalangeal joints of the fingers. Died 1801. *2887, 5438, 4491*

1710:8 Fielding **Ould**, Irish obstetrician, born; his *A treatise on midwifry*, 1742, was the first important textbook on obstetrics published in the British Isles. He did much towards the advancement of midwifery in Britain. Died 1789. *6151*

1710:9 William **Cullen**, Scottish physician and inspiring teacher, born. Instrumental in founding Glasgow Medical School. His system was based on the physiological views of Friedrich Hoffmann (1660–1742), his *Works* appeared in 1772. *76, 72*

## 1711
1711:1 **Bibliotheca Lancisiana, Rome**, founded by G.M. Lancisi

1711:2 Johann **Lieberkühn**, German anatomist, born 5 Sep; described Lieberkühn's glands or crypts in the intestine, in his *De fabrica et actione villorum tenuium hominis*, 1745. (They were discovered by Malpighi in 1688.) Died 1756. *978*

1711:3 William **Cadogan**, British paediatrician, born; his *An essay upon nursing, and the management of children, from their birth to three years of age*, 1748, filled an important need in paediatrics at a time when infant welfare was much neglected through ignorance; he laid down rules on feeding, nursing and clothing. His *Dissertation on the gout* ..., etc. attracted much attention when it appeared in 1771; he advised moderate exercise and moderation in drinking as a cure. Died 1797. *6322, 4489*

## 1712

1712:1 The specific effectiveness of **cinchona** in **malaria** finally established by the work of Francesco Torti (1658–1741); in his *Therapeutice specialis ad febres quasdam perniciosas, inopinato, ac repente lethales, una vera china china*, etc. He is also credited with the introduction of the term **malaria**. *5231*

---

1712:2 John **Fothergill**, English physician, born 8 Mar; gave the first authoritative account of both diphtheria and scarlatinal angina, in his *An account of the sore throat attended with ulcers*, 1748, but failed to differentiate between the two. Gave first description of facial neuralgia, 1776, *MOI* **5**:129; gave first accurate account of migraine, 1777, *MOI* **6**:103. Died 1780. *5049, 4516, 4517*

---

1712:3 Thomas **Dimsdale**, English physician, born 6 May; inoculated the Empress Catherine of Russia and her son against smallpox, for which he received an enormous fee and which helped in popularizing inoculation in England; he wrote *The present method for inoculating for the small-pox*, 1767. Died 1800. *5420*

## 1713

1713:1 **St Côme** amalgamated with **Académie de Chirurgie, Paris**

1713:2 **Theatrum Anatomicum** founded in **Berlin**

1713:3 **Real Academia Española, Madrid**, founded

1713:4 **Botanic Garden** at **St Petersburg**

1713:5 *Anatomy of the humane body* published by William Cheselden (1688–1752). *390*

1713:6 The **lacrimal duct** catheterized for the first time by Dominique Anel (1679–1730); in his *Observation singulière sur la fistule lacrimale*, etc. *5826*

---

1713: Govert **Bidloo** died, **born** 1649. *anatomy*

## 1714

1714:1 Daniel Gabriel **Fahrenheit** (1686–1736) constructs 212° **thermometer**

1714:2 Daniel Turner's (1667–1741) *De morbis cutaneis. A treatise of diseases incident to the skin*, is the first English text on **dermatology**; he may be regarded as the founder of English dermatology. *3981*

1714:3 Eustachius's *Tabulae anatomicae* published. Had they been published when completed in 1552 he would have ranked with Vesalius as one of the founders of modern **anatomy**. *391*

1714:4 Inoculation against **smallpox**, as practised in Constantinople, described by Emanuele Timoni (d.1718), *PT* **29**:72. *5409*

---

1714:5 Percivall **Pott**, British surgeon, born 6 Jan; gave first description of congenital hernia; in his *Treatise on ruptures*, 1756. Gave a classic description of hydrocele; in his *Practical remarks on the hydrocele or watry rupture*, 1762. His description of fistula-in-ano, in his *Remarks on the disease commonly called a fistula in ano*, 1765, is regarded as a classic of colo-rectal surgery. In his *Some few general remarks on fractures and dislocations*, 1767 he outlined methods subsequently adopted worldwide; 'Pott's fracture' is described on p. 57. His description of chimney sweep's cancer of the scrotum, in his *Chirurgical observations relative to ... the cancer of the scrotum*, 1775 (which also contained his account of senile (Pott's) gangrene), was the first description of an occupational cancer. He gave a classic description of spinal curvature due to tuberculous caries (Pott's disease) without, however recognizing its tuberculous nature; in his *Remarks on that kind of palsy of the lower limbs, which is frequently found to accompany a curvature of the spine*, 1779. Died 1788. *3576, 4164, 4165, 3242.2, 2122, 2609, 4408, 4304*

1714:6 Robert **Whytt**, British physician and neurophysiologist, born 6 Sep; first to prove that the response of the pupils to light is a reflex action, in his *Essay on the vital and other involuntary motions of animals*, 1751 ('Whytt's reflex'); wrote first important British work on neurology after Willis, his *Observations on the nature, causes and cure of those disorders which have been commonly called nervous hypochondriac, or hysteric*, etc., 1764; gave the first account of the clinical course of tuberculous meningitis in children, in his *Observations on the dropsy of the brain*, 1768. Died 1766. *1381, 4841, 4634*

1714:7 Nicolas François Joseph **Eloy**, Belgian physician, born; compiled the earliest exhaustive collection of medical biographies, *Dictionnaire historique de la médecine ancienne et moderne*, 4 vols, 1778, first published 1775. Died 1788. *6704*

1714:8 John **Hill**, British apothecary and botanist, born; first to show association of tobacco with cancer ; in his *Cautions against the immoderate use of snuff ...*, 1761. Died 1775. *2607.1*

1714: Bernardino **Ramazzini** died, **born** 1633. *occupational medicine*

1714: John **Radcliffe** died, **born** 1652. *Radcliffe Infirmary*

## 1715
1715:1 Giacomo Pylarino [Pilarini] 1659–1718) is accredited with the 'medical' discovery of **variolation**; in his *Nova et tuta variolas excitandi per transplantionem methodus* he described its practise in Constantinople. *5409.1*

1715:2 William **Watson**, British physician, born 3 Apr; gave first comprehensive account of emphysema, 1746, *PT* **54**:239. Died 1787. *3166.1*

1715: Raymond **Vieussens** died, **born** 1641. *centrum ovale, brain, nerves, heart disorders*

## 1716
1716:1 **New York** issues ordinances for **midwives**

1716:3 John **Bard**, American physician, born 1 Feb; successfully operated on a case of extrauterine pregnancy, 1764, *MOI* **2**:369. Died 1799. *6155*

1716:4 James **Lind**, British physician, born 4 Oct; the founder of naval hygiene. His classical *A treatise of the scurvy*, 1753, described important therapeutic experiments, including the use of citrus juice. His *Essay on ... preserving the health of seamen in the Royal Navy*, 1757, was instrumental in improving the conditions of sailors afloat. Died 1794. *3713, 2151*

---

1716:5 Philipp **Pfaff**, German dentist, born; published the first important German dentistry manual, *Abhandlung von den Zähnen*, 1756; in it he described the taking of impressions and the casting of models for false teeth. Died 1780. *3673*

## 1717
1717:1 **Hospital for infectious diseases** opened in **Boston**, Massachusetts

1717:2 Congenital hypertrophic **pyloric stenosis** first described by Patrick Blair (166?–1728). *3419*

1717:3 Giovanni Maria Lancisi (1654–1720) suggested that **malaria** was a poison emanating from marshes and possibly transmitted by **mosquitoes**; in his *De noxiis paludum effluviis, eorumque remediis*. *5232*

## 1718
1718:1 **Theatrum Anatomicum** founded in **Vienna**

1718:2 Lady Mary Wortley **Montagu** has son inoculated against **smallpox**

1718:3 **Nosocomium Academicum** established in **Uppsala**

1718:4 **Botanic Garden** in **Madrid**

1718:5 Lorenz Heister (1683–1758), founder of scientific **surgery** in Germany, wrote *Chirurgie in welcher alles was zur Wund-Artzney gehoret*, most popular surgical text of the 18th century. *5576*

---

1718:6 William **Hunter**, British anatomist and obstetrician, born 23 May; first recorded a case of arteriovenous aneurysm, 1757, *MOI* **1**:323; founded School of Anatomy at Gt Windmill Street, London, 1779; accurately described retroversion of the uterus, 1771, *MOI* **4**:400; **5**:388. His *Anatomia uteri humani gravidi tabulis illustrata, The anatomy of the human gravid uterus exhibited in figures*, 1774, is one of the finest anatomical atlases ever produced, containing 34 copper plates depicting the gravid uterus life-size. Recorded 3 cases of congenital heart disease, 1784, *MOI* **6**:291. His text for the atlas, *An anatomical description of the human gravid uterus and its contents*, 1794, was posthumously edited by Matthew Baillie. Died 1783. *2974, 6020, 6157, 6157.1, 2734.3*

---

1718:7 Emanuele **Timoni** died; described inoculation against smallpox, as practised in Constantinople, 1714, *PT* **29**:72. *5409*

1718: Giacinto **Cestoni** died, **born** 1663. *Sarcoptes scabiei, scabies mite*

1718: Marko **Gerbec** [Gerbezius] died, **born** 1658. *Stokes-Adams syndrome*

1718: Giacomo **Pylarino** [Pilarini] died, **born** 1659. *variolation*

## 1719
1719:1 **Hospital** at **Cambridge**, England

---

1719:2 George **Armstrong**, British paediatrician, born; his *An essay on the diseases most fatal to infants*, 1767, was one of the best works of the period on paediatrics. He founded the Dispensary for Sick Children, London, 1769, the first children's dispensary in Europe. Gave an important description of congenital hypertrophic pyloric stenosis; in his *Account of the diseases most incident to children*, 1777, p. 49. Died 1789. *6324, 3425*

1719:3 Francis **Home**, British physician, born; experimentally transmitted human measles; in his *Medical facts and experiments*, 1759, p. 266. In his *Enquiry into the nature, cause, and cure of the croup*, 1765, he gave the first clear and complete description of diphtheria. Died 1813. *5442, 5051*

**1720**
1720:1 **Westminster Hospital, London**, opened (as Westminster Dispensary)

1720:2 First **herbal** printed in North America, *Pharmacopoeia Londinensis*, Boston, by Nicholas Culpeper (1616–1654). *1828.1*

1720:3 First suggestion that **pulmonary tuberculosis** was due to a parasitic microorganism by Benjamin Marten; in his *New theory of consumptions*. *3217*

1720:4 Richard Mead's (1673–1754) advice about the **plague**, *A short discourse concerning pestilential contagion*, was later expanded to become almost a prophecy of the English **public health** system. *5123*

---

1720: Giovanni Maria **Lancisi** died, **born** 1654. *heart disease, malaria, mosquito*

1720: Frederik **Dekkers** died, **born** 1648. *albuminuria, proteinuria*

**1721**
1721:1 **Apothecaries Company of London** organized

1721:2 **University of Dijon** initiated (authorized 1723)

1721:3 Zabdiel Boylston (1679–1766) was first in America to introduce **smallpox inoculation** (Boston, 26 June 1721); *An historical account of the small-pox inoculated in New England*, 1726. Died 1766. *5415*

---

1721:4 Mark **Akenside**, British physician and poet, born 9 Nov; described multiple neurofibromatosis, 1786, *MTr* **1**:64; von Recklinghausen's classic description appeared in 1882. Died 1770. *4015.1*

1721:5 Robert **Hamilton**, British physician, born 6 Dec; gave the first modern account of mumps (epidemic parotitis), and described parotitis complicated by orchitis, 1790, *TRSE* **2**:59. Died 1793. *5523*

---

1721: James **Yonge** died, **born** 1646. *flap amputation*

**1722**
1722:1 '**Buying the smallpox**' (inoculation scabs) current custom in **Wales**

1722:2 The removal *en masse* of a **cataract** from a living subject recorded by Charles de Saint-Yves (1667–1733); in his *Nouveau traité des maladies des yeux. 5827*

---

1722:3 Pieter **Camper**, Dutch anatomist, born May 11; discovered the processus vaginalis of the peritoneum. An English translation of his collected papers appeared in 1794. Died 1789. *77*

---

1722:4 Leopold **Auenbrugger**, Austrian physician, born 19 Nov; recorded immediate percussion of the chest, as a diagnostic measure; in his *Inventum novum ex percussione thoracis humani*, 1761. Died 1809. *2672*

---

1722:5 Richard **Brocklesby** born; his *Oeconomical and medical observations ... tending to the improvement of military hospitals*, etc., 1764, was the best work of the century regarding military sanitation. Died 1797. *2153*

---

1722:6 George **Baker**, British physician, born; demonstrated that lead poisoning was the cause of 'Devonshire colic'; in his *An essay concerning the causes of epidemic colic of Devonshire*, 1767. Died 1809. *2096*

## 1723

1723:1 **Yellow fever** in **London** (from Lisbon)

1723:2 William Cheselden (1688–1752) described his method of suprapubic **lithotomy** in his *Treatise on the high operation for the stone*; he abandoned it in favour of the lateral operation in 1727, as recorded by Alexander Reid in 1746. *4282, 4284*

---

1723: Antoni van **Leeuwenhoek** died, born 1632. *bacteria, red blood corpuscles, spermatozoa, muscle, staining, protozoa*

1723: Antonio Mario **Valsalva** died, born 1666. *Valsalva's manoeuvre*

## 1724

1724:1 **Imperial Russian Academy of Sciences (St Petersburg)** founded

1724:2 *Medicina gerocomica*, first English work devoted to **geriatrics**, published by John Floyer (1649–1734). *1595*

1724:3 Catheterization of the **Eustachian tube** first attempted by Edmé Gilles Guyot (1706–1786); this was done by way of the mouth, *HARS*, p. 37. *3354*

---

1724:4 Johann Friedrich **Meckel**, the elder, German anatomist, born 31 Jul; described the sphenopalatine ('Meckel's') ganglion and Meckel's cave; in his *Tractatus anatomico-physiologicus de quinto pare nervorum cerebri*, 1748. Died 1774. *1249*

1724:5 Immanuel **Kant** born; his *Anthropologie in pragmatischer Hinsicht abgefasst*, 1798, was an attempt at a classification of mental diseases. Died 1804. *4969*

---

1724: Hendrik van **Deventer** died, born 1651. *pelvis, labour*

## 1725

1725:1 **Prussian** edict regulating the **practice of medicine**

1725:2 **Universidad Central de Venezuela** founded in **Caracas**

1725:3 **Guy's Hospital**, London, established by **Thomas Guy** (1644–1724), opened

1725:4 The first English **historian of medicine** was John Freind (1675–1728), who wrote *The history of physick, from the time of Galen to the beginning of the sixteenth century*, 2 vols, 1725–6. *6378*

## 1726
1726:1 Zabdiel Boylston (1679–1766) was first in America to introduce **smallpox inoculation** (Boston 26 June 1721); *An historical account of the small-pox inoculated in New England*, 1726). Died 1766. *5415*

---

1726:2 Anne Charles de **Lorry** born; regarded as the founder of French dermatology; his *Tractatus de morbis cutaneis*, 1777 included a classification of skin diseases on the basis of their physiological, pathological and aetiological similarities. Died 1783. *3983*

1726:3 John **Howard**, British philanthropist, born; his *State of the prisons in England and Wales*, 1777, resulted in the improvement of prison conditions. Died 1790. *1598*

---

1726: Alexis **Littré** died, **born** 1658. *Littré's glands, diverticulum hernia, intestinal obstruction, colostomy*

## 1727
1727:1 **Vasomotor nerves** discovered by François Pourfour du Petit (1664–1741), *HARS* 1. *764*

1727:2 Perforating **gastric ulcer** first reported by Christopher Rawlinson. *3420*

---

1727: Johann Conrad à **Brunner** died, **born** 1653. *diabetes mellitus*

## 1728
1728:1 Pierre Fauchard (1678–1761), the 'Father of **dentistry**', published *Le chirurgien dentiste*. *3671*

---

1728:2 John **Hunter**, British anatomist and surgeon, born 13 Feb; his classical *The natural history of the human teeth*, 1771, is a detailed and illustrated study of the mouth, jaws and teeth – this book and his *Practical treatise on the diseases of the teeth*, 1778, revolutionized the practice of dentistry. His treatment, ligation of popliteal artery for aneurysm, reported by Everard Home, 1786, *LMJ* 7:391. His *A treatise on the venereal disease*, 1786, supported the erroneous view that syphilis and gonorrhoea were caused by a single pathogen; he inoculated matter from a gonorrhoeal patient to test the theory that the venereal diseases were due to a single pathogen, unfortunately the patient also had syphilis, which developed in the inoculee, incorrectly supporting Hunter's view of a single pathogen. His *Treatise* also contains the first suggestion of lymphogranuloma venereum as a separate disease. According to Everard Home, 1799, *PT* 18:157, he suggested, in 1790, artificial insemination (actually performed by the patient's husband with a syringe). His studies on inflammation were an important contribution to the knowledge of pathology, in his *Treatise on the blood, inflammation, and gun-shot wounds*, 1794. Died 1793. *3675, 3676, 2925, 2377, 5197, 6162, 2283*

1728:3 Johann Georg **Zimmermann**, Swiss physician, born 28 Dec; wrote the first important monograph on bacillary dysentery, *Von der Ruhr unter dem Volke im Jahr 1765*, 1767. Died 1795. *5090*

---

1728:4 Charles **White**, British surgeon and obstetrician, born; introduced a method of reducing shoulder dislocation, 1762, *MOI* **2**:373. First to record excision of the head of the humerus, 1769, *PT* **59**:39. In his *A treatise on the management of pregnant and lying-in women*, 1773, he was first after Hippocrates to make any substantial contribution towards the aetiology and management of puerperal fever. He insisted on absolute cleanliness and the isolation of infected patients. In his *Inquiry into the nature and cause of that swelling, in one or both of the lower extremities, which sometimes happens to lying-in women*, 1784, he gave the first description of phlegmasia alba dolens. Died 1813. *4407, 4437, 6270, 6271*

---

1728: Patrick **Blair** died, **born** 166?. *pyloric stenosis*

1728: Guiseppe **Zambeccari** died, **born** 1665. *spleen*

1728: Daniel **Le Clerc** died, **born** 1652. *history of medicine*

1728: John **Freind** died, **born** 1675. *history of medicine*

## 1729

1729:1 **Edinburgh Royal Infirmary**, temporary 6-bed hospital, opened; permanent building, 1741

1729:2 **Iridotomy** and the construction of an artificial **pupil** carried out by William Cheselden (1688–1752) on a patient whose natural pupil had been damaged by inflammation, *PT* **35**:447. *5828*

1729:3 The first large **history of medicine**, *Histoire de la médecine*, written by Daniel Le Clerc (1652–1728), sometimes termed the 'Father of the history of medicine'. *6379*

---

1729:4 Lazzaro **Spallanzani**, Italian biologist, born 12 Jan; confirmed the solvent property of the gastric juice and discovered the action of saliva in digestion; *Dissertazioni di fisica animale e vegetabile*, 1780. Died 1799. *981*

## 1730

1730:1 **80° thermometer** introduced by René-Antoine Ferchault de **Réaumur** (1683–1757)

1730:2 **Royal Botanic Garden, Kew**, London, opened

1730:3 **Poupart's ligament**, the inguinal ligament, described by François Poupart (1661–1708), *HARS* 51. *977*

1730:4 The **pouch of Douglas** described by James Douglas (1675–1742); in his *A description of the peritonaeum* .... *1217*

1730:5 **Lithotomy** operation improved by Henri François Le Dran (1685–1770); in his *Parallèle des différentes manières de tirer la pierre hors de la vessie*; he was by some accredited with originating the lateral operation usually attributed to Cheselden. *4283*

1730:6 The first to perform **tracheotomy** for **diphtheria** was George Martine (1702–1741), *PT* **36**:448. *5048*

1730:7 A classic work on **haemorrhoids**, *De motus haemorrhoidalis et fluxus haemorrhoidum*, published by Georg Ernst Stahl (1660–1734). *3421*

1730:8 Felice **Fontana**, Italian naturalist and physiologist, born 15 Apr; his *Ricerche fisiche sopra il veleno della vipere*, 1767 was the starting point of investigations on snake venoms. Died 1805. *2103*

1730:9 Otto Friedrich **Müller**, Danish biologist, born 11 Mar; first to attempt a systematic classification of bacteria; *Animalcula infusoria fluviatilia et marina ...*, 1786. Died 1784. *2466*

1730: Johann Konrad **Amman** died, **born** 1663. *teaching of deaf-mutes*

1730: Joseph Guichard **Duverney** died, **born** 1648. *hearing*

1730: Dominique **Anel** died, **born** 1679. *lacrimal duct*

1730: Antoine **Maître-Jan** died, **born** 1650. *ophthalmology, cataract*

**1731**

1731:1 **Académie Royal de Chirurgie, Paris**, founded; after the Revolution revived as **Société Nationale de Chirurgie**

1731:2 **Philadelphia Hospital** founded

1731:3 Classic description of **chlorosis** by Friedrich Hoffmann (1660–1742); in his *De genuina chlorosis indole, origine et curatione. 3110*

1731:4 Henry **Cavendish**, British physicist and chemist, born 10 Oct; isolated hydrogen, 1766, *PT* **72**:119. Died 1810. *925*

1731:5 Erasmus **Darwin**, British naturalist, born 12 Dec; published *Zoonomia*, 1794–6. Died 1802. *105*

1731:6 (?) Matthew **Dobson** born; proved that the sweetish taste of urine in diabetes mellitus was produced by sugar; he also discovered hyperglycaemia, 1776, *MOI* **5**:298. Died 1784. *3928*

1731: Frederik **Ruysch** died, **born** 1638. *lymphatics, blood vessels*

**1732**

1732:1 **University of Göttingen** founded, 1732–1737

1732:2 Herman Boerhaave (1668–1738) was first to separate out urea from urine; in his *Elementa chemiae. 666.1*

1732:3 Thomas Dover's (1662–1742) *Ancient physician's legacy to his country* contains the original prescription for **Dover's powder**: equal quantities of **opium, ipecacuanha, liquorice,**

**saltpetre** and **tartar vitreolus** (ipecacuanha and opium powder BP, 1958), a former favourite for the relief of pain, coughs, etc.

1732:4 **Ichthyosis hystrix** apparently first described by John Machin (d.1751), *PT* **37**:299. *4013*

---

1732:5 Jean **Descemet**, French surgeon, born 20 Apr; in his *An sola lens crystallina cataracte sedes?* described the posterior membrane of the cornea ('Descemet's membrane'), 1758; it had already been noted by B. Duddell in 1729. Died 1810. *1484.1*

1732:6 Luigi **Galvani**, Italian physiologist, born 9 Sep; demonstrated the presence of electrical energy in living tissue; in his *Dell'uso e dell'attività dell arco conduttore nelle contrazioni dei muscoli*, 1794. Died 1798. *594.1*

---

1732: Walter **Harris** died, **born** 1647. *diseases of children*

**1733**

1733:1 **Library of Faculté de Médecine, Paris**, founded

1733:2 **St George's Hospital, London**, founded

1733:3 **Real Academia Nacional de Medicina, Madrid**, founded

1733:4 **Manometer** invented by Stephen Hales (1677–1761), with which he was able to measure **blood pressure**; published in his *Statical essays*. *765*

1733:5 *Osteographia* published by William Cheselden (1688–1752); a fine atlas of human and animal **bones**. *395*

1733:6 Congenital atresia of the **ileum** first reported by James Calder, *MEO* **1**:203. *3422*

1733:7 **Hypochondria** attributed by George Cheyne (1671–1743) to the moisture of the air and the variability of the weather in the British Isles; in his *The English malady*. *4840*

---

1733:8 Alexander **Monro**, Secundus, British anatomist, born 10 Mar; described the 'foramen of Monro'; in his *Structure and function of the nervous system*, 1783. Died 1817. *1385*

1733:9 Joseph **Priestley**, British chemist, born 13 Mar; isolated oxygen, 1772, *PT* **62**:147. Died 1804. *920*

---

1733:10 Caspar Friedrich **Wolff**, German embryologist, born; he published *Theoria generationis*, 1759, and other papers, 1768–9, *NCASP* **12**:43, 403; **13**:470 to support his theory of epigenesis. Died 1794. *470, 471*

1733:11 John **Millar**, British physician, born; first described laryngismus stridulus ('Millar's asthma'); in his *Observations on the asthma and the hooping cough*, 1769. Died 1805. *3167*

**1734**

1734:1 The first description in English of African **trypanosomiasis (sleeping sickness)** given by John Atkins (1685–1757); in his *The navy surgeon*, p. 364. *2148, 5265*

---

1734:2 Franz Anton **Mesmer**, German physician, born 23 May; his system of treatment under hypnosis, mesmerism, was based on his belief in animal magnetism; in his *Mémoire sur la découverte du magnétisme animale*, 1779. Died 1815. *4992.1*

1734:3 Johann Gottlieb **Walter**, German physician, born 1 Jul; accurately described peritonitis in his *Von den Krankheiten des Bauchfells und dem Schlagfluss*, 1785. Died 1818. *2279*

1734:4 Anselme Louis Bernard Berchillet **Jourdain**, French surgeon, born 28 Nov; published the first work specializing in oral surgery, *Traité des maladies et des opérations réellement chirurgicales de la bouche*, 1778. Died 1816. *3676.1*

1734:5 Antonio de **Gimbernat**, Spanish surgeon, born; described his operation for strangulated femoral hernia ('Gimbernat's operation') and the crural ligament ('Gimbernat's ligament'); in his *Nuevo método de operar en la hernia crural*, 1793. Died 1816. *3579*

1734: John **Floyer** died, **born** 1649. *geriatrics, pulse-watch, bronchial asthma*

1734: Georg Ernst **Stahl** died, **born** 1660. *haemorrhoids, lacrimal fistula*

## 1735
1735:1 **Medical Society**, **Boston**, founded

1735:2 *Systema naturae* of Linnaeus (1707–1778); first modern and logical **classification** of plants, animals and minerals. *99*

1735:3 Classical account of **purpura haemorrhagica** ('**Werlhof's disease**') by Paul Gottlieb Werlhof (1699–1767); in his *Epistologica de variolis et anthracibus*. *3052*

1735:4 The first recognizable description of **pellagra** (*mal de la rosa*) written by Gaspar Casal y Julian (1679–1759) but published posthumously: *Historia natural y medica de el Principado de Asturias*, 1762. *3750*

## 1736
1736:1 The first recorded successful **appendicectomy** performed by Claudius Amyand (168? –1740), *PT* **39**:329. *3559*

1736:2 **Mastoiditis** successfully treated by Jean Louis Petit (1674–1750); recorded in his *Traité des maladies chirurgicales …*, **1**, 153, 160, 1774. *3357*

1736:3 William Douglass (1691?–1752) gave the first adequate clinical description of **scarlet fever**; in his *Practical history of a new epidemical eruptive miliary fever, with an angina ulcusculosa*, etc. *5076*

1736:4 Considering the period in which it was written, the *De morbis veneris libri sex* of Jean Astruc (1684–1766) represents an admirable and comprehensive account of **venereal disease**. *5195*

1736:5 Domenico **Cotugno**, Spanish physician and anatomist, born 29 Jan; described labyrinthine fluid in his *De aquaeductibus auris humanae internae*, 1761; he was preceded in this by Theodor Pyl, 1742. In his *De ischiade nervosa commentarius*, 1764, he described cerebrospinal fluid, was first to associate clearly oedema with proteinuria, gave a classic description of nervous sciatica. Died 1822. *1549, 1548, 1382, 4204.2, 4515*

---

1736: Charles de **Saint-Yves** died, **born** 1667. *cataract*

**1737**
1737:1 **Royal Medical Society of Edinburgh** founded

1737:2 **Radcliffe Library**, Oxford, founded

1737:3 Bernhard Siegfried Albinus' (1697–1770) *Tabulae sceleti et musculorum corporis humani*, [1737]–1747, with its 40 large copperplate engravings established a new standard in anatomical illustration. *399*

---

1737:4 Philibert **Chabert**, French veterinary surgeon, born 6 Jan; published the first important clinical description of anthrax; in his *Description et traitement du charbon dans les animaux*, 1780. Died 1814. *4303*

1737:5 Jean Pierre **David**, French physicist and physician, born 17 Feb; described the effect of movement and rest in the treatment of diseases of joints, in his *Dissertation sur les effets du mouvement et du repos dans les maladies chirurgicales*, 1779; he included a description of **Pott's disease** (Pott, 1779). Died 1784. *4303*

---

1737:6 Michael **Underwood**, British physician, born; laid the foundation of modern paediatrics. His *Treatise on diseases of children*, 1784, was superior to anything that had previously appeared, and remained the most important treatise on the subject until the work of Charles West (1848). On p. 76 appears the first description of sclerema neonatorum ('Underwood's disease') and on p. 43 is a description of thrush (candidiasis). The second edition (1789) contains the first description of congenital heart disease to appear in a paediatric treatise, as well as (vol. 2, 53) the first consideration of poliomyelitis as an entity. Died 1820. *6326, 4015, 5516, 4662*

**1738**
1738:1 Joseph Jacob von **Plenck**, German physician, born 28 Nov; drew up a classification of skin diseases on the basis of their appearance; in his *Doctrina de morbis cutaneis*, 1776. Died 1807. *3982*

---

1738:2 Joseph Ignace **Guillotin**, French physician, born; proposed 'Guillotine' for humane execution. Died 1814.

---

1738: Caspar **Bartholin** died, **born** 1655. *salivary gland and ducts*

1738: Herman **Boerhaave** died, **born** 1668. *education, physiology, urea*

**1739**
1739:1 Special **chair of midwifery** founded at **Edinburgh**

1739:2 **Kungliga Svenska Vetenskapsakademi** founded **Stockholm** (present name adopted 1741)

---

1739:3 Heinrich **Wrisberg**, German anatomist, born 20 Jan; described the 'nerve of Wrisberg' in his *Observationes anatomicae de quinto pare nervorum encephali*, 1765. Died 1808. *1252*

1739:4 William **Hewson**, British anatomist and surgeon, born 14 Nov. His important researches on the blood included the coagulation of red blood cells and lymphocytes (*Experimental inquiry into the properties of the blood* ... Part III, 1771). In his *Experimental inquiries: Part the second. Containing a description of the lymphatics*, etc., 1774, he gave the first complete account of the lymphatics. Died 1774. *863, 1102*

## 1740
1740:1 **College** (later **University**) **of Philadelphia** founded

1740:2 **(Royal) London Hospital** founded

1740:3 Chair of **clinical medicine** established at **Edinburgh**

1740:4 First important work on clinical **thermometry** was included in *Essays medical and philosophical*, by George Martine (1702–1741). *2671*

1740:5 What is probably the first description of **myositis ossificans progressiva** given by John Freke (1688–1756), *PT* **41**:369. *4731*

1740:6 Johann Ernst **Wichmann**, German physician, born 10 May; confirmed the parasitic aetiology of scabies; in his *Aetiologie der Krätze*, 1786. Died 1892. *4016*

1740:7 Jean André **Venel**, Swiss orthopaedist, born 28 May; invented a corset and extension bed for treating deformities of the spine, 1789, *MSSPL* **2**:66, 197. Died 1791. *4305*

1740:8 Thomas **Percival**, British physician, born 29 Sep; used cod-liver oil in treatment of rheumatism, 1782, *LMJ* **3**:392; his *Medical ethics*, 1794, is the basis of current British and American codes. Died 1804. *1835, 1764*

1740:9 Thomas **Berdmore**, British dentist, born; published the first English textbook on dentistry and teeth deformities, *A treatise on the disorders and deformities of the teeth and gums*, 1768. Died 1785. *3674*

1740:10 John **Haygarth**, British physician, born; published the first monograph on rheumatism, *A clinical history of diseases. Part first .... A clinical history of the acute rheumatism*, etc., 1805. Died 1827. *4492*

1740: Claudius **Amyand** died, **born** ?1680. *appendicectomy*

## 1741
1741:1 **Foundling Hospital** established in **London** by Thomas Coram; opened 1745

1741:2 The first book on **orthopaedics**, *L'orthopédie*, was written by Nicholas Andry (1658–1742); he introduced the term. *4301*

1741:3 Joseph **Huddart**, British hydrographer, born 11 Jan; recorded the first reliable account of colour-blindness, 1777, *PT* **67**:260. Died 1816. *5832*

1741:4 William **Withering**, British physician and botanist, born 28 Mar; established action and correct dosage of digitalis; in his *Account of the foxglove*, 1785. Died 1799. *1836, 2734.31*

1741:5 Nicolas **Saucerotte**, French surgeon, born 10 Jun; first to give a clinical description of acromegaly, before the Académie de Chirurgie, Paris, 1772, recorded in his *Mélanges de chirurgie*, 1801, 407. Died 1812. *3880*

1741:6 Samuel **Farr**, British physician and botanist, born; published *Elements of medical jurisprudence*, first textbook in English on the subject, 1788. Died 1795. *1733*

1741:7 Giuseppe **Flajani**, Italian anatomist, physician and surgeon, born; gave one of the earliest accounts of exophthalmic goitre and noted cardiac disturbances in the condition; in his *Collezione d'osservazione ...*, **3**, 270–73, 1802. Died 1808. *3811*

1741: George **Martine** died, **born** 1702. *diphtheria, tracheotomy, thermometry*

1741: François **Pourfour du Petit** died, **born** 1664. *vasomotor nerves*

1741: Francesco **Torti** died, **born** 1658. *malaria, cinchona*

1741: Daniel **Turner** died, **born** 1667. *dermatology*

## 1742
1742:1 **Celsius** 100° **thermometer**; Anders Celsius (1701–1741) advocated a thermometer with 100° between freezing and boiling points of water, designating these as 100° and 0°, reversed 8 years later by M. Stromer (0° = freezing point, 100° = boiling point)

1742:2 **Kongelige Danske Videnskabernes Selskab** (Royal Danish Academy of Sciences) founded

1742:3 **Labyrinthine fluid** described by Theodor Pyl, in his *De audito in genere*; it was described by Domenico Cotugno, 1761, and named liquor Cotunnii. *1548, 1549*

1742:4 Successful operation for **intussusception** in an adult was recorded by Cornelius Henrik Velse; in his *De mutuo intestinorum ingressu. 3423*

1742:5 The first English book on children's **teeth**, *A practical treatise upon dentition; or, the breeding of teeth in children*, published by Joseph Hurlock. *3672*

1742:6 *A treatise on midwifry* by Fielding Ould (1710–1789) was the first important textbook on **obstetrics** published in the British Isles. Ould did much towards the advancement of **midwifery** in Britain. *6151*

1742:7 Samuel **Bard**, American physician, born 1 Apr; gave one of the earliest accurate descriptions of diphtheria; in his *An enquiry into the nature, cause and cure of angina suffocativa, or sore throat distemper*. 1771. Wrote *A compendium of the theory and practice of midwifery*, 1807, the first significant textbook on obstetrics written by an American. Died 1821. *5052, 6163.1*

1742:8 August Gottlieb **Richter**, German surgeon, born 13 Aug; described 'Richter's hernia (partial enterocele); in his *Abhandlung von den Brüchen*, chap. 20, 1778–9. Died 1812. *3578*

80

1742:9 Eduard **Sandifort**, Leiden pathologist, born 14 Nov; gave a good account of 'Fallot's tetralogy'; in his *Observationes anatomicae-pathologicae*, vol. 1, 1771. Died 1814. *2734.2*

1742:10 Carl Wilhelm **Scheele**, Swedish chemist, born; discovered uric acid, 1776, *SAH* **37**:327. Died 1786. *668*

1742: James **Douglas** died, **born** 1675. *Pouch of Douglas*

1742: Edmund **Halley** died, **born** 1656. *mortality rates*

1742: Nicolas **Andry** died, **born** 1658. *orthopaedics, parasitology*

1742: Friedrich **Hoffmann** died, **born** 1660. *chlorosis*

1742: Thomas **Dover** died, **born** 1662. *Dover's powder, ipecacuanha, opium*

**1743**
1743:1 **Ventilator** devised by Stephen Hales (1677–1761), inventor of artificial ventilation; in his *A description of ventilators*. *1596*

1743:2 **Tracheotomy** successfully performed for **quinsy** by Pedro Virgili (1669–1776), *MARC* **1**(3):141. *3248*

1743:3 The first book incorporating specialized **odontological** research, *Essai sur les maladies des dents*, published by Robert Bunon (1702–1748). *3672.1*

1743:4 Plastic induration of the **penis** ('**Peyronie's disease**') first described by François de La Peyronie (1678–1747), *MARC* **1**:425. *4163*

1743:5 *A medicinal dictionary*, 2 vols, 1743–45, compiled by Robert James (1705–1776), was the largest and most learned **medical dictionary** written in English prior to the early 19th century. Samuel Johnson contributed to it. *6799*

1743:6 Antoine Laurent **Lavoisier**, French chemist, born 26 Aug; isolated and defined oxygen and exploded G.E. Stahl's (1660–1734) phlogiston theory of combustion, 1775, *HARS* 520. Guillotined 1794. *922*

1743:7 François **Chopart**, French surgeon, born 30 Oct; his method of partial amputation of the foot first recorded by Lafiteau in A.F. Foucroy's *La médecine éclairée par les sciences physiques*, **4**, 85, 1792; with Desault, he was a founder of urological surgery, *Traité des maladies des voies urinaires*, 2 vols, 1791–92. Died 1795. *4439, 4165.01*

1743: George **Cheyne** died, **born** 1671. *hypochondria*

1743: Michel **Brisseau** died, **born** 1676. *cataract, glaucoma*

1743: Robert **Houstoun** died, **born** 1678. *ovarian dropsy*

**1744**
1744:1 **Académie des Sciences ... Rouen** founded

1744:2 Catheterization of the **Eustachian tube** by way of the nose carried out by Archibald Cleland, an army surgeon, *PT* **41**:848. *3355*

1744:3 The **tuberculous** nature of **kyphosis** affirmed by Zacharias Platner (1694–1747); in his *De iis, qui ex tuberculis gibberosi fiunt. 4302*

---

1744:4 Edward **Bancroft**, American inventor, born in Barbados, 31 Jan; noted the transmission of yaws by flies in his *Essay on the natural history of Guiana*, 1769, p. 385. Died 1821. *5304*

1744:5 Pierre Joseph **Desault**, French surgeon, born 6 Feb; one of the great French surgeons, his *Oeuvres chirurgicales* appeared in 3 vols, 1798–1803; he was a founder of modern vascular surgery and urological surgery. Died 1705. *4165.02, 5580*

1744:6 Henry **Park**, British surgeon, born 2 Mar; performed excision and arthrodesis in the treatment of destructive joint disease; in his *Account of a new method of treating diseases of the joints of the knee and elbow*, 1783. Died 1831. *4438*

1744:7 Michael Vincenzo Giacinto **Malacarne**, Italian physician and neurologist, born 28 Sep; in his *Della vera struttura del cervelletto umano*, 1776, gave first detailed account of the cerebellum. His *Sui gozzi e sulla stupiditá ec. dei cretini*, 1789, is probably the first important publication on cretinism and goitre. Died 1816. *1382.1, 3809*

1744:8 John Coakley **Lettsom**, British Quaker physician, born 22 Nov; founder of the Medical Society of London (1772) and the General Dispensary, Aldersgate, London (1770); gave an original account of alcoholism, 1787, *MMSL* **1**:128. *2071*

1744:9 Wilhelm Gottfried **Ploucquet**, German physician, born 30 Dec; compiled the first important classified bibliography of medicine, covering both monographs and current periodicals, *Initia bibliothecae medico-practicae et chirurgicae sive repertorii medicinae practicae et chirurgicae*, 8 vols, 1793–97. It was continued in his *Bibliotheca medico-practica et chirurgica*, 4 vols, 1799–1803, revised as *Literatura medica digesta*, 4 vols, 1808–9, with 40,000 additional citations of the *Initia bibliothecae* and the *Bibliotheca*. Died 1814. *6750–6750.2*

## 1745

1745:1 **Barbers** separated from **surgeons** in **England**; **Company of Surgeons** founded

1745:2 **Middlesex Hospital, London**, founded (as **Middlesex Infirmary**)

1745:3 **Lieberkühn's glands** or **crypts** in the intestine described by Johann Lieberkühn (1711–1756) in his *De fabrica et actione villorum tenuium hominis*. They were discovered by Malpighi in 1688. *978*

1745:4 **Aphasia** first described by Carl Linné [Linnaeus] (1707–1778), *SAH* **6**:116. *4616*

---

1745:5 Johann Peter **Frank**, German physician, born 19 Mar; considered the 'Father of public hygiene'; published *System einer vollständigen medicinischen Polizey*, 1779–1827, 9 vols, the first systematic treatise on public hygiene; first defined diabetes insipidus, in his *De curandis hominum morbis*, 1794, Lib.V., p. 38. Died 1821. *1599, 3879*

1745:6 Philippe **Pinel**, French physician, born 20 Apr; among the first to dispense with chains in the treatment of the insane, founder of the French school of psychiatry and author of the classic *Traité médico-philosophique sur l'aliénation mentale ou la manie*, 1801. Died 1826. *4922*

1745:7 (?) Pierre **Duret**, French surgeon, born; first successful construction of an artificial anus, 1798, *ReMP* **4**:45, in a child with congenital atresia. *3429*

1745:8 Valentin **Haüy**, French physician, born; founded the first school for the blind, first to emboss paper as a means of reading for the blind. His *Essai sur l'education des aveugles*, 1786, originated methods of teaching and caring for blind persons. Died 1816. *5833*

**1746**
1746:1 **College of New Jersey (Princeton University)** founded

1746:2 **London Lock Hospital** founded by William Bromfeild (1712–1792); first hospital in Britain for treatment of sick poor suffering from **venereal diseases**

1746:3 **Emphysema** first comprehensively described by William Watson (1715–1787), *PT* **54**:239. *3166.1*

1746:4 First description of **duodenal ulcer** given by Georg Erhard Hamburger (1697–1755); in his *De ruptura intestini duodeni*. *3424*

1746:5 The first work specializing in **dental prosthetics**, *Essai d'odontotechnie*, published by Claude Mouton (d.1786). *3672.2*

1746:6 Cheselden's method of lateral **lithotomy** recorded by Alexander Reid, *PT* **44**:33. *4284*

1746:7 Benjamin **Rush**, born 4 Jan; an eminent member of the medical profession in Philadelphia. Gave an important account of the 1780 Philadelphia outbreak of dengue in his *Medical enquiries and observations*, 1789, vol. 1, p. 104. Gave a classic account of the yellow fever epidemic; in his *An account of the bilious remitting yellow fever ... in Philadelphia ... in 1793*, 1794. Wrote the first American textbook on psychiatry, *Medical inquiries and observations upon the disease of the mind*, 1812. Died 1813. *5470, 5453, 4924*

1746:8 Jean Louis **Baudelocque**, French obstetrician, born 30 Nov; wrote *L'art des accouchemens*, 2 vols, 1781, invented a pelvimeter and advanced the knowledge of pelvimetry and of mechanics of labour. The external conjugate diameter is known as Baudelocque's diameter. Died 1810. *6255*

1746:9 Gaspard **Vieusseux** born; gave the first definite description of cerebrospinal meningitis, 1805, *JMCP* **11**:163. Died 1814. *4674*

**1747**
1747:1 **Inoculation** against **smallpox** advocated by Richard Mead (1673–1754) in his *De variolis et morbillis liber*. *5417*

1747:2 Albrecht von Haller (1708–1777) one of the most imposing figures in medicine, was professor of anatomy, surgery and medicine at Göttingen. His *Primae lineae physiologiae* was the first textbook of **physiology**. *438*

1747:3 A curved **obstetric forceps** introduced by André Levret (1703–1780); in his *Observations sur les causes et les accidents de plusiers accouchemens laborieux.* 6152

---

1747:4 Samuel **Stearns** born; produced and printed first herbal in the United States; *American herbal, or materia medica*, 1801. Died 1819. *1838.2*

---

1747: François de **La Peyronie** died, **born** 1678. *penis induration*

1747: Zacharias **Platner** died, **born** 1694. *tuberculous nature of kyphosis*

## 1748
1748:1 **Meckel's ganglion** and **Meckel's cave** described by Johann Friedrich Meckel, the elder (1724–1774); in his *Tractatus anatomico-physiologicus de quinto pare nervorum cerebri.* 1249

1748:2 The first authoritative account of both **diphtheria** and **scarlatinal angina** was that of John Fothergill (1712–1780), in his *An account of the sore throat attended with ulcers*, although he failed to differentiate between the two conditions. *5049*

1748:3 William Cadogan's (1711–1797) *An essay upon nursing, and the management of children, from their birth to three years of age*, filled an important need in **paediatrics** at a time when infant welfare was much neglected through ignorance. He laid down rules on feeding, nursing and clothing. *6322*

---

1748:4 Jacopo **Penada**, Italian physician, born; reported a case of perforating duodenal ulcer; in his *Saggio d'osservazioni ... sopra alcuni case singolari*, etc., 1793. Died 1828. *3428*

---

1748: Robert **Bunon** died, **born** 1702. *odontology*

## 1749
1749:1 **Medical Society** established in **New York**

---

1749:2 Benjamin **Bell**, British surgeon, born Apr; made an important classification of ulcers; in his *A treatise on the theory and management of ulcers*, 1778. First to differentiate between gonorrhoea and syphilis; in his *A treatise on gonorrhoea virulenta and lues venerea*, 1793. Died 1806. *5578, 2378, 5200*

1749:3 Edward **Jenner**, British physician, born 17 May; demonstrated that vaccination with vaccinia (cowpox) lymph matter protected against smallpox, 14 May 1796. In his *An inquiry into the causes and effects of the variolae vaccinae*, 1798, he described 23 successful vaccinations and announced one of the greatest triumphs in the history of medicine. Died 1823. *2529.3, 5423*

1749:4 Gilbert **Blane**, physician to the British Fleet, born 29 Aug; made important contributions to naval medicine and hygiene; in his *Observations on the diseases incident to seamen*, 1785. He strongly supported James Lind's views on scurvy and issued regulations for the standard use of lemon juice as a preventive in the navy. He was involved in the Quarantine Rules, 1799. Died 1834. *2158*

1749:5 Daniel **Rutherford**, British physicist, born 3 Nov.; discovered nitrogen, *De aëre fixo dicto, aut mephitico*, 1772. Died 1819. *921*

**1750**

1750:1 **City of London Lying-in Hospital** founded

1750:2 *Essay on fevers* published by John Huxham (1692–1768). *2201*

1750:3 **Typhus** shown to be identical to '**hospital fever**' by John Pringle (1707–1782); in his *Observations on the nature and cure of the hospital and jayl fevers* – he advocated better ventilation in hospitals and prisons as a preventive measure. *5374*

1750:4 (?) Guillaume **Pellier de Quengsby**, French ophthalmologist, born; wrote the first book devoted solely to ophthalmic surgery, *Précis ou cours d'opérations sur la chirurgie des yeux*, 1789–90. Died 1835. *5833.1*

1750: Jean Louis **Petit** died, **born** 1674. *bone diseases, osteomalacia, Petit's hernia and triangle*

**1751**

1751:1 **Königliche Gesellschaft für Wissenschaften, Göttingen**, founded

1751:2 Robert Whytt (1714–1766) was first to prove that the response of the **pupils** to light is a **reflex action**, in his *Essay on the vital and other involuntary motions of animals* ('**Whytt's reflex**'). *1381*

1751:3 The first to suggest the contagious nature of **puerperal fever** was John Burton (1697–1771); in his *An essay towards a complete new system of midwifery. 6268*

1751:4 John **Machin**, British mathematician, died; apparently first described ichthyosis hystrix, 1732, *PT* **37**:299. *4013*

**1752**

1752:1 **Serafimerlasarettet, Stockholm**, opened for teaching purposes

1752:2 **Pennsylvania Hospital, Philadelphia**, opened for first patients, 11 Feb; cornerstone of new building laid, opened 1754

1752:3 **Queen Charlotte's (maternity) Hospital, London**, founded

1752:4 Relation of **atmospheric conditions** to disease studied by John Huxham (1692–1768); in his *Observationes de äere et morbis epidemicis. 1675*

1752:5 The principles of **military medicine** were stated by John Pringle (1707–1782) in his *Diseases of the army. 2150*

1752:6 Tumour of the **parotid gland** first described by Carl Friedrich Kaltschmied (1706–1769); in his *De tumore scirrhoso trium cum quadrante librarum glandulae parotidis. 3424.1*

1752:7 *A treatise on the theory and practice of midwifery* written by William Smellie (1697–1763), who contributed more to the fundamentals of **obstetrics** than virtually any other individual. He accurately described the mechanism of parturition, stressing the importance of exact pelvic measurements; laid down safe rules regarding the use of **forceps**, of which he himself introduced several types; introduced the '**Smellie manoeuvre**' and published the first illustration of a **rachitic pelvis**. The celebrated atlas for his *Treatise, A sett* [sic] *of anatomical tables ...*, appeared in 1754. *6154, 6154.1*

---

1752: 8 Johann David **Schoepff**, German/American physician, born 8 Mar; compiled first full North American materia medica, 1787. Died 1800. *1837*

1752: 9 Antonio **Scarpa**, the 'Father of Italian ophthalmology', born 19 May. He made important observations on the ear and olfaction (*De structura fenestrae rotundae auris*, 1772, *De auditu et olfactu*, 1789); wrote the first textbook on ophthalmology published in Italian, *Saggio di osservazioni e d'esperienze sulle principali malattie degli occhi*, 1801; distinguished true from false aneurysm (*Sull' aneurisma*, 1804); described Scarpa's fascia and Scarpa's triangle, in his *Sull'ernie*, 1809; made valuable contributions to the knowledge of hernia, in his *Sull'ernia del perineo*, 1821. Gave the first accurate description of the pathological anatomy of talipes (club-foot); in his *Memoria chirurgica sui piedi torti congenita dei fanciulli*, 1803. His *Tabulae nevrologicae*, 1832 is considered his greatest work, in it he decisively demonstrated cardiac innervation. Died 1832. *1550, 1453, 5835, 2975, 3583, 3584, 4308, 1253*

---

1752: 10 Alexander **Gordon**, British obstetrician, born; was first to advance as a definite hypothesis the contagious nature of puerperal fever; in his *Treatise on the epidemic puerperal fever in Aberdeen*, 1795. Died 1799. *6272*

1752: 11 William **Brown**, American physician, born; compiled first original pharmacopoeia, *Pharmacopoeia simpliciorum et efficaciorum*, published in the United States, 1778. Died 1792. *1834*

---

1752: William **Douglass** died, **born** 1691. *scarlet fever*

1752: William **Cheselden** died, **born** 1688. *lithotomy, surgical anatomy, osteology, iridotomy, pupil*

**1753**
1753: 1 **British Museum and Library** founded

1753: 2 James Lind (1716–1794) wrote *A treatise of the scurvy* in which he described important therapeutic experiments, including the use of **citrus juice**. He was strongly supported by Gilbert Blane, physician to the British Fleet, who issued regulations for standard issue of **lemon juice** as a preventive in the navy. *3713*

1753: 3 The modern method of treatment of **cataract** by extraction of the lens introduced by Jacques Daviel (1693–1762), *MARC* **2**:337. *5829*

1753: 4 Several **obstetric instruments** invented and fundamental observations on **pelvic anomalies** made by André Levret (1703–1780); in his *L'art des accouchemens*. *6153*

---

1753: 5 John **Warren**, American surgeon, born 27 Jul; established first school of medicine associated with Harvard. Died 1815.

---

1753: 6 John **Heysham**, British physician and statistician, born. His Carlisle bills of mortality formed the basis of the calculations for Joshua Milne's (1776–1851) *A treatise on the valuation of annuities and assurances on lives and survivorship*, etc., 2 vols, London, 1815, the 'Carlisle Tables of Mortality'. Died 1834.

1753:7 Nicolas **Dubois de Chemant**, French dentist, born; the first dentist to manufacture artificial (porcelain) teeth; in his *Les avantages des nouvelles dents, et rateliers artificiels*, 1788. Died 1824. *3677*

**1754**
1754:1 **Botanic garden** opened in **Vienna**

1754:2 **King's College (Columbia University)** founded in **New York**

1754:3 **Scleroderma**, previously confused with leprosy and other conditions, first differentiated by Carlo Cruzio, *PT* **48**:579. *4014*

1754:4 *A sett* [sic] *of anatomical tables, with explanations, and an abridgement of the practice of midwifery*, the celebrated atlas for his *A treatise on the theory and practice of midwifery* (1752), published by William Smellie (1697–1763). *6154.1, 6154*

1754:5 Benjamin **Waterhouse**, American physician, born 4 Mar; introduced vaccination against smallpox into the US, his own child being his first case; he published *A prospect of eliminating the small-pox*, 2 pts, 1800–02. Died 1846. *5424*

1754: Richard **Mead** died, **born** 1673. *plague, smallpox, public health*

**1755**
1755:1 **University of Moscow** founded

1755:2 Samuel Thomas **Soemmerring**, Polish anatomist and naturalist, born 25 Jan. He was noted for his accuracy in anatomical illustration, especially in his *Vom Baue des menschlichen Körpers*, 5 pts, 1791–6, which includes a list of what he considered his anatomical discoveries; his inaugural dissertation, *De basi encephali et originibus nervorun cranio*, 1778, provided solid grounds for the order of the 12 cranial nerves; he gave the first description of achondroplasia; in his *Abbildungen und Beschreibungen einiger Misgeburten*, p. 30, 1791. Died 1830. *400, 1383, 4306*

1755:3 Colin **Chisholm**, British physician, born 2 Feb; apparently first to observe the mode of transmission of the guinea-worm, *Dracunculus medinensis*, causal agent in dracontiasis; in his *Essay on the malignant pestilential fever introduced into the West Indies from Boullam*, etc., 1795. Died 1825. *5336.3*

1755:4 Jean Nicolas **Corvisart des Marest**, French physician, born 15 Feb; established symptomatology of heart disease, facilitating the differentiation between cardiac and pulmonary disorders; in his *Essai sur les maladies et les lésions organiques du coeur et des gros vaisseaux*, 1896. Died 1821. *2737*

1755:5 Christian Friedrich Samuel **Hahnemann**, German physician, born 10 Apr; founded homoeopathy; published his theories in *Organon der rationellen Heilkunde*, 1810. Died 1843. *1966*

1755:6 James **Parkinson**, British surgeon and palaeontologist, born 11 Apr; first described paralysis agitans ('Parkinson's disease'); in his *Essay on the shaking palsy*, 1817. Died 1824. *4690*

1755:7 Caleb Hillier **Parry**, British physician, born 21 Oct; gave one of the first accounts of exophthalmic goitre; in his *Elements of pathology and therapeutics*, 1815. His *Collections from the unpublished medical writings of C.H. Parry*, 1825, contains, **2**, 111–29, a classic account of exophthalmic goitre, as well as his first record, **1**, 478, of facial hemiatrophy. Died 1822. *3813, 4522*

1755:8 James **Russell**, British surgeon, born; gave a detailed description of bone necrosis; in his *Practical essay on certain diseases of the bones termed necrosis*, 1794. Died 1836. *4307*

1755:9 (?)Edward **Stevens**, American physician, born Virgin Isles; isolated human gastric juice, in his *De alimentorum concoctione*, 1777. Died 1834. *980*

1755:10 (?)Thomas **Kast** born; first in America to report ligation of the femoral artery, 1790, *MCMM* 1:96. Died 1820. *2925.1*

1755: Georg Erhard **Hamburger** died, **born** 1697. *duodenal ulcer*

## 1756
1756:1 **Meath Hospital, Dublin**, founded

1756:2 First description of **congenital hernia**, by Percivall Pott (1714–1788); in his *Treatise on ruptures*. *3576*

1756:3 The first important German **dentistry** manual, *Abhandlung von den Zähnen*, published by Philipp Pfaff (1716–1780); he described the taking of impressions and the casting of models for **false teeth**. *3673*

1756:4 Everard **Home**, British physician and surgeon, born 6 May; first to describe cornu cutaneum, 1791, *PT* **81**:95; reported, 1799, *PT* **18**:157, that John Hunter suggested, in 1790, artificial insemination (actually performed by the patient's husband with a syringe). Died 1832. *4017, 6162*

1756: John **Freke** died, **born** 1688. *myositis ossificans progressiva*

1756: Johann **Lieberkühn** died, **born** 1711. *Lieberkühn's (intestinal) glands*

## 1757
1757:1 [**Royal Fredrik Hospital**], **Copenhagen**, opened

1757:2 The founder of **naval hygiene** was James Lind (1716–1794); his *Essay on ... preserving the health of seamen in the Royal Navy* was instrumental in improving the conditions of sailors afloat. *2151*

1757:3 In his *Dissertation on the malignant, ulcerous sore-throat*, John Huxham (1692–1768) gave an excellent account of **diphtheria** and was first to observe the paralysis of the soft palate, although not differentiating the disease from **scarlatinal angina**. *5050*

1757:4 First recorded case of **arteriovenous aneurysm** by William Hunter (1718–1783), *MOI* 1:323. *2974*

88

1757: 5 René Joseph Hyacinthe **Bertin**, French physician, born 10 Apr; his *Traité de la maladie vénérienne chez les enfans nouveau-nés*, 1810, was the first systematic work on congenital syphilis. Died 1828. *2378.1*

1757: 6 William Charles **Wells**, American/British physician, born 24 May; credited with first clinical report of rheumatism as cause of heart disease, 1812, *TSIM* **3**:373. First noted the presence of blood and albumin in dropsical urine and also established that dropsy occurred in the upper part of the body, 1812, *TSIM* **3**:194. Died 1817. *2740, 4205*

1757: 7 Robert **Willan**, British physician, born 12 Nov; pioneered modern dermatology and established a standard nomenclature which is more or less in use today. His *On cutaneous diseases*, 1796, includes original descriptions of prurigo mitis ('ichthyosis cornea'), p. 197, and psoriasis, p. 152. Described infantile eczema in his *On cutaneous diseases (Practical treatise on prurigo)*, 1814. Died 1812. *3985, 4018, 4021.1*

1757: 8 Johann Ludwig **Gasser** (*fl.*1757–1765) eponymized in 'Gasserian ganglion', 1765. *1251*

1757: John **Atkins** died, **born** 1685. *trypanosomiasis*

**1758**
1758: 1 **Descemet's membrane** in the **cornea** described by Jean Descemet (1732–1810), in his *An sola lens crystallina cataracte sedes?* It had already been noted by B. Duddell in 1729. *1484.1*

1758: 2 William Battie (1704–1776) was the first to teach **psychiatry** at the bedside; his *Treatise on madness* was the first textbook in English on the subject. *4919.1*

1758: 3 Franz Joseph **Gall**, German physiologist, born 9 Mar; with Johann Caspar Spurzheim made early attempt at the localization of cerebral function, in their *Anatomie et physiologie du système nerveux*, 1810–1819. The book introduced the pseudo-science of phrenology. Died 1828. *1389*

1758: Lorenz **Heister** died, **born** 1683. *surgery*

**1759**
1759: 1 **Königliche Bayerische Akademie der Wissenchaften** founded at **Munich**

1759: 2 First **public dissection** in **American Colonies** (carried out by John Bard and Peter Middleton)

1759: 3 Human **measles** experimentally transmitted by Francis Home (1719–1813); in his *Medical facts and experiments*, p. 266. *5442*

1759: 4 *Theoria generationis*, covering **embryology** and **epigenesis**, published by Caspar Friedrich Wolff (1733–1794). *470*

1759: 5 Franz Kaspar **Hesselbach**, German anatomist and surgeon, born 27 Jan; described 'Hesselbach's hernia' and 'triangle' in his *Anatomisch-chirurgische Abhandlung über den Ursprung der Leistenbrüche*, 1806. Died 1816. *3582*

1759:6 Vincenzo **Chiarugi**, Italian psychiatrist and dermatologist, born 17 Feb; the first European physician to abandon chains and fetters in the restraint of psychiatric patients; in *Regolamento dei Regi Spedali ...*, 1789. His treatment of the insane is outlined in his *Della pazzia in genre, e in specie*, 1793. Died 1820. *4920.2, 4921*

1759:7 Johann Christian **Reil**, German physician and psychiatrist, born 20 Feb; described the 'island of Reil' in the cerebral cortex; in his *Exercitationum anatomicarum ...* fasc.1, 1796; an early advocate of humane treatment of the insane, wrote *Rhapsodieen über die Anwendung der psychischen Curmethode auf Geisteszerrüttungen*, 1803, and edited the first journal devoted to mental disease – the *Magazin für Nervenheilkunde*; he is considered the founder of modern psychiatry. Died 1813. *1387, 4923*

1759:8 William **Nisbet**, British physician, born; gave the first complete description of lymphatic chancre ('Nisbet's chancre'); in his *First lines of theory and practice in venereal diseases*, 1787. Died 1822. *5198*

1759:9 Giuseppe **Baronio**, Italian surgeon, born; was among the first to attempt transplantation and experimental surgery in animals, successfully carrying out full-thickness skin grafts. He wrote *Degli innesti animali*, 1804. Died 1811. *5736*

1759:10 Friedrich Benjamin **Osiander**, German physician, born; his *Handbuch der Entbindungskunst*, 1818–1825, includes (Bd.2, Abt.II, 302) a description of his lower segment caesarean section. Died 1822. *6237*

1759: Gaspar **Casal y Julian** died, **born** 1679. *pellagra*

## 1760
1760:1 **Kongelige Norske Videnskabers Selskab** founded at **Trondheim**

1760:2 **Act** to regulate the **practice of medicine** in **New York City** passed

1760:3 The first description of **cleidocranial dysostosis** given by Sauveur-François Morand (1697–1773), *HARS* (1766), p. 47. *4302.2*

1760:4 Mathew **Carey**, Irish/American economist and publisher, born 28 Jan; in his *A short account of the malignant fever, lately prevalent in Philadelphia*, 1793, gave a graphic account of the yellow fever epidemic of 1793, with a good clinical description of the disease, mentioning the efficacy and failure of various forms of treatment. Died 1839. *5451*

1760:5 Pierre **Fine**, French surgeon, born; performed first colostomy for intestinal obstruction, 1805, *AnSMP* 6:34. Died 1814. *3430*

1760:6 Wilhelm Joseph **Schmitt**, Austrian physician, born; first reported interstitial pregnancy, 1801, *BMCW* 1:59. Died 1827. *6163*

1760:7 Thomas **Trotter**, British naval surgeon, born; his *Essay on drunkenness*, 1804, was the first printed book on alcoholism. Died 1832. *2071.1*

## 1761
1761:1 **Labyrinthine fluid** described by Domenico Cotugno (1736–1822) in his *De aquae-ductibus auris humanae internae*; he was preceded in this by Theodor Pyl, 1742. *1549, 1548*

1761:2 **Pathological anatomy**; *De sedibus et causis morborum per anatomen indagatis* published by Giovanni Battista Morgagni (1682–1771). *2276*

1761:3 Association of **tobacco** with **cancer** observed by John Hill (1714–1775); in his *Cautions against the immoderate use of snuff …. 2607.1*

1761:4 **Immediate percussion** of the **chest**, as a diagnostic measure, was introduced by Leopold Auenbrugger (1722–1809); recorded in his *Inventum novum ex percussione thoracis humani. 2672*

1761:5 Dissecting **aneurysm** of the **aorta** first described by Frank Nicholls (1699–1778), *PT* **52**:265. *2734.1*

1761:6 Nicolaus Anton **Friedreich**, German physician, born 24 Feb; gave the first description of facial paralysis; in his *De paralysi musculorum faciei rheumatici*, 1797. Died 1836. *4519*

1761:7 Matthew **Baillie**, British physician, born 27 Oct. His *Morbid anatomy of some of the most important parts of the human body*, 1793, was the first systematic textbook of pathological anatomy (he published an atlas intended to illustrate it, 1799–1803). In *Morbid anatomy* he clearly described the pulmonary lesions of tuberculosis; on p. 87 he gave the first clear description of the morbid anatomy and symptoms of gastric ulcer. In the 2nd edn, 1797, he suggested (vol. 1, p. 46) a relationship between rheumatic fever and valvular heart disease, and (vol. 2, p. 72) gave the first clinical description of chronic obstructive pulmonary oedema. In 1789 he contributed notable anatomico-pathological studies of dermoid cysts of the ovary, *PT* **79**:71. Died 1823. *2281, 2282, 3218, 3427, 3167.1, 6021*

1761:8 John **Clarke** born; gave the first account of infantile tetany and clear descriptions of tetany and laryngismus stridulus; in his *Commentaries on some of the most important diseases of children, part the first*, 1815. Died 1815. *4825, 6328*

1761:9 Mason Fitch **Cogswell**, American surgeon, born; successful ligation of the primitive carotid artery, 1803; reported in 1824, *NEJM* **13**:357. Died 1830. *2945*

1761:10 Ferdinand George **Danz**, German physician, born; first described hereditary ectodermal dysplasia, 1792, *ArGe* **4**:684. Died 1793. *6358*

1761: Stephen **Hales** died, **born** 1667. *manometer, ventilation*

1761: Pierre **Fauchard** died, **born** 1678. *dentistry*

## 1762
1762:1 **Pennsylvania Hospital Library** founded (first medical library in America)

1762:2 A classic description of **hydrocele** given by Percivall Pott (1714–1788); in his *Practical remarks on the hydrocele or watry rupture. 4164*

1762:3 A method of reducing **shoulder dislocation** introduced by Charles White (1726–1813), *MOI* **2**:373. *4407*

1762:4 The first book on **chiropody**, *Nouvelles observations, ou méthode certaine sur le traitement de cors*, written by Rousselot (d.1772). *4302.1*

1762: 5 Nathan **Smith**, American physician and surgeon, born 30 Sep; pioneer ovariotomist, performed the operation for ovarian dropsy, 1822, *AmMR* **5**:124, apparently without knowledge of the earlier operations of McDowell. In his classic account of typhoid, *A practical essay on typhous fever*, 1824, he clearly recognized the contagious nature of the disease. Gave a classic early account of osteomyelitis, 1827, *PoMoJ* **1**:11, 66. Died 1829. *6024, 6023, 5022, 4313*

1762: 6 James Carrick **Moore**, British surgeon, born 21 Dec; revived the ancient idea of using nerve compression to obtain analgesia during surgical operations; in his *A method of preventing or diminishing pain in several operations of surgery*, 1784. John Hunter used Moore's clamp successfully in a leg amputation. Died 1834. *5645.91*

1762: Jacques **Daviel** died, **born** 1693. *cataract*

## 1763
1763: 1 Secret **hospital** for the treatment of **venereal diseases** opened in **St Petersburg**

1763: 2 John **Bell** born; Scottish surgeon and brother of Charles, born 12 May; wrote *Principles of surgery*, 3 vols, 1801–9; is regarded as a founder of surgical anatomy. First to ligate the gluteal artery; reported in his *Principles*, **1**, 421. Died 1820. *5581, 2926*

1763: 3 Louis Nicolas **Vauquelin**, French chemist, born 16 May; made first complete chemical analysis of the nervous system, 1811, *AnMHN* **18**:212. Died 1829. *1389.1*

1763: 4 Georg Joseph **Beer**, Austrian ophthalmologist, born 23 Dec; the doctrines laid down in his *Lehre von den Augenkrankheiten*, 2 vols, 1813–17, dominated the practice of ophthalmology for many years. Died 1821. *5842*

1763: 5 Whitley **Stokes**, Irish physician, born; first described ecthyma terebrans, 1807, *DMPE* **1**:146. Died 1845. *4020*

1763: 6 Johan Valentin von **Hildenbrand**, Austrian physician, born; his classic description of typhus in his *Ueber den ansteckenden Typhus*, 1810, led to the eponym 'Hildenbrand's disease' in the French literature. Died 1818. *5375*

1763: William **Smellie** died, **born** 1697. *obstetrics, midwifery*

## 1764
1764: 1 **School of Surgery** founded in **Barcelona**

1764: 2 **Oedema** first clearly associated with **proteinuria** by Domenico Cotugno (1736–1822); in his *De ischiade nervosa commentarius*. The book also includes a classic description of nervous **sciatica**. *4204.2, 4515*

1764: 3 A case of **extrauterine pregnancy** successfully operated on by John Bard (1716–1799), *MOI* **2**:369. *6155*

1764: 4 Richard Brocklesby's (1722–1797) *Oeconomical and medical observations ... tending to the improvement of military hospitals*, etc., was the best work of the century regarding **military sanitation**. Died 1797. *2153*

1764:5 Robert Whytt (1714–1766) wrote the first important British work on **neurology** after Willis, his *Observations on the nature, causes and cure of those disorders which have been commonly called nervous hypochondriac, or hysteric*, etc. *4841*

1764:6 Considered by Still 'the most progressive work which has yet been written' on paediatrics, the *Underrättelser om barn-sjukdomar och deras botemedel* of Nils Rosén von Rosenstein (1706–1773) gave an impetus to research influencing the future course of **paediatrics**. English translation 1776. *6323*

1764:7 John **Abernethy**, British surgeon, born 3 Apr; a pupil of John Hunter, became a leading surgeon in London. His best work is probably his *Surgical observations on the constitutional origin and treatment of local diseases*, 1809, which contains (pp. 234–92) the report of his first ligation of the external iliac artery for aneurysm. Died 1831. *5584, 2928.*

1764:8 Joseph Constantine **Carpue**, British surgeon, born 4 May; revived the Hindu method of rhinoplasty and reported two successful cases; in his *An account of two successful operations for restoring a lost nose from the integuments of the forehead*, 1816. Died 1846. *5737*

1764:9 Thomas **Spens**, British physician, born; first reported heart block, 1792, *MCom* **7**:458. Died 1842. *2735*

## 1765
1765:1 **Medical Department** at **College of Philadelphia** (later **Pennsylvania University**) founded

1765:2 '**Nerve of Wrisberg**' described by Heinrich Wrisberg (1739–1808); in his *Observationes anatomicae de quinto pare nervorum encephali. 1252*

1765:3 The surgery of **anal fistula**, as described by Percivall Pott (1714–1788) in his *Remarks on the disease commonly called a fistula in ano* is regarded as a classic of **colo-rectal surgery**. *3242.2*

1765:4 In his *Enquiry into the nature, cause, and cure of the croup*, Francis Home (1719–1813) gave the first clear and complete description of **diphtheria**. *5051*

1765:5 '**Gasserian ganglion**' so named by A.B.R. Hirsch after Johann Ludwig Gasser (*fl.*1757–1765); in his *Pars quinti nervorum encephali .... 1251*

## 1766
1766:1 **Addenbrooke's Hospital**, Cambridge, England, opened; founded following bequest by John Addenbrooke (1618–1719)

1766:2 **Hydrogen** isolated by Henry Cavendish (1731–1810), *PT* **72**:119. *925*

1766:3 Thomas Robert **Malthus**, British political economist, born 17 Feb; his *Essay on the principle of population*, 1798, had a great influence on both Darwin and Wallace. Died 1834. *1693*

1766:4 Philip Wright **Post**, American surgeon, born 19 Feb; performed first successful ligation in America of the common carotid artery for aneurysm in America, 1814, *AmMPR* **4**:366.

First successfully to ligate the subclavian artery, outside the scalenus muscles, 1817, *TPNY* 1:387. Died 1828. *2934, 2939*

1766:5 Dominique Jean **Larrey**, 'the greatest military surgeon in history', born, France 8 Jul. Introduced 'ambulances volantes', 1793. First observed the contagious nature of trachoma (military ophthalmia, Egyptian ophthalmia), while serving in the Napoleonic campaign in Egypt; in his *Mémoire sur l'ophtalmie régnant en Egypte*, 1800. His *Mémoires de chirurgie militaire* appeared 1812–1817, and contain his report (**2**, 180) of one of the earliest successful amputations at the hip-joint. His most comprehensive treatise on surgery was *Clinique chirurgicale, excercée particulièrement dans les camps et les hôpitaux militaires depuis 1792 jusqu'en 1829*, 5 vols, 1829–36. Died 1842. *5837, 2160, 4442, 5589.1*

1766:6 Kurt Polykarp Joachim **Sprengel**, German physician and medical historian, born 3 Aug. His *Versuch einer pragmatischen Geschichte der Arzneikunde*, 5 vols, 1792–1803, is a monumental history (3rd ed. 1821–28). Died 1833. *6383*

1766:7 William Hyde **Wollaston**, British chemist and physicist, born 6 Aug; described various substances that might be found as constituents of urinary calculi, 1797, *PT* **87**:386; isolated cystine, 1810, *PT* **100**:223 (first amino acid to be isolated). Died 1828. *4287, 668.1*

1766:8 John **Dalton**, British chemist, born 6 Sep; gave the first scientific description of colour-blindness ('Daltonism'), 1798, *MLPSM* **5**, i:28. Died 1844. *5834*

---

1766: Robert **Whytt** died, **born** 1714. *reflex action, pupil, neurology, hypochondria, hysteria, tuberculous meningitis*

1766: Jean **Astruc** died, **born** 1684. *venereal disease*

1766: Zabdiel **Boylston** died, **born**, 1679. *smallpox inoculation*

## 1767
1767:1 **Library** at **Montpellier Faculté de Médecine** started by gift of 1200 books

1767:2 **Medical Department** at **King's College**, (later **Columbia University**) **New York**, founded

1767:3 **'Devonshire colic'** shown to be due to **lead-poisoned** cider by George Baker (1722–1809); in his *An essay concerning the causes of the epidemial colic of Devonshire*. *2096*

1767:4 **Snake venoms**; first modern investigation by Felice Fontana (1730–1805); in his *Ricerche fisiche sopra il veleno della vipere*. *2103*

1767:5 In *Some few general remarks on fractures and dislocations*, Percivall Pott (1714–1788) outlined methods subsequently adopted worldwide; **'Pott's fracture'** is described on p. 57. *4408*

1767:6 The first important monograph on bacillary **dysentery**, *Von der Ruhr unter dem Volke im Jahr 1765*, written by Johann Georg Zimmermann (1728–1795). *5090*

1767:7 Inoculation of the Empress Catherine of Russia and her son against **smallpox** by Thomas Dimsdale (1712–1800), for which he received an enormous fee and which helped in popularizing **inoculation** in England; he wrote *The present method for inoculating for the small-pox. 5420*

1767:8 *An essay on the diseases most fatal to infants*, by George Armstrong (1719–1789) was one of the best works of the period on **paediatrics**. Armstrong founded the Dispensary for Sick Children, London, 1769, the first children's dispensary in Europe. *6324*

1767:9 Thomas **Sutton** born; named and described alcoholic delirium tremens; in his *Tracts on delirium tremens*, 1813. He differentiated the condition from phrenitis. Died 1835. *4925*

1767:10 James **Barlow** born; reported what was apparently the first caesarean section performed in England (on 27 November 1793) from which the mother recovered; in *Medical records and researches selected from the papers of a private medical association*, 1798, p. 54. Died 1839. *6236.1*

1767: Paul Gottlieb **Werlhof** died, **born** 1699. *purpura haemorrhagica*

**1768**
1768:1 **Université de Pont-à-Mousson** moved to **Nancy**

1768:2 **Anatomical Theatre** at **Frankfurt a. Main**

1768:3 Classic description of **angina pectoris**, and introduction of the term, by William Heberden (1710–1801) in a lecture published 1772, *MTr* **2**:59. *2887*

1768:4 A successful operation for **temporo-sphenoidal abscess** recorded by Sauveur-François Morand (1697–1773); in his *Opuscules de chirurgie*, Pt. 1, p. 161. *4851*

1768:5 The first account of the clinical course of **tuberculous meningitis in children** by Robert Whytt (1714–1766); in his *Observations on the dropsy in the brain. 4634*

1768:6 The first English textbook on **dentistry** and **teeth deformities**, *A treatise on the disorders and deformities of the teeth and gums*, published by Thomas Berdmore (1740–1785). *3674*

1768:7 **Varicella** first definitely differentiated from **smallpox** by William Heberden Sr (1710–1801), *MTr* **1**:427. *5438*

1768:8 Papers on **embryology** and **epigenesis** published by Caspar Friedrich Wolff (1733–1794), *NCASP* **12**:43, 403; **13**:470. *471*

1768:9 Jean Louis Marc **Alibert**, French dermatologist, born 2 May; his *Description des maladies de la peau ...*, 1806, which includes hand-coloured illustrations, was the largest and most spectacular of the early classics of dermatology; it includes the first description of mycosis fungoides (p. 157, pl.xxxvi). The second edition, 1825, includes the first description of sycosis barbae ('Alibert's mentagra'). Gave the first accurate description of keloid ('Alibert's keloid'), 1816, *JUSM* **2**:207. Gave an important description of 'Aleppo boil' (cutaneous leishmaniasis), 1829, *RMFE* **3**:62. His *Monographie des dermatoses*, 1832, includes the first published illustration of his 'family tree' for the classification of skin diseases, never widely adopted, and an important description of dermatolysis. Died 1837. *3986, 4024, 4023, 5291, 3990.1*

1768: 10 William Potts **Dewees**, American paediatrician and gynaecologist, born 5 May; wrote the first American textbook on paediatrics, *Treatise on the medical and physical treatment of children*, 1825. Published the first American textbook on gynaecology, *A treatise on diseases of females*, 1826. Died 1841. *6331, 6026.1*

1768: 11 Philip Syng **Physick**, 'Father of American surgery', born 7 Jul. First, in 1805, to use a stomach tube for gastric lavage after poisoning; he reported this in 1812, *ER* **3**:111. Introduced several new procedures into surgery, including the use of absorbable kid and buckskin ligatures, 1816, *ER* **6**:389. Described his operation for artificial anus, 1826, *PHJMS* **13**:199. Invented the modern tonsillotome, 1828, *AmJMS* **2**:116. Died 1837. *3432, 5586, 3436, 3255*

1768: 12 Astley Paston **Cooper**, British surgeon, born 23 Aug; performed myringotomy to treat Eustachian tube obstructive deafness, 1801, *PT* **91**:435. Ligated the common carotid artery in 1805, *MCT* **1**:222; the patient died but a second case (1808) was successful, *GHR* **1**:43, 53. In his *Anatomy and surgical treatment of inguinal and congenital hernia*, 1807, he described the fascia transversalis and 'Cooper's ligament'. The second edition, 1827, included a description of 'Cooper's hernia', femoral hernia. Ligated the abdominal aorta (unsuccessfully), 1817, in his *Surgical essays ...*; published one of the earliest descriptions of hyperplastic cystic mammary disease, in his *Illustrations of the diseases of the breast*, 1829. Died 1841. *3361, 2929, 2954, 2955, 3581, 2941, 5769*

1768: 13 John Beale **Davidge**, American surgeon, born; first to report removal of the parotid gland, 1823, *BPJR* **1**:165. Died 1829. *3433.1*

1768: 14 Giuseppe Angelo **Fonzi**, Italian dentist, born; produced the first sets of individual porcelain artificial teeth mounted on a base; in his *Rapport sur les dents artificielles terro-métalliques*, 1808. Died 1840. *3679.2*

1768: John **Huxham** died, **born** 1694. *fevers, public health, epidemics, diphtheria*

## 1769
1769: 1 [**General Hospital**], **Copenhagen**, opened

1769: 2 **Laryngismus stridulus** ('**Millar's asthma**') first described by John Millar (1733–1805); in his *Observations on the asthma and the hooping cough.* *3167*

1769: 3 A powder containing calcined sponge prescribed for **goitre** by Thomas Prosser, probably the first recorded use of an **iodine** preparation in England; in his *An account and method of cure of the bronchocele or Derby neck.* *3807*

1769: 4 A corset and extension bed for treating **deformities of the spine** invented by Jean André Venel (1740–1791), *MSSPL* **2**:66, 197. *4305*

1769: 5 The first excision of the head of the **humerus** recorded by Charles White (1728–1813), *PT* **59**:39. *4437*

1769: 6 Transmission of **yaws** by flies noted by Edward Bancroft (1744–1821); in his *Essay on the natural history of Guiana*, p. 385. *5304*

1769:7 *A medical discourse, or an historical inquiry into the ancient and present state of medicine*, by Peter Middleton (d.1781), was the first American publication on **medical history**. *6380*

---

1769:8 Friedrich **Accum**, German chemist, born 29 Mar; exposed food adulteration, in his *Treatise on the adulteration of food*, 1820. Died 1838. *1604.2*

---

1769:9 Carl **Wenzel**, German physician, born; reported artificial induction of premature labour; in his *Allgemeine geburtshülfliche Betrachtungen und über die künstliche Frühgeburt*, 1818. Died 1827. *6168*

1769:10 Marie Louise **La Chapelle** born; a famous midwife, supervised 5,000 deliveries. Her vast experience was published in her *Pratique des accouchemens*, 3 vols, 1821–25, edited posthumously by her nephew. Died 1821. *6170*

---

1769: Carl Friedrich **Kaltschmied** died, **born** 1706. *parotid gland tumour*

## 1770
1770:1 **School of Anatomy** at No. 16 Great Windmill Street, **London**, founded by William Hunter (1718–1783)

1770:2 **Radcliffe Infirmary, Oxford**, opened, erected from residue of estate of John Radcliffe (1652–1714); became geriatric hospital, 1979, when the **John Radcliffe Hospital** opened on outskirts of Oxford

1770:3 **General Dispensary** in **Aldersgate Street**, London, founded by John Coakley Lettsom (1744–1815), opened

1770:4 First **medical degree in North America** conferred on Robert Tucker by **King's College, New York**

1770:5 **Pennsylvania Quarantine Act**

1770:6 The first clear description of **relapsing fever** given by John Rutty (1698–1775); in his *A chronological history of the weather and seasons and of prevailing diseases in Dublin*, p. 75. *5309*

1770:7 The first description of *Loa loa*, the African eye-worm, cause of **loaiasis** given by the French surgeon Mongin, *JMCP* **32**:338. *5336.2*

---

1770:8 John **Stearns**, American physician, born 16 May; first in America to use ergot for the induction of labour, 1808, *MRep* **5**:308. Died 1848. *6164*

---

1770:9 Alexander John Gaspard **Marcet**, Swiss physician in London, born; described alkaptonuria, 1822, *MCT* **12**:37. Died 1822. *3912*

---

1770: Mark **Akenside** died, **born** 1721. *neurofibromatosis*

1770: Bernhard Siegfried **Albinus** died, **born** 1697. *anatomy*

1770: Henri François **Le Dran** died, **born** 1685. *lithotomy*

**1771**

1771:1 First **life-table** for **actuaries (Northampton Table)** constructed by Richard Price

1771:2 **New York Hospital** chartered 12 Jul; fire and revolution delayed use of the building for its intended purpose until Jan 1791

1771:3 '**Fallot's tetralogy**' described by Eduard Sandifort (1742–1814); in his *Observationes anatomicae-pathologicae*, vol. 1. *2734.2*

1771:4 In his *Animadversiones in morbum, vulgo pellagram* Francesco Frapolli (d.1773) gave **pellagra** its present name. *3751*

1771:5 *The natural history of the human teeth*, by John Hunter (1728–1793) is a detailed and illustrated study of the mouth, jaws and teeth – this book and his *Practical treatise on the diseases of the teeth*, 1778, revolutionized the practice of **dentistry**. *3675, 3676*

1771:6 William Cadogan's (1711–1797) *Dissertation on the gout* attracted much attention; he advised moderate exercise and moderation in drinking as a cure. *4489*

1771:7 One of the earliest accurate descriptions of **diphtheria** is contained in Samuel Bard's (1742–1821) classic, *An enquiry into the nature, cause and cure of angina suffocativa, or sore throat distemper. 5052*

1771:8 **Retroversion** of the **uterus** first accurately described by William Hunter (1718–1783), *MOI* **4**:400; **5**:388. *6020*

1771:9 Important research on the **blood**, including **coagulation of red blood cells** and **lymphocytes** reported by William Hewson (1739–1774); in his *Experimental inquiry into the properties of the blood* ... III. *863*

1771:10 Albrecht von Haller (1708–1777) one of the most imposing figures in medicine, completed four great **bibliographies** of botany, anatomy, surgery and medicine, forming the most complete reference works of the time. The bibliography of **botany**, *Bibliotheca botanica*, 2 vols, was published 1771–72. *1833*

---

1771:11 Ephraim **McDowell**, American surgeon, born 11 Nov; performed the first ovariotomy, 1817, *ER* **7**:242. Died 1830. *6023*

1771:12 Marie François Xavier **Bichat**, French anatomist and physiologist, born 14 Nov. Revolutionized descriptive anatomy. His most important contribution to modern anatomy was that pathology must be based on the structure of tissues making up the organs, regardless of the location of the latter in the organism; in his *Anatomie générale*, 1802, which marks the beginning of histology. He also wrote *Traité des membranes en général*, 1800, and *Traité d'anatomie descriptive*, 5 vols, 1801–3. Died 1802. *403, 537, 404*

---

1771:13 Elisha **North**, American physician, born; his *Treatise on a malignant epidemic, commonly called spotted fever*, 1811, was the first book on cerebrospinal meningitis; in it he recommended the use of the clinical thermometer, not then in general use. Died 1843. *4676*

1771:14 John **Bostock**, British physician, born; his classical description of hay fever lead to the eponym 'Bostock's catarrh', 1819, *MCT* **10**:161. Died 1846. *2582*

1771:15 Francis **Place**, British reformer, born; one of the first to advocate birth control, 1822, but did not indicate methods, in his *Illustrations and proofs of the principle of population.* Died 1854. *1696.1*

1771: Giovanni Battista **Morgagni** died, **born** 1682. *pathological anatomy, angina pectoris*

1771: John **Burton** died, **born** 1697. *puerperal fever*

**1772**
1772:1 **Académie Royale de Belgique, Brussels**, founded

1772:2 **Nitrogen** discovered by Daniel Rutherford (1749–1819), *De aëre fixo dicto, aut mephitico. 921*

1772:3 Important observations on the **ear** and **olfaction** made by Antonio Scarpa (1752–1832); in his *De structura fenestrae rotundae auris*, 1772, and *De auditu et olfactu*, 1789. *1550, 1453*

1772:4 **Oxygen** isolated by Joseph Priestley (1733–1804), *PT* **62**:147. *920*

1772:5 The first known clinical description of **acromegaly**, by Nicolas Saucerotte (1741–1812) before the Académie de Chirurgie, Paris, was recorded in his *Mélanges de chirurgie*, 1801, 407. *3880*

1772:6 William Cullen (1710–1790) publishes his *Works. 76*

1772:7 Jean Etienne **Esquirol**, French psychiatrist, born 4 Feb; wrote the first modern textbook on psychiatry, *Des maladies mentales*, 1838, notable for its striking illustrations of insane patients. Died 1840. *4929*

1772:8 Augustin Jacob **Landré-Beauvais** born; gave the first reasonably accurate description of rheumatoid arthritis; in his *Doit-on admettre une nouvelle espèce de goutte sous la dénomination de goutte asthénique primitive?*, 1800. Died 1840. *4490*

1772:9 Carl Gustav **Himly** born; used hyoscyamine to dilate the pupil to facilitate removal of the lens; in his *Ophthalmologische Beobachtungen*, **I**, p. 97, 1801. Died 1837. *5834.1*

1772:10 **Rousselot** died; wrote the first book on chiropody, *Nouvelles observations, ou méthode certaine sur le traitement de cors*, 1762. *4302.1*

**1773**
1773:1 **Medical Society of London** founded by John Coakley Lettsom (1744–1815)

1773:2 First **insane asylum** in **US** founded at **Williamsburg**, Virginia

1773:3 John Howard (1726–1790) begins inspection of **English prisons**; leading to Act of Parliament for **sanitary** improvement. *1598*

1773:4 **University of Münster, Westphalia**, founded

1773:5 [**Royal Czech Society of Sciences**], Prague, founded

1773:6 Charles White (1726–1813), in his *A treatise on the management of pregnant and lying-in women*, was the first after Hippocrates to make any substantial contribution towards the aetiology and management of **puerperal fever**. He insisted on absolute cleanliness and the isolation of infected patients. *6270*

1773:7 Marie Anne Victoire **Boivin**, French midwife, born 9 Apr; gave a classic description of hydatidiform mole; in her *Nouvelles recherches de l'origine, la nature et le traitement de la mole vésiculaire ou grossesse hydatique*, 1827. With Antoine Dugès, practised amputation of the cervix for chronic ulceration; in their *Traité pratique des maladies de l'utérus et ses annexes*, 1833, **2**, p. 48, is the first recorded case of cancer of the female urethra. Died 1841. *6172, 6028*

1773:8 Philipp **Bozzini**, German physician, born 25 May; introduced a speculum, utilizing illumination and reflection by mirrors, 1806, *JPrH* **24**, I:107. Died 1809. *2672.1*

1773:9 Thomas **Young**, British physician and physicist, born 13 Jun; elucidated the act of accommodation in the eye, 1793, *PT* **83**:169; gave first description of astigmatism, 1801, *PT* **91**:23; established the wave theory of light, 1802, *PT* **92**:12. Died 1829. *1486, 1487, 1488*

1773:10 Abraham **Colles**, Irish surgeon, born 23 Jul; his description of the fracture of the carpal end of the radius, 1814, *EMSJ* **10**:182, led to the term 'Colles' fracture'. Ligated subclavian artery in 1811 and again in 1813, reported in 1815, *EMSJ* **11**:1. Died 1843. *4410, 2936*

1773:11 Agostino **Bassi**, Italian scientist, born 25 Sep; demonstrated the parasitic nature of the muscardine disease of silkworms, *Del mal del segno calcinaccio o moscardino*, 1835–36. He is regarded as the founder of the doctrine of pathogenic microbes. Died 1856. *2532*

1773:12 Robert **Brown**, British botanist, born 21 Dec; discovered cell nucleus, 1831, *TLS* **16**:685. Died 1858. *109*

1773:13 (?) Francesco **Frapolli** died; in his *Animadversiones in morbum, vulgo pellagram*, 1771, he gave pellagra its present name. *3751*

1773: Sauveur-François **Morand** died, **born** 1697. *temporo-sphenoidal abscess, cleidocranial dysostosis*

1773: Nils **Rosén von Rosenstein** died, **born** 1706. *paediatrics*

## 1774

1774:1 Albrecht von Haller (1708–1777) one of the most imposing figures in medicine, completed four great **bibliographies** of botany, anatomy, surgery and medicine, forming the most complete reference works of the time. The bibliographies of **anatomy** and **surgery** are respectively *Bibliotheca anatomica*, 2 vols, 1774–77; *Bibliotheca chirurgica*, 2 vols, 1774–75. *438, 5789*

1774:2 First complete account of the **lymphatics** by William Hewson (1739–1774); in his *Experimental enquiries: Part the second*. *1102*

1774:3 '**Petit's hernia**' and '**Petit's triangle**' described by Jean Louis Petit (1674–1750); in his *Traité des maladies chirurgicales*, **2**, 256. *3577*

1774:4 *Anatomia uteri humani gravidi tabulis illustrata, The anatomy of the human gravid uterus exhibited in figures,* by William Hunter (1718–1783), is one of the finest anatomical atlases ever produced, containing 34 copper plates depicting the **gravid uterus** life-size. Hunter originally trained as William Smellie's assistant. His text for the atlas, *An anatomical description of the human gravid uterus and its contents,* was published, 1794, edited by Matthew Baillie. *6157, 6157.1*

---

1774:5 John Conrad **Otto**, American physician, born 15 Mar; recognized and adequately described haemophilia, 1803, *MRep* **6**:1. Died 1844. *3054*

1774:6 Jean François **Coindet**, Swiss physician, born 12 Jul; first to administer iodine in the treatment of goitre, 1820, *AnS* **15**:49. Died 1834. *3812*

1774:7 Charles **Bell** born Nov; brother of John, distinguished as anatomist, physiologist and neurologist, was also an eminent surgeon. His works include *A system of operative surgery*, 2 vols, 1807–9. Described the long thoracic ('Bell's') nerve, and first to describe facial paralysis following a lesion of the motor nerve of the face ('Bell's palsy') 1821, *PT* **111**:398. His *Illustrations of the great operations of surgery*, 1821, is considered one of the most beautifully illustrated books in the entire literature of surgery. Died 1842. *5583, 1255, 4520, 5588*

1774:8 Georges Simon **Sérullas**, French chemist, born 2 Nov; discovered iodoform, 1822, *AnC* **20**:163. Died 1832. *1848*

---

1774:9 Jean Marie Gaspard **Itard**, French otologist, born; published the first modern text on otology, *Traité des maladies de l'oreille et de l'audition*, 1821. Died 1838. *3364*

1774:10 Joseph Claude Anthelm **Récamier**, French physician, born; first recognized cancer metastasis; in his *Recherches sur le traitement du cancer* ..., 1829. Introduced a vaginal speculum, 1843, *BuAM* **8**:661. Died 1852. *2610, 6033*

1774:11 Gaspard Laurent **Bayle**, French physician, born; his *Recherches sur la phthisie pulmonaire*, 1818, marks the beginning of modern clinical work on tuberculosis. Died 1816. *2322*

1774:12 Pierre **Blaud**, French physician, born; treated chlorosis with ferrous sulphate and potassium carbonate ('Blaud's pill'), 1832, *RMFE* **45**:337. Died 1858. *3113*

1774:13 William **Wood** born; first to describe neuroma, 1829, *TMCS* **3**:367. Died 1857. *4523*

---

1774: William **Hewson** died, **born** 1739. *blood, lymphatics, lymphocytes*

1774: Johann Friedrich **Meckel**, the elder, died, **born** 1724. *Meckel's ganglion, Meckel's cave*

## 1775
1775:1 **Botanic garden** in **Vienna**

1775:2 The first description of **occupational cancer (chimney sweeps' cancer of the scrotum)** and a description of **senile (Pott's) gangrene** given by Percivall Pott (1714–1788); in his *Chirurgical observations relative to the cataract ... the cancer of the scrotum*, etc. *2122, 2609, 4165*

1775:3 **Oxygen** isolated and defined by Antoine Laurent Lavoisier (1743–1794), thus refuting Stahl's **phlogiston** theory of combustion, *HARS* 520. *922*

---

1775:4 John Richard **Farre**, physician, born Barbados, 31 Jan; published first monograph on congenital abnormalities of the heart, *Pathological researches, Essay 1*, 1814. Died 1862. *2740.1*

---

1775:5 Johan Nepomuk **Rust**, German surgeon, born 5 Apr; his original description of tuberculous spondylitis of the cervical vertebrae led to the name 'Rust's disease'; in his *Aufsätze und Abhandlungen aus dem Gebiete der Medizin ...*, 1834. Died 1840. *4319*

---

1775:6 Adam Elias von **Siebold**, German obstetrician, born 5 Mar; gave a classic account of cancer of the uterus, *Ueber den Gebärmutterkrebs, dessen Enstehung und Verhütung*, 1824. Died 1826. *6025*

---

1775:7 Joseph **Fox**, British surgeon and dentist, born; wrote the first book on orthodontics, *Natural history of the human teeth*, 1803; his *History and treatment of diseases of the teeth*, 1890 is the first book to include illustrations of the teeth and is considered by some of more value than Hunter's *Practical treatise*, 1778. Died 1816. *3679, 3679.1*

---

1775: John **Hill** died, **born** 1714. *tobacco, cancer*

1775: John **Rutty** died, **born** 1698. *relapsing fever*

## 1776
1776:1 [**Academy of Sciences**] founded at **Agram [Zagreb]**

1776:2 First detailed account of the **cerebellum** by Michael Vincenzo Giacinto Malacarne (1744–1816); in his *Della vera struttura del cervelletto umano. 1382.1*

1776:3 First **caecostomy** performed by H. Pillore and reported by J.Z. Amussat in his *Mémoire sur la possibilité d'établir un anus artificiel ...*, 1839. *3443*

1776:4 Albrecht von Haller (1708–1777) compiled four great bibliographies, dealing with botany, anatomy, surgery, and medicine, which formed the most complete reference work of the time. The **bibliography of medicine** is the *Bibliotheca medicinae practicae*, 4 vols, 1776–88. *6747*

1776:5 The sweetish taste of urine in **diabetes mellitus** shown by Matthew Dobson (?1731–1784) to be produced by sugar; he also discovered **hyperglycaemia**, *MOI* **5**:298. *3928*

1776:6 Joseph Jacob von Plenck (1738–1807) drew up a classification of **skin diseases** on the basis of their appearance; in his *Doctrina de morbis cutaneis. 3982*

1776:7 First description of **facial neuralgia** given by John Fothergill (1712–1780), *MOI* **5**:129. *4516*

1776:8 **Uric acid** discovered by Carl Wilhelm Scheele (1742–1786), *SAH* **37**:327. *668*

---

1776:9 Walter **Brashear**, American surgeon, born 11 Feb; performed the first successful amputation of the hip-joint in the United States, 1806, *TKMS* 1853 **2**:264. Died 1860. *4462*

1776: 10 (?) François **Double**, French physician, born 11 Mar; described auscultation as a diagnostic measure; in his *Séméiologie générale*, vol. 2, 1817. Died 1842. *2672.2*

1776: 11 Conrad Johann Martin **Langenbeck**, German surgeon and ophthalmologist, born 5 Dec; introduced iridencleisis, an operation for construction of an artificial pupil; in his *Prüfung der Keratonyxis, einer neuen Methode den grauen Staar durch die Hornhaut zu reclinieren oder zu zerstückeln*, 1811. Died 1851. *5841*

1776: 12 Johann Caspar **Spurzheim**, German founder of phrenology, born 31 Dec; with Franz Joseph Gall made early attempt at the localization of cerebral function, and introduced phrenology, in their *Anatomie et physiologie du système nerveux*, 1810–1819. Died 1832. *1389*

1776: 13 Per Henrik **Ling**, Swedish founder of modern physiotherapy, born; wrote *Gymnastikens allmänna grunder*, 1834. Died 1839. *1993*

1776: 14 Joshua **Milne**, British actuary to Sun Life Assurance Co., born. He reconstructed the life tables then in use, based upon the table deduced from the burial registers of All Saints Church, Northampton, 1735–80. Milne took as the basis of his calculations the Carlisle bills of mortality which had been prepared by Dr John Heysham (1753–1834) and published *A treatise on the valuation of annuities and assurances on lives and survivorship*, etc., 2 vols, London, 1815, the 'Carlisle Tables of Mortality' [Bills of mortality: weekly statement formerly issued by parish clerks in England, showing the number of deaths (and the causes) that had occurred in each parish]. The age of the person dying was not included until the year 1778, from which year dates the 'science' of life assurance.

1776: Pedro **Virgili** died, **born** 1669. *quinsy, tracheotomy*

1776: William **Battie** died, **born** 1703. *psychiatry*

1776: Robert **James** died, **born** 1705. *medical dictionary*

## 1777

1777: 1 **Newcastle Dispensary for Smallpox Inoculation** founded; inoculation began in 1786

1777: 2 **Human gastric juice** isolated by Edward Stevens (?1755–1834), in his *De alimentorum concoctione*. *980*

1777: 3 An important description of congenital hypertrophic **pyloric stenosis** was included by George Armstrong (1719–1789) in his *Account of the diseases most incident to children*, 1777, p. 49. *3425*

1777: 4 **Prison reform** in England and Wales secured by John Howard (1726–1790); in his *State of the prisons in England and Wales. 1598*

1777: 5 Anne Charles de Lorry (1726–1783) is regarded as the founder of French **dermatology**; his *Tractatus de morbis cutaneis* included a classification of **skin diseases** on the basis of their physiological, pathological and aetiological similarities. *3983*

1777: 6 First accurate account of **migraine** given by John Fothergill (1712–1780), *MOI* **6**: 103. *4517*

1777:7 The first reliable account of **colour-blindness** recorded by Joseph Huddart (1741–1816), *PT* **67**:260. *5832*

---

1777:8 John **Cheyne**, British physician, born 3 Feb; first to describe acute hydrocephalus; in his *Essay on hydrocephalus acutus*, 1808. He believed that cerebral anaemia might be the cause of apoplexy; in his *Cases of apoplexy and lethargy*, 1812, in it he published the first illustration of a subarachnoid haemorrhage. Gave the first accurate account of 'Cheyne-Stokes respiration', 1818, *DHR* **2**:216; more fully described by William Stokes, 1854. Died 1836. *4635, 4519.1, 2743, 2760*

1777:9 Charles **Cagniard-Latour**, French biologist, born 31 May; his paper on the fermentation of wine demonstrated the true nature of yeast, 1838, *AnC* **68**:296. Died 1859. *675*

1777:10 James **Jackson**, American physician, born 3 Oct; drew attention to arthrodynia *a potu* – alcoholic neuritis, 1822, *NEJM* **2**:351. Died 1867. *4521*

1777:11 Guillaume **Dupuytren**, the best surgeon of his time in France, born 6 Oct. His greatest contributions were in the field of surgical pathology. Performed the first successful excision of the lower jaw, 1812, *JUSM* **19**:77. Successfully treated aneurysm by compression, 1818, *BFM* **6**:242. Gave the first clear description of the pathology of congenital dislocation of the hip-joint, 1826, *RGAP* **2**:82. Invented enterotome for use in his operation for artificial anus, 1828, *MARM* **1**:259. Described 'Dupuytren's abscess' of the right iliac fossa, 1828, *RMFE* **1**:367. Devised an operation for the treatment of flexion contracture deformity of the fingers ('Dupuytren's contracture'), 1831, *JUSM* **5**:352; a condition already mentioned by Felix Platter in 1614. Published a classification of burns in his *Leçons orales de clinique chirurgicale*, 4 vols, 1832–4. First to treat torticollis (wry-neck) by subcutaneous section of the sternomastoid muscle. This was recorded by C. Averill in 1823 and by Dupuytren in his *Leçons orales de clinique chirurgicales*, 2 éd., **3**, p. 455, 1839. Died 1835. *4444, 2976, 4413, 3437, 3438, 4317, 2247, 5590, 4322*

1777:12 Jacques Mathieu **Delpech**, French plastic and orthopaedic surgeon, born 12 Oct; gave the first account of rhinoplasty in France, an operation he first performed on 4 June 1823, in his *Chirurgie clinique de Montpellier*, 2 vols, 1823–28 – in the same work (**1**, 184) he described his operation of subcutaneous Achilles tenotomy for club foot; established tuberculous nature of Pott's disease, in his *De l'orthomorphie*, 2 vols, 1828, a comprehensive treatise on diseases of bones and joints. Died 1832. *5741.1, 4315*

---

1777:13 Christophe François **Delabarre**, French dentist, born; one of the first to systematize occlusal anomalies and to develop orthodontic appliances, in his *Odontologie*, 1815; published *Traité de la partie méchanique de l'art du chirurgien-dentiste*, 1820, one of the first scientifically-written textbooks on dental prosthetics. Died 1862. *3679.4, 3679.5*

1777:14 Jean George Chrétien Frédéric Martin **Lobstein**, German pathologist, born; in his *Traité de l'anatomie pathologique*, 1833, gave the first description of osteopsathyrosis ('Lobstein's disease'), a form of fragilitas ossium, **2**:204, 1833, and introduced the term arteriosclerosis (artériosclérose), **2**, 550. Died 1835. *4318, 2901*

1777:15 Antoine Germain **Labarraque**, French chemist, born; introduced a chlorine solution for disinfecting purposes; in his *De l'emploi des chlorures d'oxide de sodium et de chaux*, 1823. Died 1850. *5633*

---

1777: Albrecht von **Haller** died, **born** 1708. *bibliographies of anatomy, surgery, botany, medicine*

**1778**
1778:1 **Royal College of Surgeons of Edinburgh** assumes present name

1778:2 **University of Palermo** founded

1778:3 First United States original **pharmacopoeia**, *Pharmacopoeia simpliciorum et efficaciorum*; compiled by William Brown (1752–1792). *1834*

1778:4 '**Richter's hernia**' (partial **enterocele**) described by August Gottlieb Richter (1742–1812); in his *Abhandlung von den Brüchen*, chap. 20. *3578*

1778:5 Samuel Thomas Soemmerring's (1755–1830) inaugural dissertation, *De basi encephali et originibus nervorun cranio*, 1778, provided solid grounds for the order of the 12 **cranial nerves**. *1383*

1778:6 The first work specializing in **oral surgery** was the *Traité des maladies et des opérations réellement chirurgicales de la bouche*, by Anselme Louis Bernard Berchillet Jourdain (1734–1816). *3676.1*

1778:7 The earliest exhaustive collection of **medical biographies**, *Dictionnaire historique de la médecine ancienne et moderne*, 4 vols, 1778, first published 1775, compiled by Nicolas François Joseph Eloy (1714–1788). *6704*

1778:8 An important classification of **ulcers** made by Benjamin Bell (1749–1806); in his *A treatise on the theory and management of ulcers*. *5578*

1778:9 John Hunter's (1728–1793) *A practical treatise on the diseases of the teeth* (and his *The natural history of the human teeth*, 1771) revolutionized the practice of **dentistry**, providing a basis for later research, but also giving instruction on the dubious practice of human **dental transplantation**. *3765, 3766*

1778:10 Pierre Fidèle **Bretonneau**, French physician, born 3 Apr; in his *Des inflammations spéciales du tissu muqueux et en particulier de la diphthérite, ou inflammation pelliculaire*, 1826, demonstrated that croup, malignant angina, and 'scorbutic gangrene of the gums' were all the same disease (diphtheria). He suggested the term diphtheritis, and, later, diphthérite; he successfully performed tracheotomy for croup (p. 300). Died 1862. *5053*

1778:11 John Collins **Warren**, American surgeon, born 1 Aug; performed the first staphylorrhaphy in America in May 1824 and reported in 1828, *AmJMS* **3**:1. Published first North American book on tumours, *Surgical observations on tumours ...*, 1837. Performed the first surgical operation where ether was used for the first time to produce anaesthesia, with the anaesthetic administered by William Thomas Green Morton (1819–1868) and the operation reported by Henry Jacob Bigelow (1818–1890), 1846, *BMSJ* **35**:309, 379. Founded Massachusetts General Hospital, 1821. Died 1856. *5742, 2611.1, 5651*

1778:12 Humphry **Davy**, British chemist, born 17 Dec; discovered the anaesthetic properties of nitrous oxide; in his *Researches, chemical and philosophical, chiefly concerning nitrous* *oxide*, 1800. His suggestion that it be used during surgical operations was not immediately adopted. Died 1829. *5646*

---

1778: 13 Thomas **Bateman**, British dermatologist, born; published the most influential textbook of dermatology of the 19th century, *Practical synopsis of cutaneous diseases*, 1813; lichen urticatus is first described on p. 13. His *Delineations of cutaneous diseases ...*, 1817, which contained 72 coloured plates, may be regarded as the first atlas of dermatology. It included original descriptions of several skin diseases. Died 1821. *4021, 3988*

1778: 14 Christian Friedrich **Nasse**, German physician, born; noted immunity of females to haemophilia despite their ability to transmit the disease ('Nasse's law'), 1820, *ArMEr* 1:385. Died 1851. *3056*

1778: 15 Franz Carl **Naegele** born; his account of the mechanism of labour, 1819, *DAP* **5**:483, was the best work of its time. First described the obliquely contracted pelvis ('Naegele pelvis'); in his *Das schräg verengte Becken*, 1839. Because of its rarity and difficulty of recognition on the living, most often fatal consequences, it was unknown until his study of 37 cases. He suggested diagnostic aids for its recognition. Died 1851. *6169, 6257*

---

1778: Frank **Nicholls** died, **born** 1699. *aortic aneurysm*

1778: Carl von **Linné [Linnaeus]** died, **born** 1707. *classification, aphasia*

**1779**
1779: 1 **Academia das Sciencias (Lisbon)** founded

1779: 2 **Liverpool Medical Library** founded

1779: 3 **Hôpital Necker, Paris**, founded

1779: 4 *System einer vollständigen medicinischen Polizey*, 1779–1827, the first systematic treatise on **public hygiene** published by Johann Peter Frank (1745–1821); considered the 'Father of public hygiene'. *1599*

1779: 5 The '**Coventry treatment**' for **goitre**, which introduced the burnt sponge remedy into England, mentioned by Bradford Wilmer in his *Cases and remarks in surgery: to which is subjoined an appendix containing the method of curing the bronchocele in Coventry*, pp. 252–4. *3808*

1779: 6 A classic description of **spinal curvature** due to **tuberculous caries (Pott's disease)** was given by Percivall Pott (1714–1788) without, however recognizing its tuberculous nature; in his *Remarks on that kind of palsy of the lower limbs, which is frequently found to accompany a curvature of the spine*. *4304*

1779: 7 Several new instruments for use in suprapubic **lithotomy** were invented by Jean Baseilhac (*Frère Côme*) (1703–1781); described in his *Nouvelle méthode d'extraire la pierre de la vessie urinaire*. *4285*

1779: 8 The effect of movement and rest in the treatment of **diseases of joints** described by Jean Pierre David (1737–1784), in his *Dissertation sur les effets du mouvement et du repos* *dans les maladies chirurgicales,* he included a description of **Pott's disease** (Pott, 1779). *4303*

1779:9 **Mesmerism**, an hypnotic state induced by the operator's imposition of his will on that of the patient. Introduced by Franz Anton Mesmer (1734–1815) and based on his belief in **animal magnetism**; in his *Mémoire sur la découverte du magnétisme animale. 4992.1*

1779:10 Peter Mark **Roget**, British physician and lexicographer, born 16 Jan; best remembered for his *Thesaurus of English words and phrases*, first published in 1852 and still available. Died 1869.

**1780**
1780:1 **Chair of Clinical Medicine** founded at **Oxford**

1780:2 **University of Munster** inaugurated

1780:3 **Hôpital Cochin, Paris**, founded

1780:4 **American Academy of Arts and Sciences, Boston**, founded

1780:5 **Massachusetts Medical Society** chartered

1780:6 Lazzaro Spallanzani (1729–1799) confirmed the solvent property of the **gastric juice** and discovered the action of **saliva** in **digestion**; *Dissertazioni di fisica animale e vegetabile. 981*

1780:7 The first definite description of **dengue** given by David Bylon, who described an epidemic that occurred in the Dutch East Indies in 1779, *VBG* **2**:17. *5469*

1780:8 The first important clinical description of **anthrax** given by Philibert Chabert (1737–1814); in his *Description et traitement du charbon dans les animaux. 5162*

1780:9 Pierre Jean **Robiquet**, French chemist, born 13 Jan; isolated codeine, 1832, *AnC* **51**:225. Died 1840. *1853*

1780:10 Charles **Badham**, British physician, born 17 Apr; named bronchitis and distinguished the acute and chronic types of pneumonia and pleurisy; in his *Observations on the inflammatory affections of the mucous membrane of the bronchiae*, 1808. Died 1845. *3168*

1780:11 Philibert Joseph **Roux**, French surgeon, born 26 Apr; repaired, in 1819, the cleft palate of a medical student (*JUSM* **16**:356), John Stephenson, who described the operation in his own graduation thesis (1820). Roux published a detailed account of the operation (for which he proposed the name 'staphylorrhaphy', 1825, *ArGM* **7**:516. First to suture ruptured female perineum, 1834, *GMP* **2**:17. Died 1854. *5739.1, 5740, 5741.2, 6029*

1780:12 George **Ballingall**, British surgeon, born 2 May; first to distinguish between amoebic and bacillary dysentery; in his *Practical observations on fever, dysentery and liver complaints as they occur amongst European troops in India*, 1818. Died 1855. *5182.1*

1780:13 John **Abercrombie**, British physician, born 10 Oct; published first textbook of neuropathology, *Pathological and clinical researches on diseases of the brain and spinal cord*, 1828. Died 1844. *2285.1*

---

1780:14 Charles Louis **Derosne**, French chemist, born; isolated alkaloids from opium, 1802, *AnC* **45**:257. Died 1846. *1838.3*

---

1780:15 George **Langstaff** born; first to report carcinoma of the prostate, 1817, *MCT* **8**:272. Died 1846. *4258*

---

1780:16 John Bunnell **Davis**, British physician, born; in his *A cursory inquiry into some of the principal causes of mortality among children*, 1817, he drew attention to the high infant mortality rate, especially in London. His suggestion that poor mothers be instructed in infant care resulted in a system of health-visiting by benevolent ladies. A children's dispensary he founded in 1816 later became the Royal Waterloo Hospital for Children and Women. Died 1824. *6330*

---

1780: John **Fothergill** died, **born** 1712. *facial neuralgia, migraine, diphtheria, scarlatinal angina*

1780: Philipp **Pfaff** died, **born** 1716. *dentistry*

1780: André **Levret** died, **born** 1703. *obstetrics*

## 1781

1781:1 Jean Louis Baudelocque (1746–1810), wrote *L'art des accouchemens*, 2 vols, invented a **pelvimeter** and advanced the knowledge of pelvimetry and of the mechanics of **labour**. The external conjugate diameter is known as **Baudelocque's diameter**. *6255*

---

1781:2 René Theophile Hyacinthe **Laennec**, French physician, born 17 Feb; introduced instrumental auscultation, made possible by his invention of the stethoscope; in his *De l'auscultation médiate*, 1819. In his book he described chronic interstitial hepatitis ('Laennec's cirrhosis'), **1**, p. 368. Died 1826. *2673, 3219, 3614*

---

1781:3 Amos **Twitchell**, American surgeon, born 11 Apr; first successful ligation of carotid artery (for secondary haemorrhage), 1807; reported 1842, *NEQJ* **1**:188. Died 1850. *2959*

---

1781:4 Allan **Burns**, British surgeon, born 18 Sep; first to suggest that angina pectoris is an expression of coronary obstruction; in his *Observations on … diseases of the heart*, 1809. First to record chloroma; in his *Observations on the surgical anatomy of the head and neck*, 1811, p. 396. Died 1813. *2889, 3055*

---

1781:5 Johann Friedrich **Meckel**, the younger, German anatomist, born 17 Oct; described Meckel's diverticulum, 1809, *ArP* **9**:421. His *Tabulae anatomico-pathologicae*, 1817–26, explained many congenital abnormalities previously attributed to supernatural forces. His *System der vergleichenden Anatomie*, 5 vols, 1821–31, placed him among the greatest comparative anatomists. Died 1833. *984, 2284, 318*

---

1781:6 Laurent Théodore **Biett**, French dermatologist, born; gave a classic description of lupus erythematoides migrans ('Biett's disease'); recorded in P.L.A. Cazenave and H.E.

108

Schedel's *Abrégé pratique des maladies de la peau*, 1838, 3rd ed., pp. 11 and 45. Died 1840. *4028*

---

1781:7 Peter **Middleton** died, his *A medical discourse, or an historical inquiry into the ancient and present state of medicine* was the first American publication on medical history. *6380*

1781: Jean **Baseilhac** (*Frère Côme*) died, **born** 1703. *lithotomy*

**1782**
1782:1 **Harvard Medical School** founded; opened 7 Oct 1783

1782:2 [**Medico-Chirurgical Institute**], **Zürich**, founded

1782:3 **Società Italiana delle Scienze, Rome**, founded

1782:4 **Cod-liver oil** used in treatment of **rheumatism** by Thomas Percival (1740–1804), *LMJ* **3**:392. *1835*

---

1782:5 Philipp Franz von **Walther**, German ophthalmologist, born 3 Jan; gave first description of corneal opacity, 1845, *JCA* **34**:1. Died 1849. *5860*

1782:6 Charles **Waterton**, British naturalist, born 3 Jun; described paralysing effects of curare in his *Wanderings in South America*, 1825. Died 1865. *2074*

1782:7 James **Wardrop**, British surgeon, born 14 Aug; first to classify the various inflammations of the eye according to the structures affected. He introduced the term keratitis; in his *Essays on the morbid anatomy of the human eye*, 2 vols, 1808–18. Died 1869. *5840*

1782:8 Christian Heinrich **Bünger**, German anatomist and surgeon, born 13 Dec; carried out the first well-documented full-thickness skin graft for a rhinoplasty on a patient whose nose and forehead had been destroyed by lupus, 1822, *JCA* **4**:569. Died 1842. *5740.1*

1782:9 Anthony **White**, British surgeon, born; first to excise the head of the femur for disease of the hip-joint, 1821; in Cooper, S. *Dictionary of practical surgery*, 1838, p. 272. Died 1849. *4458*

1782:10 Samuel **Guthrie**, American chemist, born; discovered chloroform, 1832, independently of Soubeiran (1831) and Liebig (1832); he made it by distilling alcohol with chlorinated lime, *AmJSc* **21**:64, **22**:105. Died 1848. *1850, 5648, 5649, 5650*

1782: John **Pringle** died, **born** 1707. *military medicine*

**1783**
1783:1 **Harvard University School of Medicine Library** founded; amalgamated with **Boston Medical Library**, 1965, to form **Francis A. Countway Library of Medicine**

1783:2 **Austria** separates **surgeons** from barbers

1783:3 **Royal Society of Edinburgh** founded, by incorporation of Philosophical Society

1783:4 **William Hunter's Museum** bequeathed to **Glasgow University** and named **Hunterian Museum**

1783:5 The **foramen of Monro** described by Alexander Monro, *Secundus* (1733–1817); in his *Structure and function of the nervous system. 1385*

1783:6 Excision and arthrodesis in the treatment of destructive **joint disease** performed by Henry Park (1744–1831); in his *Account of a new method of treating diseases of the joints of the knee and elbow. 4438*

---

1783:7 Benjamin **Brodie**, British surgeon, born 9 Jun; first operated for varicose veins, 1814, *MCT* **7**:195. First described 'Brodie's abscess' of bone, 1828, *LMG* **2**:70. Gave the first clinical account of ankylosing spondylitis and a description of hysterical pseudofracture of the spine; in his *Pathological and surgical observations on the diseases of the joints*, 1818. Described 'Brodie's pile', 1835, *LMG* **16**:26. Described 'Brodie's tumour', a tumour of the breast, 1840, *LMG* **25**:808. First described intermittent claudication in man; in his *Lectures ... in pathology and surgery*, p. 361, 1846. Died 1862. *2994, 4314, 4311, 3440, 5770, 2902*

1783:8 Friedrich Wilhelm Adam **Sertürner**, German chemist, born 19 Jun; isolated morphine, 1805, *JPAA* 1447. Died 1841. *1839*

1783:9 William **Lawrence**, British surgeon, born 16 Jul; his *Treatise on the diseases of the eye*, 1833, was a landmark in the history of ophthalmic surgery. Died 1867. *5849*

1783:10 François **Magendie**, French physiologist, born 6 Oct; gave a classic account of deglutition and vomiting, *Mémoire sur le vomissement*, 1813. With Pierre Pelletier he isolated emetine, 1817, *AnC* **4**:172. Gave first clear description of the cerebrospinal fluid, 1827, *JPE* **5**:27; **7**:1. Produced experimental anaphylaxis, 1837; *Lectures on the blood* (1839). Described the 'foramen of Magendie' in his *Recherches sur le liquide céphalo-rachidien*, 1842; founded *Journal de Physiologie Expérimentale*, 1821. Died 1855. *985, 1843, 1392, 2585, 1397*

1783:11 John Syng **Dorsey**, American surgeon, born 23 Dec; first successful ligation of the external iliac artery in America, 1811, *ER* **2**:111. Wrote the first systematic treatise on surgery by an American, *Elements of surgery*, 1813. Died 1818. *2930, 5585.1*

1783:12 Robert **Perry** born; correctly described several of the distinctions between typhus and typhoid, 1836, *EMSJ* **45**:64. Died 1848. *5023.1*

---

1783: Anne Charles de **Lorry** died, **born** 1726. *dermatology*

1783: William **Hunter** died, **born** 1718. *heart disease, arteriovenous aneurysm, retroversion of uterus, gravid uterus, School of Anatomy*

# 1784

1784:1 **Allgemeines Krankenhaus, Vienna**, opened 16 Aug

1784:2 **Accademia dei Lincei** founded in **Rome**

1784:3 **King's College, New York**, becomes **Columbia College**

1784:4 **Royal College of Surgeons in Ireland**, founded (earlier a Guild, chartered 1577)

110

1784:5 [**Obukhhovski Hospital**], **St Petersburg**, chartered by Catherine II

1784:6 First work on **aviation medicine**, *Tentamen medicum de aerostatum* ... by Louis Leulier Duché. *2137.1*

1784:7 Three cases of **congenital heart disease** recorded by William Hunter (1718–1783), *MOI* 6:291. *2734.3*

1784:8 The ancient idea of using nerve compression to obtain **analgesia** during surgical operations revived by James Carrick Moore (1762–1834); in his *A method of preventing or diminishing pain in several operations of surgery*. John Hunter used Moore's clamp successfully in a leg amputation. *5645.91*

1784:9 In his *Inquiry into the nature and cause of that swelling, in one or both of the lower extremities, which sometimes happens to lying-in women* Charles White (1728–1813) gave the first description of **phlegmasia alba dolens**. *6271*

1784:10 Michael Underwood (1737–1820) laid the foundation of modern **paediatrics**. His *Treatise on diseases of children* was superior to anything that had previously appeared, and remained the most important work of the subject until the work of Charles West (1848). It contains a description of **thrush (candidiasis)** and on p. 76 appears the first description of **sclerema neonatorum** ('**Underwood's disease**') and the second edition (1789) contains the first description of congenital **heart disease** to appear in a paediatric treatise. *5516, 6326*

---

1784:11 Samuel **Tuke**, British philanthropist, born 13 Jul; his pioneer work advocating humane treatment of the insane is set out in his *Description of The Retreat, an institution near York, for insane persons*, 1813. Died 1857. *4925.1*

---

1784: Otto Friedrich **Müller** died, **born** 1730. *bacterial classification*

1784: Matthew **Dobson** died, **born** ?1731. *diabetes mellitus, hyperglycaemia*

1784: Jean Pierre **David** died, **born** 1737. *joint diseases, Pott's disease*

**1785**
1785:1 **Hôpital Beaujon**, **Paris**, founded

1785:2 **Royal Irish Academy**, **Dublin**, founded

1785:3 **Chair of Anatomy** founded at **University of Dublin**

1785:4 **University of Georgia (US)** founded

1785:5 **Peritonitis** accurately described by Johann Gottlieb Walter (1734–1818); *Von den Krankheiten des Bauchfells und dem Schlagfluss. 2279*

1785:6 Action and correct dosage of **digitalis** established by William Withering (1741–1799); in his *Account of the foxglove. 1836, 2734.31*

1785:7 Important contributions to **naval medicine** and hygiene by Gilbert Blane (1749–1834); in his *Observations on the diseases incident to seamen*. He strongly supported James Lind's work on **citrus juice** in prevention of **scurvy** and issued regulations for standard issue of **lemon juice** in the British Fleet. His recommendations on quarantine formed the basis of the **Quarantine Act**, 1799. *2158*

---

1785:8 Benjamin Winslow **Dudley**, American surgeon, born 12 Apr; reported the first operations on the brain performed in the US, 1823, *TrJM* **1**:9. Died 1870. *4851.1*

1785:9 George James **Guthrie**, British surgeon, born 1 May; a leading military surgeon, successfully ligated the peroneal artery, at Waterloo, 1815, *MCT* **7**:330. His *On gunshot wounds of the extremities*, 1815, is one of the most important books in the history of the subject. As reported in his *Treatise on gun-shot wounds*, 2 ed., p. 332, 1820, he successfully amputated at the hip-joint, after the Battle of Waterloo, 7 July, 1815. The earliest teacher on the surgery of the eye in Britain; he wrote *Lectures on the operative surgery of the eye*, 1823, and founded the Royal Westminster Ophthalmic Hospital. Published *On the anatomy and diseases of the neck of the bladder, and of the urethra*, 1834; this included the first description of non-prostatic obstruction of the neck of the bladder and (p. 252) a description of his prostatic catheter for use in transurethral prostatectomy. Died 1856. *2937, 2161, 4445, 5845, 4167*

1785:10 Charles **McCreary**, American physician, born 13 Jun; was reported to have performed the first resection of the clavicle in the United States, 1811, *TKMS* 1853 **2**:276. Died 1826. *4463*

1785:11 John William Keys **Parkinson**, British physician, born 11 Jul; first reported a case of appendicitis in English, 1812, *MCT* **3**:57; in it perforation was for the first time recognized as a cause of death. Died 1838. *3560*

1785:12 John Ayrton **Paris**, British physician, born 7 Aug; his *Pharmacologia*, 1820, p. 133, gave the first description of arsenic cancer. Died 1856. *2073*

1785:13 Valentine **Mott**, American surgeon, born 20 Aug; performed first ligation of the innominate artery, 1818, *MSR* **1**:9. Successfully ligated the common carotid artery, 1827, *AmJMS* **1**:156. Died 1865. *2942, 2950*

1785:14 William **Beaumont**, American surgeon, born 21 Nov; studied digestion and the movements of the stomach through a gastric fistula caused by a gunshot wound; *Experiments and observations on the gastric juice* published in 1833, his preliminary reports appeared in 1825–6, *MRecorder* **8**:14, 840; **9**:94. Died 1853. *989*

---

1785:15 Pierre Augustin **Béclard**, French anatomist, born; excised the parotid gland, 1823, *ArGM* **4**:60. Died 1825. *3434*

---

1785: Thomas **Berdmore** died, **born** 1740. *dentistry*

# 1786
1786:1 **University** buildings erected at **Budapest**

1786:2 **University of Bonn** opened

1786:3 **Botanic garden** at **Calcutta**

1786:4 **Aberdeen Medico-Chirurgical Society** founded

1786:5 **Western University of Pennsylvania** founded at **Pittsburgh**

1786:6 **Bacteria** classified systematically by Otto Friedrich Müller (1730–1784); *Animalcula infusoria fluviatilia et marina* .... *2466*

1786:7 Ligation of **popliteal artery** for **aneurysm** by John Hunter (1728–1793), reported by Everard Home, *LMJ* **7**:391. *2925*

1786:8 Mark Akenside (1721–1770) described multiple **neurofibromatosis**, *MTr* **1**:64; von Recklinghausen's classic description appeared in 1882. *4015.1*

1786:9 John Hunter (1728–1793) inoculated matter from a **gonorrhoeal** patient to test the theory that the **venereal diseases** were due to a single pathogen. Unfortunately the patient also had **syphilis**, which also developed in the inoculee, incorrectly supporting Hunter's view of a single pathogen. His *Treatise on the venereal disease* also contains the first suggestion of **lymphogranuloma venereum** as a separate disease. *2377, 5197*

1786:10 The parasitic aetiology of **scabies** confirmed by Johann Ernst Wichmann (1740–1802); in his *Aetiologie der Krätze*. *4016*

1786:11 The first school for the **blind** was founded by Valentin Haüy (1745–1822), who was first to emboss paper as a means of reading for the blind. His *Essai sur l'education des aveugles*, 1786, originated methods of teaching and caring for blind persons. *5833*

1786:12 James Cowles **Prichard**, British physician and ethnologist, born 11 Feb; gave a good account of epilepsy, in his *Treatise on diseases of the nervous system*, 1822. First to describe moral insanity; in his *Treatise on insanity*, 1835, here he also described a syndrome he called senile dementia, possibly identical with Alzheimer's disease. Died 1848. *4809, 4928*

1786:13 Walter **Channing**, American physician and obstetrician, born 15 Apr. Gave first description of pernicious anaemia of pregnancy, 1842, *NEQJ* **1**:157; an early advocate of anaesthesia in obstetrics; he wrote *A treatise on etherization in childbirth*, 1848. Died 1876. *3116, 5661*

1786:14 Jean Guillaume August **Lugol**, French physician, born 10 Aug; introduced 'Lugol's solution' of iodine for treatment of skin tuberculosis, 1829, in his *Mémoire sur l'emploi de l'iodide sur les maladies scrophuleuses*, later used for thyroid disorders. Died 1851. *1849.1*

1786:15 Michel Eugène **Chevreul**, French chemist, born 31 Aug; defined cholesterol, 1815, *AnC* **95**:5; proved that sugar in diabetic urine is glucose, 1815, *AnC* **95**:319. Died 1889. *668.2, 3931*

1786:16 Christian Andreas Justinus **Kerner**, German physician, born 18 Sep; first described botulism, 1829, in his *Neue Beobachtungen über ... den Genuss geräuchter Würste*. Died 1862. *2468*

1786:17 William **Stevens**, British surgeon, born; first successfully ligated the internal iliac artery, 1814, *MCT* **5**:422. Died 1868. *2935*

1786:18 Claude **Mouton** died; published the first work specializing in dental prosthetics, *Essai d'odontotechnie*, 1746. *3672.2*

1786: Edmé Gilles **Guyot** died, **born** 1706. *catheterization of eustachian tube*

1786: Carl Wilhelm **Scheele** died, **born** 1742. *uric acid*

**1787**
1787: 1 *Materia medica Americana*, first full North American **materia medica**, compiled by Johann David Schoepff (1752–1800). *1837*

1787: 2 **Fermentation**, first modern work by Adamo Fabbroni: *Dell'arte de fare il vino. 2467*

1787: 3 The first complete description of **lymphatic chancre** ('**Nisbet's chancre**') given by William Nisbet (1759–1822); in his *First lines of theory and practice in venereal diseases. 5198*

1787: 4 An original account of **alcoholism** given by John Coakley Lettsom (1744–1815), *MMSL* **1**: 128. *2071*

---

1787: 5 Carl Ferdinand von **Graefe**, German surgeon, born 8 Mar; reported the closure of a congenital cleft palate, 1816, *JCA* **1**: 1; revived rhinoplasty in Germany, in his *Rhinoplastik, oder die Kunst den Verlust der Nase organisch zu ersetzen*, 1818, he surveyed the Italian, Indian and 'German' methods, the last being his own variation of the Italian method; on p. 13 he described the first successful blepharoplasty. Died 1840. *5738, 5739*

1787: 6 Pierre Charles Alexandre **Louis**, French physician, born 14 Apr; his classic work on **tuberculosis**, *Recherches anatomico-pathologiques sur la phthisie*, 1825, was based on 358 dissections and 1,960 clinical case reports; introduced the term typhoid fever, in his *Recherches anatomiques, pathologiques et thérapeutiques sur la maladie connue sous les noms de … typhoïde*, etc., 1829; he first described the lenticular rose spots, and established the pathological picture. Died 1872. *3221, 5023*

1787: 7 Jules Hippolyte **Cloquet**, French physician, born 17 May; published first important work on olfaction, *Dissertation sur les odeurs*, 1815. Died 1840. *3253*

1787: 8 Jan Evangelista **Purkyně**, Bohemian physiologist, born 17 Dec; described Purkyně cells, 1837, *BVDN* **15**: 177; and Purkyně fibres, 1839, [English translation, 1845, *LMG* **36**: 1066, 1156]. Died 1869. *1396, 805*

---

1787: 9 Georg **Carabelli**, Hungarian dentist, born; first described 'Carabelli's cusps' (tuberculus anomalus), sometimes found in the upper permanent molars; in his *Systematisches Handbuch der Zahnheilkunde*, Bd.2, 1844. Died 1842. *3682*

1787: 10 John Peter **Mettauer** born; Virginian gynaecologist, believed to be the first successfully to repair a vesico-vaginal fistula, 1840, *BMSJ* **22**: 154. Died 1875. *6031*

1787: 11 William Fetherston **Montgomery**, Irish obstetrician, born; the sebaceous glands of the areola were named after him following his description in his *Exposition of the symptoms and signs of pregnancy*, 1837, although previously described by Morgagni. Died 1859. *6173*

1787: 12 Adolf Carl Peter **Callisen**, Danish surgeon and bibliographer, born; his great medical bibliography, *Medicinisches Schriftsteller-Lexicon der jetzt lebenden Aerzte, Wundärzte, Geburtshelfer, Apotheker, und Naturforscher aller gebildeten Völker*, 25 vols and 8-vol.

114

supplement, 1830–45, gives a complete view of the literature from c1780–1830 and describes over 99,000 items. Reprinted 1962–64. Died 1866. *6754*

1787:13 Ferdinand August Marie Franz **Ritgen**, German obstetrician, born; first performed extraperitoneal caesarean section, 1821, reported 1825, *HKA* **1**:263. Died 1867. *6238*

1787: William **Watson** died, **born** 1715. *emphysema*

## 1788
1788:1 **Linnean Society of London** founded

1788:2 *Elements of medical jurisprudence,* first English textbook on the subject, published by Samuel Farr (1741–1795). *1733*

1788:3 An account of **fragilitas ossium (osteogenesis imperfecta)** in three generations given by Olaus Jacob Ekman; in his doctoral thesis *Dissertatio medica descriptionem et casus aliquot osteomalaciae sistens. 4304.1*

1788:4 The first dentist to manufacture **artificial** (porcelain) **teeth** was Nicolas Dubois de Chemant (1753–1824); in his *Les avantages des nouvelles dents, et rateliers artificiels. 3677*

1788:5 A relationship between the **pancreas** and **diabetes mellitus** first suggested by Thomas Cawley, *LMJ* **9**:286. *3929*

1788:6 William **Gibson**, American surgeon, born 14 Mar; successfully ligated the common iliac artery, 1812; reported in 1820, *AmMR* **3**:185. Died 1868. *2944*

1788:7 Pierre Joseph **Pelletier**, French chemist, born 22 Mar; with François Magendie he isolated emetine, 1817, *AnC* **4**:172; with Joseph Bienaimé Caventou he isolated strychnine, 1819, *JPC* **5**:145. With Caventou, isolated quinine, 1820, *AnC* **15**:289, 337. Died 1842. *1843, 1844, 5233*

1788:8 Horatio Gates **Jameson**, American physician and surgeon, born; first to excise the superior maxilla, 1820, *AmMR* **4**:222. Died 1855. *4446*

1788: Nicolas François Joseph **Eloy** died, **born** 1714. *medical biography*

1788: Percivall **Pott** died, **born** 1714. *chimney-sweep's cancer, spinal curvature due to tuberculous caries, fractures, dislocations, hydrocele, anal fistula, congenital hernia*

## 1789
1789:1 **University of Georgetown** (DC) founded

1789:2 **Botanic garden** opened at **Sydney**, Australia

1789:3 **Medical and Chirurgical Faculty of Maryland** founded, incorporated 1799

1789:4 Reforms in the treatment of the **insane** by Vincenzo Chiarugi (1759–1820) appeared in *Regolamento dei Regi Spedali …. 4920.1*

1789:5 The first important publication on **cretinism** and **goitre** is by some considered to be *Sui gozzi e sulla stupiditá ec. dei cretini* by Michaele Vincenzo Giacinto Malacarne (1744–1816). *3809*

1789:6 Important observations on the **ear** and **olfaction** made by Antonio Scarpa (1752–1832); in his *De structura fenestrae rotundae auris*, 1772, and *De auditu et olfactu*, 1789. *1550, 1453*

1789:7 Michael Underwood (1737–1820) was the first to consider **poliomyelitis** as an entity; in his *Treatise on the diseases of children*, 2nd ed., **2**, 53, which also contains the first description of congenital **heart disease** to appear in a paediatric treatise. *6326, 4662*

1789:8 An important account of **dengue** given by Benjamin Rush (1746–1813) who described the 1780 Philadelphia outbreak in his *Medical enquiries and observations*, vol. 1, p. 104. *5470*

1789:9 Important anatomico-pathological studies on **dermoid cysts** of the **ovary** made by Matthew Baillie (1761–1823), *PT* **79**:71. *6021*

1789:10 The first book devoted solely to **ophthalmic surgery** was *Précis ou cours d'opérations sur la chirurgie des yeux*, 2 vols, 1789–90, by Guillaume Pellier de Quengsby (1750/1–1835). *5833.1*

---

1789:11 Isidore **Bricheteau**, French physician, born 3 Feb; first adequately described pneumopericardium, 1844, *ArGM* **4**:334. Died 1861. *2755*

1789:12 Peter Mere **Latham**, British physician, born 1 Jul; gave classical description of coronary thrombosis; in his *Lectures ... comprising diseases of the heart*, 2nd ed., 1846. Died 1875. *2755.1*

1789:13 Richard **Bright**, British physician, born 28 Sep; his *Reports of medical cases*, 1827–31; contain some outstanding contributions to pathology, including his description of chronic non-suppurative nephritis ('Bright's disease'). Gave the original description of acute yellow atrophy of the liver, 1836, *GHR* **1**:604, and of Jacksonian epilepsy, 1836, *GHR* **1**:36. Died 1858. *2285, 4206, 3617, 4811*

---

1789: George **Armstrong** died, **born** 1719. *diseases of children, pyloric stenosis*

1789: Fielding **Ould** died, **born** 1710. *obstetrics, midwifery*

1789: Pieter **Camper** died, **born** 1722. *anatomy*

## 1790

1790:1 Ligation of **femoral artery** first reported in America by Thomas Kast (?1755–1820), *MCMM* **1**:96. *2925.1*

1790:2 The first modern account of **mumps** (epidemic **parotitis**) given by Robert Hamilton (1721–1793), who also described parotitis complicated by orchitis, *TRSE* **2**:59. *5523*

116

1790:3 According to Everard Home, 1799, *PT* **18**:157, John Hunter (1728–1793) suggested, in 1790, **artificial insemination** (actually performed by the patient's husband with a syringe). *6162*

---

1790:4 Jean François **Reybard**, French surgeon, born 11 Jan; first to perform intestinal resection for cancer, 1844, *BuAM* **9**:1031. Died 1863. *3447*

1790:5 Johann Karl Georg **Fricke**, German surgeon, born 28 Jan; produced the first extensive publication on blepharoplasty; in his *Die Bildung neuer Augenlider (Blepharoplastik) nach Zerstörungen und dadurch hervorgebrachten Auswärtswendungen derselben*, 1829. Died 1841. *5742.1*

1790:6 Marshall **Hall**, British physiologist, born 18 Feb; established the difference between volitional action and unconscious reflexes, thus establishing reflex action, 1833, *PT* **123**:635. In his *Synopsis of cerebral and spinal seizures*, etc., 1851, was first to suggest that the paroxysmal nervous discharges of epilepsy were produced by the spinal nervous system, first to notice the connection of anaemia with epilepsy, and first to deduce that epilepsy was produced by anaemia of the medulla. Invented the Marshall Hall method of artificial respiration, 1856, *L* **1**:129. Died 1857. *1359, 4812, 2028.56*

1790:7 Jacques **Lisfranc**, French surgeon, born 2 Apr; his method of partial amputation of the foot is recorded; in his *Nouvelle méthode opératoire pour l'amputation partielle du pied*, 1815. Died 1847. *4443*

1790:8 Arthur **Jacob**, Irish ophthalmologist, born Jun; described 'Jacob's membrane', the layer containing the rods and cones of the retina, 1819, *PT* **109**:300; described 'Jacob's ulcer', a rodent ulcer attacking the face, especially the eyelids, 1827, *DHR* **4**:232. Died 1874. *1491, 4025*

1790:9 Jean Louis **Prévost**, Swiss physician, born 1 Sep; with Jean Baptiste André Dumas succeeded in transfusing blood in animals by using defibrinated blood to prevent coagulation, 1821, *AnC* **18**:281. Died 1850. *2016*

1790:10 James **Blundell**, British physician and surgeon, born 27 Dec; performed the first human-to-human blood transfusion, the patient died after 56 hours, 1819, *MCT* **9**:56; reported the successful transfusion of blood from human to human, 1828, *L* **2**:321. Died 1877. *2015.1, 2017*

---

1790:11 Wilhelm Friedrich **Ludwig** born; described 'Ludwig's angina', 1836, *MKW* **6**:21. Died 1865. *3257*

1790:12 Michael **Ferrall**, Irish ophthalmologist, born; introduced an operation for enucleation of the eyeball, 1841, *DJMS* **19**:329. Died 1860. *5854*

---

1790: John **Howard** died, **born** 1726. *prison reform*

1790: William **Cullen** died, **born** 1710. *medicine*

**1791**
1791:1 **Guillotine** proposed by Dr Joseph Ignace Guillotin (1738–1814) for humane **capital punishment**

1791:2 **Cornu cutaneum** first described by Everard Home (1756–1832), *PT* **81**:95. *4017*

1791:3 The first description of **achondroplasia** given by Samuel Thomas Soemmerring (1755–1830); in his *Abbildungen und Beschreibungen einiger Misgeburten*, p. 30. He was noted for his accuracy in **anatomical illustration**, especially in his *Vom Baue des menschlichen Körpers*, 5 pts, 1791–6, which includes a list of what he considered his anatomical discoveries. *400, 4306*

1791:4 François Chopart's (1743–1795) *Traité des maladies des voies urinaires* appeared, 2 vols, 1791–92. *4165.01*

1791:5 Jean **Cruveilhier**, French morbid anatomist, born 9 Feb; his *Anatomie pathologique du corps humain*, 1829–42, was one of the most important books on the subject. Died 1874. *2286*

1791:6 Charles Gabriel **Pravaz**, French surgeon, born 24 Mar; invented the modern galvanocautery, 1853, *CRAS* **36**:88. Died 1853. *5603*

1791:7 John **Elliotson**, British physician, born 29 Oct; showed that hay fever was due to pollen, 1831, *LMG* **8**:411, **12**:164. Proved that glanders in the horse is communicable to man, 1833, *MCT* **16**:171, **18**:201. One of the first in England to perform surgical operations with the aid of hypnosis; in his *Numerous cases of surgical operations without pain in the mesmeric state*, 1843. Died 1868. *2584, 5153, 5650.2*

1791:8 Johann Ludwig **Choulant**, German physician and medical historian, born 12 Nov; his *Handbuch der Bücherkunde für die ältere Medicin*, 1828, is one of the best **medical bibliographic** check lists of the printed works of the older medical writers. 2nd edn, 1841, last reprinted 1956. Died 1861. *6753*

1791:9 William **Wallace**, British surgeon, born; introduced potassium iodide treatment in syphilis, 1835, *L* **2**:5; gave the first description of lymphogranuloma venereum; in his *Treatise on the venereal disease and its varieties*, 1833, p. 371. Died 1837. *2379, 5215*

1791:10 Theodor **Beck**, American physician, born; published *Elements of medical jurisprudence*, 1823, first notable American text on the subject. Died 1855. *1735*

1791:11 Robert **Adams**, Irish physician, born; gave first complete description of heart block with syncopal attacks, 1827, *DHR* **4**:353; named '**Stokes-Adams syndrome**' after a further account by William Stokes, 1846. Died 1875. *2745, 2756*

1791:12 Joseph Henry **Green**, British surgeon, born; performed the first thyroidectomy, 1829, *L* **2**:351. Died 1863. *3814*

1791:13 William **Mackenzie**, British ophthalmologist, born; his *Practical treatise on diseases of the eye*, 1830, included a classic description of the symptomatology of glaucoma. He was probably the first to draw attention to increased intra-ocular pressure, characteristic of the disease. Died 1868. *5848*

1791: Jean André **Venel** died, **born** 1740. *deformities of spine*

118

**1792**

1792:1 **Law abolishing medical schools in France**

1792:2 Corporation of the **Apothecaries' Hall of Dublin** constituted

1792:3 *Vrachevnie Viedomosti*, first **Russian medical periodical**, commences publication

1792:4 **Heart block** first reported by Thomas Spens (1764–1842), *MCom* **7**:458. *2735*

1792:5 François Chopart's (1743–1795) method of partial **amputation** of the **foot** first recorded by Lafiteau in A.F. Fourcroy's *La médecine éclairée par les sciences physiques*, **4**, 85. *4439*

1792:6 Hereditary **ectodermal dysplasia** first described by Ferdinand George Danz (1761–1793), *ArGe* **4**:684. *6358*

1792:7 Kurt Polykarp Joachim Sprengel's (1766–1833) *Versuch einer pragmatischen Geschichte der Arzneikunde*, 5 vols, 1792–1803, is a monumental **history of medicine** (3rd ed. 1821–28). *6383*

---

1792:8 Johann Friedrich **Dieffenbach**, German surgeon, born 1 Feb; a pioneer in the field of plastic and orthopaedic surgery. His inaugural MD thesis, 1822, Würzburg, was entitled *Nonnula de regeneratione et transplantatione*. Successfully carried out tenotomy, rhinoplasty, and skin grafting; in his *Chirurgische Erfahrungen besonders über die Wiederherstellung zerstörter Theile des menschlichen Körpers nach neuen Methoden*, 3 vols, 1829–34. Performed cardiac catheterization, 1832, *ChA* **1**, i:86, in unsuccessful attempt to obtain blood from a cholera patient. First successfully to use Lembert's suture, 1836, *WGH* p. 401. Described his first successful attempt to treat strabismus by myotomy; in his *Ueber das Schielen und die Heilung desselben durch eine Operation*, 1842. His work encouraged the acceptance of anaesthesia in Germany; he made the first use of ether anaesthesia for plastic surgery and wrote *Die Aether gegen den Schmerz*, 1847. Died 1847. *5741, 5743, 2478.1, 3441, 5856, 5659.1, 5743*

1792:9 Karl Ernst von **Baer**, Estonian embryologist and biologist, born 17/29 Feb; announced the discovery of the mammalian ovum in his *De ovi mammalium et hominis genesi*, 1827; established the germ-layer theory, and discovered the notochord; *Ueber Entwicklungsgeschichte der Thiere*, 3 vols, 1828–88. Died 1876. *477, 479*

1792:10 Montague **Gosset**, British surgeon, born 1 Jul; repaired a vesico-vaginal fistula of 11 years' duration, using silver-gilt wire, 1835, *L* **1**:345. Died 1854. *6028.1*

1792:11 Jean **Civiale**, French genito-urinary surgeon, born 5 Jul; invented a *lithotriteur* for crushing urinary calculi inside the bladder, 1826, *ArGM* **10**:393; he placed lithotrity upon a sound basis. Died 1867. *4289*

1792:12 Pierre Saloman **Ségalas**, French urologist, born 1 Aug; introduced urethro-cystic speculum, 1827, *RMFE* **1**:157. Died 1875. *4165.1*

1792:13 Charles Henri **Ehrmann**, French surgeon, born 15 Sep; first to remove a laryngeal polyp, 1844, *CRAS* **18**:593, 709. Died 1878. *3260*

---

1792:14 Lewis **Durlacher** born; surgeon-chiropodist to Queen Victoria, gave first description of anterior metatarsalgia, in his *Treatise on corns* etc., p. 52, 1845; named 'Morton's metatarsalgia' after the description by T.G. Morton in 1876. Died 1864. *4325, 4341*

1792: William **Brown** died, **born** 1752. *pharmacopoeia*

**1793**

1793:1 Act of **accommodation** in the **eye** explained by Thomas Young (1773–1829), *PT* **83**:169. *1486*

1793:2 **Syphilis** first differentiated from **gonorrhoea** by Benjamin Bell (1749–1806), in his *Treatise on gonorrhoea virulenta and lues venerea. 2378, 5200*

1793:3 Matthew Baillie's (1761–1823) *Morbid anatomy of some of the most important parts of the human body* was the first systematic textbook of **pathological anatomy** (he published an atlas intended to illustrate it, 1799–1803). In *Morbid anatomy* he clearly described the pulmonary lesions of **tuberculosis**; on p. 87 he gave the first clear description of the morbid anatomy and symptoms of **gastric ulcer**. *2281, 2282, 3218, 3427*

1793:4 Operation for strangulated **femoral hernia** ('**Gimbernat's operation**') and the **crural ligament** ('**Gimbernat's ligament**') described by Antonio de Gimbernat (1734–1816); in his *Nuevo método de operar en la hernia crural. 3579*

1793:5 Perforating **duodenal ulcer** reported by Jacopo Penada (1748–1828); in his *Saggio d'osservazioni … sopra alcuni case singolari*, etc. *3428*

1793:6 Vincenzo Chiarugi (1759–1820) was the first European physician to abandon chains and fetters in the restraint of **psychiatric** patients; his treatment of the **insane** is outlined in his *Della pazzia in genre, e in specie. 4921*

1793:7 In his *A short account of the malignant fever, lately prevalent in Philadelphia*, Matthew Carey (1760–1839) gave a graphic account of the **yellow fever** epidemic of 1793, with a good clinical description of the disease, mentioning the efficacy and failure of various forms of treatment. *5451*

1793:8 What was apparently the first **caesarean section** performed in England (on 27 Nov) from which the mother recovered, reported by James Barlow (1767–1839) in *Medical records and researches selected from the papers of a private medical association*, 1798, p. 54. *6236.1*

1793:9 The first important classified **bibliography of medicine**, covering both monographs and current periodicals, is Wilhelm Gottfried Ploucquet's (1744–1814) *Initia bibliothecae medico-practicae et chirurgicae sive repertorii medicinae practicae et chirurgicae*, 8 vols, 1793–97. It was continued in his *Bibliotheca medico-practica et chirurgica*, 4 vols, 1799–1803, revised as *Literatura medica digesta*, 4 vols, 1808–9, with 40,000 additional citations of the *Initia bibliothecae* and the *Bibliotheca. 6750–6750.2*

1793:10 '**Ambulances volantes**' introduced by Dominique Jean Larrey (1766–1842).

1793:11 Charles Louis Stanislas **Heurteloup**, French surgeon, born 16 Feb; designed the best contemporary lithotrite; in his *Lithotripsie*, 1833; he is amongst those accredited with the introduction of modern lithotrity. Died 1864. *4290*

1793:12 Pierre François Olive **Rayer**, French physician, born 7 Mar; gave a description of pituitary obesity, 1823, *ArGM* **3**:350. Provided a classic summary of the dermatological literature of the period in his *Traité théorique et pratique des maladies de la peau*, 1826. He was first to describe adenoma sebaceum and xanthoma multiplex and the first to differentiate between acute and chronic eczema. Showed glanders to be contagious, but not a form of tuberculosis, 1837, *MARM* **6**:625. Inoculated anthrax-infected sheep blood into other sheep and saw the anthrax bacillus (*B.anthracis*) in the blood of the infected sheep, 1850, *CRSB* **2**:141. In 1875 Davaine claimed to have written the account of the experiment and sent it to Rayer for publication. Died 1867. *3881, 3989, 5154, 5163*

1793:13 Thomas **Addison**, British physician, born Apr; first to use static electricity therapeutically, 1837, *GHR* **2**:493. In his paper on 'Addison's disease' he included a classic description of pernicious anaemia, 1843, *LMG* **43**:517. First described Addison's disease and pernicious ('Addisonian') anaemia, 1849, he later expanded his account in his *On the constitutional and local effects of disease of the supra-renal capsules*, 1855. Described 'true keloid' (scleroderma, morphoea), 1854, *MCT* **37**:27. Died 1860. *4524, 3118, 3864, 4042*

1793:14 John Kearsley **Mitchell**, American physician, born 12 May; gave the first description of the neurotic spinal arthropathies, 1831, *AmJMS* **8**:55. Made the first scientific approach to the theory of a parasite as the cause of malaria; in his *On the cryptogamous origin of malarious and epidemic fevers*, 1849. Died 1858. *4493, 5234*

1793:15 Eugène **Soubeiran**, French chemist, born 24 May; discovered chloroform, 1831, *AnC* **48**:113, independently of Guthrie (1832) and Liebig (1831). Died 1858. *1851, 5649, 5648, 5650*

1793:16 Edward **Stanley**, British surgeon, born 3 Jul; used liver puncture as a diagnostic measure, 1833, *L* **1**:189. First to describe disease of the posterior columns of the spinal cord, 1839, *MCT* **23**:80. Died 1862. *3616, 4525*

1793:17 Martin Heinrich **Rathke**, Polish physiologist and pathologist, born 25 Aug; gave an important description of the pituitary, 1838, *ArA* p. 482; described 'Rathke's pouch', a diverticulum from the embryonic mouth, *Entwicklungsgeschichte der Natter*, 1839. Died 1860. *1156, 483*

1793:18 Lemuel **Shattuck**. American public hygienist and vital statistician, born 15 Oct; his *Report on public health in the United States*, 1850, led to great improvements in public health and hygiene in the US. Died 1859. *1609*

1793:19 Carl Friedrich **Quittenbaum**, German surgeon, born 10 Nov; successfully performed splenectomy, 1829; in his *De splenis hypertrophia et exterpationis splenis hypertrophici*, published 1836. Died 1852. *3763*

1793:20 Johannes Lucas **Schönlein**, German physician, born 30 Nov; established anaphylactoid ('Schönlein-Henoch') purpura as a distinct entity; in his *Allgemeine und spezielle Pathologie und Therapie*, 1837, **3**, 48–49; mentioned earlier by William Heberden Sr (1802) and later by Eduard Heinrich Henoch (1868). Discovered the fungal cause of favus (ringworm), *Achorion (Trichophyton) schönleinii*, 1839, *ArA* p. 82; confirmed by David Gruby, 1841. Died 1864. *3058, 3053, 3065, 4029, 4030*

1793:21 George **Frick**, American ophthalmologist, born; wrote the first American textbook of ophthalmology, *Treatise on the diseases of the eye*, 1823. Died 1870. *5844*

1793:22 John Kearney **Rodgers**, American surgeon, born; successfully wired an ununited fracture of the humerus, 1827, *NYMPJ* 6:521. Died 1851. *4414*

1793:23 David **Craigie**, British physician, born; gave relapsing fever its present name, 1843, *EMSJ* 60:410. Died 1866. *5311*

---

1793: Robert **Hamilton** died, **born** 1721. *mumps*

1793: Ferdinand George **Danz** died, **born** 1761. *ectodermal dysplasia*

1793: John **Hunter** died, **born** 1728. *syphilis, gonorrhoea, aneurysm, popliteal artery ligation, blood, inflammation, gunshot wounds, teeth, artificial insemination*

## 1794
1794:1 **Board of Health** at **Philadelphia**

1794:2 **Écoles de Santé** authorized in **France**

1794:3 **University of Tennessee** founded

1794:4 Luigi Galvani (1732–1798); demonstrated the presence of **electrical energy** in **living tissue**; in his *Dell'uso e del'attività dell arco conduttore nelle contrazioni sei muscoli*. Died 1798. *594.1*

1794:5 *Zoonomia*, 1794–6, published by Erasmus Darwin (1731–1802); the first comprehensive theory of **evolution.** *105*

1794:6 *Treatise on the blood, inflammation, and gun-shot wounds*, published by John Hunter (1728–1793). *2283*

1794:7 *Medical ethics*, published by Thomas Percival (1740–1804) is the basis of current British and American codes. *1764*

1794:8 A detailed description of **bone necrosis** given by James Russell (1755–1836); in his *Practical essay on certain diseases of the bones termed necrosis*. *4307*

1794:9 The first report published in Europe concerning the Indian or Hindu method of **rhino-plasty** appeared in the *Gentleman's Magazine*, vol. 64, pt. 2, p. 891, signed 'B.L.'. *5735.1*

1794:10 A classic account of the **yellow fever** epidemic in Philadelphia given by Benjamin Rush (1746–1813), eminent member of the medical profession in Philadelphia; in his *An account of the bilious remitting yellow fever ... in Philadelphia ... in 1793. 5453*

1794:11 William Hunter's (1718–1783) *An anatomical description of the human gravid uterus and its contents* [the text for his atlas, *Anatomia uteri humani gravidi tabulis illustrata, The anatomy of the human gravid uterus exhibited in figures*, 1774] published, edited by Matthew Baillie. *6157.1*

1794: 12 **Diabetes insipidus** first defined by Johann Peter Frank (1745–1821); in his *De curandis hominum morbis*, Lib.V, p. 38. *3879*

1794: 13 An English translation of the collected papers of Pieter Camper (1722–1789), **anatomist**, appeared. *77*

---

1794: 14 Marie Jean Pierre **Flourens**, French comparative anatomist, born 13 Apr; demonstrated that the cerebrum is the organ of thought and the cerebellum controls body movement, 1823, *ArGM* **2**:321; lesion of the semicircular canals causes motor incoordination and loss of equilibrium, 1828, *AnSN* **15**:113; gave experimental proof that vision depends on the integrity of the cerebral cortex, in his *Recherches experimentales sur les propriétés et les fonctions du système nerveux*, 1824; made first announcement that chloroform had an anaesthetic effect similar to that of ether, 1847, *CRAS* **24**:340. Died 1867. *1391, 1557, 1493, 5654*

1794: 15 John **Conolly**, British physician, born 27 May; he was treating his insane patients without any form of restraint as early as 1839; published *Treatment of the insane without mechanical restraints*, 1856. Died 1866. *4933*

1794: 16 James **Marsh**, British chemist, born 2 Sep; introduced the Marsh method for the detection of arsenic, 1836, *ENPJ* **21**:229. Died 1846. *2077*

1794: 17 Robert **Liston**, British surgeon, born 28 Oct; a most dexterous and speedy surgeon, was first in Britain (21 Dec 1846) to perform a major operation with the use of an anaesthetic; wrote *Practical surgery*, 1837. Died 1847. *5593*

---

1794: 18 Pierre Adolph **Piorry**, French physician, born; pioneered mediate percussion; in his *De la percussion médiate*, 1828; he introduced the percussor and pleximeter in 1826. Died 1879. *2675*

1794: 19 Benjamin Guy **Babington**, British physician, born; demonstrated a crude 'glottiscope' in 1829, *LMG* **3**:555, paving the way for laryngoscopy. Died 1866. *3327*

1794: 20 John Rhea **Barton**, American surgeon, born; described a fracture of the radius ('Barton's fracture'), 1838, *MEx* **1**:365. Died 1871. *4415*

1794: 21 Jean Pierre **Falret**, French psychiatrist, born; first to describe manic-depressive insanity, 1853, *BuAIM* **19**:382. Died 1870. *4932*

1794: 22 John **Lizars**, British surgeon, born; performed the first (unsuccessful) ovariotomy in Britain; in his *Observations on extraction of diseased ovaria*, 1825. Died 1860. *6026*

---

1794: James **Lind** died, **born** 1716. *naval hygiene, scurvy*

1794: Caspar Friedrich **Wolff** died, **born** 1733. *embryology, epigenesis*

1794: Antoine Laurent **Lavoisier** died, **born** 1743. *oxygen*

**1795**
1795: 1 **Board of Health** established at **New York City**

1795: 2 **Institut de France** established

1795:3 **Abernethian Society** founded at **St Bartholomew's Hospital, London** (as **Medical and Physical Society**; suspended 1831, revived as Abernethian Society, 1832)

1795:4 **Hôpital St Antoine, Paris,** founded

1795:5 *Archiv für die Physiologie* commences publication in Halle

1795:6 *Journal der Practische Arzneykunde* commences publication, Jena and Berlin

1795:7 **Société de Médecine de Paris** founded 1795–96

1795:8 Surgeon General **Görcke** founds **Pepinière** in **Berlin (Kaiser-Wilhelms-Akademie)**

1795:9 An important account of various **heart disorders** given by Raymond Vieussens (1641–1715); in his *Novum vasorum corporis humani systema. 2729*

1795:10 Alexander Gordon (1752–1799) was first to advance as a definite hypothesis the contagious nature of **puerperal fever**; in his *Treatise on the epidemic puerperal fever in Aberdeen. 6272*

1795:11 The first to observe the mode of transmission of the **guinea-worm,** *Dracunculus medinensis*, causal agent in **dracontiasis**, was Colin Chisholm (1755–1825); in his *Essay on the malignant pestilential fever introduced into the West Indies from Boullam*, etc. *5336.3*

1795:12 Friedlieb Ferdinand **Runge**, German chemist, born 8 Feb; prepared carbolic acid from coal tar, 1834, *AnPh* **31**:65, 513; **32**:308. Died 1867. *1855*

1795:13 Christian Gottfried **Ehrenberg**, German chemist, born 19 Apr; in his *Infusionsthierschen ...,* 1838, he described *Bacillus subtilis*. Died 1876. *2469*

1795:14 Pierre Louis Alphée **Cazenave**, French dermatologist, born 5 May; founded the first scientific dermatological journal (*Annales des maladies de la peau et de la syphilis*), classified skin diseases on an anatomical basis. His *Leçons sur les maladies de la peau* first appeared in fascicules, 1845–56. First described pemphigus foliaceus, 1844, *AnMP* **1**:208. Described lupus erythematosus ('Cazenave's disease'), 1850, *GHZ* **2**:383. Died 1877. *3992.1, 4037, 4040*

1795:15 Alfred Armand Louis Marie **Velpeau**, French surgeon, born 18 May; his *Nouveaux éléments de médécine operatoire*, 3 vols and atlas, 1832, was the most comprehensive work on operative surgery in France. He provided a classic account of breast tumours in his *Traité des maladies du sein et de la région mammaire*, 1854. Died 1867. *5592, 5771*

1795:16 Charles Turner **Thackrah**, British physician, born 22 May; wrote *The effect of the principal arts, trades, and professions, and of civic states and habits of living on health and longevity*, 1813, the first systematic publication in England on occupational diseases. Died 1833. *2123*

1795:17 Ernst Heinrich **Weber**, German physiologist, born 24 Jun; in his *De pulsu resorptione, auditu et tactu*, 1834, showed the relationship between stimulus and sensation (Fechner-Weber law) and (p. 41) published 'Weber's hearing test'. Died 1878. *1457, 3368*

1795:18 Joseph Bienaimé **Caventou**, French chemist, born 30 Jun; in collaboration with Pierre Pelletier he isolated strychnine, 1819, *JPC* **5**:145, and isolated quinine, 1820, *AnC* **15**:289, 337. Died 1877. *1844, 5233*

1795:19 Moritz Heinrich **Romberg**, German pathologist and neurologist, born 11 Nov; gave a classic description of achondroplasia; in his graduation thesis, *De rachitide congenita*, 1817; and of facial hemiatrophy ('Romberg's disease'); in his *Klinische Ergebnisse*, p. 75, 1846. He inaugurated the modern era in the study of nervous diseases and his *Lehrbuch der Nervenkrankheiten des Menschen*, 1846, is the first formal treatise on nervous diseases; it includes (p. 795) the original description of 'Romberg's sign', pathognomonic of tabes dorsalis. Died 1873. *4310, 4527, 4528*

1795:20 Paul Antoine **Du Bois**, French obstetrician, born 9 Dec; gave a classic description of hyperemesis gravidarum, 1852, *BuAM* **17**:557. Died 1871. *6179*

1795:21 James **Braid**, British surgeon and hypnotist, born; his scientific investigation of mesmerism, in his *Satanic agency and mesmerism reviewed*, 1842, convinced him that its effects were not due to an outside force, but were natural phenomena arising from the subject's heightened suggestibility; inaugurated modern hypnosis and introduced the term, in his *Neurypnology, or the rationale of nervous sleep*, 1843. Died 1860. *4992.3, 4993*

1795: François **Chopart** died, **born** 1743. *amputation of foot, urology, surgery*

1795: Pierre Joseph **Desault** died, **born** 1744. *surgery, urology*

1795: Johann Georg **Zimmermann** died, **born** 1728. *bacillary dysentery*

1795: Samuel **Farr** died, **born** 1741. *medical jurisprudence*

**1796**
1796:1 **Botanic Garden** at **Glasnevin** founded by **Royal Dublin Society**

1796:2 **Island of Reil**, in the cerebral cortex, described by Johann Christian Reil (1759–1813); in his *Excercitationum anatomicarum* ... fasc.1. *1387*

1796:3 Ligation of the external **iliac artery** for **aneurysm** by John Abernethy (1764–1831); reported in his *Surgical observations*, 1809, 234–92. *2928*

1796:4 Modern **dermatology** was inaugurated by Robert Willan (1757–1812); he established a standard nomenclature which is more or less in use today; his *On cutaneous diseases* includes original descriptions of **prurigo mitis** ('**ichthyosis cornea**'), p. 197, and **psoriasis**, p. 152. *3985, 4018*

1796:5 **Inoculation** or **vaccination** with **vaccinia (cowpox)** lymph matter shown by Edward Jenner (1749–1823) to protect against **smallpox**, 14 May. In his *An inquiry into the causes and effects of the variolae vaccinae*, 1798, he described 23 successful vaccinations and announced one of the greatest triumphs in the history of medicine. *5423, 2529.3*

1796:6 Robert James **Graves**, Irish physician, born 27 Mar; gave the first accurate account of exophthalmic goitre (Graves' disease), 1835, *LMSJ* **7**:516. Died 1853. *3815*

1796:7 Hugh Lenox **Hodge**, American obstetrician and gynaecologist, born 27 Jun; described the Hodge pessary; in his *On diseases peculiar to women, including displacement of the uterus*, 1860, chap. 5. He also produced a fine textbook, *The principles and practice of obstetrics*, 1864; at that time he was almost blind and dictated the book to his son from memory. Died 1873. *6043.1, 6185*

1796:8 George **Catlin**, American anthropologist, born 26 Jul; first noted ill effects on respiration of mouth-breathing; in his *The breath of life* ..., 1861. Died 1872. *3267*

1796:9 Jean Baptiste **Bouillaud**, French physician, born 16 Sep; in his classic account of aphasia was first to suggest that injuries of the frontal lobe were a cause, 1825, *ArGM* **8**:25. In his *Traité clinique des maladies du coeur*, 1835, described rheumatic endocarditis (Bouillard's disease). In his *Traité clinique du rhumatisme articulaire*, 1840, he drew attention to the coincidence of acute rheumatism and heart disease. Died 1881. *4618, 2749, 4494*

1796:10 Anders Adolf **Retzius**, Swedish anatomist, born 13 Oct; described the 'cave of Retzius' near the bladder, 1849, *ArA* p. 182. Died 1860. *1221*

---

1796:11 Francis Bisset **Hawkins**, British physician, born; published first English book devoted entirely to medical statistics, *Elements of medical statistics*, 1829. Died 1894. *1697*

1796:12 Sigismund Eduard **Loewenhardt** born; published the first important account of tabes dorsalis; in his *De myelophthisie chronica vera et notha*, 1817. Died 1875. *4772*

1796:13 Germanicus **Mirault**, French surgeon, born; modified Malgaigne's two-flap method for the repair of cleft lip, 1845, *JC(M)* **2**:257; **3**:5. Died 1879. *5746.1*

1796:14 James Scarth **Combe**, British physician, born; first to describe pernicious anaemia, 1822, *TMCS* **1**:194. Died 1883. *3112*

1796:15 Jean Zuléma **Amussat**, French surgeon, born; first performed lumbar colostomy; see his *Mémoire sur la possibilité d'établir un anus artificiel* ..., 1839. Died 1856. *3442*

## 1797
1797:1 **Massachusetts Public Health Act**

1797:2 *Medical Repository*, New York, first **American medical journal**, commences publication

1797:3 **Royal Victoria Hospital, Belfast**, Ireland, started as **Fever Hospital, Belfast General Hospital** (1848); present title 1899

1797:4 Matthew Baillie's (1761–1823) *Morbid anatomy of some of the most important parts of the human body*, 1793, was the first systematic textbook of **pathological anatomy** (he published an atlas intended to illustrate it, 1799–1803). In the 2nd edn, 1797, he suggested (vol. 1, p. 46) a relationship between **rheumatic fever** and **valvular heart disease**, and (vol. 2, p. 72) gave the first clinical description of chronic **obstructive pulmonary oedema**. *2736, 3167.1*

1797:5 Various substances that might be found as constituents of **urinary calculi** described by William Hyde Wollaston (1766–1828), *PT* **87**:386. *4287*

1797:6 The first description of **facial paralysis** given by Nicolaus Anton Friedreich (1761–1836); in his *De paralysi musculorum faciei rheumatici. 4519*

1797:7 Jacob Ludwig Conrad **Schroeder van der Kolk**, Dutch pathologist born 24 Mar; confirmed the medulla as the ultimate seat of epilepsy; in his *Bau und Functionen der Medulla spinalis und oblongata*, etc., 1859. Died 1862. *4815*

1797:8 Jean Leonard Marie **Poiseuille**, French physiologist, born 22 Apr; he invented a haemodynamometer, a mercury manometer, with which he was able to measure blood pressure; in his *Recherches sur la force du coeur aortique*, 1828. Died 1869. *767*

1797:9 Nathan Ryno **Smith**, American surgeon, born 21 May; introduced an anterior or suspensory splint for use in treating fractures of the **femur**, 1860, *MVMJ* **14**:1. Died 1877. *4422*

1797:10 Friedrich Christoph **Kneisel**, German orthodontist, born 10 Jun; published the first book specializing in orthodontics; *Der Schiefstand der Zähne*, 1836. Died ?1883. *3679.8*

1797:11 Camille Melchior **Gibert**, French dermatologist, born; established pityriasis rosea as a definite clinical entity; in the second edition of his *Traité pratique des maladies de la peau*, 1860, **1**, 402. Died 1866. *4048*

1797:12 Jean Baptiste Hippolyte **Dance**, French physician, born; published an important early description of parathyroid tetany, 1831, *ArGM* **26**:190, described by Steinheim (1830). Died 1832. *4828, 4827*

1797:13 John **Stephenson**, Canadian, born; while a medical student from Montreal, he had a cleft palate repaired by P. Roux in Paris. Stephenson described the operation in his graduation thesis, *Dissertatio chirurgo-medica inauguralis de velosynthesi*, 1820. Died 1842. *5740, 5739.1*

1797:14 William **Banting**, British undertaker, born; devised a diet for the treatment of obesity ('Banting diet', Bantingism); in his *Letter on corpulence: addressed to the public*, 1863. Died 1878. *3914*

1797: William **Cadogan** died, **born** 1711. *paediatrics, gout*

1797: Richard **Brocklesby** died, **born** 1722. *military sanitation*

## 1798
1798:1 **US Marine Hospital Service** established

1798:2 **[Imperial Medico-Military Academy]**, **St Petersburg**, founded

1798:3 *Essay on the principle of population* published by Thomas Malthus (1766–1834). *1693*

1798:4 In his *An inquiry into the causes and effects of the variolae vaccinae*, 1798, Edward Jenner (1749–1823) described 23 successful **vaccinations** and announced one of the greatest triumphs in the history of medicine. *2529.3, 5423*

1798:5 An artificial **anus** first successfully constructed by Pierre Duret (b.?1745) in a child with congenital atresia, *ReMP* **4**:45. *3429*

1798:6 An attempt at a classification of **mental diseases** was Immanuel Kant's (1724–1804) *Anthropologie in pragmatischer Hinsicht abgefasst. 4969*

1798:7 The first scientific description of **colour-blindness** ('**Daltonism**') given by John Dalton (1766–1844), *MLPSM* **5**, i:28. *5834*

1798:8 The *Oeuvres chirurgicales* of Pierre Joseph Desault (1744–1795) appeared, 3 vols, 1798–1803. *4165.01*

1798:9 François **Mélier**, French physician, born 14 Jul; first to show the existence of chronic appendicitis, 1827, *JGMC* **100**:317. Died 1866. *3562*

1798:10 Thomas **Hodgkin**, British pathologist, born 17 Aug; gave the first full description of lymphadenoma, 1832, *MCT* **17**:68, named 'Hodgkin's disease' by Samuel Wilks in 1865. Died 1866. *3762*

1798:11 James **Luke**, British surgeon, born; introduced Luke's operation for femoral hernia, 1841, *LMG* **28**:863. Died 1881. *3588*

1798:12 Marie Guillaume Alphonse **Devergie**, French dermatologist, born; gave first demonstration of a fungus in eczema marginatum and a clear description of pityriasis pilaris, 1856, *GMC* **3**:197. Died 1879. *4044*

1798:13 Johann Martin **Heyfelder**, German surgeon, born; introduced ethyl chloride as an anaesthetic; in his *Die Versuche mit dem Schwefeläther und Chloroform*, 1848. Died 1869. *5662*

1798:14 Gustav Adolf **Michaelis**, German obstetrician, born; his *Das enge Becken*, 1851, was the first important work dealing with pelvic deformities since the time of van Deventer. He was among the first to differentiate between the flat pelvis and the rachitic pelvis. Died 1848. *6259*

1798: Luigi **Galvani** died, **born** 1732. *electrical energy in living tissue*

## 1799

1799:1 **Jennerian vaccination** introduced on the Continent and in Asia

1799:2 **Anderson's College of Medicine, Glasgow**, opened

1799:3 **Royal Institution of Great Britain** founded in London

1799:4 **Medical and Chirurgical Faculty of Maryland** incorporated, founded 1789

1799:5 The British **Quarantine Act** was based on the recommendations of Gilbert Blane (1749–1834). *2158*

1799:6 Matthew Baillie (1761–1823) published *A series of engravings, accompanied with explanations* ..., (1799–1803), (intended to illustrate his *Morbid anatomy of some of the most important parts of the human body*, 1793). It was the first systematic atlas of **pathological anatomy**. *2282*

1799:7 Everard Home (1756–1832) reported, *PT* **18**:157, that John Hunter (1728–1793) suggested, in 1790, **artificial insemination** (actually performed by the patient's husband with a syringe). *6162*

1799:8 Antoine Laurent Jessé **Bayle**, French physician, born 13 Jan; gave the first clear description of general paresis ('Bayle's disease'); in his *Recherches sur l'arachnitis chronique*, Paris, Thèse No. 247, 1822. Died 1858. *4795*

1799:9 Prosper **Menière**, French otologist, born 18 Jan; first described aural vertigo (Menière's syndrome), 1860, *GMP* **16**:88, 239, 379, 597. Died 1862. *3372*

1799:10 Salomon Levi **Steinheim**, German physician, born 6 Aug; credited by some German writers with the first description of parathyroid tetany, 1830, *LAGH* **17**:22; an important early description was given by Dance (1831). Died 1866. *4827, 4828*

1799:11 Carl Adolph von **Basedow**, German physician, born 8 Mar; his description of exophthalmic goitre, 1840, led to the name 'Basedow's disease' being used to describe the condition in Europe outside Great Britain, *WGH* **6**:197, 220. Died 1854. *3816*

1799:12 Friedrich August von **Ammon**, German ophthalmologist, born 10 Sep; produced a fine colour-atlas summarizing contemporary knowledge of diseases of the eye, *Klinische Darstellungen der Krankheiten und Bildungfehler des menschlichen Auges*, 1838. It is one of the greatest pre-ophthalmoscopic atlases of ophthalmology. Died 1861. *5852*

1799:13 James **Syme**, British surgeon, born 7 Nov; he first successfully performed his method of amputation at the ankle-joint, 1843, *LEMJ* **3**:93. Was (simultaneously with Pirogov) the first surgeon in Europe to adopt ether anaesthesia for surgical operations, 1847, *LEMJ* **8**:73. Died 1870. *4459, 5659, 5655*

1799:14 Henry **Burton**, British physician, born; he was first to notice 'Burton's blue line' on the gums in lead poisoning, 1840, *MCT* **23**:63. Died 1849. *2099*

1799:15 George **Bodington**, British physician, born; among the first to advocate the sanatorium treatment of pulmonary tuberculosis; in his *Essay on the treatment of and cure of pulmonary consumption*, 1840. Died 1882. *3223*

1799:16 Achille Louis François **Foville**, French physician, born; drew attention to 'Foville's syndrome', crossed paralysis of the limbs on one side of the body and of the face on the other side (with loss of ability to rotate the eye), 1858, *BSAP* **33**:393. Died 1878. *4533*

1799:17 Jacob von **Heine**, German surgeon and orthopaedist, born; gave the first description of acute anterior poliomyelitis ('Heine-Medin disease'); in his *Beobachtungen über Lähmungszustände der untern Extremitäten und deren Behandlung*, 1840. He also drew attention to spastic paraplegia ('Little's disease'). Died 1879. *4664, 4667, 4691.1*

1799:18 John Light **Atlee** born; performed the first successful oöphorectomy, 1843, *NYJM* **1**:168. Died 1885. *6034*

1799: 19 Charles **Ritchie** born; carefully differentiated the symptoms of typhoid and typhus, 1847, *MJMS* **7**:347, and introduced the term **'enteric fever'**. Died 1878. *5026*

---

1799: Alexander **Gordon** died, **born** 1752. *puerperal fever*

1799: John **Bard** died, **born** 1716. *extrauterine pregnancy*

1799: William **Withering** died, **born** 1741. *digitalis*

1799: Lazzaro **Spallanzani** died, **born** 1729. *gastric juice, saliva, digestion*

## 1800

1800: 1 **Royal College of Surgeons of England** founded as successor to **Company of Surgeons** (founded 1745)

1800: 2 **Clinical instruction** at **Montpellier University** authorized

1800: 3 **Library of Congress**, Washington, founded

1800: 4 The first reasonably accurate description of **rheumatoid arthritis** was that given by Augustin Jacob Landré-Beauvais (1772–1840); in his *Doit-on admettre une nouvelle espèce de goutte sous la dénomination de goutte asthénique primitive?* *4490*

1800: 5 The **anaesthetic** properties of **nitrous oxide** discovered by Humphry Davy (1778–1829); in his *Researches, chemical and philosophical, chiefly concerning nitrous oxide*. His suggestion that it be used during surgical operations was not immediately adopted. *5646*

1800: 6 Marie François Xavier Bichat (1771–1802) revolutionized descriptive **anatomy**, wrote *Traité des membranes en général*. *537*

1800: 7 The contagious nature of **trachoma** (military **ophthalmia**, Egyptian ophthalmia) first observed by Dominique Jean Larrey (1766–1842), the military surgeon, while serving in the Napoleonic campaign in Egypt; in his *Mémoire sur l'ophtalmie régnant en Egypte*. *5837*

1800: 8 **Vaccination** against **smallpox** introduced into the US by Benjamin Waterhouse (1754–1846) who inoculated his own child as his first case; he published *A prospect of eliminating the small-pox*, 2 pts, 1800–02. *5424*

---

1800: 9 Edwin **Chadwick**, British sanitary reformer and statistician, born 24 Jan; his *Report on sanitary conditions of the labouring population of Great Britain*, 1842, led to **public health** legislation and to great improvements in the public health; the greatest sanitary reformer of the 19th century. Died 1890. *1608*

1800: 10 Hermann Friedrich **Kilian**, German obstetrician, born 5 Feb; gave the first description of pelvis spinosa; in his *Schilderungen neuer Beckenformen und ihres Verhaltens im Leben*, 1854. In the same year he published *De spondylolisthesi gravissimae pelvangustiae causa nuper detecta*, an important study of the **spondylolisthetic pelvis**. Died 1863. *6261, 6262*

1800: 11 Franz Aloys Antoine **Pollender**, German physician, born 25 May; claimed to have discovered the anthrax bacillus (*B.anthracis*) in 1849, not reporting this until 1855, *VGOM* **8**:103. His account of the organism was more exact than Rayer's. Died 1879. *5164*

1800:12 Henry Hill **Hickman**, British physician and surgeon, born 26 May; provided proof that pain at surgical operations could be abolished by the inhalation of gas, he rendered animals unconscious through partial asphyxiation by the exclusion of air and then by inhalation of carbon dioxide; in his *Letter on suspended animation*, etc., 1800. His work was the first on surgical anaesthesia. Died 1830. *5647*

1800:13 Charles Michel **Billard**, French paediatrician, born 16 Jun; he performed several hundred autopsies on infants and children, correlated the data with clinical observations and incorporated this in his *Traité des maladies des enfans nouveau-nés et à la mamelle*, 1828. It was a pioneer work on the pathological anatomy of infants. Died 1832. *6332*

1800:14 Jean Baptiste André **Dumas**, French chemist, born 15 Jul; with Jean Louis Prévost succeeded in transfusing blood in animals by using defibrinated blood to prevent coagulation, 1821, *AnC* **18**:28. Died 1884. *2016*

1800:15 Friedrich **Wöhler**, German chemist, born 31 Jul; his synthesis of urea was the first instance of an organic compound being made from inorganic materials, 1828, *AnPh* **12**:253. Died 1882. *671*

1800:16 Willard **Parker**, American surgeon, born 2 Sep; introduced cystotomy for inflammation and rupture of the bladder, 1851, *NYJM* **7**:83; first American to operate for appendicitis, 1867, *MR* **2**:25. Died 1884. *4169, 3564*

1800:17 Philippe **Ricord**, French venereologist, born in America 10 Dec; his *Traité pratique des maladies vénériennes*, 1838, includes his description of the initial lesion in syphilis which led to the eponym 'Ricord's chancre' and an account of his repeating the experiments of John Hunter, proving syphilis and gonorrhoea to be distinct diseases . Died 1889. *2381, 5202*

1800: Johann David **Schoepff** died, **born** 1752. *materia medica*

1800: Thomas **Dimsdale** died, **born** 1712. *smallpox inoculation*

## 1801
1801:1 **Medical Society** founded at **Toulouse**

1801:2 **Astigmatism** described by Thomas Young (1773–1829), *PT* **91**:23. *1487*

1801:3 The first American book on the **teeth** was the *Treatise on the human teeth*, a 26-page pamphlet intended for the lay public, by Richard Cortland Skinner (d.*c*1834). *3678*

1801:4 First **herbal** produced and printed in the United States by Samuel Stearns (1747–1819); *American herbal, or materia medica*. *1838.2*

1801:5 Marie François Xavier Bichat (1771–1802) revolutionized **descriptive anatomy**, published *Traité d'anatomie descriptive*, 5 vols, 1801–3. *404*

1801:6 **Myringotomy** performed to treat **Eustachian tube** obstructive **deafness** by Astley Paston Cooper (1768–1841), *PT* **91**:435. *3361*

1801:7 Among the first to dispense with chains in the treatment of the **insane** was Philippe Pinel (1745–1826), founder of the French school of **psychiatry** and author of the classic *Traité médico-philosophique sur l'aliénation mentale ou la manie*. *4922*

1801:8 The first textbook on **ophthalmology** published in Italian was *Saggio di osservazioni e d'esperienze sulle principali malattie degli occhi*, by Antonio Scarpa (1752–1832), the 'Father of Italian ophthalmology'. *5835.*

1801:9 **Hyoscyamine** used to dilate the **pupil** to facilitate removal of the **lens** by Karl Gustav Himly (1772–1837); in his *Ophthalmologische Beobachtungen*, I, p. 97. *5834.1*

1801:10 **Interstitial pregnancy** first reported by Wilhelm Joseph Schmitt (1760–1827), *BMCW* **1**:59. *6163*

1801:11 John Bell (1763–1820), the Scottish surgeon, brother of Charles, wrote *Principles of surgery*, 3 vols, 1801–9; is regarded as a founder of **surgical anatomy**. *5581*

---

1801:12 James **Hope**, British physician, born 23 Feb; his *Treatise on the diseases of the heart and great vessels*, 1832, did much to advance the knowledge of heart murmurs, valvular disease and aneurysm. Died 1841. *2747*

1801:13 Gustav Theodor **Fechner**, German physicist, experimental psychologist, born 19 Apr; showed the relationship between stimulus and sensation (Fechner-Weber law), 1859, *AbL* **4**:455. Wrote the first treatise on psychophysics and the physiology of sensation, *Elemente der Psychophysik*, 1860. Died 1887. *1464, 4972*

1801:14 John **Parkin**, British surgeon, born 10 May; suggested the water-borne character of cholera, and the use of charcoal filters for water purification, 1832, *LMSJ* n.s.**2**:151. Died 1886. *5105*

1801:15 James Lomax **Bardsley**, British physician, born 7 Jul; first to record the use of emetine in treatment of amoebiasis; in his *Hospital facts and observations*, 1830, p. 149. Died 1876. *5183*

1801:16 Johannes **Müller**, German anatomist and physiologist, born 14 Jul; propounded his law of specific nerve energies in his *Zur vergleichenden Physiologie des Gesichtssinnes des Menschen und der Thiere*, 1826. Supported cell theory of tumour formation in cancer; in his *Ueber den feineren Bau und die Formen der krankhaften Geschwülste*, 1838. Died 1858. *1257, 1456, 2612*

1801:17 George Biddell **Airy**, British astronomer, born 27 Jul; first drew attention to astigmatism, 1827, a condition from which he himself suffered; he used cylindrical lenses for its correction, *TCPS* **2**:267. Died 1892. *5847*

1801:18 Armand **Trousseau**, French physician, born 14 Oct; popularized tracheotomy in diphtheria, 1833, *JCMC* **1**:5, 41. First to describe haemochromatosis; in his *Clinique médicale de l'Hôtel-Dieu*, 2 ed., **2**, 663, 1865. Died 1867. *5054, 3915*

1801:19 Charles **Clay**, British surgeon, born 27 Dec; introduced the term ovariotomy, 1842, *MTG* **7**:43, 59, 67, 83, 99, 139, 153, 270; for many years the most successful ovariotomist in

Britain, he performed 395 with a mortality of 25 per cent, 1864, *TOSL* **5**:58. Died 1893. *6032, 6054*

---

1801:20 Alfred **Donné**, French bacteriologist, born; first described *Trichomonas vaginalis*, 1836, *CRAS* **3**:385, which he originally believed to be the causal organism in gonorrhoea. Discovered the blood platelets, 1842, *CRAS* **14**:366. Briefly described leukaemia; in his *Cours de microscopie*, 1844, p. 10. Died 1878. *5207, 864, 3060.1*

1801:21 Francis **Rynd**, British physician, born; invented an instrument making possible hypodermic infusions, 1845, *DMP* **13**:167. Died 1861. *1968*

1801:22 Richard Anthony **Stafford**, British physician and surgeon, born; first to record sarcoma of the prostate, 1839, *MCT* **22**:218. Died 1854. *4259*

---

1801: William **Heberden** Sr died, **born** 1710. *varicella, smallpox, rheumatic gout, angina pectoris*

## 1802
1802:1 **Wave theory of light** established by Thomas Young (1773–1829), *PT* **92**:12. *1488*

1802:2 Marie François Xavier Bichat (1771–1802) revolutionized descriptive anatomy. His most important contribution to modern **anatomy** was that **pathology** must be based on the structure of tissues making up the organs, regardless of the location of the latter in the organism; in his *Anatomie générale*, 1802, which marks the beginning of **histology**. *403*

1802:3 **Opium** alkaloids isolated by Charles Louis Derosne (1780–1846), *AnC* **45**:257. *1838.3*

1802:4 In his *Commentarii de morborum historia*, p. 130, William Heberden Sr (1710–1801) described the form of **rheumatic gout** in which nodules ('**Heberden's nodes**') appear in the interphalangeal joints of the fingers. *4491*

1802:5 Giuseppe Flajani (1741–1808) gave one of the earliest accounts of **exophthalmic goitre** and noted cardiac disturbances in the condition; in his *Collezione d'osservazione ...*, **3**, 270–73. *3811*

---

1802:6 Julius **Bettinger**, German dermatologist, born 31 Mar; demonstrated the experimental inoculability of syphilis, 1856, *AIB* **3**:425. Died 1878. *2384*

1802:7 Heinrich Gustav **Magnus**, German chemist and physicist, born 2 May; quantitatively analysed blood gases, 1837, *AnPh* **12**:583. Died 1870. *929*

1802:8 Julius **Sichel**, German ophthalmologist, born 14 May; his *Iconographie ophtalmologique*, 1852–59, ranks with the work of Ammon as one of the greatest pre-ophthalmoscopic atlases of ophthalmology. Died 1868. *5868, 5852*

1802:9 Auguste **Bérard**, French surgeon, born 2 Aug; published the first important monograph on parotid tumours, *Maladies de la glande parotide* , 1841. Died 1846. *3444*

1802:10 Antoine Jérome **Balard**, French chemist, born 30 Sep; isolated bromine, 1826, *AnC* **32**:337; discovered amyl nitrite, 1844, *CRAS* **19**:634. Died 1876. *1848.1, 1859*

1802:11 Dominic John **Corrigan**, British physician, born 1 Dec; described 'Corrigan's pulse', 'water-hammer pulse'; in his account of aortic insufficiency, 1832, *EMSJ* **37**:225 (earlier described by Vieussens, 1705). Died 1880. *2748*

1802:12 Horace **Green**, American laryngologist, born 24 Dec; published the first American treatise on laryngology, *A treatise on diseases of the air-passages*, 1846; regarded as the 'Father of laryngology in America'. Died 1866. *3261*

1802:13 William D. **Macgill** born; successful ligation of the primitive carotid artery in continuity of both carotids, 1823, in the same subject within a month – the first American to do so, *NYMPJ* **4**:576. Died 1833. *2946*

1802:14 William **Addison**, British physician, born; made important observations on the blood corpuscles, including first description of leucocytosis; in his *Observations on inflammation*, 1843; he is by some considered the world's first haematologist. Died 1881. *3059*

1802:15 Samuel Armstrong **Lane**, British surgeon, born; treated haemophilia with blood transfusion, 1840, *L* **1**:185. Died 1892. *3058.1*

1802:16 Antoine **Lembert**, French surgeon, born; described Lembert's suture, 1826, *RGAP* **2**:100; first successfully employed by Johann Friedrich Dieffenbach, 1836. Died 1851. *3435, 3441*

1802: Johann Ernst **Wichmann** died, **born** 1740. *scabies*

1802: Erasmus **Darwin** died, **born** 1731. *evolution*

1802: Marie François Xavier **Bichat** died, **born** 1771. *anatomy, membranes, histology*

**1803**
1803:1 Successful ligation of the primitive **carotid artery** by Mason Fitch Cogswell (1761–1830); reported in 1824, *NEJM* **13**:357. *2945*

1803:2 **Haemophilia** recognized and adequately described by John Conrad Otto (1774–1844), *MRep* **6**:1. *3954*

1803:3 The first book on **orthodontics** was Joseph Fox's (1775–1816) *Natural history of the human teeth. 3679*

1803:4 The first accurate description of the pathological anatomy of **talipes (club-foot)** given by Antonio Scarpa (1752–1832); in his *Memoria chirurgica sui piedi torti congenita dei fanciulli. 4308*

1803:5 Johann Christian Reil (1759–1813), an early advocate of humane treatment of the **insane**, wrote *Rhapsodieen über die Anwendung der psychischen Curmethode auf Geisteszerrüttungen*, and edited the first journal devoted to mental disease – the *Magazin für Nervenheilkund*; he is considered the founder of modern **psychiatry**. *4923*

1803:6 Arnold Adolph **Berthold**, German anatomist, born 26 Feb; demonstrated the existence of an internal secretion, 1849, *ArA* 42. Died 1861. *1176*

1803:7 Justus von **Liebig**, German chemist, born 12 May; discovered chloroform, 1832, *AnP* **1**:182, independently of Guthrie (1832) and Soubeiran (1832). Died 1873. *1852, 5650, 5648, 5649*

1803:8 Marmaduke Burr **Wright**, American physician, born 17 Nov; introduced combined cephalic version; in his *Difficult labors and their treatment*, 1854. Died 1879. *6182*

1803:9 Joseph Friedrich **Sobernheim** born; introduced the term 'myocarditis'; in his *Praktische Diagnostik*, 1837, p. 118. Died 1846. *2750*

**1804**
1804:1 True **aneurysm** distinguished from false by Antonio Scarpa (1752–1832); in his *Sull' aneurisma*. *2975*

1804:2 First book on **alcoholism** published by Thomas Trotter (1760–1832); *Essay on drunkenness*. *2071.1*

1804:3 **Rabies** transmitted from a rabid to a normal dog, to a rabbit and to a hen, by injection of saliva, proving the disease to be infectious, by Georg Gottfried Zinke; in his *Neue Ansichten der Hundswuth, ihrer Ursachen und Folgen*. *5481*

1804:4 Giuseppe Baronio (1759–1811) was among the first to attempt **transplantation** and experimental **surgery** in animals, successfully carrying out full-thickness **skin grafts**. He wrote *Degli innesti animali*. *5736*

1804:5 Carl **Rokitansky**, Bohemian pathologist, born 19 Feb; his *Handbuch der pathologischen Anatomie*, 1842–46, was an outstanding work in the field; gave the first description of spondylolisthesis, 1839, *MJOS* **19**:41, 195. Gave a classical description of the pathology of acute yellow atrophy of the liver; in his *Handbuch*, 1842, **3**, p. 13; it was also called 'Rokitansky's disease'. Died 1878. *2293, 6258, 3618*

1804:6 Georg Friedrich **Stromeyer**, German surgeon, born 6 Mar; successfully treated talipes (club-foot) by tenotomy, 1833, *MGH* **39**:195. Died 1876. *4320*

1804:7 Josiah Clark **Nott**, American physician, born 31 Mar; carried out total eradication of the os coccygis for neuralgia, 1844, *NOMSJ* **1**:58. Advanced the theory that yellow fever was caused by minute animalcula, 1848, *NOMSJ* **4**:563. Died 1873. *4852, 5454*

1804:8 Matthias Jakob **Schleiden**, German botanist, born 5 Apr; made a vital contribution to cell theory, *Beiträge zur Phytogenesis*, 1838. Died 1881. *112*

1804:9 Richard **Owen**, British comparative anatomist and zoologist, born 20 Jul; in his *Odontography*, 2 vols, 1840–45, he dealt with the whole range of the toothed vertebrates. His *Anatomy and physiology of vertebrates*, 3 vols, 1866–68, is based entirely on personal observations. Died 1892. *329, 336, 3681.1*

1804:10 Charles Emmanuel **Sédillot**, French surgeon, born 14 Sep; first to perform gastrostomy, 1849, *GMS* **9**:366. Died 1883. *3451*

1804:11 John **Hilton**, British surgeon, born 22 Sep; in his *On the influence of mechanical and physiological rest in the treatment of accidents and surgical diseases, and the diagnostic* *value of pain*, 1863, (later editions have the title *Rest and pain*) he emphasized the importance of rest in the treatment of surgical disorders; observed what was later named *Trichinella spiralis*, in human muscle, and suggested it was a parasite, 1833, *LMG* 11:605. Died 1878. *5609, 5336.5*

1804:12 William **Stokes**, British physician, born 1 Oct; gave a classical account of heart block with syncopal attacks, 1846, *DQMS* 2:73; following description by Robert Adams, 1827, named 'Stokes-Adams syndrome'; in 1854 described Cheyne-Stokes respiration and gave first account of paroxysmal tachycardia; in his *Diseases of the heart and aorta*. Died 1878. *2745, 2756, 2760*

1804:13 Erastus Bradley **Wolcott**, American surgeon, born 18 Oct; carried out the first excision of the kidney, for renal tumour, 1861, – recorded by C.L. Stoddard, *MSRep* 7:126. Died 1880. *4210*

1804:14 Gilman **Kimball**, American surgeon, born 8 Dec; performed the first successful abdominal hysteromyomectomy, 1855, *BMSJ* 52:249. Died 1892. *6042*

1804:15 Pierre Marie Edouard **Chassaignac**, French surgeon, born 24 Dec; introduced india-rubber tubes for drainage of abscesses and put the subject of surgical drainage on a scientific and methodical basis; in his *Traité pratique de la suppuration et du drainage chirurgical*, 1859. Died 1879. *5606*

———

1804:16 Jacques-Joseph **Moreau** born; he gave a classical description of cannabis intoxication; in his *Du hachische ...*, 1845. Died 1884. *2077.2*

1804:17 Josef **Dietl**, Polish physician, born; described 'Dietl's crisis', acute ureteral colic, 1864, *WMW* 14:563, 579, 593. Died 1878. *4211*

1804:18 Pierre Charles **Huguier**, French surgeon, born; gave the name *esthiomène* to the induration and discoloration of the affected parts in lymphogranuloma venereum, 1849, *MANM* 14:501. Died 1873. *5216*

———

1804: Joseph **Priestley** died, **born** 1733. *oxygen*

1804: Thomas **Percival** died, **born** 1740. *cod-liver oil, medical ethics*

1804: Immanuel **Kant** died, **born** 1724. *classification of mental diseases*

## 1805
1805:1 The first definite description of **cerebrospinal meningitis** given by Gaspard Vieusseux (1746–1814), *JMCP* 11:163. *4674*

1805:2 The first monograph on **rheumatism**, *A clinical history of diseases. Part first .... A clinical history of the acute rheumatism*, etc. published by John Haygarth (1740–1827). *4492*

1805:3 The first use of a **stomach tube** for **gastric lavage** after poisoning was made by Philip Syng Physick (1768–1837), reported in 1812, *ER* 3:111. *3432*

1805:4 **Morphine** isolated by Friedrich Wilhelm Adam Sertürner (1783–1841), *JPAA* 1447. *1839*

1805:5 Ligation of the common **carotid artery** by Astley Paston Cooper (1768–1841), reported in 1809, *MCT* **1**:222; the patient died but a second case (1808) was successful, *GHR* **1**:43, 53. *2929, 2954, 2955*

1805:6 First **colostomy** for **intestinal obstruction** performed by Pierre Fine (1760–1814), *AnSMP* **6**:34. *3430*

1805:7 Edward **Cock**, British surgeon, born 26 Jan; performed the first pharyngotomy in England, 1856, *L* **1**:125. Died 1892. *3265*

1805:8 Manuel **Garcia**, Spanish music teacher, born 17 Mar; he introduced the modern laryngoscope, 1855, *PRS* **7**:399. Died 1906. *3329*

1805:9 Samuel David **Gross**, American surgeon, born 8 Jul; published the first American treatise on orthopaedics, *The anatomy, physiology, and diseases of the bones and joints*, 1830. His *System of surgery*, 1859, a massive work of nearly 2500 page, was his greatest work, intended to be the most elaborate treatise on the subject. Died 1884. *4316.1, 5607*

1805:10 Antonius **Mathijsen**, Dutch military surgeon, born 4 Sep; introduced the modern plaster of Paris bandage; in his *Nieuwe wijze van aanwending van het gips-verband bij beenbreuken*, 1805. Died 1878. *4328*

1805:11 Joseph **Pancoast**, American surgeon, born 23 Nov; performed first successful operation for ectopia vesicae (extroversion of the bladder), 1859, *NAMR* **3**:710. Died 1882. *4170*

1805:12 Josef **Skoda**, Bohemian physician, born 10 Dec; a distinguished leader of the Vienna medical school, wrote *Abhandlung über Perkussion und Auskultation*, 1839, in which he classified the sounds obtained on percussion according to musical pitch and tone. His work confirmed and completed that of Laennec. Died 1881. *2676*

1805: Felice **Fontana** died, **born** 1730. *snake venom*

1805: John **Millar** died, **born** 1733. *asthma, laryngismus stridulus*

**1806**
1806:1 The first successful **amputation** of the **hip-joint** in the United States performed by Walter Brashear (1776–1860), *TKMS* 1853 **2**:264. *4462*

1806:2 The *Description des maladies de la peau* ... of Jean Louis Marc Alibert (1768–1837), which includes hand-coloured illustrations, was the largest and most spectacular of the early classics of **dermatology**; it includes (p. 157, pl.xxxv) the first description of mycosis fungoides. The second edition, 1825, includes the first description of **sycosis barbae** ('**Alibert's mentagra**'). *3986, 4024*

1806:3 *History and treatment of diseases of the teeth* by Joseph Fox (1775–1816) is the first book to include illustrations of the **teeth** and is considered by some of more value than Hunter's *Practical treatise*, 1778. *3679.1*

1806:4 Descriptions of '**Hesselbach's hernia**' and '**triangle**' appear in *Anatomisch-chirurgische Abhandlung über den Ursprung der Leistenbrüche* by Franz Kaspar Hesselbach (1759–1816). *3582*

1806:5 The **speculum** introduced by Philipp Bozzini (1773–1809), utilized illumination and reflection by mirrors, *JPrH* **24, I**:107. *2672.1*

1806:6 Symptomatology of **heart disease** established by Jean Nicolas Corvisart (1755–1821), making possible the differentiation between cardiac and **pulmonary** disorders; in his *Essays sur les maladies et les lésions organiques du coeur et des gros vaisseaux. 2737*

1806:7 Joseph François **Malgaigne**, French surgeon, born 14 Feb. His *Manuel de médécine opératoire*, 1834, a considerable work on operative surgery, was translated into several European languages. He also wrote *Traité d'anatomie chirurgicale et de chirurgie experimentale*, 1838. He devised a two-flap method for the repair of cleft lip, 1844, *JC(M)* **2**:1; it was modified the following year by Mirault. Died 1865. *5746, 5746.1, 5591, 5594*

1806:8 George Hilaro **Barlow**, British physician, born 2 May; with George Owen Rees, described subacute bacterial endocarditis, 1843, *GHR* n.s.**1**:189. Died 1866. *2753*

1806:9 Chapin Aaron **Harris**, American dentist, born 6 May; published *The dental art, a practical treatise on dental surgery*, 1839, one of the most popular works on dentistry; he founded the first dental college in the world, the Baltimore College of Dental Surgery. Died 1860. *3680*

1806:10 Fredrik Theodor **Berg**, Swedish physician, born 5 Sep; discovered *Candida albicans* to be causal organism in thrush (moniliasis), 1841, *Hygiea* **3**:541. Died 1887. *5518*

1806:11 Guillaume Benjamin Amand **Duchenne de Boulogne**, French neurologist, born 17 Sep; described progressive muscular atrophy ('Aran-Duchenne disease'), 1849, *CRAS* **29**:667. The most famous of the electrotherapists, employed faradic current, and classified the electrophysiology of the muscular system, *De l'électrisation localisée et de son application à la physiologie ...*, 1855; in the 3rd edition (1872) he described (p. 357) partial brachial plexus paralysis, previously described by Smellie (1763) and later (1873) by Erb ('Duchenne-Erb palsy'). His classic account of tabes dorsalis, 1858, *ArGM* **12**:641; **13**:36, 158, 417, earned the eponym 'Duchenne's disease'. First to describe chronic progressive bulbar paralysis ('Duchenne's paralysis'), 1860, *ArGM* **16**:283, 431. Studied and photographed the expression of emotions; in his *Mécanisme de la physionomie humaine*, 1862. Published *Physiologie des mouvements*, on muscular movements, 1867. Described progressive muscular dystrophy ('Duchenne's muscular dystrophy'), 1868, *ArGM* **11**:179, 305, 421, 552, it had previously been noted by Meryon (1852). Died 1875. *4732, 614, 4543, 4548, 1995, 4774, 4736, 624, 4973, 4739, 4734.1*

1806:12 John **Adams**, British surgeon, born; first to distinguish between hypertrophy and carcinoma of the prostate; in his *Anatomy and diseases of the prostate gland*, 1851. Died 1877. *4260*

1806:13 Jean Marie **Jacquemier**, French obstetrician, born; described 'Jacquemier's sign', violet coloration of the vaginal skin, diagnostic of early pregnancy, 1838, *ArGM* **3**:165. Died 1879. *6174*

1806: Benjamin **Bell** died, **born** 1749. *ulcers, gonorrhoea, syphilis*

**1807**

1807:1 *A compendium of the theory and practice of midwifery*, by Samuel Bard (1742–1848), was the first significant textbook on **obstetrics** written by an American. *6163.1*

1807:2 Charles Bell (1774–1842), brother of John, distinguished as anatomist, physiologist and neurologist, was also an eminent **surgeon**. His works include *A system of operative surgery*, 2 vols, 1807–9. *5583*

1807:3 Astley Paston Cooper's (1768–1841) *Anatomy and surgical treatment of inguinal and congenital hernia* described the transversalis fascia and 'Cooper's ligament'. The second edition, 1827, included a description of 'Cooper's hernia', femoral hernia. *3581*

1807:4 First successful ligation of **carotid artery** (for secondary haemorrhage) by Amos Twitchell (1781–1850); reported 1842, *NEQJ* **1**:188. *2959*

1807:5 **Ecthyma terebrans** first described by Whitley Stokes (1763–1845), *DMPE* **1**:146. *4020*

---

1807:6 John **Watson**, British/American surgeon, born 9 Jan; first to perform oesophagotomy, 1844, *AmJMS* **8**:309. Died 1863. *3448*

1807:7 Isaac **Ray**, American psychiatrist, born 16 Jan; the most influential American writer of his time on forensic psychiatry, wrote *A treatise on the medical jurisprudence of insanity*, 1838. Died 1887. *4929.01*

1807:8 Pierre Ernest Antoine **Bazin**, French dermatologist, born 20 Feb; first described erythema induratum scrophulosorum ('Bazin's disease'); in his *Leçons sur la scrofule*, 2nd edition, 1861, pp. 145, 501. Died 1878. *4051*

1807:9 Gurdon **Buck**, American surgeon, born 4 May; devised 'Buck's operation' for the restoration of the ankylosed knee-joint, 1845, *AmJMS* **10**:277. Treated cancer of larynx by thyrotomy, 1853; in his *On the surgical treatment of polypi* …, 1853. Introduced an extension-traction, apparatus for the treatment of fracture of the **femur**, 1860, *BNYAM* **1**:181. Wrote the first American publication devoted exclusively to reconstructive surgery, *Contributions to reparative surgery*, 1876. Died 1877. *4324, 3263, 4419, 5754.1*

1807:10 Auguste **Nélaton**, French surgeon, born 17 Jun; gave a classic description of pelvic haematocele, 1851, *GH* **3**:573, 578, 581; **4**:45, 46. Died 1873. *6178*

1807:11 Carl Friedrich **Canstatt**, German physician, born 11 Jul; published a summary of previous knowledge of geriatrics, *Die Krankheiten des höheren Alters und ihre Heilung*, 1839. Died 1850. *1605.1*

1807:12 George **Busk**, British microscopist, born 12 Aug; drew attention of George Budd to *Fasciolopsis buski*, the fluke causing fasciolopsiasis, who described it in his *On diseases of the liver*, 2nd edn, p. 484, 1852. Died 1886. *3619*

1807:13 Eduard **Zeis**, German plastic surgeon, born 1 Oct; introduced the term 'plastic surgery' in his important *Handbuch der plastischen Chirurgie*, 1838, which covers the general principles of the speciality and describes operative techniques for the individual parts of the body. Died 1868. *5743.4*

---

1807: 14 Robert William **Smith**, Irish physician, born; described generalized neurofibromatosis; in his *Treatise on the pathology, diagnosis and treatment of neuroma*, 1849. It is also called 'Recklinghausen's disease' in recognition of the classic description by Friedrich Daniel von Recklinghausen in 1882. Died 1873. *4529, 4082*

1807: 15 John **Badham**, British physician, born; gave an important early description of poliomyelitis, 1835, *LMG* **17**:215. Died 1840. *4663*

1807: 16 Louis Daniel **Beauperthuy**, physician, born West Indies; the first to advance the theory that the mosquito was responsible for the transmission of yellow fever, 1854, *GOCu* **4**: No. 57. Died 1871. *5454.1*

1807: Joseph Jacob von **Plenck** died, **born** 1738. *classification of skin diseases*

## 1808
1808: 1 **Koninklijke Nederlandse Akademie van Wetenschappen** founded, reformed in 1855

1808: 2 The use of **ergot** for the **induction of labour** first used in America by John Stearns (1770–1848), *MRep* **5**:308. *6164*

1808: 3 Acute **hydrocephalus** first described by John Cheyne (1777–1836); in his *Essay on hydrocephalus acutus. 4635*

1808: 4 The first sets of individual porcelain **artificial teeth** mounted on a base produced by Giuseppe Angelo Fonzi (1768–1840); in his *Rapport sur les dents artificielles terro-métalliques. 3679.2*

1808: 5 James Wardrop (1782–1869) first to classify the various inflammations of the **eye** according to the structures affected. He introduced the term **keratitis**; in his *Essays on the morbid anatomy of the human eye*, 2 vols, 1808–18. *5840*

1808: 6 **Bronchitis**, so named, and distinguished from **pneumonia** and **pleurisy** by Charles Badham (1780–1845); in his *Observations on the inflammatory affections of the mucous membrane of the bronchiae. 3168*

1808: 7 Walter **Burnham**, American surgeon and gynaecologist, born 12 Jan; performed the first successful abdominal hysterectomy, 1854, *NAL* **52**:147. Died 1883. *6040*

1808: 8 Washington Lemuel **Atlee** born 12 Feb; a notable American ovariotomist, reputed to have performed this operation 387 times, 1851, *TAMA* **4**:286. He was among the first to study the surgical removal of fibroids of the uterus, in his *Surgical treatment of certain fibrous tumours of the uterus*, 1853; devised an operation for vesico-vaginal fistula, 1860, *AmJMS* **39**:67. Died 1878. *6038, 6039, 6047*

1808: 9 George **Budd**, British physician, born 25 Feb; described a form of liver cirrhosis in his *On diseases of the liver*, 1845, it was named 'Budd's disease'; described *Fasciolopsis buski*, the fluke causing fasciolopsiasis, in his *On diseases of the liver*, 2nd edn, p. 484, 1852; his attention having been drawn to it by George Busk (1807–1886). Died 1882. *3619*

1808:10 William **Fergusson**, British surgeon, born 20 Mar; designed a vaginal speculum; described in his *System of practical surgery*, 1857, 4th edn, p. 724. Died 1877. *6043*

1808:11 Carl Wilhelm **Boeck**, Norwegian dermatologist and syphilologist, born 15 Dec; first described Scabies crustosa, Norwegian itch, ('Boeck's scabies'), 1842, *NML* **4**:1, 127. With Daniel Cornelius Danielssen, published the first modern description of leprosy ('Danielssen-Boeck disease'); in *Om spedalskhed*, 1847. Died 1875. *4033, 2434*

1808:12 William **Detmold**, German/American surgeon, born 27 Dec; first opened the lateral ventricles of the brain for the treatment of cerebral abscess, 1850, *AmJMS* **19**:86. Died 1894. *4853*

1808:13 Augustin Eugène **Homolle**, French chemist, born; isolated amorphous digitalin from digitalis, 1845, *JPC* 3 sér. **7**:57. Died 1875. *1860*

1808: Heinrich **Wrisberg** died, **born** 1739. *nerve of Wrisberg*

1808: Giuseppe **Flajani** died, **born** 1741. *exophthalmic goitre*

## 1809

1809:1 John Abernethy (1764–1831), a pupil of John Hunter, became a leading **surgeon** in London. His best work is probably his *Surgical observations on the constitutional origin and treatment of local diseases*, 1809. *5584*

1809:2 **Scarpa's fascia** and **Scarpa's triangle** described by Antonio Scarpa (1752–1832); in his *Sull'ernie*. *3583*

1809:3 **Angina pectoris** attributed to coronary obstruction by Allan Burns (1781–1813); in his *Observations on ... diseases of the heart*. *2889*

1809:4 **'Meckel's diverticulum'**; Johann Friedrich Meckel, *the younger* (1781–1833), *ArP* **9**:421. *984*

1809:5 Charles Robert **Darwin**, British naturalist, born 12 Feb; published his theory of evolution in *Origin of species*, 1859; his studies of the causes, physiological and psychological, of all the fundamental emotions in man and animals were recorded in his *The expression of the emotions in man and animals*, 1872. Died 1882. *220, 4975*

1809:6 Henri **Roger**, French physician, born 13 Jun; drew attention to a congenital ventricular septal defect and an accompanying murmur ('maladie de Roger', 'Roger's murmur'), 1879, *BUAM* **8**:1074, 1189. Died 1891. *2782*

1809:7 Friedrich Gustav Jakob **Henle**, German anatomist and pathologist, born 9 Jul. His *Handbuch der systematischen Anatomie des Menschen*, 3 vols, 1855–71, is among the best of the modern systems, it includes a description of 'Henle's loop' in the kidney; his studies on epithelia of the skin and intestines (*Symbolae ad anatomiam villorum intestinalium*, 1837) created histology; many of his histological discoveries are described in his *Allgemeine Anatomie*, 1841, including his demonstration of smooth muscle in small arteries (pp. 510, 690). He laid down postulates on the aetiological relationship of microbes to disease (*Pathologische Untersuchungen*, 1840, 1–82). Died 1885. *417, 539, 543, 2533*

1809:8 William Wood **Gerhard**, American physician, born 23 Jul; gave an accurate clinical description of tuberculous meningitis, 1834, *AmJMS* **13**:313; **14**:99. Differentiated typhus from typhoid, 1837, *AJMS* **19**:289, 298, 302. Died 1872. *4636, 5024*

1809:9 Henry **Hancock**, British surgeon, born 6 Aug; first successfully to treat peritonitis due to abscess of the appendix, 1848, *LMG* **7**:547. Died 1880. *3563*

1809:10 Oliver Wendell **Holmes**, American physician, poet, novelist, and essayist, born 29 Aug; the first definitely to establish the contagious nature of puerperal fever, 1843, *NEQJ* **1**:503. Because his famous essay appeared in an unimportant journal, he enlarged it into book form, *Puerperal fever, as a private pestilence*, 1855, in which he mentions the steps already being taken by Semmelweis. Died 1894. *6274, 6276, 6275*

1809:11 Jacques Gilles Thomas **Maisonneuve**, French urologist, born 10 Nov; introduced urinary hair catheter, 1845, *CRAS* **20**:70. Died 1887. *4168*

1809:12 William James Erasmus **Wilson**, British surgeon and dermatologist, born 25 Nov; gave dermatitis exfoliativa ('Wilson's disease'), known to Hippocrates, its present name, 1870, *MTG* **1**:118. Gave original descriptions of several skin diseases (a subject on which he lectured at the Royal College of Surgeons of England) in his *Lectures on dermatology*, 1871–8. Died 1884. *4061, 3994*

1809:13 Louis **Braille**, French inventor, born; in his *Procédé pour écrire au moyen des points*, 1837, he modified the system of elevated points first suggested by Charles Barbier (1820) for enabling the blind to read by touch. Today the Braille system is used throughout the world. Died 1852. *5851*

1809:14 John Stough **Bobbs**, American surgeon, born; first to perform cholecystotomy for the removal of gallstones, 1868, *TIMS* 68. Died 1870. *3621*

1809:15 Bernhard **Mohr** born; first to describe pituitary tumour with obesity and sexual infantilism ('Fröhlich's syndrome'), 1840, *WGH* **6**:565. Died 1848. *3882*

1809:16 Edward **Meryon**, British physician, born; first described Duchenne's muscular dystrophy (1868) in 1852, *MCT* **35**:73. Died 1880. *4734.1, 4739*

1809:17 William **Wilton** born; first to report a chorionic tumour, 1840, *L* **1**:691. Died 1899. *6031.1*

1809: George **Baker** died, **born** 1722. *lead poisoning*

1809: Leopold **Auenbrugger** died, **born** 1722. *percussion of chest*

1809: Philipp **Bozzini** died, **born** 1773. *speculum*

**1810**
1810:1 **Karolinska Institutet**, Stockholm, founded

1810:2 **Homoeopathy;** publication of *Organon der rationellen Heilkunde* by Christian Friedrich Samuel Hahnemann (1755–1843). *1966*

1810:3 The classic description of **typhus** given by Johan Valentin von Hildenbrand (1763–1818) in his *Ueber den ansteckenden Typhus* led to the eponym '**Hildenbrand's disease**' in the French literature. *5375*

1810:4 Congenital **syphilis**: first systematic work, *Traité de la maladie vénérienne chez les enfans nouveau-nés*, by René Joseph Hyacinthe Bertin (1757–1828). *2378.1*

1810:5 Early attempt at the **localization of cerebral function** by Franz Joseph Gall (1758–1828) and Johann Caspar Spurzheim (1776–1832) in their *Anatomie et physiologie du système nerveux*, 1810–1819. The book gave rise to phrenology. *1389*

1810:6 **Cystine** isolated by William Hyde Wollaston (1766–1828), *PT* **100**:223 (first amino acid to be isolated). *668.1*

---

1810:7 William **Henderson**, British physician, born 17 Jan; left a good account of relapsing fever and was one of the first to differentiate it from typhus, 1844, *EMSJ* **61**:201. With Robert Paterson, described the inclusion body of molluscum contagiosum, 1841, *EMSJ* **56**:213, 279. Died 1872. *5311.1, 4031,4032*

1810:8 Hermann Franz Joseph **Naegele**, German obstetrician, born 22 Jan; carried out pioneering work in obstetric auscultation, including the sounds of the foetal heart; in his *Die geburtshülfliche Auscultation*, 1838. Died 1858. *6175*

1810:9 Marie François Eugène **Belgrand**, French hydrographic engineer, born 23 Apr; constructed the sewers of Paris (1854), in his work, *La Seine*, published 1872–1887. Died 1878. *1620*

1810:10 Christian Georg Theodor **Ruete**, German ophthalmologist, born 2 May; introduced a practical lens system for examining the inverted image, and improved the illumination of the ophthalmoscope; in his *Der Augenspiegel und das Optometer für practische Aertze*, 1852. Died 1867. *5866.1*

1810:11 Gabriel Gustav **Valentin**, German physiologist, born 8 Jul; first to discover a trypanosome (in a salmon), 1841, *ArA*: 435. Died 1883. *5267.1*

1810:12 Ludwig **Türck**, Austrian neurologist and laryngologist, born 22 Jul; first noted the correlation of retinal haemorrhage with brain tumours, 1853, *ZGA* **9**, i:214. Described laryngitis sicca – ('Türck's trachoma'); in his *Klinik der Krankheiten des Kehlkopfes ...*, p. 295, 1866. Died 1868. *5870, 3273*

1810:13 William John **Little**, British surgeon, born 7 Aug; he wrote a classic work on talipes (club-foot), a condition from which he himself suffered, *On the nature of club-foot and analogous distortions*, 1839. His classic description of congenital cerebral spastic diplegia, 1844, *L* **1**:350, led to the alternative name 'Little's disease'. He was the first eminent orthopaedic surgeon in Britain, his best work was *On the nature and treatment of the deformities of the human frame*, 1853, which (p. 14) included an early description of progressive muscular dystrophy. Founded London School of Orthopaedics and the forerunner of the Royal Orthopaedic Hospital. Died 1894. *4322, 4691.1, 4329, 4735*

1810:14 David **Gruby**, Hungarian parasitologist and medical mycologist, born 20 Aug; discovered the fungal cause of favus (ringworm), *Achorion (Trichophyton) schönleinii*, 1841,

*CRAS* **13**:72, independently of Johann Lucas Schönlein. Gave the first accurate description of *Trichophyton mentagrophytes*, the fungus causing sycosis barbae, 1842, *CRAS* **15**:512. Found *Candida albicans* to be causal organism in thrush (moniliasis), 1842, *CRAS* **14**:634, independently of Berg. Described *Microsporon audouini*, a cause of tinea capitis, 1843, *CRAS* **17**:301. Discovered trypanosomes in the frog, 1843, *CRAS* **17**:1134, he first suggested the name 'trypanosome' to describe the parasite. Discovered *Trichophyton tonsurans*, a cause of tinea capitis, 1844, *CRAS* **18**:583. Died 1898. *4030, 4034, 5519, 5518, 4035, 5268, 4036*

1810: 15 Bernhard Rudolph Conrad von **Langenbeck**, German surgeon, born 8 Nov; discovered *Candida albicans*, 1839, *NNGN* **12**:145; later found by Berg (1841) to be the causal organism in thrush (candidiasis). Devised an operation for repair of cleft palate, 1862, *ArKC* **2**:205. Founded *Archiv für klinische Chirurgie*, 1861. Died 1887. *5517, 5518, 5748*

1810: 16 Nikolai Ivanovich **Pirogov**, Russian surgeon, born 15 Nov; first (simultaneously with James Syme) to adopt ether anaesthesia, recorded in his *Recherches pratiques et physiologiques sur l'éthérization* 1847, and first to practice rectal anaesthesia with ether, 1847, *CRAS* **24**:789. Introduced a method of complete osteoplastic amputation of the foot, 1854, *VMZ* **63**, 2:83. Died 1881. *5656, 5659, 5655, 4465*

1810: 17 Theodor **Schwann**, German physiologist, born 7 Dec; described pepsin, 1836, *ArA*: p. 90; proved that putrefaction is produced by living bodies, 1837, *AnPh* **41**:184. Played vital role in the development of the cell theory, 1838, and particularly in his *Mikroskopische Untersuchungen über die Übereinstimmung in der Struktur und dem Wachsthum der Thiere und Pflanzen*, in which he also described the neurilemma (' the sheath of Schwann'), 1839. Died 1882. *991, 674, 112.1, 113*

1810: 18 Johann Ludwig **Grandidier** born; first full clinical description of haemophilia; in his *Die Haemophilie oder die Bluterkrankheit*, 1855. *3063*

1810: Jean Louis **Baudelocque** died, **born** 1746. *labour, pelvimeter*

1810: Henry **Cavendish** died, **born** 1731. *hydrogen*

1810: Jean **Descemet** died, **born** 1732. *Descemet's membrane*

**1811**
1811: 1 **School of Salerno** (first mentioned 848) closed by order of Napoleon

1811: 2 **Iridencleisis**, an operation for construction of an artificial **pupil**, introduced by Conrad Johann Martin Langenbeck (1776–1851); in his *Prüfung der Keratonyxis, einer neuen Methode den grauen Staar durch die Hornhaut zu reclinieren oder zu zerstückeln. 5841*

1811: 3 The first book on **cerebrospinal meningitis** was Elisha North's (1771–1843) *Treatise on a malignant epidemic, commonly called spotted fever*; in it he recommended the use of the clinical **thermometer**, not then in general use. *4676*

1811: 4 **Chloroma** first recorded by Allan Burns (1781–1813); in *Observations on the surgical anatomy of the head and neck*, p. 396. *3055*

1811: 5 First complete **chemical analysis of the nervous system**, by Louis Nicolas Vauquelin (1763–1829), *AnMHN* **18**:212. *1389.1*

144

1811:6 Ligation of the **subclavian artery** by Abraham Colles (1773–1843); reported in 1815, *EMSJ* **11**:1. *2936*

1811:7 Charles McCreary (1785–1826) was reported to have performed the first resection of the **clavicle** in the United States, *TKMS* 1853 **2**:276. *4463*

1811:8 First successful ligation of the external **iliac artery** in America by John Syng Dorsey (1783–1818), *ER* **2**:111. *2930*

---

1811:9 John **Hutchinson**, British physician, born 14 Jan; invented the **spirometer**, making possible the determination of the vital capacity of the lungs, 1846. Died 1861. *930*

1811:10 Heinrich **Küchler**, German ophthalmologist, born 23 Apr; introduced readings of print at a distance, for eyesight testing; in his *Schriftnummerprobe für Gesichtsleidende*, 1843. Died 1873. *5858*

1811:11 Amédée **Forget**, French surgeon, born 28 May; treated acute otitis by drainage through the antrum, 1860, *UM* **6**:193. Died 1869. *3371*

1811:12 James Young **Simpson**, British obstetrician and gynaecologist, born 7 Jun; introduced some important procedures and instruments into gynaecology, among them the uterine sound for diagnosing retroposition of the uterus, 1843, *LEMJ* **3**:547, 701, 1009; **4**:208. Discovered the advantages of chloroform over ether as an anaesthetic and was first to adopt it in midwifery, 1847, *LMG* **5**:934; *L* **2**:549. Died 1870. *6035, 5657*

1811:13 Moritz Michael **Eulenburg**, German orthopaedic surgeon, born 15 Jul; first described congenital upward displacement of the scapula ('Sprengel's deformity'), 1863, *ArKC* **4**:304. Died 1877. *4332, 4359*

1811:14 Louis Auguste **Mercier**, French urologist, born 21 Aug; introduced the coudé catheter, 1836, *GHP* **7**:13; followed by the bicoudé *c*1841; diagnosed coarctation of aorta during life, 1839, *BSAP* **14**:158. Died 1882. *4168.1, 2750.1*

1811:15 Pehr Henrik **Malmsten**, Swedish physician, born 12 Sep; discovered *Balantidium coli*, the first parasitic protozoon to be recognized as such, 1857, *Hygiea* **19**:491. With Gustav Wilhelm Johann Düben, gave an accurate account of myocardial infarction, 1859, *Hygiea* **21**:629. Died 1883. *3455, 2761.1*

1811:16 William **Budd**, British physician, born 14 Sep; in his *Typhoid fever; its nature, mode of spreading, and prevention*, 1873, he insisted that typhoid was spread by contagion; he established that infection came from the dejecta of patients. He strengthened the theory of water-borne infection. Died 1880. *5029*

1811:17 John Charles Weaver **Lever**, British obstetrician, born 28 Sep; first reported albuminous urine in connection with puerperal convulsions, 1843, *GHR* **1**:495. Died 1858. *6176*

1811:18 John M. **Riggs**, American dentist, born 21 Oct; described pyorrhoea alveolaris ('Riggs' disease'), 1876, *PJDS* **3**:99. Died 1885. *3685*

1811:19 Thomas Blizard **Curling**, British surgeon, born 7 Dec; directed attention to duodenal ulcer as a complication of burns ('Curling's ulcer'), 1842, *MCT* **25**:260. Accurately described the clinical picture of cretinism, 1850, *MCT* **33**:303, later (1878) named myxoedema by William Miller Ord. Died 1888. *3445, 3838, 3825*

1811:20 Léon **Bassereau** born; first clearly defined chancroid; in his *Traité des affections de la peau symptomatiques de la syphilis*, 1852. Died 1888. *5203*

1811:21 Jonathan Mason **Warren**, American plastic surgeon, born; performed the first rhinoplasty reported in the United States, 1837, *BMSJ* **16**:69; devised an operation for closure of complete clefts of the palate, 1843, *NEQJ* **1**:538. Died 1867. *5743.3, 5745*

1811: Giuseppe **Baronio** died, **born** 1759. *transplantation surgery*

**1812**

1812:1 The first American textbook on **psychiatry**, *Medical inquiries and observations upon the diseases of the mind*, written by Benjamin Rush (1746–1813). *4924*

1812:1.1 *New England Journal of Medicine and Surgery* commences publication; united with *Boston Medical Intelligencer*, 1828 and renamed *Boston Medical and Surgical Journal*; renamed *New England Journal of Medicine*, 1928–

1812:2 Presence of blood and albumin in **dropsical urine** noted by William Charles Wells (1757–1817) who also established that dropsy occurred in the upper part of the body, *TSIM* **3**:194. *4205*

1812:3 The first successful **excision of the lower jaw** performed by Guillaume Dupuytren (1777–1835), *JUSM* **19**:77. *4444*

1812:4 John Cheyne (1777–1836) believed that **cerebral anaemia** might be the cause of **apoplexy**; in his *Cases of apoplexy and lethargy*; in it he published the first illustration of a **subarachnoid haemorrhage**. *4519.1*

1812:5 First report of a case of **appendicitis** in English by John William Keys Parkinson (1785–1838), *MCT* **3**:57; in it perforation was for the first time recognized as a cause of death. *3560*

1812:6 Successful ligation of the common **iliac artery** by William Gibson (1788–1868); reported in 1820, *AmMR* **3**:185. *2944*

1812:7 **Rheumatism** as cause of **heart disease**, first clinical report, credited to William Charles Wells (1757–1817), *TSIM* **3**:373. *2740*

1812:8 The greatest **military surgeon** in history was Dominique Jean Larrey (1766–1842). His *Mémoires de chirurgie militaire* appeared 1812–1817 and includes (**2**, 180) an account of his early successful **amputation** at the **hip-joint**. *2160, 4442*

1812:9 Édouard **Séguin**, French/American psychiatrist, born 20 Jan; first to outline a complete plan for the training of idiots; in his *Traitement moral, hygiène et education des idiots*, 1846. He later worked in America, where he published *Idiocy and its treatment by the physiological method*, 1866. Died 1880. *4937*

1812:10 Casimir Joseph **Davaine**, French physician and microbiologist, born 19 Mar; showed that anthrax could be transmitted to sheep, horses, cattle, guinea-pigs and mice, and that in such animals *Bacillus anthracis* did not appear in the blood until 4–5 hours before death, 1863, *CRSB* **57**:220,351. First conclusively to prove that a specific disease (anthrax) was caused by a specific organism (*B. anthracis*), and was thus one of the first to prove the germ theory of disease, 1865, *CRSB* **60**:1296. Died 1882. *5165, 5166*

1812:11 Carl Ferdinand von **Arlt**, Bohemian ophthalmologist, born 18 Apr; in his *Die Krankheiten des Auges*, 3 vols, 1851–56, described granular conjunctivitis (Arlt's trachoma) and an operation for transplantation of the ciliary bulbs in the treatment of distichiasis. Died 1887. *5865*

1812:12 Filippo **Pacini**, Italian anatomist, born 25 May; described Pacini's corpuscles, the end organs of sensory nerves; in his *Nuovo organi scoperti nel corpo humano*, 1840. Described vibrios seen in the intestinal contents of cholera victims and incriminated them as the pathogen, 1854, anticipating Koch by 30 years, *GMIFT* **4**:397, 405. Died 1883. *1263, 5106.1*

1812:13 James **Bolton**, American ophthalmologist and otologist, born 5 Jun; described new instruments for the treatment of strabismus; in his *Treatise on strabismus*, 1842. Died 1869. *5855*

1812:14 Noah **Worcester**, American physician, born 29 Jul; published the first comprehensive American text on skin diseases, *Synopsis ... of the more common and important diseases of the skin*, 1845. Died 1847. *3991.1*

1812:15 Victor von **Bruns**, German surgeon, born 9 Aug; first to remove a laryngeal polyp by the bloodless method, 1862; in his *Die erste Ausrottung eines Polypen in der Kehlkopfshöhle*. Died 1883. *3268*

1812:16 John Hughes **Bennett**, British physician, born 31 Aug; in his *Treatise on the oleum jecoris aselli, or cod liver oil*, 1841, drew attention to the beneficial effects of cod-liver oil. Gave first definite description of leukaemia, 1845, *EMSJ* **64**:413. Died 1875. *1858, 3061*

1812:17 Austin **Flint**, American physician, born 20 Oct; described the 'Austin Flint murmur', present at the apex beat in aortic regurgitation, 1862, *AmJMS* **44**:29. Died 1886. *2764*

1812:18 Thomas Bevill **Peacock**, British physician, born 21 Dec; gave first comprehensive study of heart malformations; in his *On malformations, etc., of the human heart*, 1858; it included a description of the tetralogy of Fallot. Died 1882. *2761*

---

1812: August Gottlieb **Richter** died, **born** 1742. *enterocele*

1812: Nicolas **Saucerotte** died, **born** 1741. *acromegaly*

1812: Robert **Willan** died, **born** 1757. *dermatology, prurigo mitis, psoriasis, infantile eczema*

## 1813

1813:1 The doctrines laid down by Georg Joseph Beer (1763–1821) in his *Lehre von den Augenkrankheiten*, 2 vols, 1813–17, dominated the practice of **ophthalmology** for many years. *5842*

1813:2 The first systematic treatise on **surgery** written by an American was *Elements of surgery*, by John Syng Dorsey (1783–1818). It also includes some of the works of his uncle, Philip Syng Physick. *5585.1*

1813:3 A classic account of **deglutition** and **vomiting** given by François Magendie (1783–1855); on his *Mémoire sur le vomissement. 985*

1813:4 Alcoholic **delirium tremens** was so named and described by Thomas Sutton (1767–1835); in his *Tracts on delirium tremens*. He differentiated the condition from **phrenitis**. *4925*

1813:5 The pioneer work of Samuel Tuke (1784–1857) advocating humane treatment of the **insane** is set out in his *Description of The Retreat, an institution near York, for insane persons. 4925.1*

1813:6 The most influential textbook of **dermatology** of the 19th century, *Practical synopsis of cutaneous diseases*, published by Thomas Bateman (1778–1821); **lichen urticatus** is first described on p. 13. *4021*

---

1813:7 James Marion **Sims**, American gynaecological surgeon, born 25 Jan; devised an operation for treatment of vesico-vaginal fistula, 1852, *AmJMS* **23**:59; in the same paper he also described the 'Sims' position', the knee-chest position. To avoid sepsis introduced a silver wire suture, described in *Silver sutures in surgery*, 1858. Devised a method for amputating the cervix, 1861, *TNYM*, 367. Wrote the controversial *Clinical notes on uterine surgery, with reference to the management of the sterile condition*, 1866, which includes (p. 16) a description of his duck-billed speculum, and pioneering work in the treatment of infertility and record of a successful artificial insemination. Devised a cholecystotomy for dropsy of the gallbladder, 1878, *BMJ* **1**:811. Died 1883. *6037, 5605, 6049, 6057, 3625*

1813:8 John **Snow**, British physician and anaesthetist, born 15 Mar; the first specialist in anaesthesiology as well as being an epidemiologist. He invented a regulating inhaler to control the amount of ether received by the patient during surgical anaesthesia, described in his *On the inhalation of the vapour of ether in surgical operations*, 1847. Invented a chloroform inhaler, 1848, *L* **1**:177. Demonstrated the water-borne character of cholera, 1849, *LMG* **44**:730, 745, 923. Attempted carbon dioxide absorption anaesthesia, 1851, *LMG* **11**:479; **12**:622. In 1853 and 1857 he delivered Queen Victoria, using chloroform. His work *On chloroform and other anaesthetics: their action and administration*, 1858, put the administration of chloroform and ether on a scientific basis. Died 1858. *5658, 5663, 5106, 5665, 5666*

1813:9 David **Livingstone**, British physician and explorer, born 19 Mar; gave an accurate account of the tsetse fly, *Glossina morsitans*, and of the disease in cattle, trypanosomiasis, due to its bite; in his *Missionary travels and researches in South Africa*, 1857, pp. 80, 571; administered arsenic in the treatment of 'nagana', trypanosomiasis in horses, 1858, *BMJ*: 360. Died 1873. *5269, 5270*

1813:10 Hermann **Lebert**, Polish physician and pathologist, born 9 Jun; gave the first systematic account of brain abscess, 1856, *VA* **10**:78, 352. Died 1878. *4638*

1813:11 Claude **Bernard**, French physiologist, born 12 Jul; investigated the glycogenic function of the liver, 1848, *ArGM* **18**:303, completed 1855, *CRAS* **41**:461. Discovered vasomotor nerves, 1852, *CRSB* **3**:163. Described the mode of action of curare, 1856, *CRAS*

**43**:825. Discovered the role of the pancreatic juice in digestion, 1857, *ArGM* **19**:60. Discovered glycogen 1857, *CRSB* 2 sér.4:147; experimented with curare, *Leçons sur les effets des substances toxiques* ... 1857. Reported as early as 1864 that chloroform anaesthesia could be prolonged by the injection of morphine; recorded in his *Leçons sur les anesthésiques et sur l'asphyxie*, 1875. Showed that in diabetes mellitus there is primarily glycaemia followed by glycosuria; in his *Leçons sur le diabète et la glycogenèse animale*, 1877. Died 1878. *995, 1000, 996, 2079, 1320, 999.1, 1863, 5673, 3942*

1813:12 Alexander Patrick **Stewart**, British physician, born 28 Aug; typhoid and typhus were often confused, he analysed a number of cases of both, and clearly demonstrated that they were two distinct fevers, 1840, *EMSJ* **54**:289. Died 1885. *5025*

1813:13 Frank Hastings **Hamilton**, American surgeon, born 10 Sep; among the first to treat ulcers by skin grafts, as described in his *Elkoplasty, or anaplasty applied to the treatment of old ulcers*, 1854. Died 1886. *5747*

1813:14 Gaspard Adolph **Chatin**, French pharmacist, born 30 Nov; showed that endemic goitre and cretinism could be prevented by iodine, 1850, *CRAS* **30**:352. Died 1901. *3817*

1813:15 Angelo **Dubini**, Italian physician, born 8 Dec. First found the hookworm of ankylostomiasis in 1838, publishing a report in 1843 in which he named it *Agchylostoma duodenale*, an etymologically erroneous name, *AnU* **106**:5; gave the first description of electric chorea ('Dubini's chorea'), the myoclonic form of epidemic encephalitis, 1846, *AnU* **117**:5. Died 1902. *5353, 4637*

---

1813:16 Philipp Friedrich Hermann **Klencke**, German physician, born; demonstrated tuberculosis transmission by cow's milk; *Ueber die Ansteckung und Verbreitung der Scrophelkrankheit bei Menschen durch den Genuss der Kuhmilch*, 1846. Died 1881. *2323*

1813:17 Sulpice Antoine **Fauvel**, French physician, born; first described presystolic murmur in mitral stenosis, 1843, *ArGM* **1**:1. Died 1884. *2754*

1813.18 George Owen **Rees**, British physician, born; with George Hilaro Barlow, described subacute bacterial endocarditis, 1843, *GHR* n.s.1:189. Died 1889. *2753*

1813:19 James **Robinson** born; a British dentist, he wrote the first textbook on surgical anaesthesia, *A treatise on the inhalation of the vapour of ether for the prevention of pain in surgical operations*, 1847. Died 1861. *5657.1*

---

1813: Johann Christian **Reil** died, **born** 1759. *island of Reil*

1813: Allan **Burns** died, **born** 1781. *angina pectoris, chloroma*

1813: Charles **White** died, **born** 1728. *excision of head of humerus, shoulder dislocation, puerperal fever, phlegmasia alba dolens*

1813: Benjamin **Rush** died, **born** 1746. *psychiatry, yellow fever, dengue*

1813: Francis **Home** died, **born** 1719. *diphtheria, measles*

**1814**

1814:1 The description of the fracture of the carpal end of the **radius** given by Abraham Colles (1773–1843), *EMSJ* **10**:182, led to the term '**Colles' fracture**'. *4410*

1814:2 The first full-length book on **dentistry** in the United States, *A treatise on the management of the teeth*, published by Benjamin James. *3679.3*

1814:3 Infantile **eczema** described by Robert Willan (1757–1812); in his *On cutaneous diseases (Practical treatise on prurigo)*. *4021.1*

1814:4 First monograph on **congenital abnormalities** of the **heart**, *Pathological researches, Essay 1*, published by John Richard Farre (1775–1862). *2740.1*

1814:5 First successful ligation of the common **carotid artery** for **aneurysm** in America by Philip Wright Post (1766–1828), *AmMPR* **4**:366. *2934*

1814:6 First successful ligation of the internal **iliac artery** by William Stevens (1786–1868), *MCT* **5**:422. *2935*

1814:7 First surgery for **varicose veins** by Benjamin Brodie (1783–1862), *MCT* **7**:195. *2994*

---

1814:8 James **Paget**, British surgeon and pathologist, born 11 Jan; discovered trichina (*Trichinella spiralis*) in human muscle, 1835; his discovery was reported by Richard Owen in 1835 and by Paget in 1866, *TZS* **1**:315. First described eczema of the nipple, due to underlying cancer of the breast, 'Paget's disease of the nipple', 1874, *SBHR* **10**:87. Gave an important description of osteitis deformans, which led to the condition being called Paget's disease of bone, 1877, *MCT* **60**:37; **65**:225. Died 1899. *5337, 5772, 4343*

1814:9 John **Goodsir**, British anatomist and pathologist, born 20 Mar; discovered *Sarcina ventriculi*, 1842, *EMSJ* **57**:430. Died 1867. *2471*

1814:10 Adolph **Hannover**, Danish pathologist, born 24 Nov; coined the term 'epithelioma'; in his *Das Epithelioma*, 1852. Died 1894. *2615*

1814:11 Jean Nicolas **Demarquay**, French surgeon, born 14 Dec; described the embryonic stage of *Wuchereria bancrofti*, 1863, *GMP* **33**:665. Died 1875. *5344.3*

1814:12 Wenzel Leopold **Gruber**, Bohemian pathological anatomist, born 24 Dec; described internal mesogastric hernia ('Gruber's hernia'), 1863, *OZPH* **9**:325, 341. Died 1890. *3592*

1814:13 Henry Bence **Jones**, British physician, born 31 Dec; described myelopathic albumosuria (Bence-Jones proteinuria), 1847, *PT* **138**:55; he found it to be present in a patient of W. Macintyre suffering from multiple myeloma. Died 1873. *4326, 4327*

---

1814:14 François Jules **Lemaire**, French scientist, born; drew attention to the antiseptic properties of carbolic acid; in his *Du coaltar saponiné, désinfectant énergique*, 1860. Died 1886. *1864*

1814:15 Robert **Paterson**, British physician, born; with William Henderson, described the inclusion body of molluscum contagiosum, 1841, *EMSJ* **56**:213, 279. Died 1889. *4031, 4032*

1814:16 Louis **Bauer**, German/American orthopaedic surgeon, born; published the first comprehensive American textbook of orthopaedics, *Lectures on orthopaedic surgery*, 1864. Died 1898. *4334*

---

1814: Eduard **Sandifort** died, **born** 1742. *Fallot's tetralogy*

1814: Pierre **Fine** died, **born** 1760. *intestinal obstruction, colostomy*

1814: Gaspard **Vieusseux** died, **born** 1746. *cerebral meningitis*

1814: Philibert **Chabert** died, **born** 1737. *anthrax*

1814: Wilhelm Gottfried **Ploucquet** died, **born** 1744. *medical bibliography*

1814: Joseph Ignace **Guillotin** died, **born** 1738. *guillotine for humane capital punishment*

## 1815

1815:1 **'Lisfranc's amputation'** of the **foot** recorded by Jacques Lisfranc (1790–1847); in his *Nouvelle méthode opératoire pour l'amputation partielle du pied. 4443*

1815:2 *Commentaries on some of the most important diseases of children*, by John Clarke (1761–1815) includes clear descriptions of **tetany** and **laryngismus stridulus**. *4825, 6328*

1815:3 Christophe François Delabarre (1777–1862) was one of the first to systematize occlusal anomalies and to develop **orthodontic** appliances; in his *Odontologie. 3679.4*

1815:4 Caleb Hillier Parry (1755–1822) gave one of the first accounts of **exophthalmic goitre**; in his *Elements of pathology and therapeutics*; a classic account is included in the *Collections from the unpublished medical writings of C.H. Parry*, **2**, 111–29, 1825. *3813*

1815:5 First important work on **olfaction**, *Dissertation sur les odeurs*, published by Jules Hippolyte Cloquet (1787–1840). *3253*

1815:6 **Pericardiocentesis** successfully performed by Francisco Romero, *BFM* **4**:373. *3021*

1815:7 Michel Eugène Chevreul (1786–1889) proved that sugar in **diabetic urine** is **glucose**, *AnC* **95**:319. *3931*

1815:8 *On gunshot wounds of the extremities* by George James Guthrie (1785–1856) is one of the most important books in the history of the subject. As reported in the 2nd edition, *Treatise on gun-shot wounds*, p. 332, 1820, he successfully **amputated** at the **hip-joint**, after the Battle of Waterloo, 7 July 1815; at the same time he was successful in **ligation** of the **peroneal artery**, 1816, *MCT* **7**:330 *2161, 4445, 2937*

1815:9 *Carlisle Tables of Mortality* published by Joshua Milne (1776–1851), British actuary to Sun Life Assurance Co. He reconstructed the life tables then in use, based upon the table deduced from the burial registers of All Saints Church, Northampton, 1735–80. Milne took as the basis of his calculations the Carlisle bills of mortality which had been prepared by Dr John Heysham (1753–1834) and published *A treatise on the valuation of annuities and assurances on lives and survivorship*, etc., 2 vols, London, 1815, the 'Carlisle Tables of Mortality' [Bills of mortality: weekly statement formerly issued by parish clerks in England, showing the number of deaths (and the causes) that had occurred in each parish]. The age of the person dying was not included until the year 1778, from which year dates the 'science' of **life assurance**.

1815: 10 **Cholesterol** defined by Michel Eugène Chevreul (1786–1889), *AnC* **95**:5. *668.2*

---

1815: 11 Horace **Wells**, American dentist and anaesthetist, born 21 Jan; used nitrous oxide successfully as a dental anaesthetic. He wrote *A history of the discovery of the application of nitrous oxide gas, ether, and other vapours, to surgical operations*, 1847. Died 1848. *5660*

1815: 12 William **Jenner**, British physician, born 30 Jan; showed that the aetiology of typhus and typhoid were quite different, that one did not communicate with, or protect against, the other, and that epidemics of the two did not prevail simultaneously, 1849, *MJMS* **9**:663. Died 1898. *5027*

1815: 13 John **Tomes**, British dental surgeon, born 21 Mar; played an important part in the development of dental education in Britain. He wrote *Course of lectures on dental physiology and surgery*, 1848, and invented a set of anatomically correct dental forceps. Died 1895. *3683*

1815: 14 William Robert Wills **Wilde**, British surgeon, otologist and oculist, born 9 Apr; published the first modern British work on otology, *Practical observations on aural surgery* ..., 1853. Died 1876. *3369*

1815: 15 Daniel Cornelius **Danielssen**, Norwegian physician, born 4 Jul; with Carl Wilhelm Boeck, published the first modern description of leprosy ('Danielssen-Boeck disease'); in *Om spedalskhed*, 1847. Died 1894. *2434*

1815: 16 Julius Thomas **Thomsen**, Danish physician, born 19 Jul; gave the first full description of myotonia congenita, from which he himself suffered, 1876, *ArPN* **6**:702, and which later became known as 'Thomsen's disease'. Died 1896. *4744*

1815: 17 Robert **Remak**, German physiologist and neuroanatomist, born 26 Jul. He discovered the non-medullated nerve-fibres ('fibres of Remak'), 1836, *ArA* p. 145; was first to describe the intrinsic ganglia of the heart, 1844, *ArA* p. 463; he was a pioneer in galvanotherapy, published *Galvanotherapie der Nerven- und Muskelkrankheiten*, 1858. Died 1865. *1260, 806, 4534*

1815: 18 Carl **Wunderlich**, German physician, born 4 Aug; published classical work on clinical thermometry; in his *Das Verhalten der Eigenwärme in Krankheiten*, 1868. Died 1877. *2677*

1815: 19 Carl Conrad Theodor **Litzmann**, German gynaecologist, born 7 Oct; described the coxalgic, scoliotic and kyphoscoliotic forms of pelvis; in his *Das schräg-ovale Becken*, 1852. His clinical classification of pelves, in his *Die Formen des Beckens, insbesondere des engen weiblichen Beckens*, 1861, was in general use until supplanted by that of Caldwell and Moloy (1933); he described various deformities of the female pelvis. He described 'Litzmann's obliquity' or posterior parietal presentation, 1871, *ArGy* **25**:182. Died 1890. *6260, 6263, 6263.1*

1815: 20 Crawford Williamson **Long**, American surgeon and anaesthetist, born 1 Nov; although he was first, on 30 March 1842, successfully to use ether as an anaesthetic, he did not publish his results until 1849, *SMSJ* **5**:705. Died 1878. *5664*

1815:21 Joseph **Toynbee**, British aural surgeon, born 30 Dec; laid the foundations of aural pathology; in his *Diseases of the ear* ..., 1860. Died 1866. *3373*

1815:22 Raffaele **Piria**, Italian chemist, born; made salicylic acid from salicin, 1839, *CRAS* **8**:479. Died 1865. *1857*

1815:23 Lucas Anton **Dressler**, German physician, born; first described paroxysmal cold haemoglobinuria, 1854, *VA* **6**:264. Died 1896. *4169.2*

1815: John **Clarke** died, **born** 1761. *diseases of children, tetany, laryngismus stridulus*

1815: Franz Anton **Mesmer** died, **born** 1734. *mesmerism, animal magnetism*

1815: John Coakley **Lettsom** died, **born** 1744. *alcoholism, Medical Society of London, General Dispensary, Aldersgate*

## 1816
1816:1 **Royal Ear Hospital, London**, founded

1816:2 **University of Ghent** founded

1816:3 **University of Liège** founded

1816:4 **University of Warsaw** founded

1816:5 **[Polish Academy of Sciences]** founded in Cracow

1816:6 The 'Father of American surgery', Philip Syng Physick (1768–1837), introduced several new procedures into **surgery**, including the use of absorbable kid and buckskin **ligatures**, *ER* **6**:389. *5586*

1816:7 The Hindu method of **rhinoplasty** revived by Joseph Constantine Carpue (1764–1846), who reported two successful cases; in his *An account of two successful operations for restoring a lost nose from the integuments of the forehead. 5737*

1816:8 Closure of a congenital **cleft palate** reported by Carl Ferdinand von Graefe (1787–1840), *JCA* **1**:1. *5739*

1816:9 The first accurate description of **keloid** ('**Alibert's keloid**') provided by Jean Louis Marc Alibert (1768–1837), *JUSM* **2**:207. *4023*

1816:10 William **Bowman**, British ophthalmic surgeon, born 20 Jul; his classical work on the kidney led to the eponym 'Bowman's capsule', 1842, *PT* **132**:57. Devised an operation for the formation of an artificial pupil, 1852, *MTG* **4**:11, 33. Died 1892. *1231, 5867*

1816:11 Charles **West**, British physician, born 8 Aug; his *Lectures on the diseases of infancy and childhood*, 1848, was in its day the best English work on paediatrics. West was one of the founders of the Hospital for Sick Children, Gt Ormond Street, London. Died 1898. *6334*

1816:12 Ernest Charles **Lasègue**, French physician, born 5 Sep. Described persecution mania ('Lasègue's disease'), 1852, *ArGM* **28**:129; observed 'Lasègue's sign' in sciatica; it was actually reported by his pupil, J.J. Forst, 1881 (*Contribution à l'étude clinique de la sciatique*, Paris, Thèse No. 33). Died 1883. *4931, 4563*

1816:13 Ferdinand von **Hebra**, Austrian dermatologist, born 7 Sep; his classification of skin diseases, 1845, was based on their pathological anatomy, *ZGA* **2**:34, 143, 211. Gave first description of pityriasis rubra ('Hebra's pityriasis'), 1857, *AWMZ* **2**:75. First described impetigo herpetiformis, 1872, *WMW* **22**:1197; it was more exhaustively dealt with by his son-in-law, Moritz Kaposi, in 1887. Died 1880. *3991, 4045, 4062, 4091*

1816:14 Carl Ferdinand **Eichstedt**, German physician, born 17 Sep; discovered *Pityrosporum orbiculare*, the fungus causing pityriasis versicolor, 1846, *NNGN* **38**:105; **39**:265, 270. Died 1892. *4038, 4039*

1816:15 Thomas **Longmore** born 10 Oct; while serving as a British army surgeon in India he gave an important account of heatstroke, 1859, *IAMS* **6**:396. Died 1895. *2248*

1816:16 John **Simon**, British physician and surgeon, born 10 Oct; first performed uretero-intestinal anastomosis, 1852, *L* **2**:568. A great sanitary reformer; his *English sanitary institutions*, 1890, led to modern developments and legislation in public health. Died 1904. *4169.1, 1650*

1816:17 Augustus Volney **Waller**, British physiologist, born 21 Dec; established the 'law of Wallerian degeneration' of nerves, 1850, *PT* **140**:423. Died 1870. *1266*

1816:18 Carl **Ludwig**, German physiologist, born 29 Dec; wrote an important monograph on renal secretion, *Beiträge zur Lehre vom Mechanismus der Harnsekretion*, 1843; elucidated the innervation of the salivary glands, 1851, *ZRM* **1**:254; invented the kymograph, 1847, by modifying Poiseuille's haemodynamometer, *ArA* 242; introduced the idea of maintaining excised organs by means of perfusion, *Die physiologischen Leistungen des Blutdrucks*, 1865. Died 1895. *1232, 770, 998, 778*

1816:19 William Withey **Gull**, British physician, born 31 Dec; showed that the lesions of locomotor ataxia (tabes dorsalis) are located in the posterior columns of the spinal cord, 1856, *GHR* **2**:143; **4**:169. First to describe syringomyelia, 1862, *GHR* **8**:244. With Henry Gawen Sutton, gave first clear description of arteriosclerotic atrophy of the kidney, and a description of hypertensive nephrosclerosis, 1872, *MCT* **55**:273. Was among the first to ascertain the cause of myxoedema, 1873, *TCSL* **7**:180. Gave classic description of anorexia, 1874, *TCSL* **7**:22. Died 1890. *4532, 4695, 4215, 3823, 4845*

1816:20 Frederic John **Mouat**, British physician, born; introduced chaulmoogra oil into Western medicine, for the treatment of leprosy, 1854, *IAMS* **1**:646. Died 1897. 2435

1816:21 James Henry **Bennet**, British gynaecologist, born; first to differentiate between benign and malignant tumours of the uterus; in his *A practical treatise on inflammation, ulceration and induration of the neck of the uterus*, 1845. Died 1891. *6036*

1816:22 Alois **Bednař**, Austrian paediatrician, born; his description of aphthae of the palate in the newborn given in his *Die Krankheiten der Neugeborenen und Säuglinge*, 1850, **1**, 104, led to the eponym 'Bednar's aphthae'. Died 1888. *6335*

1816: Michael Vincenzo Giacinto **Malacarne** died, **born** 1744. *cerebellum, cretinism, goitre*

1816: Gaspard Laurent **Bayle** died, **born** 1774. *tuberculosis*

1816: Franz Kaspar **Hesselbach** died, **born** 1759. *Hesselbach's hernia and triangle*

1816: Antonio de **Gimbernat** died, **born** 1734. *femoral hernia, crural ligament*

1816: Joseph **Fox** died, **born** 1775. *teeth, orthodontics*

1816: Anselme Louis Bernard Berchillet **Jourdain** died, **born** 1734. *oral surgery*

1816: Joseph **Huddart** died, **born** 1741. *colour-blindness*

**1817**
1817:1 **Medical Society of the District of Columbia** founded in **Washington**

1817:2 **Congenital malformations** are an important feature of Johann Friedrich Meckel's (1781–1833) *Tabulae anatomico-pathologicae*, 1817–26. *2284*

1817:3 **Emetine** isolated by Pierre Joseph Pelletier (1788–1842) and François Magendie (1783–1855), *AnC* **4**:172. *1843*

1817:4 Unsuccessful attempt to ligate the **abdominal aorta** by Astley Paston Cooper (1768–1841); in his *Surgical essays* …. *2941*

1817:5 **Auscultation** as a diagnostic measure was described by François Joseph Double (?1776–1842); in his *Séméiologie générale*, vol. 2. *2672.2*

1817:6 First successful ligation of the **subclavian artery**, outside the scalenus muscles, by Philip Wright Post (1766–1828), *TPNY* **1**:387. *2939*

1817:7 In *A cursory inquiry into some of the principal causes of mortality among children*, John Bunnell Davis (1780–1824) drew attention to the high **infant mortality rate**, especially in London. His suggestion that poor mothers be instructed in infant care resulted in a system of **health-visiting** by benevolent ladies. A children's dispensary he founded in 1816 later became the Royal Waterloo Hospital for Children and Women. *6330*

1817:8 The first **ovariotomy** performed by the pioneer ovariotomist Ephraim McDowell (1771–1830), *ER* **7**:242. *6023*

1817:9 The first successful operation for **ectopic pregnancy** recorded by John King, *MRep* **3**:388; in the following year he published an expanded account in book form. *6166*

1817:10 **Paralysis agitans** ('**Parkinson's disease**') first described by James Parkinson (1755–1824); in his *Essay on the shaking palsy. 4690*

1817:11 The first important account of **tabes dorsalis** published by Sigismund Eduard Loewenhardt (1796–1875); in his *De myelophthisie chronica vera et notha. 4772*

1817:12 Classic description of **achondroplasia** given by Moritz Heinrich Romberg (1795–1873); in his graduation thesis, *De rachitide congenita. 4310*

1817:13 **Carcinoma** of the **prostate** first reported by George Langstaff (1780–1846), *MCT* **8**:272. *4258*

1817:14 Thomas Bateman's (1778–1821) *Delineations of cutaneous diseases* …, which contained 72 coloured plates, may be regarded as the first atlas of **dermatology**. It included original descriptions of several skin diseases. *3988*

———

1817:15 Charles Édouard **Brown-Séquard**, French physician and physiologist, born Mauritius, 8 Apr; showed that lesion of one lateral half of the spinal cord causes paralysis of motion on one side and sensory loss on the other ('Brown-Séquard's paralysis'), 1850, *CRSB* **2**:3. Produced experimental epilepsy by section of the sciatic nerve, 1856, *ArGM* **7**:143; proved the indispensability of the adrenal glands, 1856, *CRAS* **43**:422, 542. Died 1894. *4530, 4813, 1140*

1817:16 Rudolph Hermann **Lotze**, German psychologist, born 21 May; wrote *Medicinische Psychologie, oder Physiologie der Seele*, 1852, and was a pioneer in the investigation of unconscious and subconscious states. Died 1881. *4970*

1817:17 John Murray **Carnochan**, American surgeon, born 4 Jul; carried out the first excision of the superior maxillary nerve for the treatment of facial neuralgia, 1858, *AmJMS* **35**:134. Died 1887. *4854*

1817:18 Rudolf Albert von **Kölliker**, Swiss comparative anatomist, embryologist and histologist, born 6 July. He determined the cellular nature of spermatozoa, 1841, *NNGN* **19**:4. In his *Handbuch der Gewebelehre des Menschen*, 1852, appeared his classification of tissue. Published the first study of the effects of poisons on muscular contraction, 1856, *VA* **10**:3, 335. His *Entwicklungsgeschichte des Menschen und der höheren Thiere*, 1861, was the first book on comparative embryology. Died 1905. *1220, 546, 2078, 487*

1817:19 François Amilcar **Aran**, French physician, born 12 Jul; independently of Duchenne, described progressive muscular atrophy ('Aran-Duchenne disease'), 1850, *ArGM* **24**:4,132. Died 1861. *4733*

1817:20 Wilhelm **Griesinger**, German physician, born 29 Jul; considered tropical anaemia to be due to the hookworm causing ankylostomiasis, 1854, *ArPH* **13**:528. First to report splenic anaemia, in an infant, 1866, *BKW* **3**:212. Died 1868. *5355, 3766*

1817:21 August **Hirsch**, Austrian physician and medical historian, born 4 Oct; compiled one of the best sources of medical biography to 1880, *Biographisches Lexikon der hervorragenden Ärzte aller Zeiten und Völker*, 6 vols, 1884–1888. A supplement by I. Fischer appeared in 1932–33. Died 1894. *6716, 6732.*

1817:22 Alexander **Wood**, British physician, born 10 Dec; first to employ hypodermic injection as therapeutic measure, 1853, *EMSJ* **82**:265. Died 1884. *1969*

1817:23 John Charles **Bucknill**, British psychiatrist, born 25 Dec; with Daniel Hack Tuke, published *A manual of psychological medicine*, 1858, for many years the standard English work on the subject. Died 1897. *4934*

———

1817:24 Jacob Augustus Lockhart **Clarke**, British anatomist, born; with John Hughlings Jackson, published an important account of syringomyelia, 1867, *MCT* **50**:489. Died 1880. *4697*

———

156

1817: William Charles **Wells** died, **born** 1757. *rheumatism, dropsy, heart disease*

1817: Alexander **Monro**, Secundus, died, **born** 1733. *foramen of Monro*

**1818**
1818:1 **University of St Louis, Missouri,** founded

1818:2 **Charing Cross Hospital, London,** founded

1818:3 **Pepinière, Berlin,** becomes **Friedrich Wilhelms Institut**

1818:4 **Gesellschaft für Natur- und Heilkunde, Dresden,** founded

1818:5 First accurate account of **Cheyne-Stokes respiration** by John Cheyne (1777–1836), *DHR* **2**:216; more fully described by William Stokes, 1854. *2743*

1818:6 Artificial **induction of premature labour** reported by Carl Wenzel (1769–1827); in his *Allgemeine geburtshülfliche Betrachtungen und über die künstliche Frühgeburt. 6168*

1818:7 The *Handbuch der Entbindungskunst*, 1818–1825, of Friedrich Benjamin Osiander (1759–1822) includes (Bd.2, Abt.II, 302) a description of his lower segment **caesarean section**. *6237*

1818:8 In his *An analysis of the subject of extrauterine foetation and of retroversion of the gravid uterus*, John King gave an expanded account of his first successful operation for **ectopic pregnancy**. *6167*

1818:9 **Rhinoplasty** revived in Germany by Carl Ferdinand von Graefe (1787–1840). In his *Rhinoplastik, oder die Kunst den Verlust der Nase organisch zu ersetzen*, he surveyed the Italian, Indian and 'German' methods, the last being his own variation of the Italian method; on p. 13 he described the first successful **blepharoplasty**. *5738*

1818:10 The first clinical account of **ankylosing spondylitis** and a description of **hysterical pseudofracture of the spine** given by Benjamin Collins Brodie (1783–1862); in his *Pathological and surgical observations on the diseases of the joints. 4311*

1818:11 Successful treatment of **aneurysm** by compression by Guillaume Dupuytren (1777–1835), *BFM* **6**:242. *2976*

1818:12 **Tuberculosis**; early clinical studies by Gaspard Laurent Bayle (1774–1816); his *Recherches sur la phthisie pulmonaire* marks the beginning of modern clinical work on tuberculosis. *2322*

1818:13 First ligation of the **innominate artery** by Valentine Mott (1785–1865), *MSR* **1**:9. *2942*

1818:14 The distinction between **amoebic** and **bacillary dysentery** first made by George Ballingall (1780–1855); in his *Practical observations on fever, dysentery and liver complaints as they occur amongst European troops in India. 5182.1*

1818: 15 Ludwig **Traube**, German physician and pathologist, born 12 Jan; gave first clear description of the rhythmic variations in tone of the vasoconstrictor centre 'Traube-Hering waves', 1865, *ZMW* **3**:881 and of pulsus alternans, 1872, *BKW* **9**:185, 221. Died 1876. *818, 2775*

1818: 16 Thomas Spencer **Wells**, British surgeon, born 3 Feb; was among the most eminent of the ovariotomists; he wrote *Diseases of the ovaries*, 1865, and a second work with the same title in 1872; introduced a pressure forceps ('Spencer Wells forceps'), 1879, *BMJ* **1**:926; **2**:3. Died 1897. *6056, 5615*

1818: 17 Henry Jacob **Bigelow**, American surgeon, born 11 Mar; reported the first surgical operation in which ether anaesthesia was used, it was induced by William Thomas Green Morton and the operation was performed by John Collins Warren, 1846, *BMSJ* **35**:309, 379. Performed the first excision of the hip-joint in the United States, 1852, *AmJMS* **24**:90. Described the mechanism of the iliofemoral ('Bigelow's') ligament and showed its importance in the reduction of dislocation of the hip-joint by the flexion method; in his *The mechanism of dislocation and fracture of the hip*, 1869. Introduced litholapaxy (lithotrity at one sitting), 1878, *AmJMS* **75**:117. Died 1890. *5651, 4461, 4424, 4292*

1818: 18 Eugène **Bouchut**, French physician, born 18 May; gave the first adequate description of neurasthenia; in his *De l'état nerveux aigu et chronique ou nervosisme*, 1860. Died 1891. *4535*

1818: 19 Frans Cornelis **Donders**, Dutch ophthalmologist, born 27 May; in his *Astigmatisme en cilindrische glazen*, 1862, he stated 'Donders' law' – the rotation of the eye around the line of sight is not voluntary. His *On the anomalies of accommodation and refraction of the eye*, 1864, was his most important work. Included in it is his explanation of astigmatism, his definition of aphakia and hypermetropia, and his distinction between myopia and hypermetropia. The first to measure the reaction time of a psychical process, 1868, *ArA* p. 657. Died 1889. *5889, 5893, 4974*

1818: 20 Karl **Vierordt**, German physiologist, born 1 Jul; invented a sphygmograph, with which a tracing of the pulse could be made, 1854, *ArPH* **13**:284. Died 1884. *772, 2759*

1818: 21 Ignaz Philipp **Semmelweis**, Hungarian obstetrician, born 1 Jul; a pioneer of antisepsis in obstetrics, he was the first to recognize that puerperal fever is a septicaemia. He concluded that doctors and students carried the infection from the autopsy room to the maternity wards, and he instituted preventive measures, 1847, *ZGA* **4**, 2:242; **5**:64. His *Die Aetiologie, der Begriff und die Prophylaxis des Kindbettfiebers* is one of the epoch-making books in medical literature. He enlarged his earlier paper (1847), classifying puerperal fever as a septicaemia, and strove to improve conditions in the lying-in wards of Vienna and Budapest. Died 1865. *6275, 6277*

1818: 22 John Eric **Erichsen**, Danish born British surgeon, born 19 Jul; his *On railway and other injuries of the nervous system*, 1866, was the first book to discuss whiplash injuries. Died 1896. *4538.1*

1818: 23 Emil **du Bois-Reymond**, German founder of modern electrophysiology, born 7 Nov; gave the first description and definition of electrotonus, 1843, *AnPh* **58**:1; collective edition of his writings, *Untersuchungen über die thierische Elektricität*, 1848–1884. Died 1896. *609, 610*

1818: 24 Max Joseph von **Pettenkofer**, German chemist and hygienist, born 3 Dec. Developed a colour reaction for bile, 1844, *ACP* **52**:90. With Carl von Voit, carried out combined feeding-respiration experiments, being first to estimate the amounts of protein, fat and carbohydrate broken down in the body, 1862–3, *ACP* Suppl. **2**:52. Planned the sewage system of Munich; in his *Das Kanal- oder Siel-System in München*, 1869. Died 1901. *679, 938, 1618*

1818: 25 William **Moon**, British inventor, born 18 Dec; becoming blind in 1840, devised a simplified form of roman letters, embossed on paper, for use by blind readers, in 1845. Recorded in his *Light for the blind: a history of the origin of Moon's system of reading ... for the blind*, 1873. Died 1894. *5909*

1818: 26 Norman **Chevers**, British physician, born; gave first clear account of chronic constrictive pericarditis, 1842, *GHR* **7**:387. Died 1886. *2752*

1818: 27 Eduard **Jaeger**, Austrian ophthalmologist, born; introduced his sight test types; in his *Schriftskalen*, 1854. Published a fine ophthalmoscopic atlas, *Ophthalmoskopischer Hand-Atlas*, 1869. The illustrations were reproduced from Jaeger's own paintings, each of which required from 20–50 sittings of from 2–3 hours. Died 1884. *5887, 5904*

1818: Johann Gottlieb **Walter** died, **born** 1734. *peritonitis*

1818: John Syng **Dorsey** died, **born** 1783. *surgery, iliac artery ligation*

1818: Johan Valentin von **Hildenbrand** died, **born** 1763. *typhus*

**1819**
1819: 1 **University of St Petersburg** founded

1819: 2 **Harvard Medical School Library** founded

1819: 3 Jean Georges Chrétien Frédéric Martin **Lobstein** (1777–1835) appointed to **first chair of pathology (Strassburg)**

1819: 4 **Medical College of Ohio** founded

1819: 5 The account of the mechanism of **labour** by Franz Carl Naegele (1778–1851), *DAP* **5**:483, was the best work of its time. *6169*

1819: 6 **Instrumental auscultation** established as an important method of diagnosis by René Théophile Hyacinthe Laennec (1781–1826), made possible by his invention of the **stethoscope**; in his *De l'auscultation médiate*; he first described **chronic interstitial hepatitis ('Laennec's cirrhosis')** in the same work, **1**, p. 368. *3219, 2673, 3614*

1819: 7 **Hay fever** ('Bostock's catarrh'); classical description by John Bostock (1773–1846), *MCT* **10**:161. *2582*

1819: 8 Philibert Joseph Roux (1789–1854) repaired the **cleft palate** of a medical student (*JUSM* **16**:356), John Stephenson, who described the operation in his own graduation thesis (1820). Roux published a detailed account of the operation (for which he proposed the name '**staphylorrhaphy**' (1825), *ArGM* **7**:516. *5739.1, 5740, 5741.2*

1819: 9 **Jacob's membrane** in the retina described by Arthur Jacob (1790–1874), *PT* **109**:300. *1491*

1819: 10 Isolation of **strychnine** by Pierre Joseph Pelletier (1788–1842) and Joseph Bienaimé Caventou (1795–1877), *JPC* **5**:145. *1844*

1819: 11 First human-to-human **blood transfusion** by James Blundell (1790–1877), *MCT* **9**:56. *2015.1*

1819: 12 Friedrich Heinrich **Rinne**, German physician, born 24 Jan; devised a test for the measurement of hearing, 1855, *VPH* **45**:71; **46**:45. Died 1868. *3370*

1819: 13 Friedrich Theodor **Frerichs**, German pathologist, born 24 Mar; gave the first important account of multiple sclerosis, 1849, *ArGesM* **10**:334; published the first description of progressive familial hepatolenticular degeneration ('Kinnier Wilson's disease'), in his *Klinik der Leberkrankheiten*, **2**, 62, 1861. Died 1885. *4692, 4693*

1819: 14 Joseph William **Bazalgette**, British engineer, born 28 Mar; he planned the sewers of London, in his *Metropolitan Board of Works Report on experiments with respect to the ventilation of sewers*, 1866–69. Died 1891. *1615*

1819: 15 Archibald Baring **Garrod**, British physician, born 13 May. Described cystinuria, 1848, *TPS* **1**:126. He was the leading authority of his time on gout (which he separated from other forms of arthritis), introduced the 'thread test', 1854, *MCT* **31**:83; **37**:49. Published *The nature and treatment of gout and rheumatic gout*, 1859, and gave rheumatoid arthritis its present name. Died 1907. *3912.1, 4495, 4497*.

1819: 16 Ernst Wilhelm von **Brücke**, German physiologist, born 6 Jun; studied the luminosity of the eye in animals, 1845, by passing a tube through a candle flame he was able to see the fundus, *ArA* 387. Died 1892. *5859*

1819: 17 Julius Otto Ludwig **Möller**, German physician, born 7 Jun; first described acute rickets combined with scurvy ('Barlow's disease'), 1859, *KMJ* **1**:377. Died 1887. *3718, 3720*

1819: 18 Friedrich Eduard Rudolph **Voltolini**, German otolaryngologist, born 17 Jun; first to use galvanocautery in surgery of larynx; in his *Die Anwendung der Galvanokaustik …*, 1867. Performed first laryngeal operation through the mouth with external illumination, 1889, *DMW* **15**:340. Died 1889. *3275, 3302*

1819: 19 William Thomas Green **Morton**, American dentist, born 9 Aug; induced ether anaesthesia for the first time during a surgical operation performed by John Collins Warren and reported by Henry Jacob Bigelow, 1846, *BMSJ* **35**:309, 379. He tried to patent his discovery of the anaesthetic effects of ether (*Circular. Morton's Letheon*, 1846). Died 1868. *5651, 5652*

1819: 20 Carl Siegmund Franz **Credé**, German obstetrician, born 23 Dec; his method of removing the retained placenta by external manual pressure ('Credé's manoeuvre') described by him in his *De optima in partu naturali placentum amovendi ratione*, 1860. Introduced the practice of instilling silver nitrate into the eyes of newborn children as a preventive measure against ophthalmia neonatorum, 1881, *ArGy* **17**:50. Died 1892. *6183, 6195*

1819:21 Wenzel **Treitz**, Bohemian pathologist, born; described Treitz's hernia – retroperitoneal hernia through the duodeno-jejunal recess, 1857; in his *Hernia retroperitonealis*, 1857. Died 1872. *3591*

1819:22 Augustin Marie **Morvan**, French physician, born; described a form of syringomyelia ('Morvan's disease'), 1883., *GMC* **20**:580, 590, 624, 721. Died 1897. *4701*

1819: Daniel **Rutherford** died, **born** 1749. *nitrogen*

1819: Samuel **Stearns** died, **born** 1747. *herbal*

**1820**
1820:1 **Académie de Médecine** founded in **Paris**, succeeding **Académie Royale de Chirurgie et de Médecine**

1820:2 **First US Pharmacopoeia** published

1820:3 **US Botanic Garden** at **Washington DC**

1820:4 While a medical student from Montreal, John Stephenson (1797–1842) had a **cleft palate** repaired by P. Roux in Paris. Stephenson described the operation in his graduation thesis, *Dissertatio chirurgo-medica inauguralis de velosynthesi*. *5740, 5739.1*

1820:5 **Quinine** isolated by Pierre Joseph Pelletier (1788–1842) and Joseph Bienaimé Caventou (1795–1877), *AnC* **15**:289, 337. *5233*

1820:6 Excision of the superior **maxilla** first carried out by Horatio Gates Jameson (1788–1855), *AmMR* **4**:222. *4446*

1820:7 Christophe François Delabarre (1777–1862) published *Traité de la partie méchanique de l'art du chirurgien-dentiste*, one of the first scientifically-written textbooks on **dental prosthetics**. *3679.5*

1820:8 Jean François Coindet (1774–1834) first to administer **iodine** in the treatment of **goitre**, *AnS* **15**:49. *3812*

1820:9 **Immunity** of females to **haemophilia** despite their ability to transmit the disease ('**Nasse's law**') noted by Christian Friedrich Nasse (1778–1851), *ArMEr* **1**:385. *3056*

1820:10 **Arsenic cancer** first described by John Ayrton Paris (1785–1856); in his *Pharmacologia*, p. 133. *2073*

1820:11 **Food adulteration** exposed by Friedrich Accum (1769–1838), in his *Treatise on the adulteration of food*. *1604.2*

1820:12 Peter Ludwig **Panum**, Danish physiologist, born 19 Feb; gave valuable account of measles outbreak in Faeroe Islands, 1847, *Bibliothek for Laeger* 3 ser. **1**:270. Died 1885. *5443*

1820:13 Lewis Albert **Sayre**, American surgeon, born 29 Feb; reported first successful hip resection for ankylosis, 1855, *NYJM* **14**:70; was first to use plaster of Paris as a support in the treatment of tuberculosis of the spine, 1876, *TAMA* **27**:573. See also his *Spinal diseases and spinal curvature, their treatment by suspension and the use of plaster of Paris bandage*, 1877. Died 1900. *4332, 4344, 4344.1*

1820:14 Georg Richard **Lewin**, German surgeon, born 9 Apr; first to remove a laryngeal growth with the aid of the laryngoscope, 1862, *AMC* **31**:9, 33, a claim also made by Victor von Bruns. Died 1896. *3269*

1820:15 Florence **Nightingale**, British nurse and hospital reformer, born 12 May; the greatest figure in the history of nursing, she also made valuable contributions to the design of hospitals; published *Notes on hospitals*, 1859, and *Notes on nursing*, 1860. Died 1910. *1611, 1612*

1820:16 Eduard Heinrich **Henoch**, German paediatrician, born 7 Jun; described a form of purpura with abdominal symptoms, 1868, *BKW* **5**:517; first mentioned by William Heberden Sr (1802) and later by Johannes Lucas Schönlein (1837) ('Schönlein-Henoch') purpura. First to describe purpura fulminans, 1887, *BKW* **24**:8. Died 1910. *3065, 3053, 3058, 3068*

1820:17 Otto Eduard Heinrich **Wucherer**, Portuguese physician, born 7 Jul; confirmed Griesinger's view that the cause of tropical anaemia was the ankylostomiasis hookworm, 1866, *GMB* **1**:27, 39, 52, 63. Saw the embryo form of the filaria worm, 1868, *GMB* **3**:97, to which the name *Wuchereria bancrofti* was later applied. Died 1873. *5356, 5355, 5344.6, 5346*

1820:18 Hubert von **Luschka**, German anatomist, born 27 Jul; gave first authentic description of polyposis of the colon, 1861, *VA* **20**:133. Died 1875. *3460*

1820:19 John **Tyndall**, British physicist, born 2 Aug; showed that *Penicillium* had a bacteria-inhibiting effect, although *Pseudomonas pyocyanea* was resistant to it, 1876, *PT* **166**:27. Discovered fractional sterilization; *Essays on the floating-matter of the air ...*, 1877. Died 1893. *1932, 2495*

1820:20 Henry **Thompson**, British surgeon, born 6 Aug; devised operation for tumours of the bladder, 1884. Died 1904. *4180*

---

1820:21 Heinrich **Müller**, German anatomist, born; discovered visual purple (rhodopsin), 1851, *ZWZ* **3**;234. Died 1864. *1506*

1820:22 Charles Harrison **Blackley**, British physician, born; showed pollen produces hay fever in both asthmatic and catarrhal forms and also evokes skin reactions; *Experimental researches on the causes and nature of catarrhus aestivus*, 1873. Died 1900. *2588*

1820:23 Henry William **Fuller**, British physician, born; diagnosed leukaemia during life, following a blood examination, 1846, *L* **2**:43. Died 1873. *3062.1*

1820:24 Gottfried von **Rittershain**, Polish-born physician, born; first described dermatitis exfoliativa neonatorum ('Rittershain's disease'), 1870, *OJP* **1**:23. Died 1883. *4060*

---

1820: Thomas **Kast** died, **born** ?1755. *femoral artery ligation*

1820: John **Bell** died, **born** 1763. *surgical anatomy, gluteal artery ligation*

1820: Michael **Underwood** died, **born** 1737. *diseases of children, sclerema neonatorum, heart disease, candidiasis, poliomyelitis*

1820: Vincenzo **Chiarugi** died, **born** 1759. *psychiatry*

**1821**

1821:1 **McGill College and University** founded at **Montreal**

1821:2 **Massachusetts General Hospital, Boston,** founded by John Collins Warren, opened to patients

1821:3 **Philadelphia College of Pharmacy** founded

1821:4 **Royal Society of New South Wales** founded at Sydney

1821:5 **University at Buenos Aires** founded

1821:6 *Journal de Physiologie Expérimentale* founded by François Magendie (1783–1855)

1821:7 Five thousand deliveries were supervised by Marie Louise La Chapelle (1769–1821), a famous **midwife**. Her vast experience was published in her *Pratique des accouchemens*, 3 vols, 1821–25, edited posthumously by her nephew. *6170*

1821:8 Extraperitoneal **caesarean section** first performed by Ferdinand August Marie Franz Ritgen (1787–1867), reported 1825, *HKA* 1:263. *6238*

1821:9 The *Illustrations of the great operations of surgery*, by Charles Bell (1774–1842) is considered one of the most beautifully illustrated books in the entire literature of **surgery**. *5588*

1821:10 First excision of the head of the **femur** for disease of the **hip-joint** by Anthony White (1782–1849); in Cooper, S. *Dictionary of practical surgery*, 1838, p. 272. *4458*

1821:11 **'Bell's nerve'** and **'Bell's palsy'**, **facial paralysis** following a lesion of the motor nerve of the face, first described by Charles Bell (1774–1842), *PT* **111**:398. *1255, 4520*

1821:12 Valuable contributions to the knowledge of **hernia** recorded by Antonio Scarpa (1752–1832); in his *Sull'ernia del perineo*. *3584*

1821:13 The first modern text on **otology**, *Traité des maladies de l'oreille et de l'audition*, published by Jean Marie Gaspard Itard (1774–1838). *3364*

1821:14 Successful **blood transfusion** in animals using defibrinated blood to prevent coagulation, by Jean Louis Prévost (1790–1850) and Jean Baptiste André Dumas (1800–1884), *AnC* **18**:28. *2016*

1821:15 Johann Friedrich Meckel's (1781–1833) *System der vergleichende Anatomie*, 5 vols, 1821–31, place him among the greatest of the comparative **anatomists**. *318*

1821:16 Adolphe **Gubler**, French physician, born 5 Apr; described crossed hemiplegia ('Gubler's paralysis'), 1856, *GMC* **3**:749, 789, 811. The later account by Hermann David Weber (1863) led to the eponym 'Weber-Gubler syndrome'. Died 1897. *4531*

1821:17 Franz **Leydig**, German anatomist and histologist, born 21 May; described the interstitial cells of the testis, 'Leydig cells', 1850, *ZWC* **2**:1. Died 1908. *1222*

1821:18 Charles Hewitt **Moore**, British surgeon, born 1 Aug; modern surgical treatment of cancer is based on principles laid down by him, 1867, *MCT* **50**:245. Died 1870. *2619*

1821:19 Hermann Ludwig Ferdinand von **Helmholtz**, German physiologist and physicist, born 31 Aug; proposed doctrine of conservation of energy, 1847; in his *Ueber die Erhaltung der Kraft*. Measured velocity of the nervous impulse, 1850, *ArA* 71. Invented the ophthalmoscope; in his *Beschreibung eines Augen-Spiegels zur Untersuchung der Netzhaut im lebenden Auge*, 1851. Explained the mechanism of accommodation in the eye, 1855, *GAO* **1**, **ii**:1. His theory of hearing, 1863, forms the basis of modern theories of resonance; in his *Die Lehre von der Tonempfindung*. Died 1894. *611, 1265, 5866, 1509, 1562*

1821:20 Karl Georg Friedrich **Leuckart**, German zoologist and parasitologist, born 7 Oct; gave the first complete and accurate account of the life history and morphology of *Taenia echinococcus*; in his *Die menschlichen Parasiten und die von ihnen herrührenden Krankheiten*, 2 vols, 1863–1882. Died 1898. *5344*

1821:21 Rudolph Ludwig Karl **Virchow**, German pathologist, born 13 Oct; gave first clear description of thrombosis and embolism, 1846, *BEP*, **2**, 227, reprinted in his *Gesammelte Abhandlungen zur wissenschaftlichen Medicin*, 1856. Discovered the neuroglia, 1854, *VA* **6**:135. First to describe pulmonary aspergillosis, 1856, *VA* **9**:557. His classic, *Die Cellularpathologie* published 1858. Confirmed syphilis to be a disease involving all organs and tissues of the body, 1858, *VA* **15**:217. Showed the connection between famine conditions and typhus outbreaks, and emphasized the social element in the generation of the disease; in his *Ueber den Hungertyphus*, 1868. Died 1902. *3006, 1268, 3169, 2299, 2385, 5376*

1821:22 Henry Willard **Williams**, American ophthalmologist, born 11 Dec; described the non-mercurial treatment of iriditis, 1856, *BMSJ* **55**:49, 69, 92. Died 1895. *5878*

1821:23 Richard James **Mackenzie** born; modified James Syme's method of amputation at the ankle-joint, 1849, *MJMS* **9**:951. Died 1854. *4460*

1821:24 Elizabeth **Blackwell**, born Bristol, England; graduated in medicine at Geneva, NY, in 1849; returned to England and was the first woman to be registered on the Medical Register, 1859. Published *Medicine as a profession for women*, 1860. Died 1910. *6649.90*

1821: Jean Nicolas **Corvisart des Marest** died, **born** 1755. *heart disease, pulmonary disorders*

1821: Johann Peter **Frank** died, **born** 1745. *diabetes insipidus, public hygiene*

1821: Thomas **Bateman** died, **born** 1778. *dermatology, lichen urticatus*

1821: Samuel **Bard** died, **born** 1742. *diphtheria*

1821: Edward **Bancroft** died, **born** 1744. *yaws*

1821: Georg Joseph **Beer** died, **born** 1763. *ophthalmology*

1821: Marie Louise **La Chapelle** died, **born** 1769. *midwifery*

**1822**
1822:1 **Gesellschaft Deutscher Naturforscher und Aertze** founded

1822:2 **Medical Society of the County of Kings (Brooklyn)** founded

1822:3 The first well-documented full-thickness **skin graft** carried out by Christian Heinrich Bünger (1782–1842) for a **rhinoplasty** on a patient whose nose and forehead had been destroyed by **lupus**, *JCA* **4**:569. *5740.1*

1822:4 Nathan Smith (1762–1829), pioneer **ovariotomist**, performed the operation for **ovarian dropsy**, apparently without knowledge of the earlier operations of McDowell, *AmMR* **5**:124. *6024, 6023*

1822:5 Johann Friedrich Dieffenbach (1792–1847) was a pioneer in the field of **plastic** and **orthopaedic surgery**. His inaugural MD thesis, Würzburg, was entitled *Nonnula de regeneratione et transplantatione. 5741*

1822:6 The first clear description of **general paresis** ('**Bayle's disease**') given by Antoine Laurent Jessé Bayle (1799–1858); in his *Recherches sur l'arachnitis chronique*, Paris, Thèse No. 247. *4795*

1822:7 A good account of **epilepsy** given by James Cowles Prichard (1786–1848); in his *Treatise on diseases of the nervous system. 4809*

1822:8 **Torticollis (wry-neck)** first treated by subcutaneous section of the sternomastoid muscle by Guillaume Dupuytren (1777–1835). This was recorded by C. Averill in 1823 and by Dupuytren in his *Leçons orales de clinique chirurgicales*, 2 éd., **3**, p. 455, 1839. *4322*

1822:9 Attention to **arthrodynia *a potu* – alcoholic neuritis** – drawn by James Jackson (1777–1867), *NEJM* **2**:351. *4521*

1822:10 **Alkaptonuria** described by Alexander John Gaspard Marcet (1770–1822), *MCT* **12**:37. *3912*

1822:11 **Pernicious anaemia** first described by James Scarth Combe (1796–1883), *TMCS* **1**:194. *3112*

1822:12 **Iodoform** discovered by Georges Simon Sérullas (1774–1832), *AnC* **20**:163. *1848*

1822:13 **Birth control** advocated by Francis Place (1771–1854), in his *Illustrations and proofs of the principle of population. 1696.1*

---

1822:14 Francis **Galton**, British statistician, experimental psychologist and eugenicist, born 16 Feb; suggested that genius was hereditary, *Hereditary genius*, 1869, *Inquiries into human faculty*, 1883 (which included the first appearance of the word 'eugenics'). Published *Natural inheritance*, 1889, *Probability: the foundation of eugenics*, 1907 – thus founding the science of eugenics. Explained the individuality of fingerprints in identification, *Fingerprints*, 1892. Died 1911. *226, 230, 233, 1709, 186*

1822:15 Adolf **Kussmaul**, German physician, born 22 Feb. With Rudolph Maier, first described periarteritis nodosa, 1866, *DAKM* 1:484. First used the oesophagoscope clinically, 1867, but not reported until 1901 by Gustav Killian, *DZC* **58**:500. Introduced the concept of the paradoxical pulse, 1873, *BKW* **10**:433, 445, 461. In his *Die Störungen der Sprache*, 1877, he termed aphasia 'word-blindness'. Died 1902. *2906, 3521, 2776, 4624*

1822:16 Friedrich Wilhelm Felix von **Bärensprung**, German physician, born 30 Mar; first described tinea cruris (eczema marginatum); in his *Ueber die Folge und den Verlauf epidermischer Krankheiten*, 1854. Ascribed herpes zoster ascribed to a lesion of the spinal ganglia, 1861, *AnCK* **9** ii:40; **10**:37; **11**:96. Died 1864. *4043, 4640*

1822:17 Karl **Thiersch**, German surgeon, born 20 Apr; advanced epithelial-cell origin of cancer histogenesis; in his *Der Epithelialkrebs namentlich der Haut*, 1865. His split-skin grafts, 1874, developed into the Ollier-Thiersch graft, *VDGC* **3**:69. Died 1895. *2618, 5753, 5752*

1822:18 Heinrich **Meckel von Hemsbach**, Swiss-born German pathologist, born 8 Jun; gave the first account of metastatic ophthalmia, 1854, *AnCK* **5**, ii:276. Died 1856. *5875*

1822:19 Alfonso **Corti**, Italian anatomist, born 15 Jun; Organ of Corti named after him, following his important investigations of the cochlea, 1851, ZWZ **3**:109. Died 1888. *1559*

1822:20 Gregor **Mendel**, Austrian biologist and priest, born 22 Jul; published his theory of heredity, the foundation of genetics, 1865, *VNVB*, **4**:3. Died 1884. *222*

1822:21 Daniel **Ayres**, American surgeon, born 4 Oct; performed the first successful plastic operation for exstrophy of the female bladder, 1859, *AmMG* **10**:81. Died 1892. *6046*

1822:22 Louis **Pasteur**, French chemist and microbiologist, born 27 Dec; in several papers between 1857 and 1861 he demonstrated the connection between fermentation and living microorganisms; *CRAS* **45**:913; **48**:557; **50**:303; **51**:348; 675; *AnSN* 16:5. In the latter year he discovered strict anaerobiosis, *CRAS* **52**:344. In 1863 he confirmed the fact, established by Schwann in 1837, that putrefaction is a biological process, *CRAS* **56**:416, 734. In the same year he differentiated between aerobic and anaerobic organisms, *CRAS* **56**:1189. He established pasteurization on a scientific basis in 1866, *Études sur le vin*. Discovered *Clostridium septicum*, 1877, *CRAS* **85**:101. Described the haemolytic streptococcus of puerperal fever, 1879, *BuAM* **8**:505. In studies on the aetiology of anthrax with Charles Chamberland and Pierre Paul Emile Roux, first to use attenuated bacterial virus, providing active immunization against the disease, 1880, *CRAS* **91**:86. His experiments on attenuation of the infective organism and inoculation of attenuated cultures, 1880, laid the foundations of immunology, *CRAS* **90**:239. Gave recognizable descriptions of staphylococcus (so named by Ogston, 1881) and streptococcus, 1880, *CRAS* **90**:1033. Discovered the pneumococcus in a child killed by rabies, 1881, *BuAM* **10**:379, independently observed in the same year by George Miller Sternberg. His earliest studies on rabies were published with his colleagues, Chamberland, Roux and Thuillier, 1881, *CRAS* **92**:1259. With Chamberland and Roux, in an attempt to develop a variety of rabies that could be used safely for vaccination they became the first to modify the pathogenicity of a virus for its natural host, by serial intracerebral passage in another species of host, 1884, *CRAS* **98**:457, 1229. His later papers describing his rabies vaccine and results obtained with it gave further proof of the protective value of attenuated virus against infective diseases in man and animals, 1885, *CRAS* **101**:765; **102**:459, 835; **103**:777. Died 1895. *2472–2475, 2475.1, 2476–2478, 2479, 2490, 6278, 5169, 2537, 2492.1, 2541, 3172, 3173, 5481.4, 5482, 5483, 2541*

1822:23 Gustav Wilhelm Johann **Düben**, Swedish physician, born; with Pehr Henrik Malmsten, gave an accurate account of myocardial infarction, 1859, *Hygiea* **21**:629. Died 1892. *2761.1*

1822:24 William **Cumming**, British ophthalmologist, born; while still a student, he was able, by shading the eye of another student from the light, to look directly into it and to obtain both the retinal reflex and the white light from the entrance of the optic nerve, 1846, *MCT* **29**:283. Died 1855. *5861*

1822:25 Arthur **Leared**, British physician, born; introduced the binaural stethoscope, 1856, *L* **2**:138, 202. Died 1879. *2676.1*

1822: Domenico **Cotugno** died, **born** 1736. *labyrinthine fluid, cerebrospinal fluid, proteinuria, sciatica*

1822: Caleb Hillier **Parry** died, **born** 1755. *exophthalmic goitre, facial hemiatrophy*

1822: Alexander John Gaspard **Marcet** died, **born** 1770. *alkaptonuria*

1822: William **Nisbet** died, **born** 1759. *lymphatic chancre*

1822: Friedrich Benjamin **Osiander** died, **born** 1759. *caesarean section*

1822: Valentin **Haüy** died, **born** 1745. *blind*

**1823**
1823:1 *Lancet* begins publication in **London**, 5 Oct

1823:2 [**Georg General Hospital**] founded in **Hamburg**

1823:3 **Faculté de Médecine**, **Paris**, revived and reorganized

1823:4 **Società Medico-Chirurgica** at **Bologna**

1823:5 Marie Jean Pierre Flourens (1794–1867) demonstrated that the **cerebrum** is the organ of **thought** and the **cerebellum** controls body movement, 1823, *ArGM* **2**:321. *1391*

1823:6 George James Guthrie (1785–1856) was the earliest teacher on the surgery of the **eye** in Britain. He wrote *Lectures on the operative surgery of the eye*; and founded the Royal Westminster Ophthalmic Hospital. *5845*

1823:7 A **chlorine** solution for **disinfecting** purposes introduced by Antoine Germain Labarraque (1777–1850); in his *De l'emploi des chlorures d'oxide de sodium et de chaux*. *5633*

1823:8 The first American textbook of **ophthalmology** was the *Treatise on the diseases of the eye* by George Frick (1793–1870). *5844*

1823:9 The first operations on the **brain** performed in the USA reported by Benjamin Winslow Dudley (1785–1870), *TrJM* **1**:9. *4851.1*

1823:10 The first published report of removal of the **parotid gland** was by John Beale Davidge (1768–1829), *BPJR* **1**:165; although he may have been preceded by others in this operation. Pierre Augustin Béclard (1785–1825) reported in 1824 that he had done so in 1823. *3433.1, 3434*

1823:11 **Parotid gland** excised by Pierre Augustin Béclard (1785–1825), 1824, *ArGM* **4**:60. *3434*

1823:12 A description of **pituitary obesity** given by Pierre François Oliver Rayer (1793–1867), *ArGM* **3**:350. *3881*

1823:13 Successful ligation of the primitive **carotid artery** in continuity of both carotids by William D. Macgill (1802–1833), in the same subject within a month – the first American to do so, *NYMPJ* **4**:576. *2946*

1823:14 *Elements of medical jurisprudence*, first notable American text, published by Theodor Beck (1791–1855). *1735*

1823:15 Jacques Mathieu Delpech (1777–1832) gave the first account of **rhinoplasty** in France, an operation he first performed on 4 June 1823, in his *Chirurgie clinique de Montpellier*, 2 vols – in the same work (**1**, 184) he described his operation of subcutaneous **Achilles tenotomy for club foot**. *5741.1*

---

1823:16 Alfred Russel **Wallace**, British naturalist, born 8 Jan; independently of Darwin, he formulated the principles of natural selection. His paper, *JPLSZ*, 1859 **3**:53, which includes a contribution by Darwin, was the final stimulus for Darwin to publish his *Origin*. Died 1913. *219*

1823:17 Johann Friedrich August von **Esmarch**, German surgeon, born 9 Jan; introduced the Esmarch (first-aid) bandage on the battlefield; described in his *Der erste Verband auf dem Schlachtfelde*, 1869. Died 1908. *2168*

1823:18 John Braxton **Hicks**, British obstetrician, born 23 Feb; introduced bipolar version, in which the breech is made to present, a method of treatment for placenta praevia, 1864, *TOSL* **5**:219; drew attention to irregular painless contractions of the uterus during pregnancy, 'Braxton Hicks' sign', 1872, *TOSL* **13**:216. Died 1897. *6186, 6189*

1823:19 Robert **Fletcher**, British/American physician, librarian and bibliographer, born 23 Mar; with John Shaw Billings, founded and edited the *Index Medicus*, 1879, and the *Index-Catalogue of the Library of the Surgeon General's Office*, 1880. Died 1912.

1823:20 Joseph **Leidy**, American biologist, born 9 Sep; first reported trichinosis in the pig, 1846, *PANS* **3**:107. Discovered the bacterial flora of the intestines, 1849, *PANS* **4**:225. First to undertake experimental transplantation of tumours, 1851, *PANS* **5**:212. Died 1891. *5338, 3450, 2614*

1823:21 Ambroise Auguste **Liébeault**, French physician, born 16 Sep; the substitution of psychotherapy for hypnotic suggestion was due to his work; in his *Le sommeil provoqué et* *les états analogues considérés sur au point du vue de l'action du moral et de physique*, 1866. Died 1904. *4994*

1823:22 Henry Hyde **Salter**, British physician, born 2 Nov; his *On asthma*, 1860, was the best work on the subject to appear during the 19th century. Died 1871. *2586, 3169.1*

1823:23 John Cooper **Forster**, British surgeon, born 13 Nov; carried out the first gastrostomy in Britain, 1858, *GHR* **4**:13. Died 1886. *3457*

1823:24 William **Brinton**, British physician, born 20 Nov; first to describe linitis plastica ('Brinton's disease'); in his *Diseases of the stomach*, p. 310, 1859. Died 1867. *3458*

1823:25 Aristide Auguste Stanislas **Verneuil**, French surgeon, born 23 Nov; introduced forcipressure in the treatment of haemorrhage, 1875, *BMSC* **1**:17, 108, 273, 522, 646; his gastrostomy operation, 1876, *BuAM* **5**:1023, was a modification of Sédillot's method. Died 1895. *5612, 3468*

1823:26 Hermann David **Weber**, German/British physician, born 30 Dec; his account of hemiplegia associated with disease of the crura cerebri, 1863, *MCT* **46**:121, first described by Adolphe Gubler (1856), led to the eponyms 'Weber's syndrome' and 'Weber-Gubler syndrome'. Died 1918. *4538, 4531*

1823:27 Ferdinand Louis Joseph **Cuignet**, French ophthalmologist, born; introduced retinoscopy, 1873, *ReO* **1**:14. *5908*

1823:28 William Senhouse **Kirkes**, British physician, born; gave classical description of embolism, 1852, *MCT* **35**:281. Died 1864. *2758*

1823: Edward **Jenner** died, **born** 1749. *smallpox vaccination*

1823: Matthew **Baillie** died, **born** 1761. *pathological anatomy, rheumatic fever, valvular disease of heart, pulmonary tuberculosis, emphysema, gastric ulcer, dermoid cysts of ovary, pulmonary oedema*

## 1824
1824:1 **Academy of Medicine** founded at **Cleveland, Ohio**

1824:2 **Franklin Institute** founded at **Philadelphia**

1824:3 A classic account of **cancer** of the **uterus**, *Ueber den Gebärmutterkrebs, dessen Enstehung und Verhütung*, given by Adam Elias von Siebold (1775–1826). *6025*

1824:4 Proof that **pain** at **surgical operations** could be abolished by the inhalation of gas provided by Henry Hill Hickman (1800–1830); he rendered animals unconscious through partial asphyxiation by the exclusion of air and then by inhalation of carbon dioxide; in his *Letter on suspended animation*, etc. His work was the first on surgical **anaesthesia**. *5647*

1824:5 **Lymphocytic choriomeningitis** first described by Arvid Johan Wallgren (1889–1973), *AcP* **4**:158. *4687*

1824:6 Marie Jean Pierre Flourens (1794–1867) gave experimental proof that **vision** depends on the integrity of the **cerebral cortex**, in his *Recherches experimentales sur les propriétés et les fonctions du système nerveux. 1493*

1824:7 In his classic account of **typhoid**, *A practical essay on typhous fever*, Nathan Smith (1762–1829) clearly recognized the contagious nature of the disease. *5022*

1824:8 First report of the value of **cod-liver oil** in treatment of **rickets** by D. Schütte, *ArMEr* 2:79. *3730*

1824:9 The first **staphylorrhaphy** in America performed by John Collins Warren (1778–1856) in May 1824 and reported in 1828, *AmJMS* 3:1. *5742*

---

1824:10 Rudolph **Maier**, German physician, born 9 Apr; with Adolf Kussmaul, first described periarteritis nodosa, 1866, *DAKM* 1:484. Died 1888. *2906*

1824:11 Edmund **Andrews**, American anaesthetist, born 22 Apr; advocated the use of oxygen-nitrous oxide mixture as an anaesthetic, 1868, *MEx* 9:665. Died 1904. *5669*

1824:12 Gustav **Simon**, German surgeon, born 30 May; first to develop cheiloplasty; in his *Beiträge zur plastischen Chirurgie*, 1868. Carried out first successful planned nephrectomy for urinary tract fistula, 1870, *DK* 22:137. Died 1876. *5749, 4213*

1824:13 Samuel **Wilks**, British physician, born 2 Jun; first described lineae atrophicae, 1861, *GHR* 7:197. Described verrucae necrogenicae (dissecting-room warts, the cutaneous tuberculosis of Laennec), sometimes called 'Wilks's disease', 1862, *GHR* 8:263. Gave an authoritative account of lymphadenoma, 1856, *GHR* 2:114; in a later paper, 1865, *GHR* 11:56, he named it 'Hodgkin's disease'. Published a classic account of alcoholic paraplegia, 1868, *MTG* 2:470, and of osteitis deformans, 1868, *TPSL* 20:273. Gave early account of bacterial endocarditis, 1870, *GHR* 15:29. A case of 'bulbar paralysis' described by him is believed to be the first definite record of myasthenia gravis, 1877, *GHR* 22:7. Died 1911. *4052, 4053, 3764, 4539, 4338, 2769, 4745*

1824:14 François Rémy Lucien **Corvisart**, French physician, born 9 Jun; nephew of J.N. Corvisart, he introduced the term 'tétanie'; in his *De la contracture des extrémités ou tétanie*, Paris, Thèse No. 223, 1852. Died 1882. *4829*

1824:15 Pierre Paul **Broca**, French surgeon, born 28 Jun; localized the speech centre in the left frontal lobe and asserted that aphasia was associated with a lesion on the left third frontal convolution of the brain ('Broca's area'), 1861, *BSAnth* 2:235. Died 1880. *4619*

1824:16 Albrecht Theodor **Middeldorpf**, German surgeon, born 3 Jul; first to operate on tumour of oesophagus, reported in his *De polypis oesophagi*, 1857; first operation for gastric fistula, in his *De fistulis ventriculi externis et chirurgica earum sanatione*, 1859. Died 1868. *3456, 3459*

1824:17 Ernst **Reissner**, anatomist, born Riga 24 Sep; described the vestibular ('Reissner's) membrane in his *De auris internae formatione*, 1851. Died 1878. *1560*

1824: 18 Joseph Pierre **Rollet**, French physician, born 12 Nov; recognized the possibility of mixed infection of a sore with both syphilis and chancroid ('Rollet's disease'), 1866, *GML* **18**:160. Died 1894. *5204*

---

1824: 19 John Reissberg **Wolfe**, British ophthalmic surgeon, born; considered that in free-skin grafts the subcutaneous tissue at the site of the graft should be removed, leaving skin only; he is remembered for the 'Wolfe-Krause graft rest', 1875, *BMJ* **2**:360. Died 1904. *5754*

---

1824: Nicolas **Dubois de Chemant** died, **born** 1753. *artificial teeth*

1824: James **Parkinson** died, **born** 1755. *paralysis agitans*

1824: John Bunnell **Davis** died, **born** 1780. *infant mortality rate, health visiting*

**1825**
1825: 1 **University of Virginia** founded at **Charlottesville**

1825: 2 **Jefferson Medical College** founded at **Philadelphia**

1825: 3 **Magyar Tudományos Akademia** [Hungarian Academy of Sciences] founded at **Budapest**

1825: 4 The first (unsuccessful) **ovariotomy** in Britain performed by John Lizars (1794–1860); in his *Observations on extraction of diseased ovaria. 6026*

1825: 5 The first American textbook on **paediatrics** was *Treatise on the medical and physical treatment of children*, by William Potts Dewees (1768–1841). *6331*

1825: 6 Philibert Joseph Roux (1789–1854) gave the first detailed account of his operation for repair of **cleft palate**, in which he proposed the name '**staphylorrhaphy**', *ArGM* **7**:516. *5741.2, 5739.1*

1825: 7 In his classic account of **aphasia** Jean Baptiste Bouillaud (1796–1881) was first to suggest that injuries of the frontal lobe were a cause, *ArGM* **8**:25. *4618*

1825: 8 **Facial hemiatrophy** first recorded by Caleb Hillier Parry (1755–1822); see his *Collections from the unpublished writings*, **1**, 478. *4522*

1825: 9 **Curare**; paralysing effects described by Charles Waterton (1782–1865); in his *Wanderings in South America. 2074*

1825: 10 Although *Experiments and observations on the gastric juice* by William Beaumont (1785–1853), reporting his studies on digestion and the movements of the stomach through a gastric fistula caused by a gunshot wound, was published in 1833, his preliminary reports appeared in 1825–6, *MRecorder*, **8**:14, 840; **9**:94. *989, 987.1, 987.2*

1825: 11 **Tuberculosis**: *Recherches anatomico-pathologiques sur la phthisie* by Pierre Charles Alexandre Louis (1787–1872) was based on 358 dissections and 1,960 clinical case reports. *3221*

---

1825:12 Friedrich Albert **Zenker**, German pathologist, born 13 Mar; first noted the intestinal and muscular forms of trichinosis and he established their connection with the disease, 1860, *VA* **18**:561. First described pulmonary fat embolism; in his *Beiträge zur normalen und pathologischen Anatomie der Lungen*, 1862. Described dust diseases of the lungs and suggested the term 'pneumonokoniosis' to describe such conditions, 1867, *DAKM* **2**:111. Died 1898. *5342, 3007, 2125.1*

1825:13 Theodor Maximilian **Bilharz**, German physician and zoologist, born 23 Mar; discovered in Egypt *Schistosoma haematobium*, parasite causing schistosomiasis (bilharziasis), 1852, *ZWC* **4**:53. Died 1862. *5339*

1825:14 Nathan **Bozeman**, American gynaecologist, born 26 Mar; successfully treated pyelitis complicating vesical and faecal fistulae in women, 1887, *IMC* **2**:514. Treated pyelitis due to vesical and faecal fistulae by ureteral catheterization through vesico-vaginal cystotomy, 1888, *AmJMS* **95**:255, 368. *6085, 4221*

1825:15 Fessenden Nott **Otis**, American urologist, born 6 May; first to employ local anaesthesia in urology, 1884, *NYMJ* **40**:635. Died 1900. *4179*

1825:16 Pierre Carl Édouard **Potain**, French physician, born 19 Jul; published classical account of the jugular movements and murmurs, diagnostic of heart diseases, 1867, *BSMH(M)* **4**:3. Introduced a portable air sphygmomanometer, 1889, *ArPhy* **1**:556. Died 1901. *2766, 2798*

1825:17 Luigi Maria **Concato**, Italian physician, born 20 Nov; described tuberculous inflammation of serous membrane, 1881, *GilSM* **3**:1037. Died 1882. *2330*

1825:18 Jean Martin **Charcot**, French neurologist, born 29 Nov; with André Victor Cornil, gave an important account of the renal lesions in gout, 1863, *CRSB* **5**:139. With Abel Bouchard, gave the first clinical description of the electric pains in tabes dorsalis, 1866, *GMP* **21**:122. Described Charcot's arthropathy, sometimes occurring in tabes dorsalis (neuropathic joint disease); the tabetic joints he described became known as 'Charcot's joints', 1868, *ArPhy* **1**:161. Published an important description of multiple sclerosis, 1868, *GH* **41**:554, 557, 566. Pioneered research on the application of hypnosis to the psychoneuroses; in his *Leçons sur les maladies du système nerveux faites à la Salpêtrière*, 3 vols, 1872–87. Differentiated between Aran-Duchenne muscular atrophy and the rarer amyotrophic lateral sclerosis, 1874, *ProM* **2**:573. Undertook important studies of localization of functions in diseases of the brain; in his *Leçons sur les localisations dans les maladies du cerveau*, 1876–78. With Pierre Marie, first described peroneal muscular atrophy (Charcot-Marie-Tooth type), 1886, *ReM* **6**:97, which was independently described by Tooth in the same year. Died 1893. *4498, 4337, 4775, 4777, 4698, 4995, 4742, 4558, 4749, 4750*

1825:19 Joseph Thomas **Clover**, British anaesthetist, born 11 Dec; introduced gas-ether inhaler (Clover's inhaler) 1873, *BMJ* **1**:282; introduced an ether inhaler ('Clover's apparatus'), 1876, *BMJ* **2**:74. Died 1882. *5671, 5674*

1825:20 Felix **Hoppe-Seyler**, German physiological chemist, born 26 Dec; obtained haemoglobin in crystalline form, 1862, *VA* **23**:446; 1864, *VA* **29**:233, 597; and did important work on lecithin and cholesterol. Died 1895. *870, 873*

1825:21 Hans Wilhelm **Meyer**, Danish physician, born; first to give a clinical description of adenoid growths, 1868, *Hos* **11**:177. Died 1895. *3276*

172

1825:22 Jean Baptiste Emil **Vidal**, French dermatologist, born; described neurodermatitis ('Vidal's disease'), 1886, *AnD* **7**:133. Died 1893. *4088*

1825:23 Alfred **Le Roy de Méricourt** born; first to describe chromhidrosis, the secretion of coloured sweat, 1858, *BuAM* **23**:1141; **26**:773. Died 1901. *4046*

1825:24 Georg Franz **Merck**, German chemist, born; isolated papaverine from opium, 1848, *AnPh* **66**:125. Died 1873. *1861*

1825:25 James **Hobrecht** born; responsible for the construction of the sewers of Berlin, 1873–83, based on a system of canalization advocated by Virchow, in his *Die Canalisation von Berlin*, 1884. Died 1902. *1624*

1825:26 Adrian Christopher van **Trigt**, Dutch physician, born; his *Dissertatio ophthalmologica inauguralis de speculo oculi*, 1853, contain the first printed illustrations of the fundus oculi. Died 1864. *5869.1*

1825: Pierre Augustin **Béclard** died, **born** 1785. *parotid gland*

1825: Colin **Chisholm** died, **born** 1755. *dracontiasis, Dracunculus medinensis*

**1826**
1826:1 **University of Munich** founded

1826:2 **Regia Escola de Cirurgia** founded at **Lisbon**

1826:3 **University College London** founded; opened 1828

1826:4 **Zoological Society of London** founded

1826:5 **Rutgers Medical College, New Jersey**, founded

1826:6 The first American textbook of **gynaecology**, *A treatise on diseases of females*, published by William Potts Dewees (1768–1841). *6026.1*

1826:7 The pathology of **congenital dislocation of the hip-joint** first clearly described by Guillaume Dupuytren (1777–1835), *RGAP* **2**:82. *4413*

1826:8 In his *Des inflammations spéciales du tissu muqueux et en particulier de la diphthérite, ou inflammation pelliculaire*, Pierre Fidèle Bretonneau (1778–1862) demonstrated that croup, malignant angina, and 'scorbutic gangrene of the gums' were all the same disease, **diphtheria**. He suggested the term **diphtheritis**, and, later, **diphthérite**; he successfully performed **tracheotomy** for **croup** (p. 300). *5053*

1826:9 In his *Traité théorique et pratique des maladies de la peau*, Pierre François Olive Rayer (1793–1867) provided a classic summary of the **dermatological literature** of the period. He was first to describe **adenoma sebaceum** and **xanthoma multiplex** and the first to differentiate between acute and chronic **eczema**. *3989*

1826:10 A *lithotriteur* for crushing **urinary calculi** inside the bladder invented by Jean Civiale (1792–1867), *ArGM* **10**:393; he placed **lithotrity** upon a sound basis. *4289*

1826: 11 **Lembert's suture** described by Antoine Lembert (1802–1851), *RGAP* **2**:100; first successfully employed by Johann Friedrich Dieffenbach, 1836. *3435, 3441*

1826: 12 **Physick's operation** for artificial **anus** described by Philip Syng Physick (1768–1837), *PHJMS* **13**:199. *3436*

1826: 13 **Müller's law of specific nerve energies** promulgated by Johannes Müller (1801–1858); in his *Zur vergleichenden Physiologie des Gesichtssinnes des Menschen und der Thiere. 1257, 1456*

1826: 14 Isolation of **bromine** by Antoine Jérome Balard (1802–1876), *AnC* **32**:337. *1848.1*

1826: 15 Edmé Félix Alfred **Vulpian**, French physician, born 5 Jan; discovered adrenaline, 1856, *CRAS* **43**:663. Died 1887. *1141*

1826: 16 Paul Louis **Duroziez**, French physician, born 8 Jan; described the double intermittent murmur, 'Duroziez's sign', in aortic insufficiency, 1861, *ArGM* **17**:417, 588. First described congenital mitral stenosis ('Duroziez's disease'), 1877, *ArGM* **30**:32, 184. Died 1897. *2762, 2780*

1826: 17 James Matthews **Duncan**, British obstetrician, born Apr; his description of the peritoneal folds associated with the uterus, 1854, *EMSJ* **81**:321, led to the name 'Duncan's folds'. Died 1890. *6181*

1826: 18 Nikolaus **Friedreich**, German physician, born 31 Jul; first description of acute leukaemia, 1857, *VA* **12**:37. First to diagnose trichinosis in a living person, 1862, *VA* **25**:399. Gave first description of an hereditary form of ataxia ('Friedreich's ataxia'), 1863–77, *VA* **26**:391, 433; **27**:1; **68**:145; **70**:140. First described paramyoclonus multiplex ('Friedreich's disease'), 1881, *VA* **86**:421. Died 1882. *3064.1, 5344.1, 4696, 4564*

1826: 19 Karl **Gegenbaur**, German comparative anatomist, born 21 Aug; proved the unicellularity of the ovum, 1861, *ArA* 491; supported Darwin and stressed the value of comparative anatomy as the basis of the study of descent, *Gründzüge der vergleichenden Anatomie der Wirbelthiere*, 2nd edn, 1870. Died 1903. *486, 337*

1826: 20 Jean Baptiste Octave **Landry**, French physician, born 10 Oct; described acute ascending polyneuritis ('Landry's paralysis'), 1859, *GMC* **6**:472, 486. Died 1865. *4639*

1826: 21 Rocco **Gritti**, Italian surgeon, born; introduced a technique of amputation of the thigh, 1857, *AnU* **161**:5, later improved by William Stokes, 1870. Died 1920. *4466, 4470*

1826: René Theophile Hyacinthe **Laennec** died, **born** 1781. *auscultation, stethoscope, hepatitis, cirrhosis*

1826: Charles **McCreary** died, **born** 1785. *resection of clavicle*

1826: Philippe **Pinel** died, **born** 1745. *psychiatry*

1826: Adam Elias von **Siebold** died, **born** 1775. *cancer of uterus*

**1827**

1827:1 *American Journal of the Medical Sciences* founded by Isaac Hays (1796–1879)

1827:2 A classic description of **hydatidiform mole** given by Marie Anne Victoire Boivin (1773–1841); in her *Nouvelles recherches de l'origine, la nature et le traitement de la mole vésiculaire ou grossesse hydatique. 6172*

1827:3 George Biddle Airy (1801–1892) first drew attention to **astigmatism**, a condition from which he himself suffered; he used cylindrical lenses for its correction, *TCPS* **2**:267. *5847*

1827:4 The successful wiring of an ununited fracture of the **humerus** carried out by John Kearney Rodgers (1793–1851), *NYMPJ* **6**:521. *4414*

1827:5 **Hemiplegic (unilateral) epilepsy** first described by Louis François Bravais (d.1842), in his *Recherches sur les symptômes et le traitement de l'épilepsie hémiplégique*, Paris, Thèse No. 118.; the excellent account by Jackson (1863) led to the term '**Bravais-Jacksonian epilepsy**'. *4810, 4816*

1827:6 **Chronic appendicitis** first recognised by François Mélier (1798–1866), *JGMC* **100**:317. *3562*

1827:7 '**Jacob's ulcer**', a **rodent ulcer** attacking the face, especially the eyelids, described by Arthur Jacob (1790–1874), *DHR* **4**:232. *4025*

1827:8 **Urethro-cystic speculum** introduced by Pierre Saloman Ségalas (1792–1875), *RMFE* **1**:157. *4165.1*

1827:9 Classic early account of **osteomyelitis** given by Nathan Smith (1762–1829), *PoMoJ* **1**:11, 66. *4313*

1827:10 First complete description of **heart block** with **syncopal attacks** by Robert Adams (1791–1875), *DHR* **4**:353; named '**Stokes-Adams syndrome**' after a further account by William Stokes, 1846. *2745*

1827:11 Successful ligation of the common **carotid artery** by Valentine Mott (1785–1865), *AmJMS* **1**:156. *2950*

1827:12 Richard Bright (1789–1858) published *Reports of medical cases*, 1827–31; containing some outstanding contributions to **pathology**, including his description of chronic non-suppurative nephritis ('**Bright's disease**'). *2285*

1827:13 Mammalian **ovum** discovered by Karl Ernst von Baer (1792–1876), announced in his *De ovi mammalium et hominis genesi*, 1827. *477*

1827:14 **Cerebrospinal fluid** first clearly described by François Magendie (1783–1855), *JPE* **5**:27; **7**:1. *1392*

---

1827:15 Jean Antoine **Villemin**, French physician, born 28 Jan; proved tuberculosis to be a specific infection, transmissible by an inoculable agent. *Étude sur la tuberculose*, 1868. Died 1892. *2324*

1827:16 Joseph **Lister**, British surgeon, born 5 Apr; published the results of his research on inflammation, 1858, *PT* **148**:645. Introduced the antiseptic principle in surgery, using carbolic acid-impregnated dressings, 1867, *L* **1**:326, 357, 387, 507; **2**:95, 358, 668. Introduced antiseptic catgut ligature for arterial ligation, 1869, *L* **1**:451. Isolated *Bacterium lactis*, 1873, *QJMS* **13**:380, and was first to obtain a pure culture of it, 1878, *TPS* **29**:425. Died 1912. *2298, 5634, 5635, 2964, 2484, 2489*

1827:17 Daniel Hack **Tuke**, British physician, born 18 Apr; with John Charles Bucknill, published *A manual of psychological medicine*, 1858, for many years the standard English work on psychological medicine. Died 1895. *4934*

1827:18 Emil **Noeggerath**, German obstetrician and gynaecologist, born 5 Oct; devised the operation of epicystotomy, 1858, *NYJM* **4**:9. In his *Die latente Gonorrhoe im weiblichen Geschlecht*, 1872, he was first to point out the late effects of gonorrhoea in women, particularly its role in the production of sterility. Died 1895. *6044, 6064*

1827:19 Anton **Biermer**, German physician, born 18 Oct; his description of pernicious anaemia ('Biermer's anaemia'), 1868, *KBSA* **2**:15, was the first to mention the retinal haemorrhages. Died 1892. *3124*

1827:20 Jean Baptiste Auguste **Chauveau**, French physician and veterinarian, born 23 Nov; he named as 'elementary bodies' the minute bodies inside the inclusion bodies, the infective particles in the smallpox virus, 1868, *CRAS* **66**:359. Died 1917. *5425.1*

1827:21 Emanuel **Winge**, Norwegian surgeon, born 20 Dec; first suggested bacterial origin of endocarditis, 1869, *NML* **23**:78. Died 1894, *2767*

1827:23 Henry **Gray**, British anatomist, born; published first edition of his *Anatomy*, 1858, now a standard work on the subject in the English-speaking world. Died 1861. *418*

1827: Johann Peter **Frank** died, **born** 1745. *public hygiene*

1827: John **Haygarth** died, **born** 1740. *rheumatism*

1827: Carl **Wenzel** died, **born** 1769. *artificially-induced premature labour*

1827: Wilhelm Joseph **Schmitt** died, **born** 1760. *interstitial pregnancy*

**1828**
1828:1 **Royal Free Hospital, London**, founded by William Marsden (1796–1867)

1828:2 **School of Medicine** founded at **Sheffield**, England

1828:3 **Medical Department** founded at **University of Georgia, Atlanta**

1828:4 *New England Journal of Medicine and Surgery* renamed *Boston Medical and Surgical Journal*

1828:5 *Gazette des Hôpitaux* founded (as *Lancette Française*)

1828:6 *Glasgow Medical Journal* founded

1828:7 **University College London** opened

1828:8 Charles Michel Billard (1800–1832) performed several hundred autopsies on infants and children, correlated the data with clinical observations and incorporated this in his *Traité des maladies des enfans nouveau-nés et à la mamelle*. It was a pioneer work on the **pathological anatomy** of **infants**. *6332*

1828:9 The *Handbuch der Bücherkunde für die ältere Medicin*, by Johann Ludwig Choulant (1791–1861) is one of the best **medical bibliographic** check lists of the printed works of the older medical writers. 2nd ed., 1841, last reprinted 1956. *6753*

1828:10 Successful human-to-human **blood transfusion** by James Blundell (1790–1877), *L* **2**:321. *2017*

1828:11 Marie Jean Pierre Flourens (1794–1867) demonstrated that lesion of the **semicircular canals** cause **motor incoordination** and loss of **equilibrium**, 1828, *AnSN* **15**:113. *1557*

1828:12 **Brodie's abscess of bone** first described by Benjamin Collins Brodie (1783–1862), *LMG* **2**:70. *4314*

1828:13 '**Dupuytren's abscess**' of the right iliac fossa described by Guillaume Dupuytren (1777–1835), *RMFE* **1**:367. *3438*

1828:14 **Enterotome** for use in his operation for artificial **anus** invented by Guillaume Dupuytren (1777–1835), *MARM* **1**:259. *3437*

1828:15 Modern **tonsillotome** invented by Philip Syng Physick (1768–1837), *AmJMS* **2**:116. *3255*

1828:16 First textbook of **neuropathology** published by John Abercrombie (1780–1844); *Pathological and clinical researches on diseases of the brain and spinal cord*. *2285.1*

1828:17 Mediate **percussion** pioneered by Pierre Adolph Piorry (1794–1879); in his *De la percussion médiate*; he introduced the **percussor** and **pleximeter** in 1826. *2675*

1828:18 **Haemodynamometer** (a mercury **manometer**) invented by Jean Leonard Marie Poiseuille (1797–1869); in his *Recherches sur la force du coeur aortique*. *767*

1828:19 Synthesis of **urea** by Friedrich Wöhler (1800–1882); this synthesis was the first instance of an organic compound being made from inorganic materials, *AnPh* **12**:253. *671*

1828:20 '**Germ-layer theory**' and **notochord** discovered by Karl Ernst von Baer (1792–1876); in his *Ueber Entwicklungsgeschichte der Thiere*, 3 vols *479*

1828:21 **Tuberculous** nature of **Pott's disease** established by Jacques Mathieu Delpech (1777–1832); in his *De l'orthomorphie*, 2 vols, a comprehensive treatise on diseases of bones and joints. *4315*

---

1828:22 Alexander **Pagenstecher**, German ophthalmologist, born 21 Apr; his method of extraction of the lens in the closed capsule through scleral incision for the treatment of cataract was recorded in *Klinische Beobachtungen aus der Augenheilanstalt zu Wiesbaden*, Heft 3, p. 10, 1866, edited by Pagenstecher and E.T. Saemisch. Died 1879. *5896*

1828:23 Etienne Stéphane **Tarnier**, French obstetrician, born 29 Apr; invented the axis-traction forceps, 1877, *AnG* **7**:241; also his *Description de deux nouveaux forceps*. First to adopt Listerian antisepsis in obstetrics, employing carbolic acid solution as early as 1881; he wrote *De l'asepsie et antisepsie en obstétrique*, 1894. Died 1897. *6192, 5639*

1828:24 Jean Henri **Dunant**, French banker, born 8 May; his *Un souvenir de Solferino*, 1862, resulted in the Geneva Convention of 1864 and the foundation of the international Red Cross. Joint first recipient of the Nobel Peace Prize, 1901, *NPL*. Died 1910. *2166*

1828:25 Friedrich Wilhelm Ernst Albrecht von **Graefe**, German ophthalmologist, born 22 May; introduced iridectomy in the treatment of iritis and iridochoroiditis, 1855, *GAO* **2**, ii:202; described an operation for strabismus, 1857, *GAO* **3**, ii:456; **4**, ii:127; **8**, ii:242; introduced the operation of iridectomy for the treatment of glaucoma, 1857, *GAO* **5**, i:136. Discovered an important diagnostic sign in exophthalmic goitre – failure of the eyelid to follow the eye when it is rolled downward ('Graefe's sign'), 1864, *DK* **16**:158. Improved the operation for cataract by modified linear extraction, 1865, *GAO* **11**, iii:1; **12**, i:150; **14**, iii:106. Gave the first thorough account of paralysis of the eye muscles and the basis for surgical treatment, in his *Symptomenlehre der Augenmuskellähmungen*, 1867. Gave a classical account of keratoconus, 1868, *BKW* **5**:241, 249. Died 1870. *5873, 5880, 5881, 4536, 3820, 5897, 5899, 5900*

1828:26 Eugène **Koeberlé**, French surgeon and gynaecologist, born 29 May; in part responsible for the introduction of ovariotomy into France, 1863, *MAIM* **26**:321; performed the first successful excision of uterus and ovaries (for tumour), 1863, *GMS* **23**:101. Died 1915. *6051, 6052*

1828:27 Johann Nepomuk **Czermak**, Czech physiologist, born 18 Jun; demonstrated the utility of Manuel Garcia's laryngoscope, substituted artificial for natural light, and made other improvements in it, 1858, *SAW* **29**:557. Died 1873. *3331*

1828:28 Jonathan **Hutchinson**, British surgeon, born 23 Jul; he described the notched incisors ('Hutchinson's teeth') present in congenital syphilis, 1858, *TPS* **9**:449. First successfully operated upon a case of intussusception in a two-year-old infant, 1871, *MCT* **57**:31. Gave the first description and illustration of sarcoidosis and a classical description of cheiropompholyx; in his *Illustrations of clinical surgery*, 1875–8, **1**, 42, 49. First described hydradenitis destruens suppurativa, 1879; in his *Lectures on clinical surgery*, 1879, **2**, 298; it was later named 'Pollitzer's disease' after the latter's description in 1892. First described varicella gangrenosa, 1882, *MCT* **65**:1. First to describe progeria, 1886, *MCT* **69**:473. Died 1913. *2386, 3466, 4067, 4075, 5439, 3790*

1828:29 William Alexander **Hammond**, American neurologist, born 28 Aug; wrote the first American treatise on neurology, *Treatise on diseases of the nervous system*, 1871; in it he included (p. 654) the original description of athetosis ('Hammond's disease'). Died 1900. *4542*

1828:30 James Edward **Garretson**, American oral surgeon, born 4 Oct; wrote the *Treatise on the diseases and surgery of the mouth*, etc., 1869, the first modern textbook of oral surgery. Died 1895. *3684.1*

1828:31 Otto **Funke**, German physiologist, born 27 Oct; discovered haemoglobin, 1852, *ZRM* **1**:172; **2**:298. Died 1879. *866*

1828:32 John Langdon Haydon **Langdon-Down**, British physician, born 18 Nov; suggested that the physiognomonical features of certain mental defectives enabled them to be classified in ethnic groups, 1866, *CLLH* **3**:259. His classification has been abandoned, but the term mongolism (now replaced by 'Down's syndrome') was used to describe one important variety of mental retardation. Died 1896. *4936*

1828:33 Robert **Battey**, American gynaecologist, born 26 Nov; his recourse to ovariotomy for the treatment of non-ovarian conditions, 1872, *AtMJ* **10**:321; *TMAG* **24**:36, later acquired greater significance in connection with more modern work on endocrinology. Died 1895. *6062*

1828:34 Karl **Kahlbaum** born; suggested catatonia as a separate disease entity; in his *Die Katatonie*, 1874. Died 1899. *4938*

1828:35 Henry Robert **Silvester** born; invented the Silvester method of artificial respiration, 1858, *BMJ* 586. Died 1908. *2028.57*

1828:36 Benjamin Horatio **Paul** born; with Alfred Cownley, obtained emetine in pure form, 1894, *PhJ* **54**:111, 373, 690. Died 1902. *1887*

1828:37 Ferdinand Ethelbert **Junker**, Austrian surgeon, born; invented a chloroform inhaler (Junker's inhaler), 1867, *MTG* 1867, **2**:590; 1868, **1**:171. Died ?1901. *5668*

1828:38 Pierre Cyprien **Oré** born; performed the first successful human intravenous anaesthesia, 1874, *CRAS* **78**:515, 651. Died 1889. *5672*

1828:39 Thomas Addis **Emmet**, American gynecologist, born; wrote *Vesico-vaginal fistula, from parturition and other causes*, 1868, a comprehensive account of the management of vesico-vaginal fistula based on Sims' technique. Treated chronic cystitis by vaginal cystotomy, 1872, *AmP* **5**:65. Devised a technique for perineorrhaphy, 1883, reported 1884, *TAGS* **8**:198. Died 1919. *6058, 6037, 6063, 6078*

1828: Franz Joseph **Gall** died, **born** 1758. *localization of cerebral function, phrenology*

1828: René Joseph Hyacinthe **Bertin** died, **born** 1757. *syphilis*

1828: Philip Wright **Post** died, **born** 1766. *subclavian artery ligation, aneurysm, carotid artery ligation*

1828: Jacopo **Penada** died, **born** 1748. *duodenal ulcer*

1828: William Hyde **Wollaston** died, **born** 1766. *urinary calculi, cystine*

## 1829

1829:1 First **water filtration system** constructed for **Chelsea Water Company**, London

1829:2 One of the earliest descriptions of hyperplastic cystic mammary disease published by Astley Paston Cooper (1768–1841); in his *Illustrations of the diseases of the breast*. *5769*

1829:3 The first extensive publication on **blepharoplasty** was recorded by Johann Karl Georg Fricke (1790–1841) in his *Die Bildung neuer Augenlider (Blepharoplastik) nach Zerstörungen und dadurch hervorgebrachten Auswärtswendungen derselben. 5742.1*

1829:4 An important description of '**Aleppo boil**' (cutaneous **leishmaniasis**) given by Jean Louis Marc Alibert (1768–1837), *RMFE* **3**:62. *5291*

1829:5 **Pathological anatomy**; Jean Cruveilhier (1791–1874) published *Anatomie pathologique du corps humain*, 1829–42, one of the most important books on the subject. *2286*

1829:6 **Laryngoscopy** was introduced when a crude '**glottiscope**' was demonstrated by Guy Babington (1794–1866), *LMG* **3**:555. *3327*

1829:7 Dominique Jean Larrey (1766–1842) was the greatest of all military surgeons. His most comprehensive treatise on **surgery** was *Clinique chirurgicale, excercée particulièrement dans les camps et les hôpitaux militaires depuis 1792 jusqu'en 1829*, 5 vols, 1829–36. *5589.1*

1829:8 **Rubella (Rötheln)** separated from measles and scarlet fever by a German physician, Wagner, *LAGH* **13**:420. *5501*

1829:9 **Tenotomy, rhinoplasty**, and **skin grafting**, successfully carried out by Johann Friedrich Dieffenbach (1792–1856); in his *Chirurgische Erfahrungen besonders über die Wiederherstellung zerstörter Theile des menschlichen Körpers nach neuen Methoden*, 3 vols, 1829–34. *5743*

1829:10 The term **typhoid fever** introduced by Pierre Charles Alexandre Louis (1787–1872), in his *Recherches anatomiques, pathologiques et thérapeutiques sur la maladie connue sous les noms de … typhoïde*, etc.; he first described the lenticular rose spots, and established the pathological picture. *5023*

1829:11 **Neuroma** first described by William Wood (1774–1857), *TMCS* **3**:367. *4523*

1829:12 **Splenectomy** performed by Carl Friedrich Quittenbaum (1793–1852); in his *De splenis hypertrophia et historia exterpationis splenis hypertrophici*, published 1836. *3763*

1829:13 The first **thyroidectomy** is accredited to Joseph Henry Green (1791–1863), *L* **2**:351. *3814*

1829:14 First English book on **medical statistics**, *Elements of medical statistics*, published by Francis Bisset Hawkins (1796–1894). *1697*

1829:15 '**Lugol's iodine**' for treatment of **skin tuberculosis** introduced by Jean Guillaume August Lugol (1786–1851); in his *Mémoire sur l'emploi de l'iodide sur les maladies scrophuleuses*; later used for **thyroid disorders**. *1849.1*

1829:16 **Cancer metastasis** first recognized by Joseph Claude Anthelm Récamier (1774–1852); in his *Recherches sur le traitement du cancer …. 2610*

1829:17 **Botulism** described by Christian Andreas Justinus Kerner (1786–1862), in his *Neue Beobachtungen über … den Genuss geräuchter Würste. 2468*

1829:18 George **Harley**, British physician, born 12 Feb; his classic description of paroxysmal haemoglobinuria, 1865, *MCT* **48**:161, led to the term 'Harley's disease'. Died 1896. *4171*

1829:19 Silas Weir **Mitchell**, American neurologist, born 15 Feb; gave first complete description of erythromelalgia, 1872, *PhMT* **3**:81, 113. His *Injuries of nerves and their consequences*, 1872, includes the first description of ascending neuritis, as well as the treatment of neuritis by cold and splint rests. In the same year he lectured on painful affections of the feet, for which he suggested the term erythromelalgia ('Mitchell's disease'). First to describe postparalytic chorea, 1874, *AmJMS* **68**:342. Introduced the Weir Mitchell treatment, in his *On rest in the treatment of nervous disease*, 1875. Published the first account of the relation of pain to weather, in a study of traumatic neuralgia, 1877, *AmJMS* **73**:305. Died 1914. *2706, 4544, 4545, 4552, 4553, 4555*

1829:20 Ernst Leberecht **Wagner**, German pathologist, born 12 Mar; his *Der Gebärmutterkrebs*, 1858, represents the first important contribution to the knowledge of the gross pathology of cancer of the uterus. First recorded dermatomyositis, now classified as a connective-tissue disease, 1863, *ArH* **4**:282; first described colloid degeneration of the skin ('Wagner's disease'), he named it 'colloid milium', 1866, *ArH* **7**:463. Died 1888. *6045, 4054, 4056*

1829:21 Anton Friedrich von **Tröltsch**, German otologist, born 3 Apr; invented the modern otoscope, 1860, *DK* **12**:113, 121, 131, 143, 151, and introduced the modern mastoid operation, 1861, *VA* **21**:295. Died 1890. *3374, 3375*

1829:22 Theodor **Billroth**, German surgeon, born 26 Apr; his *Die allgemeine chirurgische Pathologie und Therapie*, 1863, was translated into ten languages. Carried out first resection of the oesophagus, 1872, *ArKC* **13**:65. First to make a complete excision of the larynx for cancer, 1874, *VGDC* **3**, ii:76. Performed the first resection of a bladder tumour; recorded by Carl Gussenbauer, 1875, *ArKC* **18**:411. Carried out the first successful resection of the pylorus for carcinoma (the Billroth I operation), 1881, *WMW* **31**: 161, 1427. Died 1894. *5608, 3465, 3282, 4174, 3474*

1829:23 Gustav August **Braun**, Austrian obstetrician, born 28 May; introduced a decapitation hook, 1861, *WMW* **11**:713. Died 1911. 6184

1829:24 Frederick William **Pavy**, British physician and physiologist, born 29 May; described recurrent albuminuria ('Pavy's disease'), 1885, *BMJ* **2**:789. Died 1911. *4181*

1829:25 Eduard Friedrich Wilhelm **Pflüger**, German physiologist, born 7 Jun; studied the physiology of nerve, recorded in his *Untersuchungen über die Physiologie des Electrotonus*, 1859, and worked on gaseous exchange in blood and tissue and developed the concept of 'respiratory quotient', 1866, *ZMW* **4**:305, 1868; *PfA* **1**:61. Died 1910. *621, 939, 940*

1829:26 William Overend **Priestley**, British gynaecologist, born 24 Jun; first reported cases of Mittelschmerz (intermenstrual pain), 1872, *BMJ* **2**:431. Died 1900. *6065*

1829:27 Johann Ludwig Wilhelm **Thudichum**, German emigré chemist in London, born 27 Aug; identified haematoporphyrin, the first porphyrin to be discovered, 1867, *GBMO* **10**:152. Discovered cephalins and myelins in brain tissue; recorded in his *A treatise on the chemical constitution of the brain*, 1884. Died 1901. *3914.1, 1415.1*

1829:28 Joseph **Parrot**, French physician, born 1 Nov; first described the primary lesion of pulmonary tuberculosis in children ('Ghon's primary locus'), 1876, *CRSB* **3**:308. Reported discovery of pneumococcus by Louis Pasteur, 1881, *BuAM* **10**:379. Died 1883. *3224, 3233, 3172*

1829:29 Etienne **Lancereaux**, French physician, born 27 Nov; first definitely to claim a causal relationship between pancreatic lesions and diabetes mellitus, 1877, *BuAM* **6**:1215. Died 1910. *3943*

---

1829:30 Norman William **Kingsley**, American dentist, born; published the first book on the scientific treatment of irregularities of the teeth, *Treatise on oral deformities*, 1880. Died 1913. *3685.1*

---

1829: Louis Nicolas **Vauquelin** died, **born** 1763. *chemical analysis of nervous system*

1829: Thomas **Young** died, **born** 1773. *vision, optics*

1829: John Beale **Davidge** died, **born** 1768. *parotid gland*

1829: Nathan **Smith** died, **born** 1762. *osteomyelitis, typhoid, ovarian dropsy, ovariotomy*

1829: Humphry **Davy** died, **born** 1778. *anaesthetics, nitrous oxide*

**1830**
1830:1 **Academia Nacional de Medicina** founded in **Rio de Janeiro**

1830:2 The *Medicinisches Schriftsteller-Lexicon der jetzt lebenden Aerzte, Wundärzte, Geburtshelfer, Apotheker, und Naturforscher aller gebildeten Völker*, 25 vols and 8-vol. supplement, 1830–45, the great **medical bibliography** of Adolf Carl Peter Callisen (1787–1866) gives a comprehensive view of the literature from *c*.1780–1830 and describes over 99,000 items. Reprinted 1962–64. *6754*

1830:3 Salomon Levi Steinheim (1799–1866) is credited by some German writers with the first description of **parathyroid tetany**, *LAGH* **17**:22; an important early description was given by Dance (1831). *4827, 4828*

1830:4 The *Practical treatise on diseases of the eye*, by William Mackenzie (1791–1868) included a classic description of the symptomatology of **glaucoma**. Mackenzie was probably the first to draw attention to increased intra-ocular pressure, characteristic of the disease. *5848*

1830:5 The first recorded use of **emetine** in the treatment of **amoebiasis** is in *Hospital facts and observations*, p. 149, by James Lomax Bardsley (1801–1876). *5183*

1830:6 The first American treatise on **orthopaedics**, *The anatomy, physiology, and diseases of the bones and joints*, published by Samuel David Gross (1805–1884). *4316.1*

---

1830:7 Etienne Jules **Marey**, French physiologist, born 5 Mar; invented the modern sphygmograph; in his *Recherches sur la pouls*, 1860, also *CRAS* **51**:281. He was a pioneer in the use of serial pictures as a method of studying the mechanics of locomotion, *Le mouvement*, 1894. Died 1904. *776, 643*

1830:8 Eadweard **Muybridge**, British photographer, born 9 Apr; his exhaustive photographic investigations of consecutive phases of human and animal movements demonstrated the possibilities of motion pictures; *Animals in motion*, 1899, *The human figure in motion*, 1901. Died 1904. *650, 651*

1830:9 Abraham **Jacobi**, German/American paediatrician, born 6 May; was first in the United States to specialize in paediatrics. In 1862 he founded the first paediatric clinic there (in New York). In 1887 he wrote *The intestinal diseases of infancy and childhood*. Died 1919. *6342*

1830:10 Richard **Liebreich**, German ophthalmologist, born 30 Jun; introduced lateral illumination in microscopic investigation of the living eye, 1855, *GAO* **1**, ii:351. Published *Atlas der Ophthalmoscopie*, 1863, the first atlas of the fundus oculi. Died 1917. *5877, 5892*

1830:11 August **Rothmund**, German ophthalmologist, born 1 Aug; described poikiloderma congenitale, 1868, *GAO* **14**:159. Died 1906. *4056.1*

1830:12 Richard von **Volkmann**, German surgeon, born 17 Aug; described cancer due to industrial tar and paraffin; in his *Beiträge zur Chirurgie*, 1875, p. 370. Carried out the first excision of the rectum for cancer, 1878, *SKV* **131**:1113. Described 'Volkmann's ischaemic contracture', 1881, *ZCh* **8**:801. Died 1889. *2126, 3470, 5617*

1830:13 Alfred Carl **Graefe**, German ophthalmologist, born 23 Nov; cousin of Albrecht, with Edwin Theodor Saemisch edited the great work on **eye diseases**, *Handbuch der gesamten Augenheilkunde*, 1874–1880. A second edition appeared, 15 vols [in 41], 1899–1918. Died 1909. *5944*

1830:14 Jules Emile **Péan**, French surgeon, born 29 Nov; carried out gastrectomy (unsuccessful) for carcinoma, 1879, *GH* **52**:473. Described a method of *morcellement* of the uterus for the removal of tumours, 1886, *GH* **59**:445. Carried out total replacement of a shoulder, using a prosthesis made of hardened rubber and platinum, 1894, *GH* **67**:289. Carried out first operation on bladder diverticula, 1895, *BuAM* **33**:542. Died 1898. *3472, 6084, 4364.1, 4189*

1830:15 Louis Xavier Edouard Léopold **Ollier**, French surgeon, born 2 Dec; pioneered bone allografting; in his *Traité experimentale et clinique de la régenération des os*, 1867. First obtained intermediate-thickness skin grafts, 1872, *BuAM* **1**:243, from which developed the Ollier-Thiersch graft. First described 'Ollier's disease', multiple enchondromatosis, 1889, *MSML* **29**, 2:12. Died 1900. *4336.1, 5752, 5753, 4352*

1830:16 Harald **Hirschsprung**, Danish paediatrician, born; first drew attention to congenital megacolon ('Hirschsprung's disease'), 1887, *JaK* **27**:1; established congenital hypertrophic pyloric stenosis as a distinct clinical entity, 1888, *JaK* **28**:61. Died 1916. *3489, 3489.1*

1830:17 Tomas **Salazar**, Peruvian physician, born; gave the name verruga peruana to bartonellosis (Carrión's disease, Oroya fever), caused by infection with *Bartonella bacilliformis*, 1858, *GMLi* **2**:161, 175. Died 1917. *5525*

1830:18 John Zachariah **Laurence**, British physician, born; with Robert Charles Moon, reported four cases of retinitis pigmentosa with familial developmental imperfections, 1866, *OR* **2**:32. Following further reports by A. Biedl (1922), it was named the Laurence-Moon-Biedl syndrome. Died 1874. *6368, 6369*

1830: Ephraim **McDowell** died, **born** 1771. *ovariotomy*

1830: Mason Fitch **Cogswell** died, **born** 1761. *carotid artery ligation*

1830: Samuel Thomas **Soemmerring** died, **born** 1755. *anatomical illustration, cranial nerves, achondroplasia*

1830: Henry Hill **Hickman** died, **born** 1800. *anaesthesia*

**1831**

1831:1 **University of Berlin** founded

1831:2 *Proceedings of the Royal Society of London* commences publication

1831:3 **British Association for the Advancement of Science** founded in York

1831:4 **University of the City of New York** founded

1831:5 Edmund Axmann described **osteogenesis imperfecta**, occurring in himself and his two brothers, *AnGH* **4**:58. He referred to the occurrence of articular dislocations and blue sclerotics (mentioned by Eddowes in his 1900 description of osteogenesis imperfecta). *6358.1, 6367*

1831:6 An important early description of **parathyroid tetany** given by Jean Baptiste Hippolyte Dance (1797–1832), *ArGM* **26**:190, described by Steinheim (1830). *4828, 4827*

1831:7 The first description of the **neurotic spinal arthropathies** given by John Kearsley Mitchell (1793–1858), *AmJMS* **8**:55. *4493*

1831:8 An operation for the treatment of **flexion contracture deformity of the fingers** ('**Dupuytren's contracture**') devised by Guillaume Dupuytren (1777–1835), *JUSM* **5**:352; a condition already mentioned by Felix Platter in 1614. *4317*

1831:9 **Atropine** isolated in pure form by Mein, a German chemist, *AnCP* **6**:67. *1854*

1831:10 **Chloroform** discovered by Eugène Soubeiran (1793–1858), *AnC* **48**:113, independently of Samuel Guthrie, 1832, and Justus von Liebig, 1832. *1851, 5649, 1850, 5648, 1852, 5650*

1831:11 **Hay fever** shown to be due to **pollen** by John Elliotson (1791–1868), *LMG* **8**:411; **12**:164. *2584*

1831:12 **Cell nucleus** discovered by Robert Brown (1773–1858), *TLS* **16**:685. *109.*

1831:13 The first systematic publication in England on **occupational diseases**, *The effect of the principal arts, trades, and professions and the civic states and habits of living on health and longevity*, was written by Charles Turner Thackrah (1795–1833). *2123*

---

1831:14 Johann Friedrich **Horner**, Swiss ophthalmologist, born 27 Mar; drew attention to a syndrome, ptosis of the eyelid ('Horner's syndrome'), the effect of a lesion of the cervical sympathetic nerve; proof that the sympathetic governs the pupillary, vasomotor, sudomotor and pilomotor functions, 1869, *KMA* **7**:193. Died 1886. *1328, 5903*

1831:15 Henry Vandyke **Carter**, British tropical pathologist and artist, born 22 May; gave the first modern description of mycetoma of the foot ('Madura foot', 'Carter's mycetoma'), 1860, *TMPB* **6**:184; he gave a fuller account in 1874 in his *On mycetoma, or the fungus disease of India*. His original work on Asiatic relapsing fever, recorded in his *Spirillum fever*, 1882, is remembered by the eponym 'Carter's fever' and the name *Borrelia carteri*. Reported a blood spirillum, *Spirillum minus*, in a rat, 1887, *SMI* **3**:45, later shown to be a cause of spirillary rat-bite fever. Drew the illustrations for Gray's *Anatomy*. Died 1897. *4047, 4066, 5316, 5323*

1831:16 Werner **Hagedorn**, German surgeon, born 2 Jul; his operation for the repair of unilateral cleft lip, 1884, *ZCh* **11**:756, forms the basis of most modern methods. Died 1894. *5754.3*

1831:17 Wilhelm **His** Sr, Swiss anatomist and embryologist, born 9 Jul; introduced microtome, 1870, *ArMA* **6**:229; formulated neuron theory, 1886, *AbL* **13**:477 (Forel did so independently, 1887; it was named by Waldeyer, 1891). Died 1904. *268, 1368.1*

1831:18 Valentine H. **Taliaferro**, American gynaecologist, born 24 Sep; performed the first episiotomy in America (2 December 1851), reported 1852, *SVMG* **2**:382. Died 1888. *6180*

1831:19 Alarik Frithiof **Holmgren**, Swedish physiologist, born 22 Oct; introduced the electroretinogram, 1865, *ULF* **1**:177; demonstrated retinal action currents, 1871, *ULF* **6**:419. Introduced the wool-skein test for the diagnosis of colour-blindness, 1874, *NoMA* **6** nr.24:1; nr.28:1. Made an important contribution on colour-blindness and its relation to railway and maritime traffic, 1876, *ULF* **12**:171, 267. Died 1897. *1511.1, 1514, 5911, 5916*

1831:20 Carl von **Voit**, German physiologist, born 31 Oct. With M.J. von Pettenkofer, carried out combined feeding-respiration experiments, being first to estimate the amounts of protein, fat and carbohydrates broken down in the body, 1862–3, *ACP* Suppl.2:52; he became the leading investigator of metabolism, *Handbuch der Physiologie des Gesammt-Stoffwechsels und der Fortpflanzung*, 1881. Founded Hygienic Laboratory in Munich, 1866. Died 1908. *938, 635*

1831:21 Theodore Gaillard **Thomas**, American gynaecologist and obstetrician, born 21 Nov; revived and modified Ritgen's operation of extraperitoneal caesarean section, and named it gastro-elytrotomy, 1870, *AmJOD* **3**:125. Performed the first vaginal ovariotomy, 1870, *AmJMS* **59**:387. Died 1903. *6239, 6238, 6061*

———

1831:22 Ernest **Besnier**, French dermatologist, born; described sarcoidosis (Besnier-Boeck-Schaumann disease), 1889, *AnD* **10**:333. Described 'Besnier's prurigo', 1892, *AnD* **3**:634. Died 1909. *4095, 4128, 4149, 4107*

1831:23 Pietro **Loreta**, Italian surgeon, born; first to perform the operation of pyloroplasty, 1882, *MASB* **4**:353. Died 1889. *3477*

1831:24 Thomas **Hillier**, British physician, born; performed the first successful therapeutic percutaneous nephrostomy, 1865, *PRMCS* **5**:59. Died 1868. *4211.1*

1831:25 Jeffery Allen **Marston** born; British army surgeon, first to draw attention to what later became known as Weil's disease, a severe form of leptospirosis, 1861, *AMD* **3**:486. Gave the first description of Malta fever (brucellosis) as a distinct disease, 1863, *AMD* **3**:486. Died 1911. *5330, 5097*

1831:26 George **Lawson** born; first successfully transplanted sizeable free skin grafts, as well as whole-thickness skin, 1871, *TCSL* **4**:49. Died 1908. *5751*

---

1831: John **Abernethy** died, **born** 1764. *surgery, aneurysm, iliac artery ligation*

1831: Henry **Park** died, **born** 1783. *destructive joint disease*

## 1832

1832:1 **Provincial Medical and Surgical Association** founded at Worcester, England; becomes **British Medical Association**, 1855

1832:2 **Anatomy Act** passed in **England**; providing that unclaimed bodies of dead should go to medical schools for **dissection**

1832:3 **Boston Lying-in Hospital** founded

1832:4 **Liverpool Medical Institution** founded

1832:5 *Annalen der Pharmacie* (**Chemie und Pharmacie** 1840–) founded by Justus von Liebig (1803–1873)

1832:6 **Cardiac innervation** decisively demonstrated by Antonio Scarpa (1752–1832); in what is considered his greatest work, *Tabulae nevrologicae. 1253*

1832:7 Guillaume Dupuytren (1777–1835) became the best surgeon of his time in France; his greatest contributions were in the field of **surgical pathology**. His writings include *Leçons orales de clinique chirurgicale*, 4 vols, 1832–4. *5590*

1832:8 **Chloroform** discovered independently by Samuel Guthrie (1782–1848), *AmJSc* **21**:64; **22**:105, Justus von Liebig (1803–1873), *AnP* **1**:182, and (1831) by Eugène Soubeiran. *1850, 5648, 1852, 5650, 1851, 5649*

1832:9 The water-borne character of **cholera**, and the use of **charcoal filters** for **water purification**, suggested by John Parkin (1801–1886), *LMSJ* n.s.**2**:151. *5105*

1832:10 Jean Louis Marc Alibert's (1768–1837) *Monographie des dermatoses*, includes the first published illustration of his 'family tree' for the classification of **skin diseases**, never widely adopted, and an important description of **dermatolysis**. *3990.1*

1832:11 **Chlorosis** treated with **ferrous sulphate** and **potassium carbonate** ('**Blaud's pill**') by Pierre Blaud (1774–1858), *RMFE* **45**:337. *3113*

1832:12 **Cardiac catheterization** performed by Johann Friedrich Dieffenbach (1792–1847), *ChA* **1**, i:86; in unsuccessful attempt to obtain blood from a cholera patient. *2748.1*

186

1832:13 **Corrigan's pulse**, 'water-hammer pulse' described in his account of **aortic insufficiency** by Dominic John Corrigan (1802–1880), *EMSJ* **37**:225; earlier described by Vieussens, 1705. *2748*

1832:14 **Codeine** isolated by Pierre Jean Robiquet (1780–1840), *AnC* **51**:225. *1853*

1832:15 Classification of **burns** by Guillaume Dupuytren (1777–1835); in his *Leçons orales de clinique chirurgicale*. *2247*

1832:16 **Shrapnell's membrane**, the pars placida of the tympanic membrane, described by Henry Jones Shrapnell (d.1834), *LMG* **10**:120. *1558*

1832:17 The first full description of **Hodgkin's disease** given by Thomas Hodgkin (1798–1866), *MCT* **17**:68, and so named by Samuel Wilks in 1865. *3762*

1832:18 James Hope's (1801–1841) *Treatise on the diseases of the heart and great vessels*, did much to advance the knowledge of **heart murmurs, valvular disease and aneurysm**. *2747*

1832:19 *Nouveaux éléments de médecine opératoire*, 3 vols and atlas, by Alfred Armand Louis Velpeau (1795–1867), was the most comprehensive work on **operative surgery** in France. *5592*

---

1832:20 Photinos **Panas**, Greek/French ophthalmologist, born 30 Jan; introduced an operation for congenital and paralytic ptosis of the eyelid, 1886, *ArO* **6**:1. Died 1903. *5929*

1832:21 Edward **Liveing**, British physician, born 8 Feb; gave a classic account of migraine; in his *On megrim, sick-headache, and some allied disorders*, 1873. He showed an association between migraine and tetany, asthma, and false angina. Died 1919. *4549*

1832:22 Franz **König**, German surgeon, born 10 Feb; introduced the term osteochondritis dissecans, 1888, *DZC* **27**:90. Died 1910. *4350*

1832:23 Isidor von **Neumann**, Bohemian dermatologist, born 2 Mar; first described porokeratosis and named it dermatitis circumscripta herpetiformis, 1875, *VDS* **2**:41; Mibelli's more detailed account in 1893 led to the term 'Mibelli's disease'. Described pemphigus vegetans ('Neumann's disease'), 1886, *VDS* **13**:157; a suppurative form of the disease was described by Hallopeau in 1889. Died 1906. *4068, 4114, 4087, 4101*

1832:24 Jakob Hermann **Knapp**, German/Austrian ophthalmologist, born 17 Mar; wrote a valuable monograph on curvature of the cornea, *Die Krümmung der Hornhaut des menschlichen Auges*, 1859; he became one of the leading ophthalmologists in America. Died 1911. *5884*

1832:25 August **Breisky**, Bohemian gynaecologist and obstetrician, born 25 Mar; gave an important, although not the first, account of kraurosis vulvae, 1885, *ZHe* **6**:69. Died 1889. *6082*

1832:26 Ernst von **Leyden**, German physician, born 20 Apr; first described myotonia congenita; in his *Klinik der Rückenmarks-Krankheiten*, **2**, **ii**, 550, 1876. Described acute ataxia ('Leyden's ataxia'), 1891, *ZKM* **18**:576. Died 1910. *4743, 4706.1*

1832:27 Jean Baptiste **Berenger-Féraud**, French naval surgeon, born 9 May; gave an early important account of blackwater fever; in his *De la fièvre bilieuse mélanique dans les pays chauds comparée avec la fièvre jaune*, 1874. Died 1901. *5235*

1832:28 Jean Alfred **Fournier**, French venereologist, born 12 May; stated the syphilitic origin of tabes dorsalis, a view not at first accepted, in his *De l'ataxie locomotrice d'origine syphilitique*, 1876. He introduced the concept of 'parasyphilis' and showed statistically the causal relationship of syphilis to paresis and tabes, in his *Les affections parasyphilitiques*, 1894. Died 1914. *4782, 4800*

1832:29 Wilhelm Max **Wundt**, German psychologist, born 16 Aug; the founder of experimental psychology; his principal work was *Grundzüge der physiologischen Psychologie*, 1872–4. Wrote on sensory perception, 1858–1863, *ZRM* **4**:229; **7**:279, 321; **12**:145; **14**:1; **15**:104. Died 1920. *4976, 1463*

1832:30 Léon **Labbe**, French surgeon, born 29 Sep; with E. Guyon, developed pre-anaesthetic medication, 1872, *CRAS* **74**:627. Died 1916. *5670*

1832:31 Andrew Woods **Smyth**, American surgeon, born; first successful ligation of the innominate artery, 1864, *AmJMS* **52**:289. Died 1916. *2963*

1832:32 Henry Dewey **Noyes** born; first to investigate retinitis accompanying glucosuria, 1869, *TAOS* 1867–8 (1869):71. Died 1900. *3938*

1832:33 Henry Richard Lobb **Veale**, British physician, born; introduced the term rubella to describe German measles (Rötheln), 1866, *EMJ* **12**:404. Died 1908. *5502*

1832: Johann Caspar **Spurzheim** died, **born** 1776. *localization of cerebral function, phrenology*

1832: Thomas **Trotter** died, **born** 1760. *alcoholism*

1832: Georges Simon **Sérullas** died, **born** 1774. *iodoform*

1832: Everard **Home** died, **born** 1756. *cornu cutaneum, artificial insemination*

1832: Jean Baptiste Hippolyte **Dance** died, **born** 1797. *parathyroid tetany*

1832: Jacques Mathieu **Delpech** died, **born** 1777. *rhinoplasty, Pott's disease*

1832: Antonio **Scarpa** died, **born** 1752. *ophthalmology, talipes, hernia, Scarpa's fascia and triangle, ear, olfaction, aneurysm, cardiac innervation*

1832: Charles Michel **Billard** died, **born** 1800. *pathological anatomy of children*

## 1833
1833:1 **Zürich Hochschule (Universität)** Medical Faculty opened

1833:2 **Aertzlicher Verein, Munich**, founded

1833:3 **Liver puncture** used as a diagnostic measure by Edward Stanley (1793–1862), *L* **1**:189. *3616*

1833:4 **Talipes (club-foot)** successfully treated by **tenotomy** by Georg Friedrich Stromeyer (1804–1876), *MGH* **39**:195. *4320*

1833:5 **Osteopsathyrosis**, a form of **fragilitas ossium**, 'Lobstein's disease' first described by Jean George Chrétien Frédéric Martin Lobstein (1777–1835); in his *Traité de l'anatomie pathologique*, **2**:204. *4318*

1833:6 The best contemporary **lithotrite** designed by Charles Louis Stanislas Heurteloup (1793–1864); in his *Lithotripsie*; he is amongst those accredited with the introduction of modern **lithotrity**. *4290*

1833:7 The *Treatise on the diseases of the eye* by William Lawrence (1783–1867) was a landmark in the history of **ophthalmic surgery**. *5849*

1833:8 Amputation of the **cervix** for chronic ulceration practised by Marie Anne Victoire Boivin (1773–1841) and Antoine Dugès; in their *Traité pratique des maladies de l'utérus et ses annexes*, **2**, p. 648, is the first recorded case of **cancer** of the female **urethra**. *6028*

1833:9 John Elliotson (1791–1868) proved that **glanders** in the horse is communicable to man, *MCT* **16**:171; **18**:201. *5153*

1833:10 **Tracheotomy** in **diphtheria** popularized by Armand Trousseau (1801–1867), *JCMC* **1**:5, 41. *5054*

1833:11 John Hilton (1804–1878) observed what was later named *Trichinella spiralis*, in human muscle, and suggested it was a parasite, *LMG* **11**:605. *5336.5*

1833:12 The first description of **lymphogranuloma venereum** given by William Wallace (1791–1837); in his *Treatise on the venereal disease and its varieties*, p. 371. *5215*

1833:13 First use of the term **arteriosclerosis (arteriosclérose)** by Jean Georges Chrétien Frédéric Martin Lobstein (1777–1835); in his *Traité d'anatomie pathologique*, **2**, 550. *2901*

1833:14 **Reflex action** established by Marshall Hall (1790–1857), *PT* **123**:635. *1359*

1833:15 *Experiments and observations on the gastric juice* published by William Beaumont (1785–1853); studied digestion and the movements of the stomach through a gastric fistula caused by a gunshot wound. His preliminary reports appeared in 1825–6, *MRecorder*, **8**:14, 840; **9**:94. *989, 987.1, 987.2*

1833:16 Jacob Mendes **Da Costa**, American physician, born West Indies 7 Feb; described 'Da Costa's syndrome', 1871, *AmJMS* **61**:17, the 'effort syndrome' of Lewis (1917), first mentioned by Myers (1870). Died 1900. *2770*

1833:17 Carl Friedrich Otto **Westphal**, German psychiatrist, born 23 Mar; first described agoraphobia, 1871, *ArPN* **3**:138. Used the knee-jerk as a diagnostic measure in tabes dorsalis, 1875, *ArPN* **5**:803, diagnostic value discovered simultaneously by Erb. Described cerebrospinal pseudosclerosis ('Westphal's pseudosclerosis'), 1883, *ArPN* **14**:87; a later account by Strümpell (1898) led to the term 'Westphal-Strümpell disease'. Died 1890. *4844, 4781, 4780, 4702, 4709*

1833:18 Thomas **Smith**, British pathologist, born 23 Mar; first to report craniohypophyseal xanthomatosis, 1865, *TPS* **16**:224; **27**:219, later to be associated with the Hand-Schüller-Christian syndrome. Died 1909. *6359–6363*

1833:19 Julius **Althaus**, German physician, born 31 Mar; introduced Duchenne's methods of electrotherapy into England; used electrolysis for medical purposes; *On the electrolytic treatment of tumors ...*, 1867. Died 1900. *1996.3*

1833:20 Theodor Hermann **Meynert**, German neurologist and psychiatrist, born 15 Jun; first described several structures in the brain, *Der Bau der Grosshirnrinde*, 1868; wrote on insanity and described amentia, *Klinik der Erkrankungen ded Vorderhirns*, 1884. Died 1892. *1403, 4942*

1833:21 Emanuel **Zaufal**, Bohemian otologist, born 12 Jul; improved the mastoid operation devised by Schwartze and Eysell, 1884, *PMW* **9**:474. Died 1910. *3388*

1833:22 Wilhelm Alexander **Freund**, German gynaecologist, born 26 Aug; carried out the first successful abdominal hysterectomy for cancer, 1878, *BKW* **15**:417. Died 1918. *6070*

1833:23 Edwin Theodor **Saemisch**, German ophthalmologist, born 30 Sep; first described serpiginous ulcer of the cornea ('Saemisch's ulcer'); in his *Das Ulcus corneae serpens und seine Therapie*, 1870. With Alfred Carl Graefe edited the great work on **eye diseases**, *Handbuch der gesammten Augenheilkunde*, 1874–1880, it included the first description of vernal conjunctivitis, 1876, **4**, Theil 2, 29. A second edition appeared, 15 vols [in 41], 1899–1918. Died 1909. *5905, 5914, 5944*

1833:24 Paul **Bert**, French physiologist, born 17 Oct; published *La pression barométrique*, an important work in the history of altitude physiology, 1878. Died 1886. *944*

1833:25 Joseph Janvier **Woodward**, US Army medical officer, born 30 Oct; wrote the greatest single monograph on dysentery, 'Diarrhoea and dysentery', contributed to *US War Dept.: Medical and surgical history of the War of the Rebellion*, 1879, pt. 2, **1**, 1–869. The author saw Lösch's amoeba without recognizing its significance. Died 1884. *5185, 5184*

1833:26 Friedrich Daniel von **Recklinghausen**, German pathologist, born 2 Dec; gave a classic description of neurofibromatosis ('Recklinghausen's disease'); in his *Über der Haut und ihre Beziehung zu den multiplen Neuromen*, 1882. Described generalized osteitis fibrosa ('Recklinghausen's disease of bone'), in *Festschrift R. Virchow*, 1891, but was preceded by G. Engel (1864). Died 1910. *4082, 4358, 4335*

1833:27 Carlos Juan **Finlay**, Cuban physician, born 3 Dec; first suggested that the mosquito transmitted yellow fever from man to man, 1881, *AnRA* **18**:147. Died 1915. *5455*

1833:28 Abel **Bouchard**, French psychiatrist, born 18 Dec; with Jean Martin Charcot, gave the first clinical description of the electric pains in tabes dorsalis, 1866, *GMP* **21**:122. Died 1899. *4775*

1833:29 Charles Jules Alphonse **Gayet**, French physician, born 18 Dec; first to describe acute superior haemorrhagic polioencephalitis, 1875, *ArPhy* **2**:341. Died 1904. *4641*

1833:30 Rudolph **Berlin**, German ophthalmologist, born; first suggested the term 'dyslexia'; in his *Eine besondere Art der Wortblindheit*, 1887. Died 1897. *4627*

1833: Johann Friedrich **Meckel**, the younger, died, **born** 1781. *congenital malformations, Meckel's diverticulum*

1833: William D. **Macgill** died, **born** 1802. *carotid artery ligation*

1833: Charles Turner **Thackrah** died, **born** 1795. *occupational diseases*

1833: Kurt Polycarp Joachim **Sprengel** died, **born** 1766. *history of medicine*

**1834**
1834:1 **University of Berne** founded

1834:2 **University of Brussels** founded

1834:3 **Westminster School of Medicine** opened at **Westminster Hospital, London**

1834:4 **Tulane University** founded at **New Orleans**

1834:5 *Archiv für Anatomie, Physiologie und Wissenschaftliche Medicin* founded by Johannes Peter **Müller** (1801–1858)

1834:6 **Medical Society of Lisbon** founded

1834:7 **Finska Läkäkesällskapet** founded at **Helsinki**

1834:8 **Middlesex Hospital, London,** founded

1834:9 First suture of ruptured female **perineum** by Philbert Joseph Roux (1780–1854), *GMP* **2**:17. *6029*

1834:10 An accurate clinical description of **tuberculous meningitis** given by William Wood Gerhard (1809–1872), *AmJMS* **13**:313; **14**:99. *4636*

1834:11 **Tuberculous spondylitis of the cervical vertebrae** named '**Rust's disease**' after the original description by Johan Nepomuk Rust (1775–1840); in his *Aufsätze und Abhandlungen aus dem Gebiete der Medizin* .... *4319*

1834:12 George James Guthrie (1785–1856) published *On the anatomy and diseases of the neck of the bladder, and of the urethra*; it included the first description of non-prostatic obstruction of the neck of the **bladder** and (p. 252) a description of his **prostatic catheter** for use in transurethral **prostatectomy**. *4167*

1834:13 **Sphygmomanometer** invented, to record **blood pressure,** by Jules Hérisson; in his *Le sphygmomètre*. *2748.2*

1834:14 **Carbolic acid** prepared from coal tar by Friedlieb Ferdinand Runge (1795–1867), *AnPh* **31**:65, 513; **32**:308. *1855*

1834: 15 Modern **physiotherapy** initiated by Per Henrik Ling (1776–1839), founder of modern gymnastics and therapeutic massage; *Gymnastikens allmänna grunder. 1993*

1834: 16 **Fechner-Weber law** on stimulus and sensation; Ernst Heinrich Weber (1795–1878) showed the relationship between stimulus and sensation, in his *De pulsu resorptione, auditu et tactu*; 'Weber's hearing test' appears on p. 41. *1457, 3368*

1834: 17 *Manuel de médecine opératoire* by Joseph François Malgaigne (1806–1865) was a considerable work on **operative surgery**, translated into several European languages. *5591*

1834: 18 August Friedrich Leopold **Weissman**, German biologist, born 17 Jan; he located the germ plasm within the nucleus and elaborated the theory of the continuity of germ plasm; *Das Keimplasma. Eine Theorie der Vererbung*, 1892. Died 1914. *236*

1834: 19 Ernst **Neumann**, Bohemian pathologist, born 30 Jan; first to note bone-marrow changes in leukaemia and introduced the term 'myelogenous leukaemia', 1870, *ArH* **11**:1. Died 1918. *3066*

1834: 20 Theodor Albrecht Edwin **Klebs**, German pathologist and bacteriologist, born 6 Feb; produced experimental tuberculosis in cattle by feeding infected milk, 1873, *ArEP* **1**:163. Inoculated syphilis into apes, 1878, *ArEP* **10**:161. Gave a classic description of glomerulonephritis ('Klebs' disease'); in his *Handbuch der pathologischen Anatomie*, I Abt., p. 644, 1879. It is possible that he saw the typhoid bacillus, *Salmonella typhi*, before Eberth, reporting it later, 1881, *ArEP* **13**:381. Discovered *Corynebacterium diphtheriae*, causal organism in diphtheria, 1883, *VKD* **2**:139, also called Klebs-Loeffler bacillus following its cultivation by Loeffler (1884). Died 1913. *2327, 2392, 4212, 5031, 5055, 5056*

1834: 21 Ernst Heinrich Philipp August **Haeckel**, German morphologist, born 16 Feb; he accepted the principles of Darwinism, which he carried into Germany. His most important work is *Generelle Morphologie der Organismen*, 1866. Died 1919. *223*

1834: 22 Herman **Snellen**, Dutch ophthalmologist, born 19 Feb; his sight test types ('Optotypi') introduced in his *Probebuchstaben zur Bestimmung der Sehschärfe*, 1862, soon gained acceptance in the civilized world. Died 1908. *5890*

1834: 23 Philipp Jakob Wilhelm **Henke**, German anatomist, born 18 Jun; first described congenital metatarsus varus, 1863, *ZRM* **17**:188. Died 1896. *4333*

1834: 24 Karl Edwin Konstantin **Hering**, German physiologist, born 5 Aug; stated his law on binocular vision, 1868, in his *Die Lehre vom binokularen Sehen*; published his theory of colour sense, 1872–1875, *SAW* 3 Abt.**66**:5; **68**:186, 229; **69**:85, 179; **70**:169. Died 1875. *1513.1, 1515*

1834: 25 Maurice **Raynaud**, French physician, born 10 Aug; first described Raynaud's disease, intermittent pallor or cyanosis of the extremities; in his *De l'asphyxie locale ...*, 1862. Died 1881. *2704*

1834: 26 Hugh Owen **Thomas**, British manipulative surgeon, born 23 Aug; described the 'Thomas splint' in his *Diseases of the hip, knee and ankle joints*, 1875. He was the founder of orthopaedics in Britain; see his *Contributions to medicine and surgery*, 1883–90. Died 1891. *4340, 4348*

1834:27 William Miller **Ord**, British physician, born 23 Sep; introduced the term myxoedema for the condition described by Curling (1850) and Gull (1873), 1878, *MCT* **61**:57. Died 1902. *3825*

1834:28 Otto Friedrich Carl **Deiters**, German histologist, born 15 Nov; described 'Deiters' cells' (glia cells) and 'Deiters' nucleus' in his *Gehirn und Ruckenmark des Menschen*, 1865. Died 1863. *1271*

1834:29 Sydney **Ringer**, British physician and physiologist, born; introduced 'Ringer's solution', 1882, *JP* **3**:195. Died 1922. *826*

1834:30 Albert **Niemann**, German physician, born; isolated cocaine from coca leaf; in his *Ueber eine neue organische Base in den Cocablättern*, 1859. Died 1861. *1865*

1834:31 George Walter **Caldwell**, American otolaryngologist, born; devised operation for abscess of the maxillary sinus, 1893, *NYJM* **58**:526; named 'Caldwell-Luc operation', acknowledging earlier work by Henri Luc. Died 1918. *3305, 3301*

1834:32 Louis Alexis **Normond** born; found *Strongyloides stercoralis*, causal parasite of strongyloidiasis, 1876, *CRAS* **83**:316. Died ?1885. *5344.11*

1834:33 Henry Jones **Shrapnell** died; described Shrapnell's membrane, the pars placida of the tympanic membrane, 1832, *LMG* **10**:120. *1558*

1834:34 (*c.*) Richard Cortland **Skinner** died; wrote the first American book on the teeth, *Treatise on the human teeth*, 1801, a 26-page pamphlet intended for the lay public. *3678*

1834: Edward **Stevens** died, **born** ?1755. *gastric juice*

1834: Thomas **Malthus** died, **born** 1766. *population*

1834: Gilbert **Blane** died, **born** 1749. *naval medicine, scurvy, quarantine*

1834: Jean François **Coindet** died, **born** 1774. *goitre*

1834: James Carrick **Moore** died, **born** 1762. *surgical analgesia*

1834: John **Heysham** died, **born** 1753. *Carlisle Tables of Mortality*

**1835**
1835:1 **University of Athens** founded

1835:2 The use of **silver nitrate** for the treatment of **gonococcal ophthalmia** recorded by Etienne François Julliard; in his *De l'emploi de l'excision et de la cautérisation à l'aide du nitrate d'argent fondu dans l'ophtalmie blenorrhagique. 5850*

1835:3 A **vesico-vaginal fistula** of 11 years' duration repaired by Montague Gosset (1792–1854), using silver-gilt wire, *L* **1**:345. *6028.1*

1835:4 The first description of **moral insanity** was given by James Cowles Prichard (1786–1848); in his *Treatise on insanity*. He described a syndrome he called **senile dementia**, possibly identical with **Alzheimer's disease**. *4928*

1835:5 James Paget (1814–1899) discovered **trichina** (*Trichinella spiralis*) in human muscle; his discovery was reported by Richard Owen in 1835 and by Paget in 1866, *TZS* 1:315. *5337*

1835:6 An important early description of **poliomyelitis** by John Badham (1807–1840), *LMG* 17:215. *4663*

1835:7 Robert James Graves (1796–1853) gave the first accurate account of **exophthalmic goitre** ('**Graves' disease**'), *LMSJ* 7:516. *3815*

1835:8 The parasitic nature of **scabies** was already known when Simon François Renucci demonstrated the itch-mite, *Sarcoptes scabiei*, and confirmed that it was the one cause of scabies; in his *Sur la découverte de l'insecte qui produit la contagion de la gale*, etc. Paris, Thèse No. 83. *4027*

1835:9 '**Brodie's pile**' described by Benjamin Collins Brodie (1783–1862), *LMG* 16:26. *3440*

1835:10 **Rheumatic endocarditis** (**Bouillard's disease**) described by Jean Baptiste Bouillard (1796–1881); in his *Traité clinique des maladies du coeur*. *2749*

1835:11 **Syphilis: potassium iodide** treatment introduced by William Wallace (1791–1837), *L* 2:5. *2379*

1835:12 Agostino Bassi (1773–1856) demonstrated the parasitic nature of the **muscardine disease of silkworms**, in his *Del mal del segno calcinaccio o moscardino*, 1835–36. He is regarded as the founder of the doctrine of **pathogenic microbes**. *2532*

---

1835:13 John Hughlings **Jackson**, British neurologist, born 4 Apr; demonstrated the importance of the ophthalmoscope in the investigation of nervous diseases, 1863, *OHR* 4:10, 389; 5:51, 251. Gave an excellent account of unilateral epilepsy ('Jacksonian epilepsy'), 1863, *MTG* 1:588; Bravais (1827) was the first to note the condition – also named 'Bravais-Jacksonian epilepsy'. Studied aphasia for 30 years, emphasizing its psychological aspects and laying the foundations for present knowledge of the condition, 1864, *CLLH* 1:388. With Jacob Augustus Lockhart Clarke, published an important account of syringomyelia, 1867, *MCT* 50:489. Described the syndrome of paralysis of half of the tongue, the same half of the palate, and one vocal cord ('Jackson's syndrome'), 1872, *L* 2:770. Died 1911. *4537, 4816, 4810, 4620, 4697, 4547*

1835:14 František **Chvostek**, Austrian surgeon, born 21 May; introduced a reliable diagnostic sign in latent tetany, 'Chvostek's sign', 1876, *WMP* 17:1201, 1225, 1253, 1313. Died 1884. *4833*

1835:15 John **Cleland**, British anatomist, born 15 Jun; described the Arnold-Chiari malformation (abnormal development of the cerebellum and displacement of the hind-brain and cervical cord), 1883, *JA* 17:257. In 1891 Hans Chiari described the shift of the medulla caudally, and in 1894 Julius Arnold drew attention to the abnormality of the cerebellum. Died 1925. *4566.1, 4577.1, 4581.1*

1835: 16 Robert von **Olshausen**, German gynaecologist, born 3 Jul; described an operation for retroversion of the uterus, 1886, *ZGy* **10**:698. Introduced an operation for excision of the vagina, 1895, *ZGy* **19**:1. Died 1915. *6083, 6098*

1835: 17 Moritz **Benedikt**, Hungarian physician, born 6 Jul; described 'Benedikt's syndrome' (paralysis of the oculomotor nerve on one side with intense trembling on the other side), 1889, *BuM* **3**:547. Died 1920. *4576*

1835: 18 August von **Freund**, Austrian chemist, born 30 Jul; first prepared cyclopropane (trimethylene), 1882, *MhC* **3**:625. Died 1892. *5677*

1835: 19 Carl Ludwig **Fiedler**, German physician, born 5 Aug; described acute ('Fiedler's') myocarditis, 1899. Died 1921. *2809.2*

1835: 20 Griffith **Evans**, British veterinarian, born 7 Aug; saw the first pathogenic trypanosome to be discovered, in the blood of horses suffering from 'surra', 1881, *VJ* **13**:1, 82, 180, 326. Died 1935. *5271*

1835: 21 Carl Joseph **Eberth**, German pathologist, born 21 Sep; discovered *Salmonella typhi*, causal organism of typhoid, 1880, *VA* **81**:58. Died 1926. *5030*

1835: 22 Adam **Politzer**, Hungarian, born 1 Oct; one of the greatest of all otologists. Introduced a method to effect permeability of the Eustachian tube, 1863, *WMW* **13**:84, 102, 117, 148. Was first to obtain pictures of the membrana tympani by means of illumination, in his *Die Beleuchtungsbilder des Trommelfels* ..., 1865. Described an acumeter, 1877, *ArOh* **12**:104. His *Lehrbuch der Ohrenheilkunde*, 1878–82, was for many years a standard authority on the subject. First reported otosclerosis as a separate clinical entity, 1893, *PAMC* **3**:1607. Died 1920. *3377, 3378, 3387.1, 3387, 3395*

1835: 23 August **Lucae**, German otologist, born; described an interference otoscope, 1867, *ArOh* **3**:186; first study of transmission of sounds through the cranial bones as a method of diagnosing ear disease, in his *Die Schalleitung durch die Kopfknochen* ..., 1870. Died 1911. *3378.2, 3381*

1835: 24 Wharton Peter **Hood**, British physician, born; the first physician to write on joint manipulation, published *On bone-setting (so-called), and its relation to the treatment of joints crippled by injury, rheumatism, inflammation, etc.*, 1871. Died 1916. *4339.1*

1835: 25 Julius **Arnold** born; described the abnormality of the cerebellum in what later became known as the Arnold-Chiari malformation, 1894, *BPA* **16**:1. Died 1915. *4581.1, 4577.1, 4566.1*

1835: 26 Thomas George **Morton**, American surgeon, born; gave the first complete description of anterior metatarsalgia ('Morton's metatarsalgia'), 1876, *AmJMS* **71**:37, first noted by Durlacher in 1845. Died 1903. *4341, 4325*

1835: Guillaume **Pellier de Quengsby** died, **born** ?1750. *ophthalmic surgery*

1835: Jean Georges Chrétien Frédéric Martin **Lobstein** died, **born** 1777. *arteriosclerosis, osteopsathyrosis*

1835: Guillaume **Dupuytren** died, **born** 1777. *flexion contracture deformity of the fingers, artificial anus, enterotome, Dupuytren's abscess, aneurysm, congenital dislocation of hip-joint, torticollis, excision of lower jaw, surgical pathology, burns*

1835: Thomas **Sutton** died, **born** 1767. *delirium tremens, phrenitis*

**1836**

1836:1 **University of London** founded

1836:2 **Library of Surgeon General's Office, Washington**, founded (became **Army Medical Library**, 1922, and then **National Library of Medicine**, 1956)

1836:3 **[Royal Pharmaceutic Institute]**, **Stockholm**, founded

1836:4 **Registration of Births and Deaths Act (England)**

1836:5 **Chicago sewerage** constructed 1836–1848

1836:6 Several of the distinctions between **typhus** and **typhoid** correctly described by Robert Perry (1783–1848), *EMSJ* **45**:64. *5023.1*

1836:7 ***Trichomonas vaginalis*** first described by Alfred Donné (1801–1878), who originally believed it to be the causal organism in **gonorrhoea**, *CRAS* **3**:385. *5207*

1836:8 Robert Remak (1815–1865) discovered the **non-medullated nerve-fibres** ('**fibres of Remak**'), *ArA* p. 145. *1260*

1836:9 The **coudé catheter** introduced by Louis Auguste Mercier (1811–1882), *GHP* **7**:13; followed by the bicoudé *c*1841. *4168.1*

1836:10 Although Joseph Fox (1803) had included some guidance on **orthodontics** in his *Natural history of the human teeth*, the first specialized work on the subject was *Der Schiefstand der Zähne* by Friedrich Christoph Kneisel (1797–?1883). *3679.8*

1836:11 The original description of **Jacksonian epilepsy**, *GHR* **1**:36 and acute yellow atrophy of the **liver**, *GHR* **1**:604, given by Richard Bright (1789–1858). *4811, 3617*

1836:12 **Lembert's suture** first successfully used by Johann Friedrich Dieffenbach (1792–1847), *WGH* p. 401. *3441*

1836:13 **Ludwig's angina** first described by Wilhelm Friedrich Ludwig (1790–1865), *MKW* **6**:21. *3257*

1836:14 **Arsenic** detection, **Marsh method**, introduced by James Marsh (1794–1846), *ENPJ* **21**:229. *2077*

1836:15 **Pepsin** discovered by Theodor Schwann (1810–1882), *ArA* p. 90. *991*

1836:16 **Splenectomy** was performed (1829) by Carl Friedrich Quittenbaum (1793–1852); in his *De splenis hypertrophia et historia exterpationis splenis hypertrophici*, published 1836. *3763*

1836:17 William **MacCormac**, British surgeon, born 17 Jan; introduced an operation for treatment of intraperitoneal rupture of the bladder, 1886, *L* **2**:1118. Died 1901. *4182*

1836:18 Michael **Foster**, British physiologist, born 8 Mar; founded the Cambridge school of physiology; wrote the influential textbook *Text-book of physiology*, 1876 and the charming *Lectures on the history of physiology*, 1901 (reprinted 1924 and 1970). Founded the *Journal of Physiology*, 1878. Died 1907. *631, 1575*

1836:19 Thomas Clifford **Allbutt**, British physician, Regius Professor of Physic, Cambridge, born 20 Jul. Regarded by Charles Singer as 'the most learned and distinguished physician of the last hundred years'. Introduced modern type of clinical thermometer, 1870, *BFMCR* **45**:429. Suggested the aortic genesis of angina pectoris ; in his *Diseases of the arteries, including angina pectoris*, 1915. Made several valuable contributions to the literature on the history of medicine. Died 1925. *2679, 2894*

1836:20 Heinrich Wilhelm Gottfried **Waldeyer-Hartz**, German anatomist, born 6 Oct; confirmed epithelial-cell origin of cancer histogenesis, advanced by Carl Thiersch (1865), 1872, *VA* **41**:470; **55**:67. Died 1921. *2620*

1836:21 Walter Butler **Cheadle**, British physician, born 15 Oct; differentiated infantile scurvy from rickets, 1878, *L* **2**:685. Died 1910. *3719*

1836:22 Bernhard **Fraenkel**, German laryngologist, born 17 Nov; first to report mycotic pharyngitis, 1873, *BKW* **10**:94. Established ozaena as a clinical entity, 1876, *Ziemssen's Handbuch* **4**, I:125. First successful intralaryngeal extirpation of cancer of larynx, 1887, *ArKC* **34**:281. Died 1911. *3281, 3285, 3296*

1836:23 Cesare **Lombroso**, Italian physician and anthropologist, born 18 Nov; in an important study of pellagra he upheld the maize diet theory of its origin, 1869, *RCB* **8**:289. His *L'uomo delinquente*, 1876, inaugurated the doctrine of a criminal type. Died 1909. *174, 3754*

1836:24 Wilhelm **Ebstein**, German physician and pathologist, born 27 Nov; described the remittent pyrexia occurring in lymphadenoma, 1887, *BKW* **24**:565; named 'Pel-Ebstein disease' acknowledging an earlier account by Pieter Klazes Pel. Died 1912. *3771, 3770*

1836:25 William **Cayley**, British physician, born 14 Dec; induced artificial pneumothorax, by pleural incision, in intractable haemoptysis, 1885, *TCSL* **18**:278. Died 1916. *3226*

1836:26 Georg Eduard **Rindfleisch**, German pathologist, born 15 Dec; gave first clear account of bone-marrow changes in pernicious anaemia, 1890, *VA* **121**:176. Died 1908. *3131.1*

1836:27 Ernst von **Bergmann**, Latvian surgeon, born 16 Dec; a pioneer in the evolution of asepsis; his corrosive sublimate method of antisepsis was merged into steam sterilization and the present-day ritual of asepsis, 1887, *TM* **1**:41. Developed radical mastoidectomy, 1888, *BKW* **25**:1054. Died 1907. *5638, 3391*

1836:28 Claude André **Paquelin**, French physician, born 30 Dec; introduced a thermocautery ('Paquelin's cautery'), 1877, *BGT* **93**:145. Died 1905. *5614*

---

1836:29 Austin **Flint** Jr, American physician, born; discovered coprosterol, 1862, *AmJMS* **44**:305. Died 1915. *1005*

1836:30 Benjamin **Loewenberg**, German surgeon, born; found Friedländer group bacillus in ozaena, 1984, *AnIP* **8**:292. Died 1905. *3307*

1836:31 John **Brunton**, British physician, born; devised Brunton's otoscope, 1865, *L* **2**:617. Died 1899. *3378.1*

1836:32 Jean Baptiste Nicolas Voltaire **Masius**, Belgian physician, born; with Constant Vanlair, first to suggest the concept of hereditary haemolytic anaemia, 1871, *BARM* **5**:515. Died 1912. *3766.1*

1836:33 Paul August **Sick**, German surgeon, born; first to notice symptoms of loss of thyroid function (*status thyreoprivus*) after thyroidectomy, *MKW* **37**:199; he also was first to perform total thyroidectomy, 1867. Died 1900. *3821*

1836:34 William Tilbury **Fox**, British dermatologist, born; first described impetigo contagiosa, 1864, *BMJ* **1**:78, 467, 495, 553, 607. Gave the original description of dyshidrosis (pompholyx), a disturbance of sweat secretion, 1873, *BMJ* **2**:365. First description of epidermolysis bullosa, 1879, *L* **1**:766. First description of dermatitis herpetiformis, 1880, *ArD* **6**:16; following the excellent description by Louis Adolphus Duhring (1845–1913) of the latter in 1884 it was also named 'Duhring's disease'. Died 1879. *4055, 4065, 4077, 4078, 4083*

1836:35 Simon **Duplay**, French surgeon, born; described the frozen shoulder syndrome, 1872, *ArGM* **71**:37. Died 1924. *4339.2*

1836:36 Joseph **Bancroft**, British/Australian physician, born; discovered the filaria worm, 1878, *TPS* **29**:406, later to be named *Wuchereria bancrofti*. Died 1894. *5346, 5344.6*

---

1836: James **Russell** died, **born** 1755. *bone necrosis*

1836: John **Cheyne** died, **born** 1777. *apoplexy, cerebral anaemia, subarachnoid haemorrhage, Cheyne-Stokes respiration*

1836: Nicolaus Anton **Friedreich** died, **born** 1761. *facial paralysis*

## 1837

1837:1 **School of Medicine and Surgery (Kasr-el-Aini)** founded at **Cairo**

1837:2 **University of Michigan, Ann Arbor**, founded

1837:3 **Rush Medical College, Chicago**, chartered; opened 1843

1837:4 **Kaiseriiche Königliche Gesellschaft der Aertze** founded in **Vienna**

1837:5 Friedrich Gustav Jakob Henle's (1809–1885) studies on the epithelia of the **skin** and **intestines**, *Symbolae ad anatomiam villorum intestinalium*, created **histology**. *539*

1837:6 **Montgomery's glands**, the sebaceous glands of the **areola**, previously described by Morgagni, were named following the description by William Fetherston Montgomery (1787–1859) in his *Exposition of the symptoms and signs of pregnancy.* *6173*

1837:7 The first **rhinoplasty** reported in the United States was by Jonathan Mason Warren (1811–1867), *BMSJ* **16**:69. *5743.3*

1837:8 In his *Procédé pour écrire au moyen des points*, the blind Louis Braille (1809–1852) modified the system of elevated points first suggested by Charles Barbier (1820) for enabling the **blind** to read by touch. Today the **Braille system** is used throughout the world. *5851*

1837:9 A pupil of P.C.A. Louis, William Wood Gerhard (1809–1872), differentiated **typhus** from **typhoid**, *AJMS* **19**:289, 302. *5024*

1837:10 **Static electricity** first used therapeutically by Thomas Addison (1793–1860), *GHR* **2**:493. *4524*

1837:11 Anaphylactoid ('**Schönlein-Henoch**') **purpura** established as a distinct entity by Johannes Lucas Schönlein (1793–1864), in his *Allgemeine und spezielle Pathologie und Therapie*, **3**, 48–49; mentioned earlier by William Heberden Sr (1802) and later by Eduard Heinrich Henoch (1820–1910) in 1868. *3058, 3053, 3065*

1837:12 The term **myocarditis** introduced by Joseph Friedrich Sobernheim (1803–1846); in his *Praktische Diagnostik*, p. 118. *2750*

1837:13 **Experimental anaphylaxis** produced by François Magendie (1783–1855); in his *Lectures on the blood* (1839). *2585*

1837:14 First North American book on **tumours**, *Surgical observations on tumours ...*, published by John Collins Warren (1778–1856). *2611.1*

1837:15 **Blood gases** quantitatively analysed by Heinrich Gustav Magnus (1802–1870), *AnPh* **12**:583. *929*

1837:16 **Purkyně cells** described by Jan Evangelista Purkyně (1787–1869), *BVDN* **15**:177. *1396*

1837:17 **Glanders** shown to be contagious, but not a form of **tuberculosis**, by Pierre François Olive Rayer (1793–1867), *MARM* **6**:625. *5154*

1837:18 Proof that **putrefaction** is produced by living bodies provided by Theodor Schwann (1810–1882), *AnPhy* **41**:184. *674*

1837:19 *Practical surgery* published by Robert Liston (1794–1847). *5593*

1837:20 William Williams **Keen**, American surgeon, born 19 Jan; a pioneer in linear craniotomy, and reported a new operation for spasmodic torticollis, 1891, *AmJMS* **101**:549; *AnS* **13**:44. First clinical application, for surgical diagnosis, of **X rays** in the United States, March 1896, *AmJMS* **111**:256. Died 1932. *4866, 4867, 2684.1*

1837:21 Samuel Weissel **Gross**, American surgeon, born 4 Feb; published the first comprehensive account (165 cases) of bone sarcoma, 1879, *AmJMS* **78**:17, 338. Died 1889. *4346*

1837:22 Wilhelm Friedrich [Willy] **Kühne**, German physiologist and physiological chemist, born 28 Mar; described the neuromuscular end organ ('Kühne's spindle'), in his *Ueber die peripherischen Endorgane der motorischen Nerven*, 1862, and the proprioceptive receptors in muscles, 1863, *VA* **28**:528. Isolated trypsin, 1874, *VNMV* NF **1**:194; and, with Russell Henry Chittenden, isolated and named several products of digestion, 1883, *ZBi* **19**:159. Extracted visual purple from the retina, 1878, *UPIH* **1**:15. Died 1900. *1269, 1270, 1012, 1016, 1519*

1837:23 Edward Hallaran **Bennett**, British surgeon, born 4 Apr; described 'Bennett's fracture' of the first metacarpal, 1882, *DJMS* **73**:72. Died 1907. *4426*

1837:24 Henry Charlton **Bastian**, British neurologist, born 26 Apr; gave the first detailed description of *Dracunculus medinensis*, the guinea-worm, 1863, *TLS* **24**:101. Propounded 'Bastian's law' (transverse lesion of the spinal cord above the lumbar enlargement results in abolition of the tendon reflexes of the lower extremities), 1890, *MCT* **73**:151. In his *Treatise on aphasia and other speech defects*, 1898, he localized the auditory and visual centres, and described word-blindness and word-deafness. He was a champion of the doctrine of abiogenesis. Died 1915. *5344.2, 4577, 4629*

1837:25 Henry Orlando **Marcy**, American surgeon, born 2 Jun; stressed importance of reconstruction of the internal ring following reduction of the sac in treatment of hernia, 1871, *BMSJ* **85**:315; introduced antiseptic ligatures in the radical cure of hernia, 1878, *TAMA* **29**:295; published one of the most spectacular 19th century American medical texts, *Anatomy and surgical treatment of hernia*, 1892. Died 1924. *3592.1, 3594, 3601*

1837:26 André Victor **Cornil**, French pathologist and bacteriologist, born 17 Jun; with Jean Martin Charcot, gave an important account of the renal lesions in gout, 1863, *CRSB* **5**:139; gave first description of chronic arthritis in childhood, 1864, *CRSB* **1**:3. Died 1898. *4498, 4499*

1837:27 Morell **Mackenzie**, British physician, born 7 Jul; his *Manual of diseases of the throat and nose*, 1880–84, had an important influence on the development of laryngology. Died 1892. *3287*

1837:28 Hermann Hugo Rudolf **Schwartze**, German otologist, born 7 Sep; with Adolf Eysell, revived the mastoid operation; the ear was opened by chiselling ('Schwartze's operation'), 1873, *ArOh* **1**:157. Died 1910. *3382*

1837:29 Enrico **Bottini**, Italian surgeon, born 7 Sep; introduced a galvanocautery for the treatment of prostatic obstruction, 1874, *Gal* **2**:437; described an operation for the radical treatment of prostatic hypertrophy, 1891, *IMC* **10**:3, 7 Abt.90. Died 1903. *4261, 4262*

1837:30 Samuel Siegfried von **Basch**, Czech physician, born 9 Sep; developed the modern sphygmomanometer, 1881, *ZKM* **2**:79. Died 1905. *2784*

1837:31 Moritz **Kaposi** [Kohn], Hungarian dermatologist, born 23 Oct; first described Kaposi's sarcoma, multiple idiopathic haemorrhagic sarcoma, 1872, *ArD* **4**:265. Published an excellent pathological study of xeroderma pigmentosum ('Kaposi's disease'), 1882, *MJa*, p. 619. First description of lymphoderma perniciosa (premycotic or leukaemic erythroderma), 1885, *MJa*, p. 129. First description of lichen ruber moniliformis ('Kaposi's disease'), 1886, *VDS* **13**:571. Gave a full account of impetigo herpetiformis (first described by von Hebra in 1872) and established its status, 1887, *VDS* **14**:273. Published *Pathologie und Therapie der Hautkrankheiten*, 1888, one of the most important books on dermatology; followed by a valuable collection of illustrations in dermatology; *Handatlas der Hautkrankheiten*, 1898–1900. Died 1902. *4080, 4063, 4085, 4086, 4091, 3995, 4001*

1837:32 Robert Robertovich **Wreden**, Russian otologist, born; first to draw attention to otomycosis, 1867, *ArOh* **3**:1. Died 1893. *3380*

1837:33 Henry Gawen **Sutton**, British pathologist, born; with William Withey Gull, gave first clear description of arteriosclerotic atrophy of the kidney, and a description of hypertensive nephrosclerosis, 1872, *MCT* **55**:273. Died 1891. *4215*

1837:34 Douglas Moray Cooper Lamb Argyll **Robertson**, British ophthalmic surgeon, born; first described the Argyll Robertson pupil, 1869, *EMJ* **14**:696. Gave first detailed description of *Loa loa*, the parasite in loaiasis, 1895, *TOUK* **15**:137. Died 1909. *4540, 5347.1*

1837: William **Wallace** died, **born** 1791. *syphilis, potassium iodide, lymphogranuloma venereum*

1837: Philip Syng **Physick** died, **born** 1768. *tonsillotome, artificial anus, gastric lavage, stomach tube, surgery, ligatures*

1837: Jean Louis Marc **Alibert** died, **born** 1768. *dermatology, classification of skin diseases, dermatolysis, sycosis barbae, keloid, leishmaniasis, Aleppo boil, mycosis fungoides*

1837: Carl Gustav **Himly** died, **born** 1772. *lens, hyoscyamine*

**1838**
1838:1 *Proceedings of the American Philosophical Society* commences publication

1838:2 Pioneering work in **obstetric auscultation**, including the sounds of the **foetal heart**, carried out by Hermann Franz Joseph Naegele (1810–1858); in his *Die geburtshülfliche Auscultation. 6175*

1838:3 The first modern textbook on **psychiatry** was *Des maladies mentales* by Jean Etienne Esquirol (1772–1840), notable for its striking illustrations of **insane** patients. *4929*

1838:4 **Jacquemier's sign**, violet coloration of the vaginal skin, diagnostic of **early pregnancy**, described by Jean Marie Jacquemier (1806–1879), *ArGM* **3**:165. *6174*

1838:5 The most influential American writer of his time on **forensic psychiatry**, Isaac Ray (1807–1887), wrote *A treatise on the medical jurisprudence of insanity. 4929.01*

1838:6 Angelo Dubini (1813–1902) first found the **hookworm** of **ankylostomiasis**, publishing a report in 1843 in which he named it *Agchylostoma duodenale*, an etymologically erroneous name, *AnU* **106**:5. *5353*

1838:7 Repeating the experiments of John Hunter, Philippe Ricord (1800–1889) proved **syphilis** and **gonorrhoea** to be separate diseases; in his *Traité pratique des maladies vénériennes. 5202*

1838:8 The term '**plastic surgery**' introduced by Eduard Zeis (1807–1868) in his important *Handbuch der plastischen Chirurgie*, which covers the general principles of the speciality and describes operative techniques for individual parts of the body. *5743.4*

1838:9 A fine colour-atlas summarizing contemporary knowledge of diseases of the **eye**, *Klinische Darstellungen der Krankheiten und Bildungsfehler des menschlichen Auges*, produced by Friedrich August von Ammon (1799–1861). It is one of the greatest preophthalmoscopic atlases of **ophthalmology**. *5852*

1838:10 '**Barton's fracture' of the radius** described by John Rhea Barton (1794–1871), *MEx* **1**:365. *4415*

1838:11 A classic description of **lupus erythematoides migrans** ('**Biett's disease**') given by Laurent Théodore Biett (1781–1840) was recorded in P.L.A. Cazenave and H.E. Schedel's *Abrégé pratique des maladies de la peau*, 3rd ed., pp. 11 and 45. *4028*

1838:12 Vital contribution to the **cell theory**, *Beiträge zur Phytogenesis*, by Matthias Jakob Schleiden (1804–1881). *112*

1838:13 **Syphilis**: '**Ricord's chancre**', the initial lesion, described by Philippe Ricord (1800–1889); in his *Traité pratique des maladies vénériennes*. *2381*

1838:14 Charles Cagniard-Latour (1777–1859) demonstrated in his paper on the **fermentation of wine** the true nature of **yeast**, *AnC* **68**:296. *675*

1838:15 Cell theory of **tumour** formation in **cancer** supported by Johannes Müller (1801–1858); in his *Ueber den feineren Bau und die Formen der krankhaften Geschwülste*. *2612*

1838:16 ***Bacillus subtilis*** described by Christian Gottfried Ehrenberg (1796–1876); *Infusionsthierschen* .... *2469*

1838:17 Martin Heinrich Rathke (1793–1860) gave an important description of the **pituitary**, *ArA* p. 482. *1156*

1838:18 *Traité d'anatomie chirurgicale et de chirurgie experimentale*, 2 vols, by Joseph François Malgaigne (1806–1865), was an important book on **surgical anatomy** and **experimental surgery**. *5594*

---

1838:19 Albert von **Mosetig-Moorhof**, Austrian surgeon, born 26 Jan; introduced iodoform dressing in surgery, 1882, *SKV* **211** (Chir 68): 1811; used iodoform to plug bone defects, 1903, *ZCh* **30**:433. Died 1907. *4371, 5618*

1838:20 Thomas **Annandale**, British surgeon, born 2 Feb; carried out gastrotomy for intestinal obstruction, 1871, *EMJ* **16**:700. Performed the first deliberate and planned operation for the relief of internal derangement of the knee-joint due to displaced cartilage, 1885, *BMJ* **1**:779. Died 1908. *3463.1, 4426.1*

1838:21 Eduard **Hitzig**, German neurophysiologist and psychiatrist, born 6 Feb. With Gustav Theodor Fritsch, proved the existence of functional localization in the cerebral cortex of animals, 1870, *ArA* p. 300; accurately defined the limits of the motor area in the dog and monkey, 1874, *Untersuchungen über das Gehirn*. As a psychiatrist he attempted to place the treatment of patients on a more scientific basis. Died 1907. *1405, 1408*

1838:22 Jacob da Silva **Solis-Cohen**, American otorhinolaryngologist, born 28 Feb; first successful removal of cancer of the larynx, 1867, *AmJMS* **53**:404; **54**:565. Published first American textbook on otorhinolaryngology, *Diseases of the throat* ..., 1872. Died 1927. *3274, 3280*

1838:23 Gustav Theodor **Fritsch**, German anatomist and physiologist, born 5 Mar; with Eduard Hitzig, proved the existence of functional localization in the cerebral cortex of animals, 1878, *ArA* p. 300. Died 1891. *1405*

1838:24 John Shaw **Billings**, American surgeon, librarian, and bibliographer. As Librarian of the Surgeon General's Office, Washington (later National Library of Medicine) he built up that Library to be the largest medical library in the world. With Robert Fletcher, founded and edited the *Index Medicus*, 1879, and the *Index-Catalogue of the Library of the Surgeon General's Office*, one of the finest achievements in medical bibliography, 1880. Died 1913. *6762, 6763*

1838:25 George Miller **Sternberg**, American military surgeon and bacteriologist, born 8 Jun; discovered the pneumococcus, 1881, *SBJH* **2** ii:183, in the same year as Louis Pasteur, and independently. Died 1915. *3173, 3172*

1838:26 Charles Hilton **Fagge**, British physician, born 30 Jun; differentiated sporadic from endemic goitre, 1871, *MCT* **54**:155. Gave an exhaustive account of presystolic murmurs, 1871, *GHR* **16**:247. Died 1883. *3822*

1838:27 Johann Ernst Oswald **Schmiedeberg**, Latvian pharmacologist, born 13 Oct; isolated digitoxin from digitalis, 1875, *ArEP* **3**:16. Died 1921. *1869.1*

1838:28 Johann Hermann **Baas**, German physician and medical historian, born 24 Oct; his *Grundriss der Geschichte der Medicin*, 1876, was the most important one-volume history of medicine until superseded by F.H. Garrison's *Introduction*. Died 1909. *6389*

1838:29 Aleksandr Yakovlevich **Danilevsky** born; discovered trypsin, 1862, *VA* **25**:279. Died 1923. *1004*

1838:30 Arthur Bowen Richards **Myers** born; first described the 'effort syndrome' in his *On the etiology and prevalence of diseases of the heart among soldiers*, 1870 ('Da Costa's syndrome', 1871; Thomas Lewis's 'effort syndrome', 1917). Died 1921. *2768*

1838:31 Thomas John **Maclagan**, British physician, born; introduced salicylates in the treatment of rheumatism, 1876, *L* **1**:342, 383. Died 1903. *4501*

1838:32 James Ewing **Mears**, American surgeon, born; first to suggest Gasserian ganglionectomy for the treatment of trigeminal neuralgia, 1884, *MN* **45**:58. Died 1919. *4857*

1838: Jean Marie Gaspard **Itard** died, **born** 1774. *otology*

1838: John William Keys **Parkinson** died, **born** 1785. *appendicitis*

1838: Friedrich **Accum** died, **born** 1769. *food adulteration*

**1839**

1839:1 **Crichton Royal Hospital** opened at **Dumfries**, Scotland, for **mentally ill**; funded by bequest of James **Crichton** (1763–1823)

1839:2 **University of Missouri** founded at **Columbia**

1839:3 **Royal Microscopical Society** founded in London

1839:4 William **Farr** (1807–1883) functions as **statistics compiler, General Register Office**, 1839–1879

1839:5 **Torticollis (wry-neck)** first treated by subcutaneous section of the sternomastoid muscle by Guillaume Dupuytren (1777–1835) on 16 Jan 1822. This was recorded by C. Averill in 1823 and by Dupuytren in his *Leçons orales de clinique chirurgicale*, 2 éd., **3**, p. 455, 1839. *4322*

1839:6 Martin Heinrich Rathke (1793–1860) described '**Rathke's pouch**', a diverticulum from the **embryonic mouth**, *Entwicklungsgeschichte der Natter*. Died 1860. *483*

1839:7 The **obliquely contracted pelvis** ('**Naegele pelvis**') first described by Franz Carl Naegele (1778–1851); in his *Das schräg verengte Becken*. Because of its rarity and difficulty of recognition in the living, with its most often fatal consequences, it was unknown until his study of 37 cases. He suggested diagnostic aids for its recognition. *6257*

1839:8 The first description of **spondylolisthesis** given by Carl von Rokitansky (1804–1878), *MJOS* **19**:41, 195. *6258*

1839:9 *Candida albicans* discovered by Bernhard Rudolph Conrad von Langenbeck (1810–1887), *NNGN* **12**:145; later found by Berg (1841) to be the causal organism in **thrush (candidiasis)**. *5517, 5518*

1839:10 William John Little (1810–1894), who suffered from **talipes (club-foot)**, wrote a classical work on the subject, *On the nature of club-foot and analogous distortions*. *4322.1*

1839:11 Disease of the posterior columns of the **spinal cord** first described by Edward Stanley (1793–1862), *MCT* **23**:80. *4525*

1839:12 The **fungal** cause of **favus (ringworm)**, *Achorion (Trichophyton) schönleinii*, discovered by Johann Lucas Schönlein (1793–1864), *ArA* p. 82; confirmed by David Gruby, 1841. *4029, 4030*

1839:13 **Sarcoma** of the **prostate** first recorded by Richard Anthony Stafford (1801–1854), *MCT* **22**:218. *4259*

1839:14 Chapin Aaron Harris (1806–1860) published *The dental art, a practical treatise on dental surgery*, one of the most popular works on **dentistry**; he founded the first dental college in the world, the Baltimore College of Dental Surgery. *3680*

1839:15 'Nasmyth's membrane' or persistent dental capsule, described by Alexander Nasmyth (d.1848), *MCT* **22**:310. *3681*

1839:16 Lumbar colostomy first performed by Jean Zuléma Amussat (1796–1856); see his *Mémoire sur la possibilité d'établir un anus artificiel* .... *3442*

1839:17 A summary of previous knowledge of geriatrics, *Die Krankheiten des höheren Alters und ihre Heilung*, published by Carl Friedrich Canstatt (1807–1850). *1605.1*

1839:18 Vital role in the development of the cell theory played by Theodor Schwann (1810–1882); particularly his *Mikroskopische Untersuchungen über die Übereinstimmung in der Struktur und dem Wachsthum der Thiere und Pflanzen*, in which he also described the neurilemma (the sheath of Schwann). *112.1, 113*

1839:19 Josef Skoda (1805–1881) published his *Abhandlung über Perkussion und Auskultation*, in which he classified the sounds obtained on percussion according to musical pitch and tone. His work confirmed and completed that of Laennec. *2676*

1839:20 Purkyně fibres described by Jan Evangelista Purkyně (1787–1869), *Rocz. Wydzialu lekar. Univ. Jagiel*, **2**:44 [English translation, 1845, *LMG* **36**:1066, 1156]. *805*

1839:21 Coarctation of aorta diagnosed during life by Louis Auguste Mercier (1811–1882), *BSAP* **14**:158. *2750.1*

1839:22 Constant Vanlair, Belgian physician, born 21 Jan; with Jean Baptiste Nicolas Voltaire Masius, first to suggest the concept of hereditary haemolytic anaemia, 1871, *BARM* **5**:515. Died 1914. *3766.1*

1839:23 Oscar Liebreich, German physician and pharmacologist, born 14 Feb; demonstrated the value of chloral hydrate as an hypnotic, 1869, *ADGP* **16**:237. Died 1908. *1869*

1839:24 Theodor Langhans, German pathologist, born 28 Feb; first to note the presence of ('Dorothy Reed') giant cells in lymphadenoma, 1872, *VA* **54**:509. Died 1915. *3767*

1839:25 William Stokes, British surgeon, born 10 Mar; improved the method of amputation of the thigh (introduced by Rocco Gritti in 1857), ('Gritti-Stokes amputation'), 1870, *MCT* **53**:175. Died 1900. *4470, 4466*

1839:26 Louis Emile Javal, French ophthalmologist, born 5 May; invented the astigmometer, 1867, *AnO* **57**:39. Invented an ophthalmometer, 1881, *AnOc* **86**:5. Died 1907. *5901, 5920*

1839:27 George Miller Beard, American physician, born 8 May; first described neurasthenia ('Beard's disease'), 1869, *BMSJ* **80**:217; published the more detailed *Practical treatise on nervous exhaustion (neurasthenia)*, 1880. Died 1883. *4843, 4846*

1839:28 John Davidson Rockefeller, American industrialist and philanthropist, born 8 Jul; he founded the Rockefeller Institute for Medical Research, 1904, and in 1913 endowed the Rockefeller Foundation 'to promote the well-being of mankind throughout the world'. Died 1937.

1839:29 Julius **Cohnheim**, German pathologist, born 20 Jul; published important investigations on inflammation; *Neue Untersuchungen über die Entzündung*, 1873. Successfully inoculated tuberculosis into the rabbit eye, 1877; reported in his *Die Tuberkulose ... Infectionslehre*, 1880. Died 1884. *2302, 2329*

1839:30 Ludwig **Laqueur**, German ophthalmologist, born 25 Jul; introduced the use of physostigmine in the treatment of glaucoma, 1876, *ZMW* **14**:421. Died 1909. *5913*

1839:31 Samuel Jones **Gee**, British physician, born 13 Sep; first to describe idiopathic steatorrhoea (nontropical sprue, coeliac disease), 1888; a more extensive study by Thorald Einar Hess Thaysen, in 1929, led to the eponym 'Gee-Thaysen disease', *SBHR* **24**:17. Died 1911. *3491, 3550*

1839:32 Johan Anton **Waldenström**, Swedish physician, born 17 Sep; with Adolf Fredrik Lindstedt, first to record an operation for the treatment of volvulus, 1879, *ULF* **14**:513. Died 1879. *3469*

1839:33 William Morrant **Baker**, British surgeon, born 20 Oct; first described erythema serpens, 1873, *SBHR* **9**:198. First described 'Baker's cysts' of the knee-joint, 1877, *SBHR* **13**:245; **21**:177. Died 1896. *4064, 4342*

---

1839:34 Ernst Georg Ferdinand von **Küster** born; treated empyema by thoracotomy, 1889, *DMW* **15**:185. Developed radical mastoidectomy, 1889, *DMW* **15**:254. Carried out the first successful plastic operation for the relief of hydronephrosis, 1892, *ZCh* **19**: Suppl.110. Died 1930. *3177, 3392, 4223*

1839:35 Robert Fulton **Weir**, American plastic surgeon, born; introduced reduction rhinoplasty by the endonasal approach, 1892, *NYMJ* **56**:449. Died 1927. *5754.6*

---

1839: Per Henrik **Ling** died, **born** 1776. *physiotherapy*

1839: Mathew **Carey** died, **born** 1760. *yellow fever*

1839: James **Barlow** died, **born** 1767. *caesarean section*

## 1840
1840:1 **Free Vaccination Act**, England

1840:2 **'Brodie's tumour'**, a tumour of the **breast**, described by Benjamin Collins Brodie (1783–1862), *LMG* **25**:808. *5770*

1840:3 The first clinical description of **rat-bite fever** given by Whitman Willcox, *AmJMS* **26**:245. *5322*

1840:4 **Typhoid** and **typhus** were often confused. Alexander Patrick Stewart (1813–1883) analysed a number of cases of both, and clearly demonstrated that they were two distinct fevers, *EMSJ* **54**:289. *5025*

1840:5 Jacob von Heine (1799–1879) gave the first description of **acute anterior poliomyelitis** (**'Heine-Medin disease'**); in his *Beobachtungen über Lähmungszustände der untern*

*Extremitäten und deren Behandlung.* He also drew attention to **spastic paraplegia** ('**Little's disease**'). *4664, 4667, 4691.1*

1840:6 In his *Traité clinique du rhumatisme articulaire*, Jean Baptiste Bouillaud (1796–1881) drew attention to the coincidence of **acute rheumatism** and **heart disease**. *4494*

1840:7 The description of **exophthalmic goitre** by Carl Adolph von Basedow (1799–1854) led to the name '**Basedow's disease**' being used to describe the condition in Europe outside Gt Britain, *WGH* **6**:197, 220. *3816*

1840:8 In his *Odontography*, 2 vols, 1840–45, Richard Owen (1804–1892) dealt with the whole range of the toothed vertebrates. *3681.1*

1840:9 **Pituitary tumour** with **obesity** and **sexual infantilism** ('**Fröhlich's syndrome**') first described by Bernhard Mohr (1809–1848), *WGH* **6**:565. *3882*

1840:10 Sanatorium treatment for **pulmonary tuberculosis** advocated by George Bodington (1799–1882); in his *Essay on the treatment of and cure of pulmonary consumption. 3223*

1840:11 Postulates by Friedrich Gustav Jakob Henle (1809–1885) on the aetiological relationship of **microbes** to disease appear in his *Pathologische Untersuchungen*, 1–82. *2533*

1840:12 **Haemophilia** treated by **blood transfusion** by Samuel Armstrong Lane (1802–1892), *L* **1**:185. *3058.1*

1840:13 '**Pacini's corpuscles**' described by Filippo Pacini (1812–1883); in his *Nuovo organi scoperti nel corpo humano. 1263*

1840:14 '**Burton's blue line**' on the gums, diagnostic of **lead poisoning**, noted by Henry Burton (1799–1849), *MCT* **23**:63. *2099*

1840:15 A **chorionic tumour** first reported by William Wilton (1809–1899), *L* **1**:691. *6031.1*

1840:16 John Peter Mettauer (1787–1875), a Virginian gynaecologist, believed to be the first successfully to repair a **vesico-vaginal fistula**, *BMSJ* **22**:154. *6031*

---

1840:17 Johann Karl **Proksch**, German venereologist, born 1 Feb; compiled a bibliography of the literature on venereal disease from the end of the 16th century to 1900; *Die Litteratur über die venerischen Krankheiten von der ersten Schriften über Syphilis aus dem Ende des fünfzehnten Jahrhunderts bis zum Jahre 1889. (Suppl. Bd. 1: Enthalt die Litteratur von 1889–1900 und Nachträge aus früherer Zeit).* 5 vols, 1889–1900. Died 1923. *5226*

1840:18 Theodor **Leber**, German ophthalmologist, born 29 Feb; gave the first description of hereditary optic atrophy ('Leber's optic atrophy'), 1871, *GAO* **17** ii:249. Made important investigations of disorders of the eye in diabetes, 1875, *GAO* **21** iii:206. Died 1917. *5906, 3941*

1840:19 Henry Pickering **Bowditch**, American physiologist, born 4 Apr; demonstrated indefatigability of nerve ('Bowditch's law), 1890, *ArA* 505. Died 1911. *1282*

1840:20 Thomas Smith **Clouston**, British psychiatrist, born 22 Apr; recognized the relationship between general paresis and congenital syphilis, 1877, *JMS* **23**:419, he reported the condition in a patient aged sixteen. Died 1915. *4799*

1840:21 Arnold **Heller**, German pathologist, born 1 May; established syphilis as a cause of aortic aneurysm, 1899, *MMW* **46**:1669. Died 1913. *2987*

1840:22 Giuseppe **Profeta**, Italian venereologist, born 7 Jul; he stated that a non-syphilitic child of syphilitic parents is immune to the disease – 'Profeta's law', 1865, *Spe* **15**:328, 339. Died 1911. *2390*

1840:23 Kenneth **Macleod**, British military surgeon, born 23 Jul; first to draw attention to granuloma inguinale, 1882, *IMG* **17**:113. Died 1922. *5204.1*

1840:24 Frank Fontaine **Maury**, American surgeon, born 9 Aug; first in America to carry out gastrostomy for stricture of the oesophagus, 1870, *AmJMS* **59**:365. Died 1879. *3464*

1840:25 Richard von **Krafft-Ebing**, German psychiatrist, born 14 Aug; wrote a classical work on sexual deviation, *Psychopathia sexualis*, 1905, and textbooks on clinical psychiatry and forensic psychopathology. Died 1926. *4950*

1840:26 Désiré Magloire **Bourneville**, French physician, born 21 Oct; described tuberose sclerosis (epiloia, 'Bourneville's disease'), 1880, *ArN* **1**:69. Died 1909. *4700*

1840:27 Joseph **Grünfeld**, Bohemian physician, born 19 Nov; successfully catheterized the ureter under endoscopic vision, 1876, *WMP* **17**:919, 949. Died 1910. *4174.1*

1840:28 Wilhelm Heinrich **Erb**, German neurologist, born 30 Nov; introduced 'Erb's sign', diagnostic of latent tetany, 1873, *ArPN* **4**:271. Described 'Erb's palsy', partial brachial plexus paralysis, 1873, *VNMV* **1**:130; it had previously been described by Smellie (1763) and by Duchenne (1872). Described spastic spinal paralysis ('Erb-Charcot disease'), 1875, *BKW* **12**:357. First used the knee-jerk as a diagnostic measure in tabes dorsalis, 1875, *ArPN* **5**:792, diagnostic value discovered simultaneously by Westphal; gave original descriptions of several nervous disorders, especially the muscular dystrophies, in his *Handbuch der Krankheiten des Nervensystems*, 1876–78. Described myasthenia pseudoparalytica, 1879, *ArPN* **9**:172; the later account by Goldflam (1893) led to the term 'Erb-Goldflam symptom complex'; published an account of progressive muscular dystrophy ('Erb's muscular atrophy'), 1884, *DAKM* **34**:467. Gave a classic description of syphilitic spinal paralysis, sometimes referred to as 'Erb's disease', 1892, *NZ* **11**:161. Died 1921. *4832, 4548, 4543, 4556, 4780, 4781, 4557, 4746, 4757, 4747, 4788*

1840:29 Odilon Marc **Lannelongue**, French surgeon, born 4 Dec; carried out the first thyroid transplantation (for the treatment of cretinism), 1890, *BuM* **4**:225. Died 1911. *3837*

1840:30 Vladimir Mikhailovich **Kernig**, Russian physician, born; he drew attention to a flexor contracture of the leg on attempting to extend it on the thigh ('Kernig's sign') an important diagnostic sign almost always present in cerebrospinal meningitis, 1882, *SPMW* **7**:398. Died 1917. *4677*

1840:31 Friedrich **Lösch**, German physician, born; discovered *Entamoeba histolytica*, infective agent in amoebiasis, 1875, *VA* **65**:196. Died 1903. *5184*

208

1840:32 Sophia Louisa **Jex-Blake**, British physician, born; studied medicine under Elizabeth Blackwell in New York, rejected for medical training by Edinburgh University; founded London School of Medicine for Women, 1874; in 1877 (by then MD Berne) permitted to practise. In 1878 she settled in Edinburgh and founded the Women's Hospital and School of Medicine. Died 1912.

1840: Pierre Jean **Robiquet** died, **born** 1780. *codeine*

1840: Jules Hippolyte **Cloquet** died, **born** 1787. *olfaction*

1840: Giuseppangelo **Fonzi** died, **born** 1768. *artificial teeth*

1840: Laurent Théodore **Biett** died, **born** 1781. *lupus erythematoides nigrans*

1840: Augustin Jacob **Landré-Beauvais** died, **born** 1772. *rheumatoid arthritis*

1840: Johan Nepomuk **Rust** died, **born** 1775. *tuberculous spondylitis*

1840: John **Badham** died, **born** 1807. *poliomyelitis*

1840: Jean Etienne **Esquirol** died, **born** 1772. *psychiatry*

1840: Carl Ferdinand von **Graefe** died, **born** 1787. *rhinoplasty, blepharoplasty, cleft palate*

## 1841
1841:1 **Association of Medical Officers of Asylums and Hospitals for the Insane** founded in London

1841:2 **Académie Royale de Médecine de Belgique** founded

1841:3 An operation for enucleation of the **eyeball** introduced by Joseph Michael Ferrall (1790–1860), *DJMS* **19**:329. *5854*

1841:4 *Candida albicans* discovered to be causal organism in **thrush (candidiasis)** by Fredrik Theodor Berg (1806–1887), *Hygiea* **3**:541. *5518*

1841:5 The **inclusion body** of **molluscum contagiosum** described by William Henderson (1810–1872) and Robert Paterson (1814–1889), *EMSJ* **56**:213, 279. *4031, 4032*

1841:6 The cellular nature of **spermatozoa** determined by Rudolf Albert von Kölliker (1817–1905), *NNGN* **19**:4. *1220*

1841:7 The **fungal** cause of **favus (ringworm)**, *Achorion (Trichophyton) schönleinii*, discovered by David Gruby (1810–1898), *CRAS* **13**:72, independently of Johann Lucas Schönlein (1839). *4030, 4029*

1841:8 The first important monograph on **parotid tumours**, *Maladies de la glande parotide*, was published by Auguste Bérard (1802–1846). *3444*

1841:9 In his *Treatise on the oleum jecoris aselli, or cod-liver oil*, John Hughes Bennett (1812–1875) drew attention to the beneficial effects of **cod-liver oil**. *1858*

1841:10 Many of the **histological** discoveries of Friedrich Gustav Jakob Henle (1809–1885) are described in his *Allgemeine Anatomie*, including his demonstration of **smooth muscle** in **small arteries** (pp. 510, 690). *543*

1841:11 Gabriel Gustav Valentin (1810–1883) was first to discover a **trypanosome** (in a salmon), *ArA*: 435. *5267.1*

1841:12 An operation for **femoral hernia** introduced by James Luke (1798–1881), *LMG* **28**:863. *3588*

———————

1841:13 Albert Freeman Africanus **King**, American physician, born 18 Jan; first to advance a reasoned argument in support of the belief in the transmission of malaria by the mosquito, 1883, *PSM* **23**:644. Died 1914. *5237*

1841:14 Eduard **Albert**, Bohemian surgeon, born 20 Jan; first to describe arthrodesis of an ankle-joint for paralytic foot, 1882, *WMP* **23**:725. He introduced the concept of arthrodesis into orthopaedic surgery. Died 1900. *4347*

1841:15 Thomas Richard **Fraser**, British pharmacologist, born 5 Feb; isolated physostigmine (eserine), 1866, *TRSE* **24**:715. Introduced strophanthus, 1890, *TRSE* **35**:955; **36**:343. Died 1919. *1866.1, 1885*

1841:16 George **Oliver**, British physician and physiologist, born 13 Apr; with Edward Albert Sharpey-Schafer demonstrated a pressor substance, later named adrenaline, in the adrenal medulla, 1895, *JP* **18**:230. Died 1915. *1143*

1841:17 Gerhard Henrik Armauer **Hansen**, Norwegian bacteriologist, born 29 Jul; discovered leprosy bacillus, 28 February 1873, *NML* **4**, ix:1. Died 1873. *2436*

1841:18 Emil Theodor **Kocher**, Swiss surgeon, born 25 Aug; notable for his method of reduction of subluxation of the shoulder-joint, 1870, *BKW* **7**:101. Pioneered thyroidectomy for goitre, 1878, *KBSA* **8**:702 (Awarded Nobel Prize (Physiology or Medicine), 1909, for this work, *NPL*). Devised an operation for the radical extirpation of the tongue for carcinoma, 1880, *DZC* **13**:134; his pioneer work in the field led to a better understanding of its cause. Used the term 'cachexia strumipriva' to describe the myxoedema following on total thyroidectomy, 1883, *ArKC* **29**:254. Introduced silk sutures, 1888, *CBSA* **18**:3. Devised an operation for the radical cure of hernia, 1892, *KBSA* **22**:96. Died 1917. *4425, 3826, 3473, 5619.1, 3827, 3600*

1841:19 Timothy Richards **Lewis**, British bacteriologist, born 31 Aug; like Demarquay and Wucherer, he saw microfilariae in body fluids, 1871, *ARSCI* **8** App.E:241; he was first to use the term *Filaria sanguinis hominis*. First description of a trypanosome in a mammal (*Trypanosoma lewisi*), 1878, *ARSCI* **14B**:157. Died 1886. *5344.8, 5270.1*

1841:20 Carl Wilhelm Hermann **Nothnagel**, Austrian physician, born 28 Sep; described unilateral oculomotor paralysis combined with cerebellar ataxia ('Nothnagel's syndrome'); in his *Topische Diagnostik der Gehirnkrankheiten*, 1879. Died 1905. *4560*

1841:21 Joseph P. **O'Dwyer**, American physician, born 12 Oct; perfected the operation of laryngeal intubation in croup, 1885, *NJMJ* **42**:245. Died 1898. *5057*

210

1841:22 Arthur von **Hippel**, German ophthalmologist, born 24 Oct; modern keratoplasty is based on the technique introduced by him, 1888, *GAO* **34** i:108. Died 1917. *5933*

1841:23 Gustav **Nepveu**, German pathological anatomist, born 14 Nov; first to see trypanosomes in human blood, 1891, *CRSB* **43**:39. Died 1903. *5272*

1841:24 Georges **Hayem**, French physician, born 24 Nov; gave classic description of chronic interstitial hepatitis, 1874, *ArPhy* **1**:126. First accurately counted blood platelets, 1878, *ArPhy* **5**:692. His account of chlorosis placed the knowledge of the condition on a firm basis, in his *Du sang et ses altérations anatomiques*, p. 614, 1889. Drew attention to acquired haemolytic anaemia, 1898, *JMI* **2**:116. Following Widal and Abrami's account, 1907, the condition was named 'Hayem-Widal disease' and 'Widal-Abrami disease'. Died 1933. *3623, 879, 3130, 3777, 3783*

1841:25 Charles Eugène **Quinquaud**, French physician, born 26 Dec; described folliculitis decalvans, 1888, *RCSL* **9**:17. Died 1894. *4094*

1841:26 Mstislav **Novinsky**, Russian oncologist, born; successfully transplanted tumours in dogs, 1876, *MV* **16**:289. Died 1914. *2620.1*

1841:27 Julius **Krauss**, German gastroenterologist, born; published the first comprehensive study of duodenal ulcer; in his *Das perforirende Geschwür im Duodenum*, 1865. *3461*

1841:28 Eugen **Hahn** born; devised the operation of nephropexy for the relief of mobile kidney, 1881, *ZCh* **8**:449. Died 1902. *4218*

1841: Friedrich Wilhelm Adam **Sertürner** died, **born** 1783. *morphine*

1841: Jean Louis **Petit** died, **born** 1674. *mastoiditis*

1841: Astley Paston **Cooper** died, **born** 1768. *deafness, myringotomy, hernia, breast diseases, abdominal artery ligation, carotid artery ligation*

1841: Johann Karl Georg **Fricke** died, **born** 1790. *blepharoplasty*

1841: William Potts **Dewees** died, **born** 1768. *gynaecology, paediatrics*

1841: Marie Anne Victoire **Boivin** died, **born** 1773. *amputation of cervix, cancer of urethra, hydatidiform mole*

1841: James **Hope** died, **born** 1801. *heart murmurs, valvular disease, aneurysm*

**1842**
1842:1 **Brompton Hospital** (for consumption and diseases of the chest) opened at Manor House, Chelsea, **London**; moved to present site in Brompton Road, 1846

1842:2 **School of Pharmacy (Pharmaceutical Society of Great Britain)** opened in **London**

1842:3 **Anatomical Institute and New Canton Hospital, Zürich**, opened

1842:4 The first successful attempt to treat **strabismus** by myotomy described by Johann Friedrich Dieffenbach (1792–1847); in his *Ueber das Schielen und die Heilung desselben durch eine Operation.* *5856*

1842:5 The term **ovariotomy** introduced by Charles Clay (1801–1893), British ovariotomist, *MTG* **7**:43, 59, 67, 83, 99, 139, 153, 270. *6032*

1842:6 The first use of **hypnosis** as a form of **anaesthesia** during a major operation (**amputation**) in England was made by W. Squire Ward, with W. Topham, a lawyer interested in mesmerism, performing the hypnosis; in *Account of a case of successful amputation of the thigh during the mesmeric state.* *5650.1*

1842:7 Although Crawford Williamson Long (1815–1878) was first, on 30 March 1842, successfully to use **ether** as an **anaesthetic**, he did not publish his results until 1849, *SMSJ* **5**:705. *5664*

1842:8 David Gruby (1810–1898) found *Candida albicans* to be the causal organism in **thrush** (**candidiasis**), *CRAS* **14**:634, independently of Berg (1841). *5519, 5518*

1842:9 Scientific investigation of **mesmerism** by James Braid (1795–1860), in his *Satanic agency and mesmerism reviewed*, convinced him that its effects were not due to an outside force, but were natural phenomena arising from the subject's heightened suggestibility. *4992.3*

1842:10 **Scabies crustosa**, **Norwegian itch**, ('**Boeck's scabies**') first described by Carl Wilhelm Boeck (1808–1875), *NML* **4**:1, 127. *4033*

1842:11 The first accurate description of *Trichophyton mentagrophytes*, the fungus causing **sycosis barbae** given by David Gruby (1810–1898), *CRAS* **15**:512. *4034*

1842:12 Carl von Rokitansky (1804–1878) gave a classical description of the pathology of acute yellow atrophy of the **liver**; in his *Handbuch der pathologischen Anatomie*, **3**, p. 13; it was also called '**Rokitansky's disease**'. *3618*

1842:13 '**Curling's ulcer**' – duodenal ulcer as a complication of **burns** – reported by Thomas Blizard Curling (1811–1888), *MCT* **25**:260. *3445*

1842:14 **Pernicious anaemia of pregnancy** first described by Walter Channing (1786–1876), *NEQJ* **1**:157. *3116*

1842:15 **Pathological anatomy**; *Handbuch der pathologischen Anatomie*, 1842–46, published by Carl Rokitansky (1804–1878); an outstanding work in the field. *2293*

1842:16 *Report on sanitary conditions of the labouring population of Great Britain* by Edwin Chadwick (1800–1890) led to public health legislation and to great improvements in the **public health**. *1608*

1842:17 New instruments for the treatment of **strabismus** described by James Bolton (1812–1869); in his *Treatise on strabismus.* *5855*

1842:18 **Bowman's capsule** named after William Bowman (1816–1892) following his account of the Malpighian bodies, *PT* **132**:57. *1231*

1842:19 **Blood platelets** discovered by Alfred Donné (1801–1878), *CRAS* **14**:366. *864*

1842:20 First clear account of **chronic constrictive pericarditis** by Norman Chevers (1818–1886), *GHR* **7**:387. *2752*

1842:21 **Foramen of Magendie** described by François Magendie (1783–1855) in his *Recherches sur le liquide céphalo-rachidien. 1397*

1842:21.1 *Sarcina ventriculi* discovered by John Goodsir (1814–1867), *EMSJ* **57**:430. *2471*

1842:22 William **James** born, 11 Jan; the founder of the American school of experimental psychology; he wrote *The principles of psychology*, 1890. Died 1910. *4977.2*

1842:23 Josef **Breuer**, Austrian physician and psychologist, born 15 Jan; with Sigmund Freud, introduced psychoanalysis, 1893; the foundation stone was their *Studien über Hysterie*, 1895. Died 1925. *4977.3, 4978*

1842:24 François Henri **Hallopeau**, French dermatologist, born 17 Jan; described a suppurative form of pemphigus vegetans, 1889, *CRDS*, p. 344. Died 1919. *4101*

1842:25 Friedrich **Bezold**, German otologist, born 9 Feb; gave first clear description of mastoiditis, 1877, *ArOh* **13**:26. Died 1908. *3386*

1842:26 Albert **Ladenburg,** German chemist, born 2 Jul; isolated scopolamine, 1881, *AnCP* **206**:274. Died 1911. *1873*

1842:27 Robert William **Taylor**, American dermatologist, born 11 Aug; first described acrodermatitis chronica atrophicans ('Taylor's disease'), 1875, *ArDS* **2**:114; it was given its name by Herxheimer and Hartmann in 1902. Died 1906. *4069, 4138*

1842:28 Heinrich Irenaeus **Quincke**, German physician, born 26 Aug; observed aneurysm of hepatic artery, 1870, *BKW* **8**:349. Gave an excellent (but not the first) account of angioneurotic oedema ('Quincke's oedema'), 1882, *MPD* **1**:129. Introduced lumbar puncture, independently of Wynter, using it for both diagnostic and therapeutic purposes, 1891, *BKW* **28**:929. With Ernst Roos, distinguished *Entamoeba histolytica* from *Escherichia coli*, 1893, *BKW* **30**:1089. Died 1922. *2982, 4081, 4869, 4868, 5188*

1842:29 Jacques-Louis **Reverdin**, Swiss surgeon, born 28 Aug; carried out important work on the transplantation of free skin, 1869, *BSIC* **10**:511. Produced myxoedema by total or partial thyroidectomy, 1882, *RMSR* **2**:539. Died 1929. *5750, 3828*

1842:30 Edoardo **Porro**, Italian surgeon, born 17 Sep; performed caesarean section with excision of the uterus and adnexa ('Porro's operation'), 1876, *AnU* **237**:289. Died 1902. *6240*

1842:31 Vincenz **Czerny**, Czech surgeon, born 19 Nov; carried out the first total hysterectomy by the vaginal route, 1879, *WMW* **29**:1171; introduced the operation of enucleation of subperitoneal fibroids of the uterus, by the vaginal route, 1881, *WMW* **31**:501, 525. Died 1916. *6072, 6073*

1842:32 Anton Julius Friedrich **Rosenbach**, German bacteriologist and surgeon, born 16 Dec; differentiated Streptococcus and Staphylococcus, and *Staphylococcus aureus* and *Staph. albus*;

in his *Mikro-Organismen bei den Wund-Infections-Krankheiten des Menschen*, 1884. Died 1923. *5619*

---

1842:33 Louis Charles **Malassez**, French physiologist, born; designed haemocytometer, 1874, *ArPhy* 2 sér. **1**:32, (so named by W.R. Gowers). Died 1909. *876*

1842:34 Berthold Ernest **Hadra**, German/American surgeon, born; first to perform spinal surgical immobilization and fusion, 1891, *MTR* **22**:423; *TAOrA* **4**:206. Died 1903. *4359.1, 4359.2*

1842:35 Heinrich **Sellerbeck**, German ophthalmic surgeon, born; first to use human donor cornea for transplants, 1878, *GAO* **24** iv:1, 321. *5916.1*

---

1842:36 Louis François **Bravais** died; first described hemiplegic (unilateral) epilepsy, in his *Recherches sur les symptômes et le traitement de l'épilepsie hémiplégique*, Paris, Thèse No. 118, 1827; the excellent account by Jackson (1863) led to the term 'Bravais-Jacksonian epilepsy'. *4810, 4816*

1842: Charles **Bell** died, **born** 1774. *surgery, Bell's nerve, facial palsy*

1842: Dominique Jean **Larrey** died, **born** 1766. *military surgery, amputation at hip-joint, ophthalmia, trachoma*

1842: Thomas **Spens** died, **born** 1764. *heart block*

1842: François **Double** died, **born** ?1776. *auscultation*

1842: Georg **Carabelli** died, **born** 1787. *Carabelli's cusps (tuberculus anomalus)*

1842: Pierre Joseph **Pelletier** died, **born** 1788. *quinine, emetine*

1842: John **Stephenson** died, **born** 1797. *cleft palate*

1842: Christian Heinrich **Bünger** died, **born** 1782. *rhinoplasty*

## 1843
1843:1 **Sydenham Society** founded in **London**

1843:2 **Société de Chirurgie**, **Paris**, founded

1843:3 **Albuminous urine** in connection with **puerperal convulsions** first reported by John Charles Weaver Lever (1811–1858), *GHR* **1**:495. *6176*

1843:4 The first definitely to establish the contagious nature of **puerperal fever** was Oliver Wendell Holmes (1809–1894), *NEQJ* **1**:503. *6274*

1843:5 Among important procedures and instruments introduced into **gynaecology** by James Young Simpson (1811–1870) was the **uterine sound** for diagnosing **retroposition of the uterus**, *LEMJ* **3**:547, 701, 1009; **4**:208. *6035*

1843:6 The first successful **oöphorectomy** performed by John Light Atlee (1799–1885), *NYJM* 1:168. *6034*

1843:7 A **vaginal speculum** introduced by Joseph Claude Anselme Récamier (1774–1852), *BuAM* **8**:661. *6033*

1843:8 Test readings of print at a distance, for **eyesight testing** introduced by Heinrich Küchler (1811–1873); in his *Schriftnummerprobe für Gesichtsleidende. 5858*

1843:9 An operation for complete closure of **clefts** of the **palate** devised by Jonathan Mason Warren (1811–1867), *NEQJ* 1:538. *5745*

1843:10 One of the first in England to perform surgical operations with the aid of **hypnosis** was John Elliotson (1791–1868); in his *Numerous cases of surgical operations without pain in the mesmeric state. 5650.2*

1843:11 **Trypanosomes** discovered in the frog by David Gruby (1810–1898), he first suggested the name 'trypanosome' to describe the parasite, *CRAS* **17**:1134. *5268*

1843:12 **Relapsing fever** so named by David Craigie (1793–1866), *EMSJ* **60**:410. *5311*

1843:13 Modern **hypnosis** inaugurated by James Braid (1795–1860), he introduced the term in his *Neurypnology, or the rationale of nervous sleep. 4993*

1843:14 A classic description of **pernicious anaemia** given by Thomas Addison (1793–1860) in his paper on the condition later known as '**Addison's disease**', *LMG* **43**:517. *3118*

1843:15 Important observations on the **blood corpuscles**, including first description of **leucocytosis,** by William Addison (1802–1881); in his *Observations on inflammation. 3059*

1843:16 The first accurate description of *Microsporon audouini*, a cause of **tinea capitis**, given by David Gruby (1810–1898), *CRAS* **17**:301. *4035*

1843:17 '**Syme's amputation**' at the **ankle-joint** first successfully performed by James Syme (1799–1870), *LEMJ* **3**:93. *4459*

1843:18 Emil du Bois-Reymond (1818–1896), German founder of modern **electrophysiology**, gave the first description and definition of **electrotonus**, *AnPh* **58**:1. *609*

1843:19 **Subacute bacterial endocarditis** described by George Hilaro Barlow (1806–1866) and George Owen Rees (1813–1889), *GHR* n.s. **1**:189. *2753*

1843:20 **Presystolic murmur** in **mitral stenosis** first described by Sulpice Antoine Fauvel (1813–1884), *ArGM* **1**:1. *2754*

1843:21 Carl Ludwig (1816–1896) wrote an important monograph on **renal secretion**, *Beiträge zur Lehre vom Mechanismus der Harnsekretion. 1232*

1843:22 John S. **Parry**, American pathologist, born 4 Jan; his *Extra-uterine pregnancy*, 1876, was regarded by Lawson Tait as the first authoritative work on ectopic pregnancy. Died 1876. *6191*

1843:23 Johann Otto Leonhard **Heubner**, German paediatrician, born 21 Jan; first to isolate the meningococcus from cerebrospinal fluid, 1896, *JaK* **43**:1. Contributed important work on infant feeding, including determination of caloric requirement. His *Lehrbuch der Kinderheilkunde*, 3 vols, appeared in 1903–6. Died 1926. *4680, 6343*

1843:24 Otto Hugo Franz **Obermeier**, German bacteriologist, born 13 Feb; discovered *Borrelia recurrentis* (*obermeieri*), causal organism in relapsing fever, 1860, reported in 1873, *ZMW* **11**:145. Died 1873. *5314*

1843:25 Otto **Bollinger**, German pathologist, born 3 Apr; gave the first effective description of actinomycosis in cattle, 1877, *ZMW* **15**:481. He gave his botanical colleague C.O. Harz a specimen of the microparasite and Harz named it (p. 485) *Actinomyces bovis*. Died 1909. *5510*

1843:26 Julius **Hirschberg**, German ophthalmologist, born 18 Apr; introduced the electromagnet into ophthalmology; in his *Der Electromagnet in der Augenheilkunde*, 1885. Died 1925. *5927*

1843:27 Walther **Flemming**, German cytologist, born 21 Apr; discovered the centrosome, 1877, *ArMA* **13**:693. Published classic account of cell division, 1879, *ArMA* **16**:302; 1880, **18**:151. Died 1905. *498, 122*

1843:28 David **Ferrier**, British neurophysiologist, born 13 Jun; his *Functions of the brain*, 1876, laid the foundations of our knowledge of cortical localization. Died 1928. *1409*

1843:29 Camillo **Golgi**, Italian cytologist, born 7 Jul; described 'Golgi cells', 1880, *ArSM* **4**:221; described the development of the parasite of quartan malaria, 1886, *ArSM* **10**:109; described the difference between the parasites of tertian and quartan malaria, 1889, *ArSM* **13**:173. For his contribution to knowledge of neuroanatomy he shared the Nobel Prize (Physiology or Medicine) with Santiago Ramón y Cajal in 1906, *NPL*. Died 1926. *1277, 5239, 5240*

1843:30 Just Marcellin **Lucas-Championnière**, French surgeon, born 15 Aug; one of the first to adopt the antiseptic principle in surgery; he wrote *Chirurgie antiseptique*, 1876, the first authoritative text on the subject. Died 1913. *5636*

1843:31 David Douglas **Cunningham**, British pathologist and bacteriologist, born 29 Sep; saw and described what were almost certainly Leishman-Donovan bodies in tissue from Delhi boil (cutaneous leishmaniasis), 1885, *SMI* **1**:21. Died 1914. *5293*

1843:32 Robert **Koch**, German bacteriologist, born 11 Dec; first to obtain pure cultures of *Bacillus anthracis*, 1876, *BBP* **2**:277. Continuing the work of C.J. Davaine (1863, 1865), he proved that infectious diseases are caused by living reproductive microorganisms. Demonstrated the role of bacteria in the aetiology of wound infection; in his *Untersuchungen über die Aetiologie der Wundinfectionskrankheiten*, 1878 ('Koch's postulates'). His methods of culturing, fixing and staining bacteria, 1881, *MKG* **1**:1, are the bases on which bacteriology largely rests. Showed that mercuric chloride was superior to carbolic acid as an antiseptic, and that live steam surpassed hot air in sterilizing power, 1881, *MKG* **1**:234. Discovered the tubercle bacillus, 24 March 1882, *MKG* **19**:221. Discovered the Koch-Weeks bacillus in Egyptian conjunctivitis (Egyptian ophthalmia), 1883, *WMW* **33**:1548; in 1886 J.E. Weeks discovered the same organism in 'pink eye' and it was later given its present name. Isolated the cholera vibrio in pure culture, 1884, *DMW* **10**:725. Described his tuberculin skin test, the resulting inflammatory reaction ('Koch's phenomenon') in tuberculous patients and introduced tuberculin in the treatment of tuberculosis 1890, *DMW* **16**:1029; 1891, **17**:101, 1189. Prophylactic measures for the control of typhoid proposed in his *Die Bekämpfung der Typhus*, 1910, were adopted almost everywhere. Nobel Prize (Physiology or Medicine) 1905, for his work on tuberculosis, *NPL*. Died 1910. *5167, 2536, 2495.1, 5636.1, 2331, 5923, 5108, 2544.1, 2332, 5040*

1843:33 John Wickham **Legg**, British physician, born 28 Dec; first to describe multiple hereditary telangiectasis, later named 'Rendu-Osler-Weber disease', following three later accounts, 1876, *L* **2**:856. Died 1921. *2707*

1843:34 Adolf **Mayer**, German phytopathologist, born; described and named the mosaic disease of tobacco, 1886, *LV* **32**:450. Ivanovski, in 1892, described its filter-passing ability, initiating research into virus diseases. *2503.1*

1843:35 Friedrich Georg Rudolph **Wegner**, German pathologist, born; described osteochondritic separation of the epiphyses in congenital syphilis ('Wegner's disease'), 1870, *VA* **50**:305. Died 1917. *4339*

1843:36 Waren **Tay**, British surgeon and ophthalmologist, born; described amaurotic familial idiocy – dealing mainly with ocular manifestations, 1880, *TOUK* **1**:55; the cerebral changes were more fully described by Sachs (1887), 'Tay-Sachs disease'. Died 1927. *5918, 4705*

1843: Christian Friedrich Samuel **Hahnemann** died, **born** 1755. *homoeopathy*

1843: Abraham **Colles** died, **born** 1773. *subclavian artery ligation, fracture of radius*

1843: Elisha **North** died, **born** 1771. *cerebral meningitis*

**1844**
1844:1 **Association of Medical Superintendents for the Insane** organized (now **American Psychiatric Association**)

1844:2 **New York Pathological Society** founded (incorporated 1886)

1844:3 **Royal College of Veterinary Surgeons, London,** founded

1844:4 [**Association of Obstetricians and Gynaecologists**], **Berlin** founded

1844:5 A two-flap method for the repair of **cleft lip** devised by Joseph François Malgaigne (1806–1865), *JC(M)* **2**:1. It was modified the following year by Mirault. *5746, 5746.1*

1844:6 William Henderson (1810–1872) left a good account of **relapsing fever** and was one of the first to differentiate it from **typhus**, *EMSJ* **61**:201. *5311.1*

1844:7 A classic description of **congenital cerebral spastic diplegia** by William John Little (1810–1894), *L* **1**:350, led to the alternative name '**Little's disease**'. *4691.1*

1844:8 Robert Remak (1815–1865) was first to describe the intrinsic **ganglia** of the **heart**, *ArA* p. 463. *806*

1844:9 Discovery of *Trichophyton tonsurans*, a cause of **tinea capitis**, by David Gruby (1810–1898), *CRAS* **18**:583. *4036*

1844:10 First description of **pemphigus foliaceus** by Pierre Louis Alphée Cazenave (1795–1877), *AnMP* **1**:208. *4037*

1844:11 **'Carabelli's cusps'** (tuberculus anomalus), sometimes found in the upper permanent molars, first described by Georg Carabelli (1787–1842); in his *Systematisches Handbuch der Zahnheilkunde*, Bd.2. *3682*

1844:12 **Oesophagotomy** first performed by John Watson (1807–1863) for stricture of the oesophagus, *AmJMS* **8**:309. *3448*

1844:13 Max Joseph von Pettenkofer (1818–1901) developed a colour reaction for **bile**, *ACP* **52**:90 *679*

1844:14 **Intestinal resection** for **cancer** first carried out by Jean François Reybard (1790–1863), *BuAM* **9**:1031. *3447*

1844:15 **Laryngeal polyp** first removed by Charles Henri Ehrmann (1792–1878), *CRAS* **18**:593, 709. *3260*

1844:16 **Leukaemia** briefly described by Alexander Donné (1801–1878); in his *Cours de microscopie*, p. 10. *3060.1*

1844:17 **Pneumopericardium** first adequately described by Isidore Bricheteau (1789–1861), *ArGM* **4**:334. *2755*

1844:18 **Amyl nitrite** discovered by Antoine Jerome Balard (1802–1876), *CRAS* **19**:634. *1859*

1844:19 Total eradication of the os coccygis for **neuralgia** carried out by Josiah Clark Nott (1804–1873), *NOMSJ* **1**:58. *4852*

---

1844:20 Henry **Morris**, British surgeon, born 7 Jan; introduced nephrolithotomy – removal of renal calculus by lumbar incision, 1888, *TCSL* **14**:30. Died 1926. *4292.1*

1844:21 Wilhelm **Filehne**, Polish pharmacologist, born 12 Feb; introduced antipyrine, 1884, *ZKM* **7**:641; aminopyrine (pyramidon), 1896, *BKW* **33**:1061. Died 1927. *1878, 1889*

1844:22 Thomas Lauder **Brunton**, British physician, born 14 Mar; introduced amyl nitrite in management of angina pectoris, 1867, *L* **2**:97. Died 1916. *2890*

1844:23 Henri Alexandre **Danlos**, French dermatologist, born 26 Mar; with P. Bloch, first used radium in the treatment of lupus erythematosus, 1901, *BSED* **12**:438. In his description of cutis laxa ('Ehlers-Danlos syndrome'), 1908, *BSFD* **19**:70, he noted the subcutaneous tumours sometimes occurring in this condition. Died 1912. *4003, 4132, 4144*

1844:24 Martin **Bernhardt**, German neurologist, born 10 Apr; reported meralgia paraesthetica in the leg, due to disease of the external cutaneous nerve of the thigh ('Bernhardt's disease'), 1878, *DAKM* **22**:362. Died 1915. *4559*

1844:25 Edoardo **Bassini**, Italian surgeon, born 14 Apr; modified Hahn's operation of nephropexy, 1882, *AnU* **261**:281. Devised the modern method for the radical cure of inguinal hernia, 1887, *ACMI* **2**:179, almost simultaneously with William Stewart Halsted. Published a method for the cure of femoral hernia, in his *Nuovo metodo operativo per la cura dell' ernia crurale*, 1893. Died 1924. *4219, 3598, 3602*

1844:26 Alexander **Ogston**, British surgeon, born 19 Apr; discovered and named *Staphylococcus aureus* and differentiated *Staphylococcus* from *Streptococcus*, 1881, *BMJ* **1**:369. Died 1929. *2494*

1844:27 Theodor **Puschmann**, German physician and medical historian, born 4 May; his *Handbuch der Geschichte der Medizin*, 3 vols, 1902–5, is one of the most important histories of medicine. Died 1899. *6398*

1844:28 Max **Wolff**, German mycologist, born 6 May; with James Israel, isolated *Actinomyces bovis*, 1891, *VA* **126**:11. Died 1923. *5514*

1844:29 Friedrich **Trendelenburg**, German surgeon, born 24 May; performed endotracheal anaesthesia by means of tracheostomy, 1871, *ArKC* **12**:112. In a paper on the repair of vesico-vaginal fistula described an elevated pelvic position ('Trendelenburg position), 1890, *SKV* **355**:3372, first described by his pupil, W. Meyer, in 1885, *ArKC* **31**:494. Attempted the treatment of hydronephrosis by a plastic operation, 1890, *SKV* **355**:3372 – the first recorded surgical intervention for the relief of the condition. Treated varicose veins by ligation of great saphenous vein ('Trendelenburg's operation'), 1890, *BKC* **7**:195. Described 'Trendelenburg's sign' of congenital dislocation of the hip-joint, 1895, *DMW* **21**:21. Died 1924. *5669.1, 6091, 4222, 2997, 4428*

1844:30 Victor Charles **Hanot**, French physician, born 6 Jul; gave the first description of hypertrophic cirrhosis of the liver with icterus ('Hanot's disease'); in his *Étude sur une form de cirrhose hypertrophique du foie*, 1875. Died 1896. *3624*

1844:31 Henri Jules Louis **Rendu**, French physician, born 24 Jul; described multiple hereditary telangiectasis ('Rendu-Osler-Weber disease'), 1896, *GH* **69**:1322. Died 1902. *2710*

1844:32 David Tod **Gilliam**, American surgeon, born 3 Aug; used round-ligament ventrosuspension of the uterus in his operation for prolapse, 1900, *AmJOD* **41**:299. Died 1923. *6111*

1844:33 Johann Friedrich **Miescher**, Swiss physiologist, born 13 Aug; discovered nuclein (nucleoprotein), later shown to be the hereditary genetic material, 1871; in: Hoppe-Seyler, F. *Med.-chem. Untersuchungen*, Heft 4, 441. Died 1895. *695*

1844:34 Hubert **Sattler**, Austrian ophthalmologist, born 3 Sep; described 'Sattler's layer' of the choroid, 1876, *GAO* **22ii**:1. Died 1928. *1518*

1844:35 Patrick **Manson**, British physician and parasitologist, born 3 Oct; 'Father of modern tropical medicine'. Showed that *Wuchereria bancrofti*, cause of filarial elephantiasis in man, develops in, and is transmitted by, the *Culex* mosquito – the first proof that infective diseases are spread by animal vectors, 1877, *MRpt* **13**:30; **14**:1. Described the aetiology of paragonimiasis and its parasite, *Paragonimus ringeri*, 1880, *MRpt* **20**:10. First proposed his mosquito-malaria hypothesis, 1894, *BMJ* **1**:695, 751, 831. Published first edition of his textbook, *Tropical diseases*, 1898. Provided experimental proof of the mosquito-malaria theory by allowing infected mosquitoes to bite a volunteer who developed malaria 15 days later and was cured by quinine, 1900, *BMJ* **2**:949. Died 1922. *5345, 5345.1, 5346.2, 5245, 2266, 5252.2*

1844:36 Ernst Leopold **Salkowski**, German physiologist and chemical pathologist, born 11 Oct; first to describe pentosuria, 1895, *BKW* **32**:364. Died 1923. *3918*

1844:37 Stephen **Mackenzie**, British physician, born 14 Oct; described 'Mackenzie's syndrome' (paralysis of the tongue, soft palate, and vocal cord on the same side), 1886, *TCSL* **19**:317. Died 1909. *4571*

1844:38 Edward Emanuel **Klein**, Austrian/British histologist and pathologist, born 31 Oct; a report by him contains the first suggestion of the streptococcal origin of scarlet fever, 1886, *Report of Medical Officer, Local Government Board, London*, 1885, p. 90. Died 1925. *5080*

1844:39 Nicholas **Senn**, Swiss/American physician and surgeon, born 31 Oct; showed that partial removal of the pancreas was feasible and justifiable, 1886, *TASA* **4**:99. Introduced a test for detection of intestinal perforation by the rectal insufflation of hydrogen, 1888, *JAMA* **10**:767. Died 1908. *3629, 3494*

1844:40 Emil **Ponfick**, German pathologist, born 3 Nov; recognized the causative role of the fungus *Actinomyces* in human actinomycosis and established the identity of the human and animal forms, 1880, *BKW* **17**:660. Died 1913. *5512*

1844:41 Oscar **Löw** born; with Rudolph Emmerich prepared pyocyanase, an antibiotic, prepared from *Pseudomonas pyocyanea*, 1889, *ZHyg* **31**:1. *1932.2*

1844:42 Nagajosi **Nagai**, Japanese pharmacologist, born; isolated ephedrine, 1887, *PhaZ* **32**:700. Died 1929. *1883.1*

1844:43 William **Alexander**, British surgeon, born; carried out a suspension operation for retroversion of the uterus, 1881, reported 1882, *MTG* **1**:327. First to attempt the surgical treatment of epilepsy, he removed the superior sympathetic ganglia; in his *Treatment of epilepsy*, 1889. Died 1919. *6077, 4861*

1844:44 Alexei Pavlovich **Fedchenko**, Russian parasitologist, born; elucidated the life cycle of *Dracunculus medinensis*, the parasite of dracontiasis, 1869, *IOLE* **8**:71. Died 1873. *5344.7*

1844:45 John Davies **Thomas**, Australian physician, born; transmitted *Taenia echinococcus* to the dog from human sources, 1885, *PRS* **38**:449. Died 1893. *5347*

1844:46 Robert Charles **Moon**, American ophthalmologist, born; with John Zachariah Laurence, reported four cases of retinitis pigmentosa with familial developmental imperfections, 1866, *OR* **2**:32. Following further reports by A. Biedl (1922), the condition was named the Laurence-Moon-Biedl syndrome. Died 1914. *6368, 6369*

1844: John **Abercrombie** died, **born** 1780. *neuropathology*

1844: John **Dalton** died, **born** 1766. *colour-blindness*

1844: John Conrad **Otto** died, **born** 1774 *haemophilia*

**1845**

1845:1 **Queen's College**, **Belfast**, founded

1845:2 **University of Honduras** founded in **Tegucigalpa**, opened 1847

1845:3 **Academia Médico-Quirurgica Española** founded in **Madrid**

1845:4 **St Mary's Hospital**, **London**, founded as **Paddington and St Marylebone Hospital**, opened 1852

1845:5 The **luminosity** of the **eye** in animals studied by Ernst Wilhelm von Brücke (1819–1892); by passing a tube through a candle flame he was able to see the **fundus**, *ArA* 387. *5859*

1845:6 A simplified form of roman letters, embossed on paper, for use by **blind** readers, devised by William Moon (1818–1894), himself blind, in 1845. Recorded in his *Light for the blind: a history of the origin of Moon's system of reading … for the blind*, 1873. *5909*

1845:7 The first to differentiate between benign and malignant **tumours** of the **uterus** was James Henry Bennet (1816–1891); in his *A practical treatise on inflammation, ulceration and induration of the neck of the uterus*. *6036*

1845:8 The first description of **corneal opacity** given by Philipp Franz von Walther (1782–1849), *JCA* **34**:1. *5860*

1845:9 Malgaigne's two-flap method for the repair of **cleft lip** modified by Germanicus Mirault (1796–1879), *JC(M)* **2**:257; **3**:5. *5746.1*

1845:10 First description of **anterior metatarsalgia** given by Lewis Durlacher (1792–1864), **surgeon-chiropodist** to Queen Victoria; in his *Treatise on corns* etc., p. 52; named '**Morton's metatarsalgia**' after the description by T.G. Morton in 1876. *4325, 4341*

1845:11 **Buck's operation** on the **ankylosed knee-joint** performed by Gurdon Buck (1807–1877), *AmJMS* **10**:277. *4324*

1845:12 The classification of **skin diseases** by Ferdinand von Hebra (1816–1880) was based on their pathological anatomy, *ZGA* **2**:34, 143, 211. *3991*

1845:13 The first comprehensive American text on **skin diseases** was Noah Worcester's (1812–1847) *Synopsis … of the more common and important diseases of the skin*. *3991.1*

1845:14 **Urinary hair catheter** introduced by Jacques Gilles Thomas Maisonneuve (1809–1887), *CRAS* **20**:70. *4168*

1845:15 A form of **liver cirrhosis** was described by George Budd (1808–1882) in his *On diseases of the liver*; it was named '**Budd's disease**'. *3619*

1845:16 **Leukaemia** first definitely described by John Hughes Bennett (1812–1875), *EMSJ* **64**:413. *3061*

1845:17 **Hypodermic infusions** made possible by Francis Rynd (1801–1861), *DMP* **13**:167.

1845:17 **Hypodermic infusions** made possible by Francis Rynd (1801–1861), *DMP* **13**:167. *1968*

1845:18 **Cannabis** intoxication described by Jacques-Joseph Moreau (1804–1884); in his *Du hachische* …. *2077.2*

1845:19 **Digitalin** isolated from digitalis by Augustin Eugène Homolle (1808–1875), *JPC* 3 sér. **7**:57. *1860*

---

1845:20 Anton **Weichselbaum**, Austrian pathologist, born 8 Feb; discovered the meningococcus, *Neisseria meningitidis*, causal organism of cerebrospinal meningitis, 1887, *FM* **5**:573, 620. Died 1920. *4678*

1845:21 Charles **McBurney**, American surgeon, born 19 Feb; defined 'McBurney's point' in appendicitis, 1889, *NYMJ* **50**:676. Died 1913. *3570*

1845:22 Edward **Nettleship**, British ophthalmic surgeon and pathologist, born 3 Mar; his description of urticaria pigmentosa, 1869, *BMJ* **2**:323, led to the eponym 'Nettleship's disease'. Died 1913. *4057*

1845:23 Carl **Weigert**, German pathologist and histologist, born 19 Mar; introduced staining methods for bacteria, 1871, *ZMW* **9**:609. First described myocardial infarction, 1880, *VA* **79**:87. Noted the connection of myasthenia gravis with hypertrophy of the thymus, 1901, *NZ* **20**:597. Died 1904. *2482, 2783*

1845:24 William Richard **Gowers**, British neurologist, born 20 Mar; demonstrated the dorsal spinocerebellar tract and introduced the terms 'myotatic' and 'knee-jerk'; in his *Diagnosis of diseases of the spinal cord*, 1880. In his *Epilepsy and other chronic convulsive diseases*, 1881, was first to note the tetanic nature of the epileptic convulsion. First described panatrophy; in his *Manual of diseases of the nervous system*, **1**, 365, 1886. With Victor Alexander Horsley, founder of neurosurgery in England, recorded first successful operation for removal of an extramedullary tumour of the spinal cord, 1888, *MCT* **71**:377. Recorded a distal form of progressive muscular dystrophy ('distal myopathy of Gowers'), 1902, *BMJ* **2**:89. Died 1915. *4562, 4818, 4751, 4860, 4762*

1845:25 Wilhelm Conrad **Röntgen**, German physicist, born 27 Mar; discovered x rays (Röntgen rays), 8 November 1895, *SPKG:*132, 1896:11; first recipient of Nobel Prize (Physics) 1901 for this work, *NPL*. Died 1923. *2683*

1845:26 Louis Théophile Joseph **Landouzy**, French physician, born 27 Mar; gave an early account of leptospirosis icterohaemorrhagica ('Weil's disease'), 1883, *GH* **56**:809. First to suggest the infective nature of herpes zoster, 1884, *JCMP* **6**:19, 26, 37, 44, 52. With Joseph Jules Dejerine, described the 'Landouzy-Dejerine type' of (scapulo-humeral) progressive muscular atrophy, 1886, *CRSB* **3**:478. Died 1917. *5331, 4642, 4752*

1845:27 Robert Lawson **Tait**, British gynaecologist, born 1 May; reported that he had performed Battey's operation (ovariotomy) for the treatment of non-ovarian cases, 16 days before Battey, 1879, *BMJ* **1**:813. The first British surgeon to diagnose acute appendicitis and to treat it by appendicectomy, 1880, *BMR* **27**:26, 76. Carried out oöphorectomy, 1881, *BMJ* **1**:766. He was among the greatest of the ovariotomists, his work in this field is summarized in his *General summary of conclusions from one thousand cases of abdominal section*, 1884.

Performed the first successful operation for ruptured ectopic pregnancy on 1 March 1883, reported 1884, *BMJ* 1:1250. Devised a flap-splitting operation for rectocele, 1887, *BGT* 3:367; 7:195. Performed caesarean section in cases of placenta praevia ('Tait-Porro operation'), 1890, *BMJ* 1:657. Apparently the first to describe Meigs' syndrome (ovarian fibroma combined with pleural effusion), 1892, *MCT* 75:109; later described by Meigs, 1934. Died 1899. *6071, 6062, 3570.1, 6075, 6081, 6196, 6087, 6245, 6093.1, 6132.01*

1845:28 Elie **Metchnikoff**, Russian pathologist, bacteriologist and immunologist, born 16 May; originated the theory of phagocytosis, 1884, *VA* 96:177. Published important investigations on inflammation, *Lektsii o sravnitelnoi patologii vospaleniy*, 1892. His classic *L'immunité dans les maladies infectieuses*, 1901, elaborated his views on the mechanisms concerned in specific antibacterial immunity. Shared the Nobel Prize (Physiology or Medicine), 1908, with Paul Ehrlich, for his work on immunity, *NPL.* Died 1916. *2538, 2307*

1845:29 Charles Louis Alphonse **Laveran**, French physician and parasitologist, born 18 Jun; first saw the malaria parasite on 20 October 1880; report published 1881, *BSMH* 17:158. First described the parasite *Toxoplasma*, 1896, *CRSB* 52:19. Awarded Nobel Prize (Physiology or Medicine), 1907, for his work on pathogenic protozoa, *NPL.* Died 1922. *5236, 5530.2*

1845:30 William James **Morton**, American neurologist and radiologist, born 3 Jul; took the first dental radiograph in the United States, 1896, *DeC* 38:478. Died 1920. *2684.3, 3689*

1845:31 Andrew Rose **Robinson**, Canadian/American dermatologist, born 31 Jul; published the first description of hydrocystoma, 1884, *TADA*, p. 14. Died 1924. *4084*

1845:32 Thomas **Barlow**, British physician, born 4 Sep; his classic description of infantile scurvy, 1883, *MCT* 66:159, led to the eponym '**Barlow's disease**'. Died 1945. *3720*

1845:33 Caesar Peter Moeller **Boeck**, Norwegian dermatologist, born 28 Sep; established the syndrome of benign sarcoid (Boeck's sarcoid), 1899, *NML* 14:1321; the earlier account by Besnier and the later one by Schaumann led to the name 'Besnier-Boeck-Schaumann disease'. Died 1917. *4095, 4128, 4149*

1845:34 Hans **Kundrat**, Austrian physician, born 6 Oct; described 'Kundrat's' lymphosarcoma, 1893, *WKW* 6:211, 234. Died 1893. *2623*

1845:35 Otto Michael **Leichtenstern**, American physician, born 14 Oct; first described subacute combined degeneration of the spinal cord in tabes, 1883, *DMW* 10:849. First to describe subacute combined degeneration of the spinal cord, which he termed progressive pernicious anaemia of tabetics, 1884, *DMW* 10:849. Died 1900. *4783, 3128*

1845:36 Victor **Galtier**, French veterinarian, born 15 Oct; his demonstration of the transmissibility of rabies from dog to rabbit, 1879, *AnMV* 28:627, and his subsequent immunization of sheep by the inoculation of rabid saliva, 1881, *CRAS* 93:284, aroused the interest of Louis Pasteur in the disease. Died 1908. *5481.2, 5481.3*

1845:37 Angelo **Maffucci**, Italian physician, born 17 Oct; first described Maffucci's syndrome (cavernous haemangioma with enchondromatosis), 1881, *MMC* 3:399. Died 1903. *4079*

1845:38 Charles Karsner **Mills**, American neurologist, born 4 Dec; his *The nervous system and its diseases*, 1898, was the foremost American neurological text of the nineteenth century and the only one of the period to contain a section on the chemistry of the nervous system. First described unilateral progressive ascending paralysis ('Mills' disease'), 1900, *JNMD* **27**:195. First described unilateral descending paralysis, 1906, *JAMA* **47**:1638. Died 1931. *4586.1, 4711*

1845:39 Ludwig **Lichtheim**, German physician, born 7 Dec; described subcortical sensory aphasia ('Lichtheim's disease'), 1885, *DAKM* **36**:204. Died 1928. *4626*

1845:40 Louis Adolphus **Duhring**, American dermatologist, born 23 Dec; his best work in dermatology was his grouping of several eruptive conditions under the term dermatitis herpetiformis ('Duhring's disease'), 1884, *JAMA* **3**:225; first described by William Tilbury Fox in 1880. Died 1913. *4083, 4079*

---

1845:41 Henry **Moon**, British dental surgeon, born; described the irregular and defective first molars in congenital syphilitics, 1877, *TOSG* **22**:223. Died 1892. *2391*

1845:42 George Alexander **Turner**, British dermatologist, born; first described tinea imbricata ('Tokelau ringworm'), 1870, *GMJ* **2**:510. Died 1900. *4059*

1845:43 Paul **Berger**, French surgeon, born; introduced interscapulothoracic amputation ('Berger's operation'), 1883, *BSCP* **9**:656. Introduced the gauze face mask into operative surgery, 1897, *BSCP* **25**:187. Died 1908. *4471, 5641*

---

1845: Charles **Badham** died, **born** 1780. *bronchitis*

1845: Whitley **Stokes** died, **born** 1763. *ecthyma terebrans*

## 1846
1846:1 **New York Academy of Medicine** founded

1846:2 [**Royal Saxon Academy of Sciences**], **Leipzig**, founded

1846:3 **American Medical Association** organized (first meeting Philadelphia, 5 May 1847)

1846:4 **Pathological Society of London** founded

1846:5 **Ether** used for the first time to produce **anaesthesia** during a surgical operation, performed by John Collins Warren (1778–1856), with the anaesthetic administered by William Thomas Green Morton (1819–1868) and the operation reported by Henry Jacob Bigelow (1818–1890), *BMSJ* **35**:309, 379. *5651*

1846:6 William Thomas Green Morton (1819–1868) attempted to patent his discovery of the **anaesthetic** effects of **ether** (*Circular. Morton's Letheon*). *5652*

1846:7 On 21 Dec, Robert Liston (1794–1847) was the first in Britain to perform a major operation with the aid of an **anaesthetic**. *5593*

1846:8 While still a student, William Cumming (1822–1855), by shading the **eye** of another student from the light, was able to look directly into it and to obtain both the **retinal reflex** and the white light from the entrance of the **optic nerve**, *MCT* **29**:283. *5861*

1846:9 **Trichinosis** in the pig first reported by Joseph Leidy (1823–1891), *PANS* **3**:107. *5338*

1846:10 The first to outline a complete plan for the training of **idiots** was Édouard Séguin (1812–1880); in his *Traitement moral, hygiène et education des idiots*. He later worked in America, where he published *Idiocy and its treatment by the physiological method*, 1866. *4937*

1846:11 **Electric chorea** ('**Dubini's chorea**'), the myoclonic form of **epidemic encephalitis** first described by Angelo Dubini (1813–1902), *AnU* **117**:5. *4637*

1846:12 *Pityrosporum orbiculare*, the fungus causing **pityriasis versicolor**, discovered by Carl Ferdinand Eichstedt (1816–1892), *NNGN* **38**:105; **39**:265, 270. *4038, 4039*

1846:13 The first formal treatise on **nervous diseases**, *Lehrbuch der Nervenkrankheiten des Menschen*, published by Moritz Heinrich Romberg (1795–1873); on p. 795 is the original description of '**Romberg's sign**', pathognomonic of **tabes dorsalis**. A classical description of **facial hemiatrophy** ('**Romberg's disease**') given by him in his *Klinische Ergebnisse*, p. 75. *4528, 4527*

1846:14 **Leukaemia** was diagnosed during life following a blood examination by Henry William Fuller (1820–1873), *L* **2**:43. *3062.1*

1846:15 First American treatise on **laryngology**, *A treatise on diseases of the air-passages*, published by Horace Green (1802–1866), regarded as the 'Father of laryngology' in America. *3261*

1846:16 First clear description of **thrombosis** and **embolism** by Rudolph Virchow (1821–1902), *BEP* **2**:227; reprinted in his *Gesammelte Abhandlungen zur wissenschaftlichen Medicin*, 1856. *3006*

1846:17 **Intermittent claudication** first described in man by Benjamin Collins Brodie (1783–1862); in his *Lectures ... in pathology and surgery*, p. 361. *2902*

1846:18 Classical account of **heart block** with **syncopal attacks** by William Stokes (1804–1878), *DQMS* **2**:73; followed description by Robert Adams, 1827; named '**Stokes-Adams syndrome**'. *2745, 2756*

1846:19 **Tuberculosis** transmission by cow's milk demonstrated by Philipp Friedrich Hermann Klencke (1813–1881); *Ueber die Ansteckung und Verbreitung der Scrophelkrankheit bei Menschen durch den Genuss der Kuhmilch*. *2323*

1846:20 Classical description of **coronary thrombosis** by Peter Mere Latham (1789–1875); in his *Lectures ... comprising diseases of the heart*, 2nd edn *2755.1*

1846:21 Invention of the **spirometer**, making possible the determination of the vital capacity of the lungs, by John Hutchinson (1811–1861). *930*

1846:22 Hans **Eppinger**, Bohemian physician, born 17 Feb; first reported nocardiosis, 1891, *BPA* **9**:287; he isolated *Nocardia asteroides* from a patient with pseudotuberculosis. Died 1916. *5513.1*

1846:23 Adolf **Eysell**, German physician, born 17 Feb; with Hermann Hugo Rudolf Schwartze, revived the mastoid operation; the ear was opened by chiselling ('Schwartze's operation'), 1873, *ArOh* **1**:157. *3382*

1846:24 Emil **Pfeiffer**, German physician, born 1 Mar; accredited by some with the first description of infectious mononucleosis ('Pfeiffer's disease'), 1889, *JaK* **29**:257. Died 1921. *5486*

1846:25 Edouard van **Beneden**, Belgian zoologist and cytologist, born 5 Mar. Published the first detailed description of the segmentation of the mammalian ovum, 1875, *BARS* **40**:686; discovered the centrosome, independently of Walther Flemming, 1876, *BARS* **41**:38. Died 1910. *496, 497*

1846:26 Giulio Cesare **Bizzozero**, Italian histologist, born 20 Mar; demonstrated that erythropoiesis and leucopoiesis take place in the bone marrow, 1868, *RIL* 2 ser **1**:815; named the blood platelets and discovered that they play a part in blood coagulation, 1882, *Osservatore* **17**:785; **18**:97. Died 1901. *873.1, 881*

1846:27 John Brown **Buist**, British physician, born 4 May; one of the first to demonstrate an animal virus particle; he recognized, and demonstrated microscopically, the elementary bodies of the vaccinia virus, 1886, *PRSE* **13**:603. Their rediscovery by Paschen (1906) led to the term Paschen elementary bodies. Died 1915. *5427*

1846:28 Dagobert **Schwabach**, German otologist, born 6 May; devised the Schwabach hearing test, 1885, *ZOh* **14**:61. Died 1920. *3389*

1846:29 Otto Wilhelm **Madelung**, German surgeon, born 15 May; described a growth deformity of the wrist joint ('Madelung's deformity'), 1878, *VDGC* **7**, 2:259. Died 1926. *4345*

1846:30 Angelo **Mosso**, Italian physiologist, born 31 May; devised sphygmomanometer, for measuring blood-pressure in the finger, 1895, *ArIB* **23**:177. Died 1910. *2801*

1846:31 Paul **Bruns**, German surgeon, born 2 Jul; first to describe plexiform neurofibroma; in his *Das Rankenneurom*, 1870. Died 1916. *4541*

1846:32 Carl Johann August **Langenbuch**, German surgeon, born 20 Aug; carried out the first nephrectomy for malignant disease, 1877, *BKW* **14**:337. First successfully to remove the gallbladder, 1882, *BKW* **19**:725. Died 1901. *4216.1, 3627*

1846:33 Bernhard Moritz Carl Ludwig **Riedel**, German surgeon, born 18 Sep; described 'Riedel's lobe' of the liver, 1888, *BKW* **25**:577, 602; and 'Riedel's thyroiditis', a type of chronic thyroiditis, 1896, *VDK* **25**:101. Died 1916. *3631, 3841*

1846:34 Julius **Dreschfeld**, German/British physician, born Oct; differentiated lymphosarcoma from lymphadenoma (Hodgkin's disease), 1892, *BMJ* **1**:893. Died 1907. *3772*

1846:35 William Henry **Allchin**, British physician, born 16 Oct; gave the first detailed description of ulcerative colitis, 1885, *TPS* **36**:199. Died 1912. *3482.2*

1846:36 Eugen **Baumann**, German chemist, born 12 Dec; prepared sulphonal, 1884, *BDCG* **19**:2806. Demonstrated iodine in the thyroid, 1896, *HSZ* **21**:319, 481; **22**:1. Died 1896. *1882, 1131*

_____

1846:37 Ludwig **Heusner**, German surgeon, born; successfully sutured a perforated gastric ulcer, 1892, *BKW* **29**:1244, 1280; the first recorded case. Died 1916. *3505*

1846:38 Arthur Ferguson **McGill** born; recorded suprapubic prostatectomy, 1888, *TCSL* **21**:52; the operation was pioneered by him and he first performed it in 1887. Died 1890. *4262.1*

1846:39 Ernst **Münchmeyer**, German physician, born; first described progressive ossifying myositis ('Münchmeyer's disease'), 1869, *ZRM* **34**:9. Died 1880. *4741*

1846:40 Felix Jacob **Marchand**, German pathologist, born; advanced a theory concerning the histogenesis of choriocarcinoma (chorionepithelioma), 1895, *MonG* **1**:419, 513. Gave first description of pathology of carotid body tumours, 1891, *Festschrift R.Virchow* **1**:547. Died 1928. *6097.1, 3791*

_____

1846: James **Marsh** died, **born** 1794. *arsenic*

1846: Charles Louis **Derosne** died, **born** 1700. *opium*

1846: John **Bostock** died, **born** 1771. *hay fever*

1846: Joseph Friedrich **Sobernheim** died, **born** 1803. *myocarditis*

1846: Auguste **Bérard** died, **born** 1802. *parotid tumours*

1846: George **Langstaff** died, **born** 1780. *prostate carcinoma*

1846: John **Cheyne** died, **born** 1777. *hydrocephalus*

1846: Benjamin **Waterhouse** died, **born** 1754. *smallpox vaccination*

1846: Joseph Constantine **Carpue** died, **born** 1764. *rhinoplasty*

## 1847
1847:1 *Archiv für Pathologische Anatomie* founded by Rudolf Ludwig Karl Virchow (1821–1902)

1847:2 **Poor Law Board (England)** established from **Poor Law Commission**

1847:3 **Österreichische Akademie der Wissenschaften, Vienna**, founded

1847:4 **New York Academy of Medicine** incorporated

1847:5 **Warren Anatomical Museum, Harvard**

1847:6 Carl Ludwig (1816–1896) invented the **kymograph**, by modifying Poiseuille's **haemodynamometer**, *ArA* 242. *770*

1847:7 A pioneer of **antisepsis** in **obstetrics**, Ignaz Philipp Semmelweis (1818–1865) was the first to recognize that **puerperal fever** is a septicaemia. He concluded that doctors and students carried the infection from the autopsy room to the maternity wards, and he instituted preventive measures, *ZGA* **4**, 2:242; **5**:64. *6275*

1847:8 James Syme (1799–1870) was (simultaneously with Pirogov) the first surgeon in Europe to adopt **ether anaesthesia** for surgical operations, *LEMJ* **8**:73. *5659, 5655*

1847:9 The first use of **ether anaesthesia** for **plastic surgery** made by Johann Friedrich Dieffenbach (1792–1847), whose work encouraged the acceptance of anaesthesia in Germany. He wrote *Die Aether gegen den Schmerz*. *5659.1*

1847:10 **Nitrous oxide** successfully used as a dental **anaesthetic** by Horace Wells (1815–1848), a Hartford, Conn. dentist. He wrote *A history of the discovery of the application of nitrous oxide gas, ether, and other vapours, to surgical operations*. *5660*

1847:11 John Snow (1813–1858) was the first specialist in **anaesthesiology** as well as being an **epidemiologist**. He invented a regulating inhaler to control the amount of **ether** received by the patient during surgical **anaesthesia**, described in his *On the inhalation of the vapour of ether in surgical operations*. *5658*

1847:12 First announcement that **chloroform** had an **anaesthetic** effect similar to that of **ether** by Marie Jean Pierre Flourens (1794–1867), *CRAS* **24**:340. *5654*

1847:13 The first textbook on surgical **anaesthesia** was *A treatise on the inhalation of the vapour of ether for the prevention of pain in surgical operations*, by James Robinson (1813–1861), a British dentist. *5657.1*

1847:14 The advantages of **chloroform** over **ether** as an **anaesthetic** discovered by James Young Simpson (1811–1870) who was first to adopt it in midwifery, *LMG* **5**:934; *L* **2**:549. *5657*

1847:15 Rectal **anaesthesia** with **ether** first practised by Nikolai Ivanovich Pirogov (1810–1881), *CRAS* **24**:789. *5655*

1847:16 The symptoms of **typhoid** and **typhus** carefully differentiated by Charles Ritchie (1799–1878), *MJMS* **7**:347, who introduced the term '**enteric fever**'. *5026*

1847:17 **Myelopathic albumosuria (Bence-Jones proteinuria)**, named after Henry Bence Jones (1814–1873), *PT* **138**:55, who found it to be present in a patient of W. Macintyre suffering from **multiple myeloma**. *4326, 4327*

1847:18 **Leprosy**; first modern description by Daniel Cornelius Danielssen (1815–1894) and Carl Wilhelm Boeck (1808–1875) ('Danielssen-Boeck disease'); in *Om spedalskhed*. *2434*

1847:19 Doctrine of **conservation of energy**, of Hermann Ludwig Ferdinand von Helmholtz (1821–1894); in his *Ueber die Erhaltung der Kraft*. *611*

1847:20 A valuable account of **measles** outbreak in Faeroe Islands given by Peter Ludwig Panum (1820–1885), *Bibliothek for Laeger*, 3 ser. **1**:270. *5443*

1847:21 Johannes **Orth**, German pathologist, born 14 Feb; first to describe kernicterus, 1875, *VA* **63**:447. Died 1923. *3067*

1847:22 Salomon Eberhard **Henschen**, Swedish physiologist, born 28 Feb; located the visual centre in the cerebral cortex, 1888, *ULF* **27**:507, 601. Died 1930. *1521*

1847:23 Hans von **Hebra**, Austrian dermatologist, born 24 May; described rhinoscleroma, 1870, *WMW* **20**:1. Died 1902. *3277*

1847:24 Carlo **Forlanini**, Italian physician, born 11 Jun; induced artificial pneumothorax in pulmonary tuberculosis, 1888, *GOC* **3**:537, 585, 601, 609, 617, 625, 641, 657, 665, 689, 705, having first discussed it in 1882. Died 1918. *3225*

1847:25 Viktor **Janovsky**, Czech dermatologist, born 2 Jul; with Sigmund Pollitzer, first illustrated acanthosis nigricans; in their *Atlas seltener Hautkrankheiten*, 1890; it was described by Darier in 1893. Died 1925. *4102, 4113*

1847:26 William **Rose**, British surgeon, born 18 Jul; carried out Gasserian ganglionectomy for trigeminal neuralgia, suggested by Mears (1884), 1890, *L* **2**:914. Died 1910. *4863*

1847:27 Paul **Langerhans**, German pathologist, born 25 Jul; described 'Islands of Langerhans' in the pancreas, in his *Beiträge zur mikroskopischen Anatomie der Bauchspeicheldrüse*, 1869. (They were named after him in 1893.) Died 1888. *1009*

1847:28 Edmond **Delorme**, French surgeon, born 2 Aug; introduced decortication of the lung for chronic empyema, 1894, *GH* **67**:94. Died 1929. *3180*

1847:29 Walter Holbrook **Gaskell**, British physiologist, born 1 Nov; his research included the effects of nerve action on muscle arteries, the myogenic theory of the heart's action, the involuntary nervous system, the origin of vertebrates, 1882, *PT* **173**:993; 1883, *JP* **4**:43; 1916, *The involuntary nervous system*. Died 1914. *829, 830, 1331*

1847:30 Oscar Thorvald **Bloch**, Danish surgeon, born 15 Nov; first to employ the two-stage (Mikulicz) operation for colon cancer, 1892, *NoMA* **2**, i, 1; **2**, ii, 1. Died 1926. *3502*

1847:31 Karl **Friedländer**, German pathologist, born 19 Nov; discovered *Klebsiella pneumoniae* ('Friedländer's bacillus'), 1882, *VA* **87**:319. Died 1887. *3174*

1847:32 Charles **Creighton**, British physician, born 22 Nov; founder of modern epidemiology; his *History of epidemics in Britain* appeared in 1891–1894. Died 1927. *1680*

1847:33 Christine **Ladd-Franklin**, American psychologist, born 1 Dec; proposed the Ladd-Franklin theory of colour vision, 1893, *ZPPS* **4**:221. Died 1930. *1522*

---

1847:34 Adolf Fredrik **Lindstedt**, Swedish surgeon, born; with Johan Anton Waldenström, first to record an operation for the treatment of volvulus, 1879, *ULF* **14**:513. Died 1915. *3469*

1847:35 Endre **Högyes**, Hungarian physician, born; described rotational nystagmus, 1886, *PMCP* **22**:765, 787, 807, 827. Died 1906. *3389.1*

1847:36 Oskar **Medin**, Swedish physician, born; first noted the epidemic character of poliomyelitis, 1890, *Hygiea* **52**:657; it is also known as 'Heine-Medin disease'. Died 1927. *4667, 4664*

1847:37 Leo **Leistikow** born; first reported cultivation of the gonococcus, 1880, *CA* **7**:750. Died 1917. *5209*

1847:38 Nil Feodorovich **Filatov**, Russian paediatrician, born; probably gave the first description of infectious mononucleosis (glandular fever), under the name of idiopathic adenitis ('Filatov's disease'); in his *Lectures on acute infectious diseases of children* [in Russian], 2 vols, 1885–7. Died 1902. *5485*

1847:39 Fernand **Henrotin** born; described a method of vaginal hysterectomy, 1892, *AmJOD* **26**:448. Died 1906. *6095*

1847:40 Paul **Reclus** born; gave the classic description of chronic cystic mastitis, 1883, *BSAP* **58**:428, led to the term 'Reclus's disease'. Died 1914. *5774*

1847:41 Ettore **Marchiafava** born; with Angelo Celli, gave the first accurate description of the malaria parasite, *Plasmodium*, 1885, *FM* **3**:787. With Amico Bignami, described degeneration of the corpus callosum in alcoholism ('Marchiafava-Bignami disease'), 1903, *RPN* **8**:544. Died 1935. *5238, 4955*

1847:42 Alexander **Kolisko** born; with Carl Breus, gave a classic description and classification of pelvic deformities; in their *Die pathologischen Beckenformen*, 1900–14. Died 1918. *6265*

---

1847: Johann Friedrich **Dieffenbach** died, **born** 1792. *cardiac catheterization, plastic surgery, orthopaedic surgery, anaesthesia, ether, strabismus, Lembert's suture*

1847: Noah **Worcester** died, **born** 1812. *skin diseases*

1847: Jacques **Lisfranc** died, **born** 1790. *amputation of foot*

1847: Robert **Liston** died, **born** 1794. *surgery*

**1848**
1848:1 **Société de Biologie (Paris)** founded

1848:2 **University of Wisconsin** established at **Madison**

1848:3 **American Association for the Advancement of Science** founded

1848:4 **Public Health Act, England**, creating **General Board of Health** (1848–1858) and local boards of health

1848:5 The theory that **yellow fever** was caused by minute animalcula advanced by Josiah Clark Nott (1804–1873), *NOMSJ* **4**:563. *5454*

1848:6 **Glycogenic function of liver** investigated by Claude Bernard (1813–1878), *ArGM* **18**:303; completed 1855, *CRAS* **41**:461. *995, 1000*

1848:7 *Lectures on the diseases of infancy and childhood*, by Charles West (1816–1898) was in its day the best English work on **paediatrics**. West was one of the founders of the Hospital for Sick Children, Gt Ormond Street, London. *6334*

1848:8 The collective edition of the writings of Emil du Bois-Reymond (1818–1896), German founder of modern **electrophysiology**, *Untersuchungen über thierische Elektricität*, 1848–1884. *610*

1848:9 Besides his **ether** inhaler John Snow (1813–1858) invented a **chloroform** inhaler, *L* **1**:177. *5663*

1848:10 An early advocate of **anaesthesia** in **obstetrics** was Walter Channing (1786–1876); he wrote *A treatise on etherization in childbirth*. *5661*

1848:11 **Ethyl chloride** introduced as an **anaesthetic** by Johann Martin Heyfelder (1798–1869); in his *Die Versuche mit dem Schwefeläther und Chloroform*. *5662*

1848:12 **Papaverine** isolated from opium by Georg Franz Merck (1825–1873), *AnPh* **66**:125. *1861*

1848:13 John Tomes (1815–1895) played an important part in the development of **dental education** in Britain. He wrote *Course of lectures on dental physiology and surgery* and invented a set of anatomically correct dental **forceps**. *3683*

1848:14 **Peritonitis** due to abscess of the **appendix** first successfully treated by Henry Hancock (1809–1880), *LMG* **7**:547. *3563*

1848:15 **Cystinuria** described by Alfred Baring Garrod (1819–1907), *TPS* **1**:126. *3912.1*

---

1848:16 Franz von **Soxhlet**, Czechoslovakian physiologist, born 13 Jan; contributed a great deal to the knowledge of milk. He wrote on milk droplets, estimated its specific gravity with his lactodensimeter, described an apparatus for the sterilization of milk, and devised a test for the estimation of fats in milk, 1886, *MMW* **33**:253, 276. Died 1926. *6341*

1848:17 Wilhelm **Wagner**, German surgeon, born 14 Jan; devised an osteoplastic flap operation, making a large area of the brain more easily accessible than by trephining, 1889, *ZCh* **16**:833. Died 1900. *4862*

1848:18 William **Macewen**, British surgeon, born 22 Jan; first performed endotracheal anaesthesia by the administration of chloroform through a tracheal tube introduced through the mouth, 1880, *BMJ* **2**:122, 163. Reported the first allograft transplantation of bone in a human, 1881, *PRS* **32**:232. Introduced a method for the radical cure of oblique inguinal hernia, 1886, *AnS* **4**:89. His greatest work was in connection with brain surgery, *Pyogenic infective diseases of the brain*, 1894. Removed left lung for tuberculosis, 1895; reported 1906, *BMJ* **2**:1, the patient was alive in 1940. Died 1924. *5676, 4346.2, 3596, 4872, 3229*

1848:19 James **Israel**, German surgeon, born 2 Feb; reported the first human case of actinomycosis, 1878, *VA* **74**:15. In his paper he included drawings of the fungus *Actinomyces* made in 1845 by Bernard Rudolph Conrad von Langenbeck (1810–1887). With Max Wolff, isolated *Actinomyces bovis*, 1891, *VA* **126**:11. Carried out the first rhinoplasty using a free bone graft to the nose, 1896, *ArKC* **53**:255. Died 1926. *5511, 5514, 5755.1*

1848:20 Adolf **Weil**, German physician, born 7 Feb; in his classic description of leptospirosis icterohaemorrhagica, he differentiated it from other types of acute jaundice, 1886, *DAKM* **39**:209; it is also known as 'Weil's disease'. Died 1916. *5332*

1848:21 Hugo Marie de **Vries**, Dutch plant physiologist and geneticist, born 16 Feb. Like Correns and Tschermak von Seysenegg, he 're-discovered' Mendel's laws of inheritance, 1900, *BDBG* **18**:83; first advanced the theory of mutation, *Die Mutationstheorie*, 2 vols, 1901–3. Died 1935. *239.01, 240*

1848:22 Leonardo **Bianchi**, Italian psychiatrist, born 15 Apr; demonstrated that bilateral destruction of the frontal lobes caused character changes; in his *La mecanica del cervello e la funzione dei lobe frontale*, 1920. Died 1919. *4891*

1848:23 August **Gaertner**, German bacteriologist and hygienist, born 18 Apr; discovered *Salmonella enteritidis* (Gaertner's bacillus) in infected meat, 1888, *KAAV* **17**:573. Died 1934. *2506*

1848:24 Carl **Wernicke**, Polish neuropsychiatrist, born 15 May; described sensory aphasia ('Wernicke's aphasia'), in *Der aphasische Symptomencomplex*, 1874, and did important work on the localization of aphasia. His description of acute superior haemorrhagic polioencephalitis in his *Lehrbuch der Gehirnkrankheiten*, **2**, 229, resulted in the eponym 'Wernicke's encephalopathy', 1881. Died 1905. *4623, 4641*

1848:25 George Thomas **Beatson**, British surgeon, born 28 May; treated breast cancer by oöphorectomy, 1896, *L* **2**:104, 162; later combined with thyroid extract, 1901, *BMJ* **2**:1145. Died 1933. *5778.1, 5779*

1848:26 Camille Louis Antoine **Champetier de Ribes**, French obstetrician, born 3 Jun; introduced the 'Champetier de Ribes bag', used for dilating the neck of the uterus, 1888, *AnGO* **30**:401. Died 1935. *6198*

1848:27 Bernhard Laurits Frederik **Bang**, Danish veterinary pathologist and bacteriologist, born 7 Jun; discovered *Brucella abortus*, a cause of brucellosis in cattle, 1897, *ZT* **1**:241. Died 1932. *5099*

1848:28 Friedrich **Schultze**, German neurologist, born 17 Aug; described the simple ('Schultze's') form of acroparaesthesia, 1893, *DZN* **3**:300. Died 1934. *2709*

1848:29 Auguste Henri **Forel**. Swiss psychologist and neurologist, born 1 Sep; formulated the neuron theory, 1887, *ArPN* **18**:162; this had already been done by Wilhelm His in the previous year. Died 1931. *1368.2*

1848:30 Max **Nitze**, German urologist, born 18 Sep; devised an electrically lighted cystoscope, making possible great improvements in bladder surgery, 1877, *WMW* **29**:649, 688, 713, 776, 896; devised an operative cystoscope, which made it possible to excise bladder tumours *in situ*, 1897, *ZKH* **8**:8. Died 1906. *4175, 4190*

1848:31 Richard **Fleischer**, German physician, born 22 Sep; first described march haemoglobinuria, 1881, *BKW* **18**:691. *4176*

1848:32 Ephraim Fletcher **Ingals**, American physician, born 29 Sep; devised the operation of partial excision of the nasal septum for correction of deflection, 1882, *TALA* **4**:61. Died 1918. *3289*

1848:33 George Ryerson **Fowler**, American surgeon, born 25 Dec; first to perform thoracoplasty, 1893, *MR* **44**:838; described the 'Fowler' position (elevated head and trunk posture) to facilitate drainage into the pelvis, 1900, *MR* **57**:617, 1029. Died 1906. *3179, 5623*

1848:34 Ivan Romanovich **Tarchanoff**, Russian physiologist, born; described psychogalvanic reflex, 1890, *PfA* **46**:46. Died 1909. *1471*

1848:35 Alexander Hughes **Bennett**, British neurologist, born; with Rickman John Godlee, first diagnosed, accurately localized, and removed a cerebral tumour, 1884, *MCT* **68**:243. Died 1915. *4858*

1848:36 Jean Albert **Pitres**, French physician, born; published classic accounts of agraphia, 1884, *ReM* **4**:855, and paraphrasia, 1895, *ReM* **15**:873. Died 1928. *4625, 4628*

1848:37 Alexander **Nasmyth** died; described 'Nasmyth's membrane' or persistent dental capsule, 1839, *MCT* **22**:310. *3681*

1848: Gustav Adolf **Michaelis** died, **born** 1798. *pelvic deformities*

1848: Bernhard **Mohr** died, **born** 1809. *Fröhlich's syndrome*

1848: James Cowles **Prichard** died, **born** 1786. *psychiatry, senile dementia, epilepsy, Alzheimer's disease*

1848: Robert **Perry** died, **born** 1783. *typhus, typhoid*

1848: Horace **Wells** died, **born** 1815. *anaesthesia, nitrous oxide*

1848: Samuel **Guthrie** died, **born** 1782. *chloroform*

1848: Samuel **Bard** died, **born** 1742. *midwifery, obstetrics*

1848: John **Stearns** died, **born** 1770. *labour, ergot*

**1849**
1849:1 Elizabeth **Blackwell**, British/American, **first woman to qualify in medicine** (New York) and to be admitted to British Medical Register (1859)

1849:2 [**Physico-Medical Society**], **Würzburg**

1849:3 **Central Board of Health, Canada**

1849:4 **Royal Canadian Institute, Toronto**

1849:5 The first scientific approach to the theory of a parasite as the cause of **malaria** was made by John Kearsley Mitchell (1793–1858); in his *On the cryptogamous origin of malarious and epidemic fevers*. *5234*

1849:6 The induration and discoloration of the affected parts in **lymphogranuloma venereum** named **esthiomène** by Pierre Charles Huguier (1804–1873), *MANM* **14**:501. *5216*

1849:7 The water-borne character of **cholera** demonstrated by John Snow (1813–1858), *LMG* **44**:730, 745, 923. *5106*

1849:8 The aetiology of **typhus** and **typhoid** shown to be quite different by William Jenner (1815–1898), who also showed that one did not communicate with, or protect against, the other, and that epidemics of the two did not prevail simultaneously, *MJMS* **9**:663. *5027*

1849:9 Although Carswell is credited with the first description of **multiple sclerosis**, the first important account was given by Friedrich Theodor Frerichs (1819–1885), *ArGesM* **10**:334. *4692*

1849:10 Generalized **neurofibromatosis** described by Robert William Smith (1807–1873); in his *Treatise on the pathology, diagnosis and treatment of neuroma*. It is also called '**Recklinghausen's disease**' in recognition of the classic description by Friedrich Daniel von Recklinghausen in 1882. *4529, 4082*

1849:11 **Addison's disease** and **pernicious** ('**Addisonian**') **anaemia** first described by Thomas Addison (1793–1860), who later expanded his account in his *On the constitutional and local effects of disease of the supra-renal capsules*, 1855. *3864*

1849:12 **Gastrostomy** first performed by Charles Emmanuel Sédillot (1804–1883), *GMS* **9**:366. *3451*

1849:13 **Bacterial flora** of the **intestines** discovered by Joseph Leidy (1823–1891), *PANS* **4**:225. *3450*

1849:14 The '**cave of Retzius**' near the **bladder** described by Anders Adolf Retzius (1796–1860), *ArA*. p. 149. *1221*

1849:15 Existence of an **internal secretion** demonstrated by Arnold Adolph Berthold (1803–1861), *ArA* 42. *1176*

1849:16 Richard James Mackenzie (1821–1854) modified James Syme's method of amputation at the **ankle-joint**, *MJMS* **9**:951. *4460*

1849:17 **Progressive muscular atrophy** ('**Aran-Duchenne disease**') described by Guillaume Benjamin Amand Duchenne (1806–1875), *CRAS* **29**:667, and independently by François Amilcar Aran (1850). *4732, 4733*

1849:18 Crawford Williamson Long (1815–1878) was the first, on 30 March 1842, successfully to use **ether** as an **anaesthetic**, but did not publish his results until 1849, *SMSJ* **5**:705. *5664*

---

1849:19 Arthur **Hartmann**, German otolaryngologist, born 1 Jan; introduced the first audiometer, 1878, *ArAP* 155. Died 1931. *3387.2*

1849:20 Otto **Kahler**, Bohemian physician, born 8 Jan; gave the first complete description of syringomyelia, 1888, *PMW* **13**:45, 63. Died 1893. *4706*

1849:21 Erwin **Baelz**, German physician in Far East, born 13 Jan; with Kawakami, gave an early scientific account of scrub typhus (tsutsugamushi disease), 1879, *VA* **78**:373, 528. Died 1913. *5376.1*

1849:22 Karel **Pawlik**, Bohemian surgeon, born 12 Mar; carried out the first successful total cystectomy, 1891, *WMW* **41**:184. Died 1914. *4184.1*

1849:23 Felix **Balzer**, French dermatologist and syphilologist, born 4 Apr; first to suggest bismuth in treatment of syphilis, 1889, *4CRSB* **1**:537. Died 1929. *2394*

1849:24 Ludwig Mettler **Rehn**, German surgeon, born 13 Apr; performed the first thyroidectomy for exophthalmic goitre, 1880, reported in 1884, *BKW* **21**:163. Performed first successful human heart suture, 1896, *ZCh* **23**:1048; *ArKC* **55**:315; marked the beginning of cardiac surgery. Died 1930. *3833, 3023, 3023.1*

1849:25 Rickman John **Godlee**, British surgeon, born 15 Apr; with Alexander Hughes Bennett, first diagnosed, accurately localized, and removed a cerebral tumour, 1884, *MCT* **68**:243. Died 1925. *4858*

1849:26 Wilhelm August Oscar **Hertwig**, German embryologist and cytologist, born 21 Apr. Demonstrated the mechanism of fertilization – entrance of the spermatozoon into the ovum and union of the nuclei of the male and female sex cells, 1876, *MoJ* **1**:346. With his brother Richard he carried out important work on embryology and cytology, *Die Coelomtheorie*, 1881; *Untersuchungen zur Morphologie und Physiologie der Zelle*, 1884–90; *Die Zelle und die Gewebe*, 1893–8. Died 1922. *495, 502, 555, 556*

1849:27 William **Osler**, Canadian physician, born 12 Jul; his textbook, *The principles and practice of medicine*, first published 1892, was the best English work of its time. With William Gardner, gave the first complete account of progressive pernicious anaemia, 1877, *CMSJ* **5**:383. Gave a comprehensive account of subacute bacterial endocarditis, 1885, *BMJ* **1**:467, 522, 577. Described multiple hereditary telangiectasis ('Rendu-Osler-Weber disease'), 1901, *JHB* **12**:333. In 1903 described polycythaemia vera (erythraemia), *AmJMS* **126**:187, but acknowledged the priority of Vaquez ('Vaquez-Osler disease'). Gave first definite clinical description of subacute bacterial endocarditis, 1909, *QJM* **2**:219, in which he described 'Osler's nodes', first seen by him in 1888. Gave a classic account of severe anaemias of pregnancy, with a classification, 1919, *BMJ* **1**:1. Died 1919. *2231, 3125.2, 2790, 2711, 3073, 3070, 2827, 3136*

1849:28 Joseph Jules **Dejerine**, Swiss neurologist, born 3 Aug; with Louis Théophile Joseph Landouzy, described the 'Landouzy-Dejerine type' of (scapulo-humeral) progressive muscular atrophy, 1886, *CRSB* **3**:478. Gave the first description of peripheral neuritis ('Dejerine's neurotabes'), 1887, *CRSB* **4**:137; in his *Sur l'atrophie musculaire des ataxiques*, 1889. Described tabetic muscular atrophies and separated peripheral from medullary tabes. With Jules Sottas, gave the first description of hypertrophic progressive interstitial neuritis ('Dejerine-Sottas disease'), 1893, *CRSB* **45**:63. With André Thomas, first described olivo-pontocerebellar atrophy, 1912, *NIS* **25**:223. Died 1917. *4752, 4784, 4785, 4580, 4716.1*

1849:29 Paul **Fürbringer**, German physician, born 7 Aug; demonstrated the diagnostic value of spinal puncture, 1895, BKW **32**:272. Died 1930. *4873*

1849:30 Domenico **Majocchi**, Italian dermatologist, born 15 Aug; first described purpura annularis telangiectodes, 1896, *GIMV* **31**:242. Died 1929. *4125*

1849:31 Ivan Petrovich **Pavlov**, Russian physiologist, born 14 Sep; made valuable contributions to knowledge concerning the physiology of digestion, for which he was awarded the Nobel Prize (Physiology or Medicine), 1904, *NPL*; his *Lectures* on the subject appeared in 1897. His important investigations on conditioned reflexes were published under the title *Lectures on conditioned reflexes*, 1928–1941. Died 1936. *1022, 1445*

1849:32 Maximilian **Oberst**, German surgeon, born 6 Oct; his method of conduction anaesthesia was recorded by his pupil Ludwig Pernice in 1890, *DMW* **16**:287. Died 1925. *5681*

1849:33 Felix **Semon**, German-born British laryngologist, born 8 Dec; rightly contended that cachexia strumipriva, myxoedema, and cretinism were all due to loss of thyroid function, 1883, *BMJ* **2**:1072. Died 1921. *3831*

1849:34 Joseph von **Mering**, German physician, born 28 Dec; with Oscar Minkowski, produced experimental diabetes mellitus by removing the pancreas of a dog, proving the role of the pancreas in diabetes, 1890, *ArEP* **26**:371. Synthesized barbitone, with Emil Fischer, 1903, *TGe* **44**:97. Died 1908. *3950, 1892*

---

1849:35 Vasili Parmenovich **Obraztsov** born; with Nikolai Dmitrievich Strazhesko, gave the first comprehensive description of coronary thrombosis, diagnosed before death and confirmed at necroscopy, 1910, *ZKM* **71**:116. Died 1920. *2835*

1849:36 Friedrich Alexander **Hilsmann**, German physician, born; reported first pericardiocentesis for suppurative pericarditis, 1849, *SKU* Diss. no. 2. *3022*

1849:37 Charles-Emile **François-Franck**, French physician, born; carried out experimental cardiac valvulotomy in dogs, 1882, *CRSB* **4**:108. Died 1921. *3022.1*

1849:38 Thomas Rushmore **French**, American laryngologist, born; obtained first good photographs of the larynx, 1882, *TALA* **4**:32. Died 1929. *3290*

1849:39 Kanehiro **Takaki**, Japanese physician, born; showed conclusively that beriberi is of dietary origin, 1885, *TSIK* **4**:29. Died 1915. *3740*

1849:40 Antonin **Poncet** born; described tuberculous rheumatism ('Poncet's disease'), 1897, *GH* **70**:1219. Died 1913. *4504*

1849:41 Antonio **Placido da Costa** born; introduced the keratoscope, 1882, *ZPAu* **6**:30. Died 1916. *5922*

---

1849: Henry **Burton** died, **born** 1799. *lead poisoning*

1849: Anthony **White** died, **born** 1782. *excision of head of femur*

1849: Philipp Franz von **Walther** died, **born** 1782. *corneal opacity*

**1850**

1850:1 **Northwestern University, Chicago**, founded

1850:2 **Female Medical College of Pennsylvania** founded at **Philadelphia**; name changed to **Medical College of Pennsylvania**, 1969, with admission of male students

1850:3 **Epidemiological Society of London** founded

1850:4 Pierre François Olive Rayer (1793–1867) inoculated **anthrax**-infected sheep blood into other sheep and saw the anthrax bacillus (*B.anthracis*) in the blood of the infected sheep, *CRSB* **2**:141. In 1875 Davaine claimed to have written the account of the experiment and sent it to Rayer for publication. *5163*

1850:5 The lateral ventricles of the **brain** first opened for the treatment of **brain abscess** by William Detmold (1808–1894), *AmJMS* **19**:86. *4853*

1850:6 **Progressive muscular atrophy** ('**Aran-Duchenne disease**') described by François Amilcar Aran (1817–1861), *ArGM* **24**:4, 132. *4733*

1850:7 The description of **aphthae of the palate** in the newborn given by Alois Bednař (1816–1888) in his *Die Krankheiten der Neugeborenen und Säuglinge*, **1**, 104, led to the eponym '**Bednař's aphthae**'. *6335*

1850:8 **Multiple myeloma** first described by W. Macintyre, *MCT* **33**:211. *4327*

1850:9 **Lupus erythematosus** ('**Cazenave's disease**') described by Pierre Louis Alphé Cazenave (1795–1877), *GHZ* **2**:383. *4040*

1850:10 It was shown by Gaspard Adolph Chatin (1813–1901) that endemic **goitre** and **cretinism** could be prevented by **iodine**, *CRAS* **30**:352. *3817*

1850:11 Thomas Blizard Curling (1811–1888) accurately described the clinical picture of **cretinism**, *MCT* **33**:303, later named **myxoedema** by William Miller Ord in 1878. *3818, 3825*

1850:12 *Report on public health in the United States* by Lemuel Shattuck (1793–1859) led to great improvements in public health and hygiene in the USA. *1609*

1850:13 **Leydig cells** of the testis described by Franz Leydig (1821–1908), *ZWC* **2**:1. *1222*

1850:14 Charles Édouard Brown-Séquard (1817–1894) showed that lesion of one lateral half of the **spinal cord** causes paralysis of motion on one side and sensory loss on the other ('**Brown-Séquard's paralysis**'), *CRSB* **2**:3. *4530*

1850:15 **Velocity of the nervous impulse** measured by Hermann von Helmholtz (1821–1894), *ArA* **71**. *1265*

1850:16 Law of **Wallerian degeneration of nerve** established by Augustus Volney Waller (1816–1870), *PT* **140**:423. *1266*

---

1850:17 William Augustus **Hardaway**, American physician, born 8 Jan; first description of prurigo nodularis, 1879, *ArD* **5**:385; **6**:129. Died 1923. *4076*

1850:18 Anton **Wölfler**, Bohemian surgeon, born 12 Jan; perfected the operation of gastro-enterostomy, 1881, *ZCh* **8**:705. Classified thyroid tumours and was also first to describe foetal adenoma, 1883, *ArKC* **29**:1. Died 1917. *3476, 3832*

1850:19 Edmond Isidore Etienne **Nocard**, French veterinarian, born 22 Jan; first to describe a pathogenic aerobic actinomycete, 1888, *AnIP* **2**:293, later named *Nocardia farcinica*. Died 1903. *5512.1*

1850:20 James Fairchild **Baldwin**, American gynaecologist, born 12 Feb; devised a method of forming an artificial vagina by intestinal transplantation, 1904, *AnS* **40**:398. Died 1936. *6117*

1850:21 Adolph **Jarisch**, Austrian dermatologist, born 15 Feb; introduced Jarisch-Herxheimer reaction in syphilis, 1895, *WMW* **45**:720. Died 1902. *2396*

1850:22 Georg **Gaffky**, German bacteriologist, born 17 Feb; first to grow pure cultures of *Salmonella typhi* and showed it to be the true activator of typhoid, 1884, *MKJ* **2**:372. Died 1918. *5032*

1850:23 William Henry **Welch**, American pathologist and microbiologist, born 8 Apr; discovered *Staphylococcus epidermidis alba* and its relation to wound infection, 1892, *TCAP* **2**:1 and *Clostridium perfringens*, the gas gangrene bacillus (Welch bacillus), with George Henry Falkiner Nuttall, 1892, *JHB* **3**:81. Died 1934. *5621, 2508*

1850:24 George **Huntington**, American physician, born 9 Apr; gave a classic, but not the first, description of chronic degenerative hereditary chorea ('Huntington's chorea'), 1872, *MSRep* **26**:317. Died 1916. *4699*

1850:25 Johann von **Mikulicz-Radecki**, Polish surgeon, born 16 May; was among the first to use the electric oesophagoscope (invented by Leiter in 1880), 1881, *WMP* **22**: 1405, 1437, 1473, 1505, 1537, 1573, 1629. Carried out first plastic reconstruction of the oesophagus after resection for cancer, 1886, *PMW* **11**:93. Described an important operative procedure for complete rectal prolapse, 1888, *VDGC* **17**:294. First to perform enterocystoplasty, 1889, *ZCh* **26**:641. Died 1905. *3475, 3487, 3493, 4183.1*

1850:26 Edward Albert **Sharpey-Schafer**. British physiologist, born 2 Jun; with George Oliver demonstrated a pressor substance, later named adrenaline, in the adrenal medulla, 1895, *JP* **18**:230. Invented the Sharpey-Schafer method of artificial respiration, 1904, *MCT* **87**:609. Died 1935. *1143, 2028.59*

1850:27 Wilhelm **Roux**, German zoologist and embryologist, born 9 Jun; founder of the study of developmental mechanics ('Entwicklungsmechanik'), 1888, *VA* **114**:113, 246. Died 1924. *505*

1850:28 Gustav Adolf **Neuber**, German surgeon, born 24 Jun; made the first attempts at asepsis; recorded in his *Die aseptische Wundbehandlung in meinen chirurgischen Privat-Hospitälern*, 1886. Died 1932. *5637*

1850:29 Daniel Elmer **Salmon**, American veterinary pathologist, born 23 Jul; with Theobald Smith isolated *Salmonella cholerae-suis*, 1886, *AmMM* **7**:204; the Salmonellae tribe was named after Salmon though Smith actually made the discovery. Died 1914. *2505*

1850:30 Ludwik **Rydygier**, Polish surgeon, born 21 Aug; recorded the extirpation of a carcinomatous pylorus, the patient died after 12 hours, 1880, *PrzL* **19**:637. Died 1920. *3473.1*

1850:31 Charles Robert **Richet**, French physiologist, born 26 Aug; with Paul Portier, published first full description of anaphylaxis (which he named), 1902, *CRSB* **54**:170. Awarded Nobel Prize (Physiology or Medicine), 1913, for his work on anaphylaxis, *NPL*. Died 1935. *2590*

1850:32 Paul Gerson **Unna**, German dermatologist, born 8 Sep; introduced ichthammol (ichthyol) and resorcinol, 1886, *MDP* Suppl.1. Described 'Unna's seborrhoeic eczema', 1887, *MPD* **6**:827. His *Die Histopathologie der Hautkrankheiten*, 1894, is a landmark in the history of dermatology; the first description of the acne bacillus appears on p. 357. Died 1929. *1883, 4092, 4000*

1850:33 Karl Wilhelm Theodor Richard von **Hertwig**, German embryologist, protozoologist and zoologist, born 23 Sep. With his brother Wilhelm he published works on cells and tissue, and on the 'coelom theory', *Die Coelomtheorie*, 1881; *Untersuchungen zur Morphologie und Physiologie der Zelle*, 1884–90; *Die Zelle und die Gewebe*, 1893–8. Died 1937. *502, 555, 556*

1850:34 Etienne Louis Arthur **Fallot**, French physician, born 29 Sep; described 'tetralogy of Fallot', a form of congenital heart disease, 1888, *MM* **25**:77, 138, 207, 270, 341, 403. Died 1911. *2792*

1850:35 Eugen **Bostroem**, German pathologist, born 30 Sep; isolated *Actinomyces graminis* from human actinomycosis, 1890, *BPA* **9**:1, and introduced a staining method for *Actinomyces*. Died 1928. *5513*

1850:36 Paul Albert **Grawitz**, German pathologist, born 1 Oct; his important work on the origin of hypernephroma, 1884, *VDGC* **13** ii:28, led to the condition being called '**Grawitz tumour**'. Died 1932. *4220*

1850:37 Carle **Gessard**, French bacteriologist, born 3 Oct; isolated *Pseudomonas aeruginosa*, 1882, *CRAS* **94**:536. Died 1925. *2497*

1850:38 Robert Henry **Clarke**, British neurophysiologist, born 9 Oct; with Victor Alexander Haden Horsley, devised the stereotactic apparatus for the accurate location of electrodes in the brain and opened the way to stereotactic surgery of that organ, 1908, *Brain* **31**:45. Died 1926. *1435.1, 4879.1*

1850:39 Alfred **Eddowes**, British dermatologist, born 26 Nov; his description, 1900, *BMJ* **2**:222, of blue sclerotics and fragility of the bones, occurring as a familial syndrome, osteogenesis imperfecta, previously described by Axmann, led to the eponym 'Eddowes's syndrome'. Died 1946. *6367, 6358.1*

1850:40 Achille **Breda**, Italian dermatologist, born 8 Dec; described Brazilian yaws (framboesia), 1895, *ArD* **33**:3, also called 'Breda's disease'. Died 1935. *5293.1*

1850:41 Hans Ernst **Buchner**, German bacteriologist, born 16 Dec; discovered complement (alexin), 1889, *ZBP* **6**:561. Died 1902. *2543*

1850:42 Edward R. **Henry**, British Police Commissioner, born; introduced fingerprint classification system in 1900; in his *Classification and use of fingerprints*. Died 1931. *189*

1850:43 William Joseph **Dibdin**, British chemist, born; introduced sewage purification by bacterial system, 1897; in his *Purification of sewage and water*. Died 1925. *1631*

1850:44 David **Lowson**, British surgeon, born; performed partial lobectomy in pulmonary tuberculosis, 1893, *BMJ* **1**:1152. Died 1907. *3227*

1850:45 Charles **Girard** born; performed the first successful hindquarter amputation, 1895, *PVC* **9**:823. Died 1916. *4473*

1850:46 Friedrich **Pelizaeus**, German neurologist, born; described familial centrolobar sclerosis ('Pelizaeus-Merzbacher disease'), 1885, *ArPN* **16**:698; a later account given by Merzbacher (1908). Died 1917. *4703, 471, 6335*

1850:47 Edward Talbot **Ely** born; reported the first operation for otoplasty, 1881, *ArOt(NY)* **10**:97. Died 1885. *5754.2*

1850:48 William Allen **Sturge**, British neurologist, born; described an association of a port-wine naevus with a vascular abnormality of the meninges on the same side, 1879, *TCSL* **12**:162; it was also described by Parkes Weber (1922), leading to the term 'Sturge-Weber syndrome'. Died 1919. *4560.1, 4605.2*

---

1850: Carl Friedrich **Canstatt** died, **born** 1807. *geriatrics*

1850: Jean Louis **Prévost** died, **born** 1790. *blood transfusion*

1850: Amos **Twitchell** died, **born** 1781. *carotid artery ligation*

1850: Antoine Germain **Labarraque** died, **born** 1777. *disinfection, chlorine*

**1851**
1851:1 **University of Minnesota, Minneapolis**, founded

1851:2 **First International Sanitary Conference**, Paris

1851:3 **Cancer Hospital (Free), London** (later **Royal Marsden Hospital**) established by William **Marsden** (1796–1867)

1851:4 **Medical Faculty of Georgetown University** (DC) founded

1851:5 *Wiener Medizinische Wochenschrift* begins publication

1851:6 Carl Ludwig (1816–1896) elucidated the innervation of the **salivary glands**, *ZRM* **1**:254. *998*

1851:7 The first important work dealing with **pelvic deformities** since the time of van Deventer was *Das enge Becken*, by Gustav Adolf Michaelis (1798–1848). He was among the first to differentiate between the flat pelvis and the **rachitic** pelvis. *6259*

1851:8 A classic description of **pelvic haematocele** given by Auguste Nélaton (1807–1873), *GH* **3**:573, 578, 581; **4**:45, 46. *6178*

1851:9 The first **episiotomy** in America (2 December 1851) performed by Valentine H. Taliaferro (1831–1888), reported 1852, *SVMG* **2**:382. *6180*

1851:10 The American gynaecologist Washington Lemuel Atlee (1808–1878) was said to have performed **ovariotomy** 387 times; he firmly established this operation in the USA, *TAMA* **4**:286. *6038*

1851:11 The **ophthalmoscope** invented by Hermann Ludwig Ferdinand von Helmholtz (1821–1894); in his *Beschreibung eines Augen-Spiegels zur Untersuchung der Netzhaut im lebenden Auge*. *5866*

1851:12 In his *Die Krankheiten des Auges*, 3 vols, 1851–56, Carl Ferdinand von Arlt (1812–1887) described **granular conjunctivitis (Arlt's trachoma)** and an operation for **transplantation** of the **ciliary bulbs** in the treatment of **distichiasis**. *5865*

1851:13 John Snow (1813–1858) attempted **carbon dioxide** absorption **anaesthesia**, *LMG* **11**:479; **12**:622. *5665*

1851:14 In his *Synopsis of cerebral and spinal seizures*, etc., Marshall Hall (1790–1857) was first to suggest that the paroxysmal nervous discharges of **epilepsy** were produced by the spinal nervous system, first to notice the connection of **anaemia** with epilepsy, and first to deduce that epilepsy was produced by anaemia of the **medulla**. *4812*

1851:15 The distinction between hypertrophy and **carcinoma** of the **prostate** first made by John Adams (1806–1877); in his *Anatomy and diseases of the prostate gland*. *4260*

1851:16 **Cystotomy** for inflammation and rupture of the **bladder** introduced by Willard Parker (1800–1884), *NYJM* **7**:83. *4169*

1851:17 Experimental transplantation of **tumours** by Joseph Leidy (1823–1891), *PANS* **5**:212. *2614*

1851:18 **Reissner's membrane** described by Ernst Reissner (1824–1878) in his *De auris internae formatione*. *1560*

1851:19 **Visual purple (rhodopsin)** discovered by Heinrich Müller (1820–1864), *ZWZ* **3**:234. *1506*

1851:20 **Organ of Corti** so named following investigations of the **cochlea** by Alfonso Corti (1822–1888), *ZWZ* **3**:109. *1559*

---

1851:21 Hans **Chiari**, Austrian pathologist, born 1 Feb; first reported chorionepithelioma, 1877, *MJa*, 34. Drew attention to the shift of the medulla caudally in what later became known as the Arnold-Chiari malformation, 1891, *BMW* **17**:1172. Died 1916. *6066.1, 4577.1, 4581.1, 4566.1*

1851:22 Charles **Chamberland**, French bacteriologist, born 12 Mar; in studies on the aetiology of anthrax with Louis Pasteur and Pierre Paul Emile Roux, first to use attenuated bacterial virus, providing active immunization against the disease, 1880, *CRAS* **91**:86. With Pasteur, Pierre Roux and T. Thuillier, published Pasteur's earliest studies on rabies, 1881, *CRAS* **92**:1259. With Pasteur and Roux, in an attempt to develop a variety of rabies that could be used safely for vaccination they became the first to modify the pathogenicity of a virus for its natural host, by serial intracerebral passage in another species of host, 1884, *CRAS* **98**:457, 1229. Introduced the Chamberland filter for removal of bacteria from liquids, 1884, *CRAS* **99**:247. Died 1908. *5169, 5481.4, 5482, 2498.1*

1851:23 Samuel James **Meltzer**, Russian/American physician, born 22 Mar; with John Auer, carried out experimental work on intratracheal insufflation anaesthetization, 1909, *JEM* **11**:622, which led to modern endotracheal anaesthesia; considered bronchial asthma to be a phenomenon of anaphylaxis, 1910, *JAMA* **55**:1021. *5694, 2600.1*

1851:24 Robert **Abbe**, American surgeon, born 13 Apr; carried out posterior rhizotomy (surgical division of a nerve root), 1889, *MR* **35**:149; the operation was also performed by William Henry Bennett in the same year. Introduced a lip-switch flap, transferring a full-thickness flap from one lip to the other for the repair of double cleft lip, 1898), *MR* **53**:477. Died 1928. *4860.1, 4861.1, 5755.2*

1851:25 Marius Hans Erik **Tscherning**, German physician, born 5 May; introduced the photometric spectacle lens, 1922, *AnO* **159**:625. Died 1939. *5967*

1851:26 Paul **Kraske**, German surgeon, born 2 Jun; introduced sacral method of resection of the rectum for carcinoma, 1887, *BKW* **24**:899. Died 1930. *3490*

1851:27 Jacques Arsène **d'Arsonval**, French physicist born 8 Jun; introduced high-frequency currents into electrotherapy, 1892, *ArPhy* **4**:69. Died 1940. *1999*

1851:28 Oliver **Lodge**, British physicist, born 12 Jun; with Robert Jones, probably published first clinical use of x rays to locate a bullet in the wrist, 22 February 1896, *L* **1**:476. Died 1940. *2684*

1851:29 Ernst **Fuchs**, Austrian ophthalmologist, born 14 Jun; described peripheral atrophy of the optic nerve, 1885, *GAO* **31**, 1:177. First described epidemic **keratoconjunctivitis**, 1889, *WKW* **2**:837. Died 1930. *5926, 5934*

1851:30 Arnold **Pick**, Czechoslovakian neurophysiologist, born 20 Jul; described 'Pick's bundle', fibres of the pyramidal tract of the medulla oblongata, 1890, *ArPN* **21**:636. Described circumscribed atrophy of the brain with development of aphasia and presenile dementia ('Pick's disease'), 1892, *PMW* **17**:165. Died 1924. *1420, 4707*

1851:31 Graham **Steell**, British physician, born 27 Jul; described the pulmonary diastolic ('Graham Steell') murmur, 1888, *MCh* **9**:182. Died 1942. *2794*

1851:32 Emile Pierre Marie van **Ermengem**, Belgian bacteriologist, born 15 Aug; discovered *Clostridium botulinum* in cases of food poisoning, 1897, *ArPha* **3**:213, 499. Died 1932. *2510*

1851:33 Walter **Reed**, American physician, born 13 Sep; with James Carroll, Aristide Agramonte y Simoni and Jesse William Lazear, provided the first definite proof that the causal agent in yellow fever is transmitted to man by the mosquito, *Aedes aegypti*, 1900, *PhMeJ* **6**:790. Died 1902. *5457*

1851:34 Arthur Henry **Downes**, British physician, born 11 Oct; with Thomas Porter Blunt, demonstrated the bactericidal action of sunlight, 1877, *PRS* **26**:488. Died 1938. *1997*

1851:35 André **Chantemesse**, French bacteriologist, born 13 Oct; with Georges Fernand Isidor Widal, carried out experimental anti-typhoid inoculation, 1888, *AnIP* **2**:54. With Widal, isolated the dysentery bacillus, *Shigella*, 1888, *BuAM* **19**:522, but did not establish its aetiological relationship to bacillary dysentery. Died 1919. *5034, 5090.1*

1851:36 Frank Thomas **Paul**, British surgeon, born 3 Dec; introduced 'Paul's tube' for intestinal drainage, 1891, *BMJ* **2**:118. Devised extra-abdominal resection of the colon ('Paul's operation'), 1895, *BMJ* **1**:1136. Died 1941. *3499, 3515*

1851:37 Mikolaj **Reichmann**, Polish gastroenterologist, born; first to describe gastrosuccorrhoea ('Reichmann's disease'), 1882, *GL* **2**:516. Died 1918. *3478*

1851:38 Charles Lucien de **Beurmann**, French dermatologist born; with Henri Gougerot, first described sporotrichosis ('de Beurmann-Gougerot disease'); in their *Les sporotrichoses*, 1912. Died 1923. *4147*

1851: Jean Guillaume August **Lugol** died, **born** 1786. *iodine, skin diseases, thyroid disorders*

1851: Christian Friedrich **Nasse** died, **born** 1778. *haemophilia*

1851: Antoine **Lembert** died, **born** 1802. *Lembert's suture*

1851: John Kearney **Rodgers** died, **born** 1793. *humerus fracture wiring*

1851: Conrad Johann Martin **Langenbeck** died, **born** 1776. *iridencleisis, pupil*

1851: Franz Carl **Naegele** died, **born** 1778. *obliquely contracted pelvis, labour*

1851: Joshua **Milne** died, **born** 1815. *mortality statistics, life insurance*

**1852**
1852:1 **International Congress of Hygiene, Brussels**

1852:2 **Hospital for Sick Children, Gt Ormond St., London**, first hospital for children in England, opened. Founded on inspiration of Dr Charles **West** (1816–1898), in Richard **Mead's** house

1852:3 **Obstetrical Society, London**, founded

1852:4 **Pharmacy Act 1852**, governing education, qualifications, standards, conduct and control of **pharmaceutical profession** in the UK; later Acts 1868, 1954

1852:5 [**School of Military Medicine**] at **Val-de-Grâce, Paris**

1852:6 **Mercy Hospital, Chicago**, chartered

1852:7 **Tufts College, Medford**, Mass., founded; medical school, 1893

1852:8 **St Mary's Hospital, London,** founded

1852:9 The coxalgic, scoliotic and kyphoscoliotic forms of **pelvis** described by Carl Conrad Theodor Litzmann (1815–1890); in his *Das schräg-ovale Becken.* *6260*

1852:10 A classic description of **hyperemesis gravidarum** given by Paul Antoine Du Bois (1795–1871), *BuAM* **17**:557. *6179*

1852:11 The *Iconographie ophtalmologique,* 1852–59, of Julius Sichel (1802–1868) ranks with the work of Ammon as one of the greatest pre-ophthalmoscopic atlases of **ophthalmology.** *5868, 5852*

1852:12 Rudolf Albert von Kölliker's (1817–1905) *Handbuch der Gewebelehre des Menschen* included his **classification of tissue.** *546*

1852:13 An operation for the formation of an artificial **pupil** devised by William Bowman (1816–1892), *MTG* **4**:11, 33. *5867*

1852:14 Christian Georg Theodor Ruete (1810–1867) introduced a practical lens system for examining the inverted image, and improved the illumination of the **ophthalmoscope**; in his *Der Augenspiegel und das Optometer für practische Aertze. 5866.1*

1852:15 *Schistosoma haematobium,* parasite causing **schistosomiasis (bilharziasis)** discovered in Egypt by Theodor Maximilian Bilharz (1825–1862), *ZWC* **4**:53. *5339*

1852:16 **Vasomotor nerves** discovered by Claude Bernard (1813–1878), *CRSB* **3**:163. *1320*

1852:17 **Chancroid** first clearly defined by Léon Bassereau (1811–1888); in his *Traité des affections de la peau symptomatiques de la syphilis. 5203*

1852:18 **Persecution mania ('Lasègue's disease')** described by Ernest Charles Lasègue (1816–1883), *ArGM* **28**:129. *4931*

1852:19 **Duchenne's muscular dystrophy** (1868) first described by Edward Meryon (1809–1880), *MCT* **35**:73. *4734.1, 4739*

1852:20 The term **'tétanie'** introduced by François Rémy Lucien Corvisart (1824–1882), nephew of J.N. Corvisart; in his *De la contracture des extrémités ou tétanie,* Paris, Thèse No. 223. *4829*

1852:21 The first excision of the **hip-joint** in the United States performed by Henry Jacob Bigelow (1818–1890), *AmJMS* **24**:90. *4461*

1852:22 The modern **plaster of Paris bandage** introduced by Antonius Mathijsen (1805–1878); in his *Nieuwe wijze van aanwending van het gips-verband bij beenbreuken. 4328*

1852:23 **Uretero-intestinal anastomosis** first performed by John Simon (1816–1904), *L* **2**:568. *4169.1*

1852:24 *Fasciolopsis buski*, the **fluke** causing **fasciolopsiasis**, described by George Budd (1808–1882) in his *On diseases of the liver*, 2nd ed., p. 484; his attention having been drawn to it by George Busk (1807–1886). *3619*

1852:25 Classical description of **embolism** by William Senhouse Kirkes (1823–1864), *MCT* **35**:281. *2758*

1852:26 Rudolph Hermann Lotze (1817–1881), who wrote *Medicinische Psychologie, oder Physiologie der Seele*, was a pioneer in the investigation of **unconscious** and **subconscious** states. *4970*

1852:27 **Epithelioma** so named by Adolph Hannover (1814–1894); in his *Das Epithelioma*. *2615*

1852:28 **Salicylic acid** synthesized by H. Gerland, *JCS* **5**:133. *1861.1*

1852:29 **Haemoglobin** discovered by Otto Funke (1828–1879), *ZRM* **1**:172; **2**:298. *866*

1852:30 Operation for **vesico-vaginal fistula** devised by James Marion Sims (1813–1883), *AmJMS* **23**:59; in the same paper he also described the '**Sims' position**', the knee-chest position. *6037*

1852:31 Dr Peter Mark **Roget** (1779–1869) published his ***Thesaurus of English words and phrases***.

---

1852:32 Samuel Vulvovich **Goldflam**, Polish physician, born 22 Feb; described myasthenia pseudoparalytica, 1893, *DZN* **1**:96; **3**:427; it had previously been described by Erb (1879) and was named 'Erb-Goldflam symptom complex'. Died 1932. *4757, 4746*

1852:33 Pieter Klazes **Pel**, Dutch physician, born 23 Feb; described the remittent pyrexia occurring in lymphadenoma, 1885, *BKW* **22**:3; named 'Pel-Ebstein disease' following a later account by Wilhelm Ebstein. Died 1919. *3770, 3771*

1852:34 Felix von **Winiwater**, Austrian physician, born 28 Feb; described thrombo-angiitis obliterans in 1879, *ArKC* **23**:202; named 'Buerger's disease' following the account by Leo Buerger in 1908. Died 1931. *2907*

1852:35 William Henry **Bennett**, British surgeon, born 20 Mar; carried out posterior rhizotomy (surgical division of a nerve root), 1889, *MCT* **72**:329. The operation was also performed by Robert Abbe in the same year. Died 1931. *4861.1, 4860.1*

1852:36 Ivar Victor **Sandström**, Swedish anatomist, born 22 Mar; gave first systematic account of the parathyroid glands, 1880, *ULF* **15**:441. Died 1889. *1127*

1852:37 Carl **Breus**, Austrian obstetrician and gynaecologist, born 12 Apr; first described the 'Breus mole' (tuberous mole), the aborted products of conception; in his *Das tuberöse subchoriale Hämatom der Decidua*, 1892. With Alexander Kolisko, gave a classic description and classification of pelvic deformities; in their *Die pathologischen Beckenformen*, 1900–14. Died 1914. *6202, 6265*

1852:38 Francis Henry **Williams**, American radiologist, born 15 Apr; introduced the fluoroscope, 1896, *BMSJ* **135**:335. Introduced heart fluoroscopy, 1896, *BMSJ* **135**:335; the first application of x rays in cardiology. Died 1936. *2686.1, 2804.1*

1852:39 Nikolai Evgenievich **Vvedensky**, Russian physiologist, born 28 Apr; studied the reaction of living tissue to various stimulants and demonstrated the indefatigability of nerve, 1884, *ZMW* **22**:65; confirmed by Bowditch. Died 1922. *1280, 1281*

1852:40 Santiago **Ramón y Cajal**, Spanish neuroanatomist and histologist, born 1 May. His *Textura del sistema nervioso del hombre y de los vertebrados*, 2 vols [in 3], 1899–1904, a monumental work, expounds the cytological and histological foundations of modern neurology. In its time his *Estudios sobre la degeneración y regeneración del sistema nervioso*, 2 vols, 1913–14 (English translation, 1928), was the most complete work on the subject. He became one of the greatest of all histologists and shared the Nobel Prize (Physiology or Medicine), 1906, with Golgi, for his contribution to the knowledge of neuroanatomy, *NPL*. Died 1934. *1293.1, 560.1*

1852:41 Edmund **Jelinek**, Bohemian physician, born 14 May; first to use cocaine as an anaesthetic in laryngology, 1884, *WMW* **34**:1334, 1364. Died 1928. *3292*

1852:42 Guido **Banti**, Italian physician, born 18 Jun; his account of splenic anaemia, in his *Dell'anemia splenica*, 1882, led to the eponym 'Banti's disease'. Described splenomegalic anaemia ('Banti's syndrome'), 1894, *Spe* **48**:Com 447; Sez.b. 407. Died 1925. *3126, 3774*

1852:43 Friedrich August Johann **Loeffler**, German bacteriologist, born 24 Jun; discovered *Pfeifferella mallei*, causative organism in glanders, 1882, *DMW* **8**:707; *AKG* (1886) **1**:141. Successfully cultivated *Corynebacterium diphtheriae* (Klebs-Loeffler bacillus), causal organism in diphtheria, 1884, *MKG* **2**:421. Isolated *Salmonella typhi-murium*, 1892, *ZBP* **11**:129. With Paul Frosch showed foot-and-mouth disease to be due to a filter-passing virus (first recognition of such a virus as a cause of animal disease), 1898, *ZBP* I, **23**:371. Died 1915. *5156, 5056, 2507, 2511*

1852:44 Dittmar **Finkler**, German bacteriologist and hygienist, born 25 Jul; with J. Prior, isolated *Vibrio proteus*, a cholera-like vibrio, in a case of acute gastroenteritis, 1884, *DMW* **10**:579. Died 1912. *3481*

1852:45 Henry Rose **Carter**, American sanitarian, born 25 Aug; his determination of the incubation period of yellow fever, 1900, *NOMSJ* **52**:617, decided the direction of Walter Reed's later researches, which in turn led to the discovery of the virus. Compiled an epidemiological and historical study of yellow fever; *Yellow fever: an epidemiological and historical study of its place of origin*, 1931, edited after his death by L.A. Carter and W.H. Frost. Died 1925. *5456, 5468*

1852:46 Rudolph **Emmerich**, German bacteriologist, born 19 Sep; with Oscar Löw prepared pyocyanase, an antibiotic, prepared from *Pseudomonas pyocyanea*, 1889, *ZHyg* **31**:1. Died 1914. *1932.2*

1852:47 William Stewart **Halsted**, American surgeon, born 23 Sep; made the first experiments on local (infiltration) anaesthesia, 1885, *NYMJ* **42**:294. Devised the modern operation (Halsted I repair) for the radical cure of inguinal hernia, 1889, *JHB* **1**:12, 112, almost simultaneously with Edoardo Bassini. His method of radical mastectomy was one of the greatest contributions

246

to the treatment of breast cancer, 1890, *JHR* **2**:255; **4**:297. First successful ligation of left subclavian artery, with extirpation of subclavio-axillary aneurysm, 1892, *JHB* **3**:393. Introduced rubber gloves into operative surgery, 1894, *JHR* **4**:297. Died 1922. *5679, 3599, 5776, 2966, 5640*

1852:48 Emil **Fischer**, German chemist, born 9 Oct; synthesized barbitone, with Joseph von Mering, 1903, *TGe* **44**:97. Died 1919. *1892*

1852:49 Otto **Purtscher**, Austrian ophthalmologist, born 18 Oct; first described traumatic angiopathy of the retina ('Purtscher's disease'), 1912, *GAO* **82**:347. Died 1927. *5962*

1852:50 Viktor von **Hacker**, Austrian surgeon, born 21 Oct; gave the first account of the Billroth II operation for resection of the pylorus, 1885, *VDGC* **14**II:62; *ArKC* **32**:616; introduced his method of gastrostomy, 1886, *WMW* **36**:1073, 1110. Died 1933. *3483, 3486*

1852:51 John Newport **Langley**, British physiologist, born 2 Nov; mapped out much of the involuntary nervous system, *The autonomic nervous system*, 1921; edited *Journal of Physiology*, 1894 until his death. Died 1925. *1332*

1852:52 Charles **Sajous**, French/American physician, born 13 Dec; his *The internal secretions*, 2 vols, 1903–7 was the first treatise on endocrinology. Died 1929. *3793*

1852:53 Shibasaburo **Kitasato**, Japanese bacteriologist, born 20 Dec; first to obtain a pure culture of the tetanus bacillus, *Clostridium tetani*, 1889, *ZHyg* **7**:225. With Emil Adolf von Behring, discovered antitoxins and their immunizing power, 1890, *DMW* **16**:1113, 1145, through their work on diphtheria and tetanus immunity, and laid the foundation of all future treatment with antitoxins. Died 1931. *5149, 5060, 2544*

1852:54 Otto Gerhard **Sprengel**, German surgeon, born 27 Dec; described congenital upward displacement of the scapula, 1891, *ArKC* **42**:545; the condition was named 'Sprengel's deformity', despite the earlier description by M.M. Eulenburg in 1863. Died 1915. *4359, 4332, 4427*

---

1852:55 Antoine Henri **Becquerel**, French physicist, born; discovered radioactivity, 1896, *CRAS* **122**:420. Awarded Nobel Prize (Physics), 1903, jointly with Pierre Curie and Marie Curie for discovery of radioactivity, *NPL*. Died 1908. *2001, 2684.2*

1852:56 Richard Julius **Petri**, German bacteriologist, born; introduced the Petri dish, 1887, *ZBP* **1**:279. Died 1921. *2505.1*

1852:57 Hermann **Kümmell**, German surgeon, born; described a form of traumatic spondylitis ('Kümmell's disease'), 1891, *VGDA*, p. 282. Died 1937. *4357*

1852:58 Stephanos **Kartulis**, Greek physician, born; discovered amoebae in liver abscess, 1886, *VA* **105**:521; it was principally through his work that amoebae came to be considered a cause of dysentery (amoebiasis) in man. Died 1920. *5186*

1852:59 Masanori **Ogata**, Japanese physician, born; considered the flea to be the principal, if not the sole, vector of bubonic plague infection, 1897, *ZBP* I, **21**:769. Died 1919. *5128*

1852:60 Vasili Iakovlevich **Danilevski** born; discovered the malaria parasite, *Plasmodium*, in birds, *BZ* **5**:529. Died 1934. *5238.1*

1852:61 Vasili Konstantinovich **Anrep** born; suggested cocaine as a local anaesthetic, 1880, *PfA* **21**:38. *5675*

---

1852: Joseph Claude Anthelme **Récamier** died, **born** 1774. *cancer metastasis, vaginal speculum*

1852: Carl Friedrich **Quittenbaum** died, **born** 1793. *splenectomy*

1852: Louis **Braille** died, **born** 1809. *Braille system*

**1853**

1853:1 **University of Melbourne** founded

1853:2 *Association Medical Journal* succeeds *Provincial Medical and Surgical Journal* and is renamed (1857) *British Medical Journal*

1853:3 **Washington University, St Louis**, founded

1853:4 **Crimean War**, 1853–1856; Florence **Nightingale** (1820–1910) revolutionized **nursing services**

1853:5 The first printed illustrations of the **fundus oculi** appear in the *Dissertatio ophthalmologica inauguralis de speculo oculi* of Adrian Christopher van Trigt (1825–1864). *5869.1*

1853:6 Among the first to study the surgical removal of **fibroids** of the **uterus** was Washington Lemuel Atlee (1808–1878); in his *Surgical treatment of certain fibrous tumours of the uterus*. *6039*

1853:7 The correlation of **retinal haemorrhage** with **brain tumours** first noted by Ludwig Türck (1810–1868), *ZGA* **9**, i:214. *5870*

1853:8 **Circular (manic-depressive) insanity** first described by Jean Pierre Falret (1794–1870), *BuAIM* **19**:382. *4932*

1853:9 William John Little (1810–1894), who suffered from **talipes (club-foot)** was the first eminent **orthopaedic** surgeon in Britain; his best work was *On the nature and treatment of the deformities of the human frame*, which included, p. 14, an early description of **progressive muscular dystrophy**. *4329, 4735*

1853:10 **Retrocaecal hernia (Rieux's hernia)** first described by Léon Rieux; in his *Considérations sur l'étranglement de l'intestin dans la cavité abdominale*. *3590*

1853:11 The first modern British work on **otology**, *Practical observations on aural surgery* ..., published by William Robert Wills Wilde (1815–1876). *3369*

1853:12 **Cancer** of **larynx** treated by **thyrotomy** by Gurdon Buck (1807–1877); in his *On the surgical treatment of polypi* .... *3263*

1853:13 **Hypodermic injections of drugs** used as therapeutic measure by Alexander Wood (1817–1884), *EMSJ* **82**:265. *1969*

1853:14 The modern **galvanocautery** invented by Charles Gabriel Pravaz (1791–1853), *CRAS* **36**:88. *5603*

1853:15 Frederick **Treves**, British surgeon, born 15 Feb; recorded a case of true haemophilia in a female, 1886, *L* **2**:553. Died 1923. *3067.1*

1853:16 Robert Adolf Armand **Tigerstedt**, Finnish physiologist, born 23 Feb; showed, with Per Gustav Bergman, that a pressor substance (renin) was produced by the kidney, 1898, *SkAP* **8**:223. Died 1923. *1236*

1853:17 Alexander Hugh **Ferguson**, American surgeon, born 27 Feb; devised operation for hernia; in his *Technic of modern operations for hernia*, 1907. Died 1912. *3608.1*

1853:18 Karel **Maydl**, Bohemian surgeon, born 10 Mar; carried out the first successful colostomy, 1888, *ZCh* **15**:433. Devised operation for uretero-intestinal anastomosis, 1894, *WMW* **41**:1113, 1169, 1209, 1256, 1297. Died 1913. *3492, 4188.1*

1853:19 Max **Sänger**, German gynaecologist, born 14 Mar; he reported 'Sänger's operation', the so-called 'classic caesarean section'; in his *Der Kaiserschnitt bei Uterusfibromen nebst vergleichender Methodik der Sectio Caesarea und der Porro-Operation*, 1882. Published a classification of chorionic tumours and a review of the relevant literature, 1893, *ArGy* **44**:89. Died 1903. *6242, 6094*

1853:20 James **Mackenzie**, British physician, born 12 Apr; published his classic work, *The study of the pulse*, 1902; it included a description of his polygraph. Reported the action of digitalis in auricular fibrillation, 1905, *BMJ* **1**:519, 587, 702, 759, 812. Died 1925. *2812, 2819*

1853:21 Alphonse **Bertillon**, French anthropologist, born 23 Apr; introduced method of identification by means of selected measurements ('Bertillonage'); in his *Les signalements anthropométriques* 1886. Died 1914. *181*

1853:22 George Michael **Edebohls**, American surgeon, born 8 May; in the nephropexy operation he devised, 1893, flaps of the capsule of the kidney were utilized, *AmJMS* **105**:247, 417; carried out first operation on the kidney for the relief of chronic nephritis, 1899, *MN* **74**:481; introduced operation of renal decortication for the treatment of chronic nephritis, 1901, *MR* **60**:961. Died 1908. *4224, 4228, 4229*

1853:23 Ernst Adolph Gustav Gottfried **Strümpell**, German neurologist, born 28 Jun; gave an excellent description of ankylosing spondylitis (the 'spondylose rhizomélique of Pierre Marie), in his *Lehrbuch der speciellen Pathologie und Therapie der inneren Krankheiten*, **2**, ii, 152, 1884; it led to the term 'Strümpell's disease'. Described polioencephalomyelitis ('Strümpell's disease'), 1885, *JaK* **22**:173. Described hereditary spastic spinal paralysis ('Strümpell's disease'), 1886, *ArPN* **17**:217; it had previously been noted by Erb and by Charcot. His account of pseudosclerosis of the brain, 1898, *DZN* **12**:115, followed an earlier description by Westphal (1883) and led to the term 'Westphal-Strümpell disease'. Died 1925. *4349, 4643, 4704, 4709, 4702*

1853:24 Max **Gruber**, Austrian bacteriologist, born 6 Jul; with Herbert Edward Durham, discovered bacterial agglutination, 1896, *MMW* **43**:285, realizing its value in the identification of typhoid. Died 1927. *2549, 5036*

1853:25 Francis **Gotch**, British physiologist, born 13 Jul; obtained first correct electroretinogram, 1903, *JP* **29**:388. Died 1913. *1525.1*

1853:26 Willoughby Dayton **Miller**, American dentist and stomatologist, born 1 Aug; his *The micro-organisms of the human mouth*, 1890, made an important contribution to the knowledge on dental bacteriology. Died 1907. *3687*

1853:27 John Elmer **Weeks**, American ophthalmologist, born 9 Aug; discovered an organism in 'pink eye', 1886, *ArOp* **15**:441. The organism, already seen by Robert Koch in Egyptian ophthalmia, was later named 'Koch-Weeks bacillus'. Died 1949. *5930*

1853:28 Henry Solomon **Wellcome**, American/British pharmacist, born 21 Aug. In 1880 he founded the pharmaceutical firm of **Burroughs Wellcome** and in 1924 endowed the **Wellcome Foundation**. At his death in 1936 the **Wellcome Trust** was formed to support research in medicine in the UK, including the Wellcome Institute for the History of Medicine, containing one of the best medico-historical libraries in Europe

1853:29 Pierre **Marie**, French neurologist, born 9 Sep; with Jean Martin Charcot, first described peroneal muscular atrophy (Charcot-Marie-Tooth type), 1886, *ReM* **6**:97, which was independently described by Tooth in the same year. Gave first complete clinical description of acromegaly, 1886, *ReM* **6**:297. Gave the name 'spondylose rhizomélique' to ankylosing spondylitis, 1898, *ReM* **18**:285, already described by Strümpell in 1884; with Paul Sainton, gave cleidocranial dysostosis its present name, 1898, *ReN* **6**:835, already described by Morand in 1760. He disclaimed Broca's theory concerning the location of the speech centre, classified aphasia into three groups: anarthria (defects of articulation), Broca's aphasia (motor aphasia), and Wernicke's aphasia (sensory aphasia), 1906, *SMP* **26**:241. Died 1940. *4749, 4750, 3884, 4368, 4349, 4302.2, 4630*

1853:30 Hans Christian Joachim **Gram**, Danish bacteriologist, born 13 Sep; introduced the method of staining bacteria named after him and widely used today, 1884, *FM* **2**:185. Died 1938. *2499*

1853:31 Karl Martin Leonhard Albrecht **Kossel**, German biochemist, born 16 Sep; studied the chemistry of the cell and cell nucleus, *HSZ* 1882–87, **7**:7; **10**:248; **22**:167. Awarded Nobel Prize (Physiology or Medicine), 1910, *NPL*. Died 1927. *702*

1853:32 Heinrich **Unverricht**, German neurologist, born 18 Sep; first described familial myoclonus epilepsy ('Unverricht's disease'); in his *Die Myoclonie*, 1891. Died 1912. *4819*

1853:33 Eugen **Fraenkel**, German pathologist, born 28 Sep; showed the gonococcus to be the cause of vulvovaginitis in children, 1885, *VA* **99**:251. Died 1925. *5210.1*

1853:34 James Rutherford **Morison**, British surgeon, born 10 Oct; introduced 'Bipp' (an antiseptic paste), in the treatment of wounds, 1916, *L* **2**:268. Died 1939. *5644*

1853:35 Werner **Körte**, German surgeon, born 21 Oct; first successfully to treat bronchiectasis by removal of the bronchiectatic lobes, 1908, *VBMG* **39**:5. Died 1937. *3187*

1853:36 Constantin von **Monakow**, Russian neurologist, born 4 Nov; described 'Monakow's bundle', the rubrospinal tract, 1910, *AHI* **3**:51; **4**:103. Localization of cerebral function mapped in his *Die Lokalisation im Grosshirn*, 1914. Died 1930. *1375, 1438.2*

1853:37 Stephane Armand Nicolas **Leduc**, French physician, born 9 Nov; introduced ionic medication, 1900; his work on the application of galvanic current to the brain, 1903, *RIER* **13**:143, led to the introduction of electric convulsion therapy in 1938. Died 1939. *2003.1, 2003.2*

1853:38 Karl Friedrich Jakob **Sudhoff**, German physician and historian of medicine, born 26 Nov; his main research was in ancient, medieval and Renaissance medicine. Edited several important periodicals and founded (1908) the *Archiv für Geschichte der Medizin*, later named *Sudhoff's Archiv*. Died 1938. *6666*

1853:39 William **Murrell**, British physician, born 26 Nov; introduced Trinitrin (nitroglycerine) in treatment of angina pectoris, 1879, *L* **1**:113, 151, 225. Died 1912. *2892*

1853:40 Pierre Paul Emile **Roux**, French bacteriologist, born 17 Dec; in studies on the aetiology of anthrax with Pasteur and Charles Chamberland, first to use attenuated bacterial virus, providing active immunization against the disease, 1880, *CRAS* **91**:86. With Louis Pasteur, Chamberland and T. Thuillier, published Pasteur's earliest studies on rabies, 1881, *CRAS* **92**:1259. With Pasteur and Chamberland, in an attempt to develop a variety of rabies that could be used safely for vaccination they became the first to modify the pathogenicity of a virus for its natural host, by serial intracerebral passage in another species of host, 1884, *CRAS* **98**:457, 1229. With Alexandre Yersin, confirmed the work of Loeffler on *Corynebacterium diphtheriae* and demonstrated the exotoxin in diphtheria, 1888, *AnIP* **2**:629, **3**:273; **4**:385; their work marks the starting point of the development of an immunizing serum. With André Martin, showed how Behring's specific diphtheria antitoxin could be produced on a large scale, 1894, *AnIP* **8**:609. Died 1933. *5169, 5481.4, 5482 5059, 5063*

1853:41 Frederic Samuel **Eve**, British surgeon, born; first definitely authenticated a case of intersigmoid hernia, 1885, *BMJ* **1**:1195. Died 1916. *3595*

1853:42 Francis Sedgwick **Watson**, American urological surgeon, born; carried out medial perineal prostatectomy, 1889 – reported in 1905, *AnS* **41**:507. Died 1942. *4266*

1853:43 André Louis François Justin **Martin** born; with Pierre Paul Emile Roux, showed how Behring's specific diphtheria antitoxin could be produced on a large scale, 1894, *AnIP* **8**:609. Died 1921. *5063*

1853:44 George Howard **Monks**, American plastic surgeon, born; developed the modern treatment of rhinophyma, 1898, *BMSJ* **139**:262. Died 1933. *5755.4*

1853: William **Beaumont** died, **born** 1785. *gastric juice*

1853: Robert James **Graves** died, **born** 1796. *exophthalmic goitre*

1853: Charles Gabriel **Pravaz** died, **born** 1791. *galvanocautery*

# 1854
1854:1 **California Academy of Sciences, San Francisco**, founded

1854:2 **Children's Hospital and Nursery** opened at **New York**

1854:3 **Universities of Marseilles, Clermont-Ferrand and Nancy** founded

1854:4 **Boston Medical Library** founded

1854:5 *Aertzliches Intelligenz-Blatt* founded *(Münchener Medizinische Wochenschrift*, 1886)

1854:6 *Archiv für Ophthalmologie* founded by Albrecht von Graefe (1828–1870)

1854:7 The **sewers** of Paris constructed by Marie François Eugène Belgrand (1810–1878); described in his work, *La Seine*, published 1872–1887. *1620*

1854:8 The first account of metastatic **ophthalmia** given by Heinrich Meckel von Hemsbach (1821–1856), *AnCK* **5**, ii:276. *5875*

1854:9 **Combined cephalic version** introduced by Marmaduke Burr Wright (1803–1879); in his *Difficult labors and their treatment. 6182*

1854:10 The first description of **pelvis spinosa** given by Hermann Friedrich Kilian (1800–1863); in his *Schilderungen neuer Beckenformen und ihres Verhaltens im Leben*. His *De spondylolisthesi gravissimae pelvangustiae causa nuper detecta* was an important study of the **spondylolisthetic pelvis**. *6261, 6262*

1854:11 **Duncan's folds**, the peritoneal folds associated with the **uterus**, named after the description by James Matthews Duncan (1826–1890), a leading Edinburgh obstetrician, *EMSJ* **81**:321. *6181*

1854:12 **Sight test types** introduced by Eduard Jaeger (1818–1884); in his *Schriftskalen*. *5887*

1854:13 The first successful abdominal **hysterectomy** performed by Walter Burnham (1808–1883), *NAL* **52**:147. *6040*

1854:14 A classic account of **breast tumours** provided by Alfred Armand Louis Marie Velpeau (1795–1867); in his *Traité des maladies du sein et de la région mammaire. 5771*

1854:15 Among the first to treat **ulcers** by **skin grafts** was Frank Hastings Hamilton (1813–1886), as described in his *Elkoplasty, or anaplasty applied to the treatment of old ulcers. 5747*

1854:16 The first protagonist of the **mosquito** transmission of **yellow fever** was Louis Daniel Beauperthuy (1807–1871), *GOCu* **4**: No. 57. *5454.1*

1854:17 **Tropical anaemia** considered by Wilhelm Griesinger (1817–1868) to be due to the **hookworm** causing **ankylostomiasis**, *ArPH* **13**:528. *5355*

1854:18 Archibald Baring Garrod (1819–1907), the leading authority of his time on **gout** (which he separated from other forms of **arthritis**), introduced the 'thread test', *MCT* **31**:83; **37**:49. *4495*

1854:19 **Tinea cruris (eczema marginatum)** first described by Friedrich Wilhelm Felix von Bärensprung (1822–1864); in his *Ueber die Folge und den Verlauf epidermischer Krankheiten. 4043*

1854:20 '**True keloid' (scleroderma, morphoea)** described by Thomas Addison (1793–1860), *MCT* **37**:27. *4042*

1854:21 **Paroxysmal cold haemoglobinuria** first described by Lucas Anton Dressler (1815–1896), *VA* **6**:264. *4169.2*

1854:22 A method of complete **osteoplastic amputation** of the **foot** introduced by Nikolai Ivanovich Pirogov (1810–1881), *VMZ* **63**, 2:83. *4465*

1854:23 In his *Diseases of the heart and aorta* William Stokes (1804–1878) described **Cheyne-Stokes respiration** (p. 320), previously noted by John Cheyne, 1818, and **paroxysmal tachycardia** (p. 161). *2760, 2743*

1854:24 **Sphygmograph** invented by Karl Vierordt (1818–1884); the first instrument with which a tracing of the pulse could be made, *ArPH* **13**:284. *772, 2759*

1854:25 **Chaulmoogra oil** treatment of **leprosy** introduced into Western medicine by Frederic John Mouat (1816–1897), *IAMS* **1**:646. *2435*

1854:26 An early account of **decompression sickness ('caisson disease')** was given by B. Pol and T.J.J. Watelle, *AnH* **1**:241. *2124*

1854:27 Filippo Pacini (1812–1883) described **vibrios** seen in the intestinal contents of **cholera** victims and incriminated them as the pathogen, *GMIFT* **4**:397, 405. *5106.1*

1854:28 **Neuroglia** discovered by Rudolph Virchow (1821–1902), *VA* **6**:135. *1268*

1854:29 William Thomas **Councilman**, American pathologist, born 1 Jan; with Henri Amadée Lafleur, introduced the term 'amoebic dysentery' in their important investigation of the condition, 1891, *JHR* **2**:395. Died 1933. *5187*

1854:30 Sergei Sergeievich **Korsakoff**, Russian neurologist and psychiatrist, born 22 Jan; drew attention to alcoholic polyneuritis ('Korsakoff's psychosis' or syndrome), 1887, *VKP* **4** (2):1. Died 1900. *4945*

1854:31 Paul Julius **Möbius**, German psychiatrist, born 24 Jan; described ophthalmoplegic migraine ('Möbius's disease'), 1884, *BKW* **21**:604. Died 1907. *4567*

1854:32 Vincenzo **Cervello**, Italian pharmacologist, born 13 Mar; used paraldehyde as a narcotic, 1884, *ArIB* **6**:113. Died 1919. *1877*

1854:33 Paul **Ehrlich**, German bacteriologist, chemist, immunologist and founder of chemotherapy, born 14 Mar; gave the first account of the reticulocyte, 1881, *BKW* **17**:405. Introduced methylene blue as a bacterial stain, 1881, *ZKM* **2**:710. Stated his 'side-chain' theory of antibody formation; in his *Die Sauerstoff-Bedürfniss der Organismen*, 1885. (Shared Nobel Prize (Physiology or Medicine), 1908, with Elie Metchnikoff, for his work on immunity, *NPL*.) First to distinguish aplastic anaemia, 1888, *Charité-Ann* **13**:300. With Paul Guttmann, demonstrated that methylene blue is lethal *in vitro* for the malaria parasite, 1891, *BKW* **28**:953, marking the beginning of Ehrlich's work on chemotherapy. His methods of staining blood cells enabled him to differentiate lymphatic and myelogenous leukaemia; in his *Farbenanalytische Untersuchungen zur Histologie und Klinik*, 1891. Improved Behring's diphtheria antitoxin through quantitative titration, 1897, *KJ* **6**:299. He established an international standard for this and other antitoxins, initiating the concept of biological standardization. Cured experimental trypanosomiasis with his 'Trypanrot', 1907, *BKW* **44**:233, 280, 310, 341, the work led him eventually to the production of salvarsan. With Sahachiro Hata, introduced salvarsan ('606'), specific in treatment of syphilis and yaws ; *Die experimentelle Chemotherapie der Spirillosen ...*, 1910; introduced neosalvarsan (neoarsphenamine), 1912, *CZ* **36**:637. Died 1915. *3125.5, 2493, 2540, 3129, 5241.1, 3069.1, 5064, 5281, 2403, 2405*

1854:34 Emil Adolf von **Behring**, German bacteriologist and immunologist, born 15 Mar; with Shibasaburo Kitasato, discovered antitoxins and their immunizing power, 1890, *DMW* **16**:1113, 1145, through their work on diphtheria and tetanus immunity, and laid the foundation of all future treatment with antitoxins. With Kitasato discovered diphtheria and tetanus antitoxins, 1890, *DMW* **16**:1113. Introduced toxin-antitoxin for diphtheria immunization, 1913, *DMW* **39**:873; **40**:1139. Awarded Nobel Prize (Physiology or Medicine), 1901, (first recipient) for his work on antitoxins – the basis of serotherapy, *NPL*. Died 1917. *5060, 2544, 5067*

1854:35 Giovanni Battista **Grassi**, Italian parasitologist, born 27 Mar; with co-workers, first to carry out faecal diagnosis of ankylostomiasis, 1878, *GMI* **5**:193. With Amico Bignami, showed that the malaria parasite, *Plasmodium*, undergoes its sexual phase in the *Anopheles* mosquito, 1899, *AnIS* **9**:258. The best illustrations of the various stages of the malaria parasite, published up to that time, appear in his *Studi di uno zoologo sulla malaria*, 1900. Died 1925. *5357, 5252, 5252.1*

1854:36 Friedrich **Neelsen**, German pathologist, born 29 Mar; introduced Ziehl-Neelsen stain for staining *Mycobacterium tuberculosis*, 1882, *ZMW* **21**:497. Died 1894. *2331.2*

1854:37 Antonio **Carle**, Italian surgeon, born 3 May; with Giorgio Rattone, demonstrated the transmissibility of tetanus by inoculation into rabbits of pus from a human case, 1884, *GAMT* **32**:174. Died 1927. *5147*

1854:38 Max **Rubner**, German physiologist and hygienist, born 2 Jun; clarified the specific dynamic effect of foodstuffs and established the validity of the principle of the conservation of energy in living organisms; in his *Die Gesetze des Energieverbrauchs bei der Ernährung*, 1902. Died 1932. *1025*

1854:39 James **Carroll**, British-born American physician, born 5 Jun; with Walter Reed, Aristide Agramonte y Simoni and Jesse William Lazear, provided the first definite proof that the causal agent in yellow fever is transmitted to man by the mosquito, *Aedes aegypti*, 1900, *PhMeJ* **6**:790. Died 1907. *5457*

1854:40 Charles Edward **Beevor**, British neurologist, born 12 Jun; with Victor Alexander Haden Horsley investigated localization of cerebral function, 1887, *PTB* **176**:153. Died 1907. *1416.1*

1854:41 Philippe Charles Ernest **Gaucher**, French dermatologist and syphilologist, born 26 Jul; his excellent account of familial splenic anaemia led to the eponym 'Gaucher's disease'; in his *De l'epithélioma primitif de la rate*. Paris, Thèse, 1882. Died 1918. *3127, 3769*

1854:42 Victor **Babès**, Austrian bacteriologist, born 28 Jul; introduced the mallein reaction for the diagnosis of glanders, 1891, *ArMEA* **3**:619. Died 1926. *5158*

1854:43 Adolf **Lorenz**, Austrian orthopaedic surgeon, born 21 Aug; suggested a bloodless method for closed reduction of congenital dislocation of the hip-joint, 1895, *TAOrS* **7**:99. Died 1946. *4365*

1854:44 William Crawford **Gorgas**, American surgeon and sanitarian, born 3 Oct; the sanitation methods he employed against yellow fever in Havana were so successful that in three months the disease was practically eradicated, 1909, *JAMA* **52**:1075. Died 1920. *5460*

1854:45 Jokichi **Takamine**, Japanese chemist and pharmacologist, born 3 Nov; isolated adrenaline, 1901, *AmJPm* **73**:523. Died 1922. *1146*

1854:46 Friedrich **Fehleisen**, German surgeon, born; discovered *Streptococcus pyogenes*, 1882, *DZC* **16**:391. Died 1924. *2496*

1854:47 Vasiliy Isayevich **Isayev** [Issayaeff] born; with Richard Friedrich Johannes Pfeiffer recorded immune bacteriolysis ('Pfeiffer phenomenon') in cholera vibrio, 1894, *ZHyg* **17**:355; **18**:1. Died 1911. *2546*

1854:48 James **Brown**, American urologist, born; performed the first catheterization of the male ureters, 1893, *JHB* **4**:73. Died 1895. *4185.1*

1854:49 Gustav **Fütterer**, German physician, born; with Bernhard Anton, first demonstrated *Salmonella typhi* in the gallbladder in cases of typhoid, 1888, *MMW* **35**:315. Died 1922. *5033*

1854: Carl Adolph von **Basedow** died, **born** 1799. *exophthalmic goitre*

1854: Richard Anthony **Stafford** died, **born** 1801. *sarcoma of prostate*

1854: Francis **Place** died, **born** 1771. *birth control*

1854: Montague **Gosset** died, **born** 1792. *vesico-vaginal fistula*

1854: Philibert Joseph **Roux** died, **born** 1780. *perineal suture, cleft palate*

1854: Richard James **Mackenzie** died, **born** 1821. *amputation at ankle-joint*

## 1855

1855:1 **Hospital for Women's Diseases, New York**, founded by James Marion **Sims** (1813–1883)

1855:2 **Children's Hospital, Philadelphia**, opened

1855:3 **Koninklijke Nederlandse Akademie van Wetenschappen** re-formed (founded 1808)

1855:4 **British Medical Association**, formerly **Provincial Medical and Surgical Association**, founded

1855:5 **Water filtration** becomes compulsory in **London**

1855:6 Lateral illumination in microscopic investigation of the living **eye** introduced by Richard Liebreich (1830–1917), *GAO* **1**, ii:351. *5877*

1855:7 The first successful abdominal **hysteromyomectomy** performed by Gilman Kimball (1804–1892), *BMSJ* **52**:249. *6042*

1855:8 **Iridectomy** in the treatment of **iritis** and **iridochoroiditis** introduced by Friedrich Wilhelm Ernst Albrecht von Graefe (1828–1870), *GAO* **2**, ii:202. *5873*

1855:9 Because his famous essay on **puerperal fever** was published (1843) in an unimportant journal, Oliver Wendell Holmes (1809–1894) enlarged it into book form, *Puerperal fever, as a private pestilence*, in which he mentions the steps already being taken by Semmelweis. *6274, 6276, 6275*

1855:10 Franz Aloys Antoine Pollender (1800–1879) claimed to have discovered the **anthrax** bacillus (***B.anthracis***) in 1849, not reporting this until 1855, *VGOM* **8**:103. His account of the organism was more exact than Rayer's. *5164*

1855:11 **Osteoperiostitis of the metatarsals** first described by Breithaupt, *MZ* **24**:169, 175. A later description by G.P. Busquet, 1897, led to the term '**Busquet's disease**'). *4330*

1855:12 First successful **hip resection** for **ankylosis** reported by Lewis Albert Sayre (1820–1900), *NYJM* **14**:70. *4332*

1855:13 '**Rinne's test for hearing**' devised by Friedrich Heinrich Rinne (1819–1868), *VPH* **45**:71; **46**:45. *3370*

1855:14 The modern **laryngoscope** introduced by Manuel Garcia (1805–1906), a singing teacher, *PRS* **7**:399. *3329*

1855:15 First full clinical description of **haemophilia** by Johann Ludwig Grandidier (b.1810); in his *Die Haemophilie oder die Bluterkrankheit. 3063*

1855:16 Friedrich Gustav Jakob Henle's (1809–1885) *Handbuch der systematischen Anatomie des Menschen*, 3 vols, 1855–71, is among the best of the modern systems and includes a description of '**Henle's loop**' in the **kidney**. *417*

1855:17 Guillaume Benjamin Amand Duchenne de Boulogne (1806–1875) was a pioneer of **electrotherapy**; his *De l'électrisation localisée et de son application à la physiologie* ... included a classification of the **electrophysiology** of the **muscular system**. *614, 1995*

1855:18 Mechanism of **accommodation** in the eye explained by Hermann von Helmholtz (1821–1894), *GAO* **1**, ii:1. *1509*

1855:19 Henri **Luc**, French laryngologist, born 6 Jan; devised operation for abscess of the maxillary sinus ('**Caldwell-Luc operation**' following later work by George Walter Caldwell); in his *Des abscès du sinus maxillaire*, 1889. Died 1925. *3301*

1855:20 Morris **Simmonds**, Danish pathologist, born 14 Jan; described pituitary cachexia (Simmonds' disease), 1914, *DMW* **40**:322; *VA* **217**:226. Died 1925. *3901*

1855:21 Albert Ludwig Siegmund **Neisser**, German dermatologist and bacteriologist, born 22 Jan; discovered the gonococcus, causal organism in gonorrhoea, 1879, *ZMW* **17**:497, and later named *Neisseria gonorrhoeae*. With tissue obtained from Gerhard Hansen and using aniline dyes, demonstrated the leprosy bacillus (*Mycobacterium leprae*) better than Hansen, 1879, *JANVB* **57**:65. With August von Wassermann and C. Bruck, introduced a specific diagnostic blood test for syphilis, the 'Wassermann reaction', 1906, *DMW* **32**:745. Died 1916. *5208, 2436.1, 2402*

1855:22 Moritz Wilhelm Hugo **Ribbert**, German pathologist, born 1 Mar; the modern protagonist of the embryonal theory of cancer, *Die Entstehung des Carcinoms*, 1905. Died 1920. *2632*

1855:23 Luther Emmett **Holt**, American paediatrician, born 4 Mar; isolated heparin with William Henry Howell, 1919, *AmJPh* **47**:328. Died 1924. *905*

1855:24 William Chapman **Jarvis**, American laryngologist, born 13 May; introduced the Jarvis nasal snare in nasal surgery, 1881, *TALA* **2**:130. Died 1895. *3286*

1855:25 David **Bruce**, Australian bacteriologist, born 29 May; showed that brucellosis (Malta fever) was due to a micrococcus, *Brucella melitensis*, 1887, *Prac* **39**:161. In his *Preliminary report on the tsetse fly disease or nagana, in Zululand*, 1895, showed that it was due to a trypanosome, *Trypanosoma brucei*. Sent to Africa, with D.N. Nabarro, by the Royal Society of London to study sleeping sickness, reported (*Report of the Sleeping Sickness Commission of the Royal Society, 1903–1912*, 17 pts, 1903–19) that the tsetse fly was the vector of the trypanosome. Died 1931. *5098, 5273, 5277*

1855:26 Edward Hartley **Angle**, American orthodontist, born 1 Jun; through his work the speciality of orthodontics was considerably advanced, 1887, *IMC 9* **5**:565. Died 1930. *3686*

1855:27 Karl Gottfried Paul **Döhle**, German pathologist, born 6 Jun; defined specific syphilitic lesion as a cause of aortic aneurysm, 1895, *DAKM* **55**:190. Died 1928. *2985.1*

1855:28 Rudolph von **Jaksch**, Bohemian paediatrician, born 16 Jul; his classic description of infantile pseudoleukaemic anaemia led to the term 'von Jaksch's disease', 1889, *WKW* **2**:435, 456. Died 1947. *3131*

1855:29 Anatole Marie Emile **Chauffard**, French physician, born 22 Aug; gave an important description of pseudoxanthoma elasticum, 1889, *BSMH* **6**:412. Described familial haemolytic jaundice ('Minkowski-Chauffard disease'), 1907, *SMP* **27**:25; it had already been described by Minkowski in 1900. Died 1932. *4096.1, 3781, 3779*

1855:30 James Leonard **Corning**, American neurologist, born 26 Aug; introduced spinal anaesthesia, 1885, *NYMJ* **42**:483. Died 1923. *5680*

1855:31 Arnold **Netter**, French physician, born 20 Sep; with Constantin Levaditi, discovered antibodies in human poliomyelitis convalescent serum, 1910, *CRSB* **68**:855. Died 1953. *4670.2*

1855:32 Adolpho **Lutz**, Brazilian physician, born 18 Dec; first described South American blastomycosis, 1908, *BrM* **22**:121, 141. Died 1940. *5532.1*

1855:33 Hubert Montague **Murray**, British physician, born; reported in 1907 a case of asbestosis observed in 1899; in *Report of Departmental Committee on Compensation for Industrial Diseases*, Col. 3495–6. Died 1907. *2130*

1855:34 William Henry **Battle**, British surgeon, born; devised operation for the repair of femoral hernia, 1901, *L* **1**:302. Died 1936. *3606*

1855:35 Jaroslav **Hlava**, Czech physician and pathological anatomist, born; induced experimental amoebiasis induced in cats by the intrarectal inoculation of stools, 1887, *CLC* **26**:70. Died 1924. *5186.1*

1855: Theodor **Beck** died, **born** 1791. *medical jurisprudence*

1855: François **Magendie** died, **born** 1783. *emetine, anaphylaxis, cerebrospinal fluid, foramen of Magendie*

1855: Horatio Gates **Jameson** died, **born** 1788. *excision of superior maxilla*

1855: William **Cumming** died, **born** 1822. *eye*

1855: George **Ballingall** died, **born** 1780. *amoebic and bacillary dysentery*

**1856**
1856:1 **Berlin water supply filtered**

1856:2 **Pandemic diphtheria** 1856–1859

1856:3 **Adrenaline** discovered in the adrenal medulla by Edmé Félix Alfred Vulpian (1826–1887), *CRAS* **43**:663. *1141*

1856:4 The **non-mercurial** treatment of **iriditis** described by Henry Willard Williams (1821–1895), *BMSJ* **55**:49, 69, 92. *5878*

1856:5 *Treatment of the insane without mechanical restraints* published by John Conolly (1794–1866); he was treating his **insane** patients without any form of restraint as early as 1839. *4933*

1856:6 Charles Édouard Brown-Séquard (1817–1894) produced experimental **epilepsy** by section of the **sciatic nerve**, *ArGM* **7**:143 and proved indispensability of the **adrenal glands**, *CRAS* **43**:422, 452. *4813, 1140*

1856:7 The first systematic account of **brain abscess** given by Hermann Lebert (1813–1878), *VA* **10**:78, 352. *4638*

1856:8 The lesions of **locomotor ataxia (tabes dorsalis)** shown by William Withey Gull (1816–1890) to be located in the posterior columns of the spinal cord, *GHR* **2**:143; **4**:169. *4532*

1856:9 **Crossed hemiplegia** ('**Gubler's paralysis**') described by Adolphe Gubler (1821–1897), *GMC* **3**:749, 789, 811. The later account by Hermann David Weber (1863) led to the eponym '**Weber-Gubler syndrome**'. *4531*

1856:10 Pierre Louis Alphée Cazenave (1795–1877), who founded the first scientific **dermatological** journal (*Annales des Maladies de la Peau et de la Syphilis*), classified **skin diseases** on an anatomical basis. His *Leçons sur les maladies de la peau* first appeared in fascicules, 1845–56. *3992.1*

1856:11 First demonstration of a **fungus** in **eczema marginatum** and a clear description of **pityriasis pilaris** given by Marie Guillaume Alphonse Devergie (1798–1879), *GMC* **3**:197. *4044*

1856:12 Samuel Wilks (1824–1911) gave an authoritative account of **lymphadenoma**, *GHR* **2**:114; in a later paper, 1865, he named it '**Hodgkin's disease**'. *3764*

1856:13 Binaural **stethoscope** introduced by Arthur Leared (1822–1879), *L* **2**:138, 202. *2676.1*

1856:14 Rudolf Albert von Kölliker (1817–1905) published the first study of the effects of **poisons** on **muscular contraction**, 1856, *VA* **10**:3, 335. *2078*

1856:15 Pulmonary **aspergillosis** first described by Rudolf Virchow (1821–1902), *VA* **9**:557. *3169*

1856:16 The first **pharyngotomy** in England performed by Edward Cock (1805–1892), *L* **1**:125. *3265*

1856:17 **Syphilis:** inoculability demonstrated experimentally by Julius Bettinger (1802–1878), *AIB* **3**:425. *2384*

1856:18 Mode of action of **curare** described by Claude Bernard (1813–1878), *CRAS* **43**:825. *2079*

1856:19 **Blood pressure** first accurately estimated by Jean Faivre, *ASML*, 2 sér **4**:180. *773*

1856:20 **Artificial respiration**, Marshall Hall (1790–1857) method introduced, *L* **1**:129. *2028.56*

---

1856:21 Louis Anne Jean **Brocq**, French dermatologist, born 1 Feb; described parasporosis, previously described under other names, 1902, *AnD* **3**:313, 433; also called 'Brocq's disease'. Died 1928. *4135*

1856:22 Emil **Kraepelin**, German psychiatrist, born 15 Feb; evolved a new classification of insanity; in his *Einführing in die psychiatrische Klinik*, 1901. He introduced the concepts of dementia praecox (schizophrenia) and manic-depressive insanity. Died 1926. *4952*

1856:23 Alfred **Einhorn**, German chemist, born 27 Feb; synthesized procaine (novocaine), 1899, *MMW* **46**:1218, 1254. Died 1917. *5685*

1856:24 Howard Henry **Tooth**, British physician, born 22 Apr; published *The peroneal type of progressive muscular atrophy*, 1886, the same year as it was independently described by Charcot and Marie (Charcot-Marie-Tooth type of peroneal muscular atrophy). Died 1925. *4750, 4749*

1856:25 Jean **Darier**, Swiss/French dermatologist, born 26 Apr; his excellent description of keratosis follicularis (dyskeratosis), 1889, *AnD* **10**:597, earned the eponym 'Darier's disease'; it was first described by Lutz and later by J.C. White. Described acanthosis nigricans, 1893, *AnD* **4**:865; it had been illustrated by Pollitzer and Janovsky in 1890. Introduced the term *tuberculides* to describe the skin eruptions associated with tuberculosis, 1896, *AnD* **7**:1431. Died 1938. *4050, 4093, 4097, 4113, 4102, 4112*

1856:26 Sigmund **Freud**, Austrian psychiatrist and psychologist, born 6 May; in his *Zur Auffassung der Aphasien*, 1891, he refuted the doctrines of Wernicke and Lichtheim. He distinguished between defects in naming objects ('asymbolic aphasia') and defects in recognizing objects ('agnosia'). With Josef Breuer, introduced psychoanalysis, 1893, the foundation stone was their *Studien über Hysterie*, 1895. The interpretation of dreams, *Die Traumdeutung*, 1900, was his greatest work. Used the 'cathartic method' in hysterical patients as a basis for development of the method of free association and of the essential psychoanalytic concepts of the unconscious, repression and transference; in *Studien über Hysterie*, 1895. Gave an excellent description of the various forms of cerebral palsy, with precise classification of the different spastic symptoms; in his *Die infantile Cerebrallähmung*, 1897. Died 1939. *4627.1, 4977.3, 4978, 4980, 4999, 4708.2*

1856:27 Hermann **Sahli**, Swiss physician, born 23 May; introduced 'Sahli's test' for estimating the functional activity of the stomach, 1891, *KBSA* **21**:65. Died 1933. *3500*

1856:28 Frank **Hartley**, American neurosurgeon, born 10 Jun; introduced the operation of intracranial neurectomy for facial neuralgia (Hartley-Krause operation), 1892, *NYMJ* **55**:317, independently of Fedor Krause. Died 1913. *4870, 4871*

1856:29 William Arbuthnot **Lane**, British surgeon, born 4 Jul; introduced mastoidectomy for middle-ear suppuration drainage (antrectomy), 1892, *ArOt* **21**:118. Introduced a method of treatment of fractures by 'osteosynthesis' – the perfect re-apposition of the affected parts by operative intervention, 1894, *TCSL* **27**:167; described 'Lane's plates and screws' for the union of fractures, 1907, *BMJ* **1**:1037. Treated chronic constipation by short-circuiting the intestine; in his *The operative treatment of chronic constipation*, 1909. Died 1943. *3394.2, 4428, 4430, 3531*

1856:30 Augustus Désiré **Waller**, French physiologist, born 12 Jul; using electrodes, he demonstrated the action currents of the heart, preparing the ground for electrocardiography, 1887, *JP* **8**:229. He obtained the first electrocardiogram in man. Died 1922. *833*

1856:31 Francis Xavier **Dercum**, American neurologist, born 10 Aug; first to describe adiposis dolorosa ('Dercum's disease'), 1888, *UMM* **1**:140. Died 1931. *3917*

1856:32 Fritz **Frank**, German gynaecologist, born 17 Aug; introduced suprasymphyseal transperitoneal caesarean section, 1907, *ArGy* **81**:46. Died 1923. *6247*

1856:33 Charles Alfred **Ballance**, British neurosurgeon, born 30 Aug; in his *Some points on the surgery of the brain and its membranes*, 1907, recognized chronic subdural haematoma and described it with great accuracy, he operated for it and for subdural hydroma and fully discussed brain abscess and brain tumours. With Charles David Green, published the classic *Essays on the surgery of the temporal bone*, 1919. With Arthur Baldwin Duel, treated facial palsy by nerve grafts into the Fallopian canal and by other intratemporal methods, 1932, *ArOt(C)* **15**:1. Died 1936. *4879.01, 3403.1, 4889.1, 4899*

1856:34 Gustav Adolf **Walcher**, German obstetrician and gynaecologist, born 21 Sep; described the 'Walcher position', 1889, *ZGy* **13**:892. Died 1935. *6200*

1856:35 Edmund Beecher **Wilson**, American cytologist, histologist and geneticist, born 19 Oct; studied cell lineage, germinal localization, and the chromosomal theory of sex determination; in his *The cell in development and inheritance*, 1896; 3rd edn, *The cell in development and heredity*, 1925. Died 1939. *238*

1856:36 Pietro **Canalis**, Italian malariologist, born 27 Oct; in his studies on malaria, demonstrated and clearly differentiated *Plasmodium falciparum* from *P.vivax* and *P.malariae*, 1890, *ArIB* **13**:262. Died 1939. *5240.1*

1856:37 Alfred **Kast**, German physician, born; with Oscar Hinsberg, introduced phenacetin, 1887, *ZMW* **25**:145; he also introduced sulphonal, previously prepared by Eugen Baumann, 1888, *BKW* **25**:309. Died 1903. *1883.3, 1884*

1856:38 Gustav **Hauser**, German bacteriologist, born; isolated *Proteus vulgaris*, 1885; in his *Fäulnissbacterien*. Died 1935. *2502*

1856:39 William **Pasteur**, British physician, born; first discovered and described massive collapse of the lung, 1908, *L* **2**:1351. Died 1943. *3188*

1856:40 Charles Barrett **Lockwood**, British surgeon, born; published his operation for the radical cure of femoral hernia, 1893, *L* **2**:1297. Died 1914. *3604*

1856:41 Richard John **Hall**, Irish/American physician, born; first to report a case of survival after removal of perforated appendix, 1886, *NYMJ* **43**:662. Died 1897. *3568*

1856:42 Russell Henry **Chittenden**, American biochemist and nutritionist, born; with Wilhelm Friedrich [Willy] Kühn, isolated and named several products of digestion, 1883, *ZBi* **19**:159. Died 1943. *1016*

1856: John Ayrton **Paris** died, **born** 1785. *arsenic cancer*

1856: John Collins **Warren** died, **born** 1778. *tumours, anaesthesia, ether, staphylorrhaphy, Massachusetts General Hospital*

1856: Jean Zuléma **Amussat** died, **born** 1796. *artificial anus, colostomy* ⸳

1856: George James **Guthrie** died, **born** 1785. *bladder obstruction, prostatectomy, amputation at hip-joint, ophthalmic surgery, gunshot wounds, peroneal artery ligation*

1856: Heinrich **Meckel von Hemsbach** died, **born** 1821. *ophthalmia*

1856: Agostino **Bassi** died, **born** 1773. *muscardine disease of silkworms, pathogenic microbes*

**1857**

1857:1 *British Medical Journal* replaces *Association Medical Journal*

1857:2 **University of Chicago** founded

1857:3 **Universities of Calcutta and Madras** founded

1857:4 **Pathological Society of Philadelphia** founded

1857:5 The operation of **iridectomy** for the treatment of **glaucoma** introduced by Albrecht von Graefe (1828–1870), *GAO* **5**, i:136. *5881*

1857:6 A **vaginal speculum** designed by William Fergusson (1808–1877) described in his *System of practical surgery*, 4th edn, p. 724. *6043*

1857:7 An operation for **strabismus** described by Albrecht von Graefe (1828–1870), *GAO* **3**, ii:456; **4**, ii:127; **8**, ii:242. *5880*

1857:8 An accurate account of the **tsetse fly**, *Glossina morsitans*, and of the disease in cattle, **trypanosomiasis**, due to its bite given by David Livingstone (1813–1873); in his *Missionary travels and researches in South Africa*, pp. 80, 571. *5269*

1857:9 **Potassium bromide** first used in the treatment of **epilepsy** by William O'Connor (d.1880), *L* **1**:525. *4814*

1857:10 A technique of **amputation** of the **thigh** introduced by Rocco Gritti (1826–1920), *AnU* **161**:5, later improved by William Stokes, 1870. *4466, 4470*

1857:11 First description of **pityriasis rubra** ('**Hebra's pityriasis**') given by Ferdinand von Hebra (1816–1880), *AWMZ* **2**:75. *4045*

1857:12 The presence of **acetone** in **diabetic urine** demonstrated by Wilhelm Petters, *VPH* **55**:81. *3935*

1857:13 *Balantidium coli*, the first **parasitic protozoon** to be recognized as such, discovered by Pehr Henrik Malmsten (1811–1883), *Hygiea* **19**:491. *3455*

1857:14 **Treitz's hernia – retroperitoneal hernia** through the **duodenal-jejunal recess** described by Wenzel Treitz (1819–1872); in his *Hernia retroperitonealis*. *3591*

1857:15 The first operation for **tumour** of the **oesophagus** was performed by Albrecht Theodor Middeldorpf (1824–1868); reported in his *De polypis oesophagi*. *3456*

1857:16 Acute **leukaemia** first described by Nikolaus Friedreich (1826–1882), *VA* **12**:37. *3064.1*

1857:17 Experiments with **curare** carried out by Claude Bernard (1813–1878); reported in his *Leçons sur les effets des substances toxiques et médicamenteuses. 1863*

1857:18 Connection between **fermentation** and living microorganisms demonstrated by Louis Pasteur (1822–1895), considered the beginning of **bacteriology** as a modern science; *CRAS* **45**:913; **48**:557; **50**:303; **51**:348, 675; *AnSN* **16**:5. *2472–2475*

1857:19 **Glycogen** discovered by Claude Bernard (1813–1878), *CRSB*, 2 sér. **4**:147. *999.1*

1857:20 Digestive action of the **pancreatic juice** discovered by Claude Bernard (1813–1878), *ArGM* **19**:60. *996*

---

1857:21 Vladimir Michailovich **Bechterev**, Russian neuropsychiatrist, born 20 Jan; he was one of several authors to give an early description of ankylosing spondylitis, 1892, *Vrach* **13**:899, and one of its several eponyms was 'Bechterev's disease'. Died 1927. *4360*

1857:22 Wilhelm Ludvig **Johannsen**, Danish biologist, born 3 Feb; supported the Mendelian law of inheritance, *Ueber Erblichkeit in Populationen und in reinen Linien*, 1903, and introduced the concepts of 'gene', 'genotype' and 'phenotype'. Died 1927. *242*

1857:23 Julius **Wagner von Jauregg**, Austrian psychiatrist, born 7 Mar; inoculated paretics with malaria to induce pyrexia, 1918, *PNW* **20**:132, 251, a form of treatment he first used in 1887, *JaP* **7**:94, to study the effect of fevers upon psychotic conditions. For this work he received the Nobel Prize (Physiology or Medicine), 1927, *NPL*. Died 1940. *4806, 4946*

1857:24 Fedor **Krause**, German neurosurgeon, born 10 Mar; popularized the use of whole-thickness skin grafts, 1893, *VDGC* **22** ii:46. Introduced the operation of intracranial neurectomy for facial neuralgia (Hartley-Krause operation), 1892, *ArKC* **44**:821, independently of Frank Hartley. With Macewen, Cushing and Ballance, was a pioneer of neurosurgery as a speciality; his most comprehensive work is *Chirurgie des Gehirns und Rückenmarks*, 2 vols, 1908–11. With Hermann Küttner, devised an operation for gastric crises in tabes, 1909, *BKC* **63**:245; with Hermann Oppenheim, successfully removed a pineal tumour, 1913, *BKW* **50**:2316. Died 1937. *5755, 4871, 4880.2, 4881, 4884.1*

1857:25 Angelo **Celli**, Italian physician and malariologist, born 25 Mar; with Ettore Marchiafava, gave the first accurate description of the malaria parasite, *Plasmodium*, 1885, *FM* **3**:787. Died 1914. *5238*

1857:26 Théodore **Tuffier**, French surgeon, born 26 Mar; treated pulmonary tuberculosis by removal of lung apex; in his *Chirurgie du poumon* ..., 1897. Attempted to visualize the urinary tract by a combination of an opaque ureteral styletted catheter and radiography, 1899; in Duplay, S.& Reclus, P. *Traité de chirurgie*, **7**:448. Introduced a method of extrapleural pneumolysis, 1910, *BSCP* **36**:529. Carried out first successful experimental surgical treatment for chronic valvular disease, 1914, *BuAM* **71**:293. Died 1929. *3228, 4191.1, 3191, 3029*

1857:27 Franz **Ziehl**, German physician, born 13 Apr; introduced Ziehl-Neelsen stain for staining *Mycobacterium tuberculosis*, 1882, *DMW* **8**:451. Died 1926. *2331.1*

1857:28 Victor Alexander Haden **Horsley**, British surgeon, born 14 Apr; founder of neurosurgery in England. With Charles Edward Beevor investigated localization of cerebral function, 1887, *PTB* **176**:153. With William Richard Gowers, recorded first successful operation for removal of an extramedullary tumour of the spinal cord, 1888, *MCT* **71**:377. With Robert Henry Clarke, devised the stereotactic apparatus for the accurate location of electrodes in the brain opening the way to stereotactic surgery of that organ, 1908, *Brain*

**31**:45. Demonstrated that athetosis could be abolished by removal of precentral area of the brain, 1909, *BMJ* **2**:125. Died 1916. *1416.1, 4860, 1435.1, 4879.1, 4882*

1857:29 Paul Eugen **Bleuler**, Swiss psychiatrist, born 30 Apr; introduced the concept of schizophrenia and showed, in his *Dementia praecox oder die Gruppe der Schizophrenien*, 1911, that dementia praecox should include all the schizophrenias. Died 1939. *4957*

1857:30 Louis **Bard**, French pathologist, born 10 May; with Adrien Pic, described Bard-Pic syndrome, a complication of pancreatic carcinoma, 1888, *ReM* **8**:257, 363. Died 1930. *3630*

1857:31 Ronald **Ross**, British physician and malariologist, born 13 May; provided proof that the mosquito is responsible for the transmission of malaria, 1897, *BMJ* **2**:1786, he found *Plasmodium* in the stomach of *Anopheles* after it had been fed on the blood of malaria patients. Provided the last link in the chain demonstrating the complete life-cycle of the parasite of bird malaria, 1898, *L* **2**:488. Awarded Nobel Prize (Physiology or Medicine), 1901, *NPL*. Died 1932. *5247, 5251*

1857:32 John Jacob **Abel**, American physiological chemist and pharmacologist, born 19 May; obtained crystalline insulin, 1926, *PNAS* **12**:132. Died 1938. *1206, 3971*

1857:33 Pierre Félix **Lagrange**, French ophthalmologist, born 22 Jun; introduced sclerectomy for the treatment of glaucoma, 1907, *GSMB* **28**:2. Died 1928. *5953*

1857:34 Frederic William **Hewitt**, British anaesthetist, born 2 Jul; did much to develop the use of ether and advanced the knowledge of the pharmacology of anaesthetics, introducing the first practical gas and oxygen apparatus in 1892. Wrote *Anaesthetics and their administration*, 1893; described a nitrous oxide/oxygen stopcock, 1894, *JBDA* **15**:380. Died 1916. *5682, 5682.1*

1857:35 Alfred **Binet**, French psychologist, born 8 Jul; with Théodore Simon, devised the Binet-Simon intelligence tests; in their *La mésure du developpement de l'intelligence chez les jeunes enfants*, 1911. Binet had published a plan for studying intelligence as early as 1895. Died 1911. *4985*

1857:36 Daniel Alcides **Carrión**, Peruvian physician, born 13 Aug; in order to prove or disprove the connection between Oroya fever and verruca peruviana, Carrión had himself inoculated with blood from a patient suffering from verruca peruviana and died from the disease soon afterwards. Oroya fever was also named Carrión's disease by Ernesto Odriozola, 1895, *MonM* **10**:309. Died 1885. *5530*

1857:37 Georges **Gilles de la Tourette**, French neuropsychiatrist, born 30 Oct; described a syndrome consisting of generalized tics, motor incoordination, coprolalia and echolalia, 'Gilles de la Tourette syndrome', 1884, *ArN* **8**:68. Died 1904. *4848*

1857:38 Joseph François Félix **Babinski**, French neurologist, born 17 Nov; described the extensor plantar response which occurs in pyramidal-tract disease ('Babinski reflex'), 1896, *CRSB* **48**:207. Described pituitary tumour and sexual infantilism without acromegaly ('Fröhlich's syndrome') one year before Fröhlich, 1900, *ReN* **8**:531. With Jean Nageotte, described a syndrome of multiple medullary lesions of vascular origin involving the medullary tract and other structures ('syndrome of Babinski-Nageotte'), 1902, *ReN* **10**:358. Described and named anosognosia (unconcern for, or denial of, striking neurological disorders), 1914, *ReN* **22**:845. Died 1932. *4583, 3887, 4589, 4596.2*

1857:39 Archibald Edward **Garrod**, British physician, born 25 Nov; described overt disease due to congenital biochemical abnormalities in *Inborn errors of metabolism*, 1909. Died 1936. *244.1, 3921*

1857:40 Charles Scott **Sherrington**, British neurophysiologist, born 27 Nov. Made many valuable contributions to knowledge of the nervous system; including an investigation of the reciprocal innervation of muscle, 1892, *JP* **13**:621, 1893; *PRS* **53**:407; the proprioceptive system, 1906, *Brain* **29**:467; investigation of the stretch reflex (with E.G.T. Liddell), 1924–5, *PRSB* **96**:212; **97**:267. His most influential publication is probably *The integrative action of the nervous system*, 1906. He shared the Nobel Prize (Physiology or Medicine) with Edgar Douglas Adrian, 1932, for the isolation and functional analysis of the motor unit (motor cell in the spinal cord, *NPL*. Died 1952. *1288, 1288.1, 1300.1, 1443, 1432*

1857:41 Theodor **Escherich**, German paediatrician and bacteriologist, born 29 Nov; in his *Die Darmbakterien des Säuglings*, 1886, he gave the first description of *Bact. coli* infection; the genus was later named *Escherichia coli* after him. Died 1911. *6340*

1857:42 Carl **Koller**, Bohemian ophthalmologist, born 3 Dec; the first to demonstrate the practical value of cocaine, as a local anaesthetic in ophthalmology, 1884, *KMA* **22** B:60. Died 1944. *5678, 5925*

1857:43 John Benjamin **Murphy**, American surgeon, born 21 Dec; introduced 'Murphy's button' for gastric and intestinal anastomosis, 1892, *MR* **42**:665. First successful suture of femoral artery, end-to-end anastomosis, 1896, *MR* **51**:73. Died 1916. *3507, 2967*

1857:44 Oscar Heinrich **Hinsberg**, German physician, born; with Alfred Kast, introduced phenacetin, 1887, *ZMW* **25**:145. Died 1939. *1883.3*

1857:45 John Templeton **Bowen**, American dermatologist, born; described 'Bowen's disease' in 1912, a type of intra-epidermal basal-cell epithelioma, named after Bowen although described a year earlier by Queyrat, *JCGU* **30**:241. Died 1940. *4148, 4146*

1857:46 Johann **Hoffmann**, German neurologist, born; described an infantile familial form of progressive muscular atrophy, 1891, *DZN* **1**:95; **3**:427, and independently in the same year by Werdnig and named ('Werdnig-Hoffmann muscular atrophy'). Died 1919. *4756, 4755*

1857: Marshall **Hall** died, **born** 1790. *reflex action, artificial respiration, epilepsy*

1857: William **Wood** died, **born** 1774. *neuroma*

1857: Samuel **Tuke** died, **born** 1784. *psychiatry*

## 1858
1858:1 **Public Health and Local Government Acts** in **England** (transfer of functions of **General Board of Health** to Privy Council and Home Secretary)

1858:2 **Medical Act, UK**, regulating status of qualified and registered medical practitioners

1858:3 **General Medical Council**, UK, established by Medical Act, 1858; its duties include maintenance of high standard of professional conduct and behaviour, supervision of medical education, publication of an annual *Medical Register* (1859) of those qualified to practise, and publication of the *British Pharmacopoeia*

1858:4 Wilhelm Max Wundt (1832–1920) commenced his series of publications on **sensory perception**, 1858–1863, ZRM **4**:229; **7**:279, 321; **12**:145; **14**:1; **15**:104. *1463*

1858:5 The operation of **epicystotomy**, for **bladder stone**, devised by Emil Noeggerath (1827–1895), NYJM **4**:9. *6044*

1858:6 First edition of Gray's *Anatomy* published by Henry Gray (1827–1861). *418*

1858:7 *Der Gebärmutterkrebs*, by Ernst Leberecht Wagner (1829–1888) represents the first important contribution to the knowledge of the gross pathology of **cancer** of the **uterus**. *6045*

1858:8 **Verruga peruana** was the name given by Tomas Salazar (1830–1917) to **bartonellosis** (**Carrión's disease, Oroya fever**), caused by infection with *Bartonella bacilliformis*, GMLi **2**:161, 175. *5525*

1858:9 John Snow (1813–1858) was the first specialist in **anaesthesiology**; he delivered Queen Victoria in 1853 and 1857, using **chloroform**. His *On chloroform and other anaesthetics: their action and administration*, put the administration of chloroform and ether on a scientific basis. *5666*

1858:10 David Livingstone (1813–1873) administered **arsenic** in the treatment of '**nagana**', a disease in horses due to the bite of the **tsetse fly**, *Glossina morsitans*, BMJ 360. *5270*

1858:11 *A manual of psychological medicine*, by the British neurologists John Charles Bucknill (1817–1897) and Daniel Hack Tuke (1827–1895) was for many years the standard English work on **psychological medicine**. *4934*

1858:12 First excision of the superior **maxillary nerve** for the treatment of **facial neuralgia** carried out by John Murray Carnochan (1817–1887), AmJMS **35**:134. *4854*

1858:13 **Galvanotherapy** pioneered by Robert Remak (1815–1865); published *Galvanotherapie der Nerven- und Muskelkrankheiten. 4534*

1858:14 The classic account of **tabes dorsalis** given by Guillaume Benjamin Amand Duchenne (1806–1875), ArGM **12**:641; **13**:36, 158, 417, earned the eponym '**Duchenne's disease**'. *4774*

1858:15 '**Foville's syndrome**', crossed **paralysis of the limbs** on one side of the body and of the face on the other side (with loss of ability to rotate the eye), reported by Achille Louis François Foville (1799–1878), BSAP **33**:393. *4533*

1858:16 **Chromidrosis**, the secretion of coloured **sweat**, first described by Alfred Le Roy de Méricourt (1825–1901), BuAM **23**:1141; **26**:773. *4046*

1858:17 The first **gastrostomy** in Britain carried out by John Cooper Forster (1823–1886), GHR **4**:13. *3457*

1858:18 **Laryngoscope** improved by Johann Nepomuk Czermak (1828–1873), *SAW* **29**:557. *3331*

1858:19 First comprehensive study of **heart malformations** by Thomas Bevill Peacock (1812–1882); in his *On malformation, etc., of the human heart. 2761*

1858:20 **Syphilis: 'Hutchinson's teeth'**, the notched incisors present in congenital syphilis, described by Jonathan Hutchinson (1828–1913), *TPS* **9**:449. *2386*

1858:21 **Artificial respiration**; Silvester method invented by Henry Robert Silvester (1828–1908), *BMJ* 586. *2028.57*

1858:22 **Inflammation**; Joseph Lister's (1827–1912) researches published, *PT* **148**:645. *2298*

1858:23 **Syphilis** shown by Rudolf Virchow (1821–1902) to be a disease involving all organs and tissues, *VA* **15**:217. *2385*

1858:24 **Pathology**; *Die Cellularpathologie* published by Rudolph Virchow (1821–1902). *2299*

1858:25 To avoid **sepsis** in surgery James Marion Sims (1813–1883) introduced a **silver wire suture**; *Silver sutures in surgery. 5605*

---

1858:26 Hermann **Oppenheim**, German neurologist, born 1 Jan; first described amyotonia congenita ('Oppenheim's disease'), 1900, *MonP* **8**:232. With Fedor Krause, successfully removed a pineal tumour, 1913, *BKW* **50**:2316. Died 1919. *4760, 4884.1*

1858:27 Bernard **Sachs**, American neurologist, born 2 Jan; described cerebral changes in amaurotic familial idiocy **'Tay-Sachs disease'**, 1887, *JNMD* **14**:541. Died 1944. *4705, 5918*

1858:28 Oscar **Minkowski**, Russian-born pathologist, born 13 Jan; discovered beta-oxybutyric acid in the urine in diabetes mellitus, 1884, *ArEP* **18**:35. First pointed out the constancy of pituitary enlargement in acromegaly, 1887, *BKW* **24**:371. With Joseph von Mering, produced experimental diabetes mellitus by removing the pancreas of a dog, proving the role of the pancreas in diabetes, 1890, *ArEP* **26**:371. Described familial haemolytic jaundice ('Minkowski-Chauffard disease'), 1900, *VDK* **18**:316. Died 1931. *3947, 3885, 3950, 3779*

1858:29 Howard Atwood **Kelly**, American gynaecologist, born 20 Feb; professor at Pennsylvania and Johns Hopkins University and a leader in the field, published *Operative gynecology*, 1899, 2 vols. Introduced the aeroscopic examination of the bladder and catheterization of the ureters under direct inspection, 1893, *JHB* **4**:101. Published method of uretero-ureteral anastomosis using the catheter as a temporary ureteral splint, 1894, *AnS* **27**:475. Tipped catheter with wax so that it registered any pressure from renal and ureteral calculi, 1901, *AmJOD* **44**:441. Died 1943. *6108, 4187, 4188, 4295*

1858:30 Richard Friedrich Johannes **Pfeiffer**, German bacteriologist, born 29 Mar; discovered a bacillus (*Haemophilus influenzae*), then believed to be the causal organism in (bacterial) influenza, 1892, *DMW* **18**:28. With Vasiliy Isayevich Isayev [Issayaeff] recorded immune bacteriolysis ('Pfeiffer phenomenon') in *Cholera vibrio*, 1894, *ZHyg* **17**:355; **18**:1. Died 1945. *5490, 2546*

1858:31 Janos **Bokay**, Hungarian paediatrician, born 19 Apr; first suggested an aetiological relationship between varicella and herpes zoster, 1892, *MOA*: Nov. 3. Died 1937. *5439.1*

1858:32 Arthur Nathan **Hanau**, German physician, born 11 May; successfully transplanted cancer in mammals, 1889, *FM* **7**:321. Died 1900. *2621*

1858:33 Ismar Isidor **Boas**, Polish gastroenterologist, born 28 May; introduced duodenal aspiration, 1889, *ZenKM* **10**:97. Died 1938. *3496*

1858:34 Maurice **Klippel**, French neurologist, born 30 May; with Paul Trenaunay, described the Klippel-Trenaunay syndrome (angio-osteohypertrophy), 1900, *ArGM* **185**:642; with André Feil, first reported absence or incomplete development of cervical vertebrae ('Klippel-Feil syndrome'), 1912, *NIS* **25**:223. Died 1942. *4131*

1858:35 Bernard Jean Antonin **Marfan**, French paediatrician, born 23 Jun; first described Marfan's syndrome, 1896, *BSMH* **13**:220, although he described only the skeletal deformities (arachnodactyly, dolichostenomelia); eye and vascular system complications were recorded by later writers. Died 1942. *4365.1*

1858:36 Robert **Jones**, British orthopaedic surgeon, born 28 Jun; with Oliver Lodge, clinical use of x rays to locate a bullet in the wrist, 22 February 1896, *L* **1**:476. Became one of the greatest figures in British orthopaedics; with R.W. Lovett wrote *Orthopaedic surgery*, 1923. Died 1933. *2684, 4391*

1858:37 Harry **Swift**, British/Australian physician, born 7 Aug; gave the first full description of acrodynia ('pink disease', 'Swift's disease'), 1914, *TAMC* **10**:547. Died 1937. *6348*

1858:38 Christiaan **Eijkman**, Dutch physician, born 11 Aug; showed that beriberi is due to a diet of over-milled rice, 1896, *GTNI* **30**:295; **32**:353; **36**:214. He shared the Nobel Prize (Physiology or Medicine), 1929, with Frederick Gowland Hopkins, for his work on disease of dietary deficiency origin, *NPL*. Died 1930. *3741*

1858:39 Michael Idvorsky **Pupin**, Bohemian/American physicist, born 4 Oct; introduced the intensifying screen into radiography, 1896, *EI* **10**:68. Died 1935. *2685*

1858:40 Hugo Karl **Plaut**, German physician, born 12 Oct; described 'Plaut's angina', the association of fusiform bacilli in ulcerating tonsillar lesions, 1894, *DMW* **20**:920, later described more comprehensively by Jean Hyacinthe Vincent. Died 1928. *3308.1*

1858:41 Henry **Koplik**, American physician, born 28 Oct; first noted the buccal spots ('Koplik's spots'), an early diagnostic sign in measles, 1896, *ArPe* **13**:918. Died 1927. *5444*

1858:42 Karl Bernhard **Lehmann**, Swiss industrial hygienist, born 27 Nov; introduced trichlorethylene as an anaesthetic, 1911, *ArHyg* **74**:1. Died 1940. *5696*

1858:43 Frederick Lucius **Kilborne**, American bacteriologist, born; with Theobald Smith, discovered parasite of Texas cattle fever, *Babesia bigemina*, and proved its transmission by the cattle tick, *Boophilus annulatus* – the first demonstration of arthropod transmission of disease, *Investigations into ... Texas or Southern cattle fever*, 1893 (US Bureau of Animal Industry, Bulletin No. 1). Died 1936. *5529*

1858:44 Ernst Gottlob **Orthmann**, German gynaecologist, born; first to describe an ovarian tumour (the 'Brenner tumour'), 1899, *MonG* **9**:771, named after Fritz Brenner, who described it in 1907. Died 1922. *6109.1, 6118*

---

1858: Johannes **Müller** died, **born** 1801. *tumours, cell theory, specific nerve energies*

1858: Robert **Brown** died, **born** 1773. *cell nucleus*

1858: Richard **Bright** died, **born** 1789. *pathology, nephritis, chlorosis, epilepsy, yellow atrophy of liver*

1858: Pierre **Blaud** died, **born** 1774. *chlorosis*

1858: John Kearsley **Mitchell** died, **born** 1793. *malaria, neurotic spinal arthropathies*

1858: Antoine Laurent Jessé **Bayle** died, **born** 1799. *general paresis*

1858: Eugène **Soubeiran** died, **born** 1793. *chloroform*

1858: John **Snow** died, **born** 1813. *epidemiology, cholera, anaesthesia, ether*

1858: Hermann Franz Joseph **Naegele** died, **born** 1810. *obstetric auscultation*

1858: John Charles Weaver **Lever** died, **born** 1811. *puerperal convulsions*

**1859**
1859:1 First **sanatorium for tuberculous patients** opened in **Görbersdorf**, Germany

1859:2 **American Dental Association** founded

1859:3 Elizabeth Blackwell (1821–1910) was the first woman to be registered on the British **Medical Register**.

1859:4 Alfred Russel Wallace (1823–1913), British naturalist, independently of Darwin, formulated the principles of **natural selection**. His paper, *JPLSZ* **3**:53, which includes a contribution by Darwin, was the final stimulus for Darwin to publish his *Origin*. Died 1913. *219*

1859:5 *Origin of species*, theory of **evolution**, published by Charles Darwin (1809–1882). *220*

1859:6 The first successful **plastic operation** for **exstrophy** of the female **bladder** performed by Daniel Ayres (1822–1892), *AmMG* **10**:81. *6046*

1859:7 A valuable monograph on curvature of the **cornea**, *Die Krümmung der Hornhaut des menschlichen Auges*, written by Jakob Hermann Knapp (1832–1911), who became one of the leading ophthalmologists in America. *5884*

1859:8 The **medulla** confirmed as the ultimate seat of **epilepsy** by Jacob Ludwig Conrad Schroeder van der Kolk (1797–1862); in his *Bau und Functionen der Medulla spinalis und oblongata*, etc. *4815*

1859:9 Acute ascending **polyneuritis** ('**Landry's paralysis**') described by Jean Baptiste Octave Landry (1826–1865), *GMC* 6:472, 486. *4639*

1859:10 Archibald Baring Garrod (1819–1907) published *The nature and treatment of gout and rheumatic gout* and gave **rheumatoid arthritis** its present name. *4497*

1859:11 The first operation for **gastric fistula** was recorded by Albrecht Theodor Middeldorpf (1824–1868); reported in his *De fistulis ventriculi externis et chirurgica earum sanatione.* *3459*

1859:12 **Linitis plastica** ('**Brinton's disease**') first described by William Brinton (1823–1867); in his *Diseases of the stomach*, p. 310. *3458*

1859:13 **Myocardial infarction** accurately described by Pehr Henrik Malmsten (1811–1883) and Gustav Wilhelm Johann Düben (1822–1892), *Hygiea* **21**:629. *2761.1*

1859:14 **Heat-stroke** described by Thomas Longmore (1816–1895), *IAMS* **6**:396. *2248*

1859:15 **Cocaine** isolated from coca leaf by Albert Niemann (1834–1861); in his *Ueber eine neue organische Base in den Cocablättern. 1865*

1859:16 *Notes on hospitals* published by Florence Nightingale (1820–1910). *1611*

1859:17 **Fechner-Weber law** on stimulus and sensation; Gustav Theodor Fechner (1801–1887) showed the relationship between stimulus and sensation, *AbL* **4**:455. *1464*

1859:18 Acute **rickets** combined with **scurvy** ('**Barlow's disease**') first described by Julius Otto Ludwig Möller (1819–1887), *KMJ* **1**:377. *3718, 3720*

1859:19 First successful operation for **ectopia vesicae** (extroversion of the **bladder**) by Joseph Pancoast (1805–1882), *NAMR* **3**:710. *4170*

1859:20 **Sewage disposal** in London planned by Joseph William Bazalgette (1819–1891); in *Metropolitan Board of Works Report on experiments with respect to the ventilation of sewers*, 3 parts, 1886–1869. *1615*

1859:21 The physiology of **nerve** studied by Eduard Friedrich Wilhelm Pflüger (1829–1910) and recorded in his *Untersuchungen über die Physiologie des Electrotonus. 621*

1859:22 *System of surgery* by Samuel David Gross (1805–1884) was a massive work of nearly 2500 pages; it was his greatest work, intended to be the most elaborate treatise on the subject. *5607*

1859:23 **India-rubber tubes** for **drainage** of **abscesses** introduced by Pierre Marie Edouard Chassaignac (1804–1879). He put the subject of surgical drainage on a scientific and methodical basis, *Traité pratique de la suppuration et du drainage chirurgicale. 5606*

1859:24 Sigmund **Pollitzer**, American dermatologist, born 12 Jan; with Viktor Janovsky, first illustrated acanthosis nigricans; in their *Atlas seltener Hautkrankheiten*, 1890; it was described by Darier in 1893. Died 1937. *4102, 4113*

1859:25 Henry Havelock **Ellis**, British sexologist, born 2 Feb; devoted a lifetime to the study of the psychology of sex; his seven-volume *Studies in the psychology of sex*, begun in 1900, was completed in 1928. Died 1939. *4981*

1859:26 Gustav **Paul**, Bohemian public health officer, born 13 Feb; introduced a test for the diagnosis of smallpox, 1915, *ZPB* I Abt.**75**:518. Died 1933. *5431*

1859:27 Pierre **Curie**, French physicist, born 15 Mar; with Marie Curie isolated radium from pitchblende, 1898, *CRAS* **127**:175, 1215. They were jointly awarded the Nobel Prize (Physics), 1903, with Antoine Henri Becquerel for their discovery of radioactivity, *NPL*. Died 1906. *2003*

1859:28 Frederick William **Andrewes**, British pathologist, born 31 Mar; discovered *Shigella alkalescens*, an organism causing bacillary dysentery, 1918, *L* 1:560. Died 1932. *3542*

1859:29 Jacques **Loeb**, German/American physiologist and biologist, born 7 Apr; he founded the theory of 'tropisms', as the basis of the psychology of the lower forms of life, *Der Heliotropismus der Tiere*, 1890; succeeded in achieving artificial fertilization, 1899, *AmJPh* **3**:135. Died 1924. *125, 515.1*

1859:30 Ludwig **Stacke**, German otorhinolaryngologist, born 14 Apr; introduced the operation of excision of the auditory ossicles, 1890, *IMC* **4**, xi Abt.:3; introduced important modifications in the radical mastoidectomy operation of von Bergmann and Küster, 1892, *BKW* **29**:68. Died 1918. *3393, 3394*

1859:31 Clemens von **Kahlden**, German pathologist, born 29 May; first described granulosa cell tumour of the ovary, 1895, *ZAP* **6**:257. Died 1903. *6097*

1859:32 Pierre Marie Félix **Janet**, French psychiatrist, born 30 May; first described psychasthenia; in his *Les obsessions et la psychasthénie*, 1903. Died 1947. *4954*

1859:33 Karl Wilhelm Arthur **Heffter**, German pharmacologist, born 15 Jun; isolated mescaline, 1898; one of the earliest investigations of a psychedelic drug, *ArEP* **40**:385. Died 1925. *1890.1*

1859:34 George Tully **Vaughan**, American surgeon, born 27 Jun; first successful ligation of abdominal aorta, 1921, *AnS* **74**:308. Died 1948. *2970*

1859:35 Carl Ludwig **Schleich**, German physician, born 19 Jul; developed infiltration (local) anaesthesia, pioneered by Halsted, 1892, *VDGC* **21**:121. Died 1922. *5683, 5679*

1859:36 Theobald **Smith**, American bacteriologist and immunologist, born 31 Jul; discovered that immunity against live virus can be induced by dead virus, 1884, *PBSW* **3**:29. With Daniel Elmer Salmon isolated *Salmonella cholerae-suis*, 1886, *AmMM* **7**:204; the Salmonellae tribe was named after Salmon though Smith actually made the discovery. With Frederick Lucius Kilborne, discovered parasite of Texas cattle fever, *Babesia bigemina*, and proved its transmission by the cattle tick, *Boophilus annulatus* – the first demonstration of arthropod transmission of disease, *Investigations into ... Texas or Southern cattle fever*, 1893 (US Bureau of Animal Industry, Bulletin No. 1). Differentiated between the bovine and human types of *Mycobacterium tuberculosis*, 1898, *JEM* **3**:451. Died 1934. *2539, 2505, 5529, 2335*

1859:37 Thomas Burr **Osborne**, American biochemist, born 5 Aug; with L.B. Mendel, showed, like McCollum and Davis the same year, the necessity in diet of a factor later to be named vitamin A, 1913, *JBC* **23**:181. Died 1929. *1050*

1859:38 Edward **Martin**, American surgeon, born 14 Aug; with William Gibson Spiller, relieved intractable pain by spinal cordotomy, 1912, *JAMA* **58**:1489. Died 1938. *4883*

1859:39 Giuseppe **Gradenigo**, Italian otologist, born 29 Sep; introduced a test for tone decay in hearing, 1892, *GOC* **13**:1126; recorded the syndrome of acute otitis media followed by abductor paralysis ('Gradenigo's syndrome'), 1904, *GAMT* **10**:59. Died 1926. *3394.1, 3398*

1859:40 Alois **Pick**, Bohemian physician, born 15 Oct; generally credited with the first description of phlebotomus (pappataci) fever, 1886, *WMW* **36**:1141, 1168. Died 1945. *5476*

1859:41 John **Macintyre**, British laryngologist and radiologist, born 2 Nov; took the first radiogram of a kidney calculus, 1896, *L* **2**:118. Introduced X ray cinematography, 1897, *ArSk* **1**:37. Died 1928. *4293, 2687*

1859:42 Alwin Karl **Mackenrodt**, German gynaecologist, born 12 Nov; described operation for the plastic reconstruction of the vagina, 1896, *ZGy* **20**:546. Died 1925. *6102*

1859:43 Pierre Eugène **Menetrier**, French physician and medical historian, born 7 Dec; described giant hypertrophic gastritis ('Menetrier's disease'), 1888, *ArPhy* **20**:32, 236. Died 1935. *3492.1*

1859:44 Luigi Maria **Bossi**, Italian obstetrician and gynaecologist, born 30 Dec; originated the method of induction of premature labour by means of forced dilatation of the cervix, 1892, *AnOG* **14**:881. Died 1919. *6201*

1859:45 Tage Anton Ultimus **Sjögren**, Swedish surgeon, born; first successful treatment of cancer with x rays, 1899, *FSL*:208. Died 1939. *2624*

1859:46 Adolf **Passow**, German otologist, born; first attempted treatment of otosclerosis by fenestration, 1897, *VDOG* **6**:143. Died 1926. *3397*

1859:47 Jean Baptiste Edouard **Gélineau** born; gave first full description of narcolepsy, 1880, *GH* **53**:626, 635. *4561*

1859:48 Augusta **Dejerine-Klumpke**, American/French neurologist, born; first described atrophic paralysis of hand muscles following lesion of the brachial plexus and eighth cervical and first dorsal nerves ('Klumpke's paralysis'), 1885, *ReM* **5**:591, 739. Died 1927. *4748*

1859:49 Alexander **Rennie**, British surgeon, born; first to support, with evidence, the theory of the transmission of plague bacillus by rats, 1894, *BMJ* **2**:615. Died 1940. *5126*

1859: Lemuel **Shattuck** died, **born** 1793. *public health*

1859: William Fetherston **Montgomery** died, **born** 1878. *sebaceous glands of areola*

1859: Charles **Cagniard-Latour** died, **born** 1777. *fermentation, yeast*

**1860**

1860:1 **Berliner Medizinische Gesellschaft** founded

1860:2 **University of California** founded

1860:3 **Laws against milk adulteration** enacted in **England** and **Massachusetts**

1860:4 The method of removing the retained **placenta** by external manual pressure ('**Credé's manoeuvre**') described by Carl Siegmund Franz Credé (1819–1892); in his *De optima in partu naturali placentum amovendi ratione. 6183*

1860:5 *Medicine as a profession for women* written by Elizabeth Blackwell (1821–1910). *6649.90*

1860:6 The **Hodge pessary** described at length by Hugh Lenox Hodge (1796–1873) in his *On diseases peculiar to women, including displacement of the uterus*, chap. 5. *6043.1*

1860:7 An operation for **vesico-vaginal fistula** devised by Washington Lemuel Atlee (1808–1878), *AmJMS* **39**:67. *6047*

1860:8 The intestinal and muscular forms of **trichinosis** first noted by Friedrich Albert Zenker (1825–1898); he established their connection with the disease, *VA* **18**:561. *5342*

1860:9 The first treatise on **psychophysics** and the physiology of **sensation** was *Elemente der Psychophysik* by Gustav Theodor Fechner (1801–1887). *4972*

1860:10 **Chronic progressive bulbar paralysis** ('**Duchenne's paralysis**') first described by Guillaume Benjamin Amand Duchenne (1806–1875), *ArGM* **16**:283, 431. *4736*

1860:11 An anterior or suspensory splint for use in treating **fractures** of the **femur** introduced by Nathan Ryno Smith (1797–1877), *MVMJ* **14**:1. *4422*

1860:12 An extension-traction, apparatus for the treatment of **fractures** of the **femur** introduced by Gurdon Buck (1807–1877), *BNYAM* **1**:181. *4419*

1860:13 The first adequate description of **neurasthenia** given by Eugène Bouchut (1818–1891); in his *De l'état nerveux aigu et chronique ou nervosisme. 4535*

1860:14 Albrecht von Graefe (1828–1870) showed that most cases of **blindness** and impaired **vision** connected with cerebral disorders could be traced to **optic neuritis** rather than paralysis of the optic nerve, *GAO* **7** II Abt.:58. *4536*

1860:15 **Keratosis follicularis** first described by Henri Charles Lutz; in his *De l'hypertrophie générale du système sébacé*, Paris, Thèse No. 65. *4050*

1860:16 **Mycetoma of the foot** ('**Madura foot**', '**Carter's mycetoma**') given its first modern description by Henry Vandyke Carter (1831–1897), *TMPB* **6**:184; he gave a fuller account in 1874 in his *On mycetoma, or the fungus disease of India. 4047, 4066*

1860:17 Acute **otitis** treated by drainage through the antrum by Amédée Forget (1811–1869), *UM* **6**:193. *3371*

1860:18 '**Menière's syndrome**' (aural **vertigo**) first described by Prosper Menière (1799–1862), *GMP* **16**:88, 239, 379, 597. *3372*

1860:19 Foundations of **aural pathology** laid by Joseph Toynbee (1815–1866); in his *Diseases of the ear* .... *3373*

1860:20 The modern **otoscope** invented by Anton Friedrich von Tröltsch (1829–1890), *DK* **12**:113, 121, 131, 143, 151. *3374*

1860:21 **Carbolic acid**; attention drawn to its antiseptic properties by François Jules Lemaire (1814–1886); in his *Du coaltar saponiné, désinfectant énergique. 1864*

1860:22 First modern account of **asthma** by Henry Hyde Salter (1823–1871); *On asthma.* *2586*

1860:23 *Notes on nursing* published by Florence Nightingale (1820–1910). *1612*

1860:24 Modern **sphygmograph** introduced by Etienne Jules Marey (1830–1904); in his *Recherches sur la pouls*, also *CRAS* **51**:281. *776*

1860:25 **Pityriasis rosea** established as a definite clinical entity by Camille Melchior Gibert (1797–1866); in the second edition of his *Traité pratique des maladies de la peau*, 1, 402. *4048*

---

1860:26 Thomas Lane **Bancroft**, Australian physician and medical naturalist, born 2 Jan; first supplied evidence that *Aëdes aegypti* is a vector of dengue, 1906, *AuMG* **25**:17. Died 1933. *5472*

1860:27 Nathan Edwin **Brill**, American physician, born 13 Jan; first to describe 'Brill's disease', recrudescent typhus, 1910, *AmJMS* **139**:484. With co-workers, described follicular lymphadenopathy, 1925, *JAMA* **84**:668; later described by Douglas Symmers, 1927, and named 'Brill-Symmers disease'. Died 1925. *5382, 3786, 3787*

1860:28 Achille Alexandre **Souques**, French neurologist, born 6 Feb; with Stephen Chauvet, published a classic account of pituitary infantilism, 1913, *NIS* **26**:69. Recognized the importance of encephalitis as a cause of parkinsonism, 1921, *ReN* **28**:534. Died 1944. *3899, 4723*

1860:29 Vittorio **Mibelli**, Italian dermatologist, born 18 Feb; described porokeratosis ('Mibelli's disease'), 1893, *GIMV* **28**:313; it was first described by Neumann in 1875. Named angiokeratoma ('Mibelli's disease'), 1896, *GIMV* **26**:159, 260; first described by Cottle in 1877. Died 1910. *4068, 4114, 4105*

1860:30 William Henry **Howell**, American physiologist, born 20 Feb; isolated heparin with Luther Emmett Holt, 1919, *AmJPh* **47**:328. Died 1945. *905*

1860:31 Waldemar Mordecai Wolff **Haffkine**, Russian bacteriologist, born 15 Mar; prepared the first vaccine against cholera to meet with any success, 1892, *CRSB* **44**:636, 671. Developed an anti-bubonic plague vaccine for use in man, 1906, *BIP* **4**:825. Died 1930. *5109, 5129*

1860:32 Friedrich **Stolz**, German chemist, born 6 Apr; synthesized adrenaline, 1904, *BDCG* **37**:4149. Died 1936. *1147.1*

1860:33 George Neil **Stewart**, Canadian physiologist, born 18 Apr; with Julius Moses Rogoff, first to treat Addison's disease with adrenal cortical extract, 1929, *JAMA* **92**:1569. Died 1930. *3873*

1860:34 Clayton **Parkhill**, American surgeon, born 18 Apr; introduced external fixation in the treatment of fractures, 1898, *AnS* **27**:553. Died 1902. *4429.2*

1860:35 Archibald **Donald**, British obstetrician and gynaecologist, born May; devised an operation for complete prolapse of the uterus, 1908, *JOG* **13**:195. Died 1937. *6119*

1860:36 William Maddock **Bayliss**, British physiologist, born 2 May; with Ernest Henry Starling developed theory of hormonal control of internal secretion, 1904, *PRS* **73**:310; studied *The nature of enzyme action*, 1908. Died 1924. *1121*

1860:37 John Scott **Haldane**, British physiologist, born 3 May; devised an apparatus ('Haldane apparatus') for the analysis of respiratory gases, 1898, *JP* **22**:465. With Claude Gordon Douglas and others, reported high altitude physiological research at Pike's Peak, Colorado, 1913, *PT* (B) **203**: 185. Initiated oxygen therapy, 1917, *BMJ* **1**:161. Died 1936. *952.1, 1977*

1860:38 Walter Essex **Wynter**, British physician, born 5 May; first performed lumbar puncture for the relief of fluid pressure, 1891, *L* **1**:981. Died 1945. *4868*

1860:39 Eduard **Buchner**, German chemist, born 20 May; discovered cell-free fermentation, turning point in the study of enzymes, 1897, *BDCG* **30**:117, 1110, 2668; Nobel Prize (Chemistry), 1907, *NPL*. Died 1907. *719.1*

1860:40 Willem **Einthoven**, Dutch cardiologist, born 22 May; invented the string galvanometer, 1901, *ArNS* 2 sér. **6**:625; showed how it could be used to record electrical changes in the heart (electrocardiography), 1903, *KAWS* **6**:107; introduced phonocardiography, 1907, *PfA* **117**:461. Awarded the Nobel Prize (Physiology or Medicine), 1924, for his development of electrocardiography, *NPL*. Died 1927. *840, 842, 846*

1860:41 Gustav **Killian**, German laryngologist, born 2 Jun; introduced direct bronchoscopy (1898), *MMW* **45**:844, and suspension laryngoscopy, 1912, *ArL* **26**:277. Died 1921. *3336, 3338*

1860:42 Albert Siegmund Gustav **Döderlein**, German obstetrician and gynaecologist, born 5 Jul; in his study of the vaginal secretions in relation to puerperal fever, *Das Scheidensekret und seine Bedeutung für das Puerperalfieber*, 1892, he gave the first description of 'Döderlein's bacillus', a lactobacillus. Died 1941. *6279*

1860:43 Emile Charles **Achard**, French physician, born 24 Jul; with Raoul Bensaude, isolated *Salmonella paratyphi B*, 1896, the first use of the term paratyphoid, *BSMH* **13**:820. With Joseph Thiers, described the 'Achard-Thiers syndrome', the combination of hirsutism with diabetes, 1921, *BuAM* **86**:51. Died 1944. *5035, 3870*

1860:44 Anton von **Eiselsberg**, Austrian surgeon, born 31 Jul; produced tetany experimentally by removing the thyroid, 1892, *WKW* **5**:81. Died 1939. *3856*

1860:45 Paul **Frosch**, German pathologist, born 15 Aug; with Friedrich Albert Johann Loeffler showed foot-and-mouth disease to be due to a filter-passing virus (first recognition of such a virus as a cause of animal disease), 1898, *ZBP* I, **23**:371. Died 1928. *2511*

1860:46 Louis Henri **Vaquez**, French physician, born 27 Aug; first described polycythaemia (erythraemia), 1892, *CRSB* **44**:384; William Osler's later paper (1903) led to the term '**Vaquez-Osler disease**', Died 1936. *3070, 3073*

1860:47 Axel **Holst**, Norwegian pathologist, born 6 Sep; produced experimental scurvy in guinea-pigs, 1907, *JHyg* **7**:619. Died 1931. *3721*

1860:48 Franz **Nissl**, German neurologist and neuropathologist, born 9 Sep; introduced a stain for the localization of nerve cells, 1894, *NZ* **13**:507; described 'Nissl's granules' in the cytoplasm of nerve cells, 1894, *NZ* **13**:676, 781, 810. Died 1919. *1291, 1422*

1860:49 Rudolph **Matas**, American surgeon, born 12 Sep; performed first aneurysmorrhaphy, 1888, *MN* **53**:462. Died 1957. *2985*

1860:50 Thomas **Jonnesco**, Romanian surgeon, born 13 Sep; first to treat angina pectoris by cervical sympathectomy, 1920, *BuAM* **84**:93. Died 1926. *2895*

1860:51 Curt **Schimmelbusch**, German surgeon, born 16 Nov; first described cystadenoma of the breast ('Schimmelbusch's disease'), 1892, *ArKC* **44**:117. Died 1895. *5775*

1860:52 Niels Ryberg **Finsen**, Danish physician, born 15 Dec; founder of modern phototherapy; *Om anvendelse medicinen ...*, 1896. Pioneered the treatment of lupus vulgaris by light therapy; in *La photothérapie* etc., 1899. Awarded Nobel Prize (Physiology or Medicine), 1903, for his discovery of the therapeutic value of invisible light, *NPL*. Died 1904. *2000, 4002*

1860:53 Augusto **Ducrey**, Italian dermatologist born 22 Dec; discovered *Haemophilus ducreyi* ('Ducrey's bacillus'), causal organism in chancroid, 1889, *GiISM* **11**:44. Died 1940. *5205*

1860:54 Enrique **Paschen**, Mexican/German physician, born 30 Dec; rediscovered elementary bodies in the vaccinia virus [first described and demonstrated microscopically by J.B. Buist (1886)], 1906, *MMW* **53**:2391; they were named Paschen elementary bodies. Died 1936. *5430*

———

1860:55 Heinrich **Dreser** born; introduced acetylsalicylic acid (aspirin) into medicine, 1899, *PfA* **76**:306. Died 1925. *1891*

1860:56 Henri **Morau**, French oncologist, born; successfully transplanted epithelioma in mice through 17 generations, 1891–1893, *CRSB* **43**:289. *2622.1*

1860:57 Joaquin Maria **Albarran y Dominguez**, Cuban surgeon, born; carried out the first planned nephrostomy, 1896, *RC* **16**:882. Introduced 'Albarran's operation' for nephropexy, 1906, *PrM* **14**:253. Died 1912. *4226.1, 4233*

1860:58 Mathieu **Jaboulay**, French surgeon, born; introduced the operation of gastroduodenostomy, 1892, *ArPC* **1**:551. First to describe interilio-abdominal amputation, 1894, *LM* **75**:507. Carried out first sympathectomy for relief of vascular disease; in his *Chirurgie du grand sympathique et du corps thyroïde*, 1900. Died 1913. *3504, 4472, 3024*

1860:59 Paul **Blocq**, French neurologist, born; described astasia-abasia ('Blocq's disease'), 1888, *ArN* **15**:24, 187. Died 1896. *4573*

1860:60 George Henry **Noble**, American surgeon, born; introduced a flap operation for atresia of the vagina, 1900, *TSSA* **13**:78. *6112*

---

1860: Thomas **Addison** died, **born** 1793. *Addison's disease, pernicious anaemia, scleroderma, therapeutic use of static electricity*

1860: Chapin Aaron **Harris** died, **born** 1806. *dentistry*

1860: Walter **Brashear** died, **born** 1776. *amputation at hip-joint*

1860: John **Lizars** died, **born** 1794. *ovariotomy*

1860: Michael **Ferrall** died, **born** 1790. *eyeball*

1860: James **Braid** died, **born** 1795. *mesmerism, hypnosis*

1860: Anders Adolf **Retzius** died, **born** 1796. *'cave of Retzius'*

1860: Martin Heinrich **Rathke** died, **born** 1793. *pituitary, Rathke's pouch*

**1861**
1861:1 **Women's Hospital** founded in **Philadelphia**

1861:2 **Samaritan Hospital, New York**, founded

1861:3 **Massachusetts Institute of Technology** founded

1861:4 **Lineae atrophicae** first described by Samuel Wilks (1824–1911), *GHR* **7**:197. *4052*

1861:5 A method for amputating the **cervix** devised by James Marion Sims (1813–1883), *TNYM* 367. *6049*

1861:6 A **decapitation hook** introduced by Gustav August Braun (1829–1911), *WMW* **11**:713. *6184*

1861:7 The clinical classification of pelves devised by Carl Conrad Theodor Litzmann (1815–1890), in his *Die Formen des Beckens, insbesondere des engen weiblichen Beckens*, was in general use until supplanted by that of Caldwell and Moloy (1933). He described various deformities of the female pelvis. *6263*

1861:8 Pierre Paul Broca (1824–1880) localized the **speech centre** in the left frontal lobe and asserted that **aphasia** was associated with a lesion on the left third frontal convolution of the brain ('**Broca's area**'), *BSAnth* **2**:235. *4619*

1861:9 *Die Aetiologie, der Begriff und die Prophylaxis des Kindbettfiebers*, by Ignaz Philipp Semmelweis (1818–1865) is one of the epoch-making books in medical literature. He enlarged an earlier paper (1847), classifying **puerperal fever** as a septicaemia, and strove to improve conditions in the lying-in wards of Vienna and Budapest. *6277*

1861:10 Jeffery Allen Marston (1831–1911) was first to draw attention to what later became known as **Weil's disease**, a severe form of **leptospirosis**, *AMD* **3**:486. *5330*

1861:11 The first description of **progressive familial hepatolenticular degeneration (Kinnier Wilson's disease)** published by Friedrich Theodor Frerichs (1819–1885); in his *Klinik der Leberkrankheiten*, **2**, 62. *4693, 4717*

1861:12 Karl Gegenbaur (1826–1903) proved the unicellularity of the **ovum**, *ArA* 491. *486*

1861:13 **Herpes zoster** ascribed to a lesion of the spinal ganglia by Friedrich Wilhelm Felix von Bärensprung (1822–1864), *AnCK* **9** ii:40; **10**:37; **11**:96. *4640*

1861:14 **Erythema induratum scrophulosorum** ('Bazin's disease') first described by Pierre Ernest Antoine Bazin (1807–1878); in his *Leçons sur la scrofule*, 2nd edition, pp. 145, 501. *4051*

1861:15 Rudolf Albert von Kölliker's (1817–1905) *Entwicklungsgeschichte des Menschen und der höheren Thiere* was the first book on comparative **embryology**. *487*

1861:16 The first excision of the **kidney**, for **renal tumour**, carried out by Erastus Bradley Wolcott (1804–1880) – recorded by C.L. Stoddard, *MSRep* **7**:126. *4210*

1861:17 **Polyposis** of the **colon** described by Hubert von Luschka (1820–1875), *VA* **20**:133. *3460*

1861:18 **Duroziez's sign** in **aortic insufficiency** described by Paul Louis Duroziez (1826–1897), *ArGM* **17**:417, 588. *2762*

1861:19 Ill effects on **respiration** of **mouth-breathing** first noted by George Catlin (1796–1871); in his *The breath of life* …. *3267*

1861:20 Strict **anaerobiosis** discovered by Louis Pasteur (1822–1895), *CRAS* **52**:344. *2475.1*

1861:21 The modern **mastoid operation** introduced by Anton Friedrich von Tröltsch (1829–1890), *VA* **21**:295. *3375*

---

1861:22 Addeo **Toti**, Italian otolaryngologist, born 1 Jan; introduced dacryocystorhinostomy for the treatment of chronic suppuration of the lacrimal duct, 1904, *CM* **10**:385. *5948*

1861:23 Eugen **Steinach**, Austrian surgeon, born 27 Jan; introduced his rejuvenation operation (ligation of the vas deferens); in his *Verjüngung durch experimentelle Neubelebung der alternden Pubertätsdrüse*, 1920. Died 1944. *3796*

1861:24 Emerich **Ullmann**, Hungarian surgeon, born 23 Feb; carried out successfully kidney autotransplantation in dogs, 1902, *WKW* **15**:281. Died 1937. *4229.1*

1861:25 Arthur **Looss**, German parasitologist, born 16 Mar; elucidated the life cycle and mode of transmission of the hookworm, *Ankylostoma duodenale*, 1896, *ZBP* I Abt.**20**:865; **24**:441, 483. Discovered, by self-infection, that hookworm larvae can penetrate the skin, 1900, *ZBP* I Abt.**29**:733. Died 1923. *5361, 5632*

1861:26 Alessandro **Codivilla**, Italian surgeon, born 21 Mar; first to attempt the surgical lengthening of limbs, 1905, *AmJOrS* **2**:353. Died 1912. *4375.1*

1861:27 Achille **Sclavo**, Italian physician, born 23 Mar; produced a specific anti-anthrax serum providing passive immunization, 1895, *RISP* **6**:841. Died 1930. *5170*

1861:28 Franz **Torek**, German/American surgeon, born 14 Apr; introduced orchiopexy for the treatment of undescended testis, 1909, *NYMJ* **90**:948. First successfully to treat carcinoma of the oesophagus by resection of the thoracic portion, 1913, *SGO* **16**:614. Died 1938. *4196, 3540*

1861:29 Carl **Fraenkel**, German bacteriologist, born 2 May; produced artificial immunity to diphtheria in guinea-pigs by the injection of attenuated cultures of *Corynebacterium diphtheriae*, 1890, *BKW* **27**:1133. Died 1915. *5060.1*

1861:30 Karl **Herxheimer**, German dermatologist, born 26 Jun; Jarisch-Herxheimer reaction in syphilis, 1902, *DMW* **28**:895. Died 1944. *2397*

1861:31 William James **Mayo**, American surgeon, born 29 Jun; reported his operation for partial gastrectomy, 1900, *TASA* **18**:97. Devised an operation for the radical cure of umbilical hernia, 1901, *AnS* **34**:27. Introduced radical operation for carcinoma of the rectum, 1910, *AnS* **51**:854. Died 1939. *3522, 3607, 3534*

1861:32 Frederick Gowland **Hopkins**, British biochemist, born 30 Jun; with Sidney William Cole isolated tryptophan, 1901, *JP* **27**:418. Predicted the existence of vitamins, 1906, *Analyst* **31**:385. With Walter Morley Fletcher, explained the production of lactic acid in normal muscular contraction, 1907, *JP* **35**:247. Discovered growth-stimulating vitamins, 1912, *JP* **44**:425. Isolated glutathione, 1921, *BJ* **15**:286. Shared Nobel Prize (Physiology or Medicine), 1929, with Christiaan Eijkman, *NPL*. Died 1947. *723, 1044, 733, 1048, 745*

1861:33 Hastings **Gilford**, British physician, born 2 Jul; gave progeria its present name, 1897, *MCT* **80**:17. Died 1941. *3792*

1861:34 Henry **Head**, British neurologist, born 4 Aug; defined zones of hyperalgesia of the skin associated with visceral disease ('Head's areas'), 1893, *Brain* **16**:1; **17**:339; **19**:153. With Alfred Walter Campbell, showed herpes zoster to be a haemorrhagic inflammation of the posterior nerve roots and the homologous spinal ganglia, 1900, *Brain* **23**:353. With Gordon Holmes, he described the functions of the thalamus, 1911, *Brain* **34**:102. His *Aphasia and kindred disorders of speech*, 1926, is considered one of the most important works on the subject in English. His theory of aphasia conceived it as a disorder of symbolic formulation and expression. Died 1940. *4581, 4644, 1438.1, 4633,*

1861:35 William **Bateson**, British biologist and geneticist, born 8 Aug; made considerable contributions to genetics. He named the science 'genetics' and proved that Mendelian behaviour holds for animals as well as plants. His *Mendel's principles of heredity, a defence*, 1902, was the first English textbook of genetics (2nd edn, 1909). Died 1926. *241*

1861:36 Arthur Dean **Bevan**, American surgeon, born 9 Aug; devised operation for undescended testicle and congenital inguinal hernia, 1899, *JAMA* **33**:773. Died 1943. *4191*

1861:37 Almroth Edward **Wright**, British pathologist, born 10 Aug; first performed active inoculation against typhoid, 1896, *BMJ* **1**:122. With Frederick Smith, devised an agglutination test for the diagnosis of brucellosis, 1897, *Lancet* **1**:656. With Stewart Rankin Douglas, demonstrated opsonins (thermolabile substances in normal and immune serum), 1903, *PRSB* **72**:357; **73**:128. Died 1947. *5039, 5101, 2558*

1861:38 James Bryan **Herrick**, American physician, born 11 Aug; first to identify sickle-cell anaemia, 1910, *ArIM* **6**:517. Died 1954. *3133*

1861:39 Howard **Lilienthal**, American surgeon, born 1 Nov; performed total pneumonectomy for sarcoma in a tuberculous patient, 1933, *JTS* **2**:600. Died 1946. *3207*

1861:40 Giuliano **Vanghetti**, Italian surgeon, born 8 Oct; first to suggest kinematization of amputation stump – use of the musculature above an amputation stump to form a motor unit for an artificial limb; in his *Amputazione, disarticulazione et protesi*, 1898. Died 1940. *4474*

1861:41 Dmitriy Leonidovich **Romanovsky**, Russian physician, born 19 Oct; introduced the Romanovsky stain for the demonstration of the malaria parasite in blood films ; in his *Parasitology and treatment of malarial fever* [in Russian], 1891. Died 1921. *5242*

1861:42 August Karl Gustav **Bier**, German surgeon, born 24 Nov; introduced cocaine as a spinal anaesthetic, 1899, *DZC* **51**:361; introduced active and passive hyperaemia as an adjuvant in surgical treatment, 1903, *Hyperaemie als Heilmittel*. Died 1949. *5684, 5626*

1861:43 Thomas Bell **Aldrich**, American biochemist, born; independently of Jokichi Takamine, isolated adrenaline in crystalline form, 1901, *AmJPh* **5**:457; associated with O. Kamm et al. in the isolation of vasopressin and oxytocin, 1928. *1147, 1168.1*

1861:44 Fred **Neufeld**, German bacteriologist, born; with Willi Rimpau, named and described bacteriotropins, 1904, *DMW* **30**:1458; with Ludwig Haendel, introduced new antipneumococcus serum, 1910, *AKG* **34**:293. Died 1945. *2560, 3190*

1861: Henry **Gray** died, **born** 1827. *anatomy*

1861: Arnold Adolph **Berthold** died, **born** 1803. *internal secretion*

1861: John **Hutchinson** died, **born** 1811. *spirometer*

1861: Albert **Niemann** died, **born** 1834. *cocaine*

1861: Francis **Rynd** died, **born** 1801. *hypodermic infusions*

1861: François Amilcar **Aran** died, **born** 1817. *progressive muscular atrophy*

1861: James **Robinson** died, **born** 1813. *anaesthesia*

1861: Friedrich August von **Ammon** died, **born** 1799. *ophthalmology*

1861: Isidore **Bricheteau** died, **born** 1789. *pneumopericardium*

1861: Johann Ludwig **Choulant** died, **born** 1791. *medical bibliography*

**1862**

1862:1 **Australian Medical Association** formed

1862:2 **Training school for nurses** established at **St Thomas' Hospital, London,** by Florence **Nightingale** (1820–1910)

1862:3 **Coprosterol** discovered by Austin Flint Jr (1836–1915), *AmJMS* **44**:305. *1005*

1862:4 In his *Astigmatisme en cilindrische glazen,* Frans Cornelis Donders (1818–1889) states '**Donders' law**' – the rotation of the **eye** around the line of sight is not voluntary. *5889*

1862:5 The **sight test types** ('Optotypi') introduced by Herman Snellen (1834–1908) in his *Probebuchstaben zur Bestimmung der Sehschärfe* soon gained acceptance in the civilized world. *5890*

1862:6 An operation for repair of **cleft palate** devised by Bernhard Rudolph Conrad von Langenbeck (1810–1887), *ArKC* **2**:205. *5748*

1862:7 The first diagnosis of **trichinosis** in a living person made by Nikolaus Friedreich (1826–1882), *VA* **25**:399. *5344.1*

1862:8 **Syringomyelia** first described by William Withey Gull (1816–1890), *GHR* **8**:244. *4695*

1862:9 The expression of **emotions** studied and photographed by Guillaume Benjamin Amand Duchenne de Boulogne (1806–1875); in his *Mécanisme de la physionomie humaine. 4973*

1862:10 **Verrucae necrogenicae**, (dissecting-room **warts**, the cutaneous **tuberculosis of Laennec**), sometimes called 'Wilks's disease', described by Samuel Wilks (1824–1911), *GHR* **8**:263. *4053*

1862:11 First description of **pulmonary fat embolism** by Friedrich Albert Zenker (1825–1898); in his *Beiträge zur normalen und pathologischen Anatomie der Lungen. 3007*

1862:12 **Tumour** of **larynx** removed with the aid of the **laryngoscope** by Georg Richard Lewin (1820–1896), *AMC* **31**:9, 33, a claim also made by Victor von Bruns. *3269*

1862:13 Wilhelm Friedrich [Willy] Kühne (1837–1900) described the **neuromuscular end organ** ('**Kühne's spindle**'), in his *Ueber die peripherischen Endorgane der motorischen Nerven. 1269*

1862:14 First removal of a **laryngeal polyp** by the bloodless method by Victor von Bruns (1812–1883); in his *Die erste Ausrottung eines Polypen in der Kehlkopfshöhle. 3268*

1862:15 **Austin Flint murmur**, present in **aortic regurgitation**, described by Austin Flint (1812–1886), *AmJMS* **44**:29. *2764*

1862:16 **Raynaud's disease**, intermittent pallor or cyanosis of the extremities, first described by Maurice Raynaud (1834–1881); in his *De l'asphyxie locale …. 2704*

1862:17 Max Joseph von Pettenkofer (1818–1901), with Carl von Voit (1831–1908), carried out combined **feeding-respiration** experiments, being first to estimate the amounts of protein, fat and carbohydrates broken down in the body, *ACP* Suppl.**2**:52. *938*

1862:18 The international **Red Cross** was founded and the **Geneva Convention** of 1864 resulted from the publication of *Un souvenir de Solferino*, by Henri Dunant (1828–1910). *2166*

1862:19 **Trypsin** discovered by Aleksandr Yakovlevich Danilevsky (1838–1923), *VA* **25**:279. *1004*

---

1862:20 Heinrich Friedrich Wilhelm **Braun**, German surgeon, born 1 Jan; first to use procaine (novocaine) clinically, 1905, *DMW* **31**:1667. Died 1934. *5692*

1862:21 Claudio **Fermi**, Italian public health officer and epidemiologist, born 2 Jan; introduced a vaccine prepared by the chemical (carbolic acid) treatment of suspensions of fixed rabies virus (Fermi vaccine), 1908, *ZHyg* **58**:233. *5484.1*

1862:22 Nicolas Maurice **Arthus**, French physician, born 9 Jan; demonstrated the 'Arthus phenomenon', a diagnostic symptom of anaphylaxis, 1903, *CRSB* **55**:817. Died 1945. *2591*

1862:23 Max **Einhorn**, Russian/American physician, born 10 Jan; devised the method of exploration of the stomach with a tube – gastrodiaphany, 1889, *NYMM* **1**:559. Introduced the concept of achylia gastrica, a primary nervous functional disorder of gastric secretion, 1892, *MR* **41**:650. Died 1953. *3495, 3503*

1862:24 Eduard **Jacobi**, German dermatologist, born 20 Jan; first described poikiloderma vascularis atrophicans, 1907, *VDDG* **9**:321. Died 1915. *4141*

1862:25 Arthur **Nicolaier**, German physician and bacteriologist, born 4 Feb; discovery of the tetanus bacillus, *Clostridium tetani*, is attributed to him, 1884, *DMW* **10**:842, he did not isolate it in pure culture. With Max Dohr, introduced cinchophen in the treatment of gout, 1908, *DAKM* **93**:331. Died 1942. *5148, 4505.1*

1862:26 Georges Fernand Isidor **Widal**, French physician, born 9 Mar; with André Chantemesse, isolated the dysentery bacillus, *Shigella*, 1888, *BuAM* **19**:522, but did not establish its aetiological relationship to bacillary dysentery. With Chantemesse, carried out experimental anti-typhoid inoculation, 1888, *AnIP* **2**:54. With Arthur Sicard, developing the work of Max Gruber and Herbert Durham, demonstrated specific agglutinins in the blood of typhoid patients, 1896, *BSMH* **13**:681, making possible a diagnostic agglutination reaction ('Gruber-Widal test'). With Pierre Abrami, published an account of acquired haemolytic anaemia, 1907, *PrM* **15**:479; led to the eponym 'Widal-Abrami disease' and, because of the earlier description by Hayem (1898), 'Hayem-Widal disease'. Died 1929. *5090.1, 5034, 2550, 5037, 3777, 3783*

1862:27 Charles David **Green**, British surgeon, born 16 Mar; with Charles Alfred Ballance, published classical work, *Essays on the surgery of the temporal bone*, 1919. Died 1937. *3403.1*

1862:28 Alfred **Dührssen**, German gynaecologist, born 23 Mar; introduced vaginal caesarean section, 1898, *SKV* **232**:1365. Died 1933. *6246*

1862:29 Emile **Marchoux**, French tropical diseases physician, born 24 Mar; with A.T. Salimbeni and P.L. Simond, first employed convalescent serum in the treatment of yellow fever, 1903, *AnIP* **17**:665. Died 1943. *5459*

1862:30 Amico **Bignami**, Italian pathologist, born 15 Apr; with Giovanni Battista Grassi, showed that the malaria parasite, *Plasmodium*, undergoes its sexual phase in the *Anopheles* mosquito, 1899, *AnIS* **9**:258. With Ettore Marchiafava, described degeneration of the corpus callosum in alcoholism ('Marchiafava-Bignami disease'), 1903, *RPN* **8**:544. Died 1929. *5252, 4955*

1862:31 Allvar **Gullstrand**, Swedish ophthalmologist, born 5 Jun; his general theory of monochromatic aberrations was advanced in *Allgemeine Theorie der monochromatischen Aberrationen und ihre nächsten Ergebnisse für die Ophthalmologie*, 1900. Professor of ophthalmology at Uppsala; awarded the Nobel Prize (Physiology or Medicine), 1911, for his investigations of the dioptrics of the eye, *NPL*. Invented the slit-lamp, 1902, *BVOG* 290. Discovered the intracapsular mechanism of accommodation, in his *Methoden der Dioptrik des Auges*, 1911. Died 1930. *5945, 1525.2, 1526*

1862:32 Thomas Caspar **Gilchrist**, British dermatologist, born 15 Jun; his description of North American blastomycosis, 1896, *JHR* **1**:269, led to the alternative name 'Gilchrist's disease'. Died 1927. *5530.1*

1862:33 Giulio **Vassale**, Italian pathologist and endocrinologist, born 22 Jun; with Francesco Generali, showed that tetany follows removal of the parathyroid glands, 1896, *RPN* **1**:95. Died 1912. *3857*

1862:34 Rudolph **Frank**, Austrian surgeon, born 23 Jun; introduced an operation for gastrostomy, 1893, *WKW* **6**:231, which was independently described by J.F. Ssabanejew in the same year; and named '**Ssabanejew-Frank operation**'. Died 1913. *3508, 3512*

1862:35 Humphry Davy **Rolleston**, British physician and medical historian, born 21 June; he followed Clifford Allbutt as Regius Professor of Physic, Cambridge; his publications included *Cardiovascular disease since Harvey's discovery*, 1928, and *The endocrine organs in health and disease*, 1936. Died 1944. *3156, 3909*

1862:36 George Henry Falkiner **Nuttall**, American/British biologist, born 5 Jul; described the bactericidal action of blood, 1888, *ZHyg* **4**:353. Discovered *Clostridium perfringens*, the gas gangrene bacillus (Welch bacillus) with William Henry Welch, 1892, *JHB* **3**:81. Died 1937. *2542, 2508*

1862:37 Henry **Smith**, Indian Army surgeon, born 16 Aug; had remarkable success with his method of extraction of cataract within the capsule, 1900, *IMG* **35**:241; **36**:220; **40**:327. Died 1948. *5946*

1862:38 Knud Helge **Faber**, Danish physician, born 29 Aug; described simple achlorhydric anaemia, 1913, *BKW* **50**:958. Died 1956. *3134*

1862:39 Adrien **Pic**, French physician, born 3 Oct; with Louis Bard, described Bard-Pic syndrome, a complication of pancreatic carcinoma, 1888, *ReM* **8**:257, 363. *3630*

1862:40 Arthur **Kuttner**, German otorhinolaryngologist, born 8 Oct; published first important work on the radiology of the accessory nasal sinuses, *Die entzündlichen Nebenhöhlenerkrankungen der Nase im Röntgenbild*, 1908. *3316*

1862:41 Theodor **Boveri**, German biologist, born 12 Oct; demonstrated chromosome individuality, 1888, *JZN* **22**:685, and showed that different chromosomes perform different functions in development, 1903, *ZPMG* **35**:67. Died 1915. *231.1, 241.1*

1862:42 Jean Hyacinthe **Vincent**, French bacteriologist, born 22 Dec; isolated *Actinomyces madurae*, the parasite of Madura foot, mycetoma of the foot, 1894, *AnIP* **8**:129. Described ulcerative stomatitis due to a fusiform bacillus and a spirillum, *Borrelia vincenti*, 'Vincent's angina', 1896, *AnIP* **10**:488. Died 1950. *4117, 3309*

----

1862:43 Maurice **Nicolle**, French parasitologist, born; demonstrated passive anaphylaxis, 1907, *AnIP* **21**:128. Died 1932. *2597*

1862:44 Francisque **Déléage**, French physician, born; first described dystrophia myotonica ('Déléage's disease'); in his inaugural thesis *Étude clinique de la maladie de Thomsen*, 1890. *4754*

1862:45 Weller **Van Hook**, American surgeon, born; originated modern methods of ureteral repair, including uretero-ureterostomy, 1893, *JAMA* **21**:911, 965. Died 1933. *4186*

1862:46 Guido **Werdnig**, Austrian neurologist, born; described an infantile familial form of progressive muscular atrophy, 1891, *ArPN* **22**:437, independently noted in the same year by Hoffmann and named 'Werdnig-Hoffmann muscular atrophy'. *4755, 4756*

1862:47 Ernesto **Odriozola**, Peruvian physician, born; named bartonellosis (verruca peruviana, Oroya fever) Carrión's disease, 1895, *MonM* **10**:309, after Daniel Carrión (1857–85) who died of the disease after experiments with it. Died 1921. *5530*

1862:48 Hermann Johann **Pfannenstiel**, German gynaecologist, born; introduced a curved incision convex downwards just above the pubis, used in gynaecological surgery, ('Pfannenstiel's incision'), 1900, *SKV* **268**:1735. Gave first detailed description of familial icterus gravis neonatorum, 1908, *MMW* **55**:2169, 2223. Died 1909. *6113, 3080.1*

----

1862: Pierre Fidèle **Bretonneau** died, **born** 1778. *diphtheria*

1862: Christophe François **Delabarre** died, **born** 1777. *dentistry*

1862: Christian Andreas Justinus **Kerner** died, **born** 1786. *fermentation*

1862: Benjamin Collins **Brodie** died, **born** 1783. *intermittent claudication, varicose veins, Brodie's pile, bone abscess, ankylosing spondylitis, pseudofracture of spine, breast tumours*

1862: John Richard **Farre** died, **born** 1775. *congenital abnormalities of heart*

1862: Edward **Stanley** died, **born** 1793. *liver puncture, spinal cord disease*

1862: Prosper **Menière** died, **born** 1799. *aural vertigo*

1862: Theodor Maximilian **Bilharz** died, **born** 1825. *schistosomiasis, Schistosoma haematobium*

1862: Jacob Ludwig Conrad **Schroeder van der Kolk** died, **born** 1797. *epilepsy*

**1863**
1863:1 **Army Medical School (England)** established at **Royal Victoria Hospital**, Netley, Hampshire

1863:2 **Cook County Hospital, Chicago**, founded

1863:3 **American Veterinary Medical Association** founded

1863:4 **National Academy of Sciences, Washington**, chartered

1863:5 **University of Belgrade** founded

1863:6 The first successful excision of **uterus** and **ovaries** (for tumour) performed by Eugène Koeberlé (1828–1915), *GMS* **23**:101; he was partly responsible for the introduction of **ovariotomy** into France, *MAIM* **26**:321. *6052, 6051*

1863:7 The first atlas of the **fundus oculi** was Richard Liebreich's (1830–1917) *Atlas der Ophthalmoscopie*. *5892*

1863:8 The first complete and accurate account of the life history and morphology of *Taenia echinococcus* given by Karl Georg Friedrich Leuckart (1823–1898); in his *Die menschlichen Parasiten und die von ihnen herrührenden Krankheiten*, 2 vols, 1863–1882. *5344*

1863:9 The first detailed description of *Dracunculus medinensis*, the **guinea-worm**, given by Henry Charlton Bastian (1837–1915), *TLS* **24**:101. *5344.2*

1863:10 Embryonic stage of *Wuchereria bancrofti*, cause of **elephantiasis**, described by Nicolas Demarquay (1814–1878), *GMP* **33**:665. *5344.3*

1863:11 Wilhelm Friedrich [Willy] Kühne (1837–1900) described the **proprioceptive receptors** in **muscles**, *VA* **28**:528. *1270*

1863:12 Casimir Joseph Davaine (1812–1882) showed that **anthrax** could be transmitted to sheep, horses, cattle, guinea-pigs and mice, and that in such animals *Bacillus anthracis* did not appear in the blood until 4–5 hours before death, *CRSB* **57**:220, 351. *5165*

1863:13 The first description of **Malta fever (brucellosis)** as a distinct disease given by Jeffrey Allen Marston (1831–1911), *AMD* **3**:486. *5097*

1863:14 An excellent account of **unilateral epilepsy** ('**Jacksonian epilepsy**') given by John Hughlings Jackson (1835–1911), *MTG* **1**:588; Bravais (1827) was the first to note the condition – also named '**Bravais-Jacksonian epilepsy**', *4816, 4810*

1863:15 First description of an hereditary form of **ataxia** ('**Friedreich's ataxia**') by Nikolaus Friedreich (1826–1882), *VA* **26**:391, 433; **27**:1, 68, 145; **70**:140. *4696*

1863:16 Congenital **metatarsus varus** first described by Philipp Jakob Wilhelm Henke (1834–1896), *ZRM* **17**:188. *4333*

1863:17 The account of **hemiplegia** associated with disease of the **crura cerebri** by Hermann David Weber (1823–1918), *MCT* **46**:121, first described by Adolphe Gubler (1856), led to the eponyms '**Weber's syndrome**' and '**Weber-Gubler syndrome**'. *4538, 4531*

1863:18 Congenital upward displacement of the **scapula** ('**Sprengel's deformity**') first described by Moritz Michael **Eulenburg** (1811–1877), *ArKC* **4**:304. *4332, 4359*

1863:19 The importance of the **ophthalmoscope** in the investigation of **nervous diseases** demonstrated by John Hughlings Jackson (1835–1911), *OHR* **4**:10, 389; **5**:51, 251. *4537*

1863:20 An important account of the renal lesions in **gout** given by Jean Martin Charcot (1825–1893) and André Victor Cornil (1837–1898), *CRSB* **5**:139. *4498*

1863:21 **Dermatomyositis**, now classified as a connective-tissue disease, first recorded by Ernst Leberecht Wagner (1829–1888), *ArH* **4**:282. *4054*

1863:22 A diet for the treatment of **obesity** ('**Banting diet**', **Bantingism**) devised by William Banting (1797–1878); in his *Letter on corpulence: addressed to the public*. *3914*

1863:23 A method to effect permeability of the **Eustachian tube** was introduced by Adam Politzer (1835–1920), *WMW* **13**:84, 102, 117, 148. *3377*

1863:24 **Gruber's hernia** – internal **mesogastric hernia** – described by Wenzel Leopold Gruber (1814–1890), *OZPH* **9**:325, 341. *3592*

1863:25 Louis Pasteur (1822–1895) differentiated between **aerobic** and **anaerobic organisms**, *CRAS* **56**:1189. *2478*

1863:26 **Putrefaction** as a biological process (Schwann, 1837) confirmed by Louis Pasteur (1822–1895), *CRAS* **56**:416, 734. *2476, 2477*

1863:27 In his *On the influence of mechanical and physiological rest in the treatment of accidents and surgical diseases, and the diagnostic value of pain* (later editions have the title *Rest and pain*) John Hilton (1804–1878) emphasized the importance of **rest** in the treatment of **surgical disorders**. *5609*

1863:28 **Resonance theory of hearing** propounded by Hermann Helmholtz (1821–1894); in his *Die Lehre von der Tonempfindung*. *1562*

1863:29 Theodor Billroth's (1829–1894) **surgical** classic, *Die allgemeine chirurgische Pathologie und Therapie*, was translated into ten languages. *5608*

---

1863:30 Bernard **Krönig**, German obstetrician and gynaecologist, born 27 Jan; the first description of his operation of transperitoneal lower-segment caesarean section appears in *Operative Gynäkologie*, 3rd edn, 1912, p. 879, by Albert Siegmund Döderlein and Bernard Krönig. Died 1917. *6250*

1863:31 Katsusaburo **Yamagiwa**, Japanese physician, born 23 Feb; with Koichi Ichikawa, produced cancer experimentally by painting with a tar product, 1916, *VJPJ* **6**:169; **7**:191. Died 1930. *2643*

1863:32 Wilhelm **Latzko**, Austrian gynaecologist, born 3 Mar; described an extraperitoneal lower-segment caesarean section, 1909, *WKW* **22**:477. Died 1945. *6249*

1863:33 Bartolomeo **Gosio**, Italian bacteriologist, born 17 Mar; first to record the antibacterial effect of a penicillin (from *Penicillium glaucum*), 1896, *RISP* **7**:825, 829, 961. Died 1944. *1932.3*

1863:34 Eduard Konrad **Zirm**, Austrian ophthalmic surgeon, born 18 Mar; reported the first successful corneal transplant (keratoplasty), 1906, *GAO* **64**:580. Died 1944. *5950.1*

1863:35 Simon **Flexner**, American pathologist and bacteriologist, born 25 Mar; isolated a causal organism in bacillary dysentery differing from Shiga's bacillus and named *Shigella flexneri*, 1900, *JHB* **11**:231. With James Wesley Jobling, used antiserum in the treatment of epidemic cerebrospinal meningitis, 1907–8, *JEM* **9**:168; **10**:141. With Paul A. Lewis, demonstrated antibodies in convalescent serum in monkeys infected experimentally with poliomyelitis, 1910, *JAMA* **54**:1780. Died 1946. *5093, 4683, 468, 4670*

1863:36 Albert Frank Stanley **Kent**, British physiologist, born 26 Mar; he described the atrioventricular bundle ('Bundle of Kent'), 1893, *JP* **14**:233; it was also described by Wilhelm His, in the same year and named the 'Bundle of His'). *837*

1863:37 Hugo Karl **Liepmann**, German psychiatrist, born 9 Apr; gave the first adequate description of apraxia, 1900, *MonP* **8**:15, 102, 182. Died 1925. *4588*

1863:38 Leonardo **Gigli**, Italian gynaecologist, born 30 Apr; invented the 'Gigli saw', 1894, *AnOG* **16**:649, first used for pubiotomy; he adapted it for craniotomy, 1898, *ZCh* **25**:425. Died 1908. *6204, 4874*

1863:39 Frederick Parkes **Weber**, British physician, born 8 May; described multiple hereditary telangiectasis ('Rendu-Osler-Weber disease'), 1907, *L* **2**:160. Described an association of a port-wine naevus with a vascular abnormality of the meninges on the same side, 1922, *JNP* **3**:134, already recorded by Sturge (1879) – ('Sturge-Weber syndrome'). Reported erythro-keratoma non-suppurative nodular panniculitis ('Weber-Christian disease'), 1925; it was later recorded, in 1928, by Henry Asbury Christian. Died 1962. *2714, 4605.2, 4560.1, 4151, 4152*

1863:40 Petr Fokich **Borovskii**, Russian bacteriologist and protozoologist, born 8 Jun; gave the first description of the protozoon later named *Leishmania tropica*, causal organism in cutaneous leishmaniasis, 1898, *VMZ* **76**:925. Died 1932. *5294*

1863:41 Alfred **Kirstein**, German laryngologist, born 25 Jun; first to use direct-vision laryngoscopy, 1895, *ArL* **3**:156. Died 1922. *3335*

1863:42 Ludvig **Hektoen**, American pathologist, born 2 Jul; produced experimental cirrhosis of the liver, 1900, *JPB* **7**:214; demonstrated the suppression of antibody response by x rays, 1915, *JID* **17**:415. Died 1951. *3640, 2659*

1863:43 Léon Charles Albert **Calmette**, French physician and bacteriologist, born 12 Jul; with Alexandre Emile Jean Yersin and A. Borrel, successfully inoculated animals with anti-plague bacillus, 1895, *AnIP* **9**:589. Devised the conjunctival reaction test for the diagnosis of tuberculosis, 1907, *CRAS* **144**:1324. With C. Guérin and B. Weill-Hallé he introduced BCG vaccine in tuberculosis prophylaxis, 1924, *BuAM* **91**:787. Died 1933. *5127, 2337, 2343*

1863:44 John Sydney **Edkins**, British physiologist, born 12 Jul; described gastrin (gastric secretin), 1906, *JP* **34**:133. Died 1940. *1026*

1863:45 Sören **Holth**, Norwegian ophthalmologist, born 24 Jul; introduced the operation of iridencleisis for the treatment of glaucoma, 1907, *AnO* **137**:345. Died 1937. *5952*

1863:46 Luigi **Lucatello**, Italian pathologist, born 30 Jul; introduced liver puncture biopsy, 1895, *LCMI* **6**:327. Died 1926. *3635*

1863:47 Scipione **Riva-Rocci**, Italian physician and surgeon, born 7 Aug; modified the sphygmomanometer, 1896, *GMT* **47**:981, 1001. Died 1937. *2804*

1863:48 Anton **Elschnig**, Austrian ophthalmologist, born 22 Aug; suggested the anaphylactic theory of the pathogenesis of sympathetic ophthalmia, 1910, *GAO* **75**:459. Developed the method of corneal grafting (keratoplasty) introduced by von Hippel, with good results, 1930, *ArOp* **4**:165. Died 1939. *5957, 5975*

1863:49 Josef **Jadassohn**, German dermatologist and venereologist, born 10 Sep; maculopapular erythroderma, described by him in 1892, *VDDG* **2–3**:342, is also named 'Jadassohn's disease'. Died 1936. *4108*

1863:50 William Gibson **Spiller**, American neurologist, born 13 Sep; with Charles Harrison Frazier, introduced intracranial trigeminal neurotomy for the treatment of trigeminal neuralgia, 1901, *UPMB* **14**:342; with Edward Martin, relieved intractable pain by spinal cordotomy, 1912, *JAMA* **58**:1489. Died 1940. *4876, 4883*

1863:51 Charles **Donovan**, British officer in Indian Medical Service, born 19 Sep; found an organism considered to be a trypanosome, 1903, *BMJ* **2**:79. W.B. Leishman had found the same organism, which he also considered a trypanosome, it was later named *Leishmania donovani* (Leishman-Donovan bodies), and shown to be the causal organism in leishmaniasis. Died 1951. *5296, 5295*

1863:52 Murk **Jansen**, Dutch orthopaedic surgeon, born 22 Sep; published his theory of dissociation of bone growth; in the *Robert Jones Birthday Volume*, p. 43, 1928. Died 1935. *4395*

1863:53 Alexandre Emile Jean **Yersin**, Swiss bacteriologist, born 22 Sep; with Pierre Paul Emile Roux, confirmed the work of Loeffler on *Corynebacterium diphtheriae* and demonstrated the exotoxin in diphtheria, 1888, *AnIP* **2**:629; **3**:273; **4**:385. Their work marks the starting point of the development of an immunizing serum. Discovered the plague bacillus, *Pasteurella pestis*, 1894, *AnIP* **8**:662. With Léon Charles Albert Calmette (1863–1933) and A. Borrel, successfully inoculated animals with anti-plague bacillus, 1895, *AnIP* **9**:589. Died 1943. *5059, 5125, 5127*

1863:54 Frederick **Edridge-Green**, British ophthalmologist, born 14 Dec; his lantern test for colour-blindness described, in his *Colour-blindness and colour-perception*, 1891, p. 262, was adopted in Great Britain in 1915 in place of the Holmgren test. Died 1953. *5937*

1863:55 Wilhelm **His**, Jr, Swiss physician, born 29 Dec; described atrioventricular bundle ('Bundle of His'), 1893, *AMKI*: 14. Encountered a form of trench fever in Volhynia, Russia, and named it Volhynia fever, 1916, *BKW* **53**:322. Died 1934. *836, 5387*

1863:56 Samuel **Rideal**, British chemist, born; with J.T. Ainslie Walker devised a method for testing disinfectants, 1903, *JSI* **24**:424. Died 1929. *1893*

1863:57 Ignatz Leo **Nascher** born; published *Geriatrics; the diseases of old age and their treatment* ..., 1914, the first modern treatise on geriatrics; he coined the term in 1909. Died 1944. *1641.1*

1863:58 Harry de Riemer **Morgan**, British bacteriologist, born; isolated *Proteus morgani*, 1906, *BMJ* **1**:908. Died 1931. *2518.1*

1863:59 Edvard **Ehlers**, Danish dermatologist, born; described cutis laxa, 1901, *DeZ*, **8**:173; after Danlos's paper in 1908 it was named 'Ehlers-Danlos syndrome'. Died 1937. *4132, 4144*

1863:60 James Samuel Risien **Russell**, British physician, born; with Frederick Eustace Batten and J.S. Collier, gave the first full description of subacute combined degeneration of the spinal cord, 1900, *Brain* **23**:39. Died 1939. *4710*

1863:61 Henri Amadée **Lafleur** born; with William Thomas Councilman, introduced the term 'amoebic dysentery' in their important investigation of the condition, 1891, *JHR* **2**:395. Died 1939. *5187*

1863:62 George Ford **Petrie**, British bacteriologist and immunologist, born; with Arthur Felix, first prepared anti-typhoid serum, 1938, *JHyg* **38**:673. Died 1955. *5045.1*

1863: Otto Friedrich Carl **Deiters** died, **born** 1834. *glia cells, Deiter's nucleus*

1863: John **Watson** died, **born** 1807. *oesophagotomy*

1863: Jean François **Reybard** died, **born** 1790. *cancer, intestinal resection*

1863: Joseph Henry **Green** died, **born** 1791. *thyroidectomy*

1863: Hermann Friedrich **Kilian** died, **born** 1800. *pelvis spinosa, spondylolisthetic pelvis*

**1864**
1864:1 **Geneva Convention**, and adoption of **Red Cross** symbol

1864:2 **Association Française pour l'Avancement des Sciences** founded

1864:3 **Gray Herbarium** founded at **Harvard University**

1864:4 **Chicago Medical College** incorporated

1864:5 **St Louis College of Pharmacy** founded

1864:6 **University of Bucharest** founded

1864:7 *Berliner Klinische Wochenschrift* commences publication *(Klinische Wochenschrift,* 1922)

1864:8 *Archiv für Mikroskopische Anatomie* commences publication

1864:9 **St Luke's Hospital, Chicago,** opened

1864:10 The inventor of the **Hodge pessary,** Hugh Lenox Hodge (1796–1873), also produced a fine textbook, *The principles and practice of obstetrics.* At that time he was almost blind and dictated the book to his son from memory. *6185*

1864:11 **Bipolar version,** in which the breech is made to present, a method of treatment for **placenta praevia** introduced by John Braxton Hicks (1823–1897), *TOSL* **5**:219. *6186*

1864:12 For many years Charles Clay (1801–1897) was the most successful **ovariotomist** in Britain, he performed 395 operations, with a mortality of 25 per cent, *TOSL* **5**:58. *6054*

1864:13 Felix Hoppe-Seyler (1825–1895) obtained **haemoglobin** in crystalline form, *VA* **29**:233, 597. *873*

1864:14 **Trichloroethylene** discovered by E. Fischer, *JZN* **1**:123. *5667*

1864:15 **Aphasia** studied for 30 years by John Hughlings Jackson (1835–1911), emphasizing its psychological aspects and laying the foundations for present knowledge of the condition, *CLLH* **1**:388. *4620*

1864:16 The first description of **osteitis fibrosa cystica** ('**Engel-Recklinghausen disease**') given by Gerhard Engel in his *Ueber einen Fall von cystoider Entartung des ganzen Skelettes.* Von Recklinghausen's important description ('**von Recklinghausen's disease of bone**') appeared in 1891. *4335, 4358*

1864:17 First description of **chronic arthritis in childhood** given by André Victor Cornil (1837–1898), *CRSB* **1**:3. *4499*

1864:18 The first comprehensive American textbook of **orthopaedics,** *Lectures on orthopaedic surgery,* published by Louis Bauer (1814–1898). *4334*

1864:19 '**Dietl's crisis**', acute **ureteral colic,** described by Josef Dietl (1804–1878), *WMW* **14**:563, 579, 593. *4211*

1864:20 **Impetigo contagiosa** first described by William Tilbury Fox (1836–1879), *BMJ* **1**:78, 467, 495, 553, 607. *4055*

1864:21 Albrecht von Graefe (1828–1870) discovered an important diagnostic sign in **exophthalmic goitre** – failure of the eyelid to follow the eye when it is rolled downward ('**Graefe's sign**'), *DK* **16**:158. *3820*

1864:22 First successful ligation of the **innominate artery** by Andrew Woods Smyth (1832–1916), *AmJMS* **52**:289. *2963*

1864:23 First official *British Pharmacopoeia* published by the General Medical Council. *1866*

1864:24 *On the anomalies of accommodation and refraction of the eye*, the most important work of Frans Donders (1818–1889), includes his explanation of **astigmatism**, his definition of **aphakia** and **hypermetropia**, and his distinction between **myopia** and hypermetropia. *5893*

1864:25 Henri **Triboulet**, French paediatrician, born 1 Jan; with Amand Coyon, isolated streptococci from patients with acute rheumatism, 1898, *CRSB* **50**:124. Died 1920. *4504.1*

1864:26 Ernst **Wertheim**, Austrian gynaecologist, born 21 Feb; emphasized the significance of latent gonorrhoeal infection of the uterus, 1896, *VDGG* **6**:199. Demonstrated gonococcal infection of the bladder as a cause of acute cystitis, 1896, *ZGG* **35**:1. Introduced a radical operation for cancer of the uterus, 1902, *ArGy* **61**:627; **65**:1. Died 1920. *6099, 6103, 6114*

1864:27 Carl **Schlatter**, Swiss surgeon, born 18 Mar; performed first successful total gastrectomy, 1897, *BKC* **19**:757; **23**:589. Described lesions of the tibial tuberosity occurring in adolescence ('Osgood-Schlatter disease'), 1903, *BKC* **38**:874; it was also described by Osgood in the same year. Died 1934. *3517, 4374 4373*

1864:28 Karel Frederik **Wenckebach**, Dutch physician, born 24 Mar; described 'Wenckebach's phenomenon', a form of arrhythmia, 1899, *ZKM* **36**:181. Gave an important account of heart arrhythmias, reporting the value of quinine in paroxysmal fibrillation, 1914; in his *Die unregelmässige Herztätigkeit und ihre klinische Bedeutung*. In his *Das Beriberi-Herz*, 1934, he gave an important account of the heart in beriberi. Died 1940. *2809.1, 2844, 3747*

1864:29 Alois **Alzheimer**, German psychiatrist, born 14 Jun; presenile dementia is also called 'Alzheimer's disease' after his description of the condition, 1907, *AZP* **64**:146. Died 1915. *4956*

1864:30 Robert Henry **Elliot**, British ophthalmic surgeon, born 23 Aug; introduced the operation of sclero-corneal trephining for glaucoma, 1909, *Oph* **7**:804. Died 1927. *5955*

1864:31 Carl Franz Joseph Erich **Correns**, German botanist and geneticist, born 19 Sep; one of the rediscoverers of Mendel's laws (with de Vries and Tschermak von Seysenegg), he showed the deepest understanding of them, 1900, *BBBG* **18**:158. Died 1933. *239.1*

1864:32 Dmitri Iosifovich **Ivanovski**, Russian botanist, born 9 Nov; showed that tobacco mosaic disease agent was filter-passing, 1892, *BAIS* **3**:67; this was the starting point of research into the aetiology of virus diseases. Died 1920. *2506.2*

1864:33 George Washington **Crile**, American surgeon, born 11 Nov; made important observations on surgical shock, *An experimental research into surgical shock*, 1899. First to carry out anaesthetic blocking of nerve trunks, *An experimental and clinical research into certain problems relating to surgical operations*, 1901, p. 88. He advanced the kinetic theory of shock and the anoci-association concept in which local and general anaesthesia combined in sequence to eliminate pre-operative fear and tension, 1913, *L* **2**:7. Died 1943. *5622, 5624, 5687, 5629*

1864:34 Raymond Jacques Adrien **Sabouraud**, French dermatologist, born 24 Nov; studied the role of fungi in skin diseases, in his *Les trichophyties humaines*, 1894. First described the acne bacillus, *Corynebacterium acnes*, 1897, *AnIP* **11**:134. Used radiotherapy in the treatment of tinea (ringworm), 1904, *AnD* **5**:577. Gave a classic account of the different varieties of *Trichophyton*; in his *Pityriasis et alopécies pelliculaires*, 1904. Died 1938. *3999, 4126, 4004, 4139*

1864:35 Frederick George **Novy**, American bacteriologist, born 9 Dec; with Richard Edward Knapp, proved that the spirochaete isolated by Norris et al. from a case of American relapsing fever differed from that isolated by Obermeier, 1906, *JID* **3**:291. Died 1957. *5320*

1864:36 Georg **Avellis**, German otolaryngologist, born; recorded recurrent paralysis of the palate, ('Avellis's syndrome'), 1891, *BKl* **40**:1. Died 1916. *3303*

1864:37 Adolph **Reich**, American physician, born; first to obtain cholangiograms, 1918, *JAMA* **71**:1555. *3650*

1864:38 David Middleton **Greig**, British surgeon, born; first described hypertelorism as a separate entity, 1924, *EMJ* **31**:560. Died 1936. *4392*

1864: Adrian Christopher van **Trigt** died, **born** 1825. *fundus oculi*

1864: Heinrich **Müller** died, **born** 1820. *visual purple*

1864: William Senhouse **Kirkes** died, **born** 1823. *embolism*

1864: Johann Lucas **Schönlein** died, **born** 1793. *anaphylactoid purpura, ringworm*

1864: Charles Louis Stanislas **Heurteloup** died, **born** 1793. *lithotrity*

1864: Lewis **Durlacher** died, **born** 1792. *metatarsalgia*

1864: Friedrich Wilhelm Felix von **Bärensprung** died, **born** 1822. *herpes zoster, tinea cruris*

**1865**
1865:1 **Medico-Psychological Association** (formerly **Association of Medical Officers of Asylums and Hospitals for the Insane**), UK

1865:2 John Shaw **Billings** (1838–1913) appointed Librarian of Surgeon General's Office, Washington

1865:3 **Cornell University** founded at **Ithaca, NY**

1865:4 **Chicago Hospital for Women** founded

1865:5 **'Deiters' cells'** (**glia cells**) and **'Deiters' nucleus'** described by Otto Friedrich Carl Deiters (1834–1863) in his *Gehirn und Ruckenmark des Menschen*. *1271*

1865:6 Thomas Smith (1833–1909) was first to report **craniohypophyseal xanthomatosis**, later to be associated with the **Hand-Schüller-Christian syndrome**, *TPS* 16:224; 27:219. *6359–6363*

1865:7 Thomas Spencer Wells (1818–1897) was among the most eminent of the **ovariotomists**; he wrote *Diseases of the ovaries*, 1865, and a second work with the same title in 1872. *6056*

1865:8 The operation for **cataract** by modified linear extraction improved by Albrecht von Graefe (1828–1870), *GAO* 11, iii:1; 12, i:150; 14, iii:106. *5897*

1865:9 Casimir Joseph Davaine (1812–1882) first conclusively to prove that a specific disease (**anthrax**) was caused by a specific organism (*Bacillus anthracis*), and was thus one of the first to prove the germ theory of disease, *CRSB* 60:1296. *5166*

1865:10 The first successful therapeutic percutaneous **nephrostomy** performed by Thomas Hillier (1831–1868), *PRMCS* 5:59. *4211.1*

1865:11 A classic description of **paroxysmal haemoglobinuria** by George Harley (1829–1896), *MCT* 48:161, led to the eponym '**Harley's disease**'. *4171*

1865:12 **Haemochromatosis** first described by Armand Trousseau (1801–1867); in his *Clinique médicale de l'Hôtel-Dieu*, 2nd edn, 2, 663. *3915*

1865:13 Pictures of the **membrana tympani** by means of illumination obtained by Adam Politzer (1835–1920); in his *Die Beleuchtungsbilder des Trommelfells* …. *3378*

1865:14 An **otoscope** devised by John Brunton (1836–1899), *L* 2:617. *3378.1*

1865:15 The first comprehensive study of **duodenal ulcer** was published by Julius Krauss (b.1841); in his *Das perforirende Geschwür im Duodenum*. *3461*

1865:16 **Syphilis: Profeta's law** – a non-syphilitic child born of syphilitic parents is immune – stated by Giuseppe Profeta (1840–1911), *Spe* 15:328, 339. *2390*

1865:17 **Epithelial-cell** origin of **cancer** histogenesis advanced by Karl Thiersch (1822–1895); in his *Der Epithelialkrebs namentlich der Haut*. *2618*

1865:18 Theory of **heredity,** foundation of genetics, published by Gregor Mendel (1822–1884), *VNVB* 4:3. *222*

1865:19 The idea of maintaining excised **organs** by means of **perfusion** introduced by Carl Ludwig (1816–1895); in his *Die physiologischen Leistungen des Blutdrucks*. *778*

1865:20 **Electroretinogram** introduced by Alarik Frithiof Holmgren (1831–1897), *ULF* 1:177. *1511.1*

1865:21 The first clear description of the rhythmic variations in tone of the **vasoconstrictor centre** given by Ludwig Traube (1818–1876), *ZMW* 3:881. *818*

1865:22 Heinrich Ernst **Albers-Schönberg**, German radiologist, born 21 Jan; first described osteopetrosis fragilis (marble bones, 'Albers-Schönberg's disease'), 1903, *FGR* 7:158;

introduced compression diaphragm in radiography, in his *Die Röntgen-Technik*, 1903; gave first definite description of osteopoikilosis, a structural anomaly of the skeleton, 1915, *FGR* **23**:174. Died 1921. *4372, 2689, 4386.1*

1865:23 Herbert **Herbert**, British ophthalmic surgeon, born 25 Feb; introduced a small flap sclerotomy for glaucoma, 1910, *TOUK* **30**:199. Died 1942. *5958*

1865:24 John William Watson **Stephens**, British physician, born 2 Mar; with Harold Benjamin Fantham, discovered a new species of trypanosome, *Trypanosoma rhodesiense*, 1910, *PRS* **83**:28. First described *Plasmodium ovale*, a malaria parasite, 1922, *AnTM* **16**:383. Died 1946. *5285, 5255.2*

1865:25 Georg **Klemperer**, German physician, born 10 May; with Felix Klemperer, introduced old antipneumococcus serum, 1891, *BKW* **28**:833, 869. Died 1932. *3178*

1865:26 Keinosuke **Miyairi**, Japanese professor of hygiene, born 15 May; with M. Suzuki, confirmed snails as the intermediate hosts of *Schistosoma japonicum*, 1914, *MMFK* **1**:187. Died 1946. *5350.2*

1865:27 George Lenthal **Cheatle**, British surgeon, born 13 Jun; first to adopt the preperitoneal approach in the repair of hernia, 1920, *BMJ* **2**:68. Died 1951. *3608.3*

1865:28 Jules de **Nobele**, Belgian physician, born 17 Jul; found *Salmonella aertrycke* to be a cause of food poisoning, 1898; *ASMG* **77**:281. *2514*

1865:29 Greenfield **Sluder**, American laryngologist, born 30 Aug; first described the syndrome of sphenopalatine-ganglion neuralgia ('Sluder's neuralgia'), 1901, *AmJMS* **140**:868. Died 1928. *4595*

1865:30 Christian Archibald **Herter**, American physician, born 3 Sep; described 'Herter's infantilism', from chronic intestinal infection, 1908, in his *On infantilism from chronic intestinal infection*; identical to Gee-Thaysen disease. Died 1910. *3528*

1865:31 James Tayloe **Gwathmey**, one of the first specialists in anaesthesiology in the USA, born 10 Sep; produced anaesthesia by rectal injection of liquid ether with olive oil dissolved in it (synergistic anaesthesia), 1913, *NYMJ* **98**:1101, especially successful in midwifery; described a nitrous oxide-oxygen ether apparatus; in his *Anesthesia*, 1914, p. 334. Died 1944. *5699, 5699.1*

1865:32 Frederick Eustace **Batten**, British paediatrician and neuropathologist, born 29 Sep; with James Samuel Risien Russell and J.S. Collier, gave the first full description of subacute combined degeneration of the spinal cord, 1900, *Brain* **23**:39; described cases of juvenile amaurotic familial idiocy ('Batten-Mayou disease'), *TOUK* **23**:86, 1903. Died 1918. *4710, 4712*

1865:33 Berkeley George Andrew **Moynihan**, British surgeon, born 2 Oct; greatly advanced knowledge concerning duodenal ulcer; in his *Duodenal ulcer*, 1910. Died 1936. *3535*

1865:34 James Harry **Sequeira**, British dermatologist, born 2 Oct; with William Bulloch, first recognized the adrenogenital syndrome, 1905, *TPS* **56**:189. Died 1948. *3867*

1865:35 William Edward **Fothergill**, British gynaecologist, born 4 Oct; modified A. Donald's operation for prolapse of the uterus, 1915, *JOG* **27**:146. Died 1926. *6124, 6119*

1865:36 Chevalier **Jackson**, American laryngologist, born 4 Nov; first to remove endothelioma of the bronchus by peroral bronchoscopy, 1917, *AmJMS* **153**:371. With his son, Chevalier L. Jackson, published a comprehensive treatise on foreign bodies in air and food passages and their removal, *Diseases of the air and food passages of foreign body origin*, 1937. Died 1958. *3194, 3338.1*

1865:37 William Boog **Leishman**, British Army physician, born 6 Nov; developed a stain (Leishman's stain), 1901, a modification of Romanovsky's stain (1891), for the demonstration of the malaria parasite in blood films, *BMJ* **2**:757. Found an organism (1900) which he later described as possibly a trypanosome, 1903, *BMJ* **1**:1252; **2**:1476. C. Donovan (1903) found the same organism, which was later named *Leishmania donovani* (Leishman-Donovan bodies), and shown to be the causal organism in leishmaniasis. Died 1926. *5253, 5242, 5295, 5296*

1865:38 Ludolph **Brauer**, German physician, born; induced artificial pneumothorax, ('Brauer's method'), by injection of nitrogen, 1906, *MMW* **53**:338. First radical thoracoplasty for pulmonary tuberculosis, 1908, *PVC* **21**:569. Died 1951. *3230, 3231*

1865:39 Max **Askanazy**, German pathologist, born; first to associate osteitis fibrosa cystica with parathyroid tumours, 1904, *AGPA* **4**:398. Died 1940. *3858*

1865:40 Vard Houghton **Hulen**, American ophthalmic surgeon, born; devised a vacuum method of cataract extraction, 1911, *JAMA* **57**:188. Died 1939. *5959*

1865: Raffaele **Piria** died, **born** 1815. *salicylic acid*

1865: Ignaz Philipp **Semmelweis** died, **born** 1818. *obstetrics, antisepsis, puerperal fever*

1865: Charles **Waterton** died, **born** 1782. *curare*

1865: Valentine **Mott** died, **born** 1785. *innominate artery ligation, carotid artery ligation*

1865: Wilhelm Friedrich **Ludwig** died, **born** 1790. *Ludwig's angina*

1865: Robert **Remak** died, **born** 1815. *galvanotherapy, fibres of Remak, intrinsic ganglia of heart*

1865: Jean Baptiste Octave **Landry** died, **born** 1826. *polyneuritis*

1865: Joseph François **Malgaigne** died, **born** 1806. *surgery, cleft lip*

**1866**
1866:1 [**Academy of Natural Sciences**] founded at **Agram (Zagreb)**

1866:2 [**Society of Physicians**] founded at **Krakow**

1866:3 [**Society of Czechoslovak Physicians**] founded at **Prague** by Jan Evangelista **Purkyně**

1866:4 **Metropolitan Health Board** founded at **New York City**

1866:5 [**Hygienic Laboratory**] established in **Munich** by Carl Von Voit (1831–1908)

1866:6 The **Laurence-Moon (-Biedl) syndrome**, **retinitis pigmentosa** with familial developmental imperfections, first reported by John Zachariah Laurence (1830–1874) and Robert Charles Moon (1844–1914), *OR* 2:32. Further cases were reported by A. Biedl (1922). *6368, 6369*

1866:7 The method of extraction of the lens in the closed capsule through scleral incision for the treatment of **cataract** introduced by Alexander Pagenstecher (1828–1879); recorded in *Klinische Beobachtungen aus der Augenheilanstalt zu Wiesbaden*, Heft 3, p. 10, edited by Pagenstecher and E.T. Saemisch. *5896*

1866:8 Joseph William Bazalgette (1819–1891) plans for **sewage disposal** in London appear in the *Metropolitan Board of Works Report on experiments with respect to the ventilation of sewers*, 3 parts, (1866–1869). *1615*

1866:9 Studies of **gaseous exchange** in **blood** and **tissue** and the development of the concept of '**respiratory quotient**', recorded by Eduard Friedrich Wilhelm Pflüger (1829–1910), 1866, *ZMW* 4:305, 1868; *PfA* 1:61. *939, 940*

1866:10 The controversial *Clinical notes on uterine surgery, with reference to the management of the sterile condition*, written by James Marion Sims (1813–1883), includes a description of Sims' **duck-billed speculum** (p. 16) and pioneering work in the treatment of **infertility** and record of a successful **artificial insemination**. *6057*

1866:11 The term **rubella** introduced to describe German measles (Rötheln) by Henry Richard Lobb Veale (1832–1908), *EMJ* 12:404. *5502*

1866:12 Joseph Pierre Rollet (1824–1894) recognized the possibility of mixed infection of a sore with both **syphilis** and **chancroid** ('**Rollet's disease**'), *GML* 18:160. *5204*

1866:13 The substitution of **psychotherapy** for **hypnotic suggestion** was due to the work of Ambroise Auguste Liébeault (1823–1904); in his *Le sommeil provoqué et les états analogues considérés sur au point du vue de l'action du moral et de physique. 4994*

1866:14 Ernst Heinrich Philipp August Haeckel (1834–1919) accepted the principles of **Darwinism**, which he carried into Germany. His most important work is *Generelle Morphologie der Organismen. 223*

1866:15 The **physiognomonical** features of certain **mental defectives** suggested to John Langdon Haydon Langdon-Down (1828–1896) that they could be classified in ethnic groups, *CLLH* 3:259. His classification has been abandoned, but the term **mongolism** (now replaced by '**Down's syndrome**') is used to describe one important variety of mental retardation. *4936*

1866:16 The first clinical description of the electric pains in **tabes dorsalis** given by Jean Martin Charcot (1825–1893) and Abel Bouchard (1833–1899), *GMP* 21:122. *4775*

1866:17 Griesinger's view that the cause of **tropical anaemia** was the **ankylostomiasis hookworm** confirmed by Otto Eduard Heinrich Wucherer (1820–1873), *GMB* 1:27, 39, 52, 63. *5356, 5355*

1866:18 The **visceral crises** in **tabes dorsalis** first described by Georges Delamarre; in his *Des troubles gastriques dans l'ataxie locomotrice progressive*, Paris, Thèse No. 250. *4776*

1866:19 **Colloid degeneration of the skin** ('**Wagner's disease**') first described by Ernst Leberecht Wagner (1829–1888), *ArH* **7**:463; he named it '**colloid milium**'. *4056*

1866:20 **Whiplash injuries**, due to the increased speed of railway travel, first discussed in book form by John Eric Erichsen (1818–1896); in his *On railway and other injuries of the nervous system. 4538.1*

1866:21 Wilhelm Griesinger (1817–1868) first to report **splenic anaemia**, in an infant, *BKW* **3**:212. *3766*

1866:22 **Laryngitis sicca** – ('**Türck's trachoma**') – described by Ludwig Türck (1810–1868); in his *Klinik der Krankheiten des Kehlkopfes ...*, p. 295. *3273*

1866:23 **Periarteritis nodosa** first described by Adolf Kussmaul (1822–1902) and Rudolph Maier (1824–1888), *DAKM* **1**:484. *2906*

1866:24 **Pasteurization** scientifically established by Louis Pasteur (1822–1895); in *Études sur le vin. 2479*

1866:25 **Physostigmine (eserine)** isolated by Thomas Richard Fraser (1841–1919), *TRSE* **24**:715. *1866.1*

1866:26 Richard Owen's (1804–1892) *Anatomy and physiology of vertebrates*, 3 vols, 1866–68, is based entirely on personal observations. *336*

---

1866:27 Charles James **Martin**, British physiologist and bacteriologist, born 9 Jan; with Arthur William Bacot, demonstrated the mechanism of transmission of plague bacillus from rat to man by the rat **flea**, 1914, *JHyg* Plague Suppl.3:423. Died 1955. *5129.1*

1866:28 Ludwig **Aschoff**, German pathologist, born 10 Jan; published an important account of rheumatic myocarditis, 1904, *VDPG* **8**:46, which includes a description of the characteristic lesion ('Aschoff body'). Died 1942. *2816*

1866:29 John Whitridge **Williams**, American obstetrician, born 26 Jan; published *Obstetrics*, 1903, the foremost American textbook of **obstetrics**, still in print under modern editorship. Died 1931. *6210.1*

1866:30 Arthur **Keith**, British anatomist and anthropologist, born 5 Feb; with Martin William Flack (1882–1931) discovered the sino-auricular node – the 'pacemaker of the heart', 1907, *JA* **41**:172. Died 1955. *844*

1866:31 Jean **Nageotte**, French histopathologist, born 8 Feb; with Joseph François Félix Babinski, described a syndrome of multiple medullary lesions of vascular origin involving the medullary tract and other structures ('syndrome of Babinski-Nageotte'), 1902, *ReN* **10**:358. Died 1948. *4589*

1866:32 August von **Wassermann**, German bacteriologist, born 21 Feb; with A. Neisser and C. Bruck, introduced a specific diagnostic blood test for syphilis, the 'Wassermann reaction',

1906, *DMW* **32**:745. Applied his test to the cerebrospinal fluid in cases of general paralysis, 1906, *DMW* **32**:1769; it greatly facilitated the diagnosis of general paresis. Died 1925. *2402, 4804*

1866:33 Arthur Robertson **Cushny**, British pharmacologist, born 6 Mar; first to recognize auricular fibrillation in man (*Studies in pathology* ... ed. by W. Bulloch, 1906, p. 95); his theory of urinary secretion, *The secretion of the urine*, 1917, followed and modified that of Carl Ludwig. Reported important studies in *The action and uses in medicine of digitalis*, 1925. Died 1926. *2822, 1237, 1912*

1866:34 Herbert Edward **Durham**, British bacteriologist, born 25 Mar; with Max Gruber, discovered bacterial agglutination and used it in diagnosis, realizing its value in the identification of typhoid, 1896, *MMW* **43**:285. Found *Salmonella aertrycke* in cases of food poisoning, 1898, *BMJ* **2**:608. Died 1945. *2549, 5036, 2513*

1866:35 Ernest Henry **Starling**, British physiologist, born 17 Apr; developed theory of hormonal control of internal secretion with William Maddock Bayliss, 1904, *PRS* **73**:310 (in 1905 he introduced the term 'hormone'); stated his 'law of the heart', 1918, in his *Linacre Lecture on the law of the heart*. Died 1927. *1121, 853*

1866:36 Jesse William **Lazear**, American physician, born 2 May; with Walter Reed, James Carroll, and Aristide Agramonte y Simoni, provided the first definite proof that the causal agent in yellow fever is transmitted to man by the mosquito, *Aedes aegypti*, 1900, *PhMeJ* **6**:790. He died from the disease, having been accidentally bitten by a mosquito. Died 1900. *5457*

1866:37 Jules **Sottas**, French neurologist, born 22 May; with Joseph Jules Dejerine, gave the first description of hypertrophic progressive interstitial neuritis ('Dejerine-Sottas disease'), 1893, *CRSB* **45**:63. *4580*

1866:38 Paul **Portier**, French physiologist, born 22 May; with Charles Robert Richet, published first full description of anaphylaxis, 1902, *CRSB* **54**:170. Died 1962. *2590*

1866:39 Leonard Erskine **Hill**, British physiologist, born 6 Jun; with Harold Leslie Barnard, substituted pressure gauge for mercury manometer in the Riva-Rocci sphygmomanometer, 1897, *BMJ* **2**:904. Died 1952. *2807*

1866:40 Serge **Voronoff**, Russian physiologist, born 10 Jul; his experimental rejuvenation by testicular transplantation (1919) reported in his *Greffes testiculaires*, 1923. Died 1951. *3797*

1866:41 Robert **Robinson**, British chemist, born 13 Sep; awarded Nobel Prize (Chemistry), 1947, for research on products of biological importance, including alkaloids, sterols, sex hormones, penicillin, *NPL*. Died 1975.

1866:42 Charles Jules Henri **Nicolle**, French bacteriologist, born 21 Sep; considered infantile kala-azar to be due to a distinct species of *Leishmania*, *L.infantum*, 1909, *AnIP* **23**:361, 441. Demonstrated the transmission of typhus by the body louse, *Pediculus corporis*, and produced the disease in monkeys and guinea-pigs by the injection of infected blood, 1910, *AnIP* **24**:243; **25**:97; **26**:250, 332 (for this work he received the Nobel Prize (Physiology or Medicine), 1928, *NPL*). With co-workers, carried out filtration of the trachoma agent, *Chlamydia trachomatis*, 1912, *CRAS* **155**:241. Died 1936. *5300, 5384, 5961*

1866:43 Thomas Hunt **Morgan**, American geneticist, born 25 Sep; published *The mechanism of Mendelian heredity*, 1915, recording epoch-making work on heredity, with Alfred Henry Sturtevant, Hermann Joseph Muller and Colin Blackman Bridges. He established the chromosome theory of heredity (for which he was awarded the Nobel Prize (Physiology or Medicine) in 1933, *NPL*) and demonstrated sex-linked inheritance. Died 1945. *246, 245.1*

1866:44 Felix **Klemperer**, German physician, born 9 Oct; with Georg Klemperer, introduced old antipneumococcus serum, 1891, *BKW* **28**:833, 869. Died 1946. *3178*

1866:45 Franz **Kuhn**, German surgeon, born 12 Oct; introduced the intratracheal insufflation method of anaesthetization, *c*.1900, *DZC* 1905, **76**:148. Died 1929. *5693*

1866:46 Aldred Scott **Warthin**, American pathologist, born 21 Oct; gave classical clinical description of pulmonary fat embolism, 1913, *IC* 24 ser.4:171. Died 1931. *3015*

1866:47 Bertram Welton **Sippy**, American gastroenterologist, born 30 Oct; introduced a dietetic treatment of peptic ulcer ('Sippy diet'), 1915, *JAMA* **64**:1625. Died 1924. *3541*

1866:48 Abraham **Flexner**, American educationalist, born 13 Nov; made a study of American and Canadian medical schools – his highly critical report, *Medical education in the United States and Canada*, 1910, led to important reforms in North America. He published the first systematic and thorough comparisons of the major systems of medical education in Europe, *Medical education in Europe*, 1912, and *Medical education: a comprehensive study*, 1925. Died 1959. *1766.502–4*

---

1866:49 Holger **Nielsen**, Danish physician, born; invented 'arm-lift' method of artificial respiration, 1932, *UL* **94**:1201. Died 1955. *2028.60*

1866:50 Anton **Ghon**, Austrian bacteriologist, born; described anatomical distribution and development of lesions in pulmonary tuberculosis in children ('Ghon's primary focus'); in his *Die primäre Lungenherd bei der Tuberkulose der Kinder*; he was preceded by J. Parrot (1876). Died 1936. *3233*

1866:51 Sandor **Korány**, Hungarian physician, born; established cryoscopy of the urine as a kidney function test, 1894, *BKO*, p. 74. Died 1944. *4226*

1866:52 G. Paul **Busquet**, French physician, born; described osteoperiostitis of the metatarsals ('Busquet's disease'), 1897, *RC* **17**:1065. *4330*

1866:53 Arthur William **Bacot**, British entomologist, born; with Charles James Martin, demonstrated the mechanism of transmission of plague bacillus from rat to man by the rat flea, 1914, *JHyg* Plague Suppl.3:423. Died 1922. *5129.1*

1866:54 Ernst **Roos**, German physician, born; with Heinrich Irenaeus Quincke, distinguished *Entamoeba histolytica* from *Escherichia coli*, 1893, *BKW* **30**:1089. *5188*

1866:55 Ira Van **Gieson**, American neuropsychiatrist, born; introduced Van Gieson's acid fuchsin and picric acid stain for nerve tissue, 1889, *NYJM* **1**:57. Died 1913. *1419.1*

1866: 56 Victor **Morax**, Swiss ophthalmologist, born; independently of Axenfeld, he isolated the diplococcus responsible for chronic conjunctivitis, 1896, *AnIP* **10**:337, which was named 'Morax-Axenfeld bacillus'. Died 1935. *5942, 5941*

---

1866: Adolf Carl Peter **Callisen** died, **born** 1787. *medical bibliography*

1866: George Hilaro **Barlow** died, **born** 1806. *bacterial endocarditis*

1866: Horace **Green** died, **born** 1802. *laryngology*

1866: François **Mélier** died, **born** 1798. *appendicitis*

1866: Joseph **Toynbee** died, **born** 1815. *aural pathology*

1866: Benjamin Guy **Babington** died, **born** 1794. *glottiscope*

1866: Thomas **Hodgkin** died, **born** 1798. *lymphadenoma*

1866: Camille Melchior **Gibert** died, **born** 1797. *pityriasis rosea*

1866: Salomon Levi **Steinheim** died, **born** 1799. *parathyroid tetany*

1866: John **Conolly** died, **born** 1794. *psychiatry*

1866: David **Craigie** died, **born** 1793. *relapsing fever*

## 1867

1867: 1 **First International Medical Congress, Paris**

1867: 2 First tunnels for **Chicago water supply**

1867: 3 **Clinical Society of London** founded

1867: 4 The first thorough account of paralysis of the **eye muscles** and the basis for surgical treatment given by Albrecht von Graefe (1828–1870); in his *Symptomenlehre der Augenmuskellähmungen. 5899*

1867: 5 The **astigmometer** invented by Louis Emile Javal (1839–1907), *AnO* **57**:39. *5901*

1867: 6 The **antiseptic principle** in **surgery** introduced by Joseph Lister (1827–1912), using **carbolic acid**-impregnated dressings, *L* **1**:326, 357, 387, 507; **2**:95, 358, 668. *5634, 5635*

1867: 7 A **chloroform inhaler (Junker's inhaler)** invented by Ferdinand Ethelbert Junker (1828–?1901), *MTG* 1867, **2**:590; 1868, **1**:171. *5668*

1867: 8 An important account of **syringomyelia** published by Jacob Augustus Lockhart Clarke (1817–1880) and John Hughlings Jackson (1835–1911), *MCT* **50**:489. *4697*

1867: 9 **Bone allografting** pioneered by Louis Xavier Leopold Ollier (1830–1900); in his *Traité experimentale et clinique de la régenération des os. 4336.1*

300

1867:10 Paul August Sick (1836–1900) was first to notice symptoms of loss of thyroid function (*status thyreoprivus*) after **thyroidectomy**, *MKW* **37**:199; he was also first to perform total thyroidectomy. *3821*

1867:11 **Haematoporphyrin**, the first **porphyrin** to be discovered, identified by Johann Ludwig Wilhelm Thudichum (1829–1901), *GBMO* **10**:152. *3914.1, 3539*

1867:12 **Otomycosis** described by Robert Robertovich Wreden (1837–1893), *ArOh* **3**:1. *3380*

1867:13 An interference **otoscope** described by August Lucae (1835–1911), *ArOh* **3**:186. *3378.2*

1867:14 The **oesophagoscope** first used clinically by Adolf Kussmaul (1822–1902), but not reported until 1901 by Gustav Killian, *DZC* **58**:500. *3521*

1867:15 Classical account of the jugular movements and murmurs, **diagnostic** of **heart diseases**, by Pierre Édouard Potain (1825–1901), *BSMH(M)* **4**:3. *2766*

1867:16 First successful removal of **cancer** of the **larynx** by Jacob da Silva Solis-Cohen (1838–1927), *AmJMS* **53**:404; **54**:565. *3274*

1867:17 **Galvanocautery** first used in surgery of **larynx** by Friedrich Eduard Rudolph Voltolini (1819–1889); in his *Die Anwendung der Galvanokaustik* …. *3275*

1867:18 Principles of surgical treatment of **cancer** formulated by Charles Hewitt Moore (1821–1870), *MCT* **50**:245. *2619*

1867:19 **Amyl nitrite** introduced in management of **angina pectoris** by Thomas Lauder Brunton (1844–1916), *L***2**:97. *2890*

1839:20 **Salicylic acid** produced from salicin by Raffaele Piria (1815–1865), *CRAS* **8**:479. *1857*

1867:21 *Physiologie des mouvements*, on **muscular movements**, published by Guillaume Benjamin Amand Duchenne (1806–1875). *624*

1867:22 **Electrolysis** first used in England by Julius Althaus (1833–1900); *On the electrolytic treatment of tumors* …. *1996.3*

1867:23 **Pneumoconiosis** described by Friedrich Albert Zenker (1825–1898), *DAKM* **2**:111. *2125.1*

1867:24 The first American to operate for **appendicitis** was Willard Parker (1800–1884), *MR* **2**:25. *3564*

---

1867:25 Wilhelm August Paul **Schüffner**, American pathologist, born 2 Jan; with Herman Vervoort, introduced oil of chenopodium in the treatment of *ankylostomiasis*, 1900, reported in 1912, *ICH* **1**:734. With Arie Klarenbeek, first isolated *Leptospira canicola* from dog urine, 1933, *NTG* **77**:4271; with C.M. Dhont and Klarenbeek, first reported leptospirosis in humans due to infection with *Leptospira canicola*, 1934, *NTG* **78**:5297. Died 1949. *5367, 5335, 5336*

1867:26 Wilhelm Conrad **Rammstedt**, German surgeon, born 1 Feb; devised an operation for the treatment of congenital pyloric stenosis, 1912, *MK* **8**:1702. Died 1963. *3539*

1867:27 Johannes Andreas Grib **Fibiger**, Danish cancer researcher, born 13 Apr. Studied artificially-produced cancer and awarded Nobel Prize (Physiology or Medicine), 1926, for discovery of *Spiroptera* (a nematode) carcinoma, 1913, *ZKr* **13**:217; 1914, **14**:295, *NPL*. This particular work was not confirmed and his results are no longer accepted. Died 1928. *2640*

1867:28 Heinrich **Winterberg**, Bohemian physician, born 7 May; with Carl Julius Rothberger (and independently of Thomas Lewis) established auricular fibrillation as a cause of perpetual heart arrhythmia, 1909, *BMJ* **2**:1528; *WKW* **22**:839. Died 1929. *2830, 2831*

1867:29 Charles Wardell **Stiles**, American zoologist, born 15 May; discovered *Necator americanus*, the American species of hookworm, 1902, *AmM* **3**:777. Died 1941. *5363*

1867:30 Karl **Spiro**, German physiological chemist, born 24 Jun; with Arthur Stoll isolated ergotamine, 1921, *SMW* **2**:525. Died 1932. *1910*

1867:31 Karl Theodor Paul Polykarpos **Axenfeld**, German ophthalmologist, born 24 Jun; provided a classic description of metastatic ophthalmia, 1894, *GAO* **43**, iii:1; isolated a diplobacillus causing conjunctivitis, 1896, *BVOG* **25**:140 – this bacillus was independently isolated by V. Morax and named the Morax-Axenfeld bacillus. Died 1930. *5938, 5941, 5942*

1867:32 Edward Ernest **Maxey**, American physician, born 21 Aug; first described Rocky Mountain spotted fever, 1899, *MSe* **7**:433. Died 1934. *5377*

1867:33 Harris Peyton **Mosher**, American surgeon, born 1 Oct; initiated the modern method of trephining and draining inflammatory processes of the brain, 1916, *SGO* **23**:740. *4886*

1867:34 Joseph Colt **Bloodgood**, American surgeon, born 1 Nov; operation for inguinal hernia, 1898, *JHB* **29**:96. Died 1935. *3604.2*

1867:35 Max **Wilms**, German surgeon, born 5 Nov; described embryoma of the kidney ('Wilms' tumour'); in *Die Mischgeschwülste, 1. Niere*, 1899. Died 1918. *4227*

1867:36 Marie Sklodowska **Curie**, Polish chemist and physicist, born 7 Nov; with husband Pierre Curie isolated radium from pitchblende, 1898, *CRAS* **127**:175, 1215. She shared the Nobel Prize (Physics), 1903, with P. Curie and Antoine Henri Becquerel for the discovery of radioactivity, *NPL* and in 1911 she was awarded the Nobel Prize in Chemistry for her discovery of radium, *NPL*, the first occasion on which a scientist had received the award twice. Died 1934. *2003*

1867:37 Charles **Norris**, American physician, born 4 Dec; with co-workers, isolated the spirochaete causing the American variety of relapsing fever, 1906, *JID* **3**:266. Died 1935. *5319*

---

1867:38 Friedel **Pick**, Bohemian physician, born; described a form of constrictive pericarditis causing cirrhosis ('Pick's disease'), 1896, *ZKM* **29**:385. Died 1926. *2803*

1867:39 Otto Knut Olof **Folin**, Swedish/American chemist, born; with Hsien Wu, devised the Folin-Wu test for blood sugar, 1919, *JBC* **38**:81. Died 1934. *3922*

1867:40 Luis **Morquio**, Uruguayan physician, born; described a form of osteochondrodystrophy, 1929, *ArME* **32**:129, *BSPP* **27**:145, and it was named 'Morquio's disease'. Brailsford also described it in the same year, leading to the term 'Morquio-Brailsford disease'. Died 1935. *4397, 4397.1*

1867:41 Erich **Lexer** born; performed the first **osteoarticular joint transplant**, *MK* **4**:817. Died 1937. *4377.1*

1867:42 André **Thomas**, French neurologist, born; with Joseph Jules Dejerine, first described olivo-pontocerebellar atrophy, 1912, *NIS* **25**:223. Died 1963. *4716.1*

1867:43 Hugo **Schottmüller**, German physician, born; first to isolate *Streptococcus viridans* in bacterial endocarditis, 1910, *MMW* **57**:617, 697. Isolated *Streptobacillus muris ratti* from a case of streptobacillary rat-bite fever, 1914, *DeW* **58** Suppl.:77. Died 1936. *2836, 5325*

1867:44 Otto **Busse**, German physician, born; described European blastomycosis (cryptococcosis) in humans, 1895, *DMW* **21**:V–B 14, independently of Buschke; later named Busse-Buschke disease. Died 1922. *5529.1, 5529.2*

1867:45 Manuel **Uribe Troncoso**, American ophthalmologist, born; introduced a gonioscope, 1925, *AmJOp* **8**:433. *5967*

---

1867: Friedlieb Ferdinand **Runge** died, **born** 1795. *carbolic acid*

1867: John **Goodsir** died, **born** 1814. *Sarcina ventriculi*

1867: William **Brinton** died, **born** 1823. *linitis plastica*

1867: Armand **Trousseau** died, **born** 1881. *haemochromatosis, diphtheria, tracheotomy*

1867: Pierre François Oliver **Rayer** died, **born** 1793. *pituitary obesity, dermatology, anthrax, Bacillus anthracis, glanders*

1867: James **Jackson** died, **born** 1777. *alcoholic neuritis*

1867: Jean **Civiale** died, **born** 1792. *lithotrity*

1867: Jonathan Mason **Warren** died, **born** 1811. *rhinoplasty, cleft palate*

1867: Marie Jean Pierre **Flourens** died, **born** 1794. *anaesthesia, chloroform, ether, brain, movement, semicircular canals, vision*

1867: William **Lawrence** died, **born** 1783. *ophthalmic surgery*

1867: Christian Georg Theodor **Ruete** died, **born** 1810. *ophthalmoscope*

1867: Alfred Armand Louis Marie **Velpeau** died, **born** 1795. *surgery, breast tumours*

1867: Ferdinand August Marie Franz **Ritgen** died, **born** 1787. *caesarean section*

**1868**

1868:1 **University of Tokyo** founded

1868:2 **American Otological Society** founded in Boston

1868:3 **Pharmacy Act (England)** against unlicensed sale of poisons

1868:4 *Archiv für die Gesamte Physiologie* founded by Eduard Friedrich Wilhelm **Pflüger** (1829–1910)

1868:5 A classical account of **keratoconus** given by Albrecht von Graefe (1828–1870), *BKW* **5**:241, 249. *5900*

1868:6 Thomas Addis Emmet (1828–1919) wrote *Vesico-vaginal fistula, from parturition and other causes,* a comprehensive account of the management of **vesico-vaginal fistula** based on Sims' technique. *6058, 6037*

1868:7 **Cheiloplasty** first developed by Gustav Simon (1824–1876); in his *Beiträge zur plastischen Chirurgie.* *5749*

1868:8 Otto Eduard Heinrich Wucherer (1820–1873) saw the embryo form of the **filaria** worm, *GMB* **3**:97, to which the name *Wuchereria bancrofti* was later applied. *5344.6, 5346*

1868:9 The use of **oxygen-nitrous oxide** mixture as an **anaesthetic** advocated by Edmund Andrews (1824–1904), *MEx* **9**:665. *5669*

1868:10 The term 'elementary bodies' used by Jean Baptiste Auguste Chauveau (1827–1917) to describe the minute bodies inside the inclusion bodies, the infective particles in the **smallpox** virus, *CRAS* **66**:359. *5425.1*

1868:11 Rudolf Ludwig Karl Virchow (1821–1902) showed the connection between famine conditions and **typhus** outbreaks, and emphasized the social element in the generation of the disease; in his *Ueber den Hungertyphus. 5376*

1868:12 *Borrelia recurrentis (obermeieri),* causal organism in **relapsing fever**, discovered by Otto Hugo Franz Obermeier (1843–1873), reported in 1873, *ZMW* **11**:145. *5314*

1868:13 The first to measure the reaction time of a **psychical process** was Frans Cornelis Donders (1818–1889), *ArA* p. 657. *4974*

1868:14 **Charcot's arthropathy**, sometimes occurring in **tabes dorsalis**, described by Jean Martin Charcot (1825–1893), *ArPhy* **1**:161, the tabetic joints he described became known as '**Charcot's joints**'. *4337, 4777*

1868:15 An important description of **multiple sclerosis** given by Jean Martin Charcot (1825–1893), *GH* **41**:554, 557, 566. *4698*

1868:16 A classic account of **alcoholic paraplegia** published by Samuel Wilks (1824–1911), *MTG* **2**:470. *4539*

304

1868:17 A classic account of **osteitis deformans** given by Samuel Wilks (1824–1911), *TPSL* **20**:273. *4338*

1868:18 **Progressive muscular dystrophy** ('**Duchenne's muscular dystrophy**') described by Guillaume Benjamin Amand Duchenne (1806–1875), *ArGM* **11**:179, 305, 421, 552, it had previously been noted by Meryon (1852). *4739, 4734.1*

1868:19 **Poikiloderma congenitale** described by August Rothmund (1830–1906), *GAO* **14**:159. *4056.1*

1868:20 **Cholecystotomy** for the removal of **gallstones** performed by John Stough Bobbs (1809–1870), *TIMS* 68. *3621*

1868:21 A form of **purpura** with abdominal symptoms described by Eduard Heinrich Henoch (1820–1910); first mentioned by William Heberden Sr (1802) and later by Johannes Lucas Schönlein (1837) ('Schönlein-Henoch purpura'), *BKW* **5**:517. *3065, 3053, 3058*

1868:22 **Adenoid growths** first clinically described by Hans Wilhelm Meyer (1825–1895), *Hos* **11**:177. *3276*

1868:23 Description of **pernicious anaemia** ('**Biermer's anaemia**') by Anton Biermer (1827–1892) was the first to mention the **retinal haemorrhages**, *KBSA* **2**:15. *3124*

1868:24 Classical work on clinical **thermometry** published by Carl Wunderlich (1815–1877); in his *Das Verhalten der Eigenwärme in Krankheiten*. *2677*

1868:25 **Tuberculosis** proved to be a specific infection by Jean Antoine Villemin (1827–1892); *Étude sur la tuberculose*. *2324*

1868:26 Pharmacological action of **cocaine** studied by Thomas Moréno y Maïz ; in his *Recherches chimique et physiologique sur l'Erythroxylum coca du Pérou et la cocaïne*. *1868*

1868:27 **Hering's law on binocular vision** introduced by Karl Edwin Konstantin Hering (1834–1918), in his *Die Lehre vom binokularen Sehen*. *1513.1*

1868:28 Demonstration that **erythropoiesis** and **leucopoiesis** take place in the **bone marrow** by Giulio Cesare Bizzozero (1846–1901), *RIL* 2 ser. **1**:815. *881*

1868:29 Several structures in the **brain** first described by Theodor Hermann Meynert (1833–1892), in his *Der Bau der Grosshirnrinde*. *1403*

---

1868:30 Harold Leslie **Barnard**, British physiologist, born Jan; with Leonard Erskine Hill, substituted pressure gauge for mercury manometer in the Riva-Rocci sphygmomanometer, 1897, *BMJ* **2**:904. Died 1908. *2807*

1868:31 Alfred Walter **Campbell**, Australian neurologist, born 18 Jan; with Henry Head, showed herpes zoster to be a haemorrhagic inflammation of the posterior nerve roots and the homologous spinal ganglia, 1900, *Brain* **23**:353. With John Burton Cleland, while investigating Murray Valley encephalitis (Australian X disease), an acute polioencephalomyelitis, isolated a virus from cerebral tissue, 1917, *RDNSW* p. 150. Died 1937. *4644, 4648*

1868:32 Leonard **Rogers**, British pathologist, specialist in tropical diseases, born 18 Jan; found Leishman-Donovan bodies in kala-azar (visceral leishmaniasis), 1904, *BMJ* **1**:303. Died 1962. *5299*

1868:33 Michel **Weinberg**, Russian/French bacteriologist, born 30 Jan; isolated *Clostridium oedematiens*, 1915, *CRSB* **78**:274; and *Clostridium histolyticum*, 1916. Died 1940. *2520, 2521*

1868:34 Alfred **Hand**, American paediatrician, born 7 Feb; in his description of what later became termed the 'Hand-Schüller-Christian syndrome', 1893, *PPSS* **16**:282; *ArPe* **10**:673, he called it polyuria and tuberculosis. Died 1949. *6359–6363*

1868:35 George Frederic **Still**, British paediatrician, born 27 Feb; first described chronic articular rheumatism in children ('Still's disease'), 1896, *MCT* **80**:47. Died 1941. *4503*

1868:36 Leopold **Freund**, Bohemian physician, born 5 Apr; first to employ x rays for deep radiation therapy, 1897, *WKW* **10**:73. Died 1944. *2002*

1868:37 Erich **Hoffmann**, German syphilologist, born 25 Apr; with Fritz Richard Schaudinn, discovered the causal organism of syphilis, *Spirochaeta pallida* (later renamed *Treponema pallidum* by Schaudinn), 1905, *AKG* **22**:527. Died 1959. *2399*

1868:38 Fujiro **Katsurada**, Japanese parasitologist, born 5 May; gave first description of *Schistosoma japonicum*, a parasite in bilharziasis, 1904, *IS* **669**:1325. Died 1946. *5349.1*

1868:39 Hermann **Schloffer**, Austrian surgeon, born 13 May; first to operate successfully upon a pituitary tumour, 1906, *WKW* **20**:621, 670, 1075. Died 1937. *3891, 3892*

1868:40 Karl **Landsteiner**, Austrian pathologist, born 14 Jun; divided human blood into three groups, 1900, *ZBP* **27**:357. With Julius Donath, first described an auto-antibody and an auto-immune disease, 1904, *MMW* **51**:1590. With Erwin Popper, first transmitted poliomyelitis to monkeys, 1909, *ZI* **2**,1:379. With Constantin Levaditi, mixed serum from a monkey that had recovered from experimental poliomyelitis with a mixture containing active virus, which failed to produce paralytic disease when injected into fresh monkeys, 1910, *CRSB* **68**:311. With Philip Levine (1900–1987) discovered M, N and P blood groups, 1927, *PSEB* **24**:600, 941. Spent many years in fundamental research on antigen-antibody reactions; *Die Spezifizität der serologischen Reaktionen*, 1933. With Alexander Solomon Wiener, recognized Rh antigen, 1940, *PSEB* **43**:223. With Merrill Wallace Chase (b.1905) achieved passive cell transfer of delayed hypersensitivity, 1942, *PSEB* **49**:688. Awarded Nobel Prize (Physiology or Medicine), 1930, for his work on blood groups, *NPL*. Died 1943. *889, 2558.1, 4669, 4670.3, 910, 2576.2, 912.2, 2578.3*

1868:41 Ervin Sidney **Ferry**, American physicist, born 14 Jun; his modification (with W.T. Porter) of the Fechner-Weber law on stimulus and sensation led to the term 'Ferry-Porter law', 1892, *AmJSc* **44**:192; *PRS* **63**:347. Died 1956. *1473*

1868:42 Walter **Broadbent**, British physician, born 4 Aug; drew attention to recession of the intercostal spaces as a sign of adherent pericardium ('Broadbent's sign'), 1895, *L* **2**:200. Died 1951. *2800*

1868:43 Joseph **Nicolas**, French dermatologist, born 11 Aug; with Joseph Durand and Maurice Favre, gave the first important account of lymphogranuloma venereum, 1913, *BSMH* **35**:274. It is sometimes called 'Durand-Nicolas-Favre disease'. Died 1960. *5217*

1868:44 William **Bulloch**, British bacteriologist, born 19 Aug; with James Harry Sequeira, first recognized the adrenogenital syndrome, 1905, *TPS* **56**:189; with Paul Fildes, published the classic *Haemophilia*, 1911, in which they claimed to have established the fact of immunity in females and confirmed the Law of Nasse. Died 1941. *3867, 3081, 3056*

1868:45 Ludwig **Pick**, German pathologist and paediatrician, born 31 Aug; his account of a rare genetically-determined disorder in 1926, *EIM* **29**:519, also described by Albert Niemann (1914), led to the term 'Niemann-Pick disease'. Died 1935. *3785, 3784*

1868:46 Wilhelm **Kolle**, German bacteriologist, born 2 Nov; introduced the killed cholera vaccine, 1896, *ZBP*, I **19**:97. Died 1935. *5111*

1868:47 Korbinian **Brodmann**, German anatomist, born 17 Nov; defined 'Brodmann's area' in the cerebral cortex, 1908, *JPN* **10**:231; in the following year he published his comprehensive account of the localization of cerebral function in his *Vergleichende Lokalisationslehre der Grosshirnrinde*. Died 1918. *1434, 1435*

1868:48 Thomas Stephen **Cullen**, Canadian gynaecologist, born 20 Nov; the first clinical and pathological study of hyperplasia of the endometrium appears in his *Cancer of the uterus*, 1900. First to draw attention to discoloration of the skin about the umbilicus as a sign of ruptured ectopic pregnancy ('Cullen's sign'); in his *Embryology, anatomy, and diseases of the umbilicus*, 1916. Died 1953. *6110, 6124.1*

---

1868:49 Luis **Agote**, Argentinian physician, born; reported the use of citrated blood in transfusion, 1914, *AnIMod* **1**:24; followed, in 1915, by Richard Lewisohn. Died 1954. *2020*

1868:50 James Thomas Ainslie **Walker**, British military surgeon, born; with Samuel Rideal devised a method for testing disinfectants, 1903, *JSI* **24**:424. Died 1930. *1893*

1868:51 Rudolf **Kraus**, Austrian bacteriologist, born; devised the precipitin reaction, for qualitative estimation of antigens and antibodies, 1897, *WKW* **10**:736. Died 1932. *2550.1*

1868:52 Augustus Warren **Crane**, American radiologist, born; introduced kymography in clinical cardiology, 1916, *AmJR* **3**:513. Died 1937. *2845*

1868:53 Georg **Lotheissen**, Swiss surgeon, born; devised an operation for the radical repair of femoral hernia, 1898, *ZCh* **25**:548. *3605*

1868:54 Abraham **Buschke**, German dermatologist, born; described European blastomycosis (cryptococcosis) in humans, 1895, *DMW* **21**:V–B 14, independently of Busse; later named Busse-Buschke disease; described the scleroderma adultorum syndrome of Buschke, 1900, *BKW* **39**:955; *ArD* **53**:383. Died 1943. *5529.2, 5529.1, 4130*

1868:55 Felix **Pinkus**, German dermatologist, born; first described lichen nitidus ('Pinkus's disease') in 1901; published in 1907, *ArD* **85**:11. Died 1947. *4143*

1868:56 Paul **Sainton**, French neurologist, born; with Pierre Marie, gave cleidocranial dysostosis its present name, 1898, *ReN* 6:835; it was first described by Morand in 1760. Died 1958. *4369, 4302.2*

1868:57 John Brian **Christopherson**, British surgeon and specialist in tropical diseases, born; introduced tartar emetic (antimony) in the treatment of bilharziasis, 1918, *L* 2:325. Died 1955. *5350.6*

1868:58 Joseph Léon Marcel **Lignières** born; with J. Spitz, discovered the actinobacillus, 1902, *SMB* 9:207. Died 1933. *5531*

1868:59 Isidor **Fischer**, Austrian physician and medical biographer, born; compiled the *Biographisches Lexikon der hervorragenden Ärzte der letzen fünfzig Jahre*, 1 vol. [in 2], 1932–33, a supplement to the great source for medical biography to 1880, *Biographisches Lexikon*, 6 vols, 1884–1888, of A. Hirsch. Died 1943. *6732*

---

1868: John **Elliotson** died, **born** 1791. *hay fever, pollen, glanders, anaesthesia, hypnosis*

1868: William **Stevens** died, **born** 1786. *internal iliac artery ligation*

1868: William **Gibson** died, **born** 1788. *common iliac artery ligation*

1868: Ludwig **Türck** died, **born** 1810. *laryngitis sicca, brain tumours, retinal haemorrhage*

1868: Friedrich Heinrich **Rinne** died, **born** 1819. *hearing test*

1868: Albrecht Theodor **Middeldorpf** died, **born** 1824. *tumour of oesophagus, gastric fistula*

1868: Wilhelm **Griesinger** died, **born** 1817. *splenic anaemia, tropical anaemia, ankylostomiasis*

1868: Thomas **Hillier** died, **born** 1831. *nephrostomy*

1868: William Thomas Green **Morton** died, **born** 1819. *anaesthesia, ether*

1868: Eduard **Zeis** died, **born** 1807. *plastic surgery*

1868: Julius **Sichel** died, **born** 1802. *ophthalmology*

1868: William **Mackenzie** died, **born** 1791. *glaucoma*

**1869**
1869:1 *American Journal of Obstetrics* commences publication

1869:2 **Faculté de Médecine** at **Nancy**

1869:3 **Ceylon Medical College**, **Colombo**, founded

1869:4 **Chicago Medical College** becomes **Medical Department, Northwestern University**

1869:5 **Royal Sanitary Commission**, UK

1869:6 Max Joseph von Pettenkofer (1818–1901); planned the **sewage system** of Munich; in his *Das Kanal- oder Siel-System in München. 1618*

1869:7 A fine **ophthalmoscopic** atlas, *Ophthalmoskopischer Hand-Atlas*, published by Eduard Jaeger (1818–1884). The illustrations were reproduced from Jaeger's own paintings, each of which required from 20–50 sittings of from 2–3 hours. *5904*

1869:8 Important work on the **transplantation** of free **skin** carried out by Jacques Louis Reverdin (1842–1929), *BSIC* **10**:511. *5750*

1869:9 The life cycle of *Dracunculus medinensis*, the parasite of **dracontiasis**, elucidated by Alexei Pavlovich Fedchenko (1844–1873), *IOLE* **8**:71. *5344.7*

1869:10 **Progressive ossifying myositis** ('**Münchmeyer's disease**') first described by Ernst Münchmeyer (1846–1880), *ZRM* **34**:9. *4741*

1869:11 **Neurasthenia** ('**Beard's disease**') first described by George Miller Beard (1839–1883), *BMSJ* **80**:217. *4843*

1869:12 The mechanism of the **iliofemoral** ('**Bigelow's**') **ligament** described, and its importance in the reduction of dislocation of the **hip-joint** by the flexion method, shown by Henry Jacob Bigelow (1818–1890); in his *The mechanism of dislocation and fracture of the hip. 4424*

1869:13 The **Argyll Robertson pupil** first described by Douglas Moray Cooper Lamb Argyll (1837–1909), *EMJ* **14**:696. *4540*

1869:14 **Urticaria pigmentosa** described by Edward Nettleship (1845–1913), *BMJ* **2**:323, led to the eponym '**Nettleship's disease**'. *4057*

1869:15 **Trichorrhexis nodosa** first described by Francis Paxton (d.1924), *JCuM* **3**:133. *4058*

1869:16 The first investigation of **retinitis** accompanying **glycosuria** made by Henry Dewey Noyes (1832–1900), *TAOS* 1867–8 (1869):71. *3938*

1869:17 The *Treatise on the diseases and surgery of the mouth*, etc., by James Edward Garretson (1828–1895), was the first modern textbook of **oral surgery**. *3684.1*

1869:18 **Bacterial** origin of **endocarditis** first suggested by Emanuel Winge (1827–1894), *NML* **23**:78. *2767*

1869:19 **Antiseptic catgut ligature** introduced for **arterial ligation** by Joseph Lister (1827–1912), *L* **1**:451. *2964*

1869:20 **Islands of Langerhans** described by Paul Langerhans (1847–1888), in his *Beiträge zur mikroskopischen Anatomie der Bauchspeicheldrüse. 1009*

1869:21 **Ptosis of eyelid**, '**Horner's syndrome**', caused by lesion of the **cervical sympathetic** nerve, described by Johann Friedrich Horner (1831–1886); proof that the sympathetic governs the **pupillary**, **vasomotor**, **sudomotor** and **pilomotor functions**, *KMA* **7**:193. *1328*

1869:22 The **Esmarch (first-aid) bandage** was introduced on the battlefield by Johann Friedrich August von Esmarch (1823–1908); described in his *Der erste Verband auf dem Schlachtfelde. 2168*

1869:23 **Chloral hydrate**, use as hypnotic demonstrated by Oscar Liebreich (1839–1908), *ADGP* **16**:237. *1869*

1869:24 *Hereditary genius* published by Francis Galton (1822–1911). *226*

1869:25 In an important study of **pellagra** Cesare Lombroso (1836–190) upheld the maize theory of its origin, *RCB* **8**:289. *3754*

1869:26 William Ernest **Miles**, British surgeon, born 15 Jan; devised the operation of abdomino-perineal resection, 1908, *L* **2**:1812. Died 1947. *3528.1*

1869:27 Louis **Dartigues**, French surgeon, born 3 Feb; developed modern mammectomy, with transplantation of nipple and areola, 1928, *BCChnP* **20**:739. Died 1940. *5783*

1869:28 Max **Bielschowsky**, German neurologist, born 19 Feb; introduced silver stain for nerve fibres, 1903, *NZ* **21**:579. Died 1940. *1296*

1869:29 Otto **Josue**, Belgian physician, born 21 Feb; produced experimental arteriosclerosis, using venous injection of adrenaline, 1903, *CRSB* **44**:1374. Died 1923. *2910*

1869:30 Maude Elizabeth Seymour **Abbott**, Canadian cardiologist, born 18 Mar; compiled a classical *Atlas of congenital cardiac disease*, 1936. Died 1940. *2865*

1869:31 Harvey Williams **Cushing**, American neurosurgeon, born 8 Apr; used a route through the temporal fossa and beneath the middle meningeal artery for extirpation of the Gasserian ganglion in the treatment of trigeminal neuralgia, 1900, *JAMA* **34**:1035. Further developed local infiltration anaesthesia, initiated by Halsted, 1902, *AnS* **36**:321. Introduced a pneumatic tourniquet with a measurable degree of pressure, with especial use in craniotomy, 1904, *MN* **84**:577. Achieved successful operative intervention in the treatment of intracranial haemorrhage of the newborn, 1905, *AmJMS* **130**:563. Established cerebral hernia as a decompressive measure for inaccessible brain tumours, 1905, *SGO* **1**:297. With Samuel James Crowe and John Homans, demonstrated that hypophysectomy causes genital atrophy, 1910, *JHB* **21**:127. Published *The pituitary body and its disorders*, 1912, the first clinical monograph on the subject, and added much to the knowledge of the pituitary and its disorders. With Percival Bailey, published an important classification of glioma group tumours; in their *A classification of the tumours of the glioma group on a histogenetic basis*, 1926. Introduced electrocoagulation in neurosurgery, 1928, *SGO* **47**:751. As shown in his *Intracranial tumours*, 1932, his operative technique dramatically reduced the mortality rate in intracranial surgery. Advanced the theory that the hypothalamus is responsible for the development of peptic ulcer; in his *Papers relating to the pituitary body, hypothalamus*, etc., p. 175, 1932. Described 'Cushing's syndrome', now known to be due to adrenal disease, 1932, *BJH* **50**:137. With Louise Charlotte Eisenhardt, classified the meningiomas; *Meningiomas. Their classification*, etc., 1938, is among his best work. Died 1939. *4875, 5689, 5679, 4877.1, 4878, 4879, 3894, 3896, 4608, 4897.1, 4900, 3552, 3904, 4612, 4909.01*

1869:32 Friedrich Karl **Kleine**, German parasitologist, born 14 May; showed that the African trypanosome undergoes a developmental cycle in the tsetse fly, *Glossina*, 1909, *DMW* **35**:469. Died 1950. 5283.1

1869:33 Aristide **Agramonte y Simoni**, Cuban bacteriologist, born 3 Jun; with Walter Reed, James Carroll and Jesse William Lazear, provided the first definite proof that the causal agent in yellow fever is transmitted to man by the mosquito, *Aedes aegypti*, 1900, *PhMeJ* **6**:790. Died 1931. *5457*

1869:34 Frederick John **Poynton**, British rheumatologist, born 26 Jun, with Alexander Paine, considered a diplococcus to be the cause of rheumatic fever, 1900, *L* **2**:861, 932. Died 1943. *4505*

1869:35 Hans **Spemann**, German embryologist, born 27 Jun. Discovered a causal mechanism that makes it possible to control the direction in which a part of the embryo develop, 1924, *Roux* **100**:599. For his discovery of organizers in animal development, he was awarded the Nobel Prize (Physiology or Medicine), 1935, *NPL*. Died 1941. *530*

1869:36 Eugen von **Hippel**, German ophthalmologist, born 3 Aug; gave the first description of angiomatosis of the retina – 'Hippel's disease', 1895, *BVOG* **24**:269. Died 1931. *5940*

1869:37 Arnold Hermann **Knapp**, German ophthalmologist, born 20 Aug; introduced a method of extraction of cataract with forceps, 1915, *ArOp* **50**:426. Died 1956. *5964*

1869:38 Russell Aubra **Hibbs**, American surgeon, born 1 (or 11) Sep; introduced spinal fusion in the treatment of scoliosis, 1911, *NYMJ* **93**:1013. Died 1932. *4383.1*

1869:39 Wolfgang **Pauli**, Czechoslovakian biochemist, born 11 Sep; first noted the hypotensive action of thiocyanates, 1903, *MMW* **50**:153. Died 1955. *2712*

1869:40 Georg Clemens **Perthes**, German surgeon, born 17 Sep; pioneer in the study of the inhibitory effect of x rays on carcinoma, 1903, *ArKC* **71**:955. Described juvenile osteochondritis deformans (first mentioned by H. Waldenström in 1909), 1910, *DZC* **107**:111; independently described by Arthur Thornton Legg and Jacques Calvé and given the name 'Calvé-Legg-Perthes disease'. Died 1927. *2627.1, 4382, 4380, 4381*

1869:41 Leo **Loeb**, German pathologist, born 21 Sep; with R.B. Bassett he simultaneously isolated the thyroid-stimulating hormone of the anterior pituitary, 1929, *PSEB* **26**:860. Died 1959. *1138.01*

1869:42 Frederic Jay **Cotton**, American surgeon, born 24 Sep; with Walter Meredith Boothby, introduced the Boothby and Cotton flowmeter, for administration of nitrous oxide-oxygen-anaesthesia, 1912, *SGO* **15**:281. Died 1938. *5698*

1869:43 Artur **Biedl**, Yugoslavian endocrinologist, born 4 Oct; reported cases of what was later named the Laurence-Moon-Biedl syndrome, retinitis pigmentosa with familial developmental imperfections, 1922, *DMW* **48**:1630. Died 1933. *6369, 6368*

1869:44 Robert Calvin **Coffey**, American surgeon, born 20 Oct; carried out experimental work from which the modern technique of uretero-intestinal anastomosis developed, 1911, *JAMA* **56**:397. Died 1933. *4196.2*

1869:45 Joseph Bolivar **DeLee**, American obstetrician, born 28 Oct; described a low cervical caesarean section operation (laparotrachelotomy), 1919, *JAMA* **73**:91. Died 1942. *6251*

1869:46 Nicolas Constantin **Paulescu**, Romanian physician, born 30 Oct; isolated insulin before Banting and Best; he named it 'pancréine', 1921, *ArIPh* 17:**85**. Died 1931. *3965*

1869:47 Ludwig **Haendel**, German bacteriologist, born 31 Oct; with Fred Neufeld, introduced new antipneumococcus serum, 1910, *AKG* **34**:293; with Karl Wilhelm Joetten, introduced suramin (Bayer 205) in the treatment of trypanosomiasis, 1920, *BKW* **57**:821. Died 1939. *3190, 5286*

1869:48 Efim Semenovic **London**, Russian pathologist, born 27 Dec; with S.W. Goldberg, successfully treated cancer with radium, 1903, *DeZ* **10**:457. Died 1939. *2627*

1869:49 Albert Abraham **Hijmans van den Bergh**, Dutch physician, born; with J. Snapper, introduced the van den Bergh test for bilirubin in serum, 1913, *DAKM* **110**:540. Died 1943. *3647*

1869:50 James Emmons **Briggs**, American physician, born; introduced a distensible bag for controlling haemorrhage after suprapubic prostatectomy, 1906, *NEMG* **41**:391. Died 1942. *4267*

1869:51 Etienne **Lombard**, French otorhinolaryngologist, born; devised test for simulated unilateral deafness, 1910, *BAM* **64**:127. *3402.1*

1869:52 (?) John Henry Porteus **Graham** born; first reported a case of trench ever, a louse-borne infection, 1915, *L* **2**:703. Died.1957. *5385*

1869:53 Hippolyte **Morestin**, French surgeon, born; developed a method of mammaplasty, 1902, *PrM* **10**:975. Died 1919. *5756*

1869: Jan Evangelista **Purkyně** died, **born** 1787. *Purkyně cells, Purkyně fibres*

1869: Jean Leonard Marie **Poiseuille** died, **born** 1797. *manometer, haemodynamometer*

1869: Amédée **Forget** died, **born** 1811. *otitis*

1869: Johann Martin **Heyfelder** died, **born** 1798. *anaesthesia, ethyl chloride*

1869: James **Wardrop** died, **born** 1782. *eye inflammation, keratitis*

1869: James **Bolton** died, **born** 1812. *strabismus*

1869: Peter Mark **Roget** died, **born** 1779. *thesaurus*

**1870**
1870:1 **British Red Cross** founded (as **National Society for Aid to the Sick and Wounded**)

1870:2 **Metropolitan Asylums Board (England)**

1870:3 **University of Syracuse**, NY, founded

1870:4 **University of Cincinnati**, Ohio, founded

1870:5 Early account of **bacterial endocarditis** by Samuel Wilks (1824–1911), *GHR* **15**:29. *2769*

1870:6 The first full description of **kala-azar** (visceral **leishmaniasis**) given by Thomas Benjamin Briscoe, *PGBMD* **52**:31. *5292*

1870:7 Eduard Hitzig (1838–1907), with Gustav Theodor Fritsch (1838–1891), proved the existence of functional localization in the **cerebral cortex** of animals, *ArA* p. 300. *1405*

1870:8 Ritgen's operation of extraperitoneal **caesarean section** revived and modified by Theodore Gaillard Thomas (1831–1903), who named it **gastro-elytrotomy**, *AmJOD* **3**:125. *6239, 6238*

1870:9 The first vaginal **ovariotomy** performed by Theodore Gaillard Thomas (1831–1903), *AmJMS* **59**:387. *6061*

1870:10 Karl Gegenbaur (1826–1903) supported Darwin and stressed the value of comparative **anatomy** as the basis of the study of **descent**, *Gründzüge der vergleichenden Anatomie der Wirbelthiere*, 2nd edn. *337*

1870:11 Serpiginous ulcer of the **cornea** ('**Saemisch's ulcer**') first described by Edwin Theodor Saemisch (1833–1909); in his *Das Ulcus corneae serpens und seine Therapie*. *5905*

1870:12 Plexiform **neurofibroma** first described by Paul von Bruns (1846–1916); in his *Das Rankenneurom*. *4541*

1870:13 A notable method of reduction of subluxation of the **shoulder-joint** introduced by Emil Theodor Kocher (1841–1917), *BKW* **7**:101. *4425*

1870:14 **Osteochondritic separation of the epiphyses** in congenital **syphilis** ('**Wegner's disease**') described by Friedrich Rudolph Georg Wegner (1843–1917), *VA* **50**:305. *4339*

1870:15 First successful planned **nephrectomy** for **urinary tract fistula** carried out by Gustav Simon (1824–1876), *DK* **22**:137. *4213*

1870:16 **Dermatitis exfoliativa neonatorum** ('**Rittershain's disease**') first described by Gottfried von Rittershain (1820–1883), *OJP* **1**:23. *4060*

1870:17 **Dermatitis exfoliativa** ('**Wilson's disease**'), known to Hippocrates, given its present name by William James Erasmus Wilson (1809–1884), *MTG* **1**:118. *4061*

1870:18 **Tinea imbricata** ('**Tokelau ringworm**') first described by George Alexander Turner (1845–1900), *GMJ* **2**:510. *4059*

1870:19 **Gastrostomy** for stricture of **oesophagus** first performed in America by Frank Fontaine Maury (1840–1879), *AmJMS* **59**:365. *3464*

1870:20 First study of transmission of **sounds** through the **cranial bones** as a method of diagnosing **ear** disease by August Lucae (1835–1911); in his *Die Schalleitung durch die Kopfknochen* .... *3381*

1870:21 William Stokes (1839–1900) improved the method of **amputation** of the **thigh** (introduced by Rocco Gritti in 1857), ('Gritti-Stokes amputation'), *MCT* **53**:175. *4470, 4466*

1870:22 Modern type of clinical **thermometer** introduced by Thomas Clifford Allbutt (1836–1925), *BFMCR* **45**:429. *2679*

1870:23 **Aneurysm** of **hepatic artery** observed by Heinrich Irenaeus Quincke (1842–1922), *BKW* **8**:349. *2982*

1870:24 **Rhinoscleroma** described by Hans von Hebra (1847–1902), *WMW* **20**:1. *3277*

1870:25 Myelogenous **leukaemia** was a term introduced by Ernst Neumann (1834–1918) who was first to note bone-marrow changes in leukaemia, *ArH* **11**:1. *3066*

1870:26 **Effort syndrome** first described by Arthur Bowen Richards Myers (1838–1921); in his *On the etiology and prevalence of diseases of the heart among soldiers. 2768*

1870:27 The history of the **US War of the Rebellion** was recorded in *The medical and surgical history of the War of the Rebellion, 1861–65*, 6 vols, 1870–1888. *2171*

1870:28 **Microtome** introduced by Wilhelm His Sr (1831–1904), *ArMA* **6**:229. *268*

---

1870:29 Paul Theodor **Uhlenhuth**, German bacteriologist, born 7 Jan; demonstrated organ-specific antigens (in eye lens proteins), in *Festschrift ...R.Koch*, p. 49; with Erich August Hübener, first described *Salmonella paratyphi C*, 1908, *ZBP* **42**: I, Beil.127. Died 1957. *2557, 5041*

1870:30 Erik Adolf von **Willebrand**, Finnish physician, born 1 Feb; first reported pseudohaemophilia type B (von Willebrand's disease), an hereditary bleeding disorder affecting both sexes, 1926, *FLH* **68**:87. Died 1949. *3087.2*

1870:31 Alfred **Adler**, Austrian psychologist, born 7 Feb; introduced the concept of the inferiority complex; in his *Studie über Minderwertigkeit von Organen*, 1907. Founded the school of individual psychology and seceded from Freud's psychoanalytical group; in his *Über die nervösen Charakter*, 1912. Died 1937. *4984, 4985.1*

1870:32 Leon Konrad **Gliński**, Polish pathologist, born 15 Feb; his description of postpartum pituitary necrosis, panhypopituitarism, 1913, *PrzL* **4**:13, preceded the case of pituitary cachexia ('Simmonds' disease') described by Morris Simmonds (1914). Died 1918. *3900*

1870:33 Oskar **Vogt**, German neurologist, born 6 Apr; with Cécile Vogt, described disease of the corpora striata (status dysmyelinatus syndrome, 'Vogt syndrome'), 1920, *JPN*, Ergänz. iii:627. Died 1959. *4720*

1870:34 Georg Ludwig **Zuelzer**, German physician, born 10 Apr; isolated the pancreatic extract containing what is now known as insulin, 1908, *ZEP* **5**:307. Died 1949. *3961*

1870:35 Charles Harrison **Frazier**, American surgeon, born 19 Apr; with William Gordon Spiller, introduced intracranial trigeminal neurotomy for the treatment of trigeminal neuralgia, 1901, *UPMB* **14**:342. Died 1936. *4876*

1870:36 Géza von **Illyés**, Hungarian urologist, born 24 May; accurately demonstrated ureteral calculi by x rays with the help of an opaque indwelling catheter, 1901, *DZC* **62**:132. *4294*

1870:37 Oscar **Stoerck**, Austrian pathologist, born 29 May; with Hans Eppinger, gave the first clinical and pathological description of bundle-branch block, 1910, *ZKM* **71**:157. Died 1926. *2832*

1870:38 Jean Jules Baptiste Vincent **Bordet**, Belgian bacteriologist, born 13 Jun; showed that sensitizing antibody and complement are involved in bacteriolysis, 1895, *AnSR* **4**:455. Did important work on immune haemolysis, 1898, *AnIP* **12**:688; **13**:225. With Octave Gengou, devised the 'Bordet-Gengou complement-fixation reaction', a serological test, 1901, *AnIP* **15**:289, and discovered the causal organism of whooping cough, *Bordetella pertussis*, 1906, *AnIP* **20**:731; **21**:720. Awarded the Nobel Prize (Physiology or Medicine), 1919, for his work in immunology, *NPL*. Died 1961. *2547, 2551, 2553, 5087*

1870:39 Ernest Linwood **Walker**, American protozoologist, born 24 Jun; with Andrew Watson Sellards, determined the incubation period in amoebiasis and demonstrated that *Entamoeba tetragena* and *E. minuta* are identical with *E. histolytica*, 1913, *PhJS* B **8**:253. Died 1952. *5191*

1870:40 Jules **Gonin**, Swiss ophthalmologist, born 10 Jul; introduced ignipuncture for the treatment of detached retina, 1927, *AnO* **164**:817. Died 1935. *5972*

1870:41 Erich August **Hübener**, German immunologist, born 17 Aug; with Paul Theodor Uhlenhuth, first described *Salmonella paratyphi C*, 1908, *ZBP* **42**: I, Beil.127. *5041*

1870:42 Maria **Montessori**, first woman in Italy to qualify in medicine (1894), born 31 Aug; Italian educationalist and originator of **Montessori system** of teaching. Died 1952

1870:43 Hugh Hampton **Young**, American urological surgeon, born 18 Sep; devised an operation for conservative perineal prostatectomy, 1903, *JAMA* **41**:999; performed first radical prostatectomy for carcinoma, 1905, *JHB* **16**:315; introduced his punch prostatectomy operation, 1913, *JAMA* **60**:253. With colleagues introduced mercurochrome for the treatment of urinary tract infections, 1919, *JAMA* **73**:1483. With Charles Alexander Waters, first demonstrated vesiculography, 1920, *AmJR* **7**:16. Died 1945. *4265, 4266.1, 4270, 1908, 4198*

1870:44 George Burgess **Magrath**, American pathologist, born 2 Oct; with Walter Remsen Brinckerhoff, carried out successful inoculation of smallpox into the monkey, 1904, *JMR* **11**:230. Died 1938. *5429.1*

1870:45 Hermann **Küttner**, German surgeon, born 10 Oct; with Fedor Krause, devised an operation for tabes, 1909, *BKC* **63**:245. Died 1932. *4881*

1870:46 Friedrich **Göppert**, German paediatrician, born 25 Oct; gave first clear account of galactosaemia, 1917, *BKW* **54**:473. Died 1927. *3921.1*

1870:47 Fielding Hudson **Garrison**, American librarian (at the Library of the Surgeon General's Office, and later at Johns Hopkins University) and medical historian, born 5 Nov; his *Introduction to the history of medicine*, 1913, is one of the best single-volume histories of medicine; the 4th edition appeared in 1929. He was coeditor, with J.S. Billings, of the *Index Medicus* and editor of the *Quarterly Cumulative Index Medicus*. Died 1935. *6408*

1870:48 Jay Frank **Schamberg**, American dermatologist, born 6 Nov; first described progressive pigmentary dermatosis, 1901, *BJD* **13**:1. Died 1934. *4134*

1870:49 Julius **Donath**, Austrian physician, born 11 Nov; with Karl Landsteiner, first described an auto-antibody and an autoimmune disease, 1904, *MMW* **51**:1590. Died 1950. *2558.1*

1870:50 Ernest Marcel **Labbe**, French physician, born 4 Dec; with co-workers, described the chromaffin cell tumour of the adrenal medulla, 1922, *BSMH* **46**:982. Died 1939. *3871*

---

1870:51 Alfred Leon Joseph **Conor**, French pathologist, born; with A. Bruch, first to describe fièvre boutonneuse, a form of tick-borne typhus found in Tunisia, 1910, *BSPE* **3**:492. Died 1914. *5383*

1870:52 Alejandro **Posadas** born; described coccidioidomycosis, 1892, *AnCM* **15**:585, independently of R.J. Wernicke. Died 1902. *5528.1, 5528.2*

1870:53 Leopold **Heine** born; introduced cyclodialysis in the treatment of glaucoma, 1905, *DMW* **31**:824. His work made possible the manufacture of modern contact lenses, 1930, *MMW* **77**:6, 271. *5949, 5976*

1870:54 Claude **Regaud** born; with R. Ferroux, introduced x ray dose fractionation, 1927, *CRSB* **97**:431; devised the Paris method of radium treatment for cancer of the uterus, 1933, *RR* **3**:155. Died 1940. *2008, 6131*

1870:55 Alexander **Besredka**, Russian bacteriologist, born; with Edna Steinhardt, produced anti-anaphylaxis, 1907, *AnIP* **21**:117, 384. Died 1940. *2596*

1870:56 Joseph Edwin **Barnard**, British microscopist, born; supported with photomicrographs William Ewart Gye's theory of viral origin of cancer, 1925, *L* **2**:117. Died 1949. *2648*

1870:57 Samuel Short **Whillis**, British otorhinolaryngologist, born; with Frederick Charles Pybus, introduced reverse guillotine tonsillectomy, 1910, *L* **2**:875. Died 1953. *3318*

1870:58 Arthur Baldwin **Duel** born; with Charles Alfred Ballance, treated facial palsy by nerve grafts into the Fallopian canal and by other intratemporal methods, 1936, *ArOt(C)* **15**:1. Died 1936. *4899*

1870:59 Kiyoshi **Shiga**, Japanese bacteriologist, born; discovered the dysentery bacillus, *Shigella dysenteriae*, 1898, *ZBP* I, **24**:817, 870. Died 1957. *5091*

1870:60 Friedrich Ernst **Krukenberg**, German pathologist, born; gave the original description of mucinous carcinoma of the ovary ('Krukenberg's tumour'), 1896, *ArGy* **50**:287. Died 1946. *6101*

1870:61 Fritz **Hitschmann**, German obstetrician, born; with Ludwig Adler, first definitely described the cyclical changes in the endometrium and showed them to be normal physiological processes, 1908, *MonG* **27**:1. *1181*

---

1870: August Volney **Waller** died, **born** 1816. *Wallerian nerve degeneration*

1870: Heinrich Gustav **Magnus** died, **born** 1802. *blood gas analysis*

1870: Charles Hewitt **Moore** died, **born** 1821. *cancer surgery*

1870: John Stough **Bobbs** died, **born** 1809. *gallstones, cholecystotomy*

1870: James **Syme** died, **born** 1799. *anaesthesia, ether, amputation at ankle-joint*

1870: Benjamin Winslow **Dudley** died, **born** 1785. *brain surgery*

1870: Jean Pierre **Falret** died, **born** 1794. *manic depression*

1870: James Young **Simpson** died, **born** 1811. *anaesthesia, chloroform, ether, gynaecology*

1870: George **Frick** died, **born** 1793. *ophthalmology*

1870: Friedrich Wilhelm Ernst Albrecht von **Graefe** died, **born** 1828. *iridectomy, iritis, strabismus, glaucoma, cataract, keratoconus, eye muscle paralysis, optic neuritis, exophthalmic goitre*

**1871**
1871:1 **Local Goverment Board** established in **England**

1871:2 **Births and Deaths Registration Acts**, UK

1871:3 **Office of Public Vaccinator** established (**England and Wales**)

1871:4 '**Litzmann's obliquity**' or posterior parietal presentation described by Carl Conrad Theodor Litzmann (1815–1890), *ArGy* **25**:182. *6263.1*

1871:5 The first description of hereditary **optic atrophy** ('**Leber's optic atrophy**') given by Theodor Leber (1840–1917), *GAO* **17**, ii:249. *5906*

1871:6 **Endotracheal anaesthesia** by means of tracheostomy performed by Friedrich Trendelenburg (1844–1924), *ArKC* **12**:112. *5669.1*

1871:7 Although Reverdin (1869) **transplanted** small grafts of free **skin**, it was George Lawson (1831–1908) who first successfully transplanted sizeable free **skin grafts**, as well as whole-thickness skin, *TCSL* **4**:49. *5751*

1871:8 Like Demarquay and Wucherer, Timothy Richards Lewis (1841–1886) saw **microfilariae** in body fluids; he was first to use the term *Filaria sanguinis hominis*, *ARSCI* **8** App.E:241. *5344.8*

1871:9 **Agoraphobia** first described by Carl Friedrich Otto Westphal (1833–1890), *ArPN* **3**:138. *4844*

1871:10 The first publication by a physician on **joint manipulation**, *On bone-setting (so-called), and its relation to the treatment of joints crippled by injury, rheumatism, inflammation, etc.* was written by Wharton Peter Hood (1835–1916). *4339.1*

1871:11 The first American treatise on **neurology**, *Treatise on diseases of the nervous system*, written by William Alexander Hammond (1828–1900); in it he included (p. 654) the original description of **athetosis** ('**Hammond's disease**'). *4542*

1871:12 The concept of **hereditary haemolytic anaemia** first suggested by Constant Vanlair (1839–1914) and Jean Baptiste Nicolas Voltaire Masius (1836–1912), *BARM* **5**:515. *3766.1*

1871:13 Importance of reconstruction of the internal ring following reduction of the sac in treatment of **hernia** stressed by Henry Orlando Marcy (1837–1924), *BMSJ* **85**:315. *3592.1*

1871:14 **Intussusception** first successfully operated upon by Jonathan Hutchinson (1828–1913), *MCT* **57**:31. *3466*

1871:15 **Gastrotomy** for **intestinal obstruction** recorded by Thomas Annandale (1838–1908), *EMJ* **16**:700. *3463.1*

1871:16 Charles Hilton Fagge (1838–1883) differentiated sporadic from endemic **goitre**, *MCT* **54**:155. *3822*

1871:17 William James Erasmus Wilson (1809–1884) gave original descriptions of several **skin diseases** (a subject on which he lectured at the Royal College of Surgeons of England) in his *Lectures on dermatology*, 1871–8. *3994*

1871:18 **Da Costa's syndrome**, already mentioned by Myers (1870) and later by Thomas Lewis (**effort syndrome**) (1917), described by Jacob Mendes Da Costa (1833–1900), *AmJMS* **61**:17. *2770*

1871:19 **Presystolic heart murmurs** extensively described by Charles Hilton Fagge (1838–1883), *GHR* **16**:247. *2771*

1871:20 **Staining methods** for **bacteria** introduced by Carl Weigert (1845–1904), *ZMW* **9**:609. *2482*

1871:21 **Retinal action currents** demonstrated by Alarik Frithiof Holmgren (1831–1897), *ULF* **6**:419. *1514*

1871:22 **Nuclein (nucleoprotein)** discovered by Johann Friedrich Miescher (1844–1895), later shown to be the hereditary genetic material; in: Hoppe-Seyler, F. *Med.-chem.Untersuchungen*, Heft 4, 441. *695*

---

1871:23 Robert **Kienböck**, Austrian radiologist, born 18 Jan; described acute atrophy of bone in inflammatory conditions of the extremities ('Kienböck's atrophy'), 1901, *WMW* **51**:1346. Drew attention to traumatic cavity formation in the spinal cord ('Kienböck's disease'), 1902, *JaP* **21**:50. First described 'Kienböck's disease', slowly progressive osteonecrosis of the lunate bone of the wrist, carpal lunate malacia, 1910, *FGR* **16**:103. Died 1953. *4370, 4591, 4379*

1871:24 Karl **Leiner**, Bohemian paediatrician and dermatologist, born 23 Jan; described desquamative erythroderma of nurslings (Leiner), 1908. Died 1930. *4145*

1871:25 Howard Taylor **Ricketts**, American pathologist, born 9 Feb; showed that the wood tick, *Dermacentor occidentalis*, was the vector of Rocky Mountain spotted fever, 1906, *JAMA* **47**:358; described, in blood smears, the causal organism of Rocky Mountain spotted fever, 1909, *JAMA* **52**:379; with Russell Morse Wilder, differentiated Rocky Mountain spotted fever from typhus, 1910, *ArIM* **5**:361; demonstrated the causal organism of typhus, 1910, *JAMA* **54**:1373. Died 1910. *5378, 5379, 5380, 5380.1*

1871:26 Frank Cecil **Eve**, British physician, born 15 Feb: described a new 'rocking' method of artificial respiration, 1932, *L* **2**:995, which came to be associated with his name. Died 1952. *1979*

1871:27 Stewart Rankin **Douglas**, British pathologist, born 22 Feb; with Almroth Edward Wright, demonstrated opsonins (thermolabile substances in normal and immune serum), 1903, *PRSB* **72**:357; **73**:128. Died 1936. *2558*

1871:28 Wilhelm **Türk**, German haematologist, born 2 Apr; first to report a case of complete agranulocytosis, 1907, *ZBP* I, **46**:595. Died 1916. *3079*

1871:29 Vilray Papin **Blair**, American surgeon, born 15 Jun; introduced treatment of micrognathia or prognathism by closed ramisection of the mandible, 1909, *JAMA* **53**:178; wrote the first comprehensive text on maxillofacial surgery, *Surgery and diseases of the mouth and jaws*, 1912. With James Barrett Brown, introduced split-skin grafts for covering large areas of granulating surfaces, 1929, *SGO* **49**:82; with Brown, modified Mirault's technique for the repair of cleft palate, 1930, *SGO* **51**:81. Died 1955. *5756.2, 5756.7, 5761.1, 5762*

1871:30 Thomas Benton **Cooley**, American paediatrician, born 23 Jun; with co-workers, described thalassaemia, erythroblastic anaemia in children, 1925, *AmJDC* **34**:347. Died 1945. *3141*

1871:31 Alfred **Fröhlich**, Austrian pharmacologist, born 15 Aug; described 'Fröhlich's syndrome', pituitary tumour, obesity, dystrophia adiposogenitalis and sexual infantilism, 1901, *WKR* **15**:883, 906. Died 1953. *3889*

1871:32 Charles Albert **Elsberg**, American neurosurgeon, born 24 Aug; responsible for the clinical introduction of Meltzer and Auer's method of intractracheal insufflation anaesthetization (1909), 1910, *BKW* **47**:957. Died 1948. *5695, 5694*

1871:33 Paul **Linser**, German dermatologist, born 5 Sep; introduced injection treatment of varicose veins, 1916, *MK* **12**:897. Died 1963. *3000*

1871:34 Fritz Richard **Schaudinn**, German protozoologist, born 19 Sep; with Erich Hoffmann, discovered the causal organism of syphilis, *Spirochaeta pallida* (later renamed *Treponema pallidum* by Schaudinn), 1905, *AKG* **22**:527. Died 1959. *2399*

1871:35 William Blair **Bell**, outstanding figure in British gynaecology and a founder of the Royal College of Obstetricians and Gynaecologists, born 28 Sep. He wrote *The principles of gynaecology*, 1871. Died 1936. *6121*

1871:36 John **Zahorsky**, American paediatrician, born 13 Oct; first described roseola infantum (roseola subitum), 1910, *Ped* **22**:60. First described herpangina, 1920, *SMJ* **13**:871. *5506, 5538*

1871:37 Carl Julius **Rothberger**, Austrian cardiologist, born 14 Oct; with Heinrich Winterberg (and independently of Thomas Lewis) established auricular fibrillation as a cause of perpetual heart arrhythmia, 1909, *WKW* **22**:839; *BMJ* **2**:1528. *2831, 2830*

1871:38 Walter Bradford **Cannon**, American physiologist, born 19 Oct; introduced bismuth meal in fluoroscopy of digestive tract, 1898, *AmJPh* **1**:359; discussed the role of the sympathetic-adrenal mechanism in his *The wisdom of the body*, 1932. Died 1945. *2687.1, 3519, 664*

1871:39 Robert **Doerr**, Hungarian bacteriologist, born 1 Nov; showed the relationship of phlebotomus fever to the sandfly, *Phlebotomus*, 1908, *BKW* **45**:1847. Died 1952. *5477*

1871:40 Erich **Tschermak von Seysenegg**, Austrian botanist and geneticist, born 15 Nov; like Correns and de Vries, he 'rediscovered' Mendel's laws of inheritance, 1900, *BDBG* **18**:232. Died 1962. *239.1*

1871:41 Robert **Hutchison**, British paediatrician, born 28 Nov; isolated thyroglobulin from the thyroid, 1896, *JP* **20**:474. First described 'Hutchison's tumour', adrenal sarcoma in children, 1907, *QJM* **1**:33. Died 1960. *1131.1, 3868*

1871:42 John Preston **Maxwell**, British obstetrician, born 5 Dec; showed osteomalacia to be due to lack of vitamin D, 1930, *PRSM* **23**:639. Died 1961. *4396*

1871:43 Victor **Veau**, French surgeon, born 8 Dec; his operation for cleft palate is described in his *Division palatine*, 1931. Died 1949. *5763*

1871:44 Amand **Coyon** born; with Henri Triboulet, isolated streptococci from patients with acute rheumatism, 1898, *CRSB* **50**:124. Died 1928. *4504.1*

1871:45 Frederick Creighton **Wellman**, American professor of tropical medicine and hygiene, born; discovered – independently of Castellani – *Treponema pertenue*, causal organism of yaws, 1905, *JTM* **8**:345. Died 1960. *5307*

1871:46 Christian **Kielland** born; introduced the Kielland (obstetric) forceps, 1916, *MonG* **43**:48. Died 1941. *6219*

1871: Henry Hyde **Salter** died, **born** 1823. *asthma*

1871: John Rhea **Barton** died, **born** 1794. *fracture of radius*

1871: Louis Daniel **Beauperthuy** died, **born** 1807. *yellow fever, mosquito*

1871: Paul Antoine **Du Bois** died, **born** 1795. *hyperemesis gravidarum*

1871: George **Catlin** died, **born** 1796. *mouth breathing, respiration*

**1872**
1872:1 **University of Adelaide** founded

1872:2 **Metropolitan Water Act** (piped **water supply** to **London**)

1872:3 **American Public Health Association**, first meeting, 12 Sep

1872:4 **Presbyterian Hospital, New York**, founded

1872:5 **Deutsche Gesellschaft für Chirurgie** founded

1872:6 **Sociedad Científica Argentina** founded, Buenos Aires

1872:7 **Erythromelalgia**, first complete description by Silas Weir Mitchell (1829–1914), *PhMT* **3**:81, 113. *2706*

1872:8 In *Die latente Gonorrhoe im weiblichen Geschlecht*, Emil Noeggerath (1827–1895) was first to point out the late effects of **gonorrhoea** in women, particularly its role in the production of **sterility**. *6064*

1872:9 Cases of **Mittelschmerz (intermenstrual pain)** first reported by William Overend Priestley (1829–1900), *BMJ* **2**:431. *6065*

1872:10 Attention drawn to irregular painless contractions of the **uterus** during **pregnancy**, '**Braxton Hicks' sign**', by John Braxton Hicks (1823–1897), *TOSL* **13**:216. *6189*

1872:11 Intermediate-thickness **skin grafts** first obtained by Louis Xavier Edouard Léopold Ollier (1830–1900), *BuAM* **1**:243, from which developed the **Ollier-Thiersch graft**. *5752, 5753*

1872:12 **Ovariotomy** for the treatment of non-ovarian conditions, performed by Robert Battey (1828–1895), *AtMJ* **10**:321; *TMAG* **24**:36, later acquired greater significance in connection with more modern work on endocrinology. *6062*

1872:13 Chronic **cystitis** treated by **vaginal cystotomy** by Thomas Addis Emmet (1828–1919), *AmP* **5**:65. *6063*

1872:14 **Pre-anaesthetic medication** developed by Léon Labbe (1832–1916) and E. Guyon, *CRAS* **74**:627. *5670*

1872:15 His studies of the causes, physiological and psychological, of all the fundamental **emotions** in man and animals recorded by Charles Robert Darwin (1809–1882); in his *The expression of the emotions in man and animals*. *4975*

1872:16 The **sewers** of Paris constructed in 1854 by Marie François Eugène Belgrand (1810–1878); described in his work, *La Seine*, published 1872–1887. *1620*

1872:17 A classic, but not the first, description of chronic degenerative hereditary **chorea** ('**Huntington's chorea**') given by George Huntington (1850–1916), *MSRep* **26**:317. *4699*

1872:18 Research on the application of **hypnosis** to the **psychoneuroses** pioneered by Jean Martin Charcot (1825–1893); in his *Leçons sur les maladies du système nerveux faites à la Salpêtrière*, 3 vols, 1872–87. *4995*

1872:19 The syndrome of **paralysis** of half the **tongue**, the same half of the **palate**, and one **vocal cord** ('**Jackson's syndrome**') described by John Hughlings Jackson (1835–1911), *L* 2:770. *4547*

1872:20 The **frozen shoulder syndrome** described by Simon Duplay (1836–1924), *ArGM* 71:37. *4339.2*

1872:21 Silas Weir Mitchell's (1829–1914) *Injuries of nerves and their consequences* includes the first description of **ascending neuritis**, as well as the treatment of **neuritis** by cold and splint rests. In the same year he lectured on painful affections of the **feet**, for which he suggested the term **erythromelalgia** ('**Mitchell's disease**'). *4544, 4545*

1872:22 The classical *De l'électrisation localisée* of Guillaume Benjamin Amand Duchenne de Boulogne (1806–1875) includes (p. 357) his description of partial **brachial plexus paralysis**, previously described by Smellie (1763) and later (1873) by Erb ('**Duchenne-Erb palsy**'). *4543, 4548*

1872:23 First clear description of **arteriosclerotic atrophy** of the **kidney**, and a description of **hypertensive nephrosclerosis**, given by William Withey Gull (1816–1890) and Henry Gawen Sutton (1837–1891), *MCT* **55**:273. *4215*

1872:24 **Impetigo herpetiformis** first described by Ferdinand von Hebra (1816–1880), *WMW* **22**:1197; it was more exhaustively dealt with by his son-in-law, Moritz Kaposi, in 1887. *4062, 4091*

1872:25 **Kaposi's sarcoma**, multiple idiopathic haemorrhagic sarcoma, first described by Moritz Kaposi (1837–1902), *ArD* **4**:265. *4063*

1872:26 The presence of ('Dorothy Reed') giant cells in **Hodgkin's disease** first noted by Theodor Langhans (1839–1915), *VA* **54**:509. *3767*

1872:27 The first resection of the **oesophagus** carried out by Theodor Billroth (1829–1894), *ArKC* **13**:65. *3465*

1872:28 First American textbook on **otorhinolaryngology**, *Diseases of the throat ...*, published by Jacob da Silva Solis-Cohen (1838–1927). *3280*

1872:29 **Pulsus alternans** described by Ludwig Traube (1818–1876), *BKW* **9**:185, 221. *2775*

1872:30 Hering's theory of **colour sense** published by Karl Edwin Konstantin Hering (1834–1918), 1872–1875, *SAW* 3Abt. **66**:5; **68**:186, 229; **69**:85, 179; **70**:169. *1515*

1872:31 Epithelial-cell origin of **cancer** histogenesis, advanced by Carl Thiersch (1865), confirmed by Heinrich Wilhelm Gottfried Waldeyer-Hartz (1836–1921), *VA* **41**:470; **55**:67. *2620*

322

1872:32 Charles **Hunter**, British physician, born 7 Feb; first to describe the Hurler syndrome (lipochondrodystrophy and gargoylism) in two brothers, 1917, *PRSM* **10** Dis.Child.:104. Died 1955. *6371, 6371.2*

1872:33 Richard Pearson **Strong**, American physician for tropical medicine, born 18 Mar; discovered organisms resembling *Histoplasma capsulatum*, 1906, *PhJS* **1**:91. Died 1948. *5531.1*

1872:34 Edward **Francis**, American bacteriologist, born 27 Mar; demonstrated the transmission of tularaemia from man to rodents through insects, *JAMA* **84**:1243; he named the disease from Tulare County, California, where it was discovered. Died 1957. *5176*

1872:35 Samuel Taylor **Darling**, American pathologist, born 6 Apr; described histoplasmosis ('Darling's disease'), caused by *Histoplasma capsulatum*, 1906, *JAMA* **46**:1283. Died 1925. *5532*

1872:36 William Sampson **Handley**, British surgeon, born 12 Apr; in his *Cancer of the breast and its treatment*, 1906, he advanced the theory that breast cancer metastasis is due to lymphatic extension ('lymphatic permeation'), not dissemination by the blood stream. Died 1962. *5782*

1872:37 Rufus Ivory **Cole**, American physician, born 30 Apr; introduced monovalent antiserum in the treatment of type I lobar pneumonia, 1929, *JAMA* **93**:741. Died 1966. *3202.2*

1872:38 Franz **Volhard**, German physician, born 2 May; with Karl Theodor Fahr, gave the first full description of pure nephrosis; in their *Die Brightsche Nierenkrankheit*, 1914; with Victor Schmieden, carried out first complete pericardiectomy for constrictive pericarditis, 1923, *KW* **2**:5. Died 1950. *4238, 3031*

1872:39 Jean Athanase **Sicard**, French physician, born 23 Jun; with Jacques Forestier, introduced positive contrast myelography with iodized oil (lipiodol), 1921, *ReN* **28**:1264; greatly advanced bronchography by introduction of lipiodol as an opaque medium in radiography, 1924, *JMF* **13**:3. Died 1929. *4605, 2693, 3199*

1872:40 Charles Franklin **Craig**, American military surgeon and pathologist, born 4 Jul; demonstrated the existence of malaria carriers, 1905, *AmM* **10**:982, 109. With Percy Moreau Ashburn, showed that the causal organism in dengue is a filterable virus, 1907, *PhJS,B* **8**:93; *JID* **4**:440. Died 1950. *5255, 5473*

1872:41 Otto Ivar **Wickman**, Swedish neurologist, born 10 Jul; first to confirm the infectious nature of poliomyelitis, 1905, *APIH* **1**:109. Died 1914. *4668*

1872:42 Joseph **Barcroft**, British physiologist, born 26 Jul; his *Respiratory function of the blood*, 1913 (2 edn, 2 vols, 1925–28) recorded studies of the oxygen-carrying capacity of the blood, particularly the elucidation of the oxygen dissociation curve; with co-workers he also studied high-altitude physiology, 1931, *ArSB* **16**:609. Died 1947. *964, 2137.7*

1872:43 Percy Moreau **Ashburn**, American military surgeon, born 28 Jul; with Charles Franklin Craig, showed that the causal organism in dengue is a filterable virus, 1907, *PhJS, B* **8**:93; *JID* **4**:440. Died 1940. *5473*

1872:44 Benjamin Robinson **Schenck**, American surgeon, born 19 Aug; described a sporotrichosis due to the fungus *Sporotrichum beurmanni* (named after C.L. de Beurmann), 1898, *JHB* **9**:286. Died 1920. *4127*

1872:45 Emanuel **Libman**, American pathologist, born 22 Aug; with Benjamin Sacks, described lupus erythematosus with endocarditis ('Libman-Sacks disease'), 1924, *ArIM* **33**:701. Died 1946. *2855*

1872:46 Bernard Minge **Duggar**, American botanist, born 1 Sep; isolated and introduced aureomycin, 1948, *ANYAS* **51**:175. Died 1956. *1942*

1872:47 Fritz **Steinmann**, Swiss surgeon, born 18 Sep; introduced the Steinmann nail or pin for use in the union of fractures, 1907, *ZCh* **34**:938. Died 1932. *4431*

1872:48 Ernest **Fourneau**, French chemist and pharmacologist, born 4 Oct; introduced stovaine as an anaesthetic, 1903, *BSP* **10**:141. Died 1949. *5690*

1872:49 George Carmichael **Low**, British physician and malariologist, born 14 Oct; demonstrated the complete chain of filarial infection from man-to-mosquito-to-man, 1900, *BMJ* **1**:1456. Died 1952. *5349*

1872:50 Wilfred **Trotter**, British surgeon, born 3 Nov; performed the first planned operation for intracranial aneurysm diagnosed pre-operatively, 1924; reported by J.L. Birley (1928), *Brain* **51**:184. Died 1939. *3004.1, 4897.2*

1872:51 Richard **Otto**, German bacteriologist and immunologist, born 9 Nov; studied and described the Theobald Smith phenomenon, 1906; in *Gedenkschrift für den verstorbenen Generalstabsarzt ... von Leuthold*; it was not reported by Smith but communicated by him to Paul Ehrlich. Died 1952. *2594*

1872:52 Carl **Sternberg**, Austrian pathologist, born 20 Nov; in his classical description of lymphadenoma, 1898, he distinguished it from aleukaemic anaemia, with which it had previously been included, *ZHe* **19**:21. Described lymphogranulomatosis ('Sternberg's disease'); in his *Pathologie der Primärerkrankungen des lymphatischen und hämatopoetischen Apparates*, 1905. Died 1935. *3776, 3077*

1872:53 William Stevenson **Baer**, American orthopaedic surgeon, born 25 Nov; inaugurated treatment of osteomyelitis with maggots, 1931, *JBJS* **13**:438, ('**Baer therapy**'). Died 1931. *4399*

1872:54 Guido **Holzknecht**, Austrian radiologist, born 3 Dec; improved radiotherapy dosimetry standards, 1902, *WKR* **16**:685. Died 1931. *2688*

1872:55 Franz **Nowotny**, Polish otorhinolaryngologist, born; introduced therapeutic bronchoscopy for the treatment of asthma, 1907, *MonO* **41**:679. Died 1925. *3186*

1872:56 Christian Frederik **Heerfordt**, Danish ophthalmologist, born; described uveo-parotid fever ('Heerfordt's disease'), a form of sarcoidosis, 1909, *GAO* **70**:254. Died 1953. *4145.1*

1872:57 Auguste **Queyrat**, French dermatologist, born; described erythroplasia of Queyrat in 1911, a condition similar to the precancerous dermatosis described by J.T. Bowen in 1912

324

(now considered to be a variant of an intra-epidermal basal-cell epithelioma), 1911, *BSFD* **22**:178. *4146, 4148*

1872:58 Friedrich **Voelcker**, German surgeon, born; with Eugen Joseph, introduced the Voelcker kidney function test, 1903, *MMW* **50**:2081. With Alexander von Lichtenberg, obtained the first cystograms, 1905, *MMW* **52**:1576. With von Lichtenberg, introduced pyelography, 1906, *MMW* **53**:105. Died 1955. *4230, 4192, 4231*

1872:59 Adolpho Carlos **Lindenberg**, Brazilian bacteriologist, born; first described American mucocutaneous leishmaniasis, 1909, *BSPE* **2**:252. Died 1944. *5299.1*

1872:60 William Henry **Luckett**, American surgeon, born; developed the modern operation for the correction of protruding ears, 1910, *SGO* **10**:635. Found air in the cerebral ventricles following skull fracture, 1913, *SGO* **17**:37, this gave Dandy (1919) the idea for ventriculography. Died 1929. *5756.4, 4884, 4602*

---

1872: Wenzel **Treitz** died, **born** 1819. *retroperitoneal hernia*

1872: William **Henderson** died, **born** 1810. *molluscum contagiosum*

1872: William Wood **Gerhard** died, **born** 1809. *tuberculous meningitis, typhus, typhoid, relapsing fever, typhus*

1872: Pierre Charles Alexandre **Louis** died, **born** 1787. *tuberculosis, typhoid fever*

**1873**
1873:1 **[German Public Health Association]** founded, **Berlin**

1873:2 **Boards of Health** established in 134 **American** cities

1873:3 A simplified form of roman letters, embossed on paper, for use by **blind** readers, devised by William Moon (1818–1894), himself blind, in 1845. Recorded in his *Light for the blind: a history of the origin of Moon's system of reading … for the blind*, 1873. *5909*

1873:4 **Retinoscopy** introduced by Ferdinand Louis Joseph Cuignet (b.1823), *ReO* **1**:14. *5908*

1873:5 A **gas-ether inhaler** (**Clover's inhaler**) introduced by Joseph Thomas Clover (1825–1882), *BMJ* **1**:282. *5671*

1873:6 William Budd (1811–1880), in his *Typhoid fever; its nature, mode of spreading, and prevention*, insisted that **typhoid was** spread by contagion; he established that infection came from the dejecta of patients. He strengthened the theory of water-borne infection. *5029*

1873:7 **Experimental psychology** founded by Wilhelm Max Wundt (1832–1920); his principal work was *Grundzüge der physiologischen Psychologie*. *4976*

1873:8 A classic account of **migraine** given by Edward Liveing (1832–1919); in his *On megrim, sick-headache, and some allied disorders*. He showed an association between migraine and tetany, asthma, and false angina. *4549*

1873:9 Wilhelm Heinrich Erb (1840–1921) introduced '**Erb's sign**', diagnostic of latent **tetany**, *ArPN* **4**:271; described '**Erb's palsy**', partial **brachial plexus paralysis**, *VNMV* **1**:130, it had previously been described by Smellie (1763) and by Duchenne (1872) . *4832, 4548, 4543*

1873:10 The original description of **dyshidrosis (pompholyx)**, a disturbance of **sweat secretion** given by William Tilbury Fox (1836–1879), *BMJ* **2**:365. *4065*

1873:11 **Erythema serpens** first described by William Morrant Baker (1839–1896), *SBHR* **9**:198. *4064*

1873:12 Among the first to ascertain the cause of **myxoedema** was William Withey Gull (1816–1890), *TCSL* **7**:180. *3823*

1873:13 **Mycosis** of the **pharynx** first reported by Bernhard Fraenkel (1836–1911), *BKW* **10**:94. *3281*

1873:14 The **mastoid operation** was revived by Hermann Hugo Rudolf Schwartze (1837–1910) and Adolf Eysell (b.1846), *ArOh* **1**:157; the ear was opened by chiselling ('**Schwartze's operation**'). *3382*

1873:15 **Paradoxical pulse** described by Adolf Kussmaul (1822–1902), *BKW* **10**:433, 445, 461. *2776*

1873:16 *Bacterium lactis* isolated by Joseph Lister (1837–1912), *QJMS* **13**:380. *2484*

1873:17 **Leprosy bacillus (*Mycobacterium leprae*)** discovered by Gerhard Henrik Armauer Hansen (1841–1912) on 28 February 1873, *NML* **4**, ix:1. *2436*

1873:18 **Pollen** shown to produce hay fever in both **asthmatic** and **catarrhal** forms and also evokes skin reactions, by Charles Harrison Blackley (1820–1900); *Experimental researches on the causes and nature of catarrhus aestivus. 2588*

1873:19 **Inflammation**; Julius Cohnheim's (1839–1884) investigations published; *Neue Untersuchungen über die Entzündung. 2302*

1873:20 Experimental **tuberculosis** (bovine) produced by Theodor Albrecht Erwin Klebs (1834–1913), *ArEP* **1**:163. *2327*

---

1873:21 Rupert **Waterhouse**, British physician, born 15 Jan; described suprarenal apoplexy, 1911, *L* **1**:577, named Waterhouse-Friderichsen syndrome following the later account by Carl Friderichsen (1918). Died 1958. *4685, 4686*

1873:22 John F. **Anderson**, American physician, born 14 Mar; with Joseph Goldberger, transmitted measles to monkeys, 1911, *USPHR* **26**:847, 887. Died 1958. *5448*

1873:23 Yandell **Henderson**, American physiologist, born 23 Apr; first discussed decompression sickness in aviators, 1917, *AvAeE* **2**:145. Died 1944. *2137.3*

1873:24 Félix Hubert **d'Herelle**, French-Canadian bacteriologist, born 25 Apr; discovered and named bacteriophage, the agent involved in the transmissible lysis of bacteria by viruses

326

– Twort-d'Herelle phenomenon – (originally noted by Frederick William Twort in 1915), 1917, *CRAS* **165**:373. Died 1949. *2571, 2572*

1873:25 Charles Albert **Bentley**, British physician, born 25 Apr; demonstrated the mode of entry of *Ankylostoma duodenale* into the body, 1902, *BMJ* **1**:190. Died 1949. *5362.1*

1873:26 Johannes [Hans] **Berger**, German neurologist, born 21 May; introduced the electroencephalogram, enabling the electrical activity of the brain to be recorded, 1929, *ArPN* **87**:527. Died 1941. *1446*

1873:27 Fernand **Cathelin**, French urologist, born 27 May; introduced caudal anaesthesia, 1901, *CRSB* **53**:452. *5686*

1873:28 Otto **Loewi**, German pharmacologist, born 3 Jun; introduced pancreatic function test, 1908, *ArEP* **59**:83. He shared the Nobel Prize (Physiology or Medicine), 1936, with Henry Hallett Dale, for his work on the chemical mediation of nervous impulses, 1921–4, *HSZ* **189**: 239; **193**: 201; **203**: 408; **204**: 361, 629, *NPL*. Died 1961. *3644, 1343*

1873:29 Alexis **Carrel**, French/American surgeon and physiologist, born 28 Jun; perfected arterial suture technique, 1902, *LM* **98**:859. With Charles Claude Guthrie, carried out experimental heart transplantation, in a dog, 1905, *AmM* **10**:284, 1101. Demonstrated transplantation of blood vessels after storage, 1908, *JAMA* **51**:1662; *JEM* **12**:460. Transplanted kidney from one animal to another, 1908, *JEM* **10**:98. With Montrose Thomas Burrows, first to grow tumour tissue *in vitro*, 1910, *CRSB* **69**:332. With co-workers, introduced the Carrel-Dakin treatment of wounds, using Dakin's solution, a solution of sodium hypochlorite and boric acid, for the continuous irrigation of wounds, 1915, *BuAM* **74**:361. Awarded Nobel Prize (Physiology or Medicine), 1912, for surgical and cell culture experiments, *NPL*. Died 1944. *2909, 3025.1, 3027, 3028, 4235, 2636, 5642, 5643*

1873:30 Eugene Lindsay **Opie**, American pathologist, born 5 Jul; with William George MacCallum, discovered the sexual phase of the malaria parasite, 1898, *JEM* **3**:79, 103, 117. Established the association between failure of the islets of Langerhans and the occurrence of diabetes, 1901, *JEM* **5**:397, 527. Died 1971. *5249, 5250, 3955, 3956*

1873:31 Robert Bayley **Osgood**, American surgeon, born 6 Jul; described lesions of the tibial tuberosity occurring in adolescence ('Osgood-Schlatter disease'), 1903, *BMSJ* **148**:114; it was also described by Schlatter in the same year. Died 1956. *4373, 4374*

1873:32 Théodore **Simon**, French psychologist, born 10 Jul; with Alfred Binet, devised the Binet-Simon intelligence tests; in their *La mésure du developpement de l'intelligence chez les jeunes enfants*, 1911. Binet had published a plan for studying intelligence as early as 1895. Died 1961. *4985*

1873:33 Walter Morley **Fletcher**, British physiologist and medical research administrator, born 21 Jul; with Frederick Gowland Hopkins, explained the production of lactic acid in normal muscular contraction, 1907, *JP* **35**:247. He became first secretary of the Medical Research Committee (later Council) in 1914. Died 1933. *733*

1873:34 William David **Coolidge**, American physicist, born 23 Oct; invented the Coolidge high-vacuum x ray tube, 1913, *AmJR* **3**:115. Died 1975. *2692*

1873:35 William Thomas **Ritchie**, British physician, born 3 Nov; with William Adam Jolly, first described auricular flutter, 1910, *Heart* **2**:177; it had been recognized by Ritchie in 1906. Died 1945. *2833, 2821*

1873:36 John Bentley **Squier**, American urological surgeon, born 6 Nov; modified the operation of total suprapubic prostatectomy, 1911, *BMSJ* **164**:911. Died 1948. *4269*

1873:37 Otfrid **Foerster**, German neurosurgeon, born 9 Nov; devised the operation of rhizotomy for spastic paralysis, 1908, *ZOC* **22**:203. Died 1941. *4880*

1873:38 Joseph Louis Irénee **Abadie**, French neurologist, born 15 Dec; introduced the use of alcohol injection of the Gasserian ganglion for treatment of trigeminal neuralgia, 1903, *MSMB* 1903:59. *4877*

———

1873:39 Jan **Janskỳ**, Czech physician, born; classified blood into four groups, O, A, B, AB, 1906, *SK* **8**:85. Died 1921. *896*

1873:40 William Henry **Schultz** born; devised test for anaphylaxis, 1910, *JPET* **1**:549; similar work by Henry Hallett Dale, 1913, led to the term 'Schultz-Dale test'. Died 1947. *2600.2*

1873:41 Sahachiro **Hata**, Japanese bacteriologist, born; with Paul Ehrlich, introduced salvarsan ('606'), specific in treatment of syphilis and yaws; *Die experimentelle Chemotherapie der Spirillosen ...*, published 1910. Died 1938. *2403*

1873:42 Francis Randall **Hagner** born; devised the open operation for epididymitis, 1906, *MR* **70**:944. Died 1940. *4194*

1873:43 Alfred Leftwich **Gray**, American radiologist, born; introduced radiotherapy for the treatment of carcinoma of the bladder, 1906, *AmQR* **1**:53. Died 1932. *4194.1*

1873:44 Israel **Strauss**, American pathologist, born; with Leo Loewe, carried out the experimental transmission of epidemic encephalitis, 1919, *JAMA* **73**:1056. *4651*

1873:45 Kenzo **Futaki**, Japanese physician, born; with co-workers, found *Spirillum morsus muris*, in the lymphatics and blood stream in cases of rat-bite fever, 1916, *JEM* **23**:249; **25**:33. Died 1966. *5326*

1873:46 John Albertson **Sampson**, American gynaecologist, born 14 Aug; explained the true nature of endometrioma of the ovary, 1921, *ArSuC* **3**:245. Died 1946. *6128*

1873:47 Robert Johann **Wernicke**, Argentinian physician, born; described coccidioidomycosis, 1892, *RAMA* **1**:186, independently of A. Posadas. *5528.2, 5528.1*

———

1873: Justus von **Liebig** died, **born** 1803. *chloroform*

1873: Georg Franz **Merck** died, **born** 1825. *papaverine*

1873: Henry William **Fuller** died, **born** 1820. *leukaemia*

1873: Johann Nepomuk **Czermak** died, **born** 1828. *laryngoscope*

1873: Moritz Heinrich **Romberg** died, **born** 1795. *nervous diseases, facial hemiatrophy, tabes dorsalis, achondroplasia*

1873: Robert William **Smith** died, **born** 1807. *neurofibromatosis*

1873: Henry Bence **Jones** died, **born** 1814. *albumosuria, proteinuria*

1873: Josiah Clark **Nott** died, **born** 1804. *neuralgia, yellow fever*

1873: David **Livingstone** died, **born** 1813. *trypanosomiasis, tsetse fly, nagana, arsenic*

1873: Pierre Charles **Huguier** died, **born** 1804. *lymphogranuloma venereum*

1873: Otto Eduard Heinrich **Wucherer** died, **born** 1820. *filaria, Wuchereria bancrofti, tropical anaemia, ankylostomiasis*

1873: Alexei Pavlovich **Fedchenko** died, **born** 1844. *dracontiasis, Dracunculus medinensis*

1873: Otto Hugo Franz **Obermeier** died, **born** 1843. *relapsing fever, Borrelia recurrentis*

1873: Heinrich **Küchler** died, **born** 1811. *eyesight testing*

1873: Hugh Lenox **Hodge** died, **born** 1796. *obstetrics, Hodge pessary*

1873: Auguste **Nélaton** died, **born** 1807. *pelvic haematocele*

**1874**
1874:1 **London School of Medicine for Women** founded by Sophia Louisa Jex-Blake (1840–1912)

1874:2 [**Society of Croatian Physicians**] established at **Zagreb**

1874:3 **Mason College**, later **University of Birmingham**, founded at Birmingham by Sir Josiah Mason

1874:4 Classic description of **chronic interstitial hepatitis** by Georges Hayem (1841–1933), *ArPhy* 1:126. *3623*

1874:5 Jean Martin Charcot (1825–1893) differentiated between **Aran-Duchenne muscular atrophy** and the rarer **amyotrophic lateral sclerosis**, *ProM* 2:573. *4742*

1874:6 The wool-skein test for the diagnosis of **colour-blindness** introduced by Alarik Frithiof Holmgren (1831–1897), *NoMA* 6 nr.24:1; nr.28:1. *5911*

1874:7 Wilhelm Friedrich [Willy] Kühne (1837–1900) isolated **trypsin**, *VNMV* NF1:194. *1012*

1874:8 The first successful human **intravenous anaesthesia** carried out by Pierre Cyprien Oré (1828–1889), *CRAS* 78:515, 651. *5672*

1874: 9 The **split-skin grafts** of Karl Thiersch (1822–1895) developed into the **Ollier-Thiersch graft**, *VDGC* **3**:69. *5753, 5752*

1874: 10 Eduard Hitzig (1838–1907); accurately defined the limits of the **motor area** in the dog and monkey, in his *Untersuchungen über das Gehirn. 1408*

1874: 11 **Eczema** of the **nipple**, '**Paget's disease of the nipple**', first described by James Paget (1814–1899), *SBHR* **10**:87. *5772*

1874: 12 Alfred Carl Graefe (1830–1899), cousin of Albrecht, and Edwin Theodor Saemisch (1833–1909) edited the great work on **eye diseases**, *Handbuch der gesamten Augenheilkunde*, 1874–1880. A second edition appeared, 15 vols [in 41], 1899–1918. *5944*

1874: 13 An early important account of **blackwater fever** given by Laurent Jean Baptiste Berenger-Féraud (1832–1901); in his *De la fièvre bilieuse mélanique dans les pays chauds comparée avec la fièvre jaune. 5235*

1874: 14 **Catatonia** suggested as a separate disease entity by Karl Kahlbaum (1828–1899); in his *Die Katatonie. 4938*

1874: 15 Classic description of **anorexia nervosa** by William Withey Gull (1816–1890), *TCSL* **7**:22. *4845*

1874: 16 **Sensory aphasia** ('**Wernicke's aphasia**') described by Carl Wernicke (1848–1905), in *Der aphasische Symptomencomplex*; he recorded important work on the localization of aphasia. *4623*

1874: 17 **Postparalytic chorea** first described by Silas Weir Mitchell (1829–1914), *AmJMS* **68**:342. *4543*

1874: 18 A **galvanocautery** for the treatment of **prostatic obstruction** introduced by Enrico Bottini (1837–1903), *Gal* **2**:437. *4261*

1874: 19 First complete excision of the **larynx** for **cancer** by Theodor Billroth (1829–1894), *VGDC* **3**, ii:76. *3282*

1874: 20 **Haemocytometer** invented by Louis Charles Malassez (1842–1909), *ArPhy* 2 sér. **1**:32. *876*

---

1874: 21 Joseph **Erlanger**, American physiologist, born 5 Jan; with Herbert Spencer Gasser, devised means for use of cathode ray oscillograph for transmission of impulses through single nerve fibres, 1924, *AmJPh* **70**:624. They shared Nobel Prize (Physiology or Medicine), 1944, *NPL*. Died 1965. *1305*

1874: 22 Victor **Schmieden**, German surgeon, born 19 Jan; with Franz Volhard, carried out first complete pericardiectomy for constrictive pericarditis, 1923, *KW* **2**:5. Died 1945. *3031*

1874: 23 George John **Jenkins**, Australian aural surgeon, born 2 Feb; suggested modern operation of fenestration for otosclerosis, 1913, *IMC* **16**:609. Died 1939. *3403*

1874:24 Nicolai Sergeievich **Korotkov**, Russian physician, born 13 Feb; introduced the method of applying the stethoscope to the brachial artery during blood pressure examination, 1905, *IVMA* **11**:365. Died 1920. *2818*

1874:25 Alban **Köhler**, German radiologist, born 1 Mar; introduced teleradiography into heart radiography, 1905, *WKR* **19**:279. Died 1947. *2817*

1874:26 Henry Stanley **Plummer**, American physician, born 3 Mar; reported case of cardiospasm with oesophageal dilatation, 1912, *JAMA* **58**:2013; after a report by Porter Paisley Vinson (1919) named '**Plummer-Vinson syndrome**'. Died 1937. *3320*

1874:27 Julius **Wohlgemuth**, German physician, born 8 Mar; introduced a pancreatic function test, 1910, *BKW* **47**:92. Died 1948. *3646*

1874:28 William George **MacCallum**, Canadian pathologist, born 18 Apr; observed the mode of fertilization of the malaria parasite, 1897, *Lancet* **1**:1240. With Eugene Lindsay Opie, discovered the sexual phase of the malaria parasite, 1898, *JEM* **3**:79, 103, 117. With Carl Voegtlin, proved that calcium metabolism is controlled by the parathyroid glands, 1909, *JEM* **11**:118. Died 1944. *5246, 5250, 5249, 3859*

1874:29 Clemens Peter **Pirquet von Cesenatico**, Austrian allergologist, born 12 May; with Bela Schick, gave an excellent account of serum sickness, *Die Serumkrankheit*, 1905. Introduced the cutaneous reaction test for the diagnosis of tuberculosis, 1907, *WKW* **20**:1123. First suggested the term 'allergie' in his *Klinische Studien über Vakzination und vakzinale Allergie*, 1907. Died 1929. *2593, 2338, 2598*

1874:30 Jakob **Erdheim**, Polish pathologist, born 24 May; made important studies of the pathology of the pituitary and named pituitary dwarfism, 'nanosomia pituitaria', 1916, *BPA* **62**:302. Died 1937. *3902*

1874:31 Joseph Francis **McCarthy**, American urologist, born 12 Jun; introduced the McCarthy foroblique panendoscope for cysto-urethroscopy, 1923, *JU* **10**:519. Died 1965. *4198.1*

1874:32 Frederick Herman **Verhoeff**, American ophthalmic surgeon, born 9 Jul; employed buttonhole iridectomy for the removal of cataract within the capsule, 1927, *TAOS* **25**:54. *5974*

1874:33 Joseph **Goldberger**, Austro/American public health officer, born 16 Jul; with John F. Anderson, transmitted measles to monkeys, 1911, *USPHR* **26**:847, 887. Demonstrated the experimental production of pellagra and its prevention by proper diet, 1920, *USPHL* **120**:7; with co-workers, isolated an anti-pellagra factor related to vitamin B, 1926, *USPHR* **41**:297. Discovered vitamin $B_2$ (riboflavine), 1926, *USPHR* **41**:297. Died 1929. *5448, 3757, 3578, 1057*

1874:34 Frederick Parker **Gay**, American pathologist and bacteriologist, born 22 Jul; with William Palmer Lucas, made the first accurate cell counts of the cerebrospinal fluid in poliomyelitis, 1910, *ArIM* **6**:330. Died 1939. *4670.1*

1874:35 Constantin **Levaditi**, Romanian physician and bacteriologist, born 1 Aug; with Arnold Netter, discovered antibodies in human poliomyelitis convalescent serum, 1910, *CRSB* **68**:855. With Karl Landsteiner, mixed serum from a monkey that had recovered from experimental poliomyelitis with a mixture containing active virus, which failed to produce paralytic disease when injected into fresh monkeys, 1910, *CRSB* **68**:311. With Robert Sazerac, used bismuth tartrate in the treatment of syphilis, 1921, *CRAS* **173**:338. With A. Vaisman showed that sulphanilamide protected against experimental gonococcal infection, 1937, *PrM* **45**:1371. Died 1953. *4670.2, 4670.3, 2411, 5213.1*

1874:36 Joseph-Everett **Dutton**, British physician and biologist, born 9 Sep; first to recognize human trypanosomiasis: and named the parasite *Trypanosoma gambiense*, 1902, *TYL* **4**:455. With John Lancelot Todd, demonstrated, independently of Ross and Milne, relapsing fever in monkeys, and described the mechanisms of infection conveyed by infected ticks, *Ornithodorus moubata*, 1905, *BMJ* **2**:1259. The infecting organism was later named *Borrelia duttoni*, after Dutton, who died from the disease. Died 1905. *5275, 5318*

1874:37 Octave **Crouzon**, French neurologist, born 29 Sep; first to describe craniofacial dysostosis (hypertelorism), 1912, *BSMH* **33**:545. Died 1938. *4385*

1874:38 Auguste **Rollier**, Swedish physician, born 1 Oct; introduced heliotherapy (ultraviolet light and Alpine sunlight) in the treatment of tuberculosis; *Die Heliotherapie der Tuberkulose*, 1903. Died 1954. *2342*

1874:39 Schack August Steenberg **Krogh**, Danish physiologist, born 15 Nov; discovered the regulation of the motor mechanism of capillaries (see *The anatomy and physiology of the capillaries*, 1922), for which he was awarded the Nobel Prize (Physiology or Medicine), 1920, *NPL*. Died 1949. *793*

1874:40 Antonio Caetano de Abreu Freire **Egas Moniz**, Portuguese neurosurgeon, born 29 Nov; introduced cerebral arteriography and carotid arteriography, 1927, *ReN* **34** II, 72; *PrM* **35**:969. Treated psychotic conditions by prefrontal lobotomy, 1936, *BuAM* **115**:385; for this work he shared the Nobel Prize (Physiology or Medicine), 1949, with Walter Rudolph Hess, *NPL*. Died 1955. *4610, 4610.1, 4905*

1874:41 Samuel Alexander Kinnier **Wilson**, British neurologist, born 6 Dec; gave the classic description of the syndrome of progressive familial hepatolenticular degeneration associated with cirrhosis of the liver ('Wilson's disease'), 1912, *Brain* **34**:295, although it had been previously described by Frerichs (1861). In 1940 his monumental *Neurology* was published posthumously. Died 1937. *4717, 4693, 4614*

1874:42 Ernst **Moro**, Austrian paediatrician, born 8 Dec; isolated *Lactobacillus acidophilus*, 1900, *WKW* **13**:114. With Franz Hamburger, first described serum sickness, 1903, *WKW* **16**:445. Introduced a percutaneous tuberculin reaction test for tuberculosis, 1907, *MMW* **55**:216, 2025. Died 1951. *2515, 2591.1, 2339*

1874:43 Artur **Schüller**, Austrian neurologist, born 28 Dec; described two cases of the condition later termed the Hand-Schüller-Christian syndrome, 1915, *FGR* **23**:12. Died 1958. *6359–6363*

1874:44 Ryukichi **Inada**, Japanese bacteriologist, born; with co-workers, proved *Spirillum* (*Leptospira*) *icterohaemorrhagiae* to be causal organism in Weil's disease, 1916, *JEM* **23**:377. Died 1950. *5334*

332

1874:45 Per Gustav **Bergman**, Swedish physiologist, born; showed, with Robert Adolf Armand Tigerstedt, that a pressor substance (renin) was produced by the kidney, 1898, *SkAP* **8**:223. Died 1955. *1236*

1874:46 Bernard **Fantus**, American physician, born; reported the establishment of the first blood bank, 1937, *JAMA* **129**:108. Died 1940. *2026*

1874:47 Harold **Brunn**, American surgeon, born; introduced one-stage lung lobectomy, 1929, *ArSuC* **18**:490. Died 1950. *3202*

1874:48 Hans **Elsner**, German gastroenterologist, born; designed a straight gastroscope; in his *Die Gastroskopie*, 1911. *3535.1*

1874:49 Arthur Thornton **Legg**, American orthopaedic surgeon, born; described juvenile osteochondritis deformans (first mentioned by H. Waldenström in 1909), 1910, *BMSJ* **162**:202; independently described by Jacques Calvé and by Georg Clemens Perthes and given the name 'Calvé-Legg-Perthes disease'. Died 1939. *4380, 4381, 4382*

1874:50 Georges **Froin**, French physician, born; described 'Froin's syndrome', a coagulation of the cerebrospinal fluid, 1903, *GH* **76**:1005. *4645*

1874:51 Alfred Baker **Spalding**, American gynaecologist and obstetrician, born; first described overlapping of the fetal skull bones as a sign of fetal death *in utero* ('Spalding's sign'), 1922, *SGO* **35**:754. Died 1942. *6221.1*

---

1874: Arthur **Jacob** died, **born** 1790. *Jacob's membrane, rodent ulcer*

1874: Jean **Cruveilhier** died, **born** 1791. *pathological anatomy*

1874: John Zachariah **Laurence** died, **born** 1830. *retinitis pigmentosa*

**1875**
1875:1 **Boston Medical Library** founded by Oliver Wendell Holmes, James R. Chadwick and Henry I. Bowditch

1875:2 **Faculté de Médecine et Pharmacie** established at **Lille**

1875:3 **Imperial Hygienic Laboratory** established at **Osaka**

1875:4 **Public Health Act, England**; embodied a complete code of sanitary law

1875:5 *Deutsche Medizinische Wochenschrift* founded, Berlin

1875:6 **Food and Drugs Act, England**

1875:7 John Reissberg Wolfe (1824–1904) considered that in **free-skin grafts** the subcutaneous tissue at the site of the graft should be removed, leaving skin only; he is remembered for the '**Wolfe-Krause graft rest**', *BMJ* **2**:360. *5754*

1875:8 Discovery that **chloroform anaesthesia** could be prolonged by the injection of **morphine** by Claude Bernard (1813–1878); recorded in his *Leçons sur les anesthésiques et sur l'asphyxie*, 1875. *5673*

1875:9 The worm *Onchocerca* described by John O'Neill 50 years before it was linked with **onchocerciasis**, *L* **1**:265. *5344.10*

1875:10 *Entamoeba histolytica*, infective agent in **amoebiasis**, discovered by Friedrich Lösch (1840–1903), *VA* **65**:196. *5184*

1875:11 The **knee-jerk** first used as a diagnostic measure in **tabes dorsalis** by Wilhelm Heinrich Erb (1840–1921), *ArPN* **5**:792, and simultaneously by Carl Friedrich Otto Westphal (1833–1890), *ArPN* **5**:803. *4780, 4781*

1875:12 First description of **acute superior haemorrhagic polioencephalitis** by Charles Jules Alphonse Gayet (1833–1904), *ArPhy* **2**:341. *4641*

1875:13 The '**Thomas splint**' described by Hugh Owen Thomas (1834–1891) in his *Diseases of the hip, knee and ankle joints*. He was the founder of **orthopaedics** in Britain; see his *Contributions to medicine and surgery*, 1883–90. *4340, 4348*

1875:14 A classical description of **cheiropompholyx** and the first description and illustration of **sarcoidosis** given by Jonathan Hutchinson (1828–1913); in his *Illustrations of clinical surgery*, **1**, 42, 49. *4067*

1875:15 **Porokeratosis** first described by Isidor Neumann (1832–1906) who named it **dermatitis circumscripta herpetiformis**, *VDS* **2**:41; Mibelli's more detailed account in 1893 led to the term '**Mibelli's disease**'. *4068, 4114*

1875:16 **Spastic spinal paralysis** ('**Erb-Charcot disease**') described by Wilhelm Heinrich Erb (1840–1921), *BKW* **12**:357. *4556*

1875:17 The **Weir Mitchell treatment** introduced by Silas Weir Mitchell (1829–1914); in his *On rest in the treatment of nervous disease. 4553*

1875:18 **Acrodermatitis chronica atrophicans** ('**Taylor's disease**') first described by Robert William Taylor (1842–1906), *ArDS* **2**:114; it was given its name by Herxheimer and Hartmann in 1902. *4069, 4138*

1875:19 The first resection of a **bladder tumour** performed by Theodor Billroth (1829–1894) and recorded by Carl Gussenbauer, *ArKC* **18**:411. *4174*

1875:20 Important investigations of disorders of the **eye** in **diabetes mellitus** made by Theodor Leber (1840–1917), *GAO* **21**, iii:206. *3941*

1875:21 The first description of **hypertrophic cirrhosis** of the **liver** with **icterus** ('**Hanot's disease**') given by Victor Charles Hanot (1844–1896); in his *Étude sur une form de cirrhose hypertrophique du foie. 3624*

1875:22 **Kernicterus** first described by Johannes Orth (1847–1923), *VA* **63**:447. *3067*

1875:23 The first detailed description of the segmentation of the mammalian **ovum** published by Edouard van Beneden (1846–1910), *BARS* **40**:686. *496*

1875:24 First **pericardiocentesis** for suppurative **pericarditis** reported by Friedrich Alexander Hilsmann (b.1849), *SKU* Diss. No. 2. *3022*

1875:25 **Digitoxin** isolated from digitalis by Johann Ernst Oswald Schmiedeberg (1838–1921), *ArEP* **3**:16. *1869.1*

1875:26 **Cancer** due to industrial tar and paraffin described by Richard von Volkmann (1830–1889); in his *Beiträge zur Chirurgie*, p. 370. *2126*

1875:27 **Forcipressure** introduced in the treatment of **haemorrhage** by Aristide Auguste Stanislaus Verneuil (1823–1895), *BMSC* **1**:17, 198, 273, 522, 646. *5612*

1875:28 Albert **Schweitzer**, Alsatian physician, philosopher and missionary, born 14 Jan. Died 1965

1875:29 Charles Cassidy **Bass**, American parasitologist, born 29 Jan; with Foster Matthew Johns, cultivated the malaria parasites, *Plasmodium vivax* and *P.falciparum*, *in vitro*, 1912, *JEM* **16**:567. *5255.1*

1875:30 Ludwig **Merzbacher**, German physician, born 9 Feb; recorded cases of familial centrolobar sclerosis (already noted by Pelizaeus in 1885), 1908, *MK* **18**:161, 310, leading to the term 'Pelizaeus-Merzbacher disease'. *4715, 4703*

1875:31 Vladimir Petrovich **Filatov**, Russian surgeon, born 15 Feb; used a tubed pedicle flap as early as September 1916, *VO* **34**, 4–5:149. His earlier work on corneal transplantation, published in Russian journals, summarized in 1935, *ArOp* **13**:321. Died 1956. *5757.1, 5986*

1875:32 Frederick Percival **Mackie**, British tropical pathologist and bacteriologist, born 19 Feb; proved that relapsing fever could be conveyed by the body louse, *Pediculus corporis*, 1907, *BMJ* **2**:1706. Died 1944. *5321*

1875:33 Octave **Gengou**, Belgian bacteriologist, born 27 Feb; with Jules Jean Baptiste Bordet, devised the 'Bordet-Gengou complement-fixation reaction', a serological test, 1901, *AnIP* **15**:289. With Jules Jean Baptiste Vincent Bordet, discovered the causal organism of whooping cough, *Bordetella pertussis*, 1906, *AnIP* **20**:731; **21**:720. Died 1957. *2553, 5087*

1875:34 Jean René **Cruchet**, French neurologist, born 21 Mar; with co-workers reported 40 cases of epidemic encephalitis, 1917, *BSMH* **41**:614, 13 days before the classic description given by von Economo. Died 1959. *4649, 4650*

1875:35 John **Auer**, American physiologist and pharmacologist, born 30 Mar; with Samuel James Meltzer, carried out experimental work on intratracheal insufflation anaesthetization, 1909, *JEM* **11**:622, which led to modern endotracheal anaesthesia. With Paul A. Lewis, described anaphylactic shock, 1910, *JEM* **12**:151. Died 1948. *5694, 2600*

1875:36 Henry Edmund Gaskin **Boyle**, anaesthetist, born Barbados, 2 Apr; introduced Boyle's continuous-flow anaesthetic machine, 1917, *PRSM* **11**: Anaes.30. Died 1941. *5700*

1875:37 Heinrich **Vogt**, German neurologist, born 23 Apr; described juvenile amaurotic familial idiocy, 1905, *MonP* **18**:161, and later by Spielmayer (1904) leading to the eponym 'Spielmayer-Vogt disease'. *4713.1, 4714.1*

1875:38 John Charles Grant **Ledingham**, British bacteriologist, born 19 May; introduced a test for the diagnosis of smallpox, 1926, *JSM* **34**:125. Died 1944. *5433*

1875:39 Henry Hallett **Dale**, British physiologist, pharmacologist, and the leading figure in the establishment of international biological standardization, born 9 Jun; with George Barger and F.H. Carr, isolated ergotoxine, 1906, *BMJ* **2**:1792. With Barger he isolated histamine from an ergot extract, 1910, *JP* **41**:19, and from animal tissues, 1911, *JP* **41**:499. His work on anaphylaxis, 1913, *JPET* **4**:167, similar to that of William Henry Schultz, 1910, led to the term 'Schultz-Dale test'. He demonstrated the inhibitory action of acetylcholine on the heart, 1914, *JPET* **6**: 147; for this, and later work, he shared the Nobel Prize (Physiology or Medicine), 1936, with Otto Loewi, for their work on the chemical mediation of nervous impulses, *NPL*. Began study of the effect of histamine on the circulation with Alfred Newton Richards, 1918, *JP*, **52**:110. With Patrick Playfair Laidlaw, produced experimental shock by histamine and showed that it was similar to traumatic and surgical shock, 1919, *JP* **52**:355. Died 1968. *1895, 1898, 1901.1, 2600.5, 1340, 792, 5630*

1875:40 Ernst Ferdinand **Sauerbruch**, German thoracic surgeon, born 3 Jul; devised negative pressure chamber for the prevention of pneumothorax, 1904, *VDGC* **32**ii,105. Performed thymectomy for myasthenia gravis, 1913, *MGMC* **25**:746. Introduced phrenicotomy in the treatment of pulmonary tuberculosis, 1913, *MMW* **60**:625. First successful surgical intervention for cardiac aneurysm, 1931, *ArKC* **167**:586. Died 1951. *3185, 4764, 3234, 2990*

1875:41 Carl Gustav **Jung**, Swiss psychologist and psychiatrist, born 26 Jul; at first a supporter of Freud, he eventually broke away and founded the school of analytical psychology. His *Wandlungen*, published in 1911, appeared in English translation as *Psychology of the unconscious*, 1912. Died 1961. *4985.2*

1875:42 Ernest Edward **Tyzzer**, American pathologist, born 30 Aug; first recognized inclusion bodies in varicella, 1905, *JMR* **14**:361. With Clarence Cook Little, initiated the study of histocompatibility antigens, 1916, *JMR* **33**:393. Died 1965. *5440, 2570*

1875:43 Maxime Paul Marie **Laignel-Lavastine**, French physician and medical historian, born 12 Sep; general editor of *Histoire générale de la médecine, de la pharmacie, de l'art dentaire et de l'art vétérinaire*, 3 vols, 1936–1949, a well-produced and beautifully illustrated history of medicine, written by experts. Died 1953. *6430*

1875:44 Gunnar **Holmgren**, Swedish otorhinolaryngologist, born 27 Sep; devised fenestration operation for otosclerosis, 1923, *AcOL* **5**:460. Died 1954. *3404*

1875:45 Alfred Fabian **Hess**, American physician, born 19 Oct; provided experimental proof that rubella is caused by a virus, 1914, *ArIM* **13**:913. Showed that rickets and scurvy could be prevented by the ultraviolet irradiation of oils and foodstuffs; in his *Rickets, including osteomalacia and tetany*, 1929. Died 1933. *5506.1, 3735*

1875:46 Carl Joseph **Gauss**, German gynaecologist, born 29 Oct; developed Twilight sleep, 1906, *ArGy* **78**:579, introduced by von Steinbüchel in 1902 for the relief of labour pains. Died 1957. *6212, 6210*

1875:47 Stanislaus Joseph Matthias von **Prowazek**, German protozoologist and bacteriologist, born 12 Nov; with Ludwig Halberstaedter, gave the first description of the cytoplasmic inclusion bodies of trachoma (*Chlamydia trachomatis*), 1907, *AKG* **26**:44. Like Ricketts and Wilder, demonstrated the specific causal agent in typhus, 1910, *BKI* **4**:5. Died 1915. *5951, 5384.1, 5379, 5380.1*

1875:48 Ambrose Thomas **Stanton**, Canadian physician, born 14 Nov; identified the bacillus of melioidosis, (*Pfeifferella whitmori*), 1917, *SIMR* **14**. He reproduced the disease in animals by feeding and inoculation of cultures. Died 1938. *5159.1*

1875:49 Karl Bruno **Stargardt**, German ophthalmologist, born 4 Dec; demonstrated the inclusion bodies in ophthalmia neonatorum, 1909, *GAO* **69**:525. Died 1927. *5956*

1875:50 Francis Edward **Shipway**, British anaesthetist, born 6 Dec; introduced an apparatus for the administration of warm anaesthetic vapours (Shipway apparatus), 1916, *L* **1**:70. Died 1968. *5699.3*

1875:51 Henry Sessions **Souttar**, British surgeon, born 14 Dec; carried out first successful mitral valvulotomy for mitral stenosis, 1925, *BMJ* **2**:603. Died 1964. *3032*

1875:52 Karl Franz **Nagelschmidt**, German physician, born; introduced treatment by diathermy, 1909, *MMW* **56**:2575. Died 1952. *2007*

1875:53 Richard **Lewisohn**, American pathologist, born; used citrated blood in transfusion, 1915, *MR* **87**:141, about the same time as Luis Agote. Died 1962. *2021*

1875:54 Ernst **Frieben**, German physician, born; reported the carcinogenic effects of x rays, 1902, *DMW* **28**:VB, 335. *2625.1*

1875:55 Paul **Trenaunay**, French physician, born; with Maurice Klippel, described the Klippel-Trenaunay syndrome (angio-osteohypertrophy), 1900, *ArGM* **185**:642. *4131*

1875:56 Jacques **Calvé**, French orthopaedic surgeon, born; described juvenile osteochondritis deformans (first mentioned by H. Waldenström in 1909), 1910, *RC* **42**:54; independently described by Arthur Thornton Legg and by Georg Clemens Perthes and given the name 'Calvé-Legg-Perthes disease'. Died 1954. *4381, 4380, 4382*

1875:57 Cécile **Vogt**, German neurologist, born; with Oskar Vogt, described disease of the corpora striata (status dysmyelinatus syndrome, 'Vogt syndrome'), 1920, *JPN*, Ergänz. iii:627. Died 1962. *4720*

1875:58 Leslie Leon **Lumsden**, American epidemiologist, born; reported the *Culex* mosquito as vector of St Louis encephalitis, 1933, *USPHR* **73**:340 [published in 1958]. Died 1946. *4661.2*

1875:59 Antonio **Garcia Tapia**, Spanish neurologist, born; described palato-pharyngo-laryngeal hemiplegia ('Tapia's syndrome'), 1905, *SMM* **52**:211. Died 1950. *4594*

1875:60 Norman Beechey **Gwyn**, American gynaecologist, born; isolated *Salmonella paratyphi A*, 1898, *JHB* **9**:54. Died 1952. *5038*

1875:61 William Buchanan **Wherry**, American bacteriologist, born; with Benjamin Harrison Lamb, first isolated *Pasteurella tularensis*, causal organism of tularaemia, from lesions in humans, 1914, *JID* **15**:331. Died 1936. *5175*

1875:62 Walter Remsen **Brinckerhoff** born; with George Burgess Magrath, carried out successful inoculation of smallpox into the monkey, 1904, *JMR* **11**:230. Died 1911. *5429.1*

1875: Robert **Adams** died, **born** 1791. *heart block*

1875: Peter Mere **Latham** died, **born** 1789. *coronary thrombosis*

1875: John Hughes **Bennett** died, **born** 1812. *leukaemia, cod-liver oil*

1875: Guillaume Benjamin Amand **Duchenne de Boulogne** died, **born** 1806. *electrophysiology of the muscular system, electrotherapy, brachial plexus paralysis, progressive bulbar paralysis, tabes dorsalis, progressive muscular atrophy, expression of emotions*

1875: Augustin Eugène **Homolle** died, **born** 1808. *digitalin*

1875: Carl Wilhelm **Boeck** died, **born** 1808. *leprosy, scabies*

1875: Hubert von **Luschka** died, **born** 1820. *polyposis of colon*

1875: Pierre Saloman **Ségalas** died, **born** 1792. *urethro-cystic speculum*

1875: Sigismund Eduard **Loewenhardt** died, **born** 1796. *tabes dorsalis*

1875: John Peter **Mettauer** died, **born** 1787. *vesico-vaginal fistula*

1875: Jean Nicolas **Demarquay** died, **born** 1814. *filariasis, elephantiasis, Wuchereria*

**1876**
1876:1 **Physiological Society** founded, London

1876:2 **Johns Hopkins University** founded

1876:3 **University of Bristol** founded

1876:4 **[Royal Academy of Medicine, Rome]** founded

1876:5 **Société Française d'Hygiène, Paris** founded

1876:6 **American Dermatological Society** founded

1876:7 **American Chemical Society** founded

1876:8 The influential *Text-book of physiology* by Michael Foster (1836–1907) published. *631*

1876:9 One of the first to adopt the **antiseptic principle** in **surgery** was Just Marcellin Lucas-Championnière (1843–1913), who wrote *Chirurgie antiseptique*, the first authoritative text on the subject. *5636*

1876:10 The use of **physostigmine** in the treatment of **glaucoma** introduced by Ludwig Laqueur (1839–1909), *ZMW* **14**:421. *5913*

1876:11 **Caesarean section** with excision of the uterus and adnexa ('**Porro's operation**') performed by Edoardo Porro (1842–1902), *AnU* **237**:289. *6240*

1876:12 *Grundriss der Geschichte der Medicin*, by Johann Hermann Baas (1838–1909), was the most important one-volume **history of medicine** until superseded by Fielding H. Garrison's *Introduction to the history of medicine*. *6389*

1876:13 *Extra-uterine pregnancy*, by John S. Parry (1843–1876), was regarded by Lawson Tait as the first authoritative work on **ectopic pregnancy**. *6191*

1876:14 The first description of **vernal conjunctivitis** given by Edwin Theodor Saemisch (1833–1909); in A.C. Graefe and E.T. Saemisch's *Handbuch der gesammten Augenheilkinde*, **4**, Theil 2, 29. *5914*

1876:15 An important contribution on **colour-blindness** and its relation to railway and maritime traffic made by Alarik Frithiof Holmgren (1831–1897), *ULF* **12**:171, 267. *5916*

1876:16 The first American publication devoted exclusively to **reconstructive surgery** was *Contributions to reparative surgery*, by Gurdon Buck (1807–1877). *5754.1*

1876:17 An **ether inhaler** (**Clover apparatus**) introduced by Joseph Thomas Clover (1825–1882), *BMJ* **2**:74. *5674*

1876:18 *Strongyloides stercoralis*, causal parasite of **strongyloidiasis**, found by Louis Alexis Normond (1834–?1885), *CRAS* **83**:316. *5344.11*

1876:19 First to obtain pure cultures of ***Bacillus anthracis*** was Robert Koch (1843–1910), *BBP* **2**:277. Continuing the work of Davaine he proved that infectious diseases are caused by living reproductive microorganisms. *5167*

1876:20 **Myotonia congenita** first described by Ernst von Leyden (1832–1910); in his *Klinik der Rückenmarks-Krankheiten*, **2**, **ii**, 550. The first full description given by Asmus Julius Thomas Thomsen (1815–1896), himself a sufferer from the disease, *ArPN* **6**:702, which later became known as '**Thomsen's disease**' *4743, 4744*

1876:21 The **syphilitic** origin of **tabes dorsalis**, a view not at first accepted, stated by Jean Alfred Fournier (1832–1914); in his *De l'ataxie locomotrice d'origine syphilitique*. *4782*

1876:22 A reliable diagnostic sign in latent **tetany**, '**Chvostek's sign**', introduced by František Chvostek (1835–1884), *WMP* **17**:1201, 1225, 1253, 1313. *4833*

1876:23 The foundations of our knowledge of **cortical localization** were laid by David Ferrier (1843–1928); in his *Functions of the brain*. *1409*

1876:24 **Salicylates** introduced in the treatment of **rheumatism** by Thomas John Maclagan (1838–1903), *L* **1**:342, 383. *4501*

1876:25 Important studies of **localization of functions in diseases of the brain** published by Jean Martin Charcot (1825–1893); in his *Leçons sur les localisations dans les maladies du cerveau*, 1876–78. *4558*

1876:26 The first complete description of anterior **metatarsalgia**, first noted by Durlacher in 1845, given by Thomas George Morton (1835–1903) ('**Morton's metatarsalgia**'), *AmJMS* **71**:37. *4325, 4341*

1876:27 **Pyorrhoea alveolaris** ('**Riggs' disease**') described by John M. Riggs (1810–1885), *PJDS* **3**:99. *3685*

1876:28 Lewis Albert Sayre (1820–1900) was first to use **plaster of Paris** as a support in the treatment of **tuberculosis of the spine**, *TAMA* **27**:573. See also his *Spinal diseases and spinal curvature, their treatment by suspension and the use of plaster of Paris bandage*, 1877. *4344, 4344.1*

1876:29 Original descriptions of several **nervous disorders**, especially the **muscular dystrophies**, given by Wilhelm Heinrich Erb (1840–1921); in his *Handbuch der Krankheiten des Nervensystems*, 1876–78. *4557*

1876:30 The **ureter** successfully **catheterized** under **endoscopic** vision by Joseph Grünfeld (1840–1910), *WMP* **17**:919, 949. *4174.1*

1876:31 **Gastrostomy** operation by Aristide Auguste Stanislas Verneuil (1823–1895), *BuAM* **5**:1023, was a modification of Sédillot's method. *3468*

1876:32 The primary lesion of **pulmonary tuberculosis** in children ('**Ghon's primary locus**') first described by Joseph Parrot (1829–1883), *CRSB* **3**:308. *3224, 3233*

1876:33 **Ozaena** established as a clinical entity by Bernhard Fraenkel (1836–1911), Ziemssen's *Handbuch* **4**, I:125. *3285*

1876:34 **Multiple hereditary telangiectasis** ('Rendu-Osler-Weber disease') first described by John Wickham Legg (1843–1921), *L* **2**:856. *2707*

1876:35 **Penicillium** shown to have bacteria-inhibiting effect by John Tyndall (1820–1893), *PT* **166**:27. *1932*

1876:36 **Transplantation** of **tumours** in dogs by Mstislav Novinsky (1841–1914), *MV* **16**:289. *2620.1*

1876:37 **Sattler's layer** of the choroid described by Hubert Sattler (1844–1928), *GAO* **22ii**:1. *1518*

1876:38 The **centrosome** discovered by Edouard van Beneden (1846–1910), *BARS* **41**:38, independently of Flemming. *497, 498*

1876:39 The doctrine of a **criminal type** inaugurated by Cesare Lombroso (1836–1909); in his *L'uomo delinquente. 174*

1876:40 The mechanism of **fertilization** – entrance of the spermatozoon into the ovum and union of the nuclei of the male and female sex cells – demonstrated by Wilhelm August Oscar Hertwig (1849–1922), *MoJ* 1:346. *495*

1876:41 Arthur **Laewen**, German surgeon, born 6 Feb; first to use paravertebral injection of novocaine in the treatment of angina pectoris, 1922, *ZCh* **49**:1510. Died 1958. *2896*

1876:42 Henry Asbury **Christian**, American physician, born 17 Feb; gave a description of what later became known as the Hand-Schüller-Christian syndrome, 1919, in his paper in *Contributions to medical and biological research dedicated to Sir William Osler*, 1919, **1**, 390. Reported febrile nodular non-suppurative panniculitis ('Weber-Christian disease'), 1928, *ArIM* **42**:338; it had been earlier recorded, in 1925, by Frederic Parkes Weber. Died 1951. *4151, 4152, 6359–6363*

1876:43 Gordon Morgan **Holmes**, British neurologist, born 22 Feb; with Henry Head he described the functions of the thalamus, 1911, *Brain* **34**:102. Recorded the removal of a tumour of the adrenal cortex (by P. Sargent), with subsequent disappearance of the accompanying virilism, 1925, *QJM* **18**:143; thus establishing the relationship between sexual abnormality and adrenal tumours. Died 1965. *1438.1, 3872*

1876:44 Carl Gustav Abrahamsson **Forssell**, Swedish radiologist, born 2 Mar; the Stockholm method of radium treatment of cancer of the uterus, as carried out at the Radiumhemmet, Stockholm, followed the technique devised by him, 1917, *Hos* **10**:273. Died 1950. *6125*

1876:45 Georges **Guillain**, French physician, born 3 Mar; with Jean Alexandre Barré and A. Strohl, described acute infective polyneuritis (Guillain-Barré syndrome'), 1916, *BSMH* **40**:1462. Died 1961. *4647*

1876:46 Alfred Newton **Richards**, American pharmacologist, born 22 Mar; with Henry Hallett Dale began study of the effect of histamine on the circulation, 1918, *JP* **52**:110. Died 1966. *792*

1876:47 Edwin **Beer**, American urologist, born 28 Mar; his method of transurethral fulguration of bladder tumours, 1910, *JAMA* **54**:1768, led to the operation of transurethral prostatectomy. Died 1938. *4268*

1876:48 Fred Houdlett **Albee**, American surgeon, born 13 Apr; a pioneer of living bone graft surgery, used bone grafts as splints; he transplanted part of a tibia into the spine for Pott's disease, 1911, *JAMA* **57**:885. He wrote *Bone graft surgery*, 1915. Died 1945. *4384.1, 5757*

1876:49 Robert **Bárány**, Austrian physiologist, born 22 Apr; devised test for labyrinthine function (Bárány's caloric function test), 1906, *ArOh* **68**:1; reported a pointing test for localization of circumscribed cerebellar lesions, 1906, *MonO* **40**:193; **41**:447; recorded Bárány's syndrome – unilateral deafness, vertigo, and pain in the occipital region, 1911, *MK* **7**:1818. Awarded the Nobel Prize (Physiology or Medicine), 1914, for his work on the vestibular apparatus, *NPL*. Died 1936. *3400, 3401, 3402*

1876:50 Henri **Coutard**, French radiologist, born 27 Apr; treated carcinoma of pharynx with radiotherapy ('Coutard method'), 1921, *BAFC* **10**:160. Died 1950. *3196*

1876:51 Eugen Alexander **Pólya**, Hungarian surgeon, born 30 Apr; modified the Billroth II operation for cancer of the pylorus, 1911, *ZCh* **38**:892. Died ?1944. *3537, 3483*

1876:52 Marmaduke Stephen **Mayou**, British ophthalmologist, born 4 May; described cases of juvenile amaurotic familial idiocy, ('Batten-Mayou disease'), 1904, *TOUK* **24**:142. Died 1934. *4713, 4712*

1876:53 Alfred **Whitmore**, British pathologist and medical officer, Indian Army, born 16 May; with C.S. Krishnaswami, first described melioidosis, 1912, *IMG* **47**:262. The organism isolated later named *Pfeifferella whitmori*. Died 1946. *5159*

1876:54 George Walter **McCoy**, American bacteriologist and serologist, born 4 Jun; first recorded tularaemia (in rodents), 1911, *USPHB* **43**:53; with Charles Willard Chapin, isolated *Pasteurella tularensis*, the causal organism, 1912, *JID* **10**:61. Died 1952. *5173, 5174*

1876:55 José **Goyanes Capdevila**, Spanish surgeon, born 16 Jun; used vein grafts to restore arterial blood flow, 1906, *SMM* **53**:546, 561. Died 1964. *3025.2*

1876:56 Adelchi **Negri**, Italian pathologist, born 2 Aug; discovered inclusion bodies ('Negri bodies') in the nerve cells of humans and animals proved to have been infected with rabies, 1903, making possible prompt microscopic diagnosis, *BSMP* 1903:88, 229; 1904:22; 1905:321. Died 1912. *5484*

1876:57 Constantin von **Economo**, Austrian neurologist, born 21 Aug; gave a classic account of epidemic encephalitis (encephalitis lethargica, 'von Economo's disease'), 1917, *WKW* **30**:381. Died 1931. *4650*

1876:58 William Lorenzo **Moss**, American pathologist, born 23 Aug; classified blood into four groups, 1910, *JHB*, **21**:63. (This had already been done by Janský, but his work, published in a Czech journal, was not at that time known to Moss). Died 1957. *900*

1876:59 John James Rickard **Macleod**, British physiologist and biochemist, born 6 Sep; with Frederick Grant Banting and Charles Herbert Best, isolated a pancreatic extract which was named insulin, 1922, *AmJPh* **66**:479; *JLCM* **7**:251. Shared the Nobel Prize (Physiology or Medicine), 1923, with Banting, *NPL*. Died 1935. *3966, 3967*

1876:60 John Lancelot **Todd**, Canadian parasitologist, born 10 Sep; with John Everett Dutton, demonstrated, independently of Ross and Milne, relapsing fever in monkeys, and described the mechanisms of infection conveyed by infected ticks, *Ornithodorus moubata*, 1905, *BMJ* **2**:1259. The infecting organism was later named *Borrelia duttoni*, after Dutton, who died from the disease. Died 1949. *5318*

1876:61 George Ernest **Waugh**, British surgeon, born 26 Oct; introduced blunt dissection tonsillectomy, 1909, *L* **1**:1314. Died 1940. *3317*

1876:62 Hideyo **Noguchi**, Japanese/American bacteriologist, born 24 Nov; first to obtain a pure culture of *Treponema pallidum*, causative organism of syphilis, 1911, *JEM* **14**:99. With Joseph Waldron Moore, obtained a pure culture of *Trep. pallidum*, from a patient with dementia paralytica, 1913, *JEM* **17**:232. Obtained a pure culture of vaccinia virus, 1915, *JMR* **21**:539. Isolated *Bact. granulosis*, which he believed to be the causal organism in trachoma, 1927, *JAMA* **89**:739. With co-workers, showed *Phlebotomus* to be the vector of bartonellosis (Oroya fever, Carrión's disease), 1929, *JEM* **49**:993. Died 1928. *2404, 4805, 5430.1, 5973, 5538.1*

1876:63 Thomas Peel **Dunhill**, Australian surgeon, born 3 Dec; a pioneer in thyroid surgery, he devised a new technique for the removal of exophthalmic goitre, 1919, *BJS* **7**:195. Died 1957. *3849.1*

1876:64 Ludwig **Halberstaedter**, Polish physician, born 9 Dec; with Stanislaus Joseph Matthias von Prowazek, gave the first description of the cytoplasmic inclusion bodies of trachoma (*Chlamydia trachomatis*), 1907, *AKG* **26**:44. *5951*

1876:65 Nikolai Dmitrievich **Strazhesko**, Russian physician, born 17 Dec; with Vasili Parmenovich Obraztsov, gave the first comprehensive description of coronary thrombosis, diagnosed before death and confirmed at necroscopy, 1910, *ZKM* **71**:116. Died 1952. *2835*

1876:66 Adolf **Windaus**, German chemist, born 25 Dec; with Karl Vogt he synthesized histamine, 1907, *BDCG* **40**:3691. Awarded Nobel Prize (Chemistry), 1927, for research into the constitution of the sterols and their connection with the vitamins, *NPL*. Died 1959. *1895.1*

1876:67 George **Coats**, British ophthalmologist, born; described retinitis circinata ('Coats' disease'), 1908, *OHP* **17**:440. Died 1915. *5954*

1876:68 Karl **Imhoff**, German sanitary engineer, born; devised Imhoff system of sewage purification, 1942; in his *Fortschritte der Abwasserreinigung*. *1642*

1876:69 Otto Carl Willy **Prausnitz**, Breslau bacteriologist, born; with Heinz Küstner, demonstrated the 'Prausnitz-Küstner reaction', indicating the presence of antibodies in the serum of persons suffering from atopic diseases, 1921, *ZBP* I **86**:160. Died 1963. *2601.1*

1876:70 Kensuke **Mitsuda**, Japanese leprologist, born; introduced Mitsuda (lepromin) reaction for diagnosis of leprosy, 1919, *Hinyoka Zasshi*, **19**:697. [English translation by Mitsuda, *IJL* (1953) **21**:347.] *2440*

1876:71 Otto **Foerster** born; with co-workers, used mapharsen in treatment of syphilis, 1935, *ArDS* **32**:868. Died 1965. 2416

1876:72 Henry Peter George **Bayon**, South African bacteriologist, born; produced cancer experimentally by tar injection, 1912, *L* **2**:1579. Died 1952. *2639*

1876:73 Harold Benjamin **Fantham**, British protozoologist, born; with John William Watson Stephens, discovered a new species of trypanosome, *Trypanosoma rhodesiense*, 1910, *PRS* **83**:28. Died 1937. *5285*

1876:74 Paul **Hallopeau**, French surgeon, born; carried out first pericardiectomy for constrictive pericarditis, 1921, *BSCP* **47**:1120. Died 1924. *3030*

1876:75 Maurice **Favre**, French dermatologist, born; with Joseph Durand and Joseph Nicolas, gave the first important account of lymphogranuloma venereum, 1913, *BSMH* **35**:274. It is sometimes called 'Durand-Nicolas-Favre disease'. Died 1955. *5217*

1876:76 Mikhail **Arinkin**, Russian pathologist, born; introduced bone marrow biopsy by needle puncture, 1927, *VK* **30**:57. Died 1948. *3088*

1876:77 G. Paul **Laroque**, American surgeon, born; modified the standard operative procedures for the cure of femoral and inguinal hernia, 1919, *SGO* **29**:507. Died 1934. *3608.2*

1876:78 John Timothy **Geraghty**, American urological surgeon, born; with Leonard George Rowntree, introduced the phenolsulphonephthalein kidney function test, 1910, *JPET* **1**:579. Died 1924. *4236*

1876:79 James Wesley **Jobling** born; with Simon Flexner, used antiserum in the treatment of epidemic cerebrospinal meningitis, 1907–8, *JEM* **9**:168; **10**:141. *4683, 4684*

1876:80 Hans Heinrich Georg **Queckenstedt**, German neurologist, born; introduced a test for determining the patency of the spinal subarachnoid space ('Queckenstedt's test'), 1916, *DZN* **55**:325. Died 1918. *4600*

1876:81 Moritz **Oppenheim**, Austrian dermatologist born; with Rudolf Müller, introduced a complement fixation test for the diagnosis of gonorrhoea ('Müller-Oppenheim reaction'), 1906, *WKW* **19**:894. Died 1949. *5213*

1876:82 Philip Hedgeland **Ross**, British bacteriologist, born; with Arthur Dawson Milne, discovered that African relapsing fever (tick fever) is conveyed by *Ornithodorus moubata*, 1904, *BMJ* **2**:453. Died 1929. *5317*

1876:83 Joseph **Durand**, French dermatologist, born; with Joseph Nicolas and Maurice Favre, gave the first important account of lymphogranuloma venereum, 1913, *BSMH* **35**:274. It is sometimes called 'Durand-Nicolas-Favre disease'. *5217*

1876:84 Hans Willi **Töpfer**, German military surgeon, born; isolated *Rickettsia quintana* from lice found on patients with trench fever, 1916, *MMW* **63**:1495. *5389*

1876:85 Ludwig **Adler**, German obstetrician, born: with Fritz Hitschmann, first definitely described the cyclical changes in the endometrium and showed that they were a normal physiological process, 1908, *MonG* **27**:1. Died 1958. *1181*

---

1876: Karl von **Baer** died, **born** 1792. *ovum, germ-layer, notochord*

1876: Antoine Jérome **Balard** died, **born** 1802. *bromine, amyl nitrate*

1876: Christian Gottfried **Ehrenberg** died, **born** 1796. *Bacillus subtilis*

1876: Ludwig **Traube** died, **born** 1818. *pulsus alternans, vasoconstrictor centre*

1876: Walter **Channing** died, **born** 1786. *obstetrics, anaesthesia, pernicious anaemia of pregnancy*

1876: William Robert Wills **Wilde** died, **born** 1815. *otology*

1876: Gustav **Simon** died, **born** 1824. *urinary tract fistula, nephrectomy*

1876: Georg Friedrich **Stromeyer** died, **born** 1804. *talipes*

1876: James Lomax **Bardsley** died, **born** 1801. *amoebiasis, emetine*

1876: Gustav **Simon** died, **born** 1824. *cheiroplasty*

1876: John S. **Parry** died, **born** 1843. *ectopic pregnancy*

**1877**
1877:1 **Faculté de Médecine, Lyons**, founded

1877:2 The **axis-traction forceps** invented by Etienne Stéphane Tarnier (1828–1897), *AnG* **7**:241; also his *Description de deux nouveaux forceps. 6192*

1877:3 **Chorionepithelioma** first reported by Hans Chiari (1851–1916), *MJa*, 34. *6066.1*

1877:4 The **centrosome** discovered by Walther Flemming (1843–1905), *ArMA* **13**:693; independently of van Beneden. *498, 497*

1877:5 The first effective description of **actinomycosis** in cattle given by Otto Bollinger (1843–1909), *ZMW* **15**:481. He gave his botanical colleague, C.O. Harz, a specimen of the microparasite and Harz named it (p. 485) *Actinomyces bovis. 5510*

1877:6 Patrick Manson (1844–1922) showed that *Wuchereria bancrofti*, cause of **filarial elephantiasis** in man, develops in, and is transmitted by, the *Culex* **mosquito** – the first proof that infective diseases are spread by animal **vectors**, *MRpt* **13**:30; **14**:1. *5345, 5345.1*

1877:7 The first definite record of **myasthenia gravis** is believed to be a case of 'bulbar paralysis' described by Samuel Wilks (1824–1911), *GHR* **22**:7. *4745*

1877:8 The relationship between **general paresis** and **congenital syphilis** recognized by Thomas Smith Clouston (1840–1915), he reported the condition in a patient aged sixteen, *JMS* **23**:419. *4799*

1877:9 In his *Die Störungen der Sprache*, Adolph Kussmaul (1822–1902) termed **aphasia** 'word-blindness'. *4624*

1877:10 '**Baker's cysts**' of the **knee-joint** first described by William Morrant Baker (1839– 1896), *SBHR* **13**:245; **21**:177. *4342*

1877:11 An important description of **osteitis deformans**, '**Paget's disease of bone**,' given by James Paget (1814–1899), *MCT* **60**:37; **65**:225. *4343*

1877:12 The first account of the relation of **pain** to **weather** published by Silas Weir Mitchell (1829–1914), in a study of **traumatic neuralgia**, *AmJMS* **73**:305. *4555*

1877:13 The first **nephrectomy** for **malignant disease** carried out by Carl Langenbuch (1846– 1901), *BKW* **14**:337. *4216.1*

1877:14 An electrically lighted **cystoscope** devised by Max Nitze (1848–1906), making possible great improvements in **bladder surgery**, *WMW* **29**:649, 688, 713, 776, 896. *4175*

1877: 15 Claude Bernard (1813–1878) showed that in **diabetes mellitus** there is primarily **glycaemia** followed by **glycosuria**; in his *Leçons sur le diabète et la glycogenèse animale*. *3942*

1877: 16 Etienne Lancereaux (1829–1910) first definitely to claim a causal relationship between **pancreatic lesions** and **diabetes mellitus**, *BuAM* **6**:1215. *3943*

1877: 17 **Mastoiditis** was first clearly described by Friedrich Bezold (1842–1908), *ArOh* **13**:26. *3386*

1877: 18 An **acumeter** described by Adam Politzer (1835–1920), *ArOh* **12**:104. *3387.1*

1877: 19 First complete account of progressive **pernicious anaemia** by William Gardner and William Osler (1849–1919), *CMSJ* **5**:383. *3125.2*

1877: 20 **Congenital mitral stenosis** ('**Duroziez's disease**') first described by Paul Louis Duroziez (1826–1897), *ArGM* **30**:32, 184. *2780*

1877: 21 **Syphilis: 'Moon's molars'**, the irregular and defective first molars in congenital syphilitics, described by Henry Moon (1845–1892), *TOSG* **22**:223. *2391*

1877: 22 *Clostridium septicum* discovered by Louis Pasteur (1822–1895) and Jules François Joubert, *CRAS* **85**:101. *2490*

1877: 23 **Tuberculosis** inoculated into rabbit eye by Julius Cohnheim (1839–1884); reported in his *Die Tuberkulose*, 1880. *2329*

1877: 24 **Tyndallization** (fractional **sterilization**) discovered by John Tyndall (1820–1893); *Essays on the floating-matter of the air* .... *2495*

1877: 25 Bactericidal action of **sunlight** demonstrated by Arthur Henry Downes (1851–1938) and Thomas Porter Blunt, *PRS* **26**:488. *1997*

1877: 26 A **thermocautery** ('**Paquelin's cautery**') introduced by Claude André Paquelin (1836–1905), *BGT* **93**:145. *5614*

---

1877: 27 Lewis Madison **Terman**, American psychologist, born 15 Jan; with co-workers, revised the Binet-Simon scale for measurement of intelligence; in *The Stanford revision and extension of the Binet-Simon scale for measuring intelligence*, 1917. Died 1957. *4986*

1877: 28 Willi **Rimpau**, German bacteriologist, born 16 Jan; with Fred Neufeld, named and described bacteriotropins, 1904, *DMW* **30**:1458. *2560*

1877: 29 Edgar Otto Konrad von **Gierke**, German pathologist, born 9 Feb; described the glycogen storage disease known as 'von Gierke's disease', 1929, *BPA* **82**:497. Died 1945. *3656*

1877: 30 Holger Werfel **Scheuermann**, Danish orthopaedic surgeon, born 12 Feb; drew attention to kyphosis due to epiphyseal necrosis in vertebrae ('Scheuermann's disease'), 1921, *ZOC* **41**:305. Died 1960. *4389*

1877:31 Alexandre Emile **Brumpt**, French parasitologist, born 7 Mar; described the life cycle of *Trypanosoma cruzi*, 1912, *BSPE* **5**:360. Died 1951. *5285.3*

1877:32 Emil **Abderhalden**, Swiss physiologist and biochemist, born 9 Mar; first described cystinosis, 1903, *HSZ* **38**:557. He contributed notably to the technique and methodology of physiology and biochemistry, especially through his editorship of the *Handbuch der biologischen Arbeitsmethoden*, 107 vols, 1920–1939. Died 1950. *3920, 136*

1877:33 Walter Stanborough **Sutton**, American biologist, physician and geneticist, born 5 Apr. Formulated the theory of the chromosomal basis of Mendelism, 1903, *BB* **4**:231. Died 1916. *242.1*

1877:34 Charles **Mantoux**, French tuberculologist, born 14 May; introduced the Mantoux intradermal tuberculin test for tuberculosis, 1908, *CRAS* **147**:355. Died 1947. *2341*

1877:35 Heinrich Otto **Wieland**, German chemist, born 4 Jun; awarded Nobel Prize (Chemistry), 1928, for investigations of the constitution of the bile acids and related substances, *NPL*. Died 1957

1877:36 Hans **Sachs**, German immunologist, born 6 Jun; with Walter Georgi, introduced the Sachs-Georgi reaction for diagnosis of syphilis, 1919, *MMW* **66**:440. Died 1945. *2408*

1877:37 Hans **Finsterer**, Austrian surgeon, born 24 Jun; further modified the Billroth II gastro-enterostomy, 1918, *ZCh* **45**:434, and named the Hofmeister-Finsterer gastro-enterostomy. Died 1955. *3543,3529*

1877:38 Velyien Ewart **Henderson**, Canadian pharmacologist, born 27 Jun; with George Herbert William Lucas, introduced cyclopropane as an anaesthetic, 1929, *CMAJ* **21**:173. Died 1945. *5711*

1877:39 Bela **Schick**, Hungarian physician, born 16 Jul; with Clemens Peter Pirquet von Cesenatico, gave an excellent account of serum sickness, *Die Serumkrankheit*, 1905; introduced a cutaneous reaction test (Schick test) for the determination of susceptibility to diphtheria, 1908, *MMW* **55**:504; developed the test for use as an indication as to whether or not prophylactic injections are necessary in children already exposed to diphtheria, 1913, *MMW* **60**:2608. Died 1967. *2593, 5065, 5066.*

1877:40 John **Freeman**, British bacteriologist and allergologist, born 19 Jul; with Leonard Noon, introduced hay fever treatment by pollen injections, 1911, *L* **1**:1572; **2**:814. Died 1962. *2600.3, 2600.4*

1877:41 Johann Georg **Mönckeberg**, German cardiologist, born 5 Aug; described medial sclerosis of blood vessels of the extremities ('Mönckeberg's sclerosis'), 1903, *VA* **171**:141. Died 1925. *2911*

1877:42 Alfred **Wolff-Eisner**, German tuberculologist, born 25 Aug; introduced a conjunctival tuberculin reaction in diagnosis of tuberculosis, 1908, *ZTb* **12**:21. Died 1948. *2340*

1877:43 Aldo **Castellani**, Italian specialist in tropical medicine, born 8 Sep; in Uganda discovered *Trypanosoma gambiense* in the cerebrospinal fluid of a patient with trypanosomiasis (sleeping sickness), 1903, *PRS* **71**:501. Demonstrated *Treponema pertenue*, causal organism of yaws, in yaws tissue; finally establishing it as a distinct organism from the spirochaete of syphilis, *T.pallidum*, 1905, *BMJ* **2**:1280, 1330, 1430. First to suspect that toxoplasmosis could affect humans, 1914, *JTM* **17**:113. Described bronchospirochaetosis ('Castellani's bronchitis'), 1917, *PrM* **25**:377. Died 1971. *5276, 5306, 5535.1, 5544.1, 3193*

1877:44 Ugo **Cerletti**, Italian neuropsychiatrist, born 12 Sep; with Lucio Bini, introduced electric convulsion therapy in psychosis, 1930, *BAMR* **64**:136. Died 1963. *4962*

1877:45 Oscar **Riddle**, American biologist, born 27 Sep; with co-workers, prepared, identified and assayed prolactin, 1933, *AmJPh* **105**:191. Died 1968. *1171*

1877:46 Karl Theodor **Fahr**, German pathologist, born 3 Oct; with Franz Volhard, gave the first full description of pure nephrosis; in their *Die Brightsche Nierenkrankheit*, 1914. Died 1945. *4238*

1877:47 Thomas Renton **Elliott**, British physiologist and physician, born 11 Oct; suggested chemical mediation of nerve impulses and adrenaline as mediator, 1904, *JP* **31**:xx. Died 1961. *1336*

1877:48 Oswald Theodore **Avery**, American physician, born 21 Oct; with Michael Heidelberger, elucidated the antigenic structure of pneumococcus and separated the polysaccharide antigens, 1924, *JEM* **38**:73. With Colin Munro MacLeod and Maclyn McCarty, demonstrated that deoxyribonucleic acid (DNA) is the basic material responsible for genetic transformation, 1944, *JEM* **79**:137. Died 1955. *2573, 3198, 255.3.*

1877:49 Frederick William **Twort**, British microbiologist, born 23 Oct; noted the transmissible lysis of bacteria by viruses (Twort-d'Herelle phenomenon), 1915, *L* **2**:1241; discovered independently in 1917 by Félix Hubert d'Herelle, who named the lytic agent bacteriophage. Died 1950. *2571, 2572*

1877:50 Maurice **Villaret**, French physician, born 7 Dec; described the posterior retroparotid space syndrome ('Villaret's syndrome'), 1916, *ReN* **23**, I:188. Died 1946. *4719*

---

1877:51 Sydney William **Cole**, British biochemist, born; with Frederick Gowland Hopkins isolated tryptophan, 1901, *JP* **27**:418. Died 1952. *723*

1877:52 Percy William Leopold **Camps**, British physician, born; first to use adrenaline by the respiratory route in the treatment of asthma, 1929, *GHR* **79**:496. Died 1956. *3202.1*

1877:53 Giovanna **Ghedini**, Italian physician, born; introduced bone marrow biopsy (puncture of shaft of tibia), 1908, *CMI* **47**:724. *3080*

1877:54 John **Homans**, American surgeon, born; with Samuel James Crowe and Harvey Williams Cushing, demonstrated that hypophysectomy causes genital atrophy, 1910, *JHB* **21**:127. Died 1955. *3894*

1877:55 John Henry **Cunningham**, American urological surgeon, born; introduced urethrography for the diagnosis of urethral stricture, 1910, *TAAGS* **5**:369. *4196.1*

1877:56 Maximilian **Stern**, American surgeon, born; introduced a resectoscope for use in prostatic surgery, 1926, *IJMS* **39**:72. *4273*

1877:57 Charles Scott **Venable**, American surgeon, born; with co-workers, introduced vitallium experimentally in bone replacement, 1937, *AnS* **105**:917. *4402*

1877:58 Alberto **Ascoli** born; produced a thermoprecipitin reaction for the diagnosis of anthrax, 1911, *CV* **34**:2. Died 1957. *5171*

1877:59 Charles Willard **Chapin** born; with George Walter McCoy, isolated *Pasteurella tularensis*, the causal organism of tularaemia, 1912, *JID* **10**:61. *5174*

1877:60 Rudolf **Müller** born; with Moritz Oppenheim, introduced a complement fixation test for the diagnosis of gonorrhoea ('Müller-Oppenheim reaction'), 1906, *WKW* **19**:894. *5213*

1877:61 Allan Coats **Rankin**, Canadian bacteriologist, born; with George Herbert Hunt, named 'Trench fever', 1915, *L* **2**:1133. Died 1959. *5386*

1877:62 Fritz **Brenner**, German pathologist, born; an ovarian tumour described by him, 1907, *FZP* **1**:150, was later named 'Brenner tumour', although described previously by Orthmann (1899). *6118, 6109.1*

---

1877: Joseph Bienaimé **Caventou** died, **born** 1795. *strychnine, quinine*

1877: James **Blundell** died, **born** 1790. *blood transfusion*

1877: Carl **Wunderlich** died, **born** 1815. *thermometry*

1877: Gurdon **Buck** died, **born** 1807. *cancer of larynx, thyrotomy, ankylosed knee-joint, fracture of femur, reconstructive surgery*

1877: Pierre Louis Alphée **Cazenave** died, **born** 1795. *dermatology, classification of skin diseases, pemphigus foliaceus, lupus erythematosus*

1877: John **Adams** died, **born** 1806. *carcinoma of prostate*

1877: Nathan Ryno **Smith** died, **born** 1797. *fracture of femur*

1877: Moritz Michael **Eulenburg** died, **born** 1811. *upward displacement of scapula*

1877: William **Fergusson** died, **born** 1808. *vaginal speculum*

**1878**
1878:1 *Journal of Physiology*, London, founded by Michael Foster (1836–1907)

1878:2 **International Congress of Hygiene, Paris**

1878:3 **Women's Hospital and School of Medicine, Edinburgh**, founded by Sophia Louisa Jex-Blake (1840–1912)

1878:4 The first to use human donor **cornea** for **transplants** was Heinrich Sellerbeck (b.1842), *GAO* **24**, iv:1, 321. *5916.1*

1878:5 The first successful abdominal **hysterectomy** for **cancer** carried out by Wilhelm Alexander Freund (1833–1918), *BKW* **15**:417. *6070*

1878:6 The first human case of **actinomycosis** reported by James Israel (1848–1926), *VA* **74**:15. In his paper he included drawings of the fungus *Actinomyces* made in 1845 by Bernard Rudolph Conrad von Langenbeck (1810–1887). *5511*

1878:7 **Litholapaxy (lithotrity)** at one sitting introduced by Henry Jacob Bigelow (1818–1890), *AmJMS* **75**:117. *4292*

1878:8 Faecal diagnosis of **ankylostomiasis** first achieved by Giovanni Battista Grassi (1854–1925) and co-workers, *GMI* **5**:193. *5357*

1878:9 Wilhelm Friedrich [Willy] Kühne (1837–1900) extracted **visual purple (rhodopsin)** from the **retina**, *UPIH* **1**:15. *1519*

1878:10 The first description of a **trypanosome** in a mammal (*Trypanosoma lewisi*) made by Timothy Richard Lewis (1841–1886), *ARSCI* **14B**:157. *5270.1*

1878:11 Joseph Bancroft (1836–1894) discovered the **filaria** worm, later to be named *Wuchereria bancrofti*, *TPS* **29**:406. *5346, 5344.6*

1878:12 **Chrysarobin** introduced in **dermatology** by Alexander John Balmanno Squire (d.1908); in his *On the treatment of psoriasis by an ointment of chrysophanic acid. 4075.1*

1878:13 A growth deformity of the **wrist joint** ('**Madelung's deformity'**) described by Otto Wilhelm Madelung (1846–1926), *VDGC* **7**, 2:259. *4345*

1878:14 **Meralgia paraesthetica** in the **leg**, due to disease of the external cutaneous nerve of the thigh ('**Bernhardt's disease'**) reported by Martin Bernhardt (1844–1915), *DAKM* **22**:362. *4559*

1878:15 Emil Theodor Kocher (1841–1917) pioneered **thyroidectomy** for **goitre**, *KBSA* **8**:702. *3826*

1878:16 Infantile **scurvy** differentiated from **rickets** by Walter Butler Cheadle (1836–1910), *L* **2**:685. *3719*

1878:17 William Miller Ord (1834–1902) introduced the term **myxoedema** for the condition described by Curling (1850) and Gull (1873), *MCT* **61**:57. *3825*

1878:18 James Marion Sims (1813–1883) devised a **cholecystotomy** for **dropsy** of the **gallbladder**, *BMJ* **1**:811. *3625*

1878:19 The first excision of the **rectum** for **cancer** was carried out by Richard von Volkmann (1830–1889), *SKV* **131**:1113. *3470*

1878:20 Introduction of antiseptic ligatures in the radical cure of **hernia** by Henry Orlando Marcy (1837–1924), *TAMA* **29**:295. *3594*

1878:21 Adam Politzer's (1835–1920) textbook on **otology**, *Lehrbuch der Ohrenheilkunde*, was for many years a standard authority on the subject. *3387*

1878:22 The first **audiometer** was introduced by Arthur Hartmann (1849–1931), *ArAP* 155. *3387.2*

1878:23 Role of **bacteria** in the aetiology of wound **infection** ('**Koch's postulates**') demonstrated by Robert Koch (1843–1910); in his *Untersuchungen über die Aetiologie der Wundinfectionskrankheiten*. *2536*

1878:24 Joseph Lister (1827–1912) was first to obtain a **pure culture** of a **bacterium**, *Bact. lactis*, *TPS* **29**:425, which he had isolated in 1873. *2489*

1878:25 **Syphilis** inoculated into apes by Theodor Klebs (1834–1913), *ArEP* **10**:161. *2392*

1878:26 **Salicylic acid** used as antipyretic by Carl Emil Buss, *DAKM* **15**:457. *1869.2*

1878:27 *La pression barométrique*, an important work in the history of **altitude physiology**, published by Paul Bert (1833–1886). *944*

1878:28 **Blood platelets** first accurately counted by Georges Hayem (1841–1933), *ArPhy* **5**:692. *879*

---

1878:29 John Broadus **Watson**, American psychiatrist, born 9 Jan; the principal exponent of behaviourist psychology; *Psychology from the standpoint of a behaviorist*, 1919. Died 1958. *4987*

1878:30 Lars **Edling**, Swedish radiologist, born 4 Mar; first used x rays for the diagnosis of pregnancy, 1911, *FGR* **17**:345. *6216*

1878:31 Robert **McCarrison**, British Army physician and nutritionist, born 15 Mar; showed experimentally that bladder calculus could follow a diet deficient in vitamin A, 1927, *IJMR* **14**:895; **15**:197, 485, 801. Died 1960. *4296*

1878:32 Gordon **Gordon-Taylor**, British surgeon, born 18 Mar; with Philip Wiles, introduced the one-stage interinnomino-abdominal (hindquarter) amputation, 1935, *BJS* **22**:671. Died 1960. *4478*

1878:33 George **Barger**, British chemist, born 4 Apr; with Henry Hallett Dale and F.H. Carr, isolated ergotoxine, 1906, *BMJ* **2**:1792; with Dale, isolated histamine from an ergot extract, 1910, *JP* **41**:19, and from animal tissues, 1911, *JP* **41**:499; with Charles Robert Harington, synthesized thyroxine, 1927, *BJ* **21**:169. Died 1939. *1895, 1898, 1901.1, 1138*

1878:34 John Burton **Cleland**, Australian physician, born 22 Jun; with Alfred Walter Campbell, while investigating Murray Valley encephalitis (Australian X disease), an acute polioencephalomyelitis, isolated a virus from cerebral tissue, 1917, *RDNSW* p. 150. Died 1971. *4648*

1878:35 Edward Bright **Vedder**, American physician, born 28 Jun; demonstrated the amoebicidal action of emetine, 1911, *BMMS* **3**:48; his work led to its general adoption in the treatment of **amoebiasis**. Died 1952. *5189*

1878:36 Werner **Schultz**, German physician, born 3 Jul; with Willy Charlton, introduced the Schultz-Charlton reaction for the diagnosis of scarlet fever, 1918, *ZK* **17**:328; gave first description of agranulocytic angina ('Schultz's syndrome'), 1922, *DMW* **48**:1195. Died 1944. *5081, 3086*

1878:37 Frederick Lucian **Golla**, British neurologist, born 11 Aug; with co-workers, demonstrated changes in the electroencephalogram in epilepsy, 1937, *JMS* **83**:137. Died 1968. *4824*

1878:38 George Hoyt **Whipple**, American pathologist, born 28 Aug; first described 'Whipple's disease', which he termed 'intestinal lipodystrophy', 1907, *JHB* **18**:382. With Frieda Saur Robscheit-Robbins, demonstrated beneficial effect of raw liver in the treatment of anaemia, 1925, *AMJPh* **72**:408, paving the way for the establishment of this treatment by George Richards Minot and William Parry Murphy (1926), with whom Whipple shared the Nobel Prize (Physiology or Medicine), 1934, *NPL*. Died 1976. *3782, 3139, 3140*

1878:39 Ernst **Meinicke**, German immunologist, born 23 Sep; introduced the Meinicke diagnostic test for syphilis, 1917, *BKW* **66**:613. Died 1945. *2407*

1878:40 Selmar **Aschheim**, German gynaecologist, born 4 Oct; with Bernhard Zondek, isolated the gonadotrophic hormone of the anterior pituitary, 1927, *KW* **6**:348; **7**:831 and introduced the Aschheim-Zondek test for the diagnosis of pregnancy, 1928, *KW* **7**:8, 1404, 1453. Died 1965. *1168, 6222*

1878:41 Hans **Zinsser**, American bacteriologist, born 17 Nov; advanced the theory that Brill's disease is a recrudescence of epidemic typhus, 1934, *AmJH* **20**:513; the condition was subsequently named 'Brill-Zinsser disease'. Died 1940. *5396.4, 5382*

1878:42 Leonard **Noon**, British surgeon and immunologist, born 8 Dec; with John Freeman, introduced hay fever treatment by pollen injections, 1911, *L* **1**:1572; **2**:814. Died 1913. *2600.3, 2600.4*

1878:43 William Adam **Jolly**, British physiologist, born; with William Thomas Ritchie, first described auricular flutter, 1910, *Heart* **2**:177; it had been recognized by Ritchie in 1906. Died 1939. *2833*

1878:44 Dennis Emerson **Jackson**, American anaesthetist, born; first used trichlorethylene experimentally as an anaesthetic, 1934, *CRA* **13**:198. *5716*

1878: Alfred **Donné** died, **born** 1801. *blood platelets, leukaemia, gonorrhoea, Trichomonas vaginalis*

1878: Ernst Heinrich **Weber** died, **born** 1795. *Fechner-Weber law, hearing test*

1878: John **Hilton** died, **born** 1804. *postoperative rest, pain, Trichinella spiralis*

1878: Ernst **Reissner** died, **born** 1824. *Reissner's membrane*

1878: Claude **Bernard** died, **born** 1813. *glycogen, pancreatic juice, vasomotor nerves, curare, diabetes mellitus, anaesthesia, chloroform, morphine*

1878: Marie François Eugène **Belgrand** died, **born** 1810. *sewers*

1878: Julius **Bettinger** died, **born** 1802. *syphilis*

1878: Carl **Rokitansky** died, **born** 1804. *pathological anatomy, yellow atrophy of liver, spondylolisthesis*

1878: William **Stokes** died, **born** 1804. *heart block, Cheyne-Stokes respiration, paroxysmal tachycardia*

1878: Charles Henri **Ehrmann** died, **born** 1792. *laryngeal polyp*

1878: William **Banting** died, **born** 1797. *obesity*

1878: Pierre Ernest Antoine **Bazin** died, **born** 1807. *erythema induratum*

1878: Josef **Dietl** died, **born** 1804. *ureteral colic*

1878: Achille Louis François **Foville** died, **born** 1799. *paralysis*

1878: Antonius **Mathijsen** died, **born** 1805. *plaster of Paris bandage*

1878: Hermann **Lebert** died, **born** 1813. *brain abscess*

1878: Charles **Ritchie** died, **born** 1799. *typhoid, typhus*

1878: Crawford Williamson **Long** died, **born** 1815. *anaesthesia, ether*

1878: Washington Lemuel **Atlee** died, **born** 1808. *ovariotomy, fibroids, vesico-vaginal fistula*

**1879**
1879:1 Publication of *Index Medicus* commenced in New York, edited by John Shaw Billings (1838–1913) and Robert Fletcher (1823–1912); an important American contribution to **medical bibliography**. *6762*

1879:2 **National Board of Health, USA**

1879:3 The haemolytic **streptococcus** of **puerperal fever** described by Louis Pasteur (1822–1895), *BuAM* **8**:505. *6278*

1879:4 First total **hysterectomy** by the vaginal route carried out by Vincenz Czerny (1842–1916), *WMW* **29**:1171. *6072*

1879:5 Robert Lawson Tait (1845–1899) reported that he had performed **Battey's operation (ovariotomy)** for the treatment of non-ovarian conditions in 1872, 16 days before Battey, *BMJ* **1**:813. *6071, 6062*

1879:6 Classic accounts of **cell division** published by Walther Flemming (1843–1905), 1879, *ArMA* **16**:302; 1880, **18**:151. *122*

1879:7 Demonstration of the transmissibility of **rabies** from dog to rabbit by Victor Galtier (1845–1908), *AnMV* **28**:627, and his subsequent immunization of sheep by the inoculation of rabid saliva (1881), *CRAS* **93**:284, aroused the interest of Louis Pasteur in the disease. *5481.2, 5481.3*

1879: 8 An early scientific account of **scrub typhus (tsutsugamushi disease)** given by Erwin Baelz (1849–1913) and Kawakami, *VA* **78**:373, 528. *5376.1*

1879: 9 The first description of human **psittacosis** given by Jacob Ritter. *DAKM* **25**:53. *5527*

1879: 10 The **gonococcus**, causal organism in **gonorrhoea** discovered by Alfred Ludwig Siegmund Neisser (1855–1916), and later named *Neisseria gonorrhoeae*, *ZMW* **17**:497. *5208*

1879: 11 The monograph 'Diarrhoea and dysentery', contributed by Joseph Janvier Woodward (1833–1884) to *U.S. War Dept.: Medical and surgical history of the War of the Rebellion*, pt. 2, **1**, 1–869, is one of the greatest single monographs on **dysentery**. The author saw Lösch's amoeba without recognizing its significance. *5185, 5184*

1879: 12 **Myasthenia pseudoparalytica** ('**Erb-Goldflam symptom complex**') described by Wilhelm Heinrich Erb (1840–1921) and later by Goldflam (1893), *ArPN* **9**:172. *4746, 4757*

1879: 13 The first comprehensive account (165 cases) of **bone sarcoma** published by Samuel Weissel Gross (1837–1889), *AmJMS* **78**:17, 338. *4346*

1879: 14 An association of a port-wine **naevus** with a vascular abnormality of the **meninges** on the same side described by William Allen Sturge (1850–1919), *TCSL* **12**:162; it was also described by Parkes Weber (1922), leading to the term '**Sturge-Weber syndrome**'. *4560, 4605.2*

1879: 15 **Unilateral oculomotor paralysis** combined with **cerebellar ataxia** ('**Nothnagel's syndrome**') described by Carl Wilhelm Hermann Nothnagel (1841–1905); in his *Topische Diagnostik der Gehirnkrankheiten. 4560*

1879: 16 **Angiokeratoma** first described by Wyndham Cottle (d.1919), *SGHR* **9**:753; called '**Mibelli's disease**' after the description by the latter in 1891. *4071, 4105*

1879: 17 First description of **epidermolysis bullosa** by William Tilbury Fox (1836–1879), *L* **1**:766. *4077*

1879: 18 A classic description of **glomerulonephritis** ('**Klebs' disease**') given by Theodor Albrecht Edwin Klebs (1834–1913); in his *Handbuch der pathologischen Anatomie*, I Abt., p. 644. *4212*

1879: 19 The first description of **hydradenitis destruens suppurativa** given by Jonathan Hutchinson (1828–1913); in his *Lectures on clinical surgery*, **2**, 298; it was later named '**Pollitzer's disease**' after the latter's description in 1892. *4075*

1879: 20 The first description of **prurigo nodularis** given by William Augustus Hardaway (1850–1923), *ArD* **5**:385; **6**:129. *4076*

1879: 21 Unsuccessful **gastrectomy** for **carcinoma** carried out by Jules Emile Péan (1830–1898), *GH* **52**:473. *3472*

1879:22 An operation for the treatment of **volvulus** was first recorded by Adolf Fredrik Lindstedt (1847–1915) and Johan Anton Waldenström (1839–1879), *ULF* **14**:513. *3469*

1879:23 **Trinitrin (nitroglycerine)** introduced in treatment of **angina pectoris** by William Murrell (1853–1912), *L* **1**:113, 151, 225. *2892*

1879:24 Early description of **thrombo-angiitis obliterans** by Felix von Winiwarter (1852–1931), *ArKC* **23**:202; named '**Buerger's disease**' following the account by Leo Buerger in 1908. *2907*

1879:25 **Leprosy bacillus (*Mycobacterium leprae*)** demonstrated, with **aniline dyes**, by Albert Ludwig Siegmund Neisser (1855–1916) in tissue obtained from Gerhard Hansen, *JANVB* **57**:65. *2436.1*

1879:26 A **pressure forceps** ('**Spencer Wells' forceps**') introduced by Thomas Spencer Wells (1818–1897), *BMJ* **1**:926; **2**:3. *5615*

1879:27 Henri Roger (1809–1891) drew attention to a congenital **ventricular septal defect** and an accompanying murmur ('**maladie de Roger**', '**Roger's murmur**'), *BuAM* **8**:1074, 1189. *2782*

---

1879:28 Hans **Eppinger**, Bohemian physician, born 5 Jan; with Oscar Stoerck, gave the first clinical and pathological description of bundle-branch block, 1910, *ZKM* **71**:157. Died 1946. *2832*

1879:29 Donald Breadalbane **Blacklock**, British parasitologist, born 7 Jan; showed the vector of onchocerciasis to be *Simulium damnosum*, 1927, *BMJ* **1**:129. Died 1955. *5350.8*

1879:30 Maud **Slye**, American pathologist, born 8 Feb; published important studies on the heredity of cancer, 1928, *AnIM* **1**:951. Died 1954. *2652*

1879:31 Elmer Verney **McCollum**, American biochemist, born 3 Mar; with Marguerite Davis discovered vitamin A, 1913, *JBC* **15**:167; with co-workers discovered vitamin D, 1922, *JBC* **53**:297. Died 1967. *1049, 1054.1*

1879:32 Joseph Abraham **Long**, American endocrinologist, born 4 Mar; was associated with Herbert McLean Evans in the discovery of the growth hormone of the anterior pituitary, 1921, *AR* **21**:62. *1163*

1879:33 Fritz **Munk**, German physician, born 11 Mar; introduced the term 'lipoid nephrosis', on finding that urine in such cases contained anisotropic lipoid droplets, 1913, *ZKM* **78**:1. *4237*

1879:34 Robert Ernest **Kelly**, British surgeon, born 7 Apr; introduced an intratracheal ether anaesthesia apparatus, 1913, *BJS* **1**:90. Died 1944. *5699.2*

1879:35 Paul A. **Lewis**, American pathologist, born 14 Apr; with John Auer, described anaphylactic shock, 1910, *JEM* **12**:151; with Simon Flexner, demonstrated antibodies in convalescent serum in monkeys infected experimentally with poliomyelitis, 1910, *JAMA* **54**:1780. Died 1929. *2600, 4670*

1879:36 Walther **Spielmayer**, German psychiatrist, born 23 Apr; described juvenile amaurotic familial idiocy; in his *Klinische und anatomische Untersuchungen über eine besondere Form von familiärer amaurotische Idiotie*, 1907. Vogt had done so earlier (1905) resulting in the term 'Spielmayer-Vogt disease'. *4714.1, 4713.1*

1879:37 Eugen **Joseph**, German urologist, born 26 Apr; with Friedrich Voelcker, introduced the Voelcker kidney function test, 1903, *MMW* **50**:2081. *4230*

1879:38 Carlos Ribeiro Justiniano **Chagas**, Brazilian physician, born 9 Jul; discovered the causal organism of American trypanosomiasis ('Chagas's disease') at the Instituto Oswaldo Cruz and named *Trypanosoma cruzi*, 1909, *MIOC* **1**:159. Died 1934. *5283*

1879:39 Arthur Frederick **Hertz [Hurst]**, British physician, born 23 Jul; first to describe 'dumping syndrome', an after-effect of gastroenterostomy, 1913, *PRSM* **6** Surg:155. Died 1944. *3538*

1879:40 Wilbur Augustus **Sawyer**, American hygienist, born 7 Aug; with Wray Devere Marr Lloyd, introduced the intraperitoneal test for immunity against yellow fever, 1931, *JEM* **54**:533; with S.F. Kitchen and W.D.M. Lloyd, devised an immune serum for prophylactic inoculation against the disease, 1932, *JEM* **55**:945. Died 1931. *5464, 5465*

1879:41 Douglas **Symmers**, American pathologist, born 17 Sep; described follicular lymphadenopathy, 1927, *ArPa* **3**:816; previously described by Nathan Edwin Brill and co-workers, 1925, and named 'Brill-Symmers disease'. Died 1952. *3787, 3786*

1879:42 Shinobu **Ishihara**, Japanese ophthalmologist, born 25 Sep; devised tests for colour-blindness; in his *Tests for colour-blindness*, 1917. Died 1963. *5966*

1879:43 Francis Peyton **Rous**, American pathologist, born 5 Oct; demonstrated the transmissibility to normal hens of chicken sarcoma, 1910, *JEM* **12**:696; **13**:397. Shared the Nobel Prize (Physiology or Medicine), 1966, with Charles Brenton Huggins, for their work on hormone-dependent tumours, *NPL*. Died 1970. *2637*

1879:44 René **Leriche**, French surgeon, born 12 Oct; treated causalgia by periarterial sympathectomy, 1916, *PrM* **24**:178. With R. Fontaine, carried out lumbar sympathectomy by the anterolateral extraperitoneal approach, 1933, *PrM* **41**:1819. With Fontaine and M. Dupertuis, introduced arteriectomy for relief of arterial thrombosis, 1937, *SGO* **64**:149. Performed surgical obliteration of the abdominal aorta, 1940, *PrM* **48**:601. Died 1955. *4885, 4902, 3038, 3040*

1879:45 Martin **Kirschner**, German surgeon, born 28 Oct; introduced the Kirschner wire, for skeletal traction and stabilization of bone fragments or joint immobilization, 1909, *BKC* **64**:266. First successful treatment ('Trendelenburg's operation') for pulmonary artery embolism, 1924, *ArKC* **133**:312. First used avertin intravenously, 1929, *Ch* **1**:673. Died 1942. *4378, 3016, 5710*

1879:46 Alfred **Vogt**, Swiss ophthalmologist, born 31 Oct; introduced cyclodiathermy for glaucoma, 1937, *KMA* **99**:9. Died 1943. *5988*

1879:47 Gaston **Cotte**, French surgeon, born 14 Nov; introduced presacral neurectomy, 1925, *PrM* **33**:98. Died 1951. *4895*

1879:48 Henrique de **Rocha Lima**, Brazilian tropical diseases physician, born 24 Nov; first isolated the causal organism of typhus, 1916, *BKW* **53**:567, and named it *Rickettsia prowazeki* after Ricketts and Prowazek, both of whom had died of typhus. Died 1956. *5388, 5379, 5394.1*

1879:49 Leonard Gregory **Parsons**, British paediatrician, born 25 Nov; first treated infantile scurvy by administration of ascorbic acid, 1933, *PRSM* **26**:1533. Died 1950. *3725*

1879:50 Paul **Gelmo**, Austrian chemist, born 17 Dec; first to prepare sulphanilamide, 1908, *JPrC* **77**:369. Died 1961. *1948*

———

1879:51 Otto **Porges**, Austrian physician, born; introduced gastrophotography, 1929, *WKW* **42**:89. *3548*

1879:52 Leo **Buerger**, Austrian/American urologist, born; described thrombo-angiitis obliterans and gave it its present name; 1908, *AJMS* **136**:567. It is also called 'Buerger's disease'; introduced the Brown-Buerger cystoscope, 1909, *AnS* **49**:225. Died 1943. *2912, 4195.1*

1879:53 Frederick **Griffith**, British bacteriologist, born; carried out fundamental work on transformation of pneumococcal types, 1928, *JHyg* **27**:113, which led to the work of Avery, MacLeod and McCarty demonstrating the role of DNA. Published a serological classification of streptococci, 1934, *JHyg* **34**:542. Died 1941. *251.2, 255.1, 2524.3*

1879:54 Albert **Vander Veer**, American physician, born; with Robert Anderson Cooke, originated concept of atopy, 1916, *JI* **1**:201. *2600.6*

1879:55 Hans Christian **Jacobaeus**, Swedish surgeon, born; his adaptation of the cystoscope for the study of the interior of the body led to the introduction of the thoracoscope, 1910, *MMW* **57**:2090. Died 1937. *3189*

1879:56 Pierre **Abrami**, French physician, born; with Georges Fernand Isidor Widal, published an account of acquired haemolytic anaemia, 1907, *PrM* **15**:479; led to the eponym 'Widal-Abrami disease' and, because of the earlier description by Hayem (1898), 'Hayem-Widal disease'. Died 1945. *3777, 3783*

1879:57 Jörgen Nilsen **Schaumann**, Swedish dermatologist, born; established the systemic nature of sarcoidosis ('Besnier-Boeck-Schaumann disease'), 1917, *AnD* **6**:357. Died 1953. *4095, 4128, 4149*

1879:58 Joseph Waldron **Moore** born; with Hideyo Noguchi, obtained a pure culture of *Treponema pallidum*, from a patient with dementia paralytica, 1913, *JEM* **17**:232. *4805*

1879:59 William James **Wilson**, British professor of public health, born; described a diagnostic reaction for cerebrospinal and typhus fevers, 1909, *JHyg* **9**:316, later developed as the Weil-Felix reaction. Died 1954. *5381, 5390*

1879:60 Albert **Botteri**, Italian ophthalmologist, born; carried out filtration of the virus of inclusion conjunctivitis, 1912, *KMA* **50**i:653. Died 1955. *5960*

1879:61 Max **Knoll**, German physicist, born; with Ernst Ruska, produced first electron microscope, 1932, *AnPh* **12**:607 [Ruska awarded the Nobel Prize (Physics), 1986, for this work, *NPL*]. Died 1969. *269.3*

---

1879: Otto **Funke** died, **born** 1828. *haemoglobin*

1879: Arthur **Leared** died, **born** 1822. *stethoscope*

1879: Pierre Adolph **Piorry** died, **born** 1794. *percussor, pleximeter*

1879: Johan Anton **Waldenström** died, **born** 1839. *volvulus*

1879: Frank Fontaine **Maury** died, **born** 1840. *stricture of oesophagus, gastrostomy*

1879: William Tilbury **Fox** died, **born** 1836. *epidermolysis bullosa, dermatitis herpetiformis, dyshidrosis, impetigo contagiosa*

1879: Marie Guillaume Alphonse **Devergie** died, **born** 1798. *eczema marginatum, pityriasis pilaris*

1879: Jacob von **Heine** died, **born** 1799. *poliomyelitis, spastic paraplegia*

1879: Franz Aloys Antoine **Pollender** died, **born** 1800. *anthrax, Bacillus anthracis*

1879: Germanicus **Mirault** died, **born** 1796. *cleft lip*

1879: Alexander **Pagenstecher** died, **born** 1828. *cataract*

1879: Jean Marie **Jacquemier** died, **born** 1806. *early pregnancy, Jacquemier's sign*

1879: Marmaduke Burr **Wright** died, **born** 1803. *combined cephalic version*

1879: Pierre Marie Edouard **Chassaignac** died, **born** 1804. *surgical drainage*

## 1880

1880:1 Publication of *Index-catalogue of the Library of the Surgeon General's Office* commenced in Washington, edited by John Shaw Billings (1838–1913) and Robert Fletcher (1823–1912); one of the greatest achievements in **medical bibliography**. *6763*

1880:2 **American Surgical Association** founded

1880:3 **Ophthalmological Society of the United Kingdom** founded

1880:4 **Bronx River Conduit (New York City water supply)** constructed 1880–1885

1880:5 **Cocaine** suggested as a **local anaesthetic** by Vasili Konstantinovich Anrep (b.1852), *PfA* **21**:38. *5675*

1880:6 **Endotracheal anaesthesia** first performed by William Macewen (1848–1924), who administered **chloroform** through a tracheal tube introduced through the mouth, *BMJ* **2**:122, 163. *5676*

1880:7 Cultivation of the **gonococcus** first reported by Leo Leistikow (1847–1917), *CA* **7**:750. *5209*

1880:8 The aetiology of **paragonimiasis** and its parasite, *Paragonimus ringeri* described by Patrick Manson (1844–1922), *MRpt* **20**:10. *5346.2.*

1880:9 Emil Ponfick (1844–1913) recognized the causative role of the fungus *Actinomyces* in human **actinomycosis** and established the identity of the human and animal forms, *BKW* **17**:660. *5512*

1880:10 *Salmonella typhi*, causal organism of **typhoid** discovered by Carl Joseph Eberth (1835–1926), *VA* **81**:58. *5030*

1880:11 Charles Louis Alphonse Laveran (1845–1922) first saw the **malaria** parasite on 20 October 1880; report published 1881, *BSMH* **17**:158. *5236*

1880:12 In their studies on the aetiology of **anthrax**, Louis Pasteur (1822–1895), Charles Chamberland (1851–1908) and Pierre Paul Emile Roux (1853–1933) were first to use attenuated bacterial virus, providing active immunization against the disease, *CRAS* **91**:86. *5169*

1880:13 **Amaurotic familial idiocy** described by Waren Tay (1843–1927) – dealing mainly with ocular manifestations, *TOUK* **1**:55; the cerebral changes were more fully described by Sachs (1887), '**Tay-Sachs disease**'. *5918, 4705*

1880:14 *Practical treatise on nervous exhaustion* (**neurasthenia**) published by George Miller Beard (1839–1883). *4846*

1880:15 **Tuberose sclerosis (epiloia, 'Bourneville's disease')** described by Désiré Magloire Bourneville (1840–1909), *ArN* **1**:69. *4700*

1880:16 First full description of **narcolepsy** given by Jean Baptiste Edouard Gélineau (b.1859), *GH* **53**:626, 635. *4561*

1880:17 **Dorsal spinocerebellar tract** demonstrated and introduction of the terms **myotatic** and **knee-jerk** by William Richard Gowers (1845–1915); in his *Diagnosis of diseases of the spinal cord. 4562*

1880:18 **Nephrolithotomy** – removal of **renal calculus** by lumbar incision – introduced by Henry Morris (1844–1926), *TCSL* **14**:30. *4292.1*

1880:19 First description of **dermatitis herpetiformis** by William Tilbury Fox (1836–1879), *ArD* **6**:16; following the excellent description by Louis Adolphus Duhring (1845–1913) in 1884 it was also named '**Duhring's disease**'. *4078, 4083*

1880:20 The first book on the scientific treatment of **tooth deformities**, *Treatise on oral deformities*, published by Norman William Kingsley (1829–1913). *3685.1*

1880:21 The first **thyroidectomy** for **exophthalmic goitre** performed by Ludwig Rehn (1849–1930), reported in 1884, *BKW* **21**:163. *3833*

1880:22 Emil Theodor Kocher (1841–1917) devised an operation for the radical extirpation of the **tongue** for **carcinoma**, *DZC* **13**:134. *3473*

1880:23 The first (unsuccessful) removal of a **carcinomatous pylorus** reported by Ludwik Rydygier (1850–1920), *PrzL* **19**:637. *3473.1*

1880:24 An important influence on the development of **laryngology** was *Manual of diseases of the throat and nose* published by Morell Mackenzie (1837–1892); vol. 2 appeared in 1884. *3287*

1880:25 The first British surgeon to diagnose acute **appendicitis** and to treat it by **appendicectomy** was Robert Lawson Tait (1845–1899), *BMR* **27**:26, 76. *3570.1*

1880:26 **Myocardial infarction** first described by Carl Weigert (1845–1904), *VA* **79**:87. *2783*

1880:27 **Immunity**; experiments on attenuation of the infective organism and inoculation of attenuated cultures carried out by Louis Pasteur (1822–1895) laid the foundations of immunology, *CRAS* **90**:239. *2537*

1880:28 Moriz Kaposi [Kohn] (1837–1902) published *Pathologie und Therapie der Hautkrankheiten*, one of the most important books on **dermatology**. *3995*

1880:29 **Staphylococcus** and **streptococcus** recognizably described by Louis Pasteur (1822–1895), *CRAS* **90**:1033. *2492.1*

1880:30 '**Golgi cells**' described by Camillo Golgi (1843–1926), *ArSM* **4**:221. *1277*

1880:31 **Tuberculosis** inoculated into rabbit eye by Julius Cohnheim (1839–1884) in 1877; reported in his *Die Tuberkulose*, 1880. *2329*

1880:32 First systematic account of the **parathyroid glands** by Ivar Victor Sandström (1852–1889), *ULF* **15**:441. *1127*

---

1880:33 Alexander von **Lichtenberg**, Hungarian urologist, born 20 Jan; with Friedrich Voelcker, obtained the first cystograms, 1905, *MMW* **52**:1576. With Voelcker, introduced pyelography, 1906, *MMW* **53**:105. With Moses Swick, introduced uroselectan as a contrast medium in excretion urography, 1929, *KW* **8**:2087. Died 1949. *4192, 4231, 4200*

1880:34 William Palmer **Lucas**, American paediatrician, born 27 Jan; with Frederick Parker Gay, made the first accurate cell counts of the cerebrospinal fluid in poliomyelitis, 1910, *ArIM* **6**:330. Died 1960. *4670.1*

1880:35 Philip **Franklin**, American/British otorhinolaryngologist, born 1 Feb; introduced treatment of hay fever by zinc ionization, 1931, *BMJ* **1**:1115. Died 1951. *2604*

1880:36 William Edgar **Caldwell**, American obstetrician, born 23 Feb; with Howard Carman Moloy, devised a classification of the female pelvis, 1933, *AmJOG* **26**:479, in use today. Died 1943. *6266*

360

1880:37 Vittorio **Putti**, Italian orthopaedic surgeon, born 1 Mar; he developed and improved the kineplastic surgery suggested by Vanghetti (1898), 1918, *BMJ* 1:635. Died 1940. *4477, 4474*

1880:38 Henry Drysdale **Dakin**, British chemist, born 12 Mar; devised Dakin's solution, chloramine-T, a solution of sodium hypochlorite and boric acid, as an antiseptic, it was used by Alexis Carrel for the continuous irrigation of wounds (Carrel-Dakin treatment), 1915, *BMJ* 2:318. Died 1952. *5643, 5642, 1903.2*

1880:39 Edmund **Weil**, Austrian physician and bacteriologist, born 17 Apr; with Arthur Felix, developed the Weil-Felix reaction for the diagnosis of typhus, 1916, *WKW* 29:33. Died 1922. *5390, 5381*

1880:40 Charles Claude **Guthrie**, American physiologist and pharmacologist, born 13 May; with Alexis Carrel, carried out experimental heart transplantation, in a dog, 1905, *AmM* 10:284, 1101. Died 1963. *3025.1*

1880:41 Arthur Cecil Hamel **Rothera**, Australian biochemist, born 1 Jul; introduced Rothera's test for acetone bodies in urine, 1908, *JP* 37:491. Died 1915. *3960*

1880:42 Simeon Burt **Wolbach**, American pathologist, born 3 Jul; carried out important studies on Rocky Mountain spotted fever, he mentioned the causal agent, *Dermacentroxenus rickettsii* (later named *Rickettsia rickettsii*), 1919, *JMR* 41:1; with co-workers, confirmed *Rickettsia prowazeki* as causal agent in typhus, in his *The etiology and pathology of typhus*, 1922. Died 1954. *5391, 5393*

1880:43 Walter Meredith **Boothby**, American physician, born 28 Jul; with Frederic Jay Cotton, introduced the Boothby and Cotton flowmeter, for administration of nitrous oxide-oxygen-anaesthesia, 1912, *SGO* 15:281. With Arthur H. Bulbulian introduced BLB (Boothby-Lovelace-Bulbulian) oxygen inhalation mask, 1938, *PMC* 13:646, 654. Died 1953. *5698, 1982*

1880:44 Sofus **Wideröe**, Norwegian surgeon, born 26 Aug; introduced a method of myelography by air injection into the spinal subarachnoid space, 1921, *ZCh* 48:394. *4605.1*

1880:45 Gustav **Bucky**, German/American radiologist, born 3 Sep; introduced the Bucky diaphragm in radiography, 1913, *ArRR* 18:6, later modified by Hollis Elmer Potter (1916). Died 1963. *2691, 2692.1*

1880:46 Marie Carmichael **Stopes**, British birth control advocate, born 15 Oct; published pioneer handbook on birth control, 1923, *Contraception (birth control)*. Died 1958. *1641.1*

1880:47 Reynaldo dos **Santos**, Portuguese urologist, born 3 Dec; with co-workers, performed aortography, 1929, *MCon* 47:93. With J. Caldas, introduced thorotrast in arteriography, 1931, *MCon* 49:234. *2859, 2920*

1880:48 Hollis Elmer **Potter**, American radiologist, born; introduced Potter-Bucky grid in radiology, 1916, *AmJR* 3:142. Died 1964. *2692.1, 2691*

1880:49 Karl **Vogt** born; with Adolf Windaus he synthesized histamine, 1907, *BDCG* 40:3691. *1895.1*

1880:50 Ernest **Muir**, British tropical diseases physician, born; introduced diasone treatment of leprosy, 1944, *IJL* **12**:1. Died 1974. *2442*

1880:51 Robert Anderson **Cooke** born; with Albert Vander Veer, originated concept of atopy in immunology, 1916, *JI* **1**:201. Died 1960. *2600.6*

1880:52 Albert **Niemann**, German paediatrician, born; described a rare genetically-determined disorder, 1914, *JaK* **79**:1; later described by Ludwig Pick, 1926, and named 'Niemann-Pick disease'. Died 1921. *3784, 3785*

1880:53 William Jason **Mixter**, American neurosurgeon, born; with Joseph Seton Barr, demonstrated the causal role of intravertebral disk herniation in sciatica, 1934, *NEJM* **211**:210. Died 1958. *4435*

1880:54 Jean Alexandre **Barré**, French neurologist, born; with Georges Guillain and A. Strohl, described acute infective polyneuritis (Guillain-Barré syndrome'), 1916, *BSMH* **40**:1462. *4647*

1880:55 Allan **Kinghorn**, Canadian parasitologist, born; with Warrington Yorke, showed *Glossina morsitans* to be the transmitting fly of *Trypanosoma rhodesiense*, 1912, *AnTM* **6**:1. Died 1955. *5285.2*

1880:56 Edwin Hemphill **Place** born; with co-workers, reported Haverhill fever, a streptobacillary form of rat-bite fever, and isolated an organism, 1926, *BMSJ* **194**:285, later found to be identical with *Streptothrix muris ratti* and *Streptobacillus moniliformis*. *5328*

1880:57 Ejnar Oluf Sorenson **Sylvest**, Danish physician, born; gave the first full description of epidemic myositis ('Bornholm disease'), 1930, *UL* **92**:798. Died 1931. *5540*

1880:58 John Bright **Banister** born; with Archibald Hector McIndoe, devised an operation for the construction of an artificial vagina, 1938, *JOG* **45**:490. Died 1938. *6133*

1880:59 William **O'Connor** died; first used potassium bromide in the treatment of epilepsy, 1857, *L* **1**:525. *4814*

1880: Dominic John **Corrigan** died, **born** 1802. *aortic insufficiency*

1880: Henry **Hancock** died, **born** 1809. *appendix, peritonitis*

1880: Erastus Bradley **Wolcott** died, **born** 1804. *renal tumour*

1880: Ferdinand von **Hebra** died, **born** 1816. *classification of skin diseases, impetigo herpetiformis, pityriasis rubra*

1880: Jacob Augustus Lockhart **Clarke** died, **born** 1817. *syringomyelia*

1880: Ernst **Münchmeyer** died, **born** 1846. *progressive ossifying myositis*

1880: Pierre Paul **Broca** died, **born** 1824. *speech centre, aphasia*

1880: Edward **Meryon** died, **born** 1809. *Duchenne's muscular dystrophy*

1880: William **Budd** died, **born** 1811. *typhoid*

1880: Édouard **Séguin** died, **born** 1812. *psychiatry*

**1881**
1881:1 **Medical Board** established in Upper **Canada**

1881:2 **Government Animal Vaccination Establishment** opened in **London**

1881:3 **University College, Liverpool,** founded

1881:4 The practice of instilling **silver nitrate** into the eyes of newborn children as a preventive measure against **ophthalmia neonatorum** introduced by Carl Siegmund Franz Credé (1819–1892), *ArGy* **17**:50. *6195*

1881:5 Carl von Voit (1831–1908) the leading investigator of **metabolism**, published *Handbuch der Physiologie des Gesammt-Stoffwechsels und der Fortpflanzung. 635*

1881:6 The first report of Louis Pasteur's (1822–1895) studies on **rabies** was written with Charles Chamberland (1851–1908), Pierre Paul Emile Roux (1853–1933) and T. Thuillier, *CRAS* **92**:1259. *5481.4*

1881:7 The first suggestion that the **mosquito** transmitted **yellow fever** from man to man made by Carlos Juan Finlay (1833–1915), *AnRA* **18**:147. *5455*

1881:8 **Oöphorectomy** carried out by Robert Lawson Tait (1845–1899), in February 1881, *BMJ* **1**:766. *6075*

1881:9 A suspension operation for **retroversion of the uterus** carried out by William Alexander (1844–1919), reported 1882, *MTG* **1**:327. *6077*

1881:10 An **ophthalmometer** invented by Louis Emile Javal (1839–1907), *AnO* **86**:5. *5920*

1881:11 The operation of enucleation of subperitoneal **fibroids** of the **uterus**, by the vaginal route, introduced by Vincenz Czerny (1842–1916), *WMW* **31**:501, 525. *6073*

1881:12 The first operation for **otoplasty** reported by Edward Talbot Ely (1850–1885), *ArOt(C)* **10**:97. *5754.2*

1881:13 Listerian **antisepsis** first adopted in obstetrics by Stéphane Tarnier (1828–1897), employing carbolic acid solution as early as 1881; he wrote *De l'asepsie et antisepsie en obstétrique*, 1894. *5639*

1881:14 Immunization of sheep against **rabies** by the inoculation of rabid saliva, by Victor Galtier (1845–1908), *CRAS* **93**:284, and his earlier (1879) demonstration of its transmissibility from dog to rabbit aroused the interest of Louis Pasteur in the disease. *5481.3, 5481.2*

1881:15 Robert Koch (1843–1910) showed that **mercuric chloride** was superior to **carbolic acid** as an **antiseptic**, and that live steam surpassed hot air in **sterilizing** power, *MKG* **1**:234. *5636.1*

1881:16 The first pathogenic **trypanosome** to be discovered seen by Griffith Evans (1835–1935) in the blood of horses suffering from **'surra'**, *VJ* **13**:1, 82, 180, 326. *5271*

1881:17 It is possible that Theodor Albrecht Edwin Klebs (1834–1913) saw the **typhoid** bacillus, *Salmonella typhi*, before Eberth, reporting it later, *ArEP* **13**:381. *5031*

1881:18 Carl Wernicke's (1848–1905) description of **acute superior haemorrhagic polioencephalitis** in his *Lehrbuch der Gehirnkrankheiten*, **2**, 229, resulted in the eponym **'Wernicke's encephalopathy**. *4641*

1881:19 **'Lasègue's sign'** in **sciatica** discovered by Ernest Charles Lasègue (1816–1883); it was reported by his pupil, J.J. Forst (*Contribution à l'étude clinique de la sciatique*, Paris, Thèse No. 33). *4563*

1881:20 In his *Epilepsy and other chronic convulsive diseases*, William Richard Gowers (1845–1915) was first to note the tetanic nature of the **epileptic convulsion**. *4818*

1881:21 **March haemoglobinuria** first described by Richard Fleischer (b.1848), *BKW* **18**:691. *4176*

1881:22 The first **allograft transplantation of bone** in a human reported by William Macewen (1848–1924), *PRS* **32**:232. *4346.2*

1881:23 The operation of **nephropexy** for the relief of mobile **kidney** devised by Eugen Hahn (1841–1902), *ZCh* **8**:449. *4218*

1881:24 **Maffucci's syndrome** (cavernous **haemangioma** with **enchondromatosis**) first described by Angelo Maffucci (1845–1903), *MMC* **3**:399. *4079*

1881:25 Johann von Mikulicz-Radecki (1850–1905) was among the first to use the electric **oesophagoscope** (invented by Leiter in 1880), *WMP* **22**: 1405, 1437, 1473, 1505, 1537, 1573, 1629. *3475*

1881:26 Test for determination of **auditory ossicular fixation** described by Marie Ernest Gellé (1834–1923), *IMC* **3**:370. *3387.3*

1881:27 The first successful **resection** of the **pylorus** for **carcinoma** (the Billroth I operation) reported by Theodor Billroth (1829–1894), *WMW* **31**: 161, 1427. *3474*

1881:28 The operation of **gastro-enterostomy** perfected by Anton Wölfler (1850–1917), *ZCh* **8**:705. *3476*

1881:29 **Jarvis nasal snare** introduced in nasal surgery by William Chapman Jarvis (1855–1895), *TALA* **2**:130. *3286*

1881:30 The **pneumococcus** was probably first observed by Louis Pasteur (1822–1895), in a child killed by **rabies** – reported by Joseph Parrot (1829–1883), *BuAM* **10**:379; independently observed in the same year by George Miller Sternberg (1838–1915), *SBJH* **2** ii;183. *3172, 3173*

1881:31 **Paramyoclonus multiplex ('Friedreich's disease')** first described by Nikolaus Friedreich (1826–1882), *VA* **86**:421. *4564*

1881:32 **Reticulocyte** first described by Paul Ehrlich (1854–1915), *BKW* **17**:405. *3125.5*

1881:33 A modern **sphygmomanometer** was developed by Samuel Siegfried von Basch (1837–1905), *ZKM* **2**:79. *2784*

1881:34 **Methylene blue** introduced in bacterial staining by Paul Ehrlich (1854–1915), *ZKM* **2**:710. *2493*

1881:35 *Staphylococcus aureus* discovered, and *Staphylococcus* differentiated from *Streptococcus*, by Alexander Ogston (1844–1929), *BMJ* **1**:369. *2494*

1881:36 **Tuberculous inflammation of serous membranes** ('Concato's disease') described by Luigi Maria Concato (1825–1882), *GilSM* **3**:1037. *2330*

1881:37 **Bacteria**; culture, fixing and **staining** methods described by Robert Koch (1820–1910), *MKG* **1**:1. *2495.1*

1881:38 **Scopolamine** isolated by Albert Ladenburg (1842–1911), *AnCP* **206**:274. *1873*

1881:39 Wilhelm August Oscar Hertwig (1849–1922) and Karl Wilhelm Theodor Richard von Hertwig (1850–1937) carried out important work on **embryology** and **cytology**, *Die Coelomtheorie*. *502*

1881:40 '**Volkmann's ischaemic contracture**' described by Richard von Volkmann (1830–1889), *ZCh* **8**:801. *5617*

---

1881:41 Walter Rudolph **Hess**, Swiss physiologist, born 17 Mar. Published *Die funktionelle Organisation des vegetativen Nervensystems*, 1948. Shared Nobel Prize (Physiology or Medicine), 1949, with Antonio Caetano Abreu Freire Egas Moniz, for his discovery of the functional organization of the interbrain as a coordinator of the activities of the internal organs, *NPL*. Died 1973. *1451.1*

1881:42 Robert Thomson **Leiper**, British physician and helminthologist, born 17 Apr; identified the snail responsible for the transmission of *Schistosoma mansoni* and *S. haematobium*, 1915, *JRAMC* **25**:1, 147, 253; **27**:171; **30**:235. Died 1969. *5350.4*

1881:43 Carl Hamilton **Browning**, British pathologist and bacteriologist, born 21 May; with co-workers, introduced acriflavine, 1917, *BMJ* **1**:73. Died 1972. *1905*

1881:44 Ernest Lawrence **Kennaway**, British cancerologist, born 23 May; discovered carcinogenic properties of dibenzanthracene compounds with I. Hieger, James William Cook and W.V. Mayneord, 1932, *PRSB* **111**:455. Died 1958. *2654*

1881:45 Henri **Gougerot**, French dermatologist, born 2 Jul; with Charles Lucien de Beurmann, first described sporotrichosis ('de Beurmann-Gougerot disease'); in their *Les sporotrichoses*, 1912. Died 1955. *4147*

1881:46 Maurice Crowther **Hall**, American zoologist, born 15 Jul; introduced the carbon tetrachloride treatment of ankylostomiasis, 1921, *JAMA* **77**:1641. Died 1938. *5368*

1881:47 George Frederick **Dick**, American physician and bacteriologist, born 21 Jul; with Gladys Rowena Dick, devised the Dick test for determination of susceptibility to scarlet fever, 1924, *JAMA* **82**:265. In the same year they proved that the streptococcus is the cause of scarlet fever, *JAMA* **82**:301. Died 1967. *5082, 5082.1*

1881:48 Hans **Fischer**, German chemist, born 27 Jul; awarded Nobel Prize (Chemistry), 1930, for researches into the constitution of haemin and chlorophyll and the synthesis of haemin, *NPL*. Died 1945.

1881:49 Alexander **Fleming**, British bacteriologist, born 6 Aug; isolated lysozyme, a bacteriolytic secretion, found in tears, nasal secretions, etc., 1922, *PRSB* **93**:306. Discovered the growth-inhibiting action of a penicillin on certain bacteria, 1929, *BJEP* **10**:226. Shared the Nobel Prize (Physiology or Medicine), 1945, with Howard Walter Florey and Ernst Boris Chain, for his discovery concerning penicillin, *NPL*. Died 1955. *1920, 1933*

1881:50 Samuel Henry **Harris**, Australian surgeon, born 22 Aug; introduced 'Harris's operation', a technique of suprapubic prostatectomy with closure, 1927, *MJA* **1**:460; *AuNZ* **4**:226. Died 1936. *4275*

1881:51 Alfred **Hauptmann**, German neurologist, born 29 Aug; introduced phenobarbitone in the treatment of epilepsy, 1912, *MMW* **59**:1907. Died 1948. *4823*

1881:52 Yutako **Ido**, Japanese physician, born 8 Sep; with co-workers, showed rats to be the carriers of *Spirillum* (*Leptospira*) *icterohaemorrhagiae*, causal organism in Weil's disease, 1917, *JEM* **26**:341; showed that mice were carriers of *Leptospira hebdomadis*, causal organism in seven-day fever, 1918, *JEM* **28**:435. Died 1919. *5334.1, 5334.2*

1881:53 Patrick Playfair **Laidlaw**, British virologist, born 26 Sep; with Henry Hallett Dale, produced experimental shock by histamine and showed that it was similar to traumatic and surgical shock, 1919, *JP* **52**:355; with Christopher Howard Andrewes and Wilson Smith, recovered influenza A virus from throat washings of influenza patients, 1933, *L* **2**:66. Died 1940. *5630, 5494*

1881:54 Max **Kappis**, German surgeon, born 6 Oct; introduced paravertebral anaesthesia in urology, 1912, *ZCh* **39**:249; introduced splanchnic anaesthesia, 1928, *ZCh* **47**:98. Died 1938. *4197, 5701*

1881:55 Gladys Rowena **Dick**, American physician and bacteriologist, born 18 Dec; with George Frederick Dick, devised the Dick test for determination of susceptibility to scarlet fever, 1924, *JAMA* **82**:265. In the same year they proved that the streptococcus is the cause of scarlet fever, *JAMA* **82**:301. Died 1963. *5082, 5082.1*

1881:56 Noel **Fiessinger**, French physician, born 24 Dec; with Edgar Leroy, first described 'Reiter's syndrome', characterized by initial diarrhoea, urethritis, conjunctivitis and arthritis occurring in males, 1916, *BSMH* **40**:2030; reported by Reiter later in the same year. Died 1946. *6370, 6371*

1881:57 Thomas **Lewis**, British cardiologist, born 26 Dec; described 'effort syndrome', 1917; previously noted by A.B.R. Myers (1870) and J.M. Da Costa (1871), *MRC* 8. Independently of C.J. Rothberger and H. Winterberg, established auricular fibrillation as a cause of perpetual heart arrhythmia, 1909, *BMJ* **2**:1528; *WKW* **22**:839. Died 1945. *2847, 2830, 2831*

---

1881:58 Hans Conrad Julius **Reiter**, German bacteriologist, born; 'Reiter's syndrome', characterized by initial diarrhoea, urethritis, conjunctivitis and arthritis occurring in males, was named after his description, 1916, *DMW* **42**:1535, although he was preceded in this by Fiessinger and Leroy. Died 1969. *6371, 6370*

1881:59 Norman Strahan **Shenstone**, Canadian surgeon, born; with Robert Meredith Janes, introduced hilar tourniquet in lung surgery, 1932, *CMAJ* **27**:138. *3203.2*

1881:60 Allen Oldfather **Whipple**, American surgeon, born; introduced pancreaticoduodenectomy for cancer of the pancreas ('Whipple's operation'), 1935, *AnS* **102**:763. Died 1963. *3659.1*

1881:61 Elmer Isaac **McKesson**, American anaesthetist, born; introduced an intermittent gas-oxygen machine for administration of nitrous oxide-oxygen anaesthesia, 1911, *SGO* **13**:456. Died 1935. *5697*

---

1881: Philipp Friedrich Hermann **Klencke** died, **born** 1813. *tuberculosis*

1881: Jean Baptiste **Bouillard** died, **born** 1796. *rheumatic endocarditis, rheumatism, heart disease, aphasia*

1881: Matthias Jakob **Schleiden** died, **born** 1804. *cell theory*

1881: Maurice **Raynaud** died, **born** 1834. *Raynaud's disease*

1881: William **Addison** died, **born** 1802. *blood corpuscles, leucocytosis*

1881: James **Luke** died, **born** 1798. *femoral hernia*

1881: Nikolai Ivanovich **Pirogov** died, **born** 1810. *osteoplastic amputation of foot, anaesthesia, ether*

1881: Rudolph Hermann **Lotze** died, **born** 1817. *unconscious and subconscious states*

1881: Josef **Skoda** died, **born** 1805. *percussion*

## 1882

1882:1 **Christie Hospital (Manchester)** opened (as **Cancer Pavilion and Home**); present name assumed in 1892 – for Richard Copley Christie (1830–1901) and wife, benefactors

1882:2 **St John Ophthalmic Hospital** founded in **Jerusalem**

1882:3 **Public Health Act (Canada)**

1882:4 **Royal Academy of Medicine in Ireland** founded in **Dublin**

1882:5 **New York Postgraduate Medical School and Hospital** founded

1882:6 **Royal Society of Canada** founded

1882:7 Research on the effects of **nerve action** on **muscle arteries**, the **myogenic theory of the heart's action**, the **involuntary nervous system**, reported by Walter Holbrook Gaskell (1847–1914); 1882, *PT* **173**:993; 1883, *JP* 4:43, *The involuntary nervous system*, 1916. *829, 830, 1331*

1882:8 The **keratoscope** introduced by Antonio Placido da Costa (1849–1916), *ZPAu* **6**:30. *5922*

1882:9 **Blood platelets** named, and their role in **blood coagulation** discovered, by Giulio Cesare Bizzozero (1846–1901). *873.1, 881*

1882:10 '**Sänger's operation**', the so-called 'classic **caesarean section**' reported by Max Sänger (1853–1903); in his *Der Kaiserschnitt bei Uterusfibromen nebst vergleichender Methodik der Sectio Caesarea und der Porro-Operation. 6242*

1882:11 **Cyclopropane (trimethylene)** first prepared by August von Freund (1835–1892), *MhC* **3**:625. *5677*

1882:12 Karl Martin Leonhard Albrecht Kossel (1853–1927) studied the chemistry of the **cell** and **cell nucleus**, *HSZ*, 1882–7, **7**:7; **10**:248; **22**:167. Awarded Nobel Prize (Physiology or Medicine), 1910, *NPL. 702*

1882:13 Original work on Asiatic **relapsing fever** by Henry Vandyke Carter (1831–1897), recorded in his *Spirillum fever*, is remembered by the eponym '**Carter's fever**' and the name *Borrelia carteri. 5316*

1882:14 **Varicella gangrenosa** first described by Jonathan Hutchinson (1828–1913), *MCT* **65**:1. *5439*

1882:15 Kenneth Macleod (1840–1922) was first to draw attention to **granuloma inguinale**, *IMG* **17**:113. *5204.1*

1882:16 *Pfeifferella mallei*, causative organism in **glanders** discovered by Friedrich Loeffler (1852–1915), *DMW* **8**:707; *AKG* (1886) **1**:141. *5156*

1882:17 Vladimir Mikhailovich Kernig (1840–1917) drew attention to a flexor contracture of the leg on attempting to extend it on the thigh ('**Kernig's sign**') an important diagnostic sign almost always present in **cerebrospinal meningitis**, *SPMW* **7**:398. *4677*

1882:18 **Xeroderma pigmentosum** ('**Kaposi's disease**') well described by Moritz Kaposi (1837–1902), *MJa*, p. 619. *4080*

1882:19 '**Bennett's fracture**' of the first **metacarpal** recorded by Edward Hallaran Bennett (1837–1907), *DJMS* **73**:72. *4426*

1882:20 First description of **arthrodesis of an ankle-joint** for **paralytic foot** by Eduard Albert (1841–1900), *WMP* **23**:725. He introduced the concept of arthrodesis into **orthopaedic surgery**. *4347*

1882:21 A classic description of **neurofibromatosis** ('**Recklinghausen's disease**') given by Friedrich Daniel von Recklinghausen (1833–1910); in his *Über der Haut und ihre Beziehung zu den multiplen Neuromen*. *4082*

1882:22 Modification of Hahn's operation of **nephropexy** by Edoardo Bassini (1844–1924), *AnU* **261**:281. *4219*

1882:23 **Familial splenic anaemia** ('**Gaucher's disease**') described by Philippe Charles Ernest Gaucher (1854–1918); in his doctoral thesis, *De l'épithélioma primitif de la rate*. *3127, 3769*

1882:24 An excellent (but not the first) account of **angioneurotic oedema** ('**Quincke's oedema**') given by Heinrich Irenaeus Quincke (1842–1922), *MPD* **1**:129. *4081*

1882:25 An operation of partial excision of the **nasal septum** for correction of deflection devised by Ephraim Fletcher Ingals (1848–1918), *TALA* **4**:61. *3289*

1882:26 The first **pyloroplasty** was carried out by Pietro Loreta (1831–1889), *MASB* **4**:353. *3477*

1882:27 **Gastrosuccorrhoea** ('**Reichmann's disease**') first described by Mikolaj Reichmann (1851–1918), *GL* **2**:516. *3478*

1882:28 Jaques-Louis Reverdin (1842–1929) produced **myxoedema** by total or partial **thyroidectomy**, *RMSR* **2**:539. *3828*

1882:29 **Gallbladder** first successfully removed by Carl Johann August Langenbuch (1846–1901), *BKW* **19**:725. *3627*

1882:30 **Pancreatic necrosis** ('**Balser's fat necrosis**') first described by W. Balser, *VA* **90**:520. *3626*

1882:31 *Klebsiella pneumoniae* ('**Friedländer's bacillus**') discovered by Karl Friedländer (1847–1887), *VA* **87**:319. *3174*

1882:32 First good photographs of the **larynx** obtained by Thomas Rushmore French (1849–1929), *TALA* **4**:32. *3290*

1882:33 Account of **splenic anaemia** by Guido Banti (1852–1925), in his *Dell'anemia splenica*, led to the eponym '**Banti's disease**'. *3126*

1882:34 Experimental **cardiac valvulotomy** in dogs carried out by Charles-Emile François-Franck (1849–1921), *CRSB* **4**:108. *3022.1*

1882:35 *Pseudomonas aeruginosa* isolated by Carle Gessard (1850–1925), *CRAS* **94**:536. *2497*

1882:36 *Streptococcus pyogenes* discovered by Friedrich Fehleisen (1854–1924), *DZC* **16**:391. *2496*

1882:37 **Tuberculosis**; *Mycobacterium tuberculosis*, discovered by Robert Koch (1843–1910) on 24 March, *MKG* **19**:221. *2331*

1882:38 **Ziehl-Neelsen stain** introduced by Franz Ziehl (1857–1926) and Friedrich Neelsen (1854–1894) for staining *Mycobacterium tuberculosis*, *DMW* **8**:451; *ZMW* **21**:497. *2331.1, 2331.2*

1882:40 **'Ringer's solution'** introduced by Sydney Ringer (1834–1922), *JP* **3**:195. *826*

1882:41 **Iodoform dressing** introduced in **surgery** by Albert von Mosetig-Moorhof (1838–1907), *SKV* **211** (Chir 68):1811. *5618*

---

1882:42 William Edward **Gallie**, Canadian surgeon, born 29 Jan; with Arthur Baker LeMesurier, used fascial suture in the repair of inguinal hernia, 1923, *CMAJ* **13**:469. Died 1959. *3609*

1882:43 Martin William **Flack**, British physiologist, born 5 Feb; with Arthur Keith, discovered the sino-auricular node – the 'pacemaker of the heart', 1907, *JA* **41**:172. Died 1931. *844*

1882:44 Paul **Fildes**, British microbiologist, born 10 Feb; with William Bulloch, published *Haemophilia*, 1911, in which they claimed to have established the fact of immunity in females and confirmed the Law of Nasse. Died 1971. *3081, 3056*

1882:45 David Israel **Macht**, Russian/American pharmacologist, born 14 Feb; with Gui-ching Ting, demonstrated the antispasmodic action of theophylline on bronchial smooth muscle, 1921, leading to its use in management of asthma, *JPET* **18**:373. Died 1961. *3197.1*

1882:46 Carl Olaf **Sonne**, Danish bacteriologist, born 16 Apr; drew attention to a causal organism in bacillary dysentery, later named *Shigella sonnei*, 1915, *ZBP* I **75**:408. Died 1948. *5094*

1882:47 Alphonse Raymond **Dochez**, American physician, born 21 Apr; with Louis John Gillespie, differentiated four types of pneumococci, 1913, *JAMA* **61**:727. Died 1964. *3192.1*

1882:48 Harold Delf **Gillies**, New Zealand plastic surgeon, born 17 Jun; introduced a tubed pedicle flap, 1917 – in his *Plastic surgery of the face*, 1920; with William Kelsey Fry, introduced a new operation for the repair of cleft palate, 1921, *BMJ* **1**:335. Died 1960. *5758, 5759*

1882:49 Dallas B. **Phemister**, American surgeon, born 15 Jul; introduced epiphysiodesis to inhibit the bone growth of a longer leg, 1933, *JBJS* **15**:1. Died 1951. *4400.3*

1882:50 Donald Church **Balfour**, Canadian surgeon, born 22 Aug; introduced his method of resection of the sigmoid colon, 1910, *AnS* **51**:239. Died 1963. *3532*

1882:51 Alexander Thomas **Glenny**, British bacteriologist and immunologist, born 18 Sep; introduced alum-precipitated toxoid for active immunization against diphtheria, 1930, *BMJ* **2**:244. Died 1965. *5071*

1882:52 Herbert McLean **Evans**, American anatomist, embryologist, and endocrinologist, born 23 Sep; with Joseph Abraham Long discovered the growth hormone of the anterior pituitary, 1921, *AR* **21**:62; with Katharine Scott Bishop he discovered vitamin E, 1922, *Science* **56**:650; isolated vitamin F, 1934, *JBC* **106**:431; with co-workers isolated vitamin E, 1936, *JBC* **113**:319; with Choh Hao Li and others isolated interstitial-cell-stimulating (luteinizing) hormone, 1940, *En* **27**:803, and adrenocorticotrophic hormone (ACTH), 1943, *JBC* **149**:413. Died 1971. *1163, 1055, 1070, 1071, 1173.1, 1174*

1882:53 Frederick Charles **Pybus**, British surgeon, born 2 Nov; with Samuel Short Willis, introduced reverse guillotine tonsillectomy, 1910, *L* **2**:875. Died 1975. *3318*

1882:54 James Bourne **Ayer**, American neurologist, born 28 Dec; introduced cisternal puncture, 1920, *ArNP* **4**:529. Died 1963. *4890*

———

1882:55 Arthur James **Ewins**, British chemist, born; isolated acetylcholine in ergot, 1914, *BJ* **8**:44. Died 1957. *1341*

1882:56 Reuben **Ottenberg**, American physician, born; carried out pioneering work on blood grouping and paternity, 1921, *JAMA* **77**:682; **78**:873; **79**:2137. *1756*

1882:57 Julius **Hallervorden**, German neurologist, born; with Hugo Spatz, described a syndrome affecting the extrapyramidal system ('Hallervorden-Spatz syndrome'), 1922, *ZGN* **79**:254. Died 1965. *4724*

1882:58 Charles **Foix**, French neurologist, born; showed that the specific lesion in Parkinson's disease is located in the substantia nigra of the midbrain, 1921, *ReN* **28**:593. Died 1927. *4721*

1882:59 Claude Gordon **Douglas**, British physiologist, born; with John Scott Haldane, reported on high altitude physiological research at Pike's Peak, Colorado, 1913, *PT* (B) **203**:185. Died 1963. *957*

———

1882: Friedrich **Wöhler** died, **born** 1800. *urea synthesis*

1882: Thomas Bevill **Peacock** died, **born** 1812. *heart malformations*

1882: Theodor **Schwann** died, **born** 1810. *cell theory, pepsin, neurilemma, sheath of Schwann*

1882: George **Bodington** died, **born** 1799. *pulmonary tuberculosis*

1882: George **Budd** died, **born** 1808. *liver cirrhosis, fasciolopsiasis, Fasciolopsis buski*

1882: Joseph **Pancoast** died, **born** 1805. *ectopia vesicae*

1882: Louis Auguste **Mercier** died, **born** 1811. *catheter*

1882: Nikolaus **Friedreich** died, **born** 1826. *paramyoclonus, ataxia, leukaemia, trichinosis*

1882: François Rémy Lucien **Corvisart** died, **born** 1824. *tetany*

1882: Charles Robert **Darwin** died, **born** 1809. *evolution, expression of emotions*

1882: Casimir Joseph **Davaine** died, **born** 1812. *anthrax, Bacillus anthracis*

1882: Joseph Thomas **Clover** died, **born** 1825. *anaesthesia, gas-ether*

1882: Luigi Maria **Concato** died, born 1825. *tuberculosis*

**1883**

1883:1 *Journal of the American Medical Association* commences publication

1883:2 **Società Italiana di Chirurgia** founded in Rome

1883:3 **Faculty of Medicine** founded at **Beirut**

1883:4 The classic description of chronic **cystic mastitis** given by Paul Reclus (1847–1914), *BSAP* **58**:428, led to the term '**Reclus's disease**'. *5774*

1883:5 Francis Galton (1822–1911), founder of the science of **eugenics**, published *Inquiries into human faculty*, which included the first appearance of the word. *230*

1883:6 The **Koch-Weeks bacillus** discovered by Robert Koch (1843–1910) in Egyptian **conjunctivitis** (Egyptian **ophthalmia**), *WMW* **33**:1548. In 1886 J.E. Weeks discovered the same organism in 'pink eye' and it was later given its present name. *5923, 5930*

1883:7 A technique for **perineorrhaphy** devised by Thomas Addis Emmet (1828–1919), reported 1884, *TAGS* **8**:198. *6078*

1883:8 Wilhelm Friedrich [Willy] Kühne (1837–1900), with Russell Henry Chittenden (1856–1943), isolated and named several products of **digestion**, *ZBi* **19**:159. *1016*

1883:9 The first successful operation for ruptured **ectopic pregnancy** performed by Robert Lawson Tait (1845–1899) on 1 March 1883, reported 1884, *BMJ* **1**:1250. *6196*

1883:10 The first reasoned argument to support the belief in the transmission of **malaria** by the **mosquito** put forward by Albert Freeman Africanus King (1841–1914), *PSM* **23**:644. *5237*

1883:11 An early account of **leptospirosis icterohaemorrhagica** ('**Weil's disease**') given by Louis Théophile Joseph Landouzy (1845–1917), *GH* **56**:809. *5331*

1883:12 Emil Theodor Kocher (1841–1917) used the term '**cachexia strumipriva**' to describe the **myxoedema** following on total **thyroidectomy**, *ArKC* **29**:254, his pioneer work in the field led to a better understanding of its cause. *3827*

1883:13 Felix Semon (1849–1921) rightly contended that **cachexia strumipriva**, **myxoedema**, and **cretinism** were all due to loss of **thyroid** function, *BMJ* **2**:1072. *3831*

1883:14 *Corynebacterium diphtheriae*, causal organism in **diphtheria**, discovered by Theodor Albrecht Edwin Klebs (1834–1913), *VKD* **2**:139, also called **Klebs-Loeffler bacillus** following its cultivation by Loeffler (1884). *5055, 5056*

1883:15 A form of **syringomyelia** ('**Morvan's disease**') first described by Augustin Marie Morvan (1819–1897), *GMC* **20**:580, 590, 624, 721. *4701*

1883:16 **Cerebrospinal pseudosclerosis** ('**Westphal's pseudosclerosis**') described by Carl Friedrich Otto Westphal (1833–1890), *ArPN* **14**:87; a later account by Strümpell (1898) led to the term '**Westphal-Strümpell disease**'. *4702, 4709*

1883:17 **Interscapulothoracic amputation** ('**Berger's operation**') introduced by Paul Berger (1845–1908), *BSCP* **9**:656. *4471*

1883:18 The **Arnold-Chiari malformation** (abnormal development of the **cerebellum** and displacement of the **hindbrain** and **cervical cord**) described by John Cleland (1835–1925), *JA* **17**:257. In 1891 Hans Chiari described the shift of the medulla caudally, and in 1894 Julius Arnold drew attention to the abnormality of the cerebellum. *4566.1, 4577.1, 4581.1*

1883:19 Subacute combined **degeneration** of the **spinal cord** in **tabes** first described by Otto Michael Leichtenstern (1845–1900), *DMW* **10**:849. *4783*

1883:20 **Thyroid tumours** classified by Anton Wölfler (1850–1917), who was also first to describe foetal **adenoma**, *ArKC* **29**:1. *3832*

1883:21 A classic description of infantile **scurvy** by Thomas Barlow (1845–1945) led to the eponym '**Barlow's disease**', *MCT* **66**:159. *3720*

1883:22 The first description of **hydrocystoma** published by Andrew Rose Robinson (1845–1924), *TADA* p. 14. *4084*

---

1883:23 Isador Clinton **Rubin**, American gynaecologist, born 8 Jan; independently of Cary, he performed salpingography, 1914, *SGO* **20**:435; introduced a tubal insufflation method for diagnosis and treatment of sterility due to occlusion of the Fallopian tubes, 1920, *JAMA* **74**:1017; **75**:661. Died 1958. *6123, 6122, 6127*

1883:24 Kurt **Huldschinsky**, German paediatrician, born 24 Feb; cured rickets with ultraviolet irradiation, 1919, *DMW* **45**:712. Introduced the treatment of tetany with ultraviolet light, 1920, *ZK* **26**:207. Died 1941. *3732, 4836*

1883:25 Leonard **Colebrook**, British bacteriologist, born 2 Mar; with Méave Kenny; made an experimental study of the use of prontosil in the treatment of puerperal fever, 1936, *L* **1**:1279. Died 1967. *6281*

1883:26 Walter Norman **Haworth**, British chemist, born 19 Mar; awarded Nobel Prize (Chemistry), 1937, for investigations on carbohydrates and vitamin C, *NPL*. Died 1950.

1883:27 Evarts Ambrose **Graham**, American surgeon, born 19 Mar; with Warren Henry Cole, introduced cholecystography, 1924, *JAMA* **82**:613. With Jacob Jesse Singer, removed complete lung for carcinoma of bronchus, 1933, *JAMA* **101**:1371. With Ernest Ludwig Wynder, proved association of lung cancer with cigarette smoking by case-control study, 1950, *JAMA* **143**:329. Died 1957. *3652, 3205, 3215.1*

1883:28 Adalbert Goodman **Bettman**, American plastic surgeon, born 28 Mar; introduced the tannic acid-silver nitrate treatment of burns, 1935, *NM* **34**:46. *2259*

1883:29 Leonard George **Rowntree**, Canadian physician, born 10 Apr; with John Timothy Geraghty, introduced the phenolsulphonephthalein kidney function test, 1910, *JPET* 1:579. With Charles Alexander Waters and S. Bayne-Jones, introduced experimental use of lipiodol in bronchoscopy, 1917, *ArIM* 19:538. Died 1959. *4236, 3194.1*

1883:30 Warrington **Yorke**, British physician and parasitologist, born 11 Apr; with Allan Kinghorn, showed *Glossina morsitans* to be the transmitting fly of *Trypanosoma rhodesiense*, 1912, *AnTM* 6:1. Died 1943. *5285.2*

1883:31 Samuel James **Crowe**, American otolaryngologist, born 16 Apr; with Harvey Williams Cushing and John Homans, demonstrated that hypophysectomy causes genital atrophy, 1910, *JHB* 21:127. Died 1955. *3894*

1883:32 Arthur William Mickle **Ellis**, Canadian/British physician, born 4 May; published a classification of nephritis, 1941, *L* 1:1, 34, 72. Died 1966. *4254*

1883:33 George Nicholas **Papanicolaou**, Greek/American anatomist and physician, born 13 May; with Herbert Frederick Traut, pointed out the diagnostic value of cervical smears in carcinoma of the cervix, 1941, *AmJOG* 42:193. Died 1962. *6135*

1883:34 Kenneth Daniel **Blackfan**, American paediatrician, born 9 Sep; with Walter Edward Dandy, produced hydrocephalus experimentally, 1917, *AmJDC* 8:406; 14:43. Died 1941. *4597*

1883:35 Otto Heinrich **Warburg**, German biochemist, born 8 Oct. Studied metabolism of tumours and observed that malignant cells can grow without oxygen and utilize glucose by glycolysis; in his *Ueber den Stoffwechsel der Tumoren*, 1926. Discovered the nature and function of the respiratory ferment (Atmungsferment), 1929, *BcZ* 214:64; 1932, 254:438. For this work he received the Nobel Prize (Physiology or Medicine), 1931, *NPL*. Died 1970. *2651, 969, 970*

1883:36 Ralph Milton **Waters**, American anaesthetist, born 9 Oct; with Erwin Rudolph Schmidt, introduced the closed-circuit method of using cyclopropane anaesthesia, 1934, *JAMA* 103:975. *5718*

1883:37 Walter Abraham **Jacobs**, American chemist, born 14 Dec; with Michael Heidelberger introduced tryparsamide in the treatment of trypanosome infections, 1919, *JEM* 30:411. Died 1967. *1907*

———

1883:38 Karl Friedrich August **Lange**, German physician, born; introduced the colloidal gold test for cerebrospinal syphilis, 1913, *ZChem* 1:44. *2406*

1883:39 Irene Rosetta **Ewing**, British teacher of the deaf, born; with Alexander William Gordon Ewing, devised hearing tests for children, 1944, *JLO* 59:309. Died 1959. *3412.1*

1883:40 Thorald Einar Hess **Thaysen**, Danish physician, born; his extensive study of idiopathic steatorrhoea (nontropical sprue, coeliac disease), 1929, *L* 1:1086, previously described by Samuel Jones Gee, 1888, led to the eponym 'Gee-Thaysen disease'. Died 1936. *3550, 3491*

374

1883:41 William **Mestrezat**, French physician, born; gave the first exact description of the chemical constitution of the cerebrospinal fluid; in his *Le liquide céphalo-rachidien*, 1911. Died 1928. *4596*

1883:42 Marcus Walter **Schwalbe**, German physician, born; first described dystonia musculorum deformans (torsion spasm); in his inaugural dissertation, *Eine eigentümliche tonische Krampfform mit hysterischen Symptomen*, 1907. *4716*

1883:43 Robert **Knowles**, British protozoologist, born; with co-workers, demonstrated that *Leishmania donovani* is capable of reproduction in the **sandfly**, *Phlebotomus argentipes*, 1924, *IMG* **59**:593. Died 1936. *5301.1*

1883:44 Norio **Ogata**, Japanese bacteriologist, born; isolated the causal agent in tsutsugamushi disease (scrub typhus) in 1927; in reporting it in 1931, *ZBP* I Abt.**122**: 249, he named it *Rickettsia tsutsugamushi*. *5396.3*

1883:45 William Hollenback **Cary**, American gynaecologist, born; performed salpingography, to determine the patency of the Fallopian tubes, 1914, *AmJOD* **69**:462, independently of Rubin. *6122*

---

1883: Filippo **Pacini** died, **born** 1812. *Pacini's corpuscles, Balantidium coli, cholera, vibrios*

1883: Alexander Patrick **Stewart** died, **born** 1813. *typhus, typhoid*

1883: Pehr Henrik **Malmsten** died, **born** 1811. *myocardial infarction*

1883: Charles Hilton **Fagge** died, **born** 1838. *heart murmurs, goitre*

1883: Joseph **Parrot** died, **born** 1829. *pneumococcus, pulmonary tuberculosis*

1883: Victor von **Bruns** died, **born** 1812. *laryngeal polyp*

1883: James Scarth **Combe** died, **born** 1796. *pernicious anaemia*

1883: Charles Emmanuel **Sédillot** died, **born** 1804. *gastrostomy*

1883: James Marion **Sims** died, **born** 1813. *gallbladder dropsy, cholecystotomy, amputation of cervix, infertility, artificial insemination, vesico-vaginal fistula, silver wire suture*

1883: Friedrich Christoph **Kneisel** died, **born** 1797. *orthodontics*

1883: Gottfried von **Rittershain** died, **born** 1820. *dermatitis exfoliativa neonatorum*

1883: Ernest Charles **Lasègue** died, **born** 1816. *sciatica, persecution mania*

1883: George Miller **Beard** died, **born** 1839. *neurasthenia*

1883: Gabriel Gustav **Valentin** died, **born** 1810. *trypanosome*

1883: Walter **Burnham** died, **born** 1808. *hysterectomy*

**1884**

1884: 1 **International Health Exhibition, London**

1884: 2 **Medical Association of Montana** founded by John Shaw **Billings** (1838–1913)

1884: 3 **[Institute of Military Hygiene]** founded at **Madrid**

1884: 4 One of the best sources of **medical biography** to 1880 is the *Biographisches Lexikon der hervorragenden Ärzte aller Zeiten und Völker*, by August Hirsch (1817–1894), 6 vols, 1884–1888. A supplement by I. Fischer appeared in 1932–33. *6716, 6732.*

1884: 5 Robert Lawson Tait (1845–1899) was among the greatest of the **ovariotomists**; his work in this field is summarized in his *General summary of conclusions from one thousand cases of abdominal section. 6081*

1884: 6 Nikolai Evgenievich Vvedensky (1852–1922) studied the reaction of **living tissue** to various **stimulants**, and demonstrated the **indefatigability of nerve** (confirmed by Bowditch), *ZMW* 22:65. *1280*

1884: 7 Most modern methods of unilateral **cleft lip** repair are based on the operation introduced by Werner Hagedorn (1831–1894), *ZCh* 11:756. *5754.3*

1884: 8 The first to demonstrate the practical value of **cocaine** as a local **anaesthetic** in **ophthalmology** was Carl Koller (1857–1944), *KMA* 22 Bl.:60. *5925*

1884: 9 In an attempt to develop a variety of **rabies** that could be used safely for vaccination, Louis Pasteur (1822–1895), Charles Chamberland (1851–1908) and Pierre Paul Emile Roux (1853–1933) were first to modify the pathogenicity of a virus for its natural host, by serial intracerebral passage in another species of host, *CRAS* 98:457, 1229. *5482*

1884: 10 *Corynebacterium diphtheriae* (**Klebs-Loeffler bacillus**), causal organism in **diphtheria**, successfully cultivated by Friedrich Loeffler (1852–1915), *MKG* 2:421. *5056*

1884: 11 Robert Koch (1843–1910) isolated the **cholera vibrio** in pure culture, *DMW* 10:725. *5108*

1884: 12 Pure cultures of *Salmonella typhi* first grown by Georg Gaffky (1850–1918), who showed it to be the true activator of **typhoid**, *MKJ* 2:372. *5032*

1884: 13 Discovery of the **tetanus** bacillus, *Clostridium tetani*, attributed to Arthur Nicolaier (1862–1942), *DMW* 10:842; he did not isolate it in pure culture. *5148*

1884: 14 **Gasserian ganglionectomy** for the treatment of **trigeminal neuralgia** first suggested by James Ewing Mears (1838–1919), *MN* 45:58. *4857*

1884: 15 'Gilles de la Tourette syndrome', consisting of generalized tics, motor inco-ordination, **coprolalia** and **echolalia**, described by Georges Gilles de la Tourette (1857–1904), *ArN* 8:68. *4848*

1884: 16 Studies of **insanity** and a description of **amentia** appear in Theodor Hermann Meynert's (1833–1892) *Klinik der Erkrankungen des Vorderhirns. 4942*

1884:17 An account of **progressive muscular dystrophy** ('Erb's muscular atrophy') published by Wilhelm Heinrich Erb (1840–1921), *DAKM* **34**:467. *4747*

1884:18 **Ophthalmoplegic migraine** ('Möbius's disease') described by Paul Julius Möbius (1854–1907), *BKW* **21**:604. *4567*

1884:19 A classic account of **agraphia** published by Jean Albert Pitres (1848–1928), *ReM* **4**:855. *4625*

1884:20 The first suggestion of the infective nature of **herpes zoster** was by Louis Théophile Joseph Landouzy (1845–1917), *JCMP* **6**:19, 26, 37, 44, 52. *4642*

1884:21 Transmissibility of **tetanus** by inoculation into rabbits of pus from a human case demonstrated by Antonio Carle (1854–1927) and Giorgio Rattone, *GAMT* **32**:174. *5147*

1884:22 An excellent description of **ankylosing spondylitis** (the '**spondylose rhizomélique of Pierre Marie**') given by Ernst Adolph Gustav Gottfried Strümpell (1853–1925) in his *Lehrbuch der speciellen Pathologie und Therapie der inneren Krankheiten*, **2**, ii, 152; it led to the term '**Strümpell's disease**'. *4349*

1884:23 **Brain tumour** first diagnosed, accurately localized, and removed by Alexander Hughes Bennett (1848–1915) and Rickman John Godlee (1849–1925), *MCT* **68**:243. *4858*

1884:24 Louis Adolphus Duhring's (1845–1913) best work in **dermatology** was his grouping of several eruptive conditions under the term **dermatitis herpetiformis** ('**Duhring's disease**'), *JAMA* **3**:225, first described by William Tilbury Fox in 1880. *4083, 4078*

1884:25 Important work on the origin of **hypernephroma** by Paul Albert Grawitz (1850–1932), *VDGC* **13ii**:28, led to the condition being called '**Grawitz tumour**'. *4220*

1884:26 **Bladder tumour** operation devised by Henry Thompson (1820–1904); described in his *On tumours of the bladder*. *4180*

1884:27 **Local anaesthesia** first employed in **urology** by Fessenden Nott Otis (1825–1900), *NYMJ* **40**:635. *4179*

1884:28 Oscar Minkowski (1858–1931) discovered **beta-oxybutyric acid** in the urine in **diabetes mellitus**, *ArEP* **18**:35. *3947*

1884:29 The **mastoid** ('**Schwartze's**') **operation** improved by Emanuel Zaufal (1833–1910), *PMW* **9**:474. *3388*

1884:30 *Vibrio proteus*, a **cholera**-like vibrio, isolated in a case of acute gastroenteritis by Dittmar Finkler (1852–1912) and J. Prior, *DMW* **10**:579. *3481*

1884:31 **Cocaine** introduced as a **local anaesthetic** by Carl Koller (1857–1944), *KMA* **22**, B:60. *5678*

1884:32 First use of **cocaine** as an **anaesthetic** in **laryngology** by Edmund Jelinek (1852–1928), *WMW* **34**:1334, 1364. *3292*

1884:33 Subacute combined **degeneration of the spinal cord** first described by Otto Leichtenstern (1845–1900) who termed it progressive **pernicious anaemia in tabetics**, *DMW* 10:849. *3128*

1884:34 **Phagocytosis** theory originated by Elie Metchnikoff (1845–1916), *VA* **96**:177. *2538*

1884:35 **Sulphonal** prepared by Eugen Baumann (1846–1896), *BDCG* **19**:2806. *1882*

1884:36 The **sewers** of Berlin planned by James Hobrecht (1825–1902), in his *Die Canalisation von Berlin*. *1624*

1884:37 **Bacteria**; **Gram's** method of **staining** introduced by Hans Christian Joachim Gram (1853–1938), *FM* **2**:185. *2499*

1884:38 **Immunity** through attenuated **virus** discovered by Theobald Smith (1859–1934), *PBSW* **3**:29. *2539*

1884:39 **Chamberland filter** for removal of **bacteria** from liquids introduced by Charles Chamberland (1851–1908), *CRAS* **99**:247. *2498.1*

1884:40 **Antipyrine** introduced by Wilhelm Filehne (1844–1927), *ZKM* **7**:641. *1878*

1884:41 **Paraldehyde** used as a narcotic by Vincenzo Cervello (1854–1919), *ArIB* **6**:113. *1877*

1884:42 **Cephalins** and **myelins** discovered in brain tissue by Johann Ludwig Wilhelm Thudichum (1829–1901); recorded in his *A treatise on the chemical constitution of the brain*. *1415.1*

1884:43 Wilhelm August Oscar Hertwig (1849–1922) and his brother Karl Wilhelm Theodor Richard von Hertwig (1850–1937) carried out important work on **cytology**; *Untersuchungen zur Morphologie und Physiologie der Zelle*, 1884–90. *555*

1884:44 **Streptococcus**, **Staphylococcus**, and **Staph. aureus** and **albus** differentiated by Anton Julius Friedrich Rosenbach (1842–1923); in his *Mikro-Organismen bei den Wund-Infections-Krankheiten des Menschen*. *5619*

---

1884:45 Philip Edward **Smith**, American endocrinologist, born 1 Jan; showed experimentally that the activity of the gonads is maintained by the anterior pituitary, 1927, *AmJPh* **80**:114; *AmJA* **40**:159. Died 1970. *1166, 1167*

1884:46 Walter **Frey**, Swiss physician, born 10 Jan; showed quinidine to be the most effective cinchona alkaloid in treatment of auricular fibrillation, 1918, *BKW* **55**:450. *2848*

1884:47 Casimir **Funk**, Polish biochemist, born 23 Feb; determined the chemical nature of the substance in rice which could cure beriberi, 1911, *JP* **43**:395. Died 1967. *3744*

1884:48 Edward **Mellanby**, British physiologist, Secretary, (British) Medical Research Council, born 8 Apr; gave the first convincing evidence that rickets is a deficiency disease, 1918, *JP* **52**: xi, liii; *L* **1**:407. Died 1955. *3733, 3734*

1884:49 George Herbert **Hunt**, British physician, born 9 Apr; with Allan Coats Rankin, named 'Trench fever', 1915, *L* **2**:1133. Died 1926. *5386*

1884:50 Otto Fritz **Meyerhof**, German/American biochemist, born 12 Apr. His work on the chemistry of muscle laid the basis for the elucidation of the chemical pathway in the intracellular breakdown of glucose to provide energy for biological processes, 1918, *HSZ* **101**:165. Shared Nobel Prize (Physiology or Medicine), 1922, with Archibald Vivian Hill, *NPL*. Died 1951. *959*

1884:51 Burrill Bernard **Crohn**, American gastroenterologist, born 13 Jun; with L. Ginzburg and G.D. Oppenheimer, described the clinical and pathological features of regional ileitis ('Crohn's disease'), 1932, *JAMA* **99**:1323. Died 1983. *3551*

1884:52 Alfred Erich **Frank**, German physician, born 28 Jun; first definitely to connect the posterior pituitary with diabetes insipidus, 1912, *BKW* **49**:393. First reported ('Frank's') essential thrombopenia, 1915, *BKW* **52**:454, 490. Died 1957. *3897, 3083*

1884:53 Alfons Maria **Jakob** born 2 Jul; described spastic pseudosclerosis, 1921, already recorded by Creutzfeldt (1920), *ZGN* **64**:147; it is also named 'Creutzfeldt-Jakob disease'. Died 1931. *4722, 4719.1*

1884:54 Walter Clement **Alvarez**, American physician, born 22 Jul; with Cesare Gianturco, introduced Roentgen cinematography, 1932, *PMC* **7**:669. *2697*

1884:55 Robert **Schroeder**, German gynaecologist, born 3 Aug; first described metropathia haemorrhagica, 1919, *ArGy* **110**:633. Died 1919. *6126*

1884:56 William Ewart **Gye**, British oncologist, born 11 Aug; advanced the theory of viral origin of cancer, 1925, *L* **2**:109. Died 1952. *2647*

1884:57 Antoine Marcellin **Lacassagne**, French physician, born 29 Aug; demonstrated the carcinogenic effect of ovarian hormone, 1932, *CRAS* **195**:30. Died 1971. *5787*

1884:58 René **Lutembacher**, French cardiologist, born 21 Sep; described 'Lutembacher's syndrome', mitral stenosis with interatrial septal defect, 1916, *ArMC* **9**:237. *2846*

1884:59 Montrose Thomas **Burrows**, American surgeon, born 31 Oct; with Alexis Carrel, first to grow tumour tissue *in vitro*, 1910, *CRSB* **69**:332. Died 1947. *2636*

1884:60 Hermann **Rorschach**, Swiss psychiatrist, born 8 Nov; devised a test ('inkblot test') to determine personality traits; in his *Psychodiagnostik*, 1921. Died 1922. *4988.1*

1884:61 Julius Moses **Rogoff**, Latvian/American endocrinologist, born 17 Nov; with George Neil Stewart, first treated Addison's disease with adrenal cortical extract, 1929, *JAMA* **92**:1569. Died 1966. *3873*

1884:62 Albert Garland **Hogan**, American biochemist, born 31 Dec; with Ernest Milford Parrott he isolated vitamin $B_c$, 1940, *JBC* **132**:507. Died 1961. *1086*

1884:63 Barend Coenraad Petrus **Jansen** born; with Willem Frederik Donath, isolated vitamin B$_1$ (aneurine, thiamine), in crystalline form, lack of which causes beriberi, 1926, *CW* **23**:201, 1387. Died 1962. *1058, 3746*

1884:64 Arthur Lawrie **Tatum**, American pharmacologist, born; with Garrett Arthur Cooper, used mapharsen experimentally as an antisyphilitic agent, 1934, *JPET* **50**:198. Died 1955. *2415*

1884:65 Stanley Rossiter **Benedict**, American chemist, born; introduced Benedict's test for blood sugar, 1931, *JBC* **92**:141. Died 1936. *3923*

1884:66 Albert Mason **Stevens**, American paediatrician, born; with Frank Chambliss Johnson, described the Stevens-Johnson syndrome, a generalized eruption with fever and conjunctivitis, 1917. Died 1945. *4150*

1884:67 André **Feil**, French physician, born; with Maurice Klippel, first to report absence or incomplete development of cervical vertebrae ('Klippel-Feil syndrome'), 1912, *NIS* **25**:223. *4386*

1884:68 Leo **Mayer**, American orthopaedic surgeon, born; described his method of tendon transplantation, 1916, *SGO* **22**:182. Died 1972. *4386.3*

1884:69 Richard Edward **Knapp** born; with Frederick George Novy, proved that the spirochaete isolated by Norris et al. from a case of American relapsing fever differs from that isolated by Obermeier, 1906, *JID* **3**:291. *5320*

1884:70 Andrew Watson **Sellards**, American physician, born; with Ernest Linwood Walker, determined the incubation period in amoebiasis and demonstrated that *Entamoeba tetragena* and *E. minuta* are identical with *E. histolytica*, 1913, *PhJS* B **8**:253. Died 1941. *5191*

1884:71 Thomas Peck **Sprunt**, American pathologist, born; with Frank Alexander Evans, introduced the term 'infectious mononucleosis'; in their classic account of the condition, 1920, *BJH* **31**:410. *5486.1*

1884:72 Ignacio **Barraquer**, Spanish ophthalmic surgeon, born; invented a machine with which he extracted cataract by suction, 1917, *CO* **22**:328. Died 1965. *5965*

---

1884: Karl **Vierordt** died, **born** 1818. *sphygmograph*

1884: Gregor **Mendel** died, **born** 1822. *genetics*

1884: Jean Baptiste André **Dumas** died, **born** 1800. *blood transfusion*

1884: Alexander **Wood** died, **born** 1817. *hypodermic injection of drugs*

1884: Jacques-Joseph **Moreau** died, **born** 1804. *cannabis*

1884: Julius **Cohnheim** died, **born** 1839. *tuberculosis, inflammation*

1884: Sulpice Antoine **Fauvel** died, **born** 1813. *mitral stenosis, presystolic murmur*

1884: William James Erasmus **Wilson** died, **born** 1809. *dermatology, dermatitis exfoliativa*

1884: Willard **Parker** died, **born** 1800. *bladder, cystotomy, appendicitis*

1884: Samuel David **Gross** died, **born** 1805. *surgery, orthopaedics*

1884: Franti\u0161ek **Chvostek** died, **born** 1835. *tetany*

1884: Joseph Janvier **Woodward** died, **born** 1833. *dysentery*

1884: Eduard **Jaeger** died, **born** 1818. *sight test types, ophthalmoscopic atlas*

1884: Jean Claude de **la Courvée** died, **born** 1615. *symphysiotomy*

**1885**
1885:1 **Trudeau Sanitarium** established at **Saranac Lake** (Adirondacks) NY, by Edward Livingstone **Trudeau** (1848–1915)

1885:2 **Subcortical sensory aphasia** ('**Lichtheim's disease**') described by Ludwig Lichtheim (1845–1928), *DAKM* **36**:204. *4626*

1885:3 An elevated pelvic position ('**Trendelenburg position**') described by W. Meyer, *ArKC* **31**:494; also reported by Friedrich Trendelenburg in 1890, *SKV* **355**:3372. *6091*

1885:4 An important, although not the first, account of **kraurosis vulvae** given by August Breisky (1832–1889), *ZHe* **6**:69. *6082*

1885:5 The **electromagnet** introduced into **ophthalmology** by Julius Hirschberg (1843–1925); in his *Der Electromagnet in der Augenheilkunde. 5927*

1885:6 **Peripheral atrophy** of the **optic nerve** described by Ernst Fuchs (1851–1930), *GAO* **31**, 1:177. *5926*

1885:7 **Spinal anaesthesia** introduced by James Leonard Corning (1855–1923), *NYMJ* **42**:483. *5680*

1885:8 The first experiments on **local (infiltration) anaesthesia** made by William Stewart Halsted (1852–1922), *NYMJ* **42**:294. *5679*

1885:9 **Infectious mononucleosis (glandular fever)** probably first described by Nil Feodorovich Filatov (1847–1902), under the name of **idiopathic adenitis** ('**Filatov's disease**'); in his *Lectures on acute infectious diseases of children* [in Russian], 2 vols, 1885–7. *5485*

1885:10 **Gonococcus** shown, by Eugen Fraenkel (1853–1925), to be the cause of **vulvovaginitis** in children, *VA* **99**:251. *5210.1*

1885:11 The discovery of the **malaria** parasite, ***Plasmodium***, in birds made by Vasili Iakovlevich Danilevski (1852–1934), *BZ* **5**:529. *5238.1*

1885:12 The first accurate description of the **malaria** parasite, ***Plasmodium***, given by Ettore Marchiafava (1847–1935) and Angelo Celli (1857–1914), *FM* **3**:787. *5238*

1885:13 *Taenia echinococcus* transmitted to the dog from human sources by John Davies Thomas (1844–1893), *PRS* **38**:449. *5347*

1885:14 The operation of **laryngeal intubation** in **croup** perfected by Joseph P. O'Dwyer (1841–1898), *NJMJ* **42**:245. *5057*

1885:15 **Atrophic paralysis of hand muscles** following lesion of the brachial plexus and eighth cervical and first dorsal nerves ('**Klumpke's paralysis**') first described by Augusta Dejerine-Klumpke (1859–1927), *ReM* **5**:591, 739 *4748*

1885:16 **Polioencephalomyelitis** ('**Strümpell's disease**') described by Ernst Adolf Gustav Gottfried Strümpell (1853–1925), *JaK* **22**:173. *4643*

1885:17 The first deliberate and planned operation for the relief of internal derangement of the **knee-joint** due to displaced **cartilage** performed by Thomas Annandale (1838–1908), *BMJ* **1**:779. *4426.1*

1885:18 **Familial centrolobar sclerosis** ('**Pelizaeus-Merzbacher disease**') described by Friedrich Pelizaeus (1850–1917), *ArPN* **16**:698; a further account by Merzbacher (1908). *4703, 4715*

1885:19 The first description of **lymphoderma perniciosa (premycotic** or **leukaemic erythroderma)** given by Moritz Kaposi (1837–1902), *MJa*, p. 129. *4085*

1885:20 **Recurrent albuminuria** ('**Pavy's disease**') described by Frederick William Pavy (1829–1911), *BMJ* **2**:789. *4181*

1885:21 The remittent pyrexia occurring in **Hodgkin's disease** described by Pieter Klazes Pel (1852–1919), *BKW* **22**:3; named '**Pel-Ebstein disease**' following a later account by Wilhelm Ebstein. *3770, 3771*

1885:22 **Intersigmoid hernia** first definitely authenticated by Frederic Samuel Eve (1853–1916), *BMJ* **1**:1195. *3595*

1885:23 The first account of the **Billroth II operation** for resection of the **pylorus** given by Viktor von Hacker (1852–1933), *VDGC* **14**ii:62; *ArKC* **32**:616. *3483*

1885:24 **Beriberi** first conclusively shown to be of dietary origin by Kanehiro Takaki (1849–1915), *TSIK* **4**:29. *3740*

1885:25 The first detailed description of **ulcerative colitis** given by William Henry Allchin (1846–1912), *TPS* **36**:199. *3482.2*

1885:26 Artificial **pneumothorax** induced by pleural incision in intractable **haemoptysis** by William Cayley (1836–1916), *TCSL* **18**:278. *3226*

1885:27 **Subacute bacterial endocarditis** described by William Osler (1849–1919), *BMJ* **1**:467, 522, 577. *2790*

1885:28 **Antibody** formation; Ehrlich's 'side-chain' theory stated by Paul Ehrlich (1854–1915); in his *Die Sauerstoff-Bedürfniss der Organismen. 2540*

1885:29 Louis Pasteur's (1822–1895) papers describing his **rabies vaccine** and results obtained with it gave further proof of the protective value of attenuated virus against infective diseases in man and animals, *CRAS* **101**:765; **102**:459, 835; **103**:777. *2541, 5483*

1885:30 *Proteus vulgaris* isolated by Gustav Hauser (1856–1935); *Ueber Fäulnissbacterien*. *2502*

1885:31 The **Schwabach hearing test** introduced by Dagobert Schwabach (1846–1920), *ZOh* **14**:61. *3389*

1885:32 David Douglas Cunningham (1843–1914) saw and described what were almost certainly **Leishman-Donovan bodies** in tissue from **Delhi boil** (cutaneous **leishmaniasis**), *SMI* **1**:21. *5293*

---

1885:33 Lorenz **Böhler**, Austrian surgeon, born 15 Jan; introduced new methods and apparatus for the management of fractures; see his *Technik der Knochenbruchbehandlung*, 1929. Died 1973. *4433*

1885:34 John **Parkinson**, British cardiologist, born 10 Feb; with Louis Wolff and Paul Dudley White, described the Wolff-Parkinson-White syndrome, 1930, *AmHJ* **5**:685. Died 1976. *2860*

1885:35 Louise **Pearce**, American physician, born 5 Mar; introduced tryparsamide in the treatment of trypanosomiasis, 1921, *JEM* **34** Suppl.1. Died 1959. *5287*

1885:36 Williams McKim **Marriott**, American paediatrician, born 5 Mar; introduced the insulin-fattening method of treatment of malnutrition in infants, 1924, *JAMA* **83**:600. Died 1936. *6350*

1885:37 Gaspar Oliveira de **Vianna**, Brazilian physician, born 11 May; demonstrated the mode of reproduction of the trypanosome of American trypanosomiasis, *Trypanosoma cruzi*, 1911, *MIOC* **3**:276; introduced tartar emetic in the treatment of South American leishmaniasis, 1914, *AnPa* **2**:167. Died 1914. *5285.1, 5301*

1885:38 Holger **Møllgaard**, Danish surgeon, born 20 May; introduced sanocrysin in treatment of tuberculosis, 1925, *TB* **20**:1. *2344*

1885:39 Hans Gerhard **Creutzfeldt**, German neurologist, born 2 Jun; described spastic pseudosclerosis ('Creutzfeldt-Jakob disease'), 1920, *ZGN* **57**:1. Jakob also described it (1921). Died 1964. *4719.1, 4722*

1885:40 Norman Macdonnell **Keith**, Canadian/American physician, born 8 Jun; with Henry Patrick Wagener and N.W. Barker, devised the Keith-Wagener-Barker classification of essential hypertension, 1929, *AmJMS* **197**:332, 1939, *Medicine* **18**:317. Died 1976. *2716, 2723*

1885:41 Jacob Jesse **Singer**, British/American physician, born 12 Jul; with Evarts Ambrose Graham, removed complete lung for carcinoma of bronchus, 1933, *JAMA* **101**:1371. Died 1954. *3205*

1885:42 Albert Compton **Broders**, American physician, born 8 Aug; introduced the 'Broders classification' as an index of tumour malignancy, 1920, *JAMA* **74**:656. Died 1964. *2645*

1885:43 Arno Benedict **Luckhardt**, American physiologist and anaesthetist, born 26 Aug; with Jay Bailey Carter, introduced ethylene as an anaesthetic, 1923, *JAMA* **80**:765. Died 1957. *5705*

1885:44 John Hinchman **Stokes**, American dermatologist and syphilologist, born 1 Sep; with Stanley Owen Chambers, introduced bismarsen (bismuth arsphenamine sulphate) in the treatment of syphilis, 1927, *JAMA* **89**:1500. *2414*

1885:45 Wilhelm Siegmund **Frei**, German dermatologist, born 5 Sep; introduced the Frei skin test for the diagnosis of lymphogranuloma venereum, 1925, *KW* **4**:2148. Died 1943. *5218*

1885:46 Max Minor **Peet**, American surgeon, born 20 Oct; used resection of the trigeminal nerve, with conservation of the motor root, for the treatment of trigeminal neuralgia, 1918, *JMSMA* **17**:91. Introduced surgical treatment for hypertension ('Peet's operation'), 1935, *PCAM* **5**:58. Died 1949. *4889, 3036*

1885:47 Russell Morse **Wilder**, American physician, born 24 Nov; with Howard Taylor Ricketts, differentiated Rocky Mountain spotted fever from typhus, 1910, *ArIM* **5**:361. Died 1952. *5380*

1885:48 George Richards **Minot**, American haematologist, born 2 Dec; with William Parry Murphy, introduced the raw liver diet in the treatment of pernicious anaemia, 1926, *JAMA* **87**:470, following the demonstration of its value in anaemia by Robscheit-Robbins and Whipple (1925). Shared Nobel Prize (Physiology or Medicine), 1934, with William Parry Murphy and George Hoyt Whipple, for this work, *NPL*. Died 1950. *3140, 3139*

1885:49 Max **Lederer**, American pathologist, born; described 'Lederer's anaemia', a form of acute haemolytic anaemia, 1925, *AmJMS* **170**:500. Died 1952. *3138*

1885:50 Maurice **Sourdille**, French otologist, born; first successfully to restore hearing by fenestration in otosclerosis, 1937, *BNYA* **13**:673. Died 1981. *3408*

1885:51 Stephen **Chauvet** born; with Achille Alexandre Souques, published a classic account of pituitary infantilism, 1913, *NIS* **26**:69. Died 1950. *3899*

1885:52 Charles Alexander **Waters**, American radiologist, born; with S. Bayne-Jones and Leonard George Rowntree, introduced experimental use of lipiodol in bronchoscopy, 1917, *ArIM* **19**:538; with Hugh Hampton Young, first demonstrated vesiculography, 1920, *AmJR* **7**:16. *3194.1, 4198*

---

1885: John M. **Riggs** died, **born** 1811. *pyorrhoea alveolaris*

1885: Friedrich Theodor **Frerichs** died, **born** 1819. *multiple sclerosis, hepatolenticular degeneration*

1885: Louis Alexis **Normond** died, **born** 1834. *strongyloidiasis, Strongyloides stercoralis*

1885: Daniel **Carrión** died; **born** 1857. *bartonellosis*

1885: Edward Talbot **Ely** died, **born** 1850. *otoplasty*

1885: John Light **Atlee** died, **born** 1799. *oöphorectomy*

1885: Friedrich Gustav Jakob **Henle** died, **born** 1809. *anatomy, epithelia, histology, microbes, Henle's loop*

1885: Peter Ludwig **Panum** died, **born** 1820. *measles*

**1886**
1886:1 **Association of American Physicians** organized

1886:2 **New York Cancer Hospital** founded

1886:3 **Conseil de Santé, Quebec**

1886:4 **Royal Institute of Public Health, London,** founded

1886:5 **Rotational nystagmus** described by Endre Högyes (1847–1906), *PMCP* **22**:765, 787, 807, 827. *3389.1*

1886:6 Franz von Soxhlet (1848–1926) contributed a great deal to the knowledge on **milk**. He wrote on milk droplets, estimated its specific gravity with his **lactodensimeter**, described an apparatus for the sterilization of milk, and devised a test for the estimation of fats in milk, *MMW* **33**:253, 276. *6341*

1886:7 John Elmer Weeks (1853–1949) discovered an organism in 'pink eye'. The organism, already seen by Robert Koch in Egyptian ophthalmia, was later named '**Koch-Weeks bacillus**', *ArOp* **15**:441. *5930*

1886:8 An operation for congenital and paralytic **ptosis** of the **eyelid** introduced by Photinos Panas (1832–1903), *ArO* **6**:1. *5929*

1886:9 A method of *morcellement* of the **uterus** for the removal of **tumours** described by Jules Émile Péan (1830–1898), *GH* **59**:445. *6084*

1886:10 An operation for **retroversion of the uterus** described by Robert von Olshausen (1835–1915), *ZGy* **10**:698. *6083*

1886:11 The first description of **phlebotomus (pappataci) fever** is generally attributed to Alois Pick (1859–1945), *WMW* **36**:1141, 1168. *5476*

1886:12 The first attempts at **asepsis** made by Gustav Adolf Neuber (1850–1932); recorded in his *Die aseptische Wundbehandlung in meinen chirurgischen Privat-Hospitälern. 5637*

1886:13 The development of the parasite of quartan **malaria** described by Camillo Golgi (1843–1926), *ArSM* **10**:109. *5239*

1886:14 One of the first to demonstrate an animal **virus** particle was John Brown Buist (1846–1915) who recognized, and demonstrated microscopically, the elementary bodies of the **vaccinia** virus, *PRSE* **13**:603. Their rediscovery by Paschen (1906) led to the term **Paschen elementary bodies**. *5427*

1886:15 In his classic description of **leptospirosis icterohaemorrhagica**, Adolf Weil (1848–1916) differentiated it from other types of acute jaundice; it is also known as '**Weil's disease**', *DAKM* **39**:209. *5332*

1886:16 Amoebae discovered in liver abscess by Stephanos Kartulis (1852–1920); it was principally through his work that amoebae came to be considered a cause of dysentery (**amoebiasis**) in man, *VA* **105**:521. *5186*

1886:17 A report by Edward Emanuel Klein (1844–1925) contains the first suggestion of the **streptococcal** origin of **scarlet fever**, *Report of the Medical Officer Local Government Board, London* 1885, p. 90. *5080*

1886:18 The '**Landouzy-Dejerine type**' of (scapulo-humeral) **progressive muscular atrophy** described by Louis Théophile Joseph Landouzy (1845–1917) and Joseph Jules Dejerine (1849–1917), *CRSB* **3**:478. *4752*

1886:19 **Panatrophy** first described by William Richard Gowers (1845–1915); in his *Manual of diseases of the nervous system*, **1**, 365. *4751*

1886:20 **Peroneal muscular atrophy (Charcot-Marie-Tooth type)** first described by Jean Martin Charcot (1825–1893) and Pierre Marie (1853–1940), and independently by Tooth in the same year, *ReM* **6**:97. *4749, 4750*

1886:21 Howard Henry Tooth (1856–1925) published *The peroneal type of progressive muscular atrophy* in the same year as it was independently described by Charcot and Marie (**Charcot-Marie-Tooth type of peroneal muscular atrophy**). *4750, 4749*

1886:22 '**Mackenzie's syndrome**' (**paralysis** of the **tongue, soft palate**, and **vocal cord** on the same side) described by Stephen Mackenzie (1844–1909), *TCSL* **19**:317. *4571*

1886:23 Following the description of hereditary **spastic spinal paralysis** by Ernst Adolf Gottfried Strümpell (1853–1925), *ArPN* **17**:217, it was also called '**Strümpell's disease**', despite previous accounts by Erb and Charcot. *4704*

1886:24 **Neurodermatitis** ('**Vidal's disease**') described by Jean Baptiste Emil Vidal (1825–1893), *AnD* **7**:133. *4088*

1886:25 **Progeria** first described by Jonathan Hutchinson (1828–1913), *MCT* **69**:473. *3790*

1886:26 Pierre Marie (1853–1940) gave first complete clinical description of **acromegaly**, *ReM* **6**:297. *3884*

1886:27 **Phaeochromocytoma**, a tumour of the **adrenal medulla**, first described by Felix Fränkel, *VA* **103**:244. *3865*

1886:28 Operation for treatment of intraperitoneal rupture of the **bladder** introduced by William MacCormac (1836–1901), *L* **2**:1118. *4182*

1886:29 The first description of **lichen ruber moniliformis** ('**Kaposi's disease**') given by Moritz Kaposi (1837–1902), *VDS* **13**:571. *4086*

1886:30 **Pemphigus vegetans** ('**Neumann's disease**') described by Isidor von Neumann (1832–1906), *VDS* **13**:157; a suppurative form of the disease was described by Hallopeau in 1889. *4087, 4101*

1886:31 Partial removal of the **pancreas** shown to be feasible and justifiable by Nicholas Senn (1844–1908), *TASA* **4**:99. *3629*

1886:32 Viktor von Hacker (1852–1933) introduced his method of **gastrostomy**, *WMW* **36**:1073, 1110. *3486*

1886:33 First case of survival after removal of perforated **appendix** reported by Richard John Hall (1856–1897), *NYMJ* **43**:662. *3568*

1886:34 A method for the radical cure of oblique **inguinal hernia** introduced by William Macewen (1848–1924), *AnS* **4**:89. *3596*

1886:35 First plastic reconstruction of the **oesophagus** after resection for carcinoma by Johann Mikulicz-Radecki (1850–1905), *PMW* **11**:93. *3487*

1886:36 True **haemophilia** in a female recorded by Frederick Treves (1853–1923), *L* **2**:553. *3067.1*

1886:37 **Tobacco mosaic disease** (viral) described and named by Adolf Mayer (b.1843), *LV* **32**:450. *2503.1*

1886:38 Primary **amyloidosis** reported by Carl Wild, *BPA* **1**:175. *2306*

1886:39 *Salmonella cholerae-suis*, first member of *Salmonella* group, isolated by Daniel Elmer Salmon (1850–1914) and Theobald Smith (1859–1934), *AmMM* **7**:204. *2505*

1886:40 **Ichthammol** and **resorcinol** introduced by Paul Gerson Unna (1850–1929), *MDP* Suppl.1. *1883*

1886:41 '**Bertillonage**' method of anthropomorphic identification of persons introduced by Alphonse Bertillon (1853–1914); in his *Les signalements anthropométriques*. *181*

1886:42 **Neuron theory** formulated by Wilhelm His, Sr (1831–1904), *AbL* **13**:477. *1368.1*

1886:43 The first description of *Bact. coli* infection given by Theodor Escherich (1857–1911) in his *Die Darmbakterien des Säuglings*; the genus was later named *Escherichia* after him. *6340*

---

1886:44 Paul Ferdinand **Schilder**, Austrian psychiatrist, born 15 Feb; described encephalitis periaxialis diffusa ('Schilder's disease'), 1912, *ZGN* **10**:1. Died 1940. *4646*

1886:45 Robert Runnels **Williams**, American biochemist, born 16 Feb. Discovered and synthesized the anti-beriberi factor, vitamin B$_2$, 1928, *JBC* **78**:311; 1936, *JACS* **58**:1504. Died 1965. *1060, 1073*

1886:46 Clifford **Dobell**, British protozoologist, born 22 Feb; gave a classic account of the life-cycle of *Entamoeba histolytica*, 1928, *Para* **20**:357. Died 1949. *5194.1*

1886:47 Karl Wilhelm **Joetten**, German physician, born 4 Mar; with Ludwig Haendel, introduced suramin (Bayer 205) in the treatment of trypanosomiasis, 1920, *BKW* **57**:821. *5286*

1886:48 Edward Calvin **Kendall**, American biochemist, born 8 Mar; isolated thyroxine, the thyroid hormone, 1915, *JAMA* **64**:2042; isolated cortisone, 1936, *JBC* **114**:lvii, 613; **116**:267. Shared Nobel Prize (Physiology or Medicine), 1950, with Philip Showalter Hench and Tadeus Reichstein, for his work on cortisone, *NPL*. Died 1972. *1133, 1151*

1886:49 Edward **Hindle**, British zoologist, born 21 Mar; introduced the first vaccine for immunization against yellow fever, 1928, *BMJ* **1**:976. Died 1973. *5461*

1886:50 Renjiro **Kaneko**, Japanese physician, born 31 Mar; with Y. Aoki, distinguished Japanese encephalitis from epidemic encephalitis ('encephalitis lethargica'), 1928, *EIM* **34**:342. *4654*

1886:51 Walter Edward **Dandy**, American neurosurgeon, born 6 Apr; with Kenneth Daniel Blackfan, produced hydrocephalus experimentally, 1914, *AmJDC* **8**:406;**14**:43. Introduced cerebral ventriculography, 1918, *AnS* **68**:5; introduced extirpation of the choroid plexus of the lateral ventricles in communicating hydrocephalus, 1918, *AnS* **68**:569; introduced pneumoencephalography, 1919, *AnS* **70**:397; used intracranial section of the trigeminal nerve for the treatment of glossopharyngeal neuralgia, 1925, *BJH* **36**:105; devised operation for treatment of Menière's disease, 1928, *ArSuC* **16**:1127. Died 1946. *4597, 4602, 4888, 4603, 4896, 3406*

1886:52 Geoffrey **Jefferson**, British neurosurgeon, born 10 Apr; a fine teacher who occupied the first chair of neurosurgery in Britain (at Manchester); carried out the first successful embolectomy in Britain, 1925, *BMJ* **2**:965. Died 1961. *3017*

1886:53 John Albert **Kolmer**, American venereologist, born 24 Apr; introduced a complement-fixation ('Kolmer') test for syphilis, 1922, *AmJSy* **6**:82. Died 1962. *2413*

1886:54 Oswald Hope **Robertson**, British/American physician, born 2 Jun; performed blood transfusion with stored red cells, 1917, *MB* **1**:436. Died 1966. *2021.1*

1886:55 Paul Dudley **White**, American cardiologist, born 6 Jun; with Louis Wolff and John Parkinson, described the Wolff-Parkinson-White syndrome, 1930, *AmHJ* **5**:685. Died 1973. *2860*

1886:56 Elizabeth **Kenny**, Australian nurse, born 20 Sep; in her *Infantile paralysis and cerebral diplegia*, 1937, described the methods she used for the restoration of function in patients suffering from these conditions. Died 1952. *4671*

1886:57 Charles **Armstrong**, American pathologist and virologist, born 25 Sep; with Ralph Dougall Lillie, isolated the benign lymphocytic choriomeningitis virus, 1934, *USPHR* **49**:1019. Died 1967. *4688*

1886:58 Archibald Vivian **Hill**, British physiologist, born 26 Sep; shared the Nobel Prize (Physiology or Medicine), 1922, with Otto Meyerhof, for his discoveries in relation to production of heat in muscle, 1920, *JP* **54**:84, *NPL*. Died 1977. *659*

1886: 59 Gaston Léon **Ramon**, French bacteriologist and pathologist, born 30 Sep; modified the diphtheria toxin so that it lost its toxic properties while retaining its antigenic virtues, 1928, *AnIP* **42**:959, this antitoxin (toxoid) superseded toxin-antitoxin as an immunizing agent; with Christian Zoeller, first employed tetanus toxoid in the immunization of humans, 1933, *CRSB* **112**:347. Died 1963. *5070, 5151*

1886: 60 Ernest William **Goodpasture**, American pathologist and bacteriologist, born 17 Oct; with Claud D. Johnson, isolated the mumps virus, 1934, *JEM* **59**:1. Died 1960. *5543*

1886: 61 John Archibald Campbell **Colston**, American urologist, born 30 Oct; with John Essary Dees, used sulphanilamide in the treatment of gonorrhoea, 1937, *JAMA* **108**:1855. *5214*

1886: 62 William John **Adie**, Australian/British neurologist, born 31 Oct; described 'Adie's syndrome', a condition in which a pupil that is usually larger than its fellow and reacts poorly to light ('Adie's pupil') is associated with absent tendon reflexes, 1931, *BMJ* **1**:928. Died 1935. *4611*

1886: 63 Rolla Eugene **Dyer**, American pathologist, born 4 Nov; showed murine typhus to be caused by an organism, 1931, *USPHR* **46**:334, later named *Rickettsia mooseri*. *5396.2*

1886: 64 Grace **Medes**, Austrian physiological chemist, born 9 Nov; drew attention to tyrosinosis, an error of tyrosine metabolism, 1932, *BJ* **26**:917. Died 1967. *3923.1*

1886: 65 Marius Nygaard **Smith-Petersen**, Norwegian/American orthopaedic surgeon, born 14 Nov; introduced the Smith-Petersen nail, a three-flanged nail which prevented rotation of the femoral head during treatment of fractures of the neck of the femur, 1931, *ArSuC* **23**:719; with co-workers, introduced vitallium cup arthroplasty of the hip-joint, 1937, *JBJS* **21**:269. Died 1953. *4434, 4403*

1886: 66 Karl von **Frisch**, Austrian zoologist, born 28 Nov; shared Nobel Prize (Physiology or Medicine) with Konrad Lorenz and Nikolaas Tinbergen in 1973 for their discoveries concerning organization and elicitation of individual and social behaviour patterns, *NPL*. Died 1982.

1886: 67 Samuel Phillips **Bedson**, British pathologist and virologist, born 1 Dec; with J.O.W. Bland, gave conclusive proof that the causal agent in psittacosis is *Chlamydia psittaci*, 1932, *BJEP* **13**:461; with co-workers, devised a skin-test antigen for the diagnosis of lymphogranuloma venereum, 1949, *JCP* **2**:241. Died 1969. *5541.1, 5225*

1886: 68 James **Ewing**, American pathologist, born 25 Dec; described a rare form of bone sarcoma ('Ewing's sarcoma'), diffuse endothelioma of bone, 1921, *PNYP* **21**:17. Died 1943. *4388*

---

1886: 69 Louis John **Gillespie**, American physician, born; with Alphonse Raymond Dochez, differentiated four types of pneumococci, 1913, *JAMA* **61**:727. *3192.1*

1886: 70 Peter Kosciusko **Olitsky** born; with Albert Sabin, isolated and propagated poliomyelitis virus in pure culture, 1936, *PSEB* **34**:357. Died 1964. *4670.6*

1886: 71 Arnold Kirkpatrick **Henry**, British surgeon, born; devised operation for femoral hernia, using a midline extraperitoneal approach, 1936, *L* **1**:531. Died 1962. *3611*

1886:72 Petrus Johannes **Waardenburg**, Dutch geneticist and ophthalmologist, born; reported Waardenburg's syndrome, combining developmental anomalies of the eyelids and nose root with pigmentary defects of the iris and head hair and congenital deafness, 1951, *AmJHG* **3**:195. Died 1979. *4154.4*

1886:73 Carl **Friderichsen**, Danish physician, born; gave an account of the Waterhouse-Friderichsen syndrome, 1918, *JaK* **87**:109. *4686, 4685*

1886:74 Karl Erhard **Kassowitz**, German immunologist, born; introduced the 'scratch test', a cutaneous reaction for determination of susceptibility to diphtheria, 1924, *KW* **3**:1317. *5069*

1886:75 Claude Walter **Levinthal**, German microbiologist, born; found the causal agent of psittacosis to be *Chlamydia psittaci*, *KW* **9**:654. The same discovery was made simultaneously by A.C. Coles (*Lancet*, **1**, 1011) and R.D. Lillie (*Publ. Hlth. Rep., Wash.*, **45**, 773). Died 1963. *5539*

1886:76 Paul **Selter** born; first clearly described infantile acrodynia ('pink disease'), 1903, *VGK* **20**:45. *6344*

1886:77 Robert **Rendu**, French army surgeon, born; first described the 'Stevens-Johnson syndrome', 1916, *JPr* **30**:351. *6365*

1886: Johann Friedrich **Horner** died, **born** 1831. *Horner's syndrome, ptosis of eyelid*

1886: Paul **Bert** died, **born** 1833. *altitude physiology*

1886: François Jules **Lemaire** died, **born** 1814. *carbolic acid*

1886: Norman **Chevers** died, **born** 1818. *constrictive pericarditis*

1886: Austin **Flint** died, **born** 1812. *aortic regurgitation*

1886: George **Busk** died, **born** 1807. *Fasciolopsis buski*

1886: John **Parkin** died, **born** 1801. *cholera*

1886: Timothy Richards **Lewis** died, **born** 1841. *microfilariae, Filaria sanguinis hominis, Trypanosoma lewisi*

1886: Frank Hastings **Hamilton** died, **born** 1813. *skin grafts, ulcers*

1886: John Cooper **Forster** died, **born** 1823. *gastrostomy*

**1887**
1887:1 **St Mary's Hospital, Rochester**, Minn., purchased; later home of '**Mayo Clinic**'

1887:2 **Sloane Maternity Hospital, New York**, opened

1887:3 **American Physiological Society** founded

1887:4 **Royal Victoria Hospital, Montreal**, founded

1887:5 [**Psychological Society, Berlin**], founded

1887:6 Abraham Jacobi (1830–1919) was first in the United States to specialize in **paediatrics**. In 1862 he founded the first paediatric clinic there (in New York). In 1887 he wrote *The intestinal diseases of infancy and childhood. 6342*

1887:7 A flap-splitting operation for **rectocele** devised by Robert Lawson Tait (1845–1899), *BGT* **3**:367; **7**:195. *6087*

1887:8 **Pyelitis** complicating **vesical** and **faecal fistulae** in women successfully treated by Nathan Bozeman (1825–1905), *IMC* **2**:514. *6085*

1887:9 A pioneer in the evolution of **asepsis** was Ernst von Bergmann (1836–1907), whose **corrosive sublimate** method of **antisepsis** was merged into steam **sterilization** and the present-day ritual of asepsis, *TM* **1**:41. *5638*

1887:10 Henry Vandyke Carter (1831–1897) reported a blood spirillum, *Spirillum minus*, in a rat, *SMI* **3**:45, later shown to be a cause of spirillary **rat-bite fever**. *5323*

1887:11 **Brucellosis (Malta fever)** shown by David Bruce (1855–1931) to be due to a micrococcus, *Brucella melitensis*, *Prac* **39**:161. *5098*

1887:12 Experimental **amoebiasis** induced in cats by the intrarectal inoculation of stools by Jaroslav Hlava (1855–1924), *CLC* **26**:70. *5186.1*

1887:13 The **meningococcus**, *Neisseria meningitidis*, causal organism of **cerebrospinal meningitis**, discovered by Anton Weichselbaum (1845–1920), *FM* **5**:573, 620. *4678*

1887:14 Cerebral changes in **amaurotic familial idiocy** described by Bernard Sachs (1858–1944), *JNMD* **14**:541; the ocular manifestations of the disease were noted by Tay (1880) and the condition is also known as 'Tay-Sachs disease'. *4705, 5918*

1887:15 The effect of **fevers** on **psychotic conditions** studied by Julius Wagner von Jauregg (1857–1940), *JaP* **7**:94. *4946, 4806*

1887:16 The term **dyslexia** first suggested by Rudolph Berlin (1833–1897); in his *Eine besondere Art der Wortblindheit. 4627*

1887:17 The first description of **peripheral neuritis** ('**Dejerine's neurotabes**') given by Joseph Jules Dejerine (1849–1917), *CRSB* **4**:137. *4784*

1887:18 Oscar Minkowski (1858–1931) first pointed out the constancy of **pituitary** enlargement in **acromegaly**, *BKW* **24**:371. *3885*

1887:19 The speciality of **orthodontics** was considerably advanced through the work of Edward Hartley Angle (1855–1930), *IMC 9* **5**:565. *3686*

1887:20 **Impetigo circumpilaris infantilis** ('**Bockhart's impetigo**') first described by Max Bockhart, *MPD* **6**:450. *4089*

1887:21 Unna's seborrhoeic **eczema** described by Paul Gerson Unna (1850–1929), *MPD* 6:827. *4092*

1887:22 Moritz Kaposi (1837–1902) gave a full account of **impetigo herpetiformis** (first described by von Hebra in 1872) and established its status, *VDS* **14**:273. *4091*

1887:23 The remittent pyrexia occurring in **lymphadenoma** described by Wilhelm Ebstein (1836–1912), *BKW* **24**:565; named 'Pel-Ebstein disease' acknowledging an earlier account by Pieter Klazes Pel. *3771, 3770*

1887:24 Attention first drawn to congenital **megacolon** ('**Hirschsprung's disease**') by Harald Hirschsprung (1830–1916), *JaK* **27**:1. *3489*

1887:25 First successful intralaryngeal extirpation of **cancer** of **larynx** by Bernhard Fraenkel (1836–1911), *ArKC* **34**:281. *3296*

1887:26 The modern method for the radical cure of **inguinal hernia** devised by Edoardo Bassini (1844–1924), *ACMI* **2**:179, almost simultaneously with William Stewart Halsted. *3598*

1887:27 Sacral method of resection of the **rectum** for **carcinoma** introduced by Paul Kraske (1851–1930), *BKW* **24**:899. *3490*

1887:28 **Purpura fulminans** first described by Eduard Heinrich Henoch (1820–1910), *BKW* **24**:8. *3068*

1887:29 **Petri dish** introduced by Richard Julius Petri (1852–1921), *ZBP* **1**:279. *2505.1*

1887:30 **Phenacetin** introduced by Oscar Heinrich Hinsberg (1857–1939) and Alfred Kast (1856–1903), *ZMW* **25**:145. *1883.3*

1887:31 **Burns**; open or exposed method of treatment introduced by William Preston Copeland, *MR* **31**:518. *2250.1*

1887:32 **Action currents of the heart** demonstrated by use of electrodes by Augustus Désiré Waller (1856–1922); preparing the ground for **electrocardiography**, *JP* **8**:229. *833*

1887:33 **Acetanilide** introduced by Arnold Cahn and Paul Hepp, *PM* **5**:43. *1883.2*

1887:34 **Ephedrine** isolated by Nagajosi Nagai (1844–1929), *PhaZ* **32**:700. *1883.1*

1887:35 **Localization of cerebral function** investigated by Charles Edward Beevor (1854–1907) and Victor Alexander Haden Horsley (1857–1916), *PTB* **176**:153. *1416.1*

1887:36 **Neuron theory** stated by August Henri Forel (1848–1931), *ArPN* **18**:162. *1368.2*

1887:37 Attention drawn to **alcoholic polyneuritis** ('**Korsakoff's psychosis** or **syndrome**) by Sergei Sergeievich Korsakoff (1854–1900), *VKP* **4**(2):1. *4945*

1887:38 Arthur **Stoll**, Swiss chemist, born 8 Jan; with Karl Spiro isolated ergotamine, 1921, *SMW* **2**:525. With Albert Hoffmann, synthesized lysergic acid-diethylamide, 1943, *HCA* **26**:944. Died 1971. *1910, 1928.1*

1887:39 Wolfgang **Köhler**, Estonian psychologist, born 21 Jan; advanced the theory of gestalt psychology in his *Gestalt psychology*, 1929. Died 1967. *4991*

1887:40 Adrian **Stokes**, British bacteriologist, born 9 Feb; with co-workers, successfully transmitted yellow fever virus to the *Macacus rhesus* monkey, 1928, *AmJTM* **8**:103; Stokes died of the disease during his investigations. Died 1927. *5462*

1887:41 Harold **King**, British chemist, born 24 Feb; isolated *d*-tubocurarine chloride from curare, 1935, *Nature* **135**:469. Died 1956. *5719*

1887:42 David **Keilin**, Russian/British biochemist and parasitologist, born 21 Mar; discovered cytochrome, 1925, *PRSB* **98**:312. Died 1963. *968*

1887:43 Geoffrey Langdon **Keynes**, British surgeon and bibliographer, born 25 Mar; his successful radium treatment of cancer of the breast, 1927, *BJS* **19**:415, established this conservative method. Died 1982. *5786*

1887:44 Arthur **Felix**, Polish bacteriologist, born 3 Apr; with Edmund Weil, developed the Weil-Felix reaction for the diagnosis of typhus, 1916, *WKW* **29**:33. With R.M. Pitt, first described Vi antigen, the antigen of the typhoid bacillus, 1934, *Lancet* **2**:186. With George Ford Petrie, first prepared anti-typhoid serum, 1938, *JHyg* **38**:673. Died 1956. *5390, 5381, 5045, 5045.1*

1887:45 Einar **Meulengracht**, Danish physician, born 7 Apr; introduced Meulengracht diet for treatment of haematemesis and melaena, 1934, *AcM* Sup.59:375. *3555*

1887:46 Frank Earl **Adair**, American surgeon, born 9 Apr; gave the first description of plasma-cell mastitis, 1933, *ArSuC* **26**:735. *5788*

1887:47 Bernardo Alberto **Houssay**, Argentinian physiologist, born 10 Apr. For his researches, with co-workers, on the role of the anterior pituitary in carbohydrate metabolism, 1925, *CRSB* **92**:822, **101**:940, he shared the Nobel Prize (Physiology or Medicine), 1947, with Carl Ferdinand Cori and Gerty Theresa Cori, *NPL*. With Juan Carlos Fascioli, showed hypertension to be due to the action of a pressor substance, 1937, *RSAB* **13**:284. Died 1971. *2721*

1887:48 Henry Edward **Shortt**, British protozoologist and medical entomologist, born 15 Apr; with co-workers, cultivated the virus of phlebotomus fever, 1936, *IJMR* **23**:865; with C.S. Swaminath, showed *Phlebotomus argentipes* to be the vector of *Leishmania*, 1942, *IJMR* **30**:473; demonstrated the pre-erythrocytic stage of malaria, 1948, *BMJ* **1**:192, 547: 1949, **2**:1006. Died 1987. *5480, 5302, 5262*

1887:49 Reuben Leon **Kahn**, Lithuanian/American immunologist and serologist, born 26 Jul; introduced the Kahn precipitation test for syphilis, 1922, *ArDS* **5**:570. *2412*

1887:50 Paul **Klemperer**, Austrian/American pathologist, born 2 Aug; with co-workers he combined a number of hitherto unrelated diseases into the entity of 'diffuse collagen disease', 1942, *JAMA* **119**:331. Died 1964. 2237

1887:51 Leopold **Ruzicka**, Croatian chemist, born 13 Sep; synthesized androsterone (first complete synthesis of a sex hormone), 1934, *HCA* **17**:1395. Shared Nobel Prize (Chemistry), 1939, with Alfred Friedrich Butenandt, *NPL*. Died 1976. *1201*

1887:52 Richard Moreland **Taylor**, American virologist, born 10 Oct; recovered influenza C virus, 1949, *AmPuH* **39**:171. *5500*

1887:53 Harold Ward **Dudley**, British biochemist, born 20 Oct; with John Chassar Moir, isolated ergometrine, 1935, *BMJ* **1**:520. Died 1935. *6230*

1887:54 James Batcheller **Sumner**, American biochemist, born 19 Nov; succeeded in isolating an enzyme, crystalline urease, 1926, *JBC* **69**:435. He shared the Nobel Prize (Chemistry), 1946, with John Howard Northropp and Wendell Meredith Stanley, *NPL*. Died 1955.

1887:55 Henri **Chaoul**, German radiologist, born 14 Dec; with Albert Adam, introduced Chaoul therapy (radiotherapy) in the treatment of malignant tumours, 1933, *Str* **48**:31. *4007*

1887:56 John William **McNee**, British physician, born 17 Dec; demonstrated the origin of bile pigment, 1914, *JPB* **18**:325. Died 1984. *3648*

1887:57 Christian **Wolferth**, American physician, born; with Francis Clark Wood, introduced chest leads in the electrocardiographic diagnosis of coronary occlusion, 1933, *AmJMS* **183**:30. Died 1965. 2863

1887:58 Alfred Purvis **Hart**, Canadian physician, born; performed successful exchange blood transfusion for icterus gravis neonatorum, 1925, *CMAJ* **15**:1088. Died 1954. *3087.1*

1887:59 Edwin Clay **White** born; with Sanford Morris Rosenthal, devised the bromosulphthalein test for liver function, 1924, *JPET* **24**:265. *3653*

1887:60 Josef **Gerstmann**, Austrian neurologist, born; described a syndrome of finger agnosia, right-left disorientation and acalculia ('Gerstmann's syndrome') due to cerebral lesion, 1924, *WKKW* **37**:1010. *4605.3*

1887:61 Carl **Kling**, Swedish physician, born; with co-workers, recovered poliomyelitis virus from the intestinal tract, disproving that it was exclusively neurotropic; in *Investigations on epidemic infantile paralysis ... XVth International Congress on Hygiene and Demography*, 1912. Died 1967. *4670.4*

1887:62 Irving Freiler **Stein**, American obstetrician, born; with Michael Leo Leventhal, described amenorrhoea associated with bilateral polycystic ovaries (Stein-Leventhal syndrome), 1935, *AmJOG* **29**:181. *6132.1*

1887:63 Walter **Schiller**, Austrian/American pathologist, born; introduced a test for early diagnosis of carcinoma of the cervix uteri, 1933, *SGO* **56**:210. Died 1960. *6132*

1887: Gustav Theodor **Fechner** died, **born** 1801. *Fechner-Weber law, psychophysics, sensation*

1887: Edmé Félix Alfred **Vulpian** died, **born** 1826. *adrenaline*

1887: Karl **Friedländer** died, **born** 1847. *Klebsiella pneumoniae*

1887: Julius Otto Ludwig **Möller** died, **born** 1819. *rickets, scurvy*

1887: Jacques Gilles Thomas **Maisonneuve** died, **born** 1809. *urinary hair catheter*

1887: John Murray **Carnochan** died, **born** 1817. *facial neuralgia*

1887: Isaac **Ray** died, **born** 1807. *psychiatry*

1887: Bernhard Rudolph Conrad von **Langenbeck** died, **born** 1810. *cleft palate, thrush, Candida albicans*

1887: Fredrik Theodor **Berg** died, **born** 1806. *thrush, Candida albicans*

1887: Carl Ferdinand von **Arlt** died, **born** 1812. *conjunctivitis, distichiasis*

**1888**
1888:1 **Institut Pasteur, Paris,** founded

1888:2 **Local Government Act, England**

1888:3 **Bacteriological (Pathological) Laboratory** established at **Rhode Island**

1888:4 **[Public Health Laboratory]** established at **Rome**

1888:5 **Marine Biological Laboratory** established at **Woods Hole**, Mass.

1888:6 **Société Française d'Ophtalmologie** founded at Paris

1888:7 **École de Service de Santé Militaire** founded at **Lyons**

1888:8 **American Association of Anatomists** organized **(Baltimore)**

1888:9 **Australasian Association for the Advancement of Science (Sydney)** organized

1888:10 **Sulphonal** introduced into clinical use by Alfred Kast (1856–1903), *BKW* **25**:309 *1884*

1888:11 Congenital hypertrophic **pyloric stenosis** established as a distinct clinical entity by Harald Hirschsprung (1830–1916), *JaK* **28**:61. *3489.1*

1888:12 The '**Champetier de Ribes bag**', used for dilating the neck of the **uterus**, introduced by Camille Louis Antoine Champetier de Ribes (1848–1935), *AnGO* **30**:401. *6198*

1888:13 The individuality of **chromosomes** demonstrated by Theodor Boveri (1862–1915), *JZN* **22**:685. *231.1*

1888:14 Modern **keratoplasty** is based on the technique introduced by Arthur von Hippel (1841–1917), *GAO* **34**, i:108. *5933*

1888:15 The first pathogenic aerobic **actinomycete** to be described noted by Edmond Isidore Etienne Nocard (1850–1903), *AnIP* **2**:293, and was later named *Nocardia farcinica*. *5512.1*

1888:16 The work of Loeffler on *Corynebacterium diphtheriae* confirmed by Pierre Paul Emile Roux (1853–1933) and Alexandre Emile Jean Yersin (1863–1943), who demonstrated the exotoxin in **diphtheria**, *AnIP* **2**:629; **3**:273; **4**:385. Their work marks the starting point of the development of an immunizing serum. *5059*

1888:17 The **dysentery** bacillus, *Shigella*, isolated by André Chantemesse (1851–1919) and Georges Fernand Isidor Widal (1862–1929), *BuAM* **19**:522, although they did not establish its aetiological relationship to bacillary dysentery. They also carried out experimental **anti-typhoid** inoculation, *AnIP* **2**:54. *5090.1, 5034*

1888:18 First successful operation for removal of an extramedullary **tumour** of the **spinal cord** recorded by William Richard Gowers (1845–1915) and Victor Alexander Haden Horsley (1857–1916) – the founder of **neurosurgery** in England, *MCT* **71**:377. *4860*

1888:19 **Astasia-abasia** ('**Blocq's disease**') described by Paul Blocq (1860–1896), *ArN* **15**:24, 187. *4573*

1888:20 The first complete description of **syringomyelia** given by Otto Kahler (1849–1893), *PMW* **13**:45, 63. *4706*

1888:21 *Salmonella typhi* first demonstrated in the gallbladder in cases of **typhoid** by Bernhard Anton and Gustav Fütterer (1854–1922), *MMW* **35**:315. *5033*

1888:22 The term **osteochondritis dissecans** introduced by Franz König (1832–1910), *DZC* **27**:90. *4350*

1888:23 **Pyelitis** due to vesical and faecal **fistulae** treated by ureteral catheterization through vesico-vaginal cystotomy by Nathan Bozeman (1825–1905), *AmJMS* **95**:255, 368. *4221*

1888:24 **Folliculitis decalvans** described by Charles Eugène Quinquaud (1841–1894), *RCSL* **9**:17. *4094*

1888:25 Suprapubic **prostatectomy** recorded by Arthur Ferguson McGill (1846–1890), *TCSL* **21**:52; the operation was pioneered by him and he first performed it in 1887. *4262.1*

1888:26 **Adiposis dolorosa** ('**Dercum's disease**') first described by Francis Xavier Dercum (1856–1931), *UMM* **1**:140. *3917*

1888:27 **Bard-Pic syndrome**, a complication of **pancreatic carcinoma**, described by Louis Bard (1857–1930) and Adrien Pic (b.1862), *ReM* **8**:257, 363. *3630*

1888:28 An important operative procedure for complete **rectal prolapse** described by Johann von Mikulicz-Radecki (1850–1905), *VDGC* **17**:294. *3493*

1888:29 **Giant hypertrophic gastritis** ('**Menetrier's disease**') described by Pierre Eugène Menetrier (1859–1935), *ArPhy* **20**:32, 236. *3492.1*

1888:30 The first successful **colostomy** carried out by Karel Maydl (1853–1913), *ZCh* **15**:433. *3492*

1888:31 A test for detection of **intestinal perforation** by the **rectal insufflation** of hydrogen introduced by Nicholas Senn (1844–1908), *JAMA* **10**:767. *3494*

1888:32 Radical **mastoidectomy** developed by Ernst von Bergmann (1836–1907), *BKW* **25**:1054. *3391*

1888:33 **Idiopathic steatorrhoea** (nontropical **sprue, coeliac disease**) first described by Samuel Jones Gee (1839–1911); a more extensive study by Thorald Einar Hess Thaysen, in 1929, led to the eponym '**Gee-Thaysen disease**', *SBHR* **24**:17. *3491, 3550*

1888:34 Artificial **pneumothorax** induced in **pulmonary tuberculosis** by Carlo Forlanini (1847–1918), *GOC* **3**:537, 585, 601, 609, 617, 625, 641, 657, 665, 689, 705. *3225*

1888:35 First **aneurysmorrhaphy** performed by Rudolph Matas (1860–1957), *MN* **53**:462. *2985*

1888:36 **Aplastic anaemia** first distinguished by Paul Ehrlich (1854–1915), *Charité-Ann* **13**:300. *3129*

1888:37 **Fallot's tetralogy**, a form of **congenital heart disease** described by Etienne Louis Arthur Fallot (1850–1911), *MM* **25**:77, 138, 207, 270, 341, 403. *2792*

1888:38 *Salmonella enteritidis* (**Gaertner's bacillus**) discovered by August Gaertner (1848–1934), *KAAV* **17**:573. *2506*

1888:39 **Graham Steell murmur**, the **pulmonary diastolic murmur**, first described by Graham Steell (1851–1942), *MCh* **9**:182. *2794*

1888:40 **Bactericidal** action of **blood** ('natural **immunity**') described by George Henry Falkiner Nuttall (1862–1937), *ZHyg* **4**:353. *2542*

1888:41 **Visual centre** located in the cerebral cortex by Salomon Eberhard Henschen (1847–1930), *ULF* **27**:507, 601. *1521*

1888:42 '**Riedel's lobe of the liver**' described by Bernhard Moritz Carl Ludwig Riedel (1846–1916), *BKW* **25**:577, 602. *3631*

1888:43 **Silk sutures** introduced by Emil Theodor Kocher (1841–1917), *CBSA* **18**:3. *5619.1*

1888:44 Studies on **developmental mechanics** ('Entwicklungsmechanik') initiated by Wilhelm Roux (1850–1924), *VA* **114**:113, 246. *505*

---

1888:45 Michael **Heidelberger**, American immunochemist, born 29 Apr; with Walter James Jacobs introduced tryparsamide in the treatment of trypanosome infections, 1919, *JEM* **30**:411; with Oswald Theodor Avery, elucidated the antigenic structure of pneumococcus, 1923, *JEM* **38**:73; with Forrest E. Kendall, introduced quantitative precipitin reaction, 1929, *JEM* **50**:809. Died 1991. *1907, 2573.2, 3198, 2576.01*

1888:46 Rudolph **Schindler**, German gastroenterologist, born 10 May; made gastroscopy a 'method'; his first important work appeared in 1922, *ArV* **69**:535; introduced the flexible gastroscope, 1932, *MMW* **79**:1268. Died 1968. *3545, 3553*

1888:47 Friedrich **Breinl**, German immunologist, born 26 May; with Felix Haurowitz, proposed template or instruction theory of antibody formation, 1930, *HSZ* **192**:45. *2576.1*

1888:48 Herbert Spencer **Gasser**, physiologist, born 5 Jul; with Joseph Erlanger, devised means for use of cathode ray oscillograph for transmission of impulses through single nerve fibres, 1924, *AmJPh* **70**:624. They shared Nobel Prize (Physiology or Medicine), 1944, *NPL*. Died 1963. *1305*

1888:49 James Frederick **Brailsford**, British radiologist, born 8 Jul; described a form of osteochondrodystrophy, 1929, *AmJMS* **7**:404, similar to that recorded by Morquio in the same year; it was named 'Morquio-Brailsford disease'. Died 1961. *4397.1, 4397*

1888:50 Frits **Zernike**, Dutch physicist, born 16 Jul. For his development of phase contrast microscopy, 1935, *PhZ* **36**:848, he was awarded the Nobel Prize (Physics), 1953, *NPL*. Died 1966. *269.5*

1888:51 Louis Hopewell **Bauer**, American medical specialist in aviation medicine, born 18 Jul; published *Aviation medicine*, 1926, which included the first significant bibliography of this subject. Died 1964. *2137.6*

1888:52 Selman Abraham **Waksman**, Russian/American microbiologist, born 22 Jul; with co-workers, discovered streptomycin in 1944, *PSEB* **55**:66, and neomycin in 1949, *Science* **113**:305. Awarded Nobel Prize (Physiology or Medicine), 1952, for his discovery of streptomycin, *NPL*. Died 1973. *1935, 1944*

1888:53 Elliott Carr **Cutler**, American surgeon, born 30 Jul; with James Leavitt Stoddard, first isolated *Torula histolytica*, later found to be identical with *Cryptococcus neoformans*, causal organism in cryptococcosis, 1916, *RIM* 6. With Samuel Albert Levine, successfully carried out mitral valve section for relief of mitral stenosis, 1923, *BMSJ*, **188**:1023. Died 1947. *5537, 3030.1*

1888:54 Hugo **Spatz**, German neurologist, born 12 Sep; with Julius Hallervorden, described a syndrome affecting the extrapyramidal system ('Hallervorden-Spatz syndrome'), 1922, *ZGN* **79**:254. Died 1969. *4724*

1888:55 Clarence Cook **Little**, American geneticist, born 6 Oct; with Ernest Edward Tyzzer, initiated the study of histocompatibility antigens, 1916, *JMR* **33**:393; showed that homograft reaction in tissue transplantation was due to genetic differences between donor and recipient, 1924, *JCR* **8**:75. Died 1971. *2570, 2573.1*

1888:56 Arthur Walter **Proetz**, American otolaryngologist, born 12 Oct; introduced displacement method of treatment of nasal sinusitis, 1926, *ArOt(C)* 4:1. Died 1966. *3325*

1888:57 Oliver **Kamm**, American chemist, born 6 Dec; with co-workers, isolated vasopressin and oxytocin, 1928, *JACS* **50**:573. Died 1965. *1168.1*

———

1888:58 Katharine Scott **Bishop** born; with Herbert McLean Evans, discovered vitamin E, 1922, *Science* **56**:650. Died 1976. *1055*

1888:59 Pleikart **Stumpf**, German radiologist, born; introduced roentgenkymography, 1931, *FGR*, Erg.41. *2696*

398

1888:60 Koichi **Ichikawa** born; with Katsusaburo Yamagiwa, produced cancer experimentally by painting with a tar product, 1916, *VJPJ* **6**:169; **7**:191. Died 1948. *2643*

1888:61 Lucy **Wills**, British physician, born; observed the haemopoietic effect of folic acid, 1931, *BMJ* **1**:1059. Died 1964. *3146*

1888:62 John **Hepburn**, Canadian surgeon, born; with James Arnold Dauphinee, first successful excision of arteriovenous aneurysm of the lung, 1942, *AmJMS* **204**:681. *2992*

1888:63 Ivar Asbjørn **Følling**, Norwegian physician and biochemist, born; first to describe phenylketonuria, the first hereditary metabolic disorder shown to be responsible for mental retardation, 1934, *NoMT* **8**:1054. Died 1973. *3924*

1888:64 Douglas Burrows **Leitch**, Canadian physician, born, with James Bertram Collip, first used a parathyroid hormone ('parathormone') in the treatment of tetany, 1925, *CMAJ* **15**:59. *3862, 4837*

1888:65 Christian **Zoeller** born; with Gaston Léon Ramon, first employed tetanus toxoid in the immunization of humans, 1933, *CRSB* **112**:347. Died 1934. *5151*

1888:66 Arie **Klarenbeek**, Dutch physician, born; with Wilhelm August Paul Schüffner, first isolated *Leptospira canicola* from dog urine, 1933, *NTG* **77**:4271; with C.M. Dhont and Schüffner, first reported leptospirosis in humans due to infection with *Leptospira canicola*, 1934, *NTG* **78**:5297. *5335, 5336*

1888:67 Frederick Edward **Becker** born; first described Colorado tick fever as a separate entity and suggested that it was transmitted by the tick *Dermacentor andersoni*, 1930, *CoM* **27**:36. *5538.3, 5546.1*

1888:68 Hans Christian **Hagedorn**, Danish physician, born; with co-workers, introduced insulin combined with protamine, in order to delay its absorption rate, 1936, *JAMA* **106**:177. Died 1971. *3974*

---

1888: Alfonso **Corti** died, **born** 1822. *cochlea*

1888: Rudolph **Maier** died, **born** 1824. *periarteritis nodosa*

1888: Thomas Blizard **Curling** died, **born** 1811. *duodenal ulcer, burns, cretinism, myxoedema*

1888: Ernst Leberecht **Wagner** died, **born** 1829. *dermatomyositis, colloid milium, cancer of uterus*

1888: Paul **Langerhans** died, **born** 1847. *pancreatic islets of Langerhans*

1888: Léon **Bassereau** died, **born** 1811. *chancroid*

1888: Alois **Bednar** died, **born** 1816. *aphthae of palate*

1888: Valentine H. **Taliaferro** died, **born** 1831. *episiotomy*

**1889**

1889:1 **Johns Hopkins Hospital** founded at **Baltimore**

1889:2 **Hamburg-Eppendorf Hospital** founded

1889:3 **University of Fribourg, Switzerland**, founded

1889:4 The '**Walcher position**' described by the German **gynaecologist**, Gustav Adolf Walcher (1856–1935), *ZGy* **13**:892. *6200*

1889:5 Epidemic **keratoconjunctivitis** first described by Ernst Fuchs (1851–1930, *WKW* **2**:837. *5934*

1889:6 Some accredit Emil Pfeiffer (1846–1921) with the first description of **infectious mononucleosis** ('**Pfeiffer's disease**'), *JaK* **29**:257. *5486*

1889:7 Francis Galton (1822–1911), founder of the science of **eugenics**, published *Natural inheritance*. *233*

1889:8 **Complement (alexin)** discovered by Hans Ernst Buchner (1850–1902), *ZBP* **6**:561. *2543*

1889:9 The difference between the parasites of tertian and quartan **malaria** described by Camillo Golgi (1843–1926), *ArSM* **13**:173. *5240*

1889:10 A bibliography of the literature on **venereal disease** from the end of the 16th century to 1900 provided by Johann Karl Proksch's (1840–1923) *Die Litteratur über die venerischen Krankheiten von der ersten Schriften über Syphilis aus dem Ende des fünfzehnten Jahrhunderts bis zum Jahre 1889. (Suppl. Bd. 1: Enthalt die Litteratur von 1889–1900 und Nachträge aus früherer Zeit)*, 5 vols. *5226*

1889:11 *Haemophilus ducreyi* ('**Ducrey's bacillus**'), causal organism in **chancroid** discovered by Augusto Ducrey (1860–1940), *GilSM* **11**:44. *5205*

1889:12 An **osteoplastic flap operation**, making a large area of the **brain** more easily accessible than by trephining, devised by Wilhelm Wagner (1848–1900), *ZCh* **16**:833. *4862*

1889:13 A pure culture of the **tetanus** bacillus, *Clostridium tetani*, first obtained by Shibasaburo Kitasato (1852–1931), *ZHyg* **7**:225. *5149*

1889:14 The first attempt at surgical treatment of **epilepsy** by William Alexander (1844–1919), he removed the superior sympathetic ganglia; in his *Treatment of epilepsy*. *4861*

1889:15 '**Benedikt's syndrome**', **paralysis** of the **oculomotor nerve** on one side with intense trembling on the other side, described by Moritz Benedikt (1835–1920), *BuM* **3**:547. *4576*

1889:16 Posterior **rhizotomy** (surgical division of a **nerve root**) performed by Robert Abbe (1851–1928), *MR* **35**:149, and, in the same year, by William Henry Bennett (1852–1931), *MCT* **72**:329. *4860.1, 4861.1*

1889: 17 In his *Sur l'atrophie musculaire des ataxiques*, Joseph Jules Dejerine (1849–1917) described **tabetic muscular atrophies** and separated peripheral from medullary **tabes**. *4785*

1889: 18 Medial perineal **prostatectomy** carried out by Francis Sedgwick Watson (1853–1942) – reported in 1905, *AnS* **41**:507. *4266*

1889: 19 '**Ollier's disease**', **multiple enchondromatosis**, first described by Louis Xavier Edouard Leopold Ollier (1830–1900), *MSML* **29**, 2:12. *4352*

1889: 20 The first **enterocystoplasty** carried out by Johann von Mikulicz-Radecki (1850–1905), *ZCh* **26**:641. *4183.1, 4087*

1889: 21 A suppurative form of **pemphigus vegetans** described by François Henri Hallopeau (1842–1919), *CRDS*, p. 344. *4101*

1889: 22 **Pseudoxanthoma elasticum** described by Anatole Marie Emile Chauffard (1855–1932), *BSMH* **6**:412. *4096.1*

1889: 23 **Sarcoidosis**. J. Hutchinson first described this condition in 1875. Ernest Besnier's (1831–1909) description in 1889, *AnD* **10**:333, was followed in 1899 by Boeck's classical account, and Schaumann's further account, by which the systemic nature of sarcoidosis was recognized, 1917, led to the eponym '**Besnier-Boeck-Schaumann disease**'. *4067, 4095, 4128, 4149*

1889: 24 **Duodenal aspiration** introduced by Ismar Isidor Boas (1858–1938), *ZenKM* **10**:97. *3496*

1889: 25 The modern operation (**Halsted I repair**) for the radical cure of **inguinal hernia** devised, almost simultaneously with Edoardo Bassini, by William Stewart Halsted (1852–1922), *JHB* **1**:12, 112. *3599*

1889: 26 **Gastrodiaphany** – tubal exploration of the **stomach** – devised by Max Einhorn (1862–1953), *NYMM* **1**:559. *3495*

1889: 27 Operation for abscess of the **maxillary sinus** devised by Henri Luc (1855–1925); in his *Des abscès du sinus maxillaire*. *3301*

1889: 28 Radical **mastoidectomy** developed by Ernst Georg Ferdinand von Küster (1839–1930), *DMW* **15**:254. *3392*

1889: 29 **McBurney's point** in **appendicitis** defined by Charles McBurney (1845–1913), *NYMJ* **50**:676. *3570*

1889: 30 First **laryngeal** operation through the mouth with external illumination performed by Friedrich Eduard Rudolph Voltolini (1819–1889), *DMW* **15**:340. *3302*

1889: 31 Classic description of **infantile pseudoleukaemic anaemia** by Rudolph von Jaksch (1855–1947) led to the term '**von Jaksch's disease**', *WKW* **2**:435, 456. *3131*

1889: 32 An important account of **chlorosis** given by Georges Hayem (1841–1933); in his *Du sang et ses altérations anatomiques*, p. 614. *3130*

1889:33 **Empyema** treated by **thoracotomy** by Ernst Georg Ferdinand von Küster (1839–1930), *DMW* **15**:185. *3177*

1889:34 **Syphilis: bismuth** in treatment suggested by Felix Balzer (1849–1929), *CRSB* **1**:537. *2394*

1889:35 **Air sphygmomanometer** introduced by Pierre Carl Édouard Potain (1825–1901), *ArPhy* **1**:556. *2798*

1889:36 **Pyocyanase**, an antibiotic, prepared from *Pseudomonas pyocyanea* by Rudolph Emmerich (1852–1914) and Oscar Löw (b.1844), *ZHyg* **31**:1. *1932.2*

1889:37 **Cancer** successfully transplanted in mammals by Arthur Nathan Hanau (1858–1900), *FM* **7**:321. *2621*

1889:38 **Van Gieson's acid fuchsin** and **picric acid stain** for nerve tissue introduced by Ira Van Gieson (1866–1913), *NYJM* **1**:57. *1419.1*

1889:39 **Keratosis follicularis (dyskeratosis)**, so well described by Jean Darier (1856–1938), *AnD* **10**:597, is also known as **Darier's disease**; it was first described by Lutz and later by J.C. White. *4050, 4093, 4097*

---

1889:40 Colin Blackman **Bridges**, American geneticist, born 11 Jan; published *The mechanism of Mendelian heredity*, 1915, recording epoch-making work on heredity, with Thomas Hunt Morgan, Alfred Henry Sturtevant, and Hermann Joseph Muller. Died 1938. *246*

1889:41 Hulüsi **Behçet**, Turkish dermatologist, born 20 Feb; his description of Behçet's syndrome, 1937, *DeW* **105**:1152, was preceded by that of H. Planner and F. Remenovsky (1922). Died 1948. *6374*

1889:42 William Kelsey **Fry**, British physician and dental surgeon, born 18 Mar; with Harold Delf Gillies, introduced a new operation for the repair of cleft palate, 1921, *BMJ* **1**:335. Died 1963. *5759*

1889:43 Rudolph Albert **Peters**, British biochemist, born 13 Apr; with co-workers he developed dimercaprol, British anti-lewisite (BAL), a heavy metal antagonist, 1945, *Nature* **156**:616. Died 1982. *1929*

1889:44 Paul **Karrer**, Russian/Swiss chemist, born 21 Apr; with colleagues, synthesized vitamin E (α-tocopherol, 1938, *HCA* **21**:520. Shared Nobel Prize (Chemistry), 1937, with Walter Norman Haworth, for his researches into the constitution of carotenoids, flavonoids and vitamins, *NPL*. Died 1971. *1079*

1889:45 Frank Alexander **Evans**, American physician, born 23 Apr; with Thomas Peck Sprunt, introduced the term 'infectious mononucleosis'; in their classic account of the condition, 1920, *BJH* **31**:410. *5486.1*

1889:46 Walter **Georgi**, German serologist, born 24 Apr; with Hans Sachs, introduced the Sachs-Georgi reaction for diagnosis of syphilis, 1919, *MMW* **66**:440. Died 1920. *2408*

1889:47 Eli Kennerly **Marshall**, American physiologist and pharmacologist, born 2 May; with colleagues introduced sulphaguanidine, 1940, *BJH* **67**:163; with co-workers, used it in the treatment of bacillary dysentery, 1941, *JHB* **68**:94. Died 1966. *1954, 5096*

1889:48 Willem Frederik **Donath**, Dutch nutritionist, born 25 Jun; with Barend Coenraad Petrus Jansen, isolated vitamin B$_1$ (aneurine, thiamine) in crystalline form, lack of which causes beriberi, 1926, *CW* **23**:201, 1387. Died 1957. *1058, 3746*

1889:49 Kenneth Fuller **Maxcy**, American epidemiologist, born 27 Jul; described murine (flea-borne) typhus, 1926, *USPHR* **41**:1213, 2967. Died 1966. *5396*

1889:50 Vern Rheem **Mason**, American physician, born 8 Aug; gave sickle-cell anaemia its present name, 1922, *JAMA* **79**:1318. *3136.1*

1889:51 Jean **Oliver**, American pathologist, born 19 Aug; with co-workers, published an important account of the pathogenesis of acute kidney failure, 1951, *JCI* **30**:1305. Died 1976. *4256.11*

1889:52 Alan Churchill **Woods**, American ophthalmologist, born 20 Aug; used an intradermal pigment test in the diagnosis and treatment of sympathetic ophthalmia, 1925, *TOUK* **45**:208. Died 1963. *5969*

1889:53 Robert Benedict **Bourdillon**, British scientist, born 8 Sep; isolated calciferol from irradiated ergosterol; *The quantitative estimation of vitamin D by radiography*, 1931. Died 1971. *1065*

1889:54 Arvid Johann **Wallgren**, Swedish physician, born 5 Oct; first to describe lymphocytic choriomeningitis, 1824, *AcP* **4**:158. Died 1973. *4687*

1889:55 Robert James **Minnitt**, British anaesthetist, born 25 Oct; introduced an apparatus for the self-administration of gas-air analgesia in labour (the 'Minnitt apparatus'), 1934, *L* **1**:1278. Died 1974. *6228*

1889:56 Edgar Douglas **Adrian**, British physiologist, born 30 Nov. With Y. Zotterman, observed response of single sensory end organs to natural stimuli, 1926, *JP* **61**:151; published *The basis of sensation. The action of the sense organs*, 1928; shared Nobel Prize (Physiology or Medicine), 1932, with Charles Scott Sherrington, for the isolation and functional analysis of the motor cell in the spinal cord, *NPL*. Died 1977. *1307, 1308*

1889:57 George Washington **Corner**, American anatomist and embryologist, born 12 Dec; with Willard Myron Allen discovered progesterone, 1929, *AmJPh* **88**:326. Died 1981. *1188*

1889:58 John Alfred **Ryle**, British physician, born 12 Dec; devised 'Ryle's tube' for obtaining specimens of gastric juice, 1921, *GHR* **71**:42. Died 1950. *3544*

1889:59 Sewall **Wright**, American geneticist, born 21 Dec; advanced quantitative theory of the effect of mutation, migration, selection and population size on changes in gene frequencies in populations, 1931, *Genetics* **16**:97. Died 1988. *253.1*

---

1889:60 John Friend **Mahoney**, American physician, born; with colleagues, introduced penicillin in the treatment of syphilis, 1943, *VDI* **24**:355; *AmJPu* **33**:1387. Died 1957. *2418*

1889:61 Arthur Baker **LeMesurier**, Canadian surgeon, born; with William Edward Gallie, used fascial suture in the repair of inguinal hernia, 1923, *CMAJ* **13**:469. *3609*

1889:62 Julius Leo **Spivack**, German surgeon, born; introduced tubo-valvular gastrostomy, 1929, *BKC* **147**:308. Died 1956. *3549*

1889:63 Poul **Iverson**, Danish physician, born; with Kaj Roholm, introduced the modern method of aspiration biopsy of the liver, 1939, *AcM* **102**:1. *3664*

1889:64 Francis Eugene **Senear**, American dermatologist, born; with Barney David Usher, first noted pemphigus erythematodes ('Senear-Usher syndrome'), 1926, *ArDS* **13**:761. *4151.2*

1889:65 Karl Eitel Friedrich **Schmitz**, German hygienist, born; isolated *Shigella schmitzi*, a cause of bacillary dysentery, 1917, *ZHyg* **84**:449. *5095*

1889:66 Willy **Charlton**, German physician, born; with Werner Schultz, introduced the Schultz-Charlton reaction for the diagnosis of scarlet fever, 1918, *ZK* **17**:328. *5081*

1889:67 Benjamin Harrison **Lamb** born; with William Buchanan Wherry, first isolated *Pasteurella tularensis*, causal organism of tularaemia, from lesions in humans, 1914, *JID* **15**:331. *5175*

1889:68 Foster Matthew **Johns** born; with Charles Cassidy Bass, cultivated the malaria parasites, *Plasmodium vivax* and *P.falciparum*, *in vitro*, 1912, *JEM* **16**:567. *5255.1*

1889:69 Robert Davies **Defries**, American physician, born; with Neil E. McKinnon, introduced a diagnostic test for smallpox, 1928, *AmJH* **8**:93. *5434*

1889:70 James Leavitt **Stoddard**, American pathologist, born; with Elliott Carr Cutler, first isolated *Torula histolytica*, later found to be identical with *Cryptococcus neoformans*, causal organism in cryptococcosis, 1916, *RIM* 6. *5537*

1889:71 Fritz **Eichholtz**, German physician, born; first to use avertin (tribromethanol) experimentally as an anaesthetic, 1927, *DMW* **53**:710. It was used clinically by O. Butzinger in the same year. *5708, 5709*

1889:72 Jay Bailey **Carter**, American anaesthetist, born; with Arno Benedict Luckhardt, introduced ethylene as an anaesthetic, 1923, *JAMA* **80**:765. *5705*

---

1889: Ivar Victor **Sandström** died, **born** 1852. *parathyroid glands, cancer of rectum*

1889: Friedrich Eduard Rudolph **Voltolini** died, **born** 1819. *larynx, galvanocautery*

1889: Richard von **Volkmann** died, **born** 1830. *industrial cancer, Volkmann's ischaemic contracture*

1889: Philippe **Ricord** died, **born** 1800. *syphilis, gonorrhoea*

1889: George Owen **Rees** died, **born** 1813. *bacterial endocarditis*

1889: Pietro **Loreta** died, **born** 1831. *pyloroplasty*

1889: Michel Eugène **Chevreul** died, **born** 1786. *diabetes, cholesterol*

1889: Robert **Paterson** died, **born** 1814. *molluscum contagiosum*

1889: Samuel Weissel **Gross** died, **born** 1837. *bone sarcoma*

1889: Frans Cornelis **Donders** died, **born** 1818. *eye anomalies, eye rotation, astigmatism, psychical processes*

1889: Pierre Cyprien **Oré** died, **born** 1828. *intravenous anaesthesia*

1889: August **Breisky** died, **born** 1832. *kraurosis vulvae*

**1890**
1890:1 **University of Lausanne** founded, formerly **Académie**, 1537

1890:2 [**Imperial (State) Institute of Experimental Medicine**] founded at **St Petersburg**

1890:3 [**Czech Academy of Sciences and Arts**] founded at **Prague**

1890:4 **Institut Pasteur** established at **Saigon**

1890:5 **Biological Laboratory** established at **Cold Spring Harbor**, Long Island

1890:6 [**Dermatological Society**], **Vienna**, founded

1890:7 [**German Pharmaceutical Society**] founded at **Berlin**

1890:8 **Royal College of Physicians of Ireland** (1667) revived

1890:9 In a paper on the repair of **vesico-vaginal fistula**, Friedrich Trendelenburg (1844–1899) described an elevated pelvic position ('**Trendelenburg position**), *SKV* **355**:3372, first described by his pupil, W. Meyer, in 1885, *ArKC* **31**:494; Trendelenburg's paper also included the first recorded surgical intervention for the relief of **hydronephrosis**. *6091, 4222*

1890:10 William Stewart Halsted's (1852–1922) method of radical **mastectomy** was one of the greatest contributions to the treatment of **breast cancer**, *JHR* **2**:255; **4**:297. *5776*

1890:11 **Caesarean section** in cases of **placenta praevia** ('**Tait-Porro operation**') performed by Robert Lawson Tait (1845–1899), *BMJ* **1**:657. *6245*

1890:12 *Actinomyces graminis* isolated from human **actinomycosis** by Eugen Bostroem (1850–1928), *BPA* **9**:1, who introduced a staining method for *Actinomyces*. *5513*

1890:13 **Conduction anaesthesia** as performed by Maximilian Oberst (1849–1925) first recorded by his pupil Ludwig Pernice, *DMW* **16**:287. *5681*

1890:14 The founder of the American school of **experimental psychology** was William James (1842–1910); he wrote *The principles of psychology. 4977.2*

1890: 15 In his studies on **malaria**, Pietro Canalis (1856–1939) demonstrated and clearly differentiated *Plasmodium falciparum* from *P.vivax* and *P.malariae*, ArIB **13**:262. *5240.1*

1890: 16 **Gasserian ganglionectomy** for **trigeminal neuralgia**, suggested by Mears (1884), carried out by William Rose (1847–1910), L **2**:914. *4863*

1890: 17 Artificial immunity to **diphtheria** in guinea-pigs produced by Carl Fraenkel (1861–1915) by the injection of attenuated cultures of *Corynebacterium diphtheriae*, BKW **27**:1133. *5060.1*

1890: 18 **Antitoxins** and their **immunizing** power discovered by Emil Adolf von Behring (1854–1917) and Shibasaburo Kitasato (1852–1931) through their work on **diphtheria** and **tetanus** immunity, DMW **16**:1113, 1145; they laid the foundation of all future treatment with antitoxins. *2544, 5060*

1890: 19 'Bastian's law' (transverse lesion of the **spinal cord** above the lumbar enlargement results in abolition of the **tendon reflexes** of the lower extremities) propounded by Henry Charlton Bastian (1837–1915), MCT **73**:151. *4577*

1890: 20 **Dystrophia myotonica** ('Déléage's disease') first described by Francisque Déléage (b.1862); in his inaugural thesis *Étude clinique de la maladie de Thomsen*. *4754*

1890: 21 The epidemic character of **poliomyelitis** first noted by Oskar Medin (1847–1927), *Hygiea* **52**:657; the disease is also known as 'Heine-Medin disease'. *4667, 4664*

1890: 22 **Acanthosis nigricans** first illustrated by Sigmund Pollitzer (1859–1937) and Viktor Janovsky (1847–1925); in their *Atlas seltener Hautkrankheiten*; it was described by Darier in 1893. *4102, 4113*

1890: 23 *The micro-organisms of the human mouth* by Willoughby Dayton Miller (1853–1907) made an important contribution to the knowledge of the effect of bacteria on the **teeth**. *3687*

1890: 24 The first **thyroid transplantation** (for the treatment of **cretinism**) carried out by Odilon Marc Lannelongue (1840–1911), BuM **4**:225. *3837*

1890: 25 Joseph von Mering (1849–1908) and Oscar Minkowski (1858–1931) produced experimental **diabetes mellitus** by removing the **pancreas** of a dog, proving the role of the pancreas in diabetes, ArEP **26**:371. *3950*

1890: 26 The operation of excision of the **auditory ossicles** introduced by Ludwig Stacke (1859–1918), IMC **4**, xi Abt.:3. *3393*

1890: 27 **Varicose veins** treated by ligation of great **saphenous vein** ('Trendelenburg's operation') by Friedrich Trendelenburg (1844–1924), BKC **7**:195. *2997*

1890: 28 First clear account of **bone-marrow** changes in **pernicious anaemia** given by Georg Eduard Rindfleisch (1836–1908), VA **121**:176. *3131.1*

1890:29 **Tuberculin** introduced by Robert Koch (1843–1910) in the treatment of **tuberculosis**, and his skin test for tuberculosis and the resulting inflammatory reaction ('**Koch's phenomenon**') described by him, *DMW* **16**:1029, (1891); **17**:101, 1189. *2332, 2544.1*

1890:30 *English sanitary institutions* published by John Simon (1816–1904). *1650*

1890:31 **Strophanthus hispidus** introduced by Thomas Richard Fraser (1841–1919), *TRSE* **35**:955; **36**:343. *1885*

1890:32 '**Pick's bundle**', fibres of the pyramidal tract of the medulla oblongata, described by Arnold Pick (1851–1924), *ArPN* **21**:636. *1420*

1890:33 **Indefatigability of nerve** ('Bowditch's law') demonstrated by Henry Pickering Bowditch (1840–1911), *ArA* 505. *1282*

1890:34 **Psychogalvanic reflex** described by Ivan Romanovich Tarchanoff (1848–1909), *PfA* **46**:46. *1471*

1890:35 The theory of '**tropisms**', as the basis of the **psychology** of lower forms of life, founded by Jacques Loeb (1859–1924); *Der Heliotropismus der Tiere*. *125*

---

1890:36 Porter Paisley **Vinson**, American physician, born 24 Jan; reported a case of cardiospasm with oesophageal dilatation, 1919, *MCNA* **3**:623; a condition already noted by Henry Stanley Plummer (1912) and named '**Plummer-Vinson syndrome**'. Died 1959. *3321*

1890:37 Grantly **Dick-Read**, British obstetrician, born 26 Jan; advocated natural childbirth and demonstrated that prenatal education in methods of relaxation in many cases makes labour almost painless. He wrote *Natural childbirth*, 1933. Died 1959. *6225*

1890:38 Ronald Aylmer **Fisher**, British statistician, born 17 Feb; laid the foundations for biometric genetics, *The genetical theory of natural selection*. Died 1962. *253*

1890:39 Harry **Plotz**, American bacteriologist, born 17 Apr; cultivated the measles virus, 1938, *BuAM* **119**:598. Died 1947. *5449*

1890:40 Henry Patrick **Wagener**, American ophthalmologist, born 3 Jun; with Norman Macdonnell Keith and N.W. Barker, devised the Keith-Wagener-Barker classification of essential hypertension, 1929, *AmJMS* **197**:332, 1939, *Medicine* **18**:317. Died 1961. *2716, 2723*

1890:41 James Stevens **Simmons**, American physician, born 7 Jun; with co-workers, showed that *Aëdes albopictus* is a vector of dengue, 1931, *PhJS* **41**:215. Died 1954. *5475*

1890:42 Jules Thomas **Freund**, Hungarian/American immunologist, born 24 Jun; with Katherine McDermott, introduced Freund's adjuvant for use with antigens, 1942, *PSEB* **49**:548. Died 1960. *2578.1*

1890:43 Everitt George Dunne **Murray**, Canadian bacteriologist, born 21 Jul; with R.A. Webb and M.B.R. Swann isolated *Listeria monocytogenes*, 1926, *JPB* **29**:407. Died 1964. *2522.1*

1890:44 Jay **McLean**, American physician and oncologist, born 13 Aug; extracted what was later named heparin from dog liver, 1916, *AmJPh* **41**:250. Died 1957. *904*

1890:45 Pearl L. **Kendrick**, American bacteriologist and immunologist, born 24 Aug; with Grace Eldering, introduced a pertussis vaccine for immunization against whooping cough, 1939, *AmJH* **29B**:138. *5087.2*

1890:46 Frank Norman **Wilson**, American cardiologist, born 19 Nov; with co-workers, introduced unipolar leads into electrocardiography, 1934, *AmHJ* **9**:447. Died 1952. *2864*

1890:47 Hermann Joseph **Muller**, American geneticist, born 31 Dec; published *The mechanism of Mendelian heredity*, 1915, recording epoch-making work on heredity, with Thomas Hunt Morgan, Alfred Henry Sturtevant, and Colin Blackman Bridges. Awarded the Nobel Prize (Physiology or Medicine), 1946, for his work on the artificial transmutation of the gene by irradiation (1927, *Science* **66**:84), *NPL*. Died 1967. *246*

1890:48 Jacques **Forestier**, French physician, born; with Jean Athanase Sicard, introduced lipiodol as an opaque medium in radiography, positive contrast myelography with iodised oil, 1921, *ReN* **28**:1264, and greatly advanced bronchography, 1924, *JMF* **13**:3; introduced gold therapy in chronic rheumatism, 1929, *BSMH* p. 323. *2693, 4605, 3199, 4506.1*

1890:49 Carl Pauly **Seyfarth**, German physician, born; introduced the method of bone marrow biopsy by sternal puncture, 1923, *DMW* **49**:180. *3087*

1890:50 Randolph **West**, American physician, born; demonstrated the effectiveness of vitamin $B_{12}$ in treatment of pernicious anaemia, 1948, *Science* **107**:398. *3154*

1890:51 Erwin Rudolph **Schmidt** born; with Ralph Milton Waters, introduced the closed-circuit method of using cyclopropane anaesthesia, 1934, *JAMA* **103**:975. *5718*

1890:52 Thomas Orville **Menees**, American radiologist, born; with J.D. Miller and L.E. Holly, introduced amniography, 1930, *AmJR* **24**:363. Died 1937. *6223*

1890:53 George Henry **Hansmann**, American pathologist, born; with John Rudolph Schenken, cultivated *Histoplasma capsulatum*, 1933, *Science* **77** (No. 2002) Suppl. p. 8, 1934, *AmJPa* **10**:731. Almost simultaneously it was cultivated by DeMonbreun. *5541.2, 5542*

1890: Wenzel Leopold **Gruber** died, **born** 1814. *mesogastric hernia*

1890: Anton Friedrich von **Tröltsch** died, **born** 1829. *otoscope, mastoid operation*

1890: William Withey **Gull** died, **born** 1816. *myxoedema, kidney atrophy, nephrosclerosis, tabes dorsalis, syringomyelia, anorexia nervosa*

1890: Edwin **Chadwick** died, **born** 1800. *public health*

1890: Arthur Ferguson **McGill** died, **born** 1846. *prostatectomy*

1890: Henry Jacob **Bigelow** died, **born** 1818. *excision of hip-joint, litholapaxy, ileo-femoral ligament, anaesthesia, ether*

1890: Carl Friedrich Otto **Westphal** died, **born** 1833. *tabes dorsalis, knee-jerk, agoraphobia, cerebrospinal pseudosclerosis*

1890: Carl Conrad Theodor **Litzmann** died, **born** 1815. *pelvic deformities*

1890: James Matthews **Duncan** died, **born** 1826. *Duncan's folds*

**1891**
1891:1 [**Institute for Infectious Diseases**], **Berlin**, opened under Robert **Koch**

1891:2 **British Institute of Preventive Medicine, London**, founded; renamed **Jenner Institute of Preventive Medicine**, (1898–1903), and finally **Lister Institute of Preventive Medicine**

1891:3 **US Hygienic Laboratory** established at **Washington**

1891:4 **Instituto de Oftalmologia** established at **Lisbon**

1891:5 **Institut Pasteur, Saigon**, opened, 8 Jan

1891:6 **Stanford University, California**, founded

1891:7 **Association of American Medical Colleges**, founded at **Chicago**

1891:8 **University of Texas Dept of Medicine** founded at **Galveston**

1891:9 The **lantern test** for **colour-blindness** described by Frederick William Edridge-Green (1863–1953), in his *Colour-blindness and colour-perception*, p. 262, was adopted in Great Britain in 1915 in place of the Holmgren test. *5937*

1891:10 *Actinomyces bovis* isolated by Max Wolff (1844–1923) and James Israel (1848–1926), *VA* **126**:11. *5514*

1891:11 **Nocardiosis** first reported by Hans Eppinger (1846–1916) who isolated *Nocardia asteroides* from a patient with **pseudotuberculosis**, *BPA* 9:287. *5513.1*

1891:12 The **Romanovsky stain** for the demonstration of the **malaria** parasite in blood films introduced by Dmitriy Leonidovich Romanovsky (1861–1921); in his *Parasitology and treatment of malarial fever* [in Russian]. *5242*

1891:13 The demonstration that **methylene blue** is lethal *in vitro* for the **malaria** parasite, by Paul Guttmann and Paul Ehrlich (1854–1915), marks the beginning of Ehrlich's work on **chemotherapy**, *BKW* **28**:953. *5241.1*

1891:14 William Williams Keen (1837–1932) was a pioneer in linear **craniotomy**, and reported a new operation for spasmodic **torticollis**, *AmJMS* **101**:549; *AnS* **13**:44. *4866, 4867*

1891:15 The **mallein reaction** for the diagnosis of **glanders** introduced by Victor Babès (1854–1926), *ArMEA* **3**:619. *5158*

1891:16 **Frontal lobotomy** performed on four patients by G. Burckhardt, *AZP* **47**:463. *4864*

1891:17 **Lumbar puncture** for the relief of fluid pressure first performed by Walter Essex Wynter (1860–1945), *L* 1:981. *4868*

1891:18 **Lumbar puncture** introduced, independently of Wynter, by Heinrich Irenaeus Quincke (1842–1922), using it for both diagnostic and therapeutic purposes, *BKW* **28**:929. *4869, 4868*

1891:19 **Familial myoclonus epilepsy** ('**Unverricht's disease**') first described by Heinrich Unverricht (1853–1912); in his *Die Myoclonie. 4819*

1891:20 The term **amoebic dysentery** introduced by William Thomas Councilman (1854–1933) and Henri Amadée Lafleur (1863–1939) in their important investigation of the condition, *JHR* **2**:395. *5187*

1891:21 Acute **ataxia** ('**Leyden's ataxia**') described by Ernst von Leyden (1832–1910), *ZKM* **18**:576. *4706.1*

1891:22 An infantile familial form of **progressive muscular atrophy** described by Guido Werdnig (b.1862), *ArPN* **22**:437, and independently noted in the same year by Johann Hoffmann (1857–1919), *DZN* **1**:95; **3**:427, and named ('**Werdnig-Hoffmann muscular atrophy**'). *4755, 4756*

1891:23 In his *Zur Auffassung der Aphasien*, Sigmund Freud (1856–1939) refuted the doctrines of Wernicke and Lichtheim. He distinguished between defects in naming objects ('**asymbolic aphasia**') and defects in recognizing objects ('**agnosia**'). *4267.1*

1891:24 **Spinal surgical immobilization and fusion** first achieved by Berthold Ernest Hadra (1842–1903), *MTR* **22**:423; *TAOrA* **4**:206. *4359.1, 4359.2*

1891:25 Following the description of **congenital upward displacement** of the **scapula** by Otto Gerhard Karl Sprengel (1852–1915), *ArKC* **42**:545, the condition was named '**Sprengel's deformity**', despite the earlier description by M.M. Eulenburg in 1863. *4359, 4427, 4332*

1891:26 Hans Chiari (1851–1916) drew attention to the shift of the **medulla** caudally in what later became known as the **Arnold-Chiari malformation**, *BMW* **17**:1172. *4577.1, 4581.1, 4566.1*

1891:27 Friedrich Daniel von Recklinghausen (1833–1910) described generalized **osteitis fibrosa** ('**von Recklinghausen's disease of bone**'), in *Festschrift R.Virchow*, but was preceded in this by G. Engel (1864). *4358, 4335*

1891:28 A form of traumatic **spondylitis** ('**Kümmell's disease**') described by Hermann Kümmell (1852–1937), *VGDA*, p. 282. *4357*

1891:29 Operation for the radical treatment of **prostatic hypertrophy** described by Enrico Bottini (1837–1903), *IMC* **10**:3, 7 Abt.90. *4262*

1891:30 Recurrent paralysis of the **palate**, ('**Avellis's syndrome**'), recorded by Georg Avellis (1864–1916), *BKl* **40**:1. *3303*

1891:31 '**Sahli's test**' for estimating the functional activity of the **stomach** introduced by Hermann Sahli (1856–1933), *KBSA* **21**:65. *3500*

1891:32 'Paul's tube' for intestinal drainage introduced by Frank Thomas Paul (1851–1941), *BMJ* **2**:118. *3499*

1891:33 First description of pathology of carotid body tumours by Felix Jacob Marchand (1846–1928), *Festschrift R.Virchow* **1**:547. *3791*

1891:34 Lymphatic and myelogenous leukaemia differentiated by Paul Ehrlich (1845–1915) using his methods of staining blood cells; in his *Farbenanalytische Untersuchungen zur Histologie und Klinik*. *3069.1*

1891:35 Old anti-pneumococcus serum introduced by Georg Klemperer (1865–1932) and Felix Klemperer (1866–1946), *BKW* **28**:833, 869. *3178*

1891:36 Epithelioma transplanted in mice through 17 generations by Henri Morau (b.1860), *CRSB* **43**:289. *2622.1*

1891:37 Gustav Nepveu (1841–1903) was first to see trypanosomes in human blood, *CRSB* **43**:39. *5272*

1891:38 Ligation of gluteal artery by John Bell (1763–1820); reported in his *Principles of surgery*, **1**, 421. *2926*

1891:39 Berkefeld filter introduced by H. Nordtmeyer, *JHyg* **10**:145. *2506.1*

1891:40 Charles Creighton (1847–1927) began publication of his *History of epidemics in Britain*, 1891–1894. *1680*

1891:41 The first successful total cystectomy performed by Karel Pawlik (1849–1914), *WMW* **41**:184. *4184.1*

---

1891:42 Samuel Albert **Levine**, American physician, born 1 Jan; with Elliott Carr Cutler, successfully carried out mitral valve section for relief of mitral stenosis, 1923, *BMSJ*, **188**:1023. With Herman Ludwig Blumgart and D.D. Berlin, treated angina pectoris and congestive heart failure by thyroidectomy, 1933, *ArIM* **51**:866. Died 1966. *3030.1, 2899, 3033*

1891:43 Wilbur Willis **Swingle**, American physician and zoologist, born 11 Jan; with Joseph John Pfiffner, prepared an adrenal cortical hormone ('eschatin'), which was effective in the treatment of Addison's disease, 1932, *Medicine* **11**:371. *3874*

1891:44 Wilder Graves **Penfield**, Canadian neurosurgeon, born 26 Jan; developed cerebral cortical excision in the treatment of medically refractory focal epilepsy; in his *Epilepsy and cerebral localization*, 1951. Died 1976. *4910.1*

1891:45 Harry **Goldblatt**, American experimental pathologist, born 14 Mar; with co-workers, carried out important studies on experimental hypertension, 1934, *JEM* **59**:347. Died 1977. *2719*

1891:46 Hermann **Mooser**, Swiss bacteriologist, born 3 May; differentiated murine from epidemic typhus, 1928; the causal organism later named *Rickettsia mooseri*, *JID* **43**:241. Died 1971. *5396.1*

1891:47 Guy Henry **Faget**, American leprologist, born 15 Jun; with others introduced Promin (sodium glucosulphone) treatment of leprosy, 1943, *USPHR* **58**:1729. Died 1940. *2441*

1891:48 Julius **Lempert**, Polish/American otologist, born 4 Jul; devised one-step fenestration operation (Lempert's operation) for otosclerosis, 1938, *ArOt(C)* **28**:42. *3410*

1891:49 John Howard **Northrop**, American chemist, born 5 Jul; prepared crystalline pepsin and identified it as a protein, 1930, *JGP* **13**:739. Shared Nobel Prize (Chemistry), 1946, with Wendell Meredith Stanley, for their preparations of enzymes and viruses in a pure form, *NPL*. Died 1987. *1038.1*

1891:50 Bernhard **Zondek**, German/Israeli endocrinologist and gynaecologist, born 29 Jul; with Selmar Aschheim, isolated the gonadotrophic hormone of the anterior pituitary, 1927, *KW* **6**:348; **7**:831, and introduced the Aschheim-Zondek test for the diagnosis of pregnancy, 1928, *KW* **7**:8, 1404, 1453. Died 1966. *1168, 6222*

1891:51 Geoffrey Barrow **Dowling**, British dermatologist, born 9 Aug; with Ebenezer William Prosser Thomas, introduced calciferol in the treatment of lupus vulgaris, 1945, *PRSM* **39**:96. It was also used by Jacques Charpy in 1943, at that time isolated by the war in France. Died 1976. *4010, 4011*

1891:52 Beatrice Fay **Howitt**, American bacteriologist, born 23 Sep; recovered Western equine encephalitis virus from man, 1938, *Science* **88**:455. *4660*

1891:53 Hubert **Mann**, American cardiologist, born 15 Oct; initiated vectorcardiography, 1920, *ArIM* **25**:283. Died 1975. *2853.1*

1891:54 Joseph Hiram **Kite**, American immunologist, born 11 Nov; introduced a method of treating congenital club-foot (talipes), using a series of plaster casts and wedgings, 1939, *JBJS* **21**:595. *4403.1*

1891:55 Frederick Grant **Banting**, Canadian physician, born 14 Nov; with Charles Herbert Best and John James Rickard Macleod, isolated a pancreatic extract which was named insulin, 1922, *AmJPh* **59**:479; *JLCM* **7**:251; with co-workers, used insulin in the treatment of diabetes mellitus, 1922, *CMAJ* **12**:141. Shared Nobel Prize (Physiology or Medicine), 1923, with Macleod, *NPL*. Died 1941. *3966, 3967, 3968*

1891:56 Alfred Henry **Sturtevant**, American geneticist, born 21 Nov; published *The mechanism of Mendelian heredity*, 1915, recording epoch-making work on heredity, with Thomas Hunt Morgan, Hermann Joseph Muller and Colin Blackman Bridges. Died 1970. *246*

1891:57 James Stirling **Anderson**, British physician, born 3 Dec; with co-workers, distinguished the *gravis*, *mitis*, and intermediate types of *Corynebacterium diphtheriae*, 1931, *JPB* **34**:667. Died 1976. *5072*

———

1891:58 Alf Vilhelm **Westergren**, Swedish physician, born; introduced a method of measuring the erythrocyte sedimentation rate, 1921, *AcM* **54**:247. *3085*

1891:59 Frederic Eugen Basil **Foley**, American urologist, born; introduced plastic operation for the relief of hydronephrosis, 1937, *JU* **38**:643. Died 1966. *4250.1*

1891:60 Erik **Lysholm**, Swedish radiologist, born; introduced the Lysholm-Schönander skull table, allowing precise radiography of the skull, 1931, *AcR* Suppl.12. Died 1947. *4611.1*

1891:61 Louise Charlotte **Eisenhardt**, American physician, born; with Harvey Williams Cushing, classified the meningiomas; in their *Meningiomas. Their classification*, etc., 1938. Died 1967. *4909.01, 4612*

1891:62 Robert **Daubney**, British veterinarian, born; with John Richard Hudson, described Rift Valley fever, 1931, *JPB* **34**:545. *5541*

1891:63 Louis **Portes**, French gynaecologist, born; described the Portes operation – the classic caesarean section followed by temporary exteriorization of the uterus, 1924, *BSOG* **13**:171. Died 1950. *6252*

1891: Joseph William **Bazalgette** died, **born** 1819. *sewers*

1891: Joseph **Leidy** died, **born** 1823. *tumours, transplantation, intestinal bacterial flora, trichinosis*

1891: Gustav Theodor **Fritsch** died, **born** 1838. *functional localization in cerebral cortex*

1891: Henry Gawen **Sutton** died, **born** 1837. *kidney atrophy, nephrosclerosis*

1891: Hugh Owen **Thomas** died, **born** 1834. *orthopaedic splint*

1891: Eugène **Bouchut** died, **born** 1818. *neurasthenia*

1891: James Henry **Bennet** died, **born** 1816. *tumours of uterus*

1891: Henri **Roger** died, **born** 1809. *congenital ventricular septal defect, Roger's murmur*

**1892**
1892:1 [**State Hygienic Laboratory**] established at **Hamburg**

1892:2 **Instituto Bacteriológico de Câmara Pestana** opened at **Lisbon**

1892:3 [**Royal Japanese Institute for Infectious Diseases**] opened in **Tokyo**

1892:4 **American Psychological Association** founded, **New York**

1892:5 **Wistar Institute of Anatomy and Biology, Philadelphia**, incorporated

1892:6 **Norsk Medicinsk Selskap** established at **Christiania (Oslo)**

1892:7 **Biological Station** at **Bergen**

1892:8 In a study of the vaginal secretions in relation to **puerperal fever**, *Das Scheidensekret und seine Bedeutung für das Puerperalfieber*, Albert Siegmund Gustav Döderlein (1860–1941) gave the first description of '**Döderlein's bacillus**', a lactobacillus. *6279*

1892:9 The '**Breus mole**' (tuberous mole), the aborted products of conception, first described by Carl Breus (1852–1914); in his *Das tuberöse subchoriale Hämatom der Decidua. 6202*

1892:10 A method of vaginal **hysterectomy** described by Fernand Henrotin (1847–1906), *AmJOD* **26**:448. *6095*

1892:11 **Cystadenoma** of the **breast** ('**Schimmelbusch's disease**'), first described by Curt Schimmelbusch (1860–1895), *ArKC* **44**:117. *5775*

1892:12 **Meigs' syndrome (ovarian fibroma** combined with **pleural effusion)** was apparently first described by Robert Lawson Tait (1845–1899), *MCT* **75**:109, later described by Meigs, 1934. *6093.1, 6132.01*

1892:13 Reduction **rhinoplasty** by the endonasal approach introduced by Robert Fulton Weir (1838–1927), *NYMJ* **56**:449. *5754.6*

1892:14 **Coccidioidomycosis** described by Alejandro Posadas (1870–1902), *AnCM* **15**:585, and independently by Robert Johann Wernicke (b.1873), *RAMA* **1**:186. *5528.1, 5528.2*

1892:15 **Infiltration (local) anaesthesia**, pioneered by Halsted, developed by Carl Ludwig Schleich (1859–1922), *VDGC* **21**:121. *5683, 5679*

1892:16 Frederic William Hewitt (1857–1916) did much to develop the use of **ether** and advanced the knowledge of the pharmacology of **anaesthetics**, introducing the first practical gas and oxygen apparatus; wrote *Anaesthetics and their administration*, 1893. *5682*

1892:17 A bacillus (***Haemophilus influenzae***), then believed to be the causal organism in (bacterial) **influenza**, discovered by Richard Friedrich Johannes Pfeiffer (1858–1945), *DMW* **18**:28. *5490*

1892:18 August Friedrich Leopold Weissmann (1834–1914) located the **germ plasm** within the **nucleus**, and elaborated the theory of the continuity of the germ plasm; in his *Das Keimplasma. Eine Theorie der Vererbung. 236*

1892:19 The method of **induction of premature labour** by means of forced dilatation of the cervix originated by Luigi Maria Bossi (1859–1919), *AnOG* **14**:881. *6201*

1892:20 Circumscribed **atrophy of the brain** with development of **aphasia** and **presenile dementia** ('**Pick's disease**') described by Arnold Pick (1851–1924), *PMW* **17**:165. *4707*

1892:21 The operation of intracranial **neurectomy** for **facial neuralgia (Hartley-Krause operation)** introduced by Frank Hartley (1857–1913), *NYMJ* **55**:317, and independently by Fedor Krause (1856–1937), *ArKC* **44**:821. *4870, 4871*

1892:22 The first vaccine against **cholera** to meet with any success was prepared by Waldemar Mordecai Wolff Haffkine (1860–1930), *CRSB* **44**:636, 671. *5109*

1892:23 An aetiological relationship between **varicella** and **herpes zoster** first suggested by Janos Bokay (1858–1937), *MOA* Nov. 3. *5439.1*

1892:24 A classic description of **syphilitic spinal paralysis** given by Wilhelm Heinrich Erb (1840–1921), sometimes referred to as '**Erb's disease**', *NZ* **11**:161. *4788*

1892:25 A **tendon** was first successfully **transplanted** by P.F. Parrish, *NYMJ* **56**:402. *4363*

1892:26 The individuality of **fingerprints** in identification explained by Francis Galton (1822–1911); in his *Finger prints. 186*

1892:27 Vladimir Michailovich Bechterev (1857–1927) was one of several authors to give an early description of **ankylosing spondylitis**, *Vrach* **13**:899, and one of its several eponyms was '**Bechterev's disease**'. *4360*

1892:28 First successful plastic operation for the relief of **hydronephrosis** carried out by Ernst Georg Ferdinand von Küster (1839–1930), *ZCh* **19**: Suppl.110. *4223*

1892:29 **Maculopapular erythroderma** also named '**Jadassohn's disease**' following the description by Josef Jadassohn (1863–1936), *VDDG* **2–3**:342. *4108*

1892:30 **Besnier's prurigo** described by Ernest Besnier (1831–1909), *AnD* **3**:634. *4107*

1892:31 **Lymphosarcoma** differentiated from **Hodgkin's disease** by Julius Dreschfeld (1846–1907), *BMJ* **1**:893. *3772*

1892:32 An important 19th century American medical text, *Anatomy and surgical treatment of hernia*, published by Henry Orlando Marcy (1837–1924). *3601*

1892:33 The two-stage (**Mikulicz**) operation for **colon cancer** first employed by Oscar Thorvald Bloch (1847–1926), *NoMA* **2**, i, 1; **2**, ii, 1. *3502*

1892:34 '**Murphy's button**' for **gastric** and **intestinal anastomosis** introduced by John Benjamin Murphy (1857–1916), *MR* **42**:665. *3507*

1892:35 The first recorded case of successful suture of perforated **gastric ulcer** by Ludwig Heusner (1846–1916), *BKW* **29**:1244, 1280. *3505*

1892:36 An operation for the radical cure of **hernia** devised by Theodor Kocher (1841–1917), *KBSA* **22**:96. *3600*

1892:37 **Mastoidectomy** for **middle-ear** suppuration drainage (**antrectomy**) introduced by William Arbuthnot Lane (1856–1943), *ArOt* **21**:118. *3394.2*

1892:38 Important modifications in the radical **mastoidectomy** operation of von Bergmann and Küster introduced by Ludwig Stacke (1859–1918), *BKW* **29**:68. *3394*

1892:39 **Gradenigo's test** for tone decay in **hearing** introduced by Giuseppe Gradenigo (1859–1926), *GOC* **13**:1126. *3394.1*

1892:40 The operation of **gastroduodenostomy** introduced by Mathieu Jaboulay (1860–1913), *ArPC* **1**:551. *3504*

1892:41 **Achylia gastrica**, a primary nervous functional disorder of **gastric secretion**, was a concept introduced by Max Einhorn (1862–1953), *MR* **41**:650. *3503*

1892:42 First successful ligation of left **subclavian artery**, with extirpation of **subclavio-axillary aneurysm**, by William Stewart Halsted (1852–1922), *JHB* **3**:393. *2966*

1892:43 **Polycythaemia (erythraemia)** first described by Louis Henri Vaquez (1860–1936), *CRSB* **44**:384; William Osler's later paper (1903) led to the term '**Vaquez-Osler disease**'. *3070, 3073*

1892:44 The reciprocal **innervation** of **muscle** investigated by Charles Scott Sherrington (1857–1952), 1892, *JP* **13**:621; *PRS* **53**:407. *1288, 1288.1*

1892:45 Elie Metchnikoff's (1845–1916) classic lectures on **inflammation**, *Lektsii o sravnitelnoi patologii vospaleniy*, published. *2307*

1892:46 *Salmonella typhi-murium* isolated by Friedrich August Johann Loeffler (1852–1915), *ZBP* **11**:129. *2507*

1892:47 Discovery of *Clostridium perfringens*, the **gas gangrene** bacillus (Welch bacillus) by William Henry Welch (1850–1934) and George Henry Falkiner Nuttall (1862–1937), *JHB* **3**:81. *2508*

1892:48 *Staphylococcus epidermidis albus* and its relation to **wound infection** discovered by William Henry Welch (1850–1934), *TCAP* **2**:1. *5621*

1892:49 **Electrotherapy** with high-frequency currents introduced by Jacques Arsène d'Arsonval (1851–1940), *ArPhy* **4**:69. *1999*

1892:50 **Tetany** produced experimentally by **thyroidectomy**, by Anton von Eiselsberg (1860–1939), *WKW* **5**:81. *3856*

1892:51 **Tobacco mosaic disease** agent shown by Dmitri Iosifovich Ivanovski (1864–1920) to be a filter-passing **virus**, *BAIS* **3**:67; this was the starting-point of research into the aetiology of virus diseases. *2506.2*

1892:52 William Osler's (1849–1919) textbook, *Principles and practice of medicine*, published. *2231*

1892:53 **Ferry-Porter law**, a modification of the Fechner-Weber law by Ervin Sidney Ferry (1868–1956), *AmJSc* **44**:192; *PRS* **63**:347. *1473*

---

1892:54 William Parry **Murphy**, American physician, born 6 Feb; with George Richards Minot, introduced the raw liver diet in the treatment of pernicious anaemia, 1926, *JAMA* **87**:470, following the demonstration of its value in anaemia by Robscheit-Robbins and Whipple (1925). For this work he shared the Nobel Prize (Physiology or Medicine), 1934, with Minot and George Hoyt Whipple, *NPL*. *3140, 3139*

1892:55 Emmy **Klieneberger**, German/British bacteriologist, born 25 Feb; isolated pleuropneumonia-like organisms (mycoplasma) from *Streptobacillus moniliformis*, 1935, *JPB* **40**:93. Died 1985. *2524.4*

1892:56 Cornèille Jean François **Heymans**, Belgian physiologist, born 28 Mar; his work on the sinus-aorta mechanism in respiration, *Le sinus carotidien et la zone homologue cardio-aortique*, 1929, gained him the Nobel Prize (Physiology or Medicine), 1938, *NPL*. Died 1968. *967*

1892:57 Edgar **Allen**, American anatomist and endocrinologist, born 2 May; with Edward Adelbert Doisy, isolated oestrin, 1923, *JAMA* **81**:819. Died 1943. *1183*

1892:58 Percival **Bailey**, American neurologist, born 9 May; with Harvey Williams Cushing, published an important classification of glioma group tumours; in their *A classification of the tumours of the glioma group on a histogenetic basis*, 1926. Died 1973. *4608*

1892:59 William Smith **Tillett**, American physician, born 10 Jul; with Raymond Loraine Garner, discovered streptokinase, a fibrinolysin, 1933, *JEM* **58**:485. Died 1974. *1924.1*

1892:60 Norman McAlister **Gregg**, Australian ophthalmologist, born 27 Jul; pointed out that rubella in early pregnancy could result in congenital defects in the infant, 1941, *TOSA* **3**:35. Died 1966. *5507*

1892:61 Henry Hubert **Turner**, American physician, born 28 Aug; noted 'Turner's syndrome' (infantilism, congenital webbed neck, and cubitus valgus), 1938, *En* **23**:566. Died 1970. *3801.1*

1892:62 Joe Vincent **Meigs**, American gynaecologist, born 24 Oct; described fibroma of the ovary with pleural effusion ('Meigs' syndrome'); in his *Tumors of the female pelvic organs*, 1934, p. 262.; described earlier by Lawson Tait, 1892. *6132.01, 6093.1*

1892:63 John Burdon Sanderson **Haldane**, British biochemist and geneticist, born 5 Nov; his mathematical theory of natural selection appeared in, 1924, *TCPS* **23**:19; *PCPS* **1**:23, 26, 27, 28, and in *Gen*, 1934, **19**:412; summarized in *Causes of evolution*, 1932. Died 1964. *254*

1892:64 James Bertram **Collip**, Canadian endocrinologist, born 20 Nov; extracted a parathyroid hormone ('parathormone'), 1925, *JBC* **63**:395, and, with Douglas Burrows Leitch used it in the treatment of tetany, 1925, *CMAJ* **15**:59. Died 1965. *3861, 3862, 4837*

1892:65 William Hugh **Feldman**, British/American pathologist, born 30 Nov; with others, introduced promin (sodium glucosulphone) in treatment of tuberculosis, 1940, *PMC* **15**:295; with Horton Corwin Hinshaw, introduced streptomycin in treatment of tuberculosis, 1945, *PMC* **20**:313. Died 1974. *2349, 2350.*

1892:66 Carl Richard **Moore**, American endocrinologist, born 5 Dec; isolated androsterone, 1929, *En* **13**:367. Died 1955. *1191*

---

1892:67 Max **Aron** born; simultaneously with Leo Loeb and R.B. Bassett he isolated the thyroid-stimulating hormone of the anterior pituitary, 1929, *CRSB* **102**:682. Died 1974. *1138.02*

1892:68 Manoel de **Abreu**, Brazilian radiologist, born; introduced mass chest radiography, 1936, *RAPM* **9**:313. Died 1962. *3209.1*

1892:69 Felix **Mandl**, Austrian physician, born; successfully treated osteitis fibrosa generalisata by removal of a parathyroid tumour, 1925, *WKW* **38**:1343. Died 1957. *3863*

1892:70 Mari **Takata**, Japanese pathologist, born; with Kiyoshi Ara, devised the Takata-Ara reaction for the diagnosis of liver disease, 1925, *Far 6*, **1**:667. *3654*

1892:71 Guido **Fanconi**, Swiss paediatrician, born; drew attention to a metabolic disorder subsequently named after him, 1927, *JaK* **117**:257. Described 'Fanconi syndrome', multiple defects in renal tubular function, 1931, *JaK* **133**:257. With co-workers, first described cystic fibrosis (mucoviscidosis), 1936, *WMW* **86**:753. Died 1979. *3142, 4248, 3659.2*

1892:72 Morten Ansgar **Kveim**, Norwegian physician, born; introduced the Kveim test for sarcoidosis, 1941, *NoM* **9**:169. *4153*

1892:73 Arvid Vilhelm **Lindau**, Swedish pathologist, born; made an important histological study of haemangiomatosis retinae ('Lindau's disease'), 1926, *AcPMS* Suppl.1. *5971*

1892:74 Carl Gustav Vilhelm **Nylin**, Swedish surgeon, born; with Clarence Crafoord, pioneered, at same time as Robert Edward Gross, surgical treatment of coarctation of aorta, 1945, *JTS* **14**:347. Died 1961. *3044*

---

1892: William **Bowman** died, born 1816. *Bowman's capsule, artificial pupil*

1892: Theodor Hermann **Meynert** died, born 1833. *brain, insanity, amentia*

1892: Jean Antoine **Villemin** died, born 1827. *tuberculosis*

1892: Henry **Moon** died, born 1845. *syphilis*

1892: Anton **Biermer** died, born 1827. *pernicious anaemia*

1892: Morell **Mackenzie** died, born 1837. *laryngology*

1892: Edward **Cock** died, born 1805. *pharyngotomy*

1892: Samuel Armstrong **Lane** died, born 1802. *haemophilia, blood transfusion*

1892: Gustav Wilhelm Johann **Düben** died, born 1822. *myocardial infarction*

1892: Richard **Owen** died, born 1804. *odontography*

1892: Carl Ferdinand **Eichstedt** died, born 1816. *pityriasis versicolor*

1892: August von **Freund** died, born 1835. *anaesthesia, cyclopropane*

1892: George Biddle **Airy** died, born 1801. *astigmatism*

1892: Gilman **Kimball** died, born 1804. *hysteromyomectomy*

1892: Daniel **Ayres** died, born 1822. *exstrophy of bladder*

1892: Ernst Wilhelm von **Brücke** died, born 1819. *eye*

418

1892: Carl Siegmund Franz **Credé** died, **born** 1819. *removal of placenta, Credé's manoeuvre, ophthalmia neonatorum, silver nitrate*

## 1893
1893:1 **Undergraduate medical school** established at **Johns Hopkins Hospital**

1893:2 Consolidation of **London water supply** 1893–1899

1893:3 In his description of what later became termed the **Hand-Schüller-Christian syndrome**, Alfred Hand (1868–1949) called it **polyuria and tuberculosis**, *PPSS* **16**:282; *ArPe* **10**:673. *6359–6363*

1893:4 The use of whole-thickness **skin grafts** popularized by Fedor Krause (1857–1937), *VDGC* **22**ii:46. *5755*

1893:5 A classification of **chorionic tumours** and a review of the relevant literature provided by Max Sanger (1853–1903), *ArGy* **44**:89. *6094*

1893:6 **Ankylostomiasis** first recognized in North America by Walter L. Blickhahn, *MN* **63**:662. *5360*

1893:7 **Psychoanalysis** began with collaboration between Sigmund Freud (1856–1939) and Josef Breuer (1842–1925); the foundation stone was their *Studien über Hysterie. 4977.3, 4978*

1893:8 *Entamoeba histolytica* distinguished from *Escherichia coli* by Heinrich Irenaeus Quincke (1842–1922) and Ernst Roos (b.1866), *BKW* **30**:1089. *5188*

1893:9 Original description of **hereditary cerebellar ataxia** given by Pierre Marie (1853–1940), *SMP* **13**:444. *4708.1*

1893:10 Zones of **hyperalgesia** of the **skin** associated with **visceral disease** ('**Head's areas**') defined by Henry Head (1861–1940), *Brain* **16**:1; **17**:339; **19**:153. *4581*

1893:11 **Myasthenia pseudoparalytica** described by Samuel Vulvovich Goldflam (1852–1932), *DZN* **1**:96; **3**:427; it had previously been described by Erb (1879) and was named '**Erb-Goldflam symptom complex**. *4757, 4746*

1893:12 The first description of **hypertrophic progressive interstitial neuritis** ('**Dejerine-Sottas disease**') given by Joseph Jules Dejerine (1849–1917) and Jules Sottas (b.1866), *CRSB* **45**:63. *4580*

1893:13 **Acanthosis nigricans**, illustrated by Pollitzer and Janovsky in 1890, was described by Jean Darier (1856–1938), *AnD* **4**:865. *4113, 4102*

1893:14 The first catheterization of the male **ureters** performed by James Brown (1854–1895), *JHB* **4**:73. *4185.1*

1893:15 The aeroscopic examination of the **bladder** and catheterization of the **ureters** under direct inspection introduced by Howard Atwood Kelly (1858–1943), *JHB* **4**:101. *4187*

1893:16 **Porokeratosis** named '**Mibelli's disease**' after the description by Vittorio Mibelli (1860–1910), *GIMV* **28**:313; it was first described by Neumann in 1875. *4068, 4114*

1893:17 In the **nephropexy** operation devised by George Michael Edebohls (1853–1908) flaps of the capsule of the **kidney** were utilized, *AmJMS* **105**:247, 417. *4224*

1893:18 Modern methods of **ureteral repair**, including **uretero-ureterostomy**, originated by Weller Van Hook (1862–1933), *JAMA* **21**:911, 965. *4186*

1893:19 **Gonococcus** first isolated from **arthritic joints** by Heinrich Höck, *WKW* **6**:736. *4502.1*

1893:20 Hans Kundrat (1845–1893) differentiated **lymphosarcoma** ('**Kundrat's disease**') from other malignant tumours involving the lymphatic system, *WKW* **6**:211, 234. *2623, 3773*

1893:21 Partial lobectomy in **pulmonary tuberculosis** performed by David Lowson (1850–1907), *BMJ* **1**:1152. *3227*

1893:22 **Thoracoplasty** first performed by George Ryerson Fowler (1848–1906), *MR* **44**:838. *3179*

1893:23 Charles Barrett Lockwood's (1856–1914) operation for the radical cure of **femoral hernia** published, *L* **2**:1297. *3604*

1893:24 An operation for **gastrostomy** introduced by Rudolph Frank (1862–1913), *WKW* **6**:231, and was independently described by J.F. Ssabanejew in the same year; named '**Ssabanejew-Frank operation**'. *3508, 3512*

1893:25 Operation for abscess of the **maxillary sinus** devised by George Walter Caldwell (1834–1918), *NYJM* **58**:526; named '**Caldwell-Luc operation**' acknowledging earlier work by Henri Luc. *3305, 3301*

1893:26 **Otosclerosis** first reported as a separate clinical entity by Adam Politzer (1835–1920), *PAMC* **3**:1607. *3395*

1893:27 A method for the cure of **femoral hernia** published by Edoardo Bassini (1844–1924); in his *Nuovo metodo operativo per la cura dell' ernia crurale*. *3602*

1893:28 **Acroparaesthesia** described by Friedrich Schultze (1848–1934), *DZN* **3**:300. *2709*

1893:29 **Ladd-Franklin evolutionary theory of colour vision** proposed by Christine Ladd-Franklin (1847–1930), *ZPPS* **4**:221. *1522*

1893:30 **Atrioventricular bundle**, ('**Bundle of His**'), described by Wilhelm His Jr (1863–1934), *AMKI* 14. (In the same year it was also described by Albert Frank Stanley Kent (1839–1958), *JP* **14**:233.) *836, 837*

1893:31 Theobald Smith (1859–1934) and Frederick Lucius Kilborne (1858–1936) discovered **parasite** of **Texas cattle fever**, *Babesia bigemina*, and proved its transmission by the **cattle tick**, *Boöphilus annulatus* – the first demonstration of **arthropod transmission of disease**,

*Investigations into ... Texas or Southern cattle fever*, (US Bureau of Animal Industry, Bulletin No. 1). *5529*

1893:32 Important work on **cells** and **tissue** published by Wilhelm August Oscar Hertwig (1849–1922) and Karl Wilhelm Theodor Richard von Hertwig (1850–1937); *Die Zelle und die Gewebe*, 1893–8. *556*

---

1893:33 John Rodman **Paul**, American physician, born 18 Apr; with Walls Willard Bunnell, introduced the 'Paul-Bunnell test' for the diagnosis of infectious mononucleosis, 1932, *AmJMS* **183**:90. Died 1971. *5487*

1893:34 James William Tudor **Thomas**, British ophthalmic surgeon, born 23 May; carried out important experimental work on corneal transplantation, 1930, *TOUK* **50**:127. Died 1976. *5979*

1893:35 Earl Calvin **Padgett**, American plastic surgeon, born 8 Jul; introduced the Padgett dermatome, for cutting calibrated skin grafts, 1939, *SGO* **69**:779. Died 1946. *5763.1*

1893:36 Albert **Szent-Györgyi**, Hungarian biochemist, born 16 Sep; isolated vitamin C (ascorbic acid), 1928, *BJ* **20**:537; for this and other biochemical discoveries he received the Nobel Prize (Physiology or Medicine), 1937, *NPL*. Died 1986. *1059*

1893:37 Lester Reynold **Dragstedt**, American surgeon, born 2 Oct; with Frederick Mitchum Owens, treated peptic ulcer by vagotomy, 1943, *PSEB* **53**:152. Died 1975. *3557*

1893:38 Guy William John **Bousfield**, British physician, born 20 Oct; recorded electrocardiographic changes during an attack of angina pectoris, 1917, *L* **2**:457. Died 1974. *2894.1*

1893:39 Edward Adelbert **Doisy** born, 13 Nov; with Edgar Allen, isolated oestrin, 1923, *JAMA* **81**:819; associated with Donald William McCorquodale in the isolation of oestradiol, 1935, *JBC* **115**:435. Shared Nobel Prize (Physiology or Medicine), 1943, with Carl Peter Henrik Dam, for his discovery of the chemical structure of vitamin K, *NPL*. Died 1986. *1183, 1202*

1893:40 Cicely Delphine **Williams**, British paediatrician, born 2 Dec; gave the first accurate description of kwashiorkor, 1935, *L* **2**:1151. Died 1992. *3759*

---

1893:41 Frieda Saur **Robscheit-Robbins**, American physician, born; with George Hoyt Whipple, demonstrated beneficial effect of raw liver in the treatment of anaemia, 1925, *AMJPh* **72**:408, paving the way for the establishment of this treatment by Minot and Murphy (1926). *3139, 3140*

1893:42 Kurt **Beringer** born; gave a comprehensive account of mescaline poisoning; in his *Der Meskalinrausch*, 1927. Died 1949. *2086.1*

1893:43 Samuel Oscar **Freedlander**, American surgeon, born; carried out the first planned lobectomy in pulmonary tuberculosis, 1935, *JTS* **5**:132. *3238*

1893:44 Jaroslav **Drbohlav**, American parasitologist, born; with William Charles Boeck, evolved the first media upon which amoebae could be cultivated for indefinite periods, 1925, *AmJH* **5**:371. Died 1946. *5194*

---

1893: Hans **Kundrat** died, **born** 1845. *lymphosarcoma*

1893: Jean Baptiste Emil **Vidal** died, **born** 1825. *neurodermatitis*

1893: Jean Martin **Charcot** died, **born** 1825. *tabetic arthropathy, gout, localization of function in brain, multiple sclerosis, muscular atrophy, amyotrophic lateral sclerosis, tabes dorsalis, peroneal muscular atrophy*

1893: Otto **Kahler** died, **born** 1849. *syringomyelia, psychoneuroses, hypnosis*

1893: John **Tyndall** died, **born** 1820. *Penicillium, sterilization*

1893: Robert Robertovich **Wreden** died, **born** 1837. *otomycosis*

1893: John Davies **Thomas** died, **born** 1844. *Taenia echinococcus*

1893: Charles **Clay** died, **born** 1801. *ovariotomy*

**1894**
1894:1 **Institut Pasteur, Tunis**, founded

1894:2 **Local Government Act, England**

1894:3 Maria Montessori (1870–1952) first woman to **qualify** in **medicine** in **Italy**, developed the Montessori system of **teaching**

1894:4 **International Lending Library for the Blind (Deutsche Zentralbücherei)** established at **Leipzig**

1894:5 **Wellcome Physiological Research Laboratories (London)** founded

1894:6 **Institut Solvay (de Physiologie)** founded at **Brussels**

1894:7 **Field Museum of Natural History** founded at **Chicago**

1894:8 Franz Nissl (1860–1919) introduced **Nissl's stain** for nerve cells , *NZ* **13**:507; described 'Nissl's granules' in the cytoplasm of nerve cells, *NZ* **13**:676, 781, 810. *1291, 1422*

1894:9 The '**Gigli saw**', invented by Leonardo Gigli (1863–1908), was first used for **pubiotomy**, *AnOG* **16**:649. *6204*

1894:10 A classic account of **metastatic ophthalmia** provided by Karl Theodor Paul Polykarpos Axenfeld (1867–1930), *GAO* **43**, iii:1. *5938*

1894:11 A **nitrous oxide/oxygen** stopcock devised by Frederic William Hewitt (1857–1916), *JBDA* **15**:380. *5682.1*

1894:12 **Rubber gloves** introduced into operative **surgery** by William Stewart Halsted (1852–1922), *JHR* **4**:297. *5640*

1894:13 Patrick Manson (1844–1922) first proposed his **mosquito-malaria hypothesis**, *BMJ* 1:695, 751, 831. *5245*

1894:14 The **plague** bacillus, *Pasteurella pestis*, discovered by Alexandre Emile Jean Yersin (1863–1943), *AnIP* 8:662. *5125*

1894:15 The first to support, with evidence, the theory of the transmission of **plague** bacillus by rats was Alexander Rennie (1859–1940), *BMJ* 2:615. *5126*

1894:16 Pierre Paul Emile Roux (1853–1933) and André Louis François Justin Martin (1853–1921) showed how Behring's specific **diphtheria antitoxin** could be produced on a large scale, *AnIP* 8:609. *5063*

1894:17 The concept of '**parasyphilis**' introduced by Jean Alfred Fournier (1832–1914) in his *Les infections parasyphilitiques*; he showed statistically the causal relationship of **syphilis** to **paresis** and **tabes**. *4800*

1894:18 First description of **interilio-abdominal amputation** by Mathieu Jaboulay (1860–1913), *LM* **75**:507. *4472*

1894:19 Etienne Jules Marey (1830–1904), a pioneer in the use of serial pictures as a method of studying the mechanics of **locomotion**; in his *Le mouvement. 643*

1894:20 **Total replacement of a shoulder** carried out by Jules Émile Péan (1830–1898), using a **prosthesis** made of hardened rubber and platinum, *GH* **67**:289. *4364.1*

1894:21 A method of treatment of **fractures** by '**osteosynthesis**' – the perfect re-apposition of the affected parts by operative intervention – introduced by William Arbuthnot Lane (1856–1943), *TCSL* **27**:167. *4429*

1894:22 Julius Arnold (1835–1915) described the abnormality of the **cerebellum** in what later became known as the **Arnold-Chiari malformation**, *BPA* 16:1. *4581.1, 4577.1, 4566.1*

1894:23 *Die Histopathologie der Hautkrankheiten*, published by Paul Gerson Unna (1850–1929), is a landmark in the history of **dermatology**; the first description of the **acne bacillus** appears on p. 357. *4000*

1894:24 *Actinomyces madurae*, the parasite of **Madura foot**, **mycetoma** of the foot, isolated by Jean Hyacinthe Vincent (1862–1950), *AnIP* 8:129. *4117*

1894:25 Method of **uretero-ureteral anastomosis** using the catheter as a temporary ureteral splint published by Howard Atwood Kelly (1858–1943), *AnS* **27**:475. *4188*

1894:26 Operation for **uretero-intestinal anastomosis** devised by Karel Maydl (1853–1913), *WMW* **41**:1113, 1169, 1209, 1256, 1297. *4188.1*

1894:27 **Cryoscopy of the urine** established as a **kidney function test** by Sandor Korány (1866–1944), *BKO*, p. 74. *4226*

1894:28 Raymond Jacques Adrien Sabouraud (1864–1938) studied the role of **fungi** in **skin diseases**; in his *Les trichophyties humaines. 3999*

1894:29 **Splenomegalic anaemia** ('**Banti's syndrome**') described by Guido Banti (1852–1925), *Spe* **48**:Com. 447; Sez.b. 407. *3774*

1894:30 '**Plaut's angina**', the association of fusiform bacilli in ulcerating tonsillar lesions, described by Hugo Karl Plaut (1858–1928), *DMW* **20**:920, and more comprehensively later by Jean Hyacinthe Vincent. *3308.1*

1894:31 **Friedländer group bacillus** found in **ozaena** by Benjamin Loewenberg (1836–1905), *AnIP* **8**:292. *3307*

1894:32 **Immune bacteriolysis** ('**Pfeiffer phenomenon**') recorded in *Cholera vibrio* by Richard Friedrich Johannes Pfeiffer (1858–1945) and Vasiliy Isayevich Isayev [Issayaeff] (1854–1911), *ZHyg* **17**:355; **18**:1. *2546*

1894:33 **Emetine** obtained in pure form by Benjamin Horatio Paul (1828–1902) and Alfred John Cownley, *PhJ* **54**:111, 373, 690. *1887*

1894:34 Decortication of the **lung** for chronic **empyema** introduced by Edmond Delorme (1847–1929), *GH* **67**:94. *3180*

1894:35 *Pyogenic infective diseases of the brain* published by William Macewen (1848–1924). *4872*

---

1894:36 Neil E. **McKinnon**, Canadian epidemiologist, born 12 Jan; with Robert Davies Defries, introduced a diagnostic test for smallpox, 1928, *AmJH* **8**:93. *5434*

1894:37 William Charles **Boeck**, American physiologist and parasitologist, born 18 Feb; with Jaroslav Drbohlav, evolved the first media upon which amoebae could be cultivated for indefinite periods, 1925, *AmJH* **5**:371. *5194*

1894:38 Herbert Frederick **Traut**, American obstetrician and gynaecologist, born 3 Apr; with George Nicholas Papanicolaou, pointed out the diagnostic value of cervical smears in carcinoma of the cervix, 1941, *AmJOG* **42**:193. *6135*

1894:39 Tracy Jackson **Putnam**, American neurologist, born 14 Apr; treated hydrocephalus by endoscopic coagulation of the choroid plexus, 1934, *NEJM* **210**:1373; with Hyram Houston Merritt, introduced diphenylhydantoin in the treatment of convulsive disorders, 1938, *JAMA* **111**:1068. *4903, 4824.1*

1894:40 Frederick Roland George **Heaf**, British tuberculologist, born 21 Jun; introduced Heaf multipuncture tuberculin test for tuberculosis, 1951, *L* **2**:151. Died 1973. *2352.1*

1894:41 John Silas **Lundy**, American anaesthetist, born 6 Jul; introduced thiopentone sodium as an anaesthetic, 1935, *PMC* **10**:536. *5720*

1894:42 Armand James **Quick**, American haematologist, born 18 Jul; introduced a liver function test, 1933, *AmJMS* **185**:630. Introduced a method for prothrombin clotting time estimation ('Quick's method'), 1935, *JBC* **109**:lxxiii. With H.N. Ottenstein and H. Weltchek, introduced an intravenous hippuric acid liver-function test, 1938, *PSEB* **38**:77. Died 1977. *3659, 3095, 3663*

1894:43 Harold Randall **Griffith**, Canadian/American anaesthetist, born 25 Jul; with G. Enid Johnson, introduced curare into general anaesthesia, 1942, *Ane* **3**:418. *5724*

1894:44 Ernest Basil **Verney**, British pharmacologist, born 22 Aug; elucidated the factors involved in the release of antidiuretic hormone, 1947, *PRS* **135**:26. Died 1967. *1244.2*

1894:45 George Herbert William **Lucas**, Canadian pharmacologist, born 25 Aug; with Velyien Ewart Henderson, introduced cyclopropane as an anaesthetic, 1929, *CMAJ* **21**:173. *5711*

1894:46 Robert Meredith **Janes**, Canadian surgeon, born 6 Sep; with Norman Strahan Shenstone, introduced hilar tourniquet in lung surgery, 1932, *CMAJ* **27**:138. *3203.2*

1894:47 Franklin McCue **Hanger**, American physician, born 6 Sep; introduced cephalin-cholesterol liver-function test, 1938, *TAAP* **53**:148. Died 1971. *3662*

1894:48 Claude Schaeffer **Beck**, American surgeon, born 8 Nov; provided collateral blood supply to the heart by pericardial implantation of pectoral muscle, 1935, *AnS* **102**:801; in the same year, with V.L. Tichy, he carried out the first cardio-omentopexy for the same purpose, *AmHJ* **10**:849. With co-workers, carried out revascularization of the brain by the establishment of a cervical arteriovenous fistula, 1947, *JPe* **35**:317, and introduced treatment of ventricular fibrillation by direct application of electric shock, 1947, *JAMA* **135**:985. Died 1971. *3034, 3035, 4914, 2878.1*

1894:49 Raymond **Lewthwaite**, American pathologist and specialist in tropical; medicine, born 18 Nov; with S.R. Savoor, showed scrub typhus and tsutsugamushi disease to be identical, 1940, *L* **1**:255, 304. Died 1972. *5398.2*

1894:50 Norbert **Wiener**, American mathematician, born 26 Nov; founded the science of cybernetics; he wrote *Cybernetics: or control and communication in the animal and the machine*, 1948. Died 1966. *4991.1*

1894:51 Philip **Drinker**, American industrial hygienist, born 12 Dec; with C.F. McKhann introduced the Drinker respirator ('iron lung'), 1929, *JAMA* **92**:1658. Died 1972. *1978*

---

1894:52 Edward Clark **Davidson**, American physician, born; introduced tannic acid treatment of burns, 1925, *SGO* **41**:202. Died 1933. *2254*

1894:53 Erwin **Schliephake**, German physician, born; introduced short-wave diathermy, 1930, *KW* **9**:2333. *2009*

1894:54 David **Goldblatt**, American surgeon, born; introduced a classification of burns, 1927, *AnS* **85**:490. *2255*

1894:55 Donald Walter Gordon **Murray**, Canadian surgeon, born; with co-workers, first to use heparin clinically, 1937, *Surgery* **2**:163. First successful aortic valve homograft, 1956, *Angiology* **7**:466. Died 1976. *3019, 3047.8*

1894:56 Kiyoshi **Ara**, Japanese pathologist, born; with Mari Takata, devised the Takata-Ara reaction for the diagnosis of liver disease, 1925, *Far 6*, **1**:667. *3654*

1894:57 Frank Chambliss **Johnson**, American physician, born; with Albert Mason Stevens, described the Stevens-Johnson syndrome, a generalized eruption with fever and conjunctivitis, 1917. Died 1934. *4150*

1894:58 Hans **Theiler**, American pathologist, born; with Donald Leslie Augustine, introduced an intradermal test for the diagnosis of trichinosis, 1932, *Para* **24**:60. *5351.1*

1894:59 Leslie Tillotson **Webster**, American experimental epidemiologist, born; with Anna D. Clow, grew the rabies virus in tissue culture and uses the culture virus as anti-rabies vaccine, 1936, *Science* **84**:487. Died 1943. *5484.2*

1894:60 William Edward Mandell **Wardill**, British surgeon, born; devised an operation for the repair of cleft palate, 1928, *BJS* **16**:127. Died 1960. *5761*

1894:61 Clilian Bethany **Powell**, American obstetrician, born; with William Snow, achieved direct radiography of the placenta, 1934, *AmJR* **31**:37. *6229*

---

1894: Hermann Ludwig Ferdinand von **Helmholtz** died, **born** 1821. *conservation of energy, nerve impulse velocity, vision, hearing, ophthalmoscope*

1894: Francis Bisset **Hawkins** died, **born** 1796. *medical statistics*

1894: Adolph **Hannover** died, **born** 1814. *epithelioma*

1894: Friedrich **Neelsen** died, **born** 1854. *tuberculosis, Mycobacterium*

1894: Daniel Cornelius **Danielssen** died, **born** 1815. *leprosy*

1894: Theodor **Billroth** died, **born** 1829. *surgery, cancer of larynx, carcinoma of pylorus, resection of oesophagus, bladder tumour*

1894: Charles Eugène **Quinquaud** died, **born** 1841. *folliculitis decalvans*

1894: Charles Édouard **Brown-Séquard** died, **born** 1817. *paralysis, epilepsy, adrenal glands*

1894: Emanuel **Winge** died, **born** 1827. *bacterial endocarditis*

1894: William **Detmold** died, **born** 1808. *brain abscess surgery*

1894: William John **Little** died, **born** 1810. *cerebral spastic diplegia, progressive muscular dystrophy, talipes, orthopaedics*

1894: Joseph Pierre **Rollet** died, **born** 1824. *syphilis, chancroid*

1894: Joseph **Bancroft** died, **born** 1836. *Wuchereria bancrofti*

1894: Werner **Hagedorn** died, **born** 1831. *cleft lip*

1894: William **Moon** died, **born** 1818. *embossed type for blind*

1894: August **Hirsch** died, **born** 1817. *medical biography*

1894: Oliver Wendell **Holmes** died, **born** 1809. *puerperal fever*

**1895**
1895:1 **Friedrich-Wilhelms Institut, Berlin,** becomes **Kaiser-Wilhelms Akademie**

1895:2 **Bureau of Laboratories** established by **New York Health Dept**

1895:3 Henry Solomon **Wellcome** (1853–1936) begins collection for **Wellcome Historical Medical Library**

1895:4 **Pasteur Institute** established at **Annam** for **Indo-China**

1895:5 **Universidad Central, Quito (Ecuador)** reorganized to include **medical faculty**

1895:6 **Bacteriolysis**; involvement of sensitizing **antibody** and **complement** shown by Jean Jules Baptiste Bordet (1870–1961), *AnSR* **4**:455. *2547*

1895:7 An operation for excision of the **vagina** introduced by Robert von Olshausen (1835–1915), *ZGy* **19**:1. *6098*

1895:8 The first description of **angiomatosis** of the **retina** given by Eugen von Hippel (1869–1931) and named '**Hippel's disease**', *BVOG* **24**:269. *5940*

1895:9 A theory concerning the histogenesis of **choriocarcinoma (chorionepithelioma)** advanced by Felix von Marchand (1846–1928), *MonG* **1**:419, 513. *6097.1*

1895:10 **Granulosa cell tumour** of the **ovary** first described by Clemens von Kahlden (1859–1903), *ZAP* **6**:257. *6097*

1895:11 **Bartonellosis (verucca peruviana, Oroya fever)** named **Carrión's disease** by Ernesto Odriozola (1862–1921), *MonM* **10**:309, after Daniel Carrión (1857–85) who died of the disease after experiments with it. *5530*

1895:12 European **blastomycosis (cryptococcosis)** in humans described by Otto Busse (1867–1922), *DMW* **21**:V–B 14, and independently by Abraham Buschke (1868–1943), *DMW* **21**:V–B 14; later named **Busse-Buschke disease**. *5529.1, 5529.2*

1895:13 In his *Preliminary report on the tsetse fly disease or nagana, in Zululand*, David Bruce (1855–1931) showed that it was due to a **trypanosome,** *Trypanosoma brucei*. *5273*

1895:14 Brazilian **yaws (framboesia)** described by Achille Breda (1850–1935), *ArD* **33**:3, also called '**Breda's disease**'. *5293.1*

1895:15 First detailed description of *Loa loa*, the parasite in **loaiasis** given by Douglas Moray Cooper Lamb Argyll Robertson (1837–1909), *TOUK* **15**:137. *5347.1*

1895:16 The '**cathartic method**' used in **hysterical** patients by Sigmund Freud (1856–1939) as a basis for development of the method of free association and of the essential **psychoanalytic** concepts of the unconscious, repression and transference; in his *Studien über Hysterie*, 1895. *4999*

1895:17 Successful inoculation of animals with **anti-plague** bacillus by Alexandre Emile Jean Yersin (1863–1943), Léon Charles Albert Calmette (1863–1933) and A. Borrel, *AnIP* **9**:589. *5127*

1895:18 The diagnostic value of **cerebrospinal fluid examination** demonstrated by Paul Fürbringer (1849–1930), *BKW* **32**:272. *4873*

1895:19 A specific **anti-anthrax** serum providing passive immunization produced by Achille Sclavo (1861–1930), *RISP* **6**:841. *5170*

1895:20 A classic account of **paraphrasia** published by Jean Albert Pitres (1848–1928), *ReM* **15**:873. *4628*

1895:21 A bloodless method for closed reduction of congenital **dislocation of the hip-joint** suggested by Adolf Lorenz (1854–1946), *TAOrA* **7**:99. *4365*

1895:22 'Trendelenburg's sign' of **congenital dislocation of the hip-joint** described by Friedrich Trendelenburg (1844–1924), *DMW* **21**:21. *4428*

1895:23 **Hindquarter amputation** first successfully performed by Charles Girard (1850–1916), *PVC* **9**:823. *4473*

1895:24 First operation on **bladder diverticula** carried out by Jules Émile Péan (1830–1898), *BuAM* **33**:542. *4189*

1895:25 **Pentosuria** first described by Ernst Leopold Salkowski (1844–1923), *BKW* **32**:364. *3918*

1895:26 **Liver puncture biopsy** introduced by Luigi Lucatello (1863–1926), *LCMI* **6**:327. *3635*

1895:27 Extra-abdominal resection of the **colon** ('Paul's operation') devised by Frank Thomas Paul (1851–1941), *BMJ* **1**:1136. *3515*

1895:28 Direct-vision **laryngoscopy** introduced by Alfred Kirstein (1863–1922), *ArL* **3**:156. *3335*

1895:29 Specific **syphilitic** lesion defined as a cause of **aortic aneurysm** by Karl Gottfried Paul Döhle (1855–1928), *DAKM* **55**:190. *2985.1*

1895:30 Removal of lung for **tuberculosis** by William Macewen (1848–1924); reported 1906, *BMJ* **2**:1, the patient was alive in 1940. *3229*

1895:31 **X rays** (Röntgen rays) discovered by Wilhelm Conrad Röntgen (1845–1923), 8 November, *SPKG* 1895:132; 1896:11. *2683*

1895:32 **Diuretin** introduced in treatment of **angina pectoris** by S. Askanazy, *DAKM* **56**:209. *2893*

1895:33 **Sphygmomanometer**, for measuring blood-pressure in the finger, devised by Angelo Mosso (1846–1910), *ArIB* **23**:177. *2801*

1895:34 **Broadbent's sign** of **adherent pericardium** described by Walter Broadbent (1868–1951), *L* **2**:200. *2800*

1895:35 **Syphilis: Jarisch-Herxheimer reaction,** introduced by Adolph Jarisch (1850–1902), *WMW* **45**:720. *2396, 2397*

1895:36 A pressor substance, later named **adrenaline**, was demonstrated in the adrenal medulla by George Oliver (1841–1915) and Edward Albert Sharpey-Schafer (1850–1935), *JP* **18**:230. *1143*

1895:37 Donald Leslie **Augustine**, American parasitologist, born 1 Jan; with Hans Theiler, introduced an intradermal test for the diagnosis of trichinosis, 1932, *Para* **24**:60. *5351.1*

1895:38 Rebecca Craighill **Lancefield**, American bacteriologist, born 5 Jan; determined the different pathogenic strains of haemolytic streptococci and subdivided them into types, 1933, *JEM* **57**:571. Died 1981. *2524.2*

1895:39 Wilhelm **Raab**, Austrian/American physician, born 14 Jan; treated angina pectoris with thiouracil, 1945, *JAMA* **128**:249. Died 1969. *2900*

1895:40 Earl Dorland **Osborne**, American dermatologist, born 1 Feb; with co-workers, introduced sodium iodide as a contrast medium in uretero-pyelography, 1923, *JAMA* **80**:368. Died 1960. *4199*

1895:41 Carl Pieter Henrik **Dam**, Danish biochemist, born 21 Feb; discovered vitamin K, 1929, *BcZ* **215**:475; isolated vitamin K$_1$ with co-workers, 1939, *HCA* **22**:310. Shared Nobel Prize (Physiology or Medicine), 1943, with Edward Adelbert Doisy, *NPL*. Died 1976. *1062, 1080*

1895:42 Isaac **Starr**, American cardiologist, born 6 Mar; with co-workers, introduced the ballistocardiogram, 1939, *AmJPh* **127**:1. *2870*

1895:43 Marion Baldur **Sulzberger**, American dermatologist, born 12 Mar; showed that urticarial reactions could be caused by inhaled allergens, and coined the term 'atopic dermatitis', 1934, *JAl* **5**:554. Died 1983. *2605.1*

1895:44 Lionel Ernest Howard **Whitby**, British physician, born 8 May; showed experimentally the effectiveness of sulphapyridine (M & B 693) in pneumococcal and staphylococcal infections, 1938, *L* **1**:1210. Died 1956. *1951*

1895:45 Herman Ludwig **Blumgart**, American physician, born 19 Jul; with Samuel Albert Levine and D.D. Berlin, treated angina pectoris and congestive heart failure by thyroidectomy, 1933, *ArIM* **51**:866. *2899, 3033*

1895:46 Richard H. **Lawler**, American surgeon, born 12 Aug; with co-workers, carried out the first human kidney transplant in which the patient survived, 1950, *JAMA* **144**:844. Died 1982. *4256.1*

1895:47 André Frédéric **Cournand**, French/American physiologist, born 24 Sep; with Hilmert Albert Ranges, used the cardiac catheter as a method of clinical investigation, 1941, *PSEB*

**46**:462; for which he shared the Nobel Prize (Physiology or Medicine), 1956, with Werner Theodor Otto Forssmann and Dickinson Woodruff Roberts, *NPL*. Died 1988. *2871*

1895:48 Dickinson Woodruff **Richards** born, American physician, born 30 Oct; made important observations on catheterization of the right heart, 1957, *AmHJ* **54**:161, for which he shared the Nobel Prize (Physiology or Medicine), 1956, with André Frédéric Cournand and Werner Theodor Otto Forssmann, *NPL*. Died 1973. *2883.2*

1895:49 Gerhard **Domagk**, German pharmacologist, born 30 Oct; when research director at I.G. Farbenindustrie he introduced prontosil, the first drug containing a sulphonamide, 1935, *DMW* **61**:250; awarded Nobel Prize (Physiology or Medicine), 1939, for this work, *NPL*. With co-workers introduced thiosemicarbazone in treatment of tuberculosis, 1946, *NW* **33**:315. Died 1964. *1949, 2351*

1895:50 Walter **Freeman**, American neurologist and psychiatrist, born 14 Nov; with James Winston Watts, performed prefrontal lobotomy in treatment of certain psychotic conditions, 1936, *MADC* **5**:326. Died 1972. *4906*

1895:51 Anna **Freud**, Austrian child psychoanalyst, born 3 Dec; daughter of Sigmund Freud, made a special study of child psychoanalysis; in her *Einführung in die Technik der Kinderanalyse*, 1927. Died 1982. *4990.1*

1895:52 Charles Koran **Maytum**, American physician, born 20 Dec; reported hyperventilation syndrome, 1933, *PMC* **8**:282. *3207*

———

1895:53 Carl Boye **Semb**, Norwegian surgeon, born; introduced thoracoplasty with extrafascial apicolysis ('Semb's operation') in pulmonary tuberculosis, 1935, *AcC* Suppl.37ii:1. Died 1972. *3239*

1895:54 Hsien **Wu**, Chinese biochemist, born; with Otto Knut Olof Folin, devised the Folin-Wu test for blood sugar, 1919, *JBC* **38**:81. Died 1959. *3922*

1895:55 Louis Arthur **Milkman**, American radiologist, born; described osteomalacia with pseudofractures due to lack of calcium, 1930, *AmJR* **24**:29, and named 'Milkman's syndrome'. Died 1951. *4398*

1895:56 Augustus Roy **Felty**, American physician, born; described the combination of rheumatoid arthritis with splenomegaly and leucopenia ('Felty's syndrome'), 1924, *JHB* **35**:16. *4506*

1895:57 Paul **Durand**, French physician, born; isolated a virus (D virus) from his own blood. The resulting infection was named 'Durand's disease', 1940, *ArIP* **29**:179. Died 1961. *4661*

1895:58 Saul **Adler**, Russian/British parasitologist, born; with Mordehai Ber, proved that *Leishmania tropica*, causal organism of cutaneous leishmaniasis, is transmitted by the bite of *Phlebotomus papatasii*, 1941, *IJMR* **29**:803. Died 1966. *5301.2*

1895:59 Hugh Bethune **Maitland**, Canadian/British bacteriologist, born; with Mary Cowan Maitland, introduced 'Maitland's medium' for the cultivation of vaccinia virus, 1928, *L* **2**:596. Died 1972. *5434.1*

1895:60 Erich **Letterer**, German pathologist, born; first to describe Letterer-Siwe disease, 1924, *FZP* **30**:377. Died 1982. *6272, 6373*

---

1895: Carl **Ludwig** died, **born** 1816. *kymograph, renal secretion, salivary glands, excised organ perfusion*

1895: Johann Friedrich **Miescher** died, **born** 1844. *nuclein*

1895: Thomas **Longmore** died, **born** 1816. *heatstroke*

1895: Karl **Thiersch** died, **born** 1822. *cancer, epithelial cells, skin grafts*

1895: Louis **Pasteur** died, **born** 1822. *microorganisms, fermentation, aerobiosis, anaerobiosis, pasteurization, Clostridium septicum, staphylococcus, streptococcus, rabies vaccine, immunity, pneumococcus, anthrax immunization, puerperal fever*

1895: Hans Wilhelm **Meyer** died, **born** 1825. *adenoid growths*

1895: Aristide Auguste Stanislas **Verneuil** died, **born** 1823. *forcipressure in haemorrhage, gastrostomy*

1895: John **Tomes** died, **born** 1815. *dental education, dental forceps*

1895: James Edward **Garretson** died, **born** 1828. *oral surgery*

1895: James **Brown** died, **born** 1854. *catheterization of male ureters*

1895: Daniel Hack **Tuke** died, **born** 1827. *psychological medicine*

1895: Emil **Noeggerath** died, **born** 1827. *gonorrhoea, sterility, epicystotomy*

1895: Curt **Schimmelbusch** died, **born** 1860. *cystadenoma of breast*

1895: Robert **Battey** died, **born** 1828. *ovariotomy*

1895: Felix **Hoppe-Seyler** died, **born** 1825. *haemoglobin*

1895: William Chapman **Jarvis** died, **born** 1855. *nasal snare*

1895: Henry Willard **Williams** died, **born** 1821. *iriditis*

## 1896
1896:1 **University** founded at **Lyons**

1896:2 *Journal of Experimental Medicine* founded by William Henry **Welch**

1896:3 **[Institute for Infectious Diseases]** opened at **Berne**

1896:4 **Association Française d'Urologie** organized, **Paris**

1896:5 **Institut Pasteur de la Loire-Inférieur** founded at **Nancy**; opened 1898

1896:6 **Verein Abstinenter Aertze (Physicians' Temperance Society)** founded at **Berlin**

1896:7 **[Bacteriological Institute]** founded at **Kiev**, Ukraine

1896:8 **Röntgen Institute** opened at Stockholm

1896:9 **Medicinske Lyseninstitut (Phototherapeutic Institute)** opened at **Copenhagen** by Niels Ryberg **Finsen**

1896:10 **Gonoccocal** infection of the **bladder** as a cause of acute **cystitis** demonstrated by Ernst Wertheim (1864–1920), *ZGG* **35**:1. *6103*

1896:11 **Breast cancer** treated by **oöphorectomy** by George Thomas Beatson (1848–1933), *L* **2**:104, 162. *5778.1*

1896:12 A **diplobacillus** causing **conjunctivitis** isolated by Karl Theodor Paul Polykarpos Axenfeld (1867–1930), *BVOG* **25**:140. This bacillus was independently isolated by Victor Morax (1866–1935), *AnIP* **10**:337, and named the **Morax-Axenfeld bacillus**. *5941, 5942*

1896:13 The original description of mucinous **carcinoma** of the **ovary** ('**Krukenberg's tumour**') given by Friedrich Ernst Krukenberg (1870–1946), *ArGy* **50**:287. *6101*

1896:14 The significance of latent **gonorrhoeal infection** of the **uterus** emphasized by Ernst Wertheim (1864–1920), *VDGG* **6**:199. *6099*

1896:15 The first **rhinoplasty** using a free **bone graft** to the nose carried out by James Israel (1848–1926), *ArKC* **53**:255. *5755.1*

1896:16 Operation for the plastic reconstruction of the **vagina** described by Alwin Karl Mackenrodt (1859–1925), *ZGy* **20**:546. *6102*

1896:17 The buccal spots ('**Koplik's spots**'), an early diagnostic sign in **measles**, first noted by Henry Koplik (1858–1927), *ArPe* **13**:918. *5444*

1896:18 The parasite *Toxoplasma* first described by Charles Louis Alphonse Laveran (1845–1922), *CRSB* **52**:19. *5530.2*

1896:19 North American **blastomycosis** is also known as '**Gilchrist's disease**', following the description by Thomas Caspar Gilchrist (1862–1927), *JHR* **1**:269. *5530.1*

1896:20 **Cell lineage, germinal location**, and the **chromosomal** theory of **sex determination** studied by Edmund Beecher Wilson (1856–1939); in his *The cell in development and inheritance* (3rd edn *The cell in development and heredity*, 1925). *238*

1896:21 The life cycle and mode of transmission of the **hookworm**, *Ankylostoma duodenale*, elucidated by Arthur Looss (1861–1923), *ZBP* I Abt. **20**:865; **24**:441, 483. *5361*

1896:22 The discovery of **bacterial agglutination** made by Max Gruber (1853–1927) and Herbert Edward Durham (1866–1945), who realized its value in the identification of **typhoid**, *MMW* **43**:285. *5036*

1896:23 Killed **cholera** vaccine introduced by Wilhelm Kolle (1868–1935), *ZBP* I **19**:97. *5111*

1896:24 Specific **agglutinins** in the blood of **typhoid** patients demonstrated by Georges Fernand Isidor Widal (1862–1929) and Arthur Sicard, making possible a diagnostic **agglutination reaction** ('**Gruber-Widal test**'), *BSMH* **13**:681. *5037*

1896:25 Active inoculation against **typhoid** first performed by Almroth Edward Wright (1861–1947), *BMJ* **1**:122. *5039*

1896:26 *Salmonella paratyphi B* isolated by Emile Charles Achard (1860–1941) and Raoul Bensaude; the first use of the term **paratyphoid**, *BSMH* **13**:820. *5035*

1896:27 The extensor plantar response which occurs in **pyramidal-tract disease** ('**Babinski reflex**') described by Joseph François Félix Babinski (1857–1932), *CRSB* **48**:207. *4583*

1896:28 The **meningococcus** first isolated from cerebrospinal fluid by Johan Otto Leonhard Heubner (1843–1926), *JaK* **43**:1. *4680*

1896:29 **Marfan's syndrome** first described by Bernard Jean Antonin Marfan (1858–1942), *BSMH* **13**:220, although he described only the skeletal deformities (arachnodactyly, dolichostenomelia); eye and vascular system complications were recorded by later writers. *4365.1*

1896:30 **Chronic articular rheumatism in children** ('**Still's disease**') first described by George Frederic Still (1868–1941), *MCT* **80**:47. *4503*

1896:31 The first **radiogram** of a **kidney calculus** taken by John Macintyre (1857–1928), *L* **2**:118. *4293*

1896:32 The skin eruptions associated with **tuberculosis** grouped under the name **tuberculides** by Jean Darier (1856–1938), *AnD* **7**:1431. *4122*

1896:33 **Purpura annularis telangiectodes** first described by Domenico Majocchi (1849–1929), *GIMV* **31**:242. *4125*

1896:34 **Angiokeratoma**, first described by Cottle in 1877, was so named by Vittorio Mibelli (1860–1910), *GIMV* **26**:159, 260; it is also known as '**Mibelli's disease**'. *4105*

1896:35 A **gastroscope** introduced by Theodor Rosenheim, *BKW* **33**:275, 298, 325. *3516.1*

1896:36 A method of making **radiographs** of the **teeth** described by Frank Harrison, *JBD* **17**:624. *3688*

1896:37 The first **dental radiograph** in the United States taken by William James Morton (1845–1920), *DeC* **38**:478. *2684.3, 3689*

1896:38 **Biliary tract calculi** studied **radiographically** for the first time by J. Chappuis and H. Chauvel, *BuAM* **35**:410. *3636*

1896:39 Giulio Vassale (1862–1912) and Francesco Generali showed that **tetany** follows removal of the **parathyroid glands**, *RPN* **1**:95. *3857*

1896:40 The chief cause of **beriberi** shown by Christiaan Eijkman (1858–1930) to be a diet of over-milled rice, *GTNI* **30**:295; **32**:353; **36**:214. *3741*

1896:41 The first planned **nephrostomy** carried out by Joaquin Maria Albarran y Dominguez (1860–1912), *RC* **16**:882. *4226.1*

1896:42 **Ulcerative stomatitis** due to a fusiform bacillus and *Borrelia vincenti*, 'Vincent's angina', described by Jean Hyacinthe Vincent (1862–1950), *AnIP* **10**:488. *3309*

1896:43 First successful human **heart suture** performed by Ludwig Rehn (1849–1930), *ZCh* **23**:1048; *ArKC* **55**:315; marked the beginning of cardiac surgery. *3023, 3023.1*

1896:44 First successful suture of **femoral artery**, end-to-end anastomosis, by John Benjamin Murphy (1857–1916), *MR* **51**:73. *2967*

1896:45 **Radioactivity** discovered by Antoine Henri Becquerel (1852–1908), *CRAS* **122**:420. *2001, 2684.2*

1896:46 Intensifying screen introduced into **radiography** by Michael Idvorsky Pupin (1858–1935), *El* **10**:68. *2685*

1896:47 'Gruber-Widal' **bacterial agglutination test** developed by Georges Fernand Isidor Widal (1862–1929), *BSMH* **13**:681. *2550*

1896:48 Modified **sphygmomanometer** introduced by Scipione Riva-Rocci (1863–1937, *GMT* **47**:981, 1001. *2804*

1896:49 **Heart fluoroscopy**, the first application of **x rays** in cardiology, introduced by Francis Henry Williams (1852–1936), *BMSJ* **135**:335. *2686.1, 2804.1*

1896:50 First clinical application, for surgical diagnosis, of **x rays** in the United States by William Williams Keen (1837–1922), March, *AmJMS* **111**:256. *2684.1*

1896:51 Clinical use of **x rays**, to locate a bullet in the wrist, by Robert Jones (1858–1933) and Oliver Lodge (1851–1940), *L* **1**:476. *2684*

1896:52 **Pick's disease, constrictive pericarditis** causing cirrhosis, described by Friedel Pick (1867–1926), *ZKM* **29**:385. *2803*

1896:53 Account of **multiple hereditary telangiectasis** ('Rendu-Osler-Weber disease') by Henri Jules Louis Rendu (1844–1902), *GH* **69**:1322. *2710*

1896:54 **Bacterial agglutination** observed by Max Gruber (1853–1927) and Herbert Edward Durham (1866–1945) and used in diagnosis, *MMW* **43**:285. *2549*

1896:55 Antibacterial effect of a **penicillin** (from *Penicillium glaucum*) first recorded by Bartolomeo Gosio (1863–1944), *RISP* **7**:825, 829, 961. *1932.3*

1896:56 **Aminopyrine (pyramidon)** introduced by Wilhelm Filehne (1844–1927), *BKW* **33**:1061. *1889*

1896:57 Modern **phototherapy** introduced by Niels Ryberg Finsen (1860–1904); *Om anvendelse medicinen* .... *2000*

1896:58 **Thyroglobulin** isolated by Robert Hutchison (1871–1960), *JP* **20**:474. *1131.1*

1896:59 **Iodine** demonstrated in the thyroid by Eugen Baumann (1846–1896), *HSZ* **21**:319, 481; **22**:1. *1131*

1896:60 '**Riedel's thyroiditis**', a type of chronic thyroiditis, described by Bernhard Moritz Carl Ludwig Riedel (1846–1916), *VDK* **25**:101. *3841*

1896:61 Lee **Foshay**, American microbiologist, born 20 Jan; introduced a skin test for the diagnosis of tularaemia, 1932, *JID* **51**:286; devised a serum for treatment, 1933, *JAMA* **98**:552; **101**:1047; with A. Bernard Pasternack, used streptomycin in treatment, 1946, *JAMA* **130**:393. Died 1960. *5178, 5179, 5180*

1896:62 Joseph **Stokes**, American paediatrician, born 22 Feb; with co-workers, introduced mumps vaccine, 1946, *JEM* **84**:407. Died 1972. *5544.2*

1896:63 Philip Showalter **Hench**, American physician, born 28 Feb; with co-workers, introduced cortisone and adrenocorticotrophic hormone (ACTH) in the treatment of rheumatoid arthritis, 1949, *PMC* **24**:181, for which work he shared the Nobel Prize (Physiology or Medicine), 1950, with Edward Calvin Kendall and Tadeus Reichstein, *NPL*. Died 1965. *4508*

1896:64 Ladislaus Joseph **Meduna**, Hungarian neuropsychiatrist, born 27 Mar; introduced cardiazol (metrazol, pentylenetetrazol) convulsion therapy in the treatment of schizophrenia, 1935, *ZGN* **152**:235. Died 1965. *4961*

1896:65 Leo **Loewe**, American physician, born 15 Apr; with Israel Strauss, carried out experimental transmission of epidemic encephalitis, 1919, *JAMA* **73**:1056; with co-workers, first isolated *Rickettsia prowazeki*, causal agent in typhus, from blood, 1921, *JAMA* **77**:1967. *4651, 5392*

1896:66 Gregory **Shwartzman**, Russian/American bacteriologist, born 26 May; observed Shwartzman phenomenon, local skin reactivity to *Bacillus typhosus* filtrate, 1928, *JEM* **48**:247. Died 1965. *2576*

1896:67 Christopher Howard **Andrewes**, British virologist, born 7 Jun; introduced the diazo-colour test of kidney function, 1924, *L* **1**:590. With Wilson Smith and Patrick Playfair Laidlaw, recovered influenza A virus from throat washings of influenza patients, 1933, *L* **2**:66. Died 1988. *4244, 5494*

1896:68 Albert Markley **Snell**, American physician, born 9 Jun; with Hugh Roland Butt, used vitamin K in the treatment of haemorrhagic disease, 1938, *PMC* **13**:74. Died 1960. *3097*

1896:69 Hugh William Bell **Cairns**, British neurosurgeon, born in Australia, 26 Jun; with Charles Skinner Hallpike, described the histological changes in Menière's syndrome, 1938, *PRSM* **31**:1317. Died 1952. *3409*

1896:70 Ralph Dougall **Lillie**, American pathologist and histologist, born 1 Aug; showed that **Chlamydia psittaci** was causal agent of psittacosis, 1930, *USPHY* **45**:773; with Charles Armstrong, isolated the benign lymphocytic choriomeningitis virus, 1934, *USPHR* **49**:1019. *4688*

1896:71 Gerty Theresa **Cori**, Czech biochemist, born 8 Aug; collaborated with her husband, Carl Ferdinand Cori (1896–1984), in research on the course of catalytic transformation of glycogens and made the first *in vitro* synthesis of glycogen, 1947, *Harvey Lectures* (1945–6) **41**:253. They shared the Nobel Prize (Physiology or Medicine), 1947, with Bernardo Alberto Houssay, *NPL*. Died 1957. *751.4*

1896:72 Chauncey Depew **Leake**, American pharmacologist, born 5 Sep; with Mei-Yu Chen, first demonstrated the anaesthetic properties of divinyl ether, 1930, *PSEB* **28**:151. Died 1978. *5713*

1896:73 Rudolph **Nissen**, German surgeon, born 9 Sep; successful complete removal of bronchiectatic lung, 1931, *ZCh* **58**:3003. *3203*

1896:74 Jószef **Baló**, Hungarian physician, born 10 Nov; described encephalitis periaxialis concentrica ('Baló's disease'), 1927, *MOA* **28**:108. *4653*

1896:75 Adolphe **Franceschetti**, Swiss ophthalmologist and plastic surgeon, born 10 Nov; with Archibald McIndoe, used reciprocal skin homografts to prove the relationship of identical twins, 1950, *BJPS* **2**:283. *1757*

1896:76 Herbert Windsor **Wade**, American leprologist, born 23 Nov; introduced scraped-incision slit-skin method for diagnosis of leprosy, 1924, *JPMA* **4**:132. Died 1968. *2440.1*

1896:77 Bernard **Schlesinger**, British paediatrician, born 23 Nov; showed that haemolytic streptococcal infection was a cause of acute rheumatism in children, 1930, *ArDiC* **5**:411. Died 1984. *4507*

1896:78 Carl Ferdinand **Cori**, Czech biochemist, born 5 Dec; collaborated with his wife, Gerty Theresa Cori (1896–1957), in research on the course of catalytic transformation of glycogens and made the first *in vitro* synthesis of glycogen, *Harvey Lectures* (1945–6), 1947, **41**:253. They shared the Nobel Prize (Physiology or Medicine), 1947, with Bernardo Alberto Houssay, *NPL*. Died 1984. *751.4*

1896:79 Alexander William Gordon **Ewing**, British physician, born 6 Dec; with Irene Rosetta Ewing, devised hearing tests for children, 1944, *JLO* **59**:309. Died 1980. *3412.1*

1896:80 Walter **Kikuth**, Latvian/German physician, born 21 Dec; introduced mepacrine (atebrine, quinacrine), an antimalarial, 1932, *DMW* **58**:530. With co-workers, introduced lucanthone hydrochloride (Miracil D) for the treatment of bilharziasis, 1946, *NW* **33**:253. Died 1968. *5257, 5351.2*

---

1896:81 Hermann **Vollmer**, American paediatrician, born; with Esther White Goldberger, introduced the tuberculin patch test for tuberculosis, 1937, *AmJDC* **54**:1019. Died 1955. *2348*

1896:82 Benjamin **Sacks**, American physician, born; with Emanuel Libman, described lupus erythematosus with endocarditis ('Libman-Sacks disease'), 1924, *ArIM* **33**:701. *2855*

436

1896:83 Tenji **Taniguchi**, Japanese virologist, born; with co-workers, established a virus aetiology for Japanese B encephalitis, 1936, *JJEM* **14**:185. Died 1961. *4659*

1896:84 William Thomas **Lemmon**, American anaesthetist, born; introduced continuous spinal analgesia, 1940, *AnS* **111**:141. *5722*

---

1896: Eugen **Baumann** died, **born** 1846. *iodine, sulphonal*

1896: Georg Richard **Lewin** died, **born** 1820. *tumour of larynx, laryngoscope*

1896: Victor Charles **Hanot** died, **born** 1844. *liver cirrhosis*

1896: William Morrant **Baker** died, **born** 1839. *erythema serpens, cysts of knee-joint*

1896: George **Harley** died, **born** 1829. *paroxysmal haemoglobinuria*

1896: John **Macintyre** died, **born** 1857. *kidney calculus, radiogram*

1896: Philipp Jakob Wilhelm **Henke** died, **born** 1834. *metatarsus varus*

1896: John Eric **Erichsen** died, **born** 1818. *whiplash injuries*

1896: Paul **Blocq** died, **born** 1860. *astasia-abasia*

1896: Julius Thomas **Thomsen** died, **born** 1815. *myotonia congenita*

1896: Lucas Anton **Dressler** died, **born** 1815. *paroxysmal cold, haemoglobinuria*

1896: Emil **du Bois-Reymond** died, **born** 1818. *electrophysiology, electrotonus*

1896: John Langdon Haydon **Langdon-Down** died, **born** 1828. *mongolism, Down's syndrome*

**1897**
1897:1 **Kyoto Imperial University** founded

1897:2 **Röntgen Society** founded in **London**

1897:3 **Institut National d'Hygiene et de Bactériologie** founded at **Luxembourg**

1897:4 The gauze **face mask** introduced into operative **surgery** by Paul Berger (1845–1908), *BCSP* **25**:187. *5641*

1897:5 **Precipitin reaction**, for qualitative estimation of **antigens** and **antibodies**, devised by Rudolf Kraus (1868–1932), *WKW* **10**:736. *2550.1*

1897:6 The mode of fertilization of the **malaria** parasite observed by William George MacCallum (1874–1944), *Lancet* **1**:1240. *5246*

1897:7 Proof that the **mosquito** is responsible for the transmission of **malaria** provided by Ronald Ross (1857–1937), he found *Plasmodium* in the stomach of *Anopheles* after it had been fed on the blood of malaria patients, *BMJ* **2**:1786. *5247*

1897:8 The **flea** considered by Masanori Ogata (1852–1919) to be the principal, if not the sole, vector of bubonic **plague** infection, *ZBP* I, **21**:769. *5128*

1897:9 *Brucella abortus*, a cause of **brucellosis** in cattle, discovered by Bernhard Laurits Frederik Bang (1848–1932), *ZT* **1**:241. *5099*

1897:10 Paul Ehrlich (1854–1915) improved Behring's **diphtheria antitoxin** through quantitative titration, *KJ* **6**:299; the first exposition of Ehrlich's **side-chain theory** appeared in this paper. He established an international standard for this and other antitoxins, initiating the concept of **biological standardization**. *5064*

1897:11 An agglutination test for the diagnosis of **brucellosis** devised by Almroth Edward Wright (1861–1947) and Frederick Smith, *Lancet* **1**:656. *5101*

1897:12 An excellent description of the various forms of **cerebral palsy**, with precise classification of the different spastic symptoms, given by Sigmund Freud (1856–1939); in his *Die infantile Cerebrallähmung*. *4708.2*

1897:13 **Tuberculous rheumatism** ('**Poncet's disease**') described by Antonin Poncet (1849–1913), *GH* **70**:1219. *4504*

1897:14 Operative **cystoscope** devised by Max Nitze (1848–1906), made it possible to excise **bladder tumours** *in situ*, *ZKH* **8**:8. *4190*

1897:15 The **acne bacillus**, *Corynebacterium acnes*, first described by Raymond Jacques Adrien Sabouraud (1864–1938), *AnIP* **11**:134. *4126*

1897:16 **Osteoperiostitis of the metatarsals** ('**Busquet's disease**') described by G.P. Busquet (b.1866), *RC* **17**:1065. *4330*

1897:17 **Progeria** so named by Hastings Gilford (1861–1941), *MCT* **80**:17. *3792*

1897:18 Treatment of **otosclerosis** by **fenestration** first attempted by Adolf Passow (1859–1926), *VDOG* **6**:143. *3397*

1897:19 First successful total **gastrectomy** performed by Carl Schlatter (1864–1934), *BKC* **19**:757; **23**:589. *3517*

1897:20 **Pulmonary tuberculosis** treated by removal of lung apex by Théodore Tuffier (1857–1929); in his *Chirurgie du poumon* …. *3228*

1897:21 **X ray cinematography** introduced by John MacIntyre (1859–1928), *ArSk* **1**:37. *2687*

1897:22 **Eisenmenger syndrome** described by Victor Eisenmenger, *ZKM* **32** (Sup.) 1. *2806*

1897:23 Pressure gauge substituted for mercury manometer in the Riva-Rocci **sphygmomanometer** by Leonard Erskine Hill (1866–1952) and Harold Leslie Barnard (1868–1908), *BMJ* **2**:904. *2807*

1897:24 Bacterial system of **sewage purification** introduced by William Joseph Dibdin (1850–1925); in his *Purification of sewage and water. 1631*

1897:25 **Deep radiation therapy** with **x rays** used by Leopold Freund (1868–1944), *WKW* **10**:73. *2002*

1897:26 *Clostridium botulinum* discovered by Emile Pierre Marie van Ermengem (1851–1932) in cases of **food poisoning**, *ArPha* **3**:213, 499. *2510*

1897:27 Classical work on **digestion** published by Ivan Petrovich Pavlov (1849–1936), in his *Lectures. 1022*

1897:28 Cell-free **fermentation**, turning point in the study of **enzymes**, discovered by Eduard Buchner (1860–1910), *BDCG* **30**:117, 1110, 2668. *719.1*

---

1897:29 Claus W. **Jungeblut**, American bacteriologist and immunologist, born 12 Jan; with Murray Sanders, isolated the encephalomyocarditis virus, 1940, *JEM* **72**:407. *4661.1*

1897:30 John Franklin **Enders**, American microbiologist, born 10 Feb; with Thomas Huckle Weller and F.C. Robbins, grew poliomyelitis virus in cultures of various tissues, removing obstacles to vaccine production, 1949, *Science* **109**:85; for this work all three shared the Nobel Prize (Physiology or Medicine), 1954, *NPL*. With Thomas C. Peebles, isolated measles virus, 1954, *PSEB* **86**:277. With Samuel Lawrence Katz and M. Milovanovič, propagated the virus in cultures of chick embryo cells, 1958, *PSEB* **97**:23. With Samuel Lawrence Katz, M. Milovanovič and A. Holloway, produced a live virus vaccine, 1960, *NEJM* **263**:153. Died 1985. *4671.1, 5449.2, 5449.3, 5449.4*

1897:31 Leon Grotius **Zerfas**, American anaesthetist, born 7 Mar; with co-workers, first used sodium amytal as an intravenous anaesthetic, 1929, *PSEB* **26**:399. *5712*

1897:32 Chester Scott **Keefer**, American physician, born 3 May; with William Edward R. Greer, first described cat-scratch fever, 1951, *NEJM* **244**:545. Died 1972. *5546.2*

1897:33 Sanford Morris **Rosenthal**, American pharmacologist, born 5 May; with Edwin Clay White, devised the bromsulphthalein test for liver function, 1924, *JPET* **24**:265. *3653*

1897:34 Wilson **Smith**, British bacteriologist, born 1 Jun; with Christopher Howard Andrewes and Patrick Playfair Laidlaw, recovered influenza A virus from throat washings of influenza patients, 1933, *L* **2**:66. With Charles Herbert Stuart-Harris, reported first successful passage of influenza from animal to man, 1936, *L* **2**:121. Died 1965. *5494, 5497*

1897:35 John Frederick **Wilkinson**, British physician, born 10 Jun; with Martin Cyril Gordon Israëls, first described achrestic anaemia, 1935, *BMJ* **1**:139, 194. *3148*

1897:36 Austin Bradford **Hill**, British medical statistician, born 8 Jul; with William Richard Shaboe Doll, proved association of lung cancer with cigarette smoking (Müller, 1939; Wynder & Graham, 1950), 1950, *BMJ* **2**:139. Died 1991. *3215.2, 3213, 3215.1*

1897:37 Tadeus **Reichstein**, Polish biochemist, born 10 Jul; with co-workers synthesized vitamin C, 1933, *HCA* **16**:1019. Isolated Compound Fa (cortisone), 1936, *HCA* **19**:1107, for which work he shared the Nobel Prize (Physiology or Medicine), 1950, with Philip Showalter Hench and Edward Calvin Kendall, *NPL*. Died 1996. *1068, 1153*

1897:38 Charles Robert **Harington**, British biochemist, born 1 Aug; with George Barger, synthesized thyroxine, 1927, *BJ* **21**:169. Died 1972. *1138*

1897:39 Achile Mario **Dogliotti**, Italian surgeon, born 25 Sep; introduced the subarachnoid injection of alcohol for the relief of pain, 1931, *PrM* **39**:1249. First used surgical section of the lemniscus lateralis for the relief of severe intractable pain, 1938, *CRA* **17**:143. Died 1966. *4898, 4909*

1897:40 William Bosworth **Castle**, American physician, born 21 Oct; showed pernicious anaemia to be due to absence from the gastric juice of haemopoietin (Castle's instrinsic factor), necessary for the absorption of vitamin B$_{12}$, 1929, *AmJMS* **178**:748. *3143*

1897:41 Josep **Trueta**, Spanish surgeon, born 28 Oct; during the Spanish civil war he developed a method of treating wounds and compound fractures by the application of closed plaster after packing the excised wound with sterile vaselined gauze, which he termed the biological treatment of wounds; in his *El tratamiento de la fractura de guerra*, 1938. Died 1977. *5632, 4435.1*

1897:42 Hobart Ansteth **Reimann**, American physician, born 31 Oct; first described atypical pneumonia, 1938, *JAMA* **111**:2377. *3211*

------

1897:43 Stanley Owen **Chambers** born; with John Hinchman Stokes, introduced bismarsen (bismuth arsphenamine sulphate) in the treatment of syphilis, 1927, *JAMA* **89**:1500. *2414*

1897:44 Heinz **Küstner**, Bohemian gynaecologist, born; with Otto Carl Willy Prausnitz, demonstrated the 'Prausnitz-Küstner reaction', the presence of antibodies in the serum of persons suffering from atopic diseases, 1921, *ZBP* I **86**:160. Died 1931. *2601.1*

1897:45 Josef **Berberich**, German physician, born; with S. Hirsch, made the first angiogram of a living patient, 1923, *KW* **2**:2226. *2916*

1897:46 Manes **Kartagener**, Swiss physician, born; reported bronchiectasis associated with sinusitis and situs inversus ('Kartagener's syndrome'), 1933, *BKT* **83**:489. *3206*

1897:47 H. Lowry **Rush**, American surgeon, born; with Leslie V. Rush, introduced 'Rush pins', made of specially hardened stainless steel, for the fixation of fractures of long bones, 1949, *AmJSu* **78**:324. Died 1965. *4435.2*

1897:48 Helmut **Weese**, German anaesthetist, born; with Walther Scharpff, introduced evipan (hexobarbitone) as an anaesthetic, 1932, *DMW* **58**:1205. Died 1954. *5714*

1897:49 Cecil **Striker**, American pharmacologist, born; with co-workers, first reported human anaesthetization with trichlorethylene, 1935, *CRA* **14**:68. *5721*

1897:50 Sture August **Siwe**, Swedish physician, born; published his account of Letterer-Siwe disease in 1933, *ZK* **55**:212. *6373, 6372*

1897:51 Garwood Colvin **Richardson** born; with Gustav William Rapp, introduced a saliva test for prenatal sex determination, 1952, *Science* **115**:265. *6235*

---

1897: Alarik Frithiof **Holmgren** died, **born** 1831. *electroretinogram, retinal action currents, colour-blindness*

1897: Frederic John **Mouat** died, **born** 1816. *chaulmoogra oil, leprosy*

1897: Paul Louis **Duroziez** died, **born** 1826. *mitral stenosis, aortic insufficiency*

1897: Richard John **Hall** died, **born** 1856. *appendicectomy*

1897: Henry Vandyke **Carter** died, **born** 1831. *mycetoma, relapsing fever, Borrelia carteri, rat-bite fever, Spirillum minus*

1897: Adolphe **Gubler** died, **born** 1821. *hemiplegia*

1897: Rudolph **Berlin** died, **born** 1833. *dyslexia*

1897: Augustin Marie **Morvan** died, **born** 1819. *syringomyelia*

1897: John Charles **Bucknill** died, **born** 1817. *psychological medicine*

1897: Etienne Stéphane **Tarnier** died, **born** 1828. *antisepsis, axis-traction forceps*

1897: Thomas Spencer **Wells** died, **born** 1818. *pressure forceps, ovariotomy*

1897: John Braxton **Hicks** died, **born** 1823. *placenta praevia, bipolar version, Braxton-Hicks' sign*

**1898**
1898:1 **Rush Medical College** affiliated with **University of Chicago**

1898:2 **Cornell University Medical College (New York City)** founded

1898:3 **Faculty of Medicine** at **Porto Alegre, Brazil**, organized

1898:4 **Philippine Health Service** organized at **Manila**

1898:5 **Institute for the Study of Malignant Disease (New York)** founded

1898:6 **State Sanitariun for Tuberculosis** opened in **Massachusetts**

1898:7 **Liverpool School of Tropical Medicine** founded

1898:8 Émile **Marchoux** (1862–1943) founds **Bacteriological Laboratory for East Africa** at **St Louis, Senegal**

1898:9 **Deutsche Pathologische Gesellschaft** founded at **Dresden**

1898:10 **Washington Academy of Sciences** organized

1898:11 **Gallstones** first demonstrated **radiographically** by A. Buxbaum, *WMP* **39**:534. *3638*

1898:12 Important studies on **immune haemolysis** by Jean Jules Baptiste Vincent Bordet (1870–1961), 1898, *AnIP* **12**:688; 1899, **13**:225. *2551*

1898:13 **Haldane apparatus** for analysis of **respiratory gases** devised by John Scott Haldane (1860–1936), *JP* **22**:465. *951.1*

1898:14 Vaginal **caesarean section** introduced by Alfred Dührssen (1862–1933), *SKV* **232**:1365. *6246*

1898:15 A lip-switch flap, transferring a full-thickness flap from one lip to the other for the repair of double **cleft lip** introduced by Robert Abbe (1851–1928), *MR* **53**:477. *5755.2*

1898:16 The modern treatment of **rhinophyma** developed by George Howard Monks (1853–1933), *BMSJ* **139**:262. *5755.4*

1898:17 The last link in the chain demonstrating the complete life-cycle of the parasite of bird **malaria** provided by Ronald Ross (1857–1932), *L* **2**:488. *5251*

1898:18 Eugene Lindsay Opie (1873–1971) and William George MacCallum (1874–1944) discovered the sexual phase of the **malaria** parasite, *JEM* **3**:79, 103, 117. *5249, 5250*

1898:19 The first description of the protozoon later named *Leishmania tropica*, causal organism in cutaneous **leishmaniasis**, given by Petr Fokich Borovskii (1863–1932), *VMZ* **76**:925. *5294*

1898:20 *Salmonella paratyphi A* isolated by Norman Beechey Gwyn (1875–1952), *JHB* **9**:54. *5038*

1898:21 Leonardo Gigli (1863–1908) adapted his saw, **Gigli's saw**, for **craniotomy**, *ZCh* **25**:425. *4874*

1898:22 The **dysentery** bacillus, *Shigella dysenteriae*, discovered by Kiyoshi Shiga (1870–1957), *ZBP* I, **24**:817, 870. *5091*

1898:23 An account of **pseudosclerosis of the brain** by Ernst Adolf Gustav Gottfried Strümpell (1853–1925), *DZN* **12**:115, followed an earlier description by Westphal (1883) and led to the term '**Westphal-Strümpell disease**'. *4709, 4702*

1898:24 *The nervous system and its diseases*, by Charles Karsner Mills (1845–1931) was the foremost American **neurological** text of the nineteenth century and the only one of the period to contain a section on the chemistry of the **nervous system**. *4586.1*

1898:25 In his *Treatise on aphasia and other speech defects*, Henry Charlton Bastian (1837–1915) localized the **auditory** and **visual centres**, and described **word-blindness** and **word-deafness**. *4629*

1898:26 **Kinematization of amputation stump** – use of the musculature above an amputation stump to form a motor unit for an **artificial limb** – first suggested by Giuliano Vanghetti (1861–1940); in his *Amputazione, disarticulazione et protesi*. *4474*

1898:27 The name 'spondylose rhizomélique' given by Pierre Marie (1853–1940) to ankylosing spondylitis, *ReM* 18:285, already described by Strümpell in 1884. *4368, 4349*

1898:28 Cleido-cranial dysostosis given its present name by Pierre Marie (1853–1940) and Paul Sainton (1868–1958), *ReN* 6:835; it was first described by Morand in 1760. *4369, 4302.2*

1898:29 Isolation of streptococci from patients with acute rheumatism reported by Henri Triboulet (1864–1920) and Amand Coyon (1871–1928), *CRSB* 50:124. *4504.1*

1898:30 Moriz Kaposi [Kohn] (1837–1902) published a valuable collection of illustrations in dermatology; *Handatlas der Hautkrankheiten*, 1898–1900. *4001*

1898:31 A sporotrichosis due to the fungus *Sporotrichum beurmanni* (named after C.L. de Beurmann), described by Benjamin Robinson Schenck (1872–1920), *JHB* 9:286. 4127

1898:32 External fixation in the treatment of fractures was introduced by Clayton Parkhill (1860–1902), *AnS* 27:553. *4429.2*

1898:33 Georges Hayem (1841–1933) drew attention to acquired haemolytic anaemia, *JMI* 2:116. Following Widal and Abrami's account, 1907, the condition was named 'Hayem-Widal disease' and 'Widal-Abrami disease'. *3777, 3783*

1898:34 In his classical description of lymphadenoma, Carl Sternberg (1872–1935) distinguished it from aleukaemic anaemia, with which it had previously been included, *ZHe* 19:21. *3776*

1898:35 Georg Lotheissen (b.1868) devised an operation for the radical repair of femoral hernia, *ZCh* 25:548. *3605*

1898:36 Joseph Colt Bloodgood's (1867–1935) operation for inguinal hernia published, *JHB* 29:96. *3604.2*

1898:37 The bismuth meal introduced by Walter Bradford Cannon (1871–1945) to enable roentgenological examination of the digestive tract, *AmJPh* 1:359. *2678.1, 3519*

1898:38 Direct bronchoscopy introduced by Gustav Killian (1860–1921), *MMW* 45:844. *3336*

1898:39 Foot-and-mouth disease shown to be due to a filter-passing virus (first recognition of such a virus as a cause of animal disease) by Friedrich Albert Johann Loeffler (1852–1915) and Paul Frosch (1860–1928), *ZBP I*, 23:371. *2511*

1898:40 Tubercle bacillus; bovine and human types differentiated by Theobald Smith (1859–1934), *JEM* 3:451. *2335*

1898:41 *Salmonella aertrycke* found to be a cause of food poisoning by Herbert Edward Durham (1866–1945), *BMJ* 2:608. A similar finding was made by Jules de Nobele (b.1865); *ASMG* 77:281. *2513, 2514*

1898:42 Tropical disease; Patrick Manson (1844–1922), 'Father of modern tropical medicine', published first edition of his textbook, *Tropical diseases. 2266*

1898:43 **Mescaline** isolated by Karl Wilhelm Arthur Heffter (1859–1925); one of the earliest investigations of a psychedelic drug, *ArEP* **40**:385. *1890.1*

1898:44 **Radium** isolated by Pierre (1859–1906) and Marie Curie (1867–1934), *CRAS* **127**:175, 1215. *2003*

1898:45 A pressor substance, **renin**, shown to be produced by the kidneys by Robert Adolf Armand Tigerstedt (1853–1923) and Per Gustav Bergman (1874–1955), *SkAP* **8**:223. *1236*

---

1898:46 Grace Mary **Sickles**, American virologist, born 12 Jan; with Gilbert Julius Dalldorf, isolated the coxsackie virus from children with paralysis, 1948, *Science* **108**:61. Died 1959. *5545*

1898:47 Leo Max **Davidoff**, Latvian/American neurosurgeon, born 16 Jan; with C.G. Dyke, introduced lumbar encephalography, 1932, *BNI* **2**:75. Died 1975. *4611.3*

1898:48 Soma **Weiss**, American physiologist and pharmacologist, born 27 Jan; with James Porter Baker, first described carotid sinus syndrome, 1933, *Medicine* **12**:297. Died 1942. *2921*

1898:49 William Stewart **Duke-Elder**, British ophthalmologist, born 22 Apr; editor of *System of ophthalmology*, 19 vols, 1958–76. Died 1978.

1898:50 Helen Brooke **Taussig**, American physician, born 4 May; with Alfred Blalock, devised operation for congenital defects of the pulmonary artery ('Blalock-Taussig operation'), 1945, *JAMA* **128**:189. Died 1986. *3043*

1898:51 Lionel Sharples **Penrose**, British geneticist and medical statistician, born 11 Jun; pointed out the significance of maternal age in the aetiology of Down's syndrome; in *A clinical and genetic study of 1,280 cases of mental defect* (Spec. Rep. Ser., MRC, No. 229), 1938. Died 1972. *4962.1*

1898:52 Cornelius Packard **Rhoads**, American pathologist, born 20 Jun; with co-workers, introduced triethylene melamine (TEM) in the treatment of Hodgkin's disease, 1950, *TAAP* **63**:136. Died 1959. *3788.1*

1898:53 Donald William **McCorquodale**, American biochemist, born 30 Jun; with co-workers isolated oestradiol, 1936, *JBC* **115**:435. *1202*

1898:54 George Porter **Robb**, American cardiologist, born 8 Jul; with Israel Steinberg, introduced angiocardiography, 1938, *JCI* **17**:507. *2689*

1898:55 Warren Henry **Cole**, American physician, born 24 Jul; with Evarts Ambrose Graham, introduced cholecystography, 1924, *JAMA* **82**:613. *3652*

1898:56 Edward Holbrook **Derrick**, Australian pathologist, born 20 Sep; first described the rickettsial infection, Q (query) fever, 1937, *MJA* **2**:281. Died 1976. *5397*

1898:57 Owen Harding **Wangensteen**, American surgeon, born 21 Sep; introduced decompression apparatus for the treatment of acute intestinal obstruction, 1932, *WJS* **40**:1. Died 1981. *3554*

1898: 58 Howard Walter **Florey**, Australian pathologist, born 24 Sep; with Ernst Boris Chain, Edward Penley Abraham et al., proved the chemotherapeutic action of penicillin, 1940, *L* **2**:226. Shared the Nobel Prize (Physiology or Medicine), 1945, with Alexander Fleming and use in man, *NPL*. Died 1968. *1933.3*

1898: 59 Osker Paul **Wintersteiner**, Austrian/American chemist, born 15 Nov; isolated cortisone, 1936, *JBC* **111**:599; **116**:291. Died 1971. *1152*

1898: 60 Forrest E. **Kendall**, American immunologist, born; with Michael Heidelberger, introduced quantitative precipitin reaction, 1929, *JEM* **50**:809. *2576.01*

1898: 61 Pierre **Grabar**, French chemist, born; introduced immunoelectrophoresis, 1953, *BBA* **10**:193. Died 1986. *2578.13*

1898: 62 Max **Schmidt**, Danish psychiatrist, born; first to describe temporal arteritis, 1930, *Brain* **53**:489. *2919*

1898: 63 Louis **Wolff**, American physician, born; with John Parkinson and Paul Dudley White, described the Wolff-Parkinson-White syndrome, 1930, *AmHJ* **5**:685. *2860*

1898: 64 Jörgen **Lehmann** born; introduced *p*-aminosalicylic acid in the treatment of pulmonary tuberculosis, first specific anti-tuberculosis drug, 1946, *L* **1**:15. *3241*

1898: 65 Leslie Julius **Harris**, British biochemist, born; with Y.L. Wang, developed Wang's test for vitamin deficiency (avitaminosis), 1938, *BJ* **33**:1356. Died 1973. *3708*

1898: 66 William **Snow**, American radiologist, born; with Clilian Bethany Powell, achieved direct radiography of the placenta, 1934, *AmJR* **31**:37. *6229*

1898: Friedrich Albert **Zenker** died, **born** 1825. *pneumoconiosis, pulmonary fat embolism, trichinosis*

1898: Jules Émile **Péan** died, **born** 1830. *carcinoma, gastrectomy, bladder diverticula, shoulder prosthesis, uterine tumours*

1898: David **Gruby** died, **born** 1810. *ringworm, sycosis barbae, tinea capitis, trypanosome, thrush, Candida albicans*

1898: André Victor **Cornil** died, **born** 1837. *gout, arthritis*

1898: Louis **Bauer** died, **born** 1814. *orthopaedics*

1898: Joseph P. **O'Dwyer** died, **born** 1841. *croup, laryngeal intubation*

1898: William **Jenner** died, **born** 1815. *typhus, typhoid*

1898: Karl Georg Friedrich **Leuckart** died, **born** 1823. *Taenia echinococcus*

1898: Charles **West** died, **born** 1816. *paediatrics*

**1899**

1899:1 **London School of Tropical Medicine** founded; became London School of Hygiene and Tropical Medicine, 1924

1899:2 **Instituto Nacional de Higiene de Alfonso XIII, Madrid**, founded

1899:3 **Medical Library Association (US)** founded

1899:4 **American Anthropological Association** founded, Washington, DC

1899:5 **Cancer Commission of Harvard University** founded

1899:6 **Instituto Butantan** founded at **São Paulo** by Vital Brazil

1899:7 Howard Atwood Kelly (1858–1943) published *Operative gynecology*, 2 vols. *6108*

1899:8 An ovarian tumour, the '**Brenner tumour**', named after Fritz Brenner, who described it in 1907, first noted by Ernst Gottlob Orthmann (1858–1922), *MonG* **9**:771. *6109.1, 6118*

1899:9 The use of **cocaine** as a **spinal anaesthetic** introduced by August Karl Gustav Bier (1861–1949), *DZC* **51**:361. *5684*

1899:10 **Procaine (novocaine), local anaesthetic**, synthesized by Alfred Einhorn (1856–1917), *MMW* **46**:1218, 1254. *5685*

1899:11 Giovanni Battista Grassi (1854–1925) and Amico Bignami (1862–1929) showed that the **malaria** parasite, *Plasmodium*, undergoes its sexual phase in the *Anopheles* **mosquito**, *AnIS* **9**:258. *5252*

1899:12 **Influenzal meningitis** first described by Slawyk, *ZHyg* **32**:443. *4681*

1899:13 Nils Ryberg Finsen (1860–1904) pioneered the treatment of **lupus vulgaris** by **light therapy**; in *La photothérapie*, etc. *4002*

1899:14 Attempt to visualize the **urinary tract** by a combination of an opaque **ureteral** styletted catheter and **radiography** by Théodore Tuffier (1857–1929); in Duplay, S. & Reclus, P. *Traité de chirurgie*, **7**:448. *4191.1*

1899:15 First operation on the **kidney** for the relief of chronic **nephritis** carried out by George Michael Edebohls (1853–1908), *MN* **74**:481. *4228*

1899:16 Caesar Peter Moeller Boeck (1845–1917) established the syndrome of **benign sarcoid (Boeck's sarcoid)**, *NML* **14**:1321; the earlier account by Besnier and the later one by Schaumann led to the name '**Besnier-Boeck-Schaumann disease**'. *4095, 4128, 4149*

1899:17 Operation for **undescended testicle** and **congenital inguinal hernia** devised by Arthur Dean Bevan (1861–1943), *JAMA* **33**:773. *4191*

1899:18 **Embryoma** of the **kidney** ('**Wilms' tumour**') described by Max Wilms (1867–1918); in *Die Mischgeschwülste, 1. Niere.* *4227*

1899:19 **Syphilis** established as a cause of **aortic aneurysm** by Arnold Heller (1840–1913), *MMW* **46**:1669. *2987*

1899:20 **Acute myocarditis** ('**Fiedler's myocarditis'**) described by Carl Ludwig Fiedler (1835–1921); in his *Über akute interstitielle Myokarditis*. *2809.2*

1899:21 First successful treatment of **cancer** with **x rays** carried out by Tage Anton Ultimus Sjögren (1859–1939), *FSL*:208. *2624*

1899:22 **Arterial suture** technique introduced by Julius Dörfler, *BKC* **25**:781. *2908.2*

1899:23 **Heart arrhythmia, 'Wenckebach's phenomenon'**, described by Karel Frederik Wenckebach (1864–1940), *ZKM* **36**:181. *2809.1*

1899:24 **Acetylsalicylic acid (aspirin)** introduced into medicine by Heinrich Dreser (1860–1925), *PfA* **76**:306. *1891*

1899:25 *Animals in motion* published by Eadweard Muybridge (1830–1904). *650*

1899:26 **Rocky Mountain spotted fever** first described by Edward Ernest Maxey (1867–1934), *MSe* **7**:433. *5377*

1899:27 **Keratosis follicularis (dyskeratosis)**, so well described by Jean Darier (1856–1938), *AnD* **10**:597, is also known as **Darier's disease**; it was first described by Lutz and later by J.C. White. *4050, 4093, 4097*

1899:28 **Artificial fertilization** achieved by Jacques Loeb (1859–1924), *AmJPh* **3**:135. *515.1*

1899:29 Important observations on **surgical shock** made by George Washington Crile (1864–1843); *An experimental research into surgical shock*. *5622*

1899:30 The monumental *Textura del sistema nervioso de hombre y de los vertebrados*, 2 vols (in 3), of Santiago Ramón y Cajal (1852–1934) expounds the cytological and histological foundations of modern **neuroanatomy**. *1293.1*

---

1899:31 Paul Hermann **Müller**, Swiss chemist, born 12 Jan; with co-workers he introduced dichlorodiphenyltrichloroethane (DDT) as an insecticide, 1944, *HCA* **27**:892. For this work he was awarded the Nobel Prize (Physiology or Medicine), 1948, *NPL*. Died 1965. *1928.3*

1899:32 Max **Theiler**, South African virologist, born 30 Jan; introduced the intracerebral protection test in mice, for the diagnosis of yellow fever and for the determination of its past existence in the community, 1930, *AnTM* **24**:249. With Eugen Haagen, grew yellow fever virus in culture, 1932, *ZBP* Abt.I **125**:145. With Hugh Hollingsworth Smith, devised the method of immunization against yellow fever without the use of immune serum, 1937, *JEM* **65**:787. Awarded the Nobel Prize (Physiology or Medicine), 1951, for his work on the diagnosis of, and prophylaxis against, yellow fever, *NPL*. Died 1972. *5463, 5465.1, 5467*

1899:33 Edgar Jacob **Poth**, American physician, born 1 Feb; with Frank Louis Knotts, introduced sulphasuxidine, 1941, *PSEB* **48**:129. *1957*

1899:34 Theodor Lasater **Terry**, American ophthalmologist, born 19 Feb; first described retrolental fibroplasia, 1942, *AmJOp* **25**:203. Died 1946. *5989*

1899:35 George Christian **Henny**, American medical physiologist, born 22 Feb; with co-workers, introduced electrokymograph for recording movements of the heart, 1899, *AmJR* **57**:409. *2876*

1899:36 Charles Herbert **Best**, Canadian physiologist, born 27 Feb; with Frederick Grant Banting and John James Rickard Macleod, isolated a pancreatic extract which was named insulin, 1922, *AmJPh* **66**:479; *JLCM* **7**:251. Died 1978. *3966, 3967*

1899:37 Alfred **Blalock**, American surgeon, born 3 Apr; showed that surgical shock is due to a decrease in circulating blood volume, 1930, *ArSuC* **20**:959. Treated myasthenia gravis by thymectomy, 1939, *AnS* **110**:554. With Helen Brooke Taussig, devised operation for congenital defects of the pulmonary artery ('Blalock-Taussig operation'), 1945, *JAMA* **128**:189. Died 1964. *5630.3, 4771, 3043*

1899:38 Max **Cutler**, American surgeon, born 9 May; first to employ ovarian hormone systematically in the treatment of chronic mastitis, 1931, *JAMA* **96**:1201. Died 1984. *5785*

1899:39 Georg von **Békésy**, Hungarian physicist, born 3 Jun. His experiments on hearing first appeared in 1933, *PhZ* **34**:577; introduced the Békésy (semiautomatic) audiometer, 1947, *AcOL* **35**:411. Awarded the Nobel Prize (Physiology or Medicine), 1961, for his discoveries concerning the physical mechanisms of stimulation within the cochlea, *NPL*. Died 1972. *1570.1, 3412.3*

1899:40 Fritz Albert **Lipmann**, German/American biochemist, born 12 Jun; discovered coenzyme A, 1946, *JBC* **162**:743. Shared Nobel Prize (Physiology or Medicine), 1953, with Hans Adolf Krebs, *NPL*. Died 1986. *751.3*

1899:41 William Andrew **DeMonbreun**, American pathologist, born 12 Jul; cultivated *Histoplasma capsulatum*, 1934, *AmJTM* **14**:93, almost simultaneously with Hansmann and Schenken. *5542, 5541.2*

1899:42 Philip **Wiles**, British orthopaedic surgeon, born 17 Aug; with Gordon Gordon-Taylor, introduced the one-stage interinnomino-abdominal (hindquarter) amputation, 1935, *BJS* **22**:671. Died 1967. *4478*

1899:43 Albert **Claude**, Belgian cytologist, born 23 Aug; shared Nobel Prize (Physiology or Medicine) with Christian de Duve and George Emil Palade in 1974 for their discoveries concerning the structural and functional organization of the cell, *NPL*. Died 1983.

1899:44 Ronald **Hare**, British bacteriologist, born 30 Aug; with Laurella McClelland, discovered virus haemagglutination, 1941, *CPHJ* **32**:530, independently of George Keble Hirst. Died 1986. *2578*

1899:45 Frank Macfarlane **Burnet**, Australian immunologist and virologist, born 3 Sep; with Jean Macnamara, demonstrated immunological differences between strains of poliomyelitis virus, 1931, *BJEP* **12**:57. Successfully cultivated influenza A virus, 1935, *MJA* **2**:687. With Mavis Freeman, discovered the causal agent in Q (query) fever, *Rickettsia burneti*, 1937, *MJA* **2**:299. With Frank John Fenner, explained acquired immunological tolerance; in *The* *production of antibodies*, 1949. Proposed clonal selection theory of acquired immunity, 1957; in his *Clonal selection theory of acquired immunity*. Shared Nobel Prize (Physiology or Medicine), 1960, with Peter Brian Medawar, for their discovery of acquired immunological tolerance, *NPL*. Died 1985. *4670.5, 5496, 5398, 2578.7, 2578.31*

1899:46 James Barrett **Brown**, American plastic surgeon, born 20 Sep; with Vilray Papin Blair, introduced split-skin grafts for covering large areas of granulating surfaces, 1929, *SGO* **49**:82; with Blair, modified Mirault's technique for the repair of cleft palate, 1930, *SGO* **51**:81. Died 1971. *5761.1, 5762*

1899:47 Francis Dring Wetherill **Lukens**, American physician, born 5 Oct; with Francis Curtis Dohan, produced experimental diabetes by artificially-induced hyperglycaemia, 1948, *En* **42**:244. *3977*

1899:48 John Christian **Krantz**, American pharmacist, born 8 Oct; with co-workers, introduced fluroxene, the first fluorine-containing anaesthetic, 1953, *JPET* **108**:488. *5729.1*

1899:49 Edward Charles **Dodds**, British biochemist, born 13 Oct; with co-workers, introduced stilboestrol, the first synthetic oestrogen, 1938, *Nature* **141**:247, and dienoestrol, 1938, *Nature* **142**:34. Died 1975. *3799, 3800*

1899:50 Reginald Hammerick **Smithwick**, American surgeon, born 20 Oct; devised the 'Smithwick operation', splanchnic resection, in the treatment of essential hypertension, 1940, *Surgery* **7**:1. Died 1987. *3041*

1899:51 Maxwell Edward **Lapham**, American obstetrician, born 25 Dec; with Harold Friedman, introduced the Friedman test for the diagnosis of pregnancy, 1931, *AmJOG* **21**:405. Died 1983. *6224*

---

1899:52 Marion Herbert **Barker**, American physician, born; developed thiocyanate treatment of hypertension, 1936, *JAMA* **106**:762. Died 1947. *2720*

1899:53 Vladmir Leslie **Tichy**, Czech/American physician, born; with Claude Schaeffer Beck, carried out the first cardio-omentopexy to provide a collateral circulation to the heart, 1935, *AmHJ* **10**:849. Died 1967. *3035*

1899:54 Clarence **Crafoord**, Swedish cardiovascular surgeon, born; with Carl Gustav Vilhelm Nylin, pioneered, at same time as Robert Edward Gross, surgical treatment of coarctation of aorta, 1945, *JTS* **14**:347. Died 1984. *3044*

1899:55 Barney David **Usher**, Canadian dermatologist, born; with Francis Eugene Senear, first noted pemphigus erythematodes ('Senear-Usher syndrome'), 1926, *ArDS* **13**:761. *4151.2*

---

1899: Robert Lawson **Tait** died, **born** 1845. *appendicitis, appendicectomy, ovarian fibroma, rectocele, ovariotomy, oöphorectomy, placenta praevia, caesarean section, ectopic pregnancy*

1899: John **Brunton** died, **born** 1836. *otoscope*

1899: Friedrich Eduard Rudolph **Voltolini** died, **born** 1819. *laryngeal surgery*

1899: Georg Peter Heinrich **Krukenberg** died, **born** 1855. *mucinous carcinoma of ovary*

1899: James **Paget** died, **born** 1814. *osteitis deformans, Trichinella spiralis, eczema of nipple*

1899: Abel **Bouchard** died, **born** 1833. *tabes dorsalis*

1899: Karl **Kahlbaum** died, **born** 1828. *catatonia*

1899: Alfred Carl **Graefe** died, **born** 1830. *ophthalmology*

1899: William **Wilton** died, **born** 1809. *chorionic tumour*

1899: Friedrich **Trendelenburg** died, **born** 1844. *vesico-vaginal fistula, elevated pelvic position*

1899: Theodor **Puschmann** died, **born** 1844. *history of medicine*

## 1900

1900:1 (*c*) **St Mary's Hospital, Rochester, Minnesota**. Here worked William Worrall **Mayo** (1819–1911), British/American physician, joined in due course by his sons William James (1861–1939) and Charles Horace (1865–1939). They established a great reputation and about 1909 were spoken of as 'running the **Mayo Clinic**'

1900:2 **University of Odessa** founded

1900:3 **Hartmann-Bund (Verband der Ärzte Deutschlands)** founded at **Leipzig**

1900:4 **Institute for Medical Research, Kuala Lumpur, Malaysia**, founded

1900:5 **American Association of Pathologists and Bacteriologists** founded

1900:6 **American Röntgen Ray Society** founded

1900:7 **Yale Botanical Garden** opened at **New Haven**

1900:8 **College of Physicians and Surgeons (Chicago)** becomes **College of Medicine, University of Illinois**

1900:9 **Baylor University College of Medicine, Dallas**, founded

1900:10 **Human blood** classified into three **groups** by Karl Landsteiner (1868–1943), *ZBP* 27:357. *889*

1900:11 His general theory of **monochromatic aberrations** advanced by Allvar Gullstrand (1862–1930) in *Allgemeine Theorie der monochromatischen Aberrationen und ihre nächsten Ergebnisse für die Ophthalmologie*. Awarded the Nobel Prize (Physiology or Medicine), 1911, *NPL. 5945*

1900:12 A classic description and classification of **pelvic deformities** given by Carl Breus (1852–1914) and Alexander Kolisko (1847–1918); in their *Die pathologischen Beckenformen*, 1900–14. *6265*

1900:13 Carl Franz Joseph Erich Correns (1864–1933) was one of the leading 're-discoverers' of Mendel's laws of **inheritance**, he showed the deepest understanding, *BDBG*, **18**:158. Others were: Hugo Marie de Vries (1848–1935), *BDBG* **18**:83, who first advanced the theory of **mutation** in his *Die Mutationstheorie*, 2 vols, 1901–3; and Erich Tschermak von Seysenegg (1871–1962), *BDBG* **18**:232. *239.1, 239.01, 240, 239.2*

1900:14 Blue sclerotics and fragility of the bones, occurring as a familial syndrome, **osteogenesis imperfecta**, previously described by Axmann, named '**Eddowes's syndrome**' following the description by Alfred Eddowes (1850–1946), *BMJ* **2**:222. *6367, 6358.1*

1900:15 A curved incision convex downwards just above the pubis, used in **gynaecological surgery,** ('**Pfannenstiel's incision**'), introduced by Hermann Johann Pfannenstiel (1862–1909), *SKV* **268**:1735. *6113*

1900:16 A flap operation for atresia of the **vagina** introduced by George Henry Noble (b.1860), *TSSA* **13**:78. *6112*

1900:17 Henry Smith (1862–1948) had remarkable success with his method of extraction of **cataract** within the capsule, *IMG* **35**:241; **36**:220; **40**:327. *5946*

1900:18 The first clinical and pathological study of **hyperplasia** of the **endometrium** appears in *Cancer of the uterus* by Thomas Stephen Cullen (1868–1953). *6110*

1900:19 Round-ligament ventrosuspension of the **uterus** used by David Tod Gilliam (1844–1923) in his operation for **prolapse**, *AmJOD* **41**:299. *6111*

1900:20 The **intratracheal insufflation** method of **anaesthetization** introduced by Franz Kuhn (1866–1929), *DZC* **76**:148. *5693*

1900:21 The determination of the incubation period of **yellow fever** by Henry Rose Carter (1852–1925) decided the direction of Walter Reed's later researches, which in turn led to the discovery of the virus, *NOMSJ* **52**:617. *5456*

1900:22 The first definite proof that the causal agent in **yellow fever** is transmitted to man by the **mosquito**, *Aedes aegypti*, provided by Walter Reed (1851–1902), James Carroll (1854–1907), Aristides Agramonte y Simoni (1868–1931) and Jesse William Lazear (1866–1900), *PhMeJ* **6**:790. *5457*

1900:23 The best illustrations of the various stages of the **malaria** parasite, published up to that time, appear in *Studi di uno zoologo sulla malaria* by Giovanni Battista Grassi (1854–1925). *5252.1*

1900:24 Experimental proof of the **mosquito-malaria** theory provided by Patrick Manson (1844–1922) by allowing infected mosquitoes to bite a volunteer who developed malaria 15 days later and was cured by **quinine**, *BMJ* **2**:949. *5252.2*

1900:25 **Oil of chenopodium** introduced in the treatment of **ankylostomiasis** by Wilhelm Schüffner (1867–1949) and Herman Vervoort, reported in 1912, *ICH* **1**:734. *5367*

1900:26 The interpretation of **dreams**, *Die Traumdeutung*, was Sigmund Freud's (1856–1939) greatest work. *4980*

1900:27 Henry Havelock Ellis (1859–1939) devoted a lifetime to the study of the **psychology** of **sex**, his seven-volume *Studies in the psychology of sex*, begun in 1900, was completed in 1928. *4981*

1900:28 The complete chain of **filarial** infection from man-to-mosquito-to-man demonstrated by George Carmichael Low (1872–1952), *BMJ* **1**:1456. *5349*

1900:29 Arthur Looss (1861–1923) discovered, by self-infection, that **hookworm** larvae can penetrate the skin, *ZBP* I Abt. **29**:733. *5362*

1900:30 Harvey Williams Cushing (1869–1939) used a route through the temporal fossa and beneath the middle meningeal artery for extirpation of the **Gasserian ganglion** in the treatment of **trigeminal neuralgia**, *JAMA* **34**:1035. *4875*

1900:31 Simon Flexner (1863–1946) isolated a causal organism in bacillary **dysentery** differing from Shiga's bacillus and named *Shigella flexneri*, *JHB* **11**:231. *5093*

1900:32 **Herpes zoster** shown by Henry Head (1861–1940) and Alfred Walter Campbell (1868–1937) to be a haemorrhagic inflammation of the posterior nerve roots and the homologous spinal ganglia, *Brain* **23**:353. *4644*

1900:33 **Unilateral progressive ascending paralysis** ('**Mills' disease**') first described by Charles Karsner Mills (1845–1918), *JNMD* **27**:195. *4711*

1900:34 The first full description of **subacute combined degeneration of the spinal cord** given by James Samuel Risien Russell (1863–1939), Frederick Eustace Batten (1865–1918) and J.S. Collier, *Brain* **23**:39. *4710*

1900:35 **Apraxia** first adequately described by Hugo Karl Liepmann (1863–1925), *MonP* **8**:15, 102, 182. *4588*

1900:36 **Amyotonia congenita** ('**Oppenheim's disease**') first described by Hermann Oppenheim (1858–1919), *MonP* **8**:232. *4760*

1900:37 The cause of **rheumatic fever** considered by Frederick John Poynton (1869–1943) and Alexander Paine to be a **diplococcus**, *L* **2**:861, 932. *4505*

1900:38 **Klippel-Trenaunay syndrome (angio-osteohypertrophy)** described by Maurice Klippel (1856–1942) and Paul Trenaunay (b.1875), *ArGM* **185**:642. *4131*

1900:39 **Rhinosporidiosis** first described by Guillermo Rudolpho Seeber; in his *Un nuevo esporozoario parasíto del hombre*, Tesis, Buenos Aires. *4131.1*

1900:40 **Scleroderma adultorum syndrome of Buschke** described by Abraham Buschke (1868–1943), *BKW* **39**:955; *ArD* **53**:383. *4130*

1900:41 **Familial haemolytic jaundice** ('**Minkowski-Chauffard disease**') described by Oscar Minkowski (1858–1931), *VDK* **18**:316. *3779*

1900:42 **Liver cirrhosis** produced experimentally by Ludvig Hektoen (1863–1951), *JPB* **7**:214. *3640*

1900:43 Joseph François Félix Babinski (1857–1932) described **pituitary tumour** and **sexual infantilism without acromegaly** ('**Fröhlich's syndrome**') one year before Fröhlich, *ReN* **8**:531. *3887*

1900:44 **Partial gastrectomy** ('**Mayo's operation**') reported by William James Mayo (1861–1939), *TASA* **18**:97. *3522*

1900:45 **Sympathectomy** for relief of **vascular** disease first carried out by Mathieu Jaboulay (1860–1913); in his *Chirurgie du grand sympathique et du corps thyroïde*. *3024*

1900:46 *Lactobacillus acidophilus* isolated by Ernst Moro (1874–1951), *WKW* **13**:114. *2515*

1900:47 **Ionic medication** introduced by Stephane Armand Nicolas Leduc (1853–1939), *CRAFS* **29**:1111. *2003.1*

1900:48 **Fingerprint classification** system introduced by Edward R. Henry (1850–1931); in his *Classification and use of fingerprints. 189*

1900:49 **The 'Fowler' position** (elevated head and trunk posture) to facilitate **drainage** into the **pelvis**, described by George Ryerson Fowler (1848–1906), *MR* **57**:627, 1029. *5623*

---

1900:50 Fuller **Albright**, American endocrinologist, born Jan; with co-workers, described a syndrome characterized by osteitis fibrosa cystica with other abnormalities ('Albright's syndrome'), 1937, *NEJM* **216**:727. With H.P. Klinefelter and E.C. Reifenstein, first described the Klinefelter syndrome, an endocrine disorder, 1942, *JCE* **2**:615. Died 1969. *4401, 3804*

1900:51 Franz **Bergel**, German/British medical chemist, born 13 Feb; with J.A. Stock, introduced nitrogen mustard (melphalan), 1954, *JCS*:2409; it was later used in the chemotherapy of cancer. *2660.7*

1900:52 Gilbert Julius **Dalldorf**, American pathologist, born 12 Mar; with Grace Mary Sickles, isolated the Coxsackie virus from children with paralysis, 1948, *Science* **108**:61. *5545*

1900:53 John Henry **Gaddum**, British pharmacologist, born 31 Mar; with Ulf Svante von Euler, isolated Substance P, the first peptide neurotransmitter, 1931, *JP* **72**:74; with Wilhelm Feldberg determined action of acetylcholine in transmission of nerve impulses, 1934, *JP* **81**:305. Died 1965. *1352*

1900:54 Archibald Hector **McIndoe**, New Zealand/British plastic surgeon, born 4 May; with John Bright Banister, devised an operation for the construction of an artificial vagina, 1938, *JOG* **45**:490. With Adolphe Franceschetti, used reciprocal skin homografts to prove the relationship of identical twins, 1950, *BJPS* **2**:283. Died 1960. *6133, 1757*

1900:55 William **Dameshek**, Russian/American physician, born 22 May; with Steven Otto Schwarts, first recognition of an auto-immune disease, acquired haemolytic anaemia, 1938, *AJMS* **196**:769. Died 1969. *3787.1*

1900:56 Manfred Joshua **Sakel**, Austrian/American physician, born 6 Jun; introduced insulin shock therapy in the treatment of schizophrenia, 1934, *WMW* **84**:1211. Died 1957. *4960*

1900:57 Kenneth Stewart **Cole**, American biophysicist, born 10 Jul; with H.J. Curtis, carried out fundamental research on the electrical conductance of living cell membranes, 1938, *Nature*, **142**:209; *JGP* **22**:37, 649. Died 1984

1900:58 Thomas **Francis**, American epidemiologist, born 15 Jul; recovered influenza B virus, 1940, *Science* **92**:405, independently of T.P. Magill. Died 1969. *5498, 5499*

1900:59 Charles Skinner **Hallpike**, British otologist, born 19 Jul; with H.W. Cairns, described the histological changes in Menière's syndrome, 1938, *PRSM* **31**:1317. Died 1979. *3409*

1900:60 Harold Leeming **Sheehan**, British pathologist, born 1 Aug; described 'Sheehan's disease' – hypopituitarism due to postpartum pituitary necrosis, 1937, *JPB* **45**:189. Died 1988. *3907.1*

1900:61 Chevalier L. **Jackson**, American otorhinolaryngologist, born 19 Aug; with his father, Chevalier Jackson, published a comprehensive treatise on foreign bodies in air and food passages and their removal, *Diseases of the air and food passages of foreign body origin*, 1937. Died 1961. *3338.1*

1900:62 Hans Adolf **Krebs**, German/British biochemist, born 25 Aug; with W.A. Jackson, discovered the citric acid cycle of carbohydrate metabolism, 1937, *Enz* **4**:148. Shared Nobel Prize (Physiology or Medicine), 1953, with Fritz Albert Lipmann, *NPL*. Died 1981. *751.1*

1908:63 Lucio **Bini**, Italian neurologist, born 18 Sep; with Ugo Cerletti, introduced electric convulsion therapy in psychosis, 1930, *BAMR* **64**:136. Died 1964. *4962*

1900:64 William Ingledew **Daggett**, British otologist, born 2 Oct; introduced tympanoplasty operation for treatment of chronic suppurative otitis media, 1949, *JLO* **63**:635. Died 1980. *3412.4*

1900:65 Ragnar Arthur **Granit**, Finnish physiologist, born 30 Oct; his *Sensory mechanisms of the retina*, 1947, is an account of his researches over 20 years. Shared the Nobel Prize (Physiology or Medicine), 1967, with Haldan Keffer Hartline and George Wald, *NPL*. Died 1991. *1534*

1900:66 Hugh Leslie **Marriott**, South African physician, born 6 Nov; with Alan Kekwick, introduced the slow-drip method of blood transfusion, 1935, *L* **1**:977. Died 1963. *2023*

1900:67 Wilhelm **Feldberg**, German/British physiologist and pharmacologist, born 14 Nov; with John Henry Gaddum determined action of acetylcholine in transmission of nerve impulses, 1934, *JP* **81**:305. Died 1993. *1352*

1900:68 Francis Henry Laskey **Taylor**, British/American biochemist, born 23 Nov; with Arthur Jackson Patek, isolated antihaemophilic globulin (Factor VIII), 1937, *JCI* **16**:113. Died 1959. *3096.1*

1900:69 Richard **Kuhn**, German chemist, born 3 Dec; awarded Nobel Prize (Chemistry), 1938, for his work on carotenoids and vitamins, *NPL*. Died 1967.

454

1900:70 James Wilfred **Cook**, British chemist, born 10 Dec; discovered carcinogenic properties of dibenzanthracene compounds with I. Hieger, Ernest Lawrence Kennaway (1881–1958) and W.V. Mayneord, 1932, *PRSB* **111**:455. Died 1975. *2654*

1900:71 Arthur H. **Bulbulian**, Turkish/American maxillofacial prosthetician, born 20 Dec; with William Meredith Boothby, introduced BLB (Boothby-Lovelace-Bulbulian) oxygen inhalation mask, 1938, *PMC* **13**:646, 654. *1982*

1900:72 Laurence **O'Shaughnessy**, British thoracic surgeon, born 24 Dec; attached a pedicled graft to the surface of the heart, (cardio-omentopexy – first carried out experimentally by Beck and Tichy (1935)), thus providing a collateral circulation to that organ and an advance in the treatment of angina and cardiac ischaemia, 1936, *BJS* **23**:665. Died 1940. *3037, 3034*

1900:73 Philip **Levine**, Russian/American immunologist, born; with Karl Landsteiner, discovered M, N and P blood groups, 1927, *PSEB* **24**:600, 941; with co-workers, reported erythroblastosis foetalis due to rhesus incompatibility between mother and child, 1941, *AmJOG* **42**:925. Died 1987. *910, 3100*

1900:74 Joseph **Needham**, British biochemist, born; published classic works; *Chemical embryology*, 1931, *Biochemistry and morphogenesis*, 1942. Died 1995. *531*

1900:75 Wilhelm **Eilbott**, German physician, born; devised a bilirubin excretion test of liver function, 1927, *ZKM* **106**:529. *3655*

1900:76 Paul **Kimmelstiel**, American pathologist, born; with Clifford Wilson, first described 'Kimmelstiel-Wilson syndrome', nodular intercapillary glomerulosclerosis, 1936, *AmJPa* **12**:83. Died 1970. *4250*

1900:77 Jacques **Charpy**, French allergologist, born; introduced calciferol in the treatment of lupus vulgaris, 1943, *AnD* **8** Ser. 3:331; it was introduced independently by Geoffrey Barrow Dowling (1891–1976) and Ebenezer William Prosser Thomas in 1945. *4010, 4011*

1900:78 Walter Putnam **Blount**, American orthopaedic surgeon, born; with G.R. Clarke, introduced the use of epiphyseal stapling (Blount staple) to control bone growth, 1949, *JBJS* **31**A:464. *4404.2*

1900:79 S.R. **Savoor**, Indian pathologist, born; with Raymond Lewthwaite, showed scrub typhus and tsutsugamushi disease to be identical, 1940, *L* **1**:255, 304. Died 1980. *5398.2*

1900:80 Priscilla **White**, American physician, born; with co-workers, first reported hormone treatment in diabetic pregnancy, 1939, *AmJMS* **198**:482. *6231*

1900:81 John Chassar **Moir**, British obstetrician and gynaecologist, born; with Harold Ward Dudley, isolated ergometrine, 1935, *BMJ* **1**:520. Died 1977. *6230*

1900:82 Moses **Swick**, American radiologist born; with Alexander von Lichtenberg, introduced uroselectan as a contrast medium in excretion urography, 1929, *KW* **8**:2087; introduced hippuran (sodium ortho-hippurate), 1933, *SGO* **56**:62. *4200, 4201*

1900: Willy **Kühne** died, **born** 1837. *neuromuscular end organ, proprioceptive receptor, trypsin, digestion, visual purple*

1900: Sergei Sergeievich **Korsakoff**, died, **born** 1854. *alcoholic polyneuritis, Korsakoff's psychosis*

1900: Julius **Althaus** died, **born** 1833. *electrolysis*

1900: Charles Harrison **Blackley** died, **born** 1820. *hay fever, asthma, catarrh, pollen*

1900: Arthur Nathan **Hanau** died, **born** 1858. *cancer, transplantation*

1900: Otto Michael **Leichtenstern** died, **born** 1845. *tabes dorsalis, spinal cord degeneration, pernicious anaemia*

1900: Paul August **Sick** died, **born** 1836. *thyroidectomy, status thyreoprivus*

1900: Henry Dewey **Noyes** died, **born** 1832. *glycosuria, retinitis*

1900: Fessenden Nott **Otis** died, **born** 1825. *urology, local anaesthesia*

1900: George Alexander **Turner** died, **born** 1845. *tinea imbricata*

1900: William Alexander **Hammond** died, **born** 1828. *neurology, athetosis*

1900: Eduard **Albert** died, **born** 1841. *paralytic foot, arthrodesis of ankle-joint*

1900: William **Stokes** died, **born** 1839. *amputation of thigh*

1900: Lewis Albert **Sayre** died, **born** 1820. *tuberculosis of spine, plaster of Paris, ankylosis, hip resection*

1900: Louis Xavier Edouard Léopold **Ollier** died, **born** 1830. *skin grafts, bone allografts, dyschondroplasia*

1900: Wilhelm **Wagner** died, **born** 1848. *brain surgery*

1900: Jacob Mendes Da **Costa** died, **born** 1833. *effort syndrome*

1900: Jesse William **Lazear** died, **born** 1866. *yellow fever, mosquito*

## 1901

1901:1 **Nobel Prizes** instituted. Alfred Bernhard Nobel (1833–1896), Swedish engineer and chemist, amassed a large fortune from his various inventions and discoveries, and the exploitation of the Baku oilfields. At his death he left the bulk of this in trust for five annual prizes, to be awarded without distinction of nationality or sex, for eminence in **Physics, Chemistry, Physiology or Medicine, Literature**, and to one who rendered the greatest service to promote **International Peace**. Nobel Prizes relevant to medicine are individually recorded here in the year of their award

1901:2 **Nobel Prize** (Physiology or Medicine): Emil Adolf von Behring (1854–1917), for his discovery of **antitoxins** and introduction of **serum therapy**, especially in **diphtheria**, *NPL*. *2544*

456

1901:3 **Nobel Prize** (Physics): Wilhelm Konrad Röntgen (1845–1923), for his discovery of **x rays**, *NPL. 2544*

1901:4 **Nobel Prize** (Peace): Jean Henri Dunant (1828–1910), Swiss banker, for his initiative in the establishment of the **Red Cross**, *NPL. 2166*

1901:5 **Instituto Oswaldo Cruz, Rio de Janeiro**, opened

1901:6 **Deutsche Gesellschaft für Geschichte der Medizin, Naturwissenchaft und Technik** founded, **Leipzig**

1901:7 *Biometrika* founded

1901:8 **Hygienic Laboratory, US Public Health Service**, opened

1901:9 *Journal of Hygiene* founded

1901:10 **Anaesthetic** blocking of **nerve trunks** first carried out by George Washington Crile (1864–1943); in his *An experimental and clinical research into certain problems relating to surgical operations*, p. 88. *5624, 5687*

1901:11 **Caudal anaesthesia** introduced by Fernand Cathelin (b.1873), *CRSB* **53**:452. *5686*

1901:12 **Breast cancer** treated by **oöphorectomy** combined with thyroid extract by George Thomas Beatson (1848–1933), *BMJ* **2**:1145. *5779*

1901:13 A new classification of **insanity** evolved by Emil Kraepelin (1856–1926); in his *Einführung in die psychiatrische Klinik*. He introduced the concepts of **dementia praecox (schizophrenia)** and **manic-depressive insanity**. *4952*

1901:14 William Boog Leishman (1865–1926) developed **Leishman's stain**, a modification of Romanovsky's stain (1891), for the demonstration of the **malaria** parasite in blood films, *BMJ* **2**:757. *5253, 5242*

1901:15 **Intracranial trigeminal neurotomy** introduced by William Gordon Spiller (1863–1940) and Charles Harrison Frazier (1870–1936) for the treatment of **trigeminal neuralgia**, *UPMB* **14**:342. *4876*

1901:16 The syndrome of **sphenopalatine-ganglion neuralgia** ('**Sluder's neuralgia**') first described by Greenfield Sluder (1865–1928), *AmJMS* **140**:868. *4595*

1901:17 **Catheter** tipped with wax by Howard Atwood Kelly (1858–1943) to register any pressure from **renal** and **ureteral calculi**, *AmJOD* **44**:441. *4295*

1901:18 Acute **atrophy of bone** in inflammatory conditions of the extremities ('**Kienböck's atrophy**') described by Robert Kienböck (1871–1953), *WMW* **51**:1346. *4370*

1901:19 **Ureteral calculi** accurately demonstrated **radiographically** with the help of an opaque indwelling catheter by Géza von Illyés (b.1870), *DZC* **62**:132. *4294*

1901:20 The connection of **myasthenia gravis** with hypertrophy of the **thymus** noted by Carl Weigert (1845–1904), *NZ* **20**:597. *4761*

1901:21 **Lichen nitidus** ('**Pinkus's disease**') first described by Felix Pinkus (1868–1947) and published in 1907, *ArD* **85**:11. *4143*

1901:22 Operation of **renal decortication** introduced for the treatment of chronic **nephritis** by George Michael Edebohls (1853–1908), *MR* **60**:961. *4229*

1901:23 **Progressive pigmentary dermatosis** first described by Jay Frank Schamberg (1870–1934), *BJD* **13**:1. *4134*

1901:24 **Cutis laxa** described by Edvard Ehlers (1863–1937); after Danlos's paper in 1908 it was named '**Ehlers-Danlos syndrome**', *DeZ* **8**:173. *4132, 4144*

1901:25 **Radium** first used in the treatment of **lupus erythematosus** by Henri Alexandre Danlos (1844–1912) and P. Bloch, *BSED* **12**:438. *4003*

1901:26 Eugene Lindsay Opie (1873–1971) established the association between failure of the **islets of Langerhans** and the occurrence of **diabetes**, *JEM* **5**:397, 527. *3955, 3956*

1901:27 Alfred Fröhlich (1871–1953) described the syndrome of **pituitary tumour, obesity, dystrophia adiposogenitalis** and **sexual infantilism** ('**Fröhlich's syndrome**'), *WKR* **15**:883, 906. *3889*

1901:28 An account of William Henry Battle's (1855–1936) operation for the repair of **femoral hernia** appeared, *L* **1**:302. *3606*

1901:29 Mayo's operation for the radical cure of **umbilical hernia** devised by William James Mayo (1861–1939), *AnS* **34**:276. *3607*

1901:30 Account of **multiple hereditary telangiectasis** ('**Rendu-Osler-Weber disease**') by William Osler (1849–1918), *JHB* **12**:333. *2711*

1901:31 '**Bordet-Gengou complement-fixation reaction**', a serological test, introduced by Jules Jean Baptiste Bordet (1870–1961) and Octave Gengou (1875–1957), *AnIP* **15**:289. *2553*

1901:32 Isolation of **tryptophan** by Frederick Gowland Hopkins (1861–1947) and Sidney William Cole (1877–1952), *JP* **27**:418. *723*

1901:33 **Adrenaline** isolated by Jokichi Takamine (1854–1922) and by Thomas Bell Aldrich (b.1861), *AmJPm* **73**:523; *AmJPh* **5**:457. *1146, 1147*

1901:34 *The human figure in motion* published by Eadweard Muybridge (1830–1904). *651*

1901:35 **String galvanometer** invented by Willem Einthoven (1860–1927), *ArNS* 2 sér. **6**:625. *840*

1901:36 The mechanisms concerned in specific **antibacterial immunity** elaborated by Élie Metchnikoff (1845–1916); in his *L'immunité dans les maladies infectieuses*. *2555*

1901:37 *Lectures on the history of physiology* published by Michael Foster (1836–1907). *1575*

---

1901:38 Irvine Heinly **Page**, American physician, born 7 Jan; first described the use of sodium amytal as an anaesthetic, 1923, *JLCM* **9**:194. With O.M. Helmer, isolated angiotensin, 1940, *JEM* **71**:29; also isolated independently by Eduardo Braun-Menendez, 1940, *JP* **98**:283. *5706, 2724.1, 2742.2*

1901:39 Edward Franklin **Bland**, American cardiologist, born 21 Jan; with Richard Harwood Sweet, performed first successful pulmonary-azygos shunt for mitral stenosis, 1948, *AmPr* **2**:756. *3047*

1901:40 René Jules **Dubos**, French/American microbiologist, born 20 Feb; isolated gramicidin, 1939, *PSEB* **40**:311. Died 1982. *1933.1*

1901:41 Valy **Menkin**, Russian/American pathologist, born 26 Feb; isolated leucotaxine, factor responsible for increased capillary permeability, 1937, *PSEB* **36**:164. *2312*

1901:42 Linus Carl **Pauling**, American chemist, born 28 Feb; with co-workers, showed sickle-cell anaemia to be due to a structural haemoglobin variant (the first recognition of a haemoglobin variant), 1949, *Science* **110**:543. Awarded Nobel Prize (Chemistry), 1954, for his research into the nature of the chemical bond and its application to the elucidation of the structure of complex substances, *NPL*. Died 1994. *3154.1*

1901:43 LeRoy Dryden **Fothergill**, American physician, born 15 Apr; with co-workers, isolated the virus of Eastern equine encephalitis from man, 1938, *NEJM* **219**:411. Died 1967. *4659.1*

1901:44 Allen Dudley **Keller**, American physiologist, born 16 Apr; in association with William Kendrick Hare, located the heat-regulating mechanism in the hypothalamus, 1932, *PSEB* **29**:1069. *1446.3*

1901:45 Vincent du **Vigneaud**, American chemist, born 18 May; with others, synthesized oxytocin, 1953, *JACS* **75**:4879; vasopressin, 1954, *JACS* **76**:4751. Awarded Nobel Prize (Chemistry), 1955, *NPL*. Died 1978. *1175.3, 1175.4*

1901:46 Conrad Arnold **Elvehjem**, American biochemist, born 27 May; with co-workers, isolated nicotinic acid, a constituent of the vitamin B complex, as the pellagra-preventing factor, 1938, *JBC* **123**:137. Died 1962. *3760, 1077*

1901:47 Richard Harwood **Sweet**, American surgeon, born 30 May; with Edward Franklin Bland, performed first successful pulmonary-azygos shunt for mitral stenosis, 1948, *AmPr* **2**:756. *3047*

1901:48 Ernest **Witebsky**, German/American immunologist, born 3 Sep; with Noel Richard Rose, produced auto-immune thyroiditis experimentally, 1956, *JI* **76**:408. Died 1969. *3855.3*

1901:49 Alexander **Brunschwig**, American surgeon, born 11 Sep; introduced the operation of pancreatoduodenectomy, 1937, *SGO* **65**:681. Died 1969. *3660*

1901:50 William Henry **Sebrell**, American physician, born 11 Sep; with Roy Edwin Butler, made a preliminary report on riboflavin (vitamin B complex) deficiency, ariboflavinosis, 1938, *USPHR* **53**:2284. *3707*

1901:51 Charles Brenton **Huggins** Canadian/American, born 22 Sep; with Clarence Vernard Hodges, introduced stilboestrol in the treatment of prostatic carcinoma, 1941, *CR* **1**:293; with William Wallace Scott, introduced adrenalectomy for prostatic carcinoma, 1945, *AnS* **122**:1031. Shared the Nobel Prize (Physiology or Medicine), 1966, with Francis Peyton Rous, for work on hormone-dependent tumours, *NPL*. *4276, 4276.1*

1901:52 Francis Clark **Wood**, American cardiologist, born 1 Oct, with Christian Wolferth, introduced chest leads in the electrocardiographic diagnosis of coronary occlusion, 1933, *AmJMS* **183**:30. *2863*

1901:53 Joseph Seton **Barr**, American orthopaedic surgeon, born 14 Oct; with William Jason Mixter, demonstrated the causal role of intravertebral disk herniation in sciatica, 1934, *NEJM* **211**:210. Died 1963. *4435*

1901:54 Maxwell Myer **Wintrobe**, Canadian/American physician, born 27 Oct; with J. Walter Landsberg, introduced Wintrobe's method for determination of erythrocyte sedimentation rate, 1935, *AmJMS* **189**:102. Died 1986. *3096*

1901:55 Carl Olof **Sjöqvist**, Swedish neurosurgeon, born 9 Dec; introduced trigeminal tractotomy in the treatment of trigeminal neuralgia, 1937, *ZN* **2**:274. *4908*

1901:56 Richard Edwin **Shope**, American virologist, born 25 Dec; described a benign infectious tumour of viral origin, Shope papilloma, 1932, *JEM* **56**:793. Died 1966. *2656*

———

1901:57 Sven Curt Alfred **Hellerström**, Swedish venereologist, born; with Erik Wassén, transmitted lymphogranuloma venereum to animals and attributed it to a virus, 1931, *CRDS* 1930, p. 1147. *5220*

1901:58 Michael Leo **Leventhal**, American obstetrician and gynaecologist, born; with Irving Freiler Stein, described amenorrhoea associated with bilateral polycystic ovaries (Stein-Leventhal syndrome), 1935, *AmJOG* **29**:181. *6132.1*

———

1901: Johann Ludwig Wilhelm **Thudichum** died, **born** 1829. *cephalins, myelins, haematoporphyrin*

1901: Max Joseph von **Pettenkofer** died, **born** 1818. *colour reaction for bile, feeding-respiration experiments, sewer planning*

1901: Pierre Carl Édouard **Potain** died, **born** 1825. *heart diseases, sphygmomanometer*

1901: Carl Johan August **Langenbuch** died, **born** 1846. *gall-bladder removal, kidney cancer, nephrectomy*

1901: Gaspard Adolph **Chatin** died, **born** 1813. *goitre, cretinism*

1901: William **MacCormac** died, **born** 1836. *bladder rupture*

1901: Alfred Le Roy de **Méricourt** died, **born** 1825. *chromidrosis*

1901: Emil **Kraepelin** died, **born** 1856. *dementia praecox, manic-depression*

1901: Jean Baptiste **Berenger-Féraud** died, **born** 1832. *blackwater fever*

1901: (c) Ferdinand Ethelbert **Junker** died, **born** 1828. *anaesthesia, chloroform*

1901: William Overend **Priestley** died, **born** 1829. *intermenstrual pain*

1901: Giulio Cesare **Bizzozero** died, **born** 1846. *erythropoiesis, leucopoiesis, blood platelet role in coagulation*

**1902**
1902: 1 **Nobel Prize** (Physiology or Medicine): Ronald Ross (1857–1932), for his identification of the vector **mosquito** in **malaria** and demonstration of the life-cycle of the parasite, *NPL. 5251*

1902: 2 **Carnegie Institution of Washington** founded

1902: 3 **Royal Army Medical College, London**, founded

1902: 4 **Pan-American Sanitary Bureau** established (became regional office of WHO, 1947)

1902: 5 One of the most important **histories of medicine** is Theodor Puschmann's (1844–1899) *Handbuch der Geschichte der Medizin*, 3 vols, 1902–5. *6398*

1902: 6 **Twilight sleep**, induced by **hyoscine-morphine** injections, for the relief of **labour pains**, introduced by Richard von Steinbüchel, *ZGy* **26**:1304, and developed by C.J. Gauss. *6210, 6212*

1902: 7 A radical operation for **cancer** of the **uterus** introduced by Ernst Wertheim (1864–1920), *ArGy* **61**:627; 65:1. *6114*

1902: 8 The specific dynamic effect of **foodstuffs** clarified, and the validity of the principle of the conservation of energy in living organisms established, by Max Rubner (1854–1932); in his *Die Gesetze des Energieverbrauchs bei der Ernährung. 1025*

1902: 9 William Bateson (1861–1926) made considerable contributions to **genetics**. His *Mendel's principles of heredity, a defence* was the first English text on genetics (2nd edn, 1909). *241*

1902: 10 A method of **mammaplasty** developed by Hippolyte Morestin (1869–1919), *PrM* **10**:975. *5756*

1902: 11 The experiments on **local infiltration anaesthesia**, initiated by Halsted, further developed by Harvey Williams Cushing (1869–1939), *AnS* **36**:321. *5689, 5679*

1902: 12 The **actinobacillus** discovered by Joseph Léon Marcel Lignières (1868–1933) and J. Spitz, *SMB* **9**:207. *5531*

1902:13 Human **trypanosomiasis** first recognized, and the parasite named *Trypanosoma gambiense*, by Joseph Everett Dutton (1876–1905), *TYL* **4**:455. *5275*

1902:14 The mode of entry of *Ankylostoma duodenale* into the body demonstrated by Charles Albert Bentley (1873–1949), *BMJ* **1**:190. *5362.1*

1902:15 A syndrome of multiple medullary lesions of vascular origin involving the **medullary tract** and other structures ('**syndrome of Babinski-Nageotte**') described by Joseph François Félix Babinski (1857–1932) and Jean Nageotte (1866–1948), *ReN* **10**:358. *4589*

1902:16 *Necator americanus*, the American species of **hookworm**, discovered by Charles Wardell Stiles (1867–1941), *AmM* **3**:777. *5363*

1902:17 **Traumatic cavity formation** in the **spinal cord** ('**Kienböck's disease**') noted by Robert Kienböck (1871–1953), *JaP* **21**:50. *4591*

1902:18 A distal form of **progressive muscular dystrophy** ('**distal myopathy of Gowers**') recorded by William Richard Gowers (1845–1915), *BMJ* **2**:89. *4762*

1902:19 **Parasporosis**, previously described under other names, was so named by Louis Anne Jean Brocq (1856–1928), *AnD* **3**:313,433; also called '**Brocq's disease**'. *4135*

1902:20 Successful **kidney autotransplantation**, in dogs, carried out by Emerich Ullmann (1861–1937), *WKW* **15**:281. *4229.1*

1902:21 In her classical study of **lymphadenoma**, Dorothy Reed included a detailed histological account of '**Dorothy Reed's giant cells**', *JHR* **10**:133. *3780*

1902:22 **Arterial suture** technique perfected by Alexis Carrel (1873–1944), *LM* **98**:859. *2909*

1902:23 **Carcinogenic** effects of **x rays** reported by Ernst Frieben (b.1875), *DMW* **28**:VB, 335. *2625.1*

1902:24 **Radiotherapy** dosimetry standards improved by Guido Holzknecht (1872–1931), *WKR* **16**:685. *2688*

1902:25 *The study of the pulse* published by James Mackenzie (1853–1925); included a description of his **polygraph**. *2812*

1902:26 First full description of **anaphylaxis** by Paul Portier (1866–1962) and Charles Robert Richet (1850–1935), *CRSB* **54**:170. *2590*

1902:27 **Orthodiagraphy** introduced into **radiography** of the **heart** by Friedrich Moritz (1861–1938), *MMW* **49**:1. *2813*

1902:28 **Syphilis: Jarisch-Herxheimer reaction**, introduced by Karl Herxheimer (1861–1944), *DMW* **28**:895. *2396, 2397*

1902:29 Invention of the **slit-lamp** by Alvar Gullstrand (1862–1930), *BVOG* 290. *1525.2*

1902:30 Hyram Houston **Merritt**, American neurologist, born 12 Jan; with Tracy J. Putnam, introduced diphenylhydantoin in the treatment of convulsive disorders, 1938, *JAMA* **111**:1068. Died 1979. *4824.1*

1902:31 Alf Sven **Alving**, Swedish/American physician, born 8 Mar; with Benjamin Frank Miller, introduced the inulin clearance test for the measurement of the glomerular filtration rate, 1940, *ArIM* **66**:306. With co-workers, undertook clinical trials with pentaquine in malaria, 1948, *JCI* **27**, 3II:25. *4251, 5261.2*

1902:32 Maxwell **Finland**, Russian/American physician, born 15 Mar; with co-workers introduced sulphadiazine, 1941, *JAMA* **116**:2641. *1956*

1902:33 Wilfrid Fletcher **Gaisford**, British paediatrician, born 6 Apr; with Gladys Mary Evans, introduced M & B 693 (sulphapyridine) in the treatment of pneumonia, 1938, *L* **2**:14. Died 1988. *3210*

1902:34 Thomas Holmes **Sellors**, British surgeon, born 7 Apr; successfully divided the pulmonary valve for the treatment of pulmonary stenosis, 1947, *L* **1**:988. Died 1987. *3046.2*

1902:35 André Michael **Lwoff**, French microbiologist, born 8 May; shared Nobel Prize (Physiology or Medicine), 1965, with François Jacob and Jacques Lucien Monod for work on the genetic control of enzyme and virus synthesis, *NPL*. Died 1994.

1902:36 Louis Klein **Diamond**, American haematologist and paediatrician, born 11 May; used exchange blood transfusion in the treatment of erythroblastosis foetalis, 1948, *Ped* **2**:520. *3107.1*

1902:37 Abner **Wolf**, American neuropathologist, born 14 May; with David Cowen, first recognized toxoplasmosis in humans, 1937, *BNI* **6**:306. *5544.1*

1902:38 Barbara **McClintock**, American geneticist, born 16 Jun; awarded Nobel Prize (Physiology or Medicine), 1983, for her discovery of mobile genetic elements, *NPL*. Died 1992.

1902:39 Arne Wilhelm Kaurin **Tiselius**, Swedish biochemist, born 10 Aug; with Elvin Abraham Kabat, showed antibodies to be gamma globulins, 1939, *JEM* **69**:119. Awarded Nobel Prize (Chemistry), 1948, for research on electrophoresis and adsorption analysis, especially for his discoveries concerning the complex nature of the serum proteins, *NPL*. Died 1971. *2576.8*

1902:40 Paul Eby **Steiner**, American pathologist, born 9 Oct; with Clarence Chancelum Lushbaugh, first described amniotic fluid embolism, 1941, *JAMA* **117**:1245, 1340. *6232*

1902:41 Benedict **Cassen**, American biophysicist, born 13 Nov; with co-workers, introduced the use of scintillation counters in the location of tumours, 1950, *Nuc* **6**:78. *2660.2*

1902:42 Hugh Hollingsworth **Smith**, American virologist, born 12 Dec; with Max Theiler, devised the method of immunization against yellow fever without the use of immune serum, 1937, *JEM* **65**:787. *5467*

———

1902:43 Forest Dewey **Dodrill** born; devised first successful heart bypass apparatus, 1952, *JTS* **24**:134. *859.1*

1902:44 Robert Henry **Aldrich**, American surgeon, born; introduced the use of gentian violet in the treatment of burns, 1933, *NEJM* **208**:299. *2258*

1902:45 Horton Corwin **Hinshaw** born; with William Hugh Feldman, introduced streptomycin in treatment of tuberculosis, 1945, *PMC* **20**:313. *2350*

1902:46 Israel **Steinberg**, American physician, born; with George Porter Robb, introduced angiocardiography, 1938, *JCI* **17**:507. *2689*

1902:47 Roy Edwin **Butler**, US Public Health Service surgeon, born; with William Henry Sebrell, made a preliminary report on riboflavin (vitamin B complex) deficiency, ariboflavinosis, 1938, *USPHR* **53**:2284. *3707*

1902:48 Edward Moody **Robertson**, British gynaecologist and obstetrician, born; with Archibald Ian Macpherson, introduced triphenylchloroethylene, a synthetic oestrogen, into clinical use, 1939, *L* **2**:1362. *3803*

1902:49 Walls Willard **Bunnell**, American physician, born; with John Rodman Paul, introduced the 'Paul-Bunnell test' for the diagnosis of infectious mononucleosis, 1932, *AmJMS* **183**:90. *5487*

1902:50 Wray Devere Marr **Lloyd**, Canadian epidemiologist, born; with Wilbur Augustus Sawyer, introduced the intraperitoneal test for immunity against yellow fever, 1931, *JEM* **54**:533; with S.F. Kitchen and Sawyer, devised an immune serum for prophylactic inoculation against the disease, 1932, *JEM* **55**:945. Died 1936. *5464, 5465*

---

1902: Rudolf Ludwig Karl **Virchow** died, **born** 1821. *cellular pathology, neuroglia, syphilis, aspergillosis, thrombosis, embolism, typhus*

1902: James **Hobrecht** died, **born** 1825. *sewers*

1902: Benjamin Horatio **Paul** died, **born** 1828. *emetine*

1902: Adolph **Jarisch** died, **born** 1850. *syphilis*

1902: Henri Jules Louis **Rendu** died, **born** 1844. *telangiectasis*

1902: Adolf **Kussmaul** died, **born** 1822. *oesophagoscope, paradoxical pulse, periarteritis nodosa, aphasia*

1902: Hans von **Hebra** died, **born** 1847. *rhinoscleroma*

1902: William Miller **Ord** died, **born** 1834. *myxoedema*

1902: Moriz **Kaposi** [Kohn] died, **born** 1837. *Kaposi's sarcoma, impetigo herpetiformis, dermatology, lymphoderma perniciosa, lichen ruber moniliformis, xeroderma pigmentosum*

1902: Eugen **Hahn** died, **born** 1841. *nephropexy*

1902: Clayton **Parkhill** died, **born** 1860. *fractures*

464

1902: Angelo **Dubini** died, **born** 1813. *chorea, encephalitis, ankylostomiasis*

1902: Nil Feodorovich **Filatov** died, **born** 1847. *infectious mononucleosis*

1902: Alejandro **Posadas** died, **born** 1870. *coccidioidomycosis*

1902: Walter **Reed** died, **born** 1851. *yellow fever, mosquito*

1902: Edoardo **Porro** died, **born** 1842. *caesarean section*

1902: Hans Ernst **Buchner** died, **born** 1850. *complement, alexin*

**1903**
1903:1 **Nobel Prize** (Physiology or Medicine): Niels Ryberg Finsen (1860–1904), for his discovery of the therapeutic value of invisible **light, actinic rays**, and **ultraviolet rays**, *NPL. 2000*

1903:2 **Nobel Prize** (Physics) Pierre Curie (1859–1906) and Marie Sklodowska Curie (1867–1934), for their discovery of **radium**, shared with Antoine Henri Becquerel (1852–1908), for his discovery of **radioactivity,** *NPL. 2003, 2001*

1903:3 **[School of Tropical Medicine], Lisbon**, founded

1903:4 **Henry Phipps Institute for Tuberculosis, Baltimore**, opened

1903:5 **American Society for Tropical Medicine**, founded at **Philadelphia**

1903:6 **Wellcome Tropical Research Laboratories, Khartoum**

1903:7 **Société d'Histoire de Médecine** founded in **Paris**

1903:8 **Medical Academy** at **Osaka**

1903:9 **Smallpox vaccination** obligatory in **Spain**

1903:10 **[Bacteriological Institute]** at **Zagreb**

1903:11 **Barbitone (barbital)** introduced into medicine by Emil Fischer (1852–1919) and Joseph von Mering (1849–1908), *TGe* **44**:97. *1892*

1903:12 American obstetrician, John Whitridge Williams (1866–1931), published *Obstetrics*, the foremost American textbook of **obstetrics**, still in print under modern editorship. *6210.1*

1903:13 **Infantile acrodynia ('pink disease')** first clearly described by Paul Selter (b.1886), *VGK* **20**:45. *6344*

1903:14 Johann Otto Leonard Heubner (1843–1926), professor of **paediatrics** at Berlin, contributed important work on **infant feeding**, including determination of caloric requirement. His *Lehrbuch der Kinderheilkunde*, 3 vols, appeared in 1903–6. *6343*

1903:15 **Inclusion bodies** ('**Negri bodies**') in the nerve cells of humans and animals proved to have been infected with **rabies** discovered by Adelchi Negri (1876–1912), making possible prompt microscopic diagnosis, *BSMP* 1903:88, 229; 1904:22; 1905:321. *5484*

1903:16 **Yellow fever** convalescent serum first employed by Emile Marchoux (1862–1943), A.T. Salimbeni and P.L. Simond, *AnIP* **17**:665. *5459*

1903:17 **Stovaine** introduced as an anaesthetic by Ernest Fourneau (1872–1949), *BSP* **10**:141. *5690*

1903:18 Prophylactic measures for the control of **typhoid** suggested by Robert Koch (1843–1910), in his *Die Bekämpfung der Typhus*, were generally adopted. *5040*

1903:19 Wilhelm Ludwig Johannsen (1857–1927) supported the Mendelian law of **inheritance** in his *Ueber Erblichkeit in Populationen und in reinen Linien*. He introduced the concepts of '**gene**', '**genotype**' and '**phenotype**'. *242*

1903:20 **Psychasthenia** first described by Pierre Marie Félix Janet (1859–1947); in his *Les obsessions et la psychasthénie*. *4954*

1903:21 Degeneration of the **corpus callosum** in **alcoholism** ('**Marchiafava-Bignami disease**') described by Ettore Marchiafava (1847–1935) and Amico Bignami (1862–1929), *RPN* **8**:544. *4955*

1903:22 William Boog Leishman (1865–1926) found an organism (1900) which he later described, 1903, *BMJ* **1**:1252; **2**:1476, as possibly a **trypanosome**. In the same year Charles Donovan (1863–1951), *BMJ* **2**:79, found the same organism, later named *Leishmania donovani* (**Leishman-Donovan bodies**), and shown to be the causal organism in leishmaniasis. *5295, 5296*

1903:23 In Uganda, Aldo Castellani (1877–1971) discovered *Trypanosoma gambiense* in the cerebrospinal fluid of a patient with **trypanosomiasis (sleeping sickness)**, *PRS* **71**:501. *5276*

1903:24 David Bruce (1855–1931) and D.N. Nabarro, sent to Africa by the Royal Society of London to study **sleeping sickness**, reported (*Report of the Sleeping Sickness Commission of the Royal Society, 1903–1912*, 17 pts, 1903–19) that the **tsetse fly** was the vector of the **trypanosome**. *5277*

1903:25 Use of alcohol injection of the **Gasserian ganglion** for treatment of **trigeminal neuralgia** introduced by Joseph Louis Irénée Abadie (b.1873), *MSMB* 1903:59. *4877*

1903:26 '**Froin's syndrome**', a coagulation of the **cerebrospinal fluid**, described by Georges Froin (b.1874), *GH* **76**:1005. *4645*

1903:27 Lesions of the **tibial tuberosity** in adolescence first described almost simultaneously by both Robert Bayley Osgood (1873–1956), *BMSJ* **148**:114, and by Carl Schlatter (1864–1934), *BKC* 38:874, and called '**Osgood-Schlatter disease**'. *4373, 4374*

1903:28 The theory of the **chromosomal** basis of **Mendelism** formulated by Walter Stanborough Sutton (1877–1916), *BB* **4**:231. *242.1*

1903:29 Cases of **juvenile amaurotic familial idiocy** ('**Batten-Mayou disease**') described by Frederick Eustace Batten (1865–1918), *TOUK* **23**:86, and later by Mayou (1904). *4712, 4713*

1903:30 Theodor Boveri (1862–1915) demonstrated that different **chromosomes** perform different functions in **development**, *ZPMG* **35**:67. *241.1*

1903:31 **Iodoform** used to plug **bone defects** by Albert von Mosetig-Moorhof (1838–1907), *ZCh* **30**:433. *4371*

1903:32 **Osteopetrosis fragilis (marble bones, 'Albers-Schönberg's disease'**) first described by Heinrich Ernst Albers-Schönberg (1865–1921), *FGR* **7**:158. *4372*

1903:33 **Voelcker kidney function test** introduced by Friedrich Voelcker (1872–1955) and Eugen Joseph (b.1879), *MMW* **50**:2081. *4230*

1903:34 An operation for conservative perineal **prostatectomy** devised by Hugh Hampton Young (1870–1945), *JAMA* **41**:999. *4265*

1903:35 The first treatise on **endocrinology** was *The internal secretions ...*, 2 vols, 1903–7, by Charles Sajous (1852–1929). *3793*

1903:36 **Cystinosis** first described by Emil Abderhalden (1877–1950), *HSZ* **38**:557. *3920*

1903:37 **Polycythaemia vera (erythraemia)** described by William Osler (1849–1919), *AmJMS* **126**:187, who acknowledged the priority of Vaquez ('**Vaquez-Osler disease**'). *3073, 3070*

1903:38 Successful ligation of **hepatic artery** by Hans Kehr, *MMW* **50**:1861. *2968*

1903:39 Inhibitory effect of **x rays** on **carcinoma** reported by Georg Clemens Perthes (1869–1927), *ArKC* **71**:955. *2627.1*

1903:40 **Radium** treatment of **cancer** by S.W. Goldberg and Efim Semenovic London (1869–1939), *DeZ* **10**:457. *2627*

1903:41 Experimental **arteriosclerosis** produced, using venous injection of adrenaline, by Otto Josue (1869–1923), *CRSB* **44**:1374. *2910*

1903:42 **Medial sclerosis** of **blood vessels** of the extremities ('**Mönckeberg's sclerosis**') described by Johann Georg Mönckeberg (1877–1925), *VA* **171**:141. *2911*

1903:43 **Hypotensive** action of **thiocyanates** first reported by Wolfgang Pauli (1869–1955), *MMW* **50**:153. *2712*

1903:44 Compression diaphragm introduced in **radiography** by Heinrich Ernst Albers-Schönberg (1865–1921); in his *Die Röntgen-Technik. 2689*

1903:45 **Serum sickness** described by Franz Hamburger (1874–1954) and Ernst Moro (1874–1951), *WKW* **16**:445. *2591.1*

1903:46 **Arthus phenomenon**, a diagnostic symptom of anaphylaxis, demonstrated by Nicolas Maurice Arthus (1862–1945), *CRSB* **55**:817. *2591*

1903:47 **Heliotherapy** (ultraviolet light and Alpine sunlight) used in the treatment of **tuberculosis** by Auguste Rollier (1874–1954); *Die Heliotherapie der Tuberkulose. 2342*

1903:48 **Opsonins** (thermolabile substances in normal and **immune serum**) demonstrated by Almroth Edward Wright (1861–1947) and Stewart Rankin Douglas (1871–1936), *PRSB* **72**:357; **73**:128. *2558*

1903:49 **Electric convulsion therapy** (introduced by Cerletti and Bini in 1938) was made possible by Stephane Armand Nicolas Leduc (1853–1939) who reported the cerebral effect of galvanic current, *RIER* **13**:143. *2003.2*

1903:50 **Rideal-Walker test for disinfectants** devised by Samuel Rideal (1863–1929) and J.T. Ainslie Walker (1868–1930), *JSI* **24**:424. *1893*

1903:51 First correct **electroretinogram** obtained by Francis Gotch (1853–1913), *JP* **29**:388. *1525.1*

1903:52 **Bielschowsky's silver stain for nerve fibres** introduced by Max Bielschowsky (1869–1940), *NZ* **21**:579. *1296*

1903:53 **Electrocardiography** introduced by Willem Einthoven (1860–1927), *KAWS* **6**:107. *842*

1903:54 Active and passive **hyperaemia** introduced as an adjuvant in **surgical** treatment by August Karl Gustav Bier (1861–1949); *Hyperaemie als Heilmittel. 5626*

1903:55 **Organ-specific antigens** demonstrated, in **eye lens proteins**, by Paul Theodor Uhlenhuth (1870–1957), *Festschrift …R. Koch*, p. 49. *2557*

---

1903:56 Terence John **Millin**, British urological surgeon, born 9 Jan; introduced a new extravesical technique for retropubic prostatectomy, 1945, *L* **2**:693. Died 1980. *4277*

1903:57 James Arnold **Dauphinee**, Canadian physician, born 9 Jan; with John Hepburn, first successful excision of arteriovenous aneurysm of the lung, 1942, *AmJMS* **204**:681. *2992*

1903:58 Samuel **Gelfan**, Russian/American physiologist, born 16 Jan; with I.R. Bell, first put divinyl ether to clinical use, 1933, *JPET* **47**:1. *5715*

1903:59 John Carew **Eccles**, Australian physiologist, born 22 Jan; he shared the Nobel Prize (Physiology or Medicine), 1963, with Alan Lloyd Hodgkin and Andrew Fielding Huxley, for discoveries concerning ionic mechanisms involved in the excitation and inhibition of the nerve cell membrane in the peripheral and central nervous systems, *NPL. 1310.2*

1903:60 William Clouser **Boyd**, American immunochemist, born 4 Mar; showed blood groups to be inherited and not changed by environment, 1939, *Tab* **17**:113. Died 1983. *912*

1903:61 Adolf Friedrich Johann **Butenandt**, German biochemist, born 24 Mar; isolated androsterone, 1931, *ZAngC* **44**:905; isolated progesterone in crystalline form, 1934, *WKW*

**47**:897, 934. Shared Nobel Prize (Chemistry), 1939, with Leonard Ruzicka, *NPL*. Died 1995. *1195, 1200*

1903:62 Bernard **Benjamin**, American paediatrician, born 29 Mar; with Isador Max Tarlov, introduced plasma clot nerve suture, 1943, *SGO* **76**:366. *4912*

1903:63 Gregory Goodwin **Pincus**, American biologist, born 9 Apr; with Min Chueh Chang, demonstrated an oral contraceptive (progesterone) in the rabbit, 1953, *AcPL* **3**:177. Died 1967. *1931.2*

1903:64 Thomas Pleines **Magill**, American microbiologist, born 24 May; recovered influenza B virus, 1940, *PSEB* **45**:162, independently of T. Francis. *5499, 5498*

1903:65 Axel Hugo Teodor **Theorell**, Swedish biochemist, born 6 Jul; awarded the Nobel Prize (Physiology or Medicine), 1955, for his discoveries relating to the nature and mode of action of oxidizing enzymes, *NPL*. His work is summarized in *Festschrift Arthur Stoll*, 1957, p. 35. Died 1982. *752.5*

1903:66 Herbert John **Seddon**, British orthopaedic surgeon, born 13 Jul; published a classification of nerve injuries, 1943, *Brain* **66**:237. Died 1977. *4911*

1903:67 Robert Milton **Zollinger**, American surgeon, born 4 Sep; with Edwin Homer Ellison, described the Zollinger-Ellison syndrome, 1955, *AnS* **142**:709. *3558.2*

1903:68 John Heysham **Gibbon**, American physician, born 29 Sep; first successful use of heart-lung machine on an animal, 1939, *JLCM* **24**:1192; first to use a mechanical heart and lung apparatus (pump oxygenator) on a human, 1954, *MinnM* **37**:185. Died 1973. *3038.1, 3047.5*

1903:69 Sidney **Farber**, American pathologist, born 30 Sep; with co-workers, used TEPA (triethylenephosphoramide) in the treatment of cancer, 1953, *Cancer* **6**:135. Died 1973. *2660.5*

1903:70 George Wells **Beadle**, American geneticist, born 22 Oct; worked with Edward Lawrie Tatum on mutations induced in *Neurospora*, 1941, *PNAS* **27**:499. They shared the Nobel Prize (Physiology or Medicine), 1958, with Joshua Lederberg, for their researches on the mechanism by which the chromosomes in the cell nucleus transmit inherited characters, *NPL*. Died 1989. *254.3*

1903:71 Russell Claude **Brock**, British thoracic surgeon, born 24 Oct; introduced pulmonary valvulotomy in the treatment of congenital stenosis, 1948, *BMJ* **1**:1121. Died 1980. *3046*

1903:72 John Perry **Hubbard**, American paediatrician, born 26 Oct; with Robert Edward Gross, successful surgical repair of a patent ductus arteriosus in congenital heart disease, 193, *JAMA* **112**:7299. *3039*

1903:73 Konrad Zacharias **Lorenz**, Austrian zoologist, born 7 Nov; shared Nobel Prize (Physiology or Medicine), 1973, with Karl von Frisch and Nikolaas Tinbergen, for their discoveries concerning organization and elicitation of individual and social behaviour patterns, *NPL*. Died 1989.

1903:74 Ernest Milford **Parrott**, American nutritionist, born 17 Dec; with Albert Garland Hogan he isolated vitamin B_c, 1940, *JBC* **132**:507. *1086*

1903:75 George Davis **Snell**, American geneticist and immunologist, born 19 Dec; named genes governing transplantation as 'histocompatibility genes', 1958, *JNCI* **20**:787. For his contribution to the fundamentals of transplantation genetics he shared the Nobel Prize (Physiology or Medicine), 1980, with Baruj Benacerraf and Jean Baptiste Dausset, *NPL*. Died 1996. *2578.30*

1903:76 Haldan Keffer **Hartline**, American physiologist, born 22 Dec; his studies on the electrical discharges of the optic nerve, 1938, *AmJPh* **121**:400, continued the work of E.D. Adrian and R. Matthews. He shared the Nobel Prize (Physiology or Medicine), 1967, with Ragnar Granit and George Wald, for his work on visual mechanisms, *NPL*. Died 1983. *1532*

1903:77 Joseph John **Pfiffner**, American biochemist, born; with Wilbur Willis Swingle, prepared an adrenal cortical hormone ('eschatin'), which was effective in the treatment of Addison's disease, 1932, *Medicine* **11**:371. Isolated cortisone, 1936, *JBC* **111**:599; **116**:291. Died 1975. *3874, 1152*

1903:78 Roger **Couvelaire**, French surgeon, born; constructed an artificial bladder, 1951, *JUMC* **57**:408. Died 1986. *4203.1*

1903:79 Edward Graeme **Robertson**, Australian neurologist, born; improved the accuracy and reliability of encephalography; recorded in his *Encephalography*, 1941. *4614.1*

1903:80 Richard Homer **Fitch**, American pharmacologist, born; with co-workers, first used pentobarbitone sodium as an intravenous anaesthetic, 1930, *AmJSu* **9**:110. *5712.1*

1903:81 Machteld Elisabeth **Sano**, American physician, born; first to use fibrin glue for skin grafting, 1943, *AmJS* **61**:105. *5765*

1903:82 Eduardo **Braun-Menendez**, Argentinian physiologist, born; with co-workers, isolated angiotensin, 1940, *JP* **98**:283; also isolated independently by Irving Heinly Page and O.M. Helmer, *JEM* **71**:29. *2724.1, 2724.2*

1903:83 Howard Carman **Moloy**, Canadian obstetrician, born; with William Edgar Caldwell, devised a classification of the female pelvis, 1933, *AmJOG* **26**:479, in use today. Died 1953. *6266*

1903:84 Harold **Friedman**, American physiologist, born; with Maxwell Edward Lapham, introduced the Friedman test for the diagnosis of pregnancy, 1931, *AmJOG* **21**:405. *6224*

1903: Alfred **Kast** died, **born** 1856. *phenacetin, sulphonal*

1903: Angelo **Maffucci** died, **born** 1845. *Maffucci's syndrome, dyschondroplasia*

1903: Enrico **Bottini** died, **born** 1837. *prostate*

1903: Thomas George **Morton** died, **born** 1835. *metatarsalgia*

1903: Berthold Ernest **Hadra** died, **born** 1842. *surgical spinal immobilization and fusion*

1903: Thomas John **Maclagan** died, **born** 1838. *rheumatism, salicylates*

1903: Friedrich **Lösch** died, **born** 1840. *amoebiasis, Entamoeba histolytica*

1903: Gustav **Nepveu** died, **born** 1841. *trypanosome*

1903: Edmond Isidore Etienne **Nocard** died, **born** 1850. *Nocardia farcinica*

1903: Clemens von **Kahlden** died, **born** 1859. *ovarian tumours*

1903: Theodore Gaillard **Thomas** died, **born** 1831. *ovariotomy, caesarean section*

1903: Photinos **Panas** died, **born** 1832. *ptosis of eyelid*

1903: Max **Sanger** died, **born** 1853. *chorionic tumours, caesarean section*

1903: Karl **Gegenbaur** died, **born** 1826. *ovum, comparative anatomy in study of descent*

## 1904
1904:1 **Nobel Prize** (Physiology or Medicine): Ivan Petrovich Pavlov (1849–1936) for his contribution to the knowledge of the physiology of digestion, *NPL. 1022*

1904:2 **Imperial Cancer Research Fund Laboratories, London**, opened

1904:3 **Rockefeller Institute for Medical Research, New York**, founded by John Davidson **Rockefeller** (1839–1937)

1904:4 **University of Sofia** founded; medical faculty, 1918

1904:5 **Deutsche Physiologische Gesellschaft** founded

1904:6 **National Tuberculosis Association, New York**, founded

1904:7 **Academia Nacional de Medicina, Caracas**, founded

1904:8 **Dacryocystorhinostomy** for the treatment of chronic suppuration of the **lacrimal duct** introduced by Addeo Toti (b.1861), *CM* **10**:385. *5948*

1904:9 A method of forming an **artificial vagina** by intestinal transplantation devised by James Fairchild Baldwin (1850–1936), *AnS* **40**:398 *6117*

1904:10 **Pneumatic tourniquet** with a measurable degree of pressure, with especial use in **craniotomy**, introduced by Harvey Williams Cushing (1869–1939), *MN* **84**:577. *4877.1*

1904:11 First description of *Schistosoma japonicum*, a parasite in **bilharziasis**, given by Fujiro Katsurada (1868–1946), *IS* **669**:1325. *5349.1*

1904:12 Philip Hedgeland Ross (1876–1929) and Arthur Dawson Milne (d.1932) discovered that African **relapsing fever** (**tick fever**) is conveyed by *Ornithodorus moubata*, *BMJ* **2**:453. *5317*

1904:13 **Leishman-Donovan bodies** found in **kala-azar** (**visceral leishmaniasis**) by Leonard Rogers (1868–1962), *BMJ* **1**:303. *5299*

1904:14 Successful inoculation of **smallpox** into the monkey carried out by George Burgess Magrath (1870–1938) and Walter Remsen Brinckerhoff (1875–1911), *JMR* **11**:230. *5429.1*

1904:15 Cases of **juvenile amaurotic familial idiocy,** ('**Batten-Mayou disease**') described by Marmaduke Stephen Mayou (1876–1934), *TOUK* **24**:142. *4713, 4712*

1904:16 Raymond Jacques Adrien Sabouraud (1864–1938) used **radiotherapy** in the treatment of **tinea** (**ringworm**), *AnD* **5**:577. He gave a classic account of the different varieties of *Trichophyton*; in his *Pityriasis et alopécies pelliculaires*. *4004, 4139*

1904:17 **Osteitis fibrosa cystica** shown to be related to **parathyroid tumours** by Max Askanazy (1865–1940), *AGPA* **4**:398. *3858*

1904:18 Negative pressure chamber for the prevention of **pneumothorax** devised by Ernst Ferdinand Sauerbruch (1875–1951), *VDGC* **32**ii, 105. *3185*

1904:19 **Gradenigo's syndrome** (acute **otitis media** followed by **abductor paralysis**) reported by Giuseppe Gradenigo (1859–1926), *GAMT* **10**:59. *3398*

1904:20 The important account of **rheumatic myocarditis** by Ludwig Aschoff (1866–1942), *VDPG* **8**:46, includes a description of the characteristic lesion ('**Aschoff body**'). *2816*

1904:21 **Auto-antibody** and **auto-immune disease** demonstrated by Julius Donath (1870–1950) and Karl Landsteiner (1868–1943), *MMW* **51**:1590. *2558.1*

1904:22 **Bacteriotropins** named and described by Fred Neufeld (1861–1945) and Willi Rimpau (b.1877), *DMW* **30**:1458. *2560*

1904:23 Theory of **hormonal control of internal secretion** developed by William Maddock Bayliss (1860–1924) and Ernest Henry Starling (1866–1927), *PRS* **73**:310. *1121*

1904:24 **Artificial respiration**; Sharpey-Schafer method introduced by Edward Albert Sharpey-Schafer (1850–1935), *MCT* **87**:609. *2028.59*

1904:25 **Adrenaline** synthesized by Friedrich Stolz (1860–1936), *BDCG* **37**:4149. *1147.1*

1904:26 **Chemical mediation of nerve impulses** suggested by Thomas Renton Elliott (1877–1961), proposed adrenaline as mediator, *JP* **31**:xx. *1336*

1904:27 **Platyspondylia** first described by Pierre Nau in his *Les scolioses congénitales*, his Thèse, Paris, 1904. *4375*

---

1904:28 John Hundale **Lawrence**, American physician, born 7 Jan; with co-workers, introduced the treatment of leukaemia with radiophosphorus, 1939, *NIC* **3**:33; *Rad* **35**:51. *3098, 3099*

1904:29 James Winston **Watts**, American neurosurgeon, born 19 Jan; with Walter Freeman, performed prefrontal lobotomy in treatment of certain psychotic conditions, 1936, *MADC* **5**:326. *4906*

1904:30 John Joseph **Bittner**, American biologist and oncologist, born 25 Feb; isolated a milk factor in cancer transmission in mice, 1936, *Science*, **84**:162. Died 1961. *2658*

1904:31 Guy Frederic **Marrian**, British biochemist, born 3 Mar; isolated pregnanediol, 1929, *BJ* 23:1090; isolated oestriol in crystalline form, 1930, *BJ* **24**:435. Died 1981. *1190, 1194*

1904:32 Arthur Jackson **Patek**, American physician, born 6 May; with Francis Henry Laskey Taylor, isolated antihaemophilic globulin (Factor VIII), 1937, *JCI* **16**:113. *3096.1*

1904:33 William McDowell **Hammon**, American epidemiologist, born 20 Jul; with co-workers, carried out trials of prophylaxis of poliomyelitis by gamma globulin, 1952, *JAMA* **150**:739. *4672*

1904:34 Garrett Arthur **Cooper**, American dermatologist, born 24 Jul; with Arthur Lewis Tatum, used mapharsen experimentally as an antisyphilitic agent, 1934, *JPET* **50**:198. *2415*

1904:35 Ernest Lester **Smith**, British biochemist, born 7 Aug; independently of Rickes et al. he isolated vitamin B$_{12}$, 1948, *Nature* **162**:144. Died 1992. *1092, 1091*

1904:36 Wendell Meredith **Stanley**, American biochemist, born 16 Aug; isolated a virus, in crystalline form, later shown to be a nucleoprotein, 1935, *Science* **81**:644. Shared Nobel Prize (Chemistry), 1946, with John Howard Northrop, for their preparations of enzymes and viruses in a pure form, *NPL*. Died 1971. *2524.5*

1904:37 Ramon **Castroviejo**, Spanish/American ophthalmologist, born 24 Aug; introduced a new method of keratoplasty (corneal grafting), 1932, *AmJOp* **15**:825, 905. Died 1987. *5981*

1904:38 Werner Theodor Otto **Forssmann**, German surgeon, born 29 Aug; first to carry out cardiac catheterization on a living person (he catheterized his own heart), 1929, *KW* **8**:2085, 2287. Shared the Nobel Prize (Physiology or Medicine), 1956, with André Frédéric Cournand and Dickinson Woodruff Richards, *NPL*. Died 1979. *2858*

1904:39 William Barlow **Stillman**, American chemist, born 21 Sep; with Matthew Charles Dodd, introduced nitrofuran (nitrofurazone) as a bacteriostatic, 1944, *JPET* **82**:11. *1928.2*

1904:40 Willard Myron **Allen**, American obstetrician and gynaecologist, born 5 Nov; with George Washington Corner discovered progesterone, 1929, *AmJPh* **88**:326. *1188*

1904:41 Monroe Davies **Eaton**, American microbiologist, born 2 Dec; with co-workers, isolated Eaton agent in patients with primary atypical pneumonia, 1944, *JEM* **79**:649. *3213.1*

1904:42 Noel Francis **Maclagan**, British pathologist, born 25 Dec; used the serum colloidal gold reaction and the thymol turbidity test as liver function tests, 1944, *BJEP* **25**:15, 234. Died 1987. *3665, 3666*

———

1904:43 Celestino L. **Ruiz**, Argentinian physician, born; with co-workers, discovered the hypoglycaemic effect of certain sulphonamides, 1930, *RSAB* **6**:134. *3973*

———

1904: Wilhelm **His** Sr died, **born** 1831. *microtome, neuron theory*

1904: Etienne Jules **Marey** died, **born** 1830. *sphygmograph, serial pictures in study of locomotion*

1904: Eadweard **Muybridge** died, **born** 1830. *movement in man and animals*

1904: John **Simon** died, **born** 1816. *public health, uretero-intestinal anastomosis*

1904: Carl **Weigert** died, **born** 1845. *bacterial stains, myocardial infarction, myasthenia gravis*

1904: Nils Ryberg **Finsen** died, **born** 1860. *lupus vulgaris, light therapy*

1904: Henry **Thompson** died, **born** 1820. *bladder tumour*

1904: Charles Jules Alphonse **Gayet** died, **born** 1833. *polioencephalitis*

1904: Georges Gilles de la **Tourette** died, **born** 1857. *Gilles de la Tourette syndrome*

1904: Ambroise Auguste **Liébeault** died, **born** 1823. *hypnosis, psychotherapy*

1904: Edmund **Andrews** died, **born** 1824. *anaesthesia, oxygen-nitrous oxide*

1904: John Reissberg **Wolfe** died, **born** 1824. *skin grafts*

## 1905

1905:1 **Nobel Prize** (Physiology or Medicine): Robert Koch (1843–1910), for his work on **tuberculosis**, *NPL. 2331, 2332*

1905:2 **British Red Cross** (1870) adopts present name

1905:3 **Deutsche Röntgengesellschaft** founded in **Berlin**

1905:4 **Société de Pathologie Exotique** founded in **Paris**

1905:5 **King Edward VII College of Medicine, Singapore,** founded

1905:6 **Cyclodialysis** in the treatment of **glaucoma** introduced by Leopold Heine (b.1870), *DMW* **31**:824. *5949*

1905:7 An excellent account of **serum sickness** given by Bela Schick (1874–1929) and Clemens Peter Pirquet von Cesenatico (1877–1967); in their *Die Serumkrankheit. 2593*

1905:8 A classical work on **sexual deviation**, *Psychopathia sexualis*, published by Richard von Krafft-Ebing (1840–1926). *4950*

1905:9 In scrapings of **yaws** tissue Aldo Castellani (1877–1971) demonstrated, the causal organism, *Treponema pertenue, BMJ* **2**:1280, 1330, 1430; finally establishing it as a distinct organism from the spirochaete of **syphilis**, *T.pallidum*. It was independently discovered by Frederick Creighton Wellman (1871–1960), *JTM* **8**:345. *5306, 5307*

1905:10 **Procaine (novocaine)**, synthesized by Einhorn, first used as an **anaesthetic** by Heinrich Friedrich Wilhelm Braun (1862–1934), *DMW* **31**:1667. *5692, 5685*

1905:11 Inclusion bodies in **varicella** first recognized by Ernest Edward Tyzzer (1875–1965), *JMR* **14**:361. *5440*

1905:12 The existence of **malaria** carriers demonstrated by Charles Franklin Craig (1872–1950), *AmM* **10**:982, 109. *5255*

1905:13 Independently of Ross and Milne, John Everett Dutton (1874–1905) and John Lancelot Todd (1876–1949) demonstrated **relapsing fever** in monkeys, and described the mechanisms of infection conveyed by infected **ticks**, *Ornithodorus moubata*, *BMJ* **2**:1259. The infecting organism was later named *Borrelia duttoni*, after Dutton, who died from the disease. *5318*

1905:14 Harold Wolferstan Thomas and Anton Breinl discovered the value of **atoxyl**, an **arsenical**, in the treatment of experimental **trypanosomiasis**. This work led eventually to Ehrlich's study of arsenicals and the production of **salvarsan**; in *Report on trypanosomes, trypanosomiasis, and sleeping sickness*, etc. *5279*

1905:15 Harvey Williams Cushing (1869–1939) established **cerebral hernia** as a decompressive measure for inaccessible **brain tumours**, *SGO* **1**:297, and achieved successful operative intervention in the treatment of **intracranial haemorrhage of the newborn**, *AmJMS* **130**:563. *4879, 4878*

1905:16 **Juvenile amaurotic familial idiocy** described by Heinrich Vogt (b.1875), *MonP* **18**:161, and later by Spielmayer (1904) leading to the eponym '**Spielmeyer-Vogt disease**'. *4713.1, 4714.1*

1905:17 The infectious nature of **poliomyelitis** first confirmed by Otto Ivar Wickman (1872–1914), *APIH* **1**:109. *4668*

1905:18 **Palato-pharyngo-laryngeal hemiplegia** ('**Tapia's syndrome**') described by Antonio Garcia Tapia (1875–1950), *SMM* **52**:211. *4594*

1905:19 The first attempt at **surgical lengthening of limbs** made by Alessandro Codivilla (1861–1912), *AmJOrS* **2**:353. *4375.1*

1905:20 '**Looser's syndrome**', a form of **fragilitas ossium**, described as **osteogenesis imperfecta tarda** by Emile Looser, *VDPG*, 239. *4376.1*

1905:21 First **cystograms** obtained by Friedrich Voelcker (1872–1955) and Alexander von Lichtenberg (1880–1949), *MMW* **52**:1576. *4192*

1905:22 The **adrenogenital syndrome** first recognized by William Bulloch (1868–1941) and James Harry Sequeira (1865–1948), *TPS* **56**:189. *3867*

1905:23 First radical **prostatectomy** for **carcinoma** performed by Hugh Hampton Young (1870–1945), *JHB* **16**:315. *4266.1*

1905:24 Experimental **heart transplantation**, in a dog, carried out by Alexis Carrel (1873–1944) and Charles Claude Guthrie (1880–1963), *AmM* **10**:284, 1101. *3025.1*

1905:25 **Lymphogranulomatosis** ('**Sternberg's disease**') described by Carl Sternberg (1872–1935); in his *Pathologie der Primärerkrankungen des lymphatischen und hämatopoetischen Apparates. 3077*

1905:26 **Polycythaemia hypertonica** ('**Geisböck's disease**') described by Felix Geisböck, *DAKM* **83**:363. *3076*

1905:27 Embryonal origin of **cancer** proposed by Moritz Wilhelm Hugo Ribbert (1855–1920); in *Die Entstehung des Carcinoms. 2632*

1905:28 Action of **digitalis** in **auricular fibrillation** reported by James Mackenzie (1853–1925), *BMJ* **1**:519, 587, 702, 759, 812. *2819*

1905:29 **Teleradiography** introduced into **heart radiography** by Alban Köhler (1874–1947), *WKR* **19**:279. *2817*

1905:30 In **blood pressure examination** Nicolai Sergeievich Korotkov (1874–1920) introduced the method of applying the **stethoscope** to the brachial artery during the use of the Riva-Rocci **sphygmomanometer**, *IVMA* **11**:365. *2818*

1905:31 **Syphilis:** *Spirochaeta pallida* (*Treponema pallidum*), the causal organism, discovered by Fritz Richard Schaudinn (1871–1906) and Erich Hoffmann (1868–1959), *AKG* **22**:527. *2399*

---

1905:32 John Rudolph **Schenken**, American pathologist and bacteriologist, born 6 Jan; with George Henry Hansmann, cultivated *Histoplasma capsulatum*, 1933, *Science* **77** (No. 2002), Supplement, p. 8, 1934, *AmJPa* **10**:731. Almost simultaneously it was cultivated by DeMonbreun. *5541.2, 5542*

1905:33 Ulf Svante von **Euler**, Swedish physiologist, born 7 Feb; with John Henry Gaddum, isolated Substance P, the first peptide neurotransmitter, 1931, *JP* **72**:74. Extracted prostaglandins from seminal fluid, 1934, *ArEP* **175**:78. Showed noradrenaline to be predominant transmitter of the effects of sympathetic nerve impulses, 1946, *AcPS* **12**:73. Shared the Nobel Prize (Physiology or Medicine), 1970, with Julius Axelrod and Bernard Katz, for research on chemical neurotransmission, *NPL*. Died 1983. *1924.3, 1354.1*

1905:34 Cesare **Gianturco**, Italian/American physician, born 12 Feb; with Walter Clement Alvarez, introduced Roentgen cinematography, 1932, *PMC* **7**:669. *2697*

1905:35 Johan Albert **Levan**, Swedish chromosome cytologist, born 8 Mar; with J.H. Tjio showed the chromosome number in man to be 46, 1956, *Her* **42**:1. *256.5*

1905:36 George H. **Hitchings**, American chemotherapist, born 18 Apr; shared the Nobel Prize (Physiology or Medicine), 1988, with James W. Black and Gertrude Belle Elion, for their discoveries of important principles for drug therapy, *NPL*.

1905:37 Isador Max **Tarlov**, American neurosurgeon, born 16 May; with Bernard Benjamin, introduced plasma clot nerve suture, 1943, *SGO* **76**:366. *4912*

1905:38 Robert Edward **Gross**, American surgeon, born 2 Jul; with John Perry Hubbard, successful surgical repair of a patent ductus arteriosus in congenital heart disease, 1939,

*JAMA* **112**:729. Pioneered, at same time as Clarence Crafoord and Karl Gustav Vilhelm Nylin, surgical treatment of coarctation of aorta, 1945, *Surgery* **18**:673. Died 1988. *3039, 3044.1*

1905:39 Harry **Eagle**. American microbiologist, born 13 Jul; introduced the Eagle flocculation test for the diagnosis of syphilis, 1932, *JLCM* **17**:787. *2414.1*

1905:40 Erwin **Chargaff**, Austrian/American chemist, born 11 Aug; his chemical studies revolutionized attitudes towards DNA, 1950, *Ex* **6**:201. *255.6*

1905:41 Merrill Wallace **Chase**, American immunologist, born 17 Sep; with Karl Landsteiner, discovered passive cell transfer of delayed hypersensitivity, 1942, *PSEB* **49**:688. *2578.3*

1905:42 Severo **Ochoa**, Spanish biochemist, born 24 Sep; with Marianne Grunberg-Manago artificially synthesized nucleic acids, 1955, *JACS* **77**:3165. Shared Nobel Prize (Physiology or Medicine), 1959, with Arthur Kornberg, *NPL*. *752.3*

1905:43 Hermann **Pinkus**, German/American dermatologist, born 18 Nov; recorded follicular mucinosis, alopecia mucinosa, 1957, *ArDS* **76**:419. *4154.5*

1905:44 Geoffrey Clough **Ainsworth** born; he was among several who simultaneously discovered polymyxins, 1947, *Nature* **160**:263. *1937*

1905:45 Esther White **Goldberger** born; with Hermann Vollmer, introduced the tuberculin patch test for tuberculosis, 1937, *AmJDC* **54**:1019. *2348*

1905:46 Otto **Metz** born; developed acoustic impedance hearing test, 1946, *AcOL*, Suppl. 63. *3412.2*

1905:47 Saul **Hertz** born; with A. Roberts, treated exophthalmic goitre with radioactive iodine, 1942, *JCI* **21**:624. *3853*

1905:48 Leslie V. **Rush** born; with H. Lowry Rush, introduced 'Rush pins', made of specially hardened stainless steel, for the fixation of fractures of long bones, 1949, *AmJSu* **78**:324. *4435.2*

1905:49 Jean **Judet**, French orthopaedic surgeon, born; with Robert Louis Judet, introduced the use of an acrylic prosthesis for hip arthroplasty, 1950, *JBJS* **32B**:166. *4405*

1905:50 José Antonio **Gay Prieto**, Spanish dermato-syphilologist, born; first to see the infective agent in lymphogranuloma venereum, 1927, *ACDS* **20**:122. Died 1979. *5219*

1905:51 John Alden **Stiles**, American anaesthetist, born; with co-workers, first used cyclopropane anaesthesia clinically, 1934, *CRA* **13**:56. *5717*

1905:52 Josef **Dallos**, Hungarian ophthalmologist, born; introduced contact lenses, 1933, *KMA* **91**:640. Died 1979. *5985*

1905:53 Waldo Berry **Edwards**, American surgeon, born; with Robert Andrew Hingson, first reported continuous caudal anaesthesia during labour and delivery, 1942, *CRA* **21**:301. *6232.1*

1905: Samuel Siegfried von **Basch** died, **born** 1837. *sphygmomanometer*

1905: Johann von **Mikulicz-Radecki** died, **born** 1850. *rectal prolapse, reconstruction of oesophagus, oesophagoscope, enterocystoplasty*

1905: Benjamin **Loewenberg** died, **born** 1836. *Friedländler group bacillus, ozaena*

1905: Rudolf Albert von **Kölliker** died, **born** 1817. *spermatozoa, classification of tissue, histology, embryology, poisons and muscular contraction*

1905: Walther **Flemming** died, **born** 1843. *centrosome*

1905: Nathan **Bozeman** died, **born** 1825. *pyelitis*

1905: Carl Wilhelm Hermann **Nothnagel** died, **born** 1841. *paralysis, ataxia*

1905: Carl **Wernicke** died, **born** 1848. *polioencephalitis, aphasia*

1905: Joseph Everett **Dutton** died, **born** 1874. *relapsing fever, Ornithodorus moubata, trypanosomiasis, Trypanosoma gambiense*

1905: Claude André **Paquelin** died, **born** 1836. *thermocautery*

## 1906

1906:1 **Nobel Prize** (Physiology or Medicine): Camillo Golgi (1843–1926) and Santiago Ramón y Cajal (1852–1934), for their work on **neuroanatomy** and **histology**, *NPL. 1416, 1287*

1906:2 **Federal Food and Drugs Act**, US, passed

1906:3 **Carnegie Nutrition Laboratory, Boston** opened

1906:4 **[Institute for Experimental Cancer Research], Heidelberg**

1906:5 **American Association of Biological Chemists**, founded, **Ann Arbor**

1906:6 **Chemotherapeutisches Institut, Georg Speyer Haus**, opened at **Frankfurt am Main**

1906:7 **[State School of Tropical Medicine]** opened at **Brussels**

1906:8 **Pathological Society of Great Britain and Ireland** founded at **Cambridge**

1906:9 The first recognition of **auricular fibrillation** in man by Arthur Robertson Cushny (1866–1926); *Studies in pathology* ... ed. by W. Bulloch, p. 95. *2822*

1906:10 **Twilight sleep**, introduced by von Steinbüchel in 1902 for the relief of **labour pains**, was developed by Carl Joseph Gauss (1875–1957), *ArGy* **78**:579. *6212, 6210*

1906:11 **Histoplasmosis** ('**Darling's disease**'), caused by *Histoplasma capsulatum*, described by Samuel Taylor Darling (1872–1925), *JAMA* **46**:1283. *5532*

1906:12 The first successful **corneal transplant (keratoplasty)** reported by Eduard Konrad Zirm (1863–1944), *GAO* **64**:580. *5950.1*

1906:13 In his *Cancer of the breast and its treatment*, William Sampson Handley (1872–1962) advanced the theory that **breast cancer** metastasis is due to lymphatic extension ('lymphatic permeation'), not dissemination by the blood stream. *5782*

1906:14 The causal organism of **whooping cough**, *Bordetella pertussis*, discovered by Jules Jean Baptiste Vincent Bordet (1870–1961) and Octave Gengou (1875–1957), *AnIP* **20**:731; **21**:720. *5087*

1906:15 An anti-bubonic **plague** vaccine for use in man developed by Waldemar Mordecai Wolff Haffkine (1860–1930), *BIP* **4**:825. *5129*

1906:16 A complement fixation test for the diagnosis of **gonorrhoea** ('**Müller-Oppenheim reaction**') introduced by Rudolf Müller (b.1877) and Moritz Oppenheim (1876–1949), *WKW* **19**:894. *5213*

1906:17 **Wood tick**, *Dermacentor occidentalis*, shown to be vector of **Rocky Mountain spotted fever** by Howard Taylor Ricketts (1871–1910), *JAMA* **47**:358. *5378*

1906:18 The **Paschen elementary bodies** in the **vaccinia** virus, first described and demonstrated microscopically by J.B. Buist (1886), rediscovered by Enrique Paschen (1860–1936) and named after him, *MMW* **53**:2391. *5430*

1906:19 The **spirochaete** causing the American variety of **relapsing fever** isolated by Charles Norris (1867–1935) and co-workers, *JID* **3**:266. *5319*

1906:20 Frederick George Novy (1864–1957) and Richard Edward Knapp (b.1884) proved that the **spirochaete** isolated by Norris et al. from a case of American **relapsing fever** differed from that isolated by Obermeier, *JID* **3**:291. *5320*

1906:21 Charles Scott Sherrington (1857–1952) investigated the **proprioceptive** system, *Brain* **29**:467, and produced his most important work, *The integrative action of the nervous system*. *1432*

1906:22 Evidence that *Aëdes aegypti* is a vector of **dengue** first supplied by Thomas Lane Bancroft (1860–1933), *AuMG* **25**:17. *5472*

1906:23 Organisms resembling *Histoplasma capsulatum* discovered by Richard Pearson Strong (1872–1948), *PhJS* **1**:91. *5531.1*

1906:24 August von Wassermann (1866–1925) applied his test (for **syphilis**) to the **cerebrospinal fluid** in cases of general paralysis, *DMW* **32**:1769; it greatly facilitated the diagnosis of **general paresis**. *4804*

1906:25 **Pyknolepsy** first described by Max Friedmann, *DZN* **30**:462. *4594.1*

1906:26 **Unilateral descending paralysis** first described by Charles Karsner **Mills** (1845–1931), *JAMA* **47**:1638. *4714*

1906:27 Pierre Marie (1853–1940), who disclaimed Broca's theory concerning the location of the **speech centre**, classified **aphasia** into three groups: **anarthria** (defects of articulation),

Broca's aphasia (motor aphasia), and Wernicke's aphasia (sensory aphasia), *SMP* **26**:241. *4630*

1906:28 A distensible bag for controlling **haemorrhage** after suprapubic **prostatectomy** introduced by James Emmons Briggs (1869–1942), *NEMG* **41**:391. *4267*

1906:29 **Carcinoma** of the **bladder** treated with **radiotherapy** by Alfred Leftwich Gray (1873–1932), *AmQR* **1**:53. *4194.1*

1906:30 Open operation for **epididymitis** devised by Francis Randall Hagner (1873–1940), *MR* **70**:944. *4194*

1906:31 '**Albarran's operation**' for **nephropexy** introduced by Joaquin Maria Albarran y Dominguez (1860–1912), *PrM* **14**:253. *4233*

1906:32 **Pyelography** introduced by Friedrich Voelcker (1872–1955) and Alexander von Lichtenberg (1880–1949), *MMW* **53**:105. *4231*

1906:33 **Galactose tolerance test** introduced by Richard Bauer, *WMW* **56**:20. *3643*

1906:34 Hermann Schloffer (1868–1937) first to operate successfully upon a **pituitary tumour**, *WKW* **20**:621, 670, 1075. *3891, 3892*

1906:35 Robert Bárány (1876–1936) introduced his **caloric test** for **labyrinthine** function, *ArOh* **68**:1, and also reported his **pointing test** for localization of circumscribed **cerebellar lesions**, *MonO* **40**:193; **41**:447. *3400, 3401*

1906:36 Artificial **pneumothorax**, ('**Brauer's method**') induced by injection of nitrogen by Ludolph Brauer (1865–1951), *MMW* **53**:338. *3230*

1906:37 **Vein grafts** used to restore **arterial blood flow** by José Goyanes Capdevila (1876–1964), *SMM* **53**:546, 561. *3025.2*

1906:38 **Syphilis of aorta** reported by Karl Reuter, *MMW* **53**:778. *2824*

1906:39 **Syphilis: Wassermann reaction**, a specific diagnostic blood test, introduced by August von Wassermann (1866–1925) with Albert Ludwig Siegmund Neisser (1855–1916) and C. Bruck, *DMW* **32**:745. *2402*

1906:40 The **Theobald Smith phenomenon** was studied and described by Richard Otto (1872–1952); in *Gedenkschrift für den verstorbenen Generalstabsarzt ... von Leuthold*; it was not reported by Smith but communicated by him to Paul Ehrlich. *2594*

1906:41 *Proteus morgani* isolated by Harry de Riemer Morgan (1863–1931), *BMJ* **1**:908. *2518.1*

1906:42 Isolation of **ergotoxine** by George Barger (1878–1939), F.H. Carr and Henry Hallett Dale (1875–1968), *BMJ* **2**:1792. *1895*

1906:43 Existence of **vitamins** predicted by Frederick Gowland Hopkins (1861–1947), *Analyst* **31**:385. *1044*

1906:44 **Blood classified into four groups** by Jan Jansky (1873–1921), *SK* **8**:85. *896*

1906:45 **Gastrin** (gastric secretin) described by John Sydney Edkins (1863–1940), *JP* **34**:133. *1026*

---

1906:46 Albert **Hofmann**, Swiss chemist, born 11 Jan; with Arthur Stoll, synthesized lysergic acid-diethylamide, 1943, *HCA* **26**:944. *1928.1*

1906:47 George Widmer **Thorn**, American physician, born 15 Jan; with co-workers, introduced deoxycorticosterone acetate in the treatment of adrenal insufficiency, 1939, *BJH* **64**:155. *3877*

1906:48 Clifford **Wilson**, British physician, born 27 Jan; with Paul Kimmelstiel, first described 'Kimmelstiel-Wilson syndrome', nodular intercapillary glomerulosclerosis, 1936, *AmJPa* **12**:83. *4250*

1906:49 Alexander Carpenter **Finlay**, American biochemist and bacteriologist, born 9 Feb; with colleagues he discovered oxytetracycline (tetramycin), *Science* **111**:85, 1950. *1945.1*

1906:50 Raymond Loraine **Garner**, American biochemist, born 5 Mar; with William Smith Tillett, discovered streptokinase, a fibrinolysin, 1933, *JEM* **58**:485. *1924.1*

1906:51 Cecile **Leuchtenberger**, German/American cytologist, born 17 Mar; with co-workers, used folic acid concentrate used to inhibit tumour growth, 1944, *PSEB* **59**:204. *2659.2*

1906:52 Georges **Ungar**, Hungarian physiologist and pharmacologist, born 30 Mar; with co-workers, introduced phenformin, a hyperglycaemic biguanide, into the treatment of diabetes, 1957, *PSEB* **95**:190. *3978.3*

1906:53 Jan Gösta **Waldenström**, Swedish physician, born 17 Apr; described Waldenström's macroglobulinaemia, 1944, *AcM* **117**:216. *3924.1*

1906:54 Norman Cecil **Tanner**, British surgeon, born 13 Jun; introduced Tanner slide operation for inguinal and femoral hernia, 1942, *BJS* **29**:285. Died 1982. *3611.1*

1906:55 Ernst Boris **Chain** born 19 Jun; with Howard Walter Florey, Edward Penley Abraham et al., proved the chemotherapeutic action of penicillin, 1940, *Lancet* **2**:226; with Abraham, isolated penicillinase, an enzyme able to destroy penicillin, 1940, *Nature* **146**:837. Shared Nobel Prize (Physiology or Medicine), 1945, with Howard Walter Florey and Alexander Fleming, for the development of penicillin as an antibacterial antibiotic suitable for use in man, *NPL*. Died 1979. *1934, 1933.3*

1906:56 Nicholas Harold Lloyd **Ridley**, British ophthalmic surgeon, born 10 Jul; implanted the first intra-ocular acrylic lens, 1951, *TOUK* **71**:617. *5991*

1906:57 Vladimir **Prelog**, Yugoslav/Swiss chemist, born 23 Jul; shared Nobel Prize (Chemistry), 1975, with John Warcup Cornforth, for his work on the stereochemistry of organic molecules and reactions, *NPL*.

1906:58 Sarah Elizabeth **Stewart**, American physician, born 16 Aug; with co-workers, isolated the papovavirus, 1957, *Vir* **3**:380. *2660.10*

1906:59 Albert Bruce **Sabin**, Russian/American microbiologist, born 26 Aug; with Arthur M. Wright, reported a case of herpesvirus simiae (B virus) and isolated the virus, 1934, *JEM* **59**:115. With Peter Kosciusko Olitsky, isolated and propagated poliomyelitis virus in pure culture, 1936, *PSEB* **34**:357. With Robert Walter Schlesinger, successfully propagated dengue in mice and produced a vaccine, 1945, *Science* **101**:604. Introduced a live attenuated poliomyelitis virus vaccine, 1955, *ANYAS* **61**:924. *4658, 4670.6, 5475.1, 4672.3*

1906:60 Louis Sanford **Goodman**, American pharmacologist, born 27 Aug; with co-workers, introduced nitrogen mustard therapy (methyl-bis amine hydrochloride and methyl-tris amine hydrochloride) for Hodgkin's disease, lymphosarcoma, etc., 1946, *JAMA* **105**:475. *2659.6*

1906:61 Max **Delbrück**, German/American biologist, born 4 Sep; with W.T. Bailey, induced genetic recombination in bacteriophages, 1946, *CSHS* **11**:33. Shared Nobel Prize (Physiology or Medicine), 1969, with Alfred Day Hershey and Salvador Edward Luria, for his work on genetics and the replication of bacteria, *NPL*. Died 1981. *2578.5*

1906:62 Luis Frederico **Leloir**, Argentinian biochemist, born 6 Sep; awarded Nobel Prize (Chemistry), 1970, for his discovery of sugar nucleotides and their role in the biosynthesis of carbohydrates, *NPL*

1906:63 Geoffrey Cureton **Knight**, British neurosurgeon, born 4 Oct; carried out stereotactic tractotomy in the treatment of mental illness, 1965, *JNNP* **28**:304. *4914.3*

1906:64 George **Wald**, American biologist, born 18 Nov; shared Nobel Prize (Physiology or Medicine), 1967, with Halden Keffer Hartline and Ragnar Arthur Granit, for his research on the photosensitive pigments of the visual receptor apparatus, *NPL*. *1535*

1906:65 Per Johannes **Hedenius**, Swedish physician, born; introduced the use of heparin in blood transfusion, 1936, AcM **89**:263. *2024*

1906:66 Hilmert Albert **Ranges**, American physician, born; with André Frédéric Cournand, first used cardiac catheterization in clinical investigation, 1941, *PSEB* **46**:462. Died 1969. *2871*

1906:67 Ernst **Ruska**, German physicist, born; with Max Knoll, produced the first electron microscope, 1932, *AnPh* **12**:607. He shared the Nobel Prize (Physics), 1986, with Gerd Binnig and Heinrich Rohrer, for this work, *NPL*. *269.3*

1906: Pierre **Curie** died, **born** 1859. *radium*

1906: Fritz Richard **Schaudinn** died, **born** 1871. *syphilis, Spirochaeta*

1906: George Ryerson **Fowler** died, **born** 1848. *thoracoplasty, Fowler drainage position*

1906: Manuel **Garcia** died, **born** 1805. *laryngoscope*

1906: Endre **Högyes** died, **born** 1847. *rotational nystagmus*

1906: Isidor **Neumann** died, **born** 1832. *porokeratosis, pemphigus vegetans*

1906: Robert William **Taylor** died, **born** 1842. *acrodermatitis chronica atrophicans*

1906: Max **Nitze** died, **born** 1848. *cystocope*

1906: August **Rothmund** died, **born** 1830. *poikiloderma congenitale*

1906: Fernand **Henrotin** died, **born** 1847. *hysterectomy*

**1907**
1907:1 **Nobel Prize** (Physiology or Medicine): Charles Louis Alphonse Laveran (1844–1922), for work on pathogenic **protozoa**, including the **malaria parasite**, *NPL. 5236*

1907:2 **Nobel Prize** (Chemistry): Eduard Buchner (1860–1917), for his discovery of **cell-free fermentation**, *NPL. 719.1*

1907:3 **Office International d'Hygiène Publique, Paris**, founded

1907:4 **Royal Society of Medicine, London**, founded from amalgamation of **Royal Medico-Chirurgical Society** (1805) with others

1907:5 **University of Saskatchewan** founded at **Saskatoon** (opened 1909)

1907:6 **Tohoku Imperial University, Sendai**, opened

1907:7 **International Association of Medical Museums** founded at **Montreal**

1907:8 **International Sleeping Sickness Congress, London**

1907:9 **[Italian Society of Medical History]** founded, **Florence**

1907:10 **Notification of Births Act, England**

1907:11 Frederick Percival Mackie (1875–1944) proved that **relapsing fever** could be conveyed by the body **louse**, *Pediculus corporis, BMJ* **2**:1706. *5321*

1907:12 The **sino-auricular node** – the 'pacemaker of the heart' discovered by Arthur Keith (1866–1955) and Martin William Flack (1882–1931), *JA* **41**:172. *844*

1907:13 The production of **lactic acid** in normal **muscular contraction** explained by Frederick Gowland Hopkins (1861–1947) and Walter Morley Fletcher (1873–1933), *JP* **35**:247. *733*

1907:14 In his *Some points on the surgery of the brain and its membranes*, Charles Alfred Ballance (1856–1936). Recognized and described chronic **subdural haematoma**, he operated for it and for **subdural hydroma** and fully discussed **brain abscess** and **brain tumours**. *4879.01*

1907:15 **Sclerectomy** for the treatment of **glaucoma** introduced by Pierre Félix Lagrange (1857–1928), *GSMB* **28**:2. *5953*

1907:16 The operation of **iridencleisis** for the treatment of **glaucoma** introduced by Sören Holth (1863–1937), *AnO* **137**:345. *5952*

1907:17 The first description of the cytoplasmic **inclusion bodies** of **trachoma** (*Chlamydia trachomatis*) given by Ludwig Halberstaedter (b.1876) and Stanislaus Joseph Matthias von Prowazek (1875–1915), *AKG* **26**:44. *5951*

1907:18 An **ovarian tumour** described by Fritz Brenner (b.1877), *FZP* **1**:150, was later named 'Brenner tumour', although described previously by Orthmann (1899). *6118, 6109.1*

1907:19 Suprasymphyseal transperitoneal **caesarean section** introduced by Fritz Frank (1856–1923), *ArGy* **81**:46. *6247*

1907:20 The causal organism in **dengue** shown to be a filterable virus by Percy Moreau Ashburn (1872–1940) and Charles Franklin Craig (1872–1950), *PhJS, B* **8**:93; *JID* **4**:440. *5473*

1907:21 Experimental **trypanosomiasis** cured by Paul Ehrlich (1854–1915) with his 'Trypanrot', *BKW* **44**:233, 280, 310, 341, the work led him eventually to the production of **salvarsan**. *5281*

1907:22 **Convalescent human serum** first used in **measles** prophylaxis by Francesco Cenci, *RCP* **5**:1017. *5447*

1907:23 **Presenile dementia**, also called '**Alzheimer's disease**' after the description of the condition by Alois Alzheimer (1864–1915), *AZP* **64**:146. *4956*

1907:24 Antiserum used in the treatment of epidemic **cerebrospinal meningitis** by Simon Flexner (1863–1946) and James Wesley Jobling (b.1876), *JEM* **9**:168; **10**:141. *4683, 4684*

1907:25 **Juvenile amaurotic familial idiocy** described by Walther Spielmayer (b.1879); in his *Klinische und anatomische Untersuchungen über eine besondere Form von familiärer amaurotische Idiotie*. Vogt had done so earlier (1905) resulting in the term '**Spielmayer-Vogt disease**'. *4714.1, 4713.1*

1907:26 **Dystonia musculorum deformans (torsion spasm)** first described by Marcus Walter Schwalbe (b.1883); in his inaugural dissertation, *Eine eigentümliche tonische Krampfform mit hysterischen Symptomen*. *4716*

1907:27 '**Whipple's disease**', which he termed **intestinal lipodystrophy**, first described by George Hoyt Whipple (1878–1976), *JHB* **18**:382. *3782*

1907:28 '**Hutchison's tumour**', **adrenal sarcoma** in children, described by Robert Hutchison (1871–1960), *QJM* **1**:33. *3868*

1907:29 The account of **acquired haemolytic anaemia** by Georges Fernand Isidor Widal (1862–1929) and Pierre Abrami (1879–1945), *PrM* **15**:479, led to the eponym '**Widal-Abrami disease**' and, because of the earlier description by Hayem (1898), '**Hayem-Widal disease**'. *3777, 3783*

1907:30 A description of the **Ferguson operation** for **hernia** appeared in Alexander Hugh Ferguson's (1853–1912) *Technic of modern operations for hernia*. *3608.1*

1907:31 Therapeutic **bronchoscopy** for the treatment of **asthma** introduced by Franz Nowotny (1872–1925), *MonO* **41**:679. *3186*

1907:32 First case of complete **agranulocytosis** reported by Wilhelm Türk (1871–1916), *ZBP* I, **46**:595. *3079*

1907:33 Account of **multiple hereditary telangiectasis ('Rendu-Osler-Weber disease')** by Frederick Parkes Weber (1863–1962), *L* **2**:160. *2714*

1907:34 **Tuberculosis; Pirquet's cutaneous reaction test** for diagnosis introduced by Clemens Peter Pirquet von Cesenatico (1874–1929), *WKW* **20**:1123. *2338*

1907:35 **Tuberculosis; Calmette's conjunctival reaction test** for diagnosis devised by Léon Charles Albert Calmette (1863–1933), *CRAS* **144**:1324. *2337*

1907:36 Term **allergy** first suggested by Clemens Peter Pirquet (1874–1929); in his *Klinische Studien über Vakzination und vakzinale Allergie. 2598*

1907:37 **Anti-anaphylaxis** produced by Alexander Besredka (1870–1940) and Edna Steinhardt, *AnIP* **21**:117, 384. *2596*

1907:38 **Passive anaphylaxis** demonstrated by Maurice Nicolle (1862–1932), *AnIP* **21**:128. *2597*

1907:39 First case of **asbestosis** reported by Hubert Montague Murray (1855–1907); in *Report of Departmental Committee on Compensation for Industrial Diseases*, Col. 3495–6. *2130*

1907:40 Synthesis of **histamine** by Adolf Otto Reinhold Windaus (1876–1959) and Karl Vogt (b.1880), *BDCG* **40**:3691. *1895.1*

1907:41 **Phonocardiography** introduced by Willem Einthoven (1860–1927), *PfA* **117**:461. *846*

1907:42 The concept of the **inferiority complex** introduced by Alfred Adler (1870–1937); in his *Studie über Minderwertigkeit von Organen. 4984*

1907:43 '**Lane's plates and screws**' for the union of **fractures** described by William Arbuthnot Lane (1856–1943), *BMJ* **1**:1037. *4430*

1907:44 The **Steinmann nail** or **pin** for use in the union of **fractures** introduced by Fritz Steinmann (1872–1932), *ZCh* **34**:938. *4431*

1907:45 **Poikiloderma vascularis atrophicans** first described by Eduard Jacobi (1862–1915), *VDDG* **9**:321. *4141*

1907:46 Experimental **scurvy** produced in guinea-pigs by Axel Holst (1860–1931), *JHyg* **7**:619. *3721*

1907:47 **Familial haemolytic jaundice** ('**Minkowski-Chauffard disease**') described by Anatole Marie Emile Chauffard (1855–1932), *SMP* **27**:25; it had already been described by Minkowski in 1900. *3781, 3779*

1907:48 Joseph Edwin **Smadel**, American microbiologist, born 10 Jan; with Elizabeth B. Jackson, introduced chloramphenicol in the treatment of typhus, 1947, *Science* **106**:418. Died 1963. *5402*

1907:49 Alexander **Haddow**, British pathologist and oncologist, born 18 Jan; with co-workers, achieved regression of mammary cancer with oestrogen administration, 1944, *BMJ* **2**:393. With Geoffrey Milward Timmis, introduced treatment of chronic myeloid leukaemia with myleran, 1953, *L* **1**:207. Died 1976. *2659.3, 3108.4*

1907:50 Hans **Selye**, Austrian/Canadian physician, born 26 Jan; developed the idea that the 'general adaptation syndrome' is a reaction to stress or injury, *The physiology and pathology of exposure to stress*, 1950. Died 1982. *2238*

1907:51 William Eugene **Deacon**, American microbiologist, born 5 Feb; with co-workers, introduced fluorescent treponemal antibody test in syphilis, 1957, *PSEB* **96**:477. *2419.2*

1907:52 Herald Rea **Cox**, American virologist, born 28 Feb; with E. John Bell, introduced a typhus vaccine, 1940, *USPHR* **55**:110. *5398.1*

1907:53 Alexander Solomon **Wiener**, American immunologist, born 16 Mar; with Karl Landsteiner, recognized Rh antigen, 1940, *PSEB* **43**:223. Devised conglutination test for rhesus sensitization, 1945, *JLCM* **30**:662. Died 1976. *912.2, 3105*

1907:54 Daniel **Bovet**, Swiss pharmacologist, born 23 Mar; with the Tréfouëls and other co-workers discovered the therapeutic value of sulphanilamide, 1935, *CRSB* **120**:756. With Anne-Marie Staub, described antihistamine structure and action, 1937, *CRSB* **124**:547. With co-workers, introduced gallamine triethiodide (flaxedil) into anaesthesia, 1946, *CRAS* **223**:597; with co-workers, introduced succinylcholine chloride, an anaesthetic, 1949, *RISS* **12**:106. Awarded the Nobel Prize (Physiology or Medicine), 1957, for his discoveries in chemotherapy, *NPL*. Died 1992. *1950, 1925, 5725, 5728*

1907:55 Francis Curtis **Dohan**, American endocrinologist, born 24 Mar; with Francis Dring Wetherill Lukens, produced experimental diabetes by artificially-induced hyperglycaemia, 1948, *En* **42**:244. *3977*

1907:56 Peter Alfred **Gorer**, British immunologist, born 14 Apr; discovered antigen II and established transplantation immunology laws, 1937, *JPB* **44**:691; **47**:231. Died 1961. *2576.5*

1907:57 Nikolaas **Tinbergen**, Dutch zoologist, born 15 Apr; shared Nobel Prize (Physiology or Medicine), 1973, with Karl von Frisch and Konrad Lorenz, for their discoveries concerning organization and elicitation of individual and social behaviour patterns, *NPL*.

1907:58 Georges **Wakim**, Lebanese/American physiologist, born 17 Jun; introduced microwave radiation therapy, 1949, *JAMA* **139**:989. *2010.5*

1907:59 Robert Gwyn **Macfarlane**, British physician, born 26 Jun; with Burgess Barnett, introduced snake venom in the treatment of haemophilia, 1934, *L* **2**:985. Died 1987. *3093*

1907:60 David **Cowen**, American neuropathologist, born 29 Jul; with Abner Wolf, first recognized toxoplasmosis in humans, 1937, *BNI* **6**:306. *5544.1*

1907:61 Walter Frederick **Kvale**, American physician, born 30 Jul; with Grace M. Roth, introduced the Roth-Kvale histamine test for the diagnosis of phaeochromocytoma, 1945, *AmJMS* **210**:653. *3869*

1907:62 Mary Candace **Pangborn**, American biochemist, born 13 Aug; used cardiolipin antigen for serological diagnosis of syphilis, 1941, *PSEB* **48**:484. *2417*

1907:63 Benjamin Frank **Miller**, American physician, born 10 Sep; with Alf Sven Alving; introduced the inulin clearance test for the measurement of the glomerular filtration rate, 1940, *ArIM* **66**:306. *4251*

1907:64 Edwin Mattison **McMillan**, American physicist, born 18 Sep; introduced synchrotron, 1945, *PsR* **68**:143. *2659.4*

1907:65 Harry **Most**, American physician, born 18 Sep; with co-workers, undertook clinical trials of chloroquine in the treatment of malaria, 1946, *JAMA* **131**:963. *5261.1*

1907:66 Jerome W. **Conn**, American physician, born 24 Sep; first to record primary aldosteronism ('Conn's syndrome'), 1955, *JLCM* **45**:661. *3877.1*

1907:67 Alexander Robertus **Todd**, British chemist, born 2 Oct; isolated ß-tocopherol, vitamin E, 1937, *BJ* **31**:2557; awarded Nobel Prize (Chemistry), 1957, for his work on nucleotides and nucleotide co-enzymes, *NPL*.

1907:68 Richard Owen **Roblin**, American chemist, born 11 Dec; with co-workers, synthesized sulphamerazine, 1940, *JACS* **62**:2002. *1955*

1907:69 John **Ehrlich**, American biologist, born 13 Dec; with co-workers, produced chloramphenicol (chloromycetin), 1947, *Science* **106**:417. *1938*

1907:70 William Randolph **Lovelace**, American surgeon and aerospace physician, born 30 Dec; devised BLB (Boothby-Lovelace-Bulbulian) oxygen inhalation apparatus, 1938, *PMC* **13**:646, 654. Died 1965. *1981, 1982*

1907:71 Kendall Brooks **Corbin**, American physician, born 31 Dec; introduced Artane in the treatment of Parkinson's disease, 1949, *JAMA* **141**:377. *4729*

———

1907:72 Gunnar **Ågren**, Swedish biochemist, born; prepared crystalline secretin, 1930, *SkAP* **70**:10. *1039*

1907:73 John **Bunyan**, British naval surgeon, born; introduced the envelope ('Bunyan bag') method of treating burns, 1940, *PRSM* **34**:65. Died 1983. *2260*

1907:74 Thomas Frank **Davey**, British leprologist, born; with Gordon Currie, introduced diphenylthiourea (thiambutosine) in treatment of leprosy, 1956, *LR* **27**:94; with L.M. Hogerzeil, used ditophal (Etisul), 1959, *LR* **30**:61. Died 1983. *2442.2, 2442.3*

1907:75 J. Walter **Landsberg**, American haematologist, born; with Maxwell Myer Wintrobe, introduced a method for determination of erythrocyte sedimentation rate, 1935, *AmJMS* **189**:102. *3096*

1907:76 Sigvald **Refsum**, Norwegian psychiatrist, born; first to describe 'Refsum's syndrome', an inherited disorder of lipid metabolism, 1946, *AcPsS* Sup. 38. Died 1991. *3924.2*

1907:77 Lazar **Remen**, German neurologist, born; introduced the use of neostigmine in the treatment of myasthenia gravis, 1932, *DZN* **128**:66. *4767*

1907:78 Jean **Delay**, French psychiatrist, born; with Pierre Deniker, introduced chlorpromazine in the treatment of psychosis; in *C.R. Congr.Alien. et Neurol. de Langue Franç.*, 1952. *4962.3*

1907:79 Andrew **Yeomans**, US naval medical officer, born; with co-workers, introduced para-aminobenzoic acid in the treatment of scrub typhus, 1944, *JAMA* **126**:349. *5398.3*

---

1907: Charles Edward **Beevor** died, **born** 1854. *localization of cerebral function*

1907: Hubert Montague **Murray** died, **born** 1855. *asbestosis*

1907: David **Lowson** died, **born** 1850. *pulmonary tuberculosis*

1907: Julius **Dreschfeld** died, **born** 1846. *lymphosarcoma, lymphadenoma*

1907: Willoughby Dayton **Miller** died **born** 1854. *oral bacteria*

1907: Paul Julius **Möbius** died, **born** 1853. *migraine*

1907: Archibald Baring **Garrod** died, **born** 1819. *gout, arthritis, cystinuria*

1907: Albert von **Mosetig-Moorhof** died, **born** 1838. *bone defects, iodoform*

1907: Edward Hallaran **Bennett** died, **born** 1837. *metacarpal fracture*

1907: James **Carroll** died, **born** 1854. *yellow fever, mosquito*

1907: Louis Emile **Javal** died, **born** 1839. *astigmometer, ophthalmometer*

1907: Eduard **Hitzig** died, **born** 1838. *functional localization in the cerebral cortex, motor area, psychiatry*

1907: Ernst von **Bergmann** died, **born** 1836. *asepsis, mastoidectomy*

1907: Eduard **Buchner** died, **born** 1860. *enzymes*

1907: Michael **Foster** died, **born** 1836. *physiology*

## 1908

1908:1 **Nobel Prize** (Physiology or Medicine): Paul Ehrlich (1854–1915) and Élie Metchnikoff (1845–1916), for work on **immunity**, *NPL. 2555, 2559*

1908:2 **Peking Union Medical College** founded by **Rockefeller Institute**

1908:3 **University of the Philippines** founded (**College of Medicine**, 1910)

1908:4 **Royal Army Medical College**, Millbank, **London**, opened

1908:5 **Tropical Diseases Bureau, London**, founded

1908:6 **Asociacíon Española para el Progresso de las Ciencias** founded

1908:7 [**Psycho-Neurological Institute**], **St Petersburg** founded

1908:8 **Institut für Radiumforschung, Vienna**, founded

1908:9 **Deutsche Gesellschaft für Rassenhygiene** founded in **Berlin**

1908:10 *Archiv für Geschichte der Medizin* founded by Karl Friedrich Jakob Sudhoff (1853–1938), a distinguished **medical historian** whose main research was in ancient, medieval and Renaissance medicine; in 1929 renamed *Sudhoff's Archiv. 6666*

1908:11 **Tuberculosis; Wolff-Eisner conjunctival tuberculin reaction** introduced by Alfred Wolff-Eisner (1877–1948), *ZTb* **12**:21. *2340*

1908:12 **Retinitis circinata** ('**Coats' disease**') described by George Coats (1876–1915), *OHP* **17**:440. *5954*

1908:13 An operation for complete **prolapse** of the **uterus** introduced by Archibald Donald (1860–1937), *JOG* **13**:195. *6119*

1908:14 South American **blastomycosis** first described by Adolpho Lutz (1855–1940), *BrM* **22**:121, 141. *5532.1*

1908:15 The relationship of **phlebotomus fever** to the **sandfly**, *Phlebotomus*, shown by Robert Doerr (1871–1952), *BKW* **45**:1847. *5477*

1908:16 A vaccine prepared by the chemical (**carbolic acid**) treatment of suspensions of fixed **rabies** virus (**Fermi vaccine**) introduced by Claudio Fermi (b.1862), *ZHyg* **58**:233. *5484.1*

1908:17 The **stereotactic** apparatus devised by Victor Alexander Haden Horsley (1857–1916) and Robert Henry Clarke (1850–1926) for the accurate location of electrodes in the **brain** opened the way to **stereotactic surgery** of that organ, *Brain* **31**:45. *1435.1, 4879.1*

1908:18 A cutaneous reaction test (**Schick test**) for the determination of susceptibility to **diphtheria** introduced by Bela Schick (1877–1967), *MMW* **55**:504. *5065*

1908:19 The operation of **rhizotomy** for **spastic paralysis** devised by Otfrid Foerster (1873–1941), *ZOC* **22**:203. *4880*

1908:20 With Macewen, Cushing and Ballance, Fedor Krause (1857–1937) was a pioneer of **neurosurgery** as a speciality. His most comprehensive work is *Chirurgie des Gehirns und Rückenmarks*, 2 vols, 1908–11. *4880.2*

1908:21 Cases of **familial centrolobar sclerosis** (already noted by Pelizaeus (1885)) recorded by Ludwig Merzbacher (b.1875), *MK* **18**:161,310, leading to the term '**Pelizaeus-Merzbacher disease**'. *4715, 4703*

1908:22 *Salmonella paratyphi C* first described by Paul Theodor Uhlenhuth (1870–1957) and Erich August Hübener (b.1870), *ZBP* **42**:I, Beil.127. *5041*

1908:23 **Cinchophen** introduced in the treatment of **gout** by Arthur Nicolaier (b.1862) and Max Dohrn, *DAKM* **93**:331. *4505.1*

1908:24 The first **osteoarticular joint transplant** performed by Erich Lexer (1867–1937), *MK* **4**:817. *4377.1*

1908:25 **Rothera's test** for **acetone** bodies in **urine** introduced by Arthur Cecil Hamel Rothera (1880–1915), *JP* **37**:491. *3960*

1908:26 **Kidney transplanted** from one animal to another by Alexis Carrel (1873–1944), *JEM* **10**:98. *4235*

1908:27 **Desquamative erythroderma** of nurslings (Leiner) described by Karl Leiner (1871–1930). *4145*

1908:28 In his description of **cutis laxa** ('**Ehlers-Danlos syndrome**') Henri Alexandre Danlos (1844–1937) noted the subcutaneous tumours sometimes occurring in this condition, *BSFD* **19**:70. *4132, 4144*

1908:29 Georg Ludwig Zuelzer (1870–1949) isolated the **pancreatic extract** containing what is now known as **insulin**, *ZEP* **5**:307. *3961*

1908:30 **Pancreatic function test** introduced by Otto Loewi (1873–1961), *ArEP* **59**:83. *3644*

1908:31 '**Herter's infantilism**', from chronic intestinal infection, described by Christian Archibald Herter (1865–1910), in his *On infantilism from chronic intestinal infection*; identical to **Gee-Thaysen disease**. *3528*

1908:32 First important work on the **radiology** of the accessory **nasal sinuses**, *Die entzündlichen Nebenhöhlenerkrankungen der Nase im Röntgenbild*, published by Arthur Kuttner (b.1862). *3316*

1908:33 The operation of **abdomino-perineal resection** devised by William Ernest Miles (1869–1947), *L* **2**:1812. *3528.1*

1908:34 Treatment of **bronchiectasis** by **lobectomy** introduced by Werner Körte (1853–1937), *VBMG* **39**:5. *3187*

1908:35 Massive collapse of the **lung** was discovered and described by William Pasteur (1856–1943), *L* **2**:1351. *3188*

1908:36 **Transplantation** of **blood vessels** after storage demonstrated by Alexis Carrel (1875–1944), *JAMA* **51**:1662; *JEM* **12**:460. *3027, 3028*

1908:37 **Thrombo-angiitis obliterans** so named by Leo Buerger (1879–1943), *AJMS* **136**:567, and later termed '**Buerger's disease**' *2912*

1908:38 First radical **thoracoplasty** for **pulmonary tuberculosis** by Ludolph Brauer (1865–1951), *PVC* **21**:569. *3231*

1908:39 Familial **icterus gravis neonatorum**, first detailed description by Hermann Johann Pfannenstiel (1862–1909), *MMW* **55**:2169, 2223. *3080.1*

1908:40 **Bone marrow biopsy** (puncture of shaft of tibia) introduced by Giovanna Ghedini (b.1877), *CMI* **47**:724. *3080*

1908:41 **Tuberculosis; Mantoux intradermal tuberculin test** introduced by Charles Mantoux (1877–1947), *CRAS* **147**:355. *2341*

1908:42 **Tuberculosis; Moro's percutaneous tuberculin reaction** for diagnosis introduced by Ernst Moro (1874–1951), *MMW* **55**:216, 2025. *2339*

1908:43 **Sulphanilamide** prepared by Paul Gelmo (1879–1961), *JPrC* **77**:369. *1948*

1908:44 '**Brodmann's area**' in the cerebral cortex defined by Korbinian Brodmann (1868–1918), *JPN* **10**:231. *1434*

1908:45 The cyclical changes in the **endometrium** were first definitely described by Fritz Hitschmann (1870–1926) and Ludwig Adler (1876–1958), and shown to be a normal physiological process, *MonG* **27**:1. *1181*

---

1908:46 William Kendrick **Hare**, American paediatrician, born 6 Jan; in association with Allen Dudley Keller, located the heat-regulating mechanism in the hypothalamus, 1932, *PSEB* **29**:1069. *1446.3*

1908:47 Albert **Gilman**, American pharmacologist, born 5 Feb; with Frederick Stanley Philips, introduced nitrogen mustard in the treatment of Hodgkin's disease, 1946, *Science* **103**:409. *3788*

1908:48 Max Leonard **Rosenheim**, British physician, born 15 Mar; introduced mandelic acid in the treatment of urinary infections, 1935, *L* **1**:1032. Died 1972. *4202*

1908:49 Frank George **Young**, British biochemist, born 25 Mar; produced permanent experimental diabetes by anterior pituitary injections (anterior pituitary diabetogenic hormone), 1937, *L* **2**:372. Died 1988. *1173, 3976*

1908:50 Ernst Trier **Morch**, Danish/American surgeon, born 14 May; established the fact that chondrodystrophy may be inherited; in his *Chondrodystrophic dwarfism in Denmark*, 1941. *4404*

1908:51 Robert Bews **Kerr**, Canadian physician, born 30 Aug; with co-workers combined zinc with insulin, and later also with protamine, to form protamine zinc insulin, to delay the absorption rate, 1936, *CMAJ* **34**:400. *3975*

1908:52 Min Chueh **Chang**, Chinese/American biologist, born 10 Oct; with Gregory Goodwin Pincus, demonstrated an oral contraceptive (progesterone) in the rabbit, 1953, *AcPL* **3**:177. *1931.2*

1908:53 Robley Cook **Williams**, American biophysicist, born 13 Oct; with Heinz Ludwig Fraenkel-Conrat reconstituted active tobacco mosaic virus, 1955, *PNAS* **41**:690. *2527*

1908:54 Alfred Day **Hershey**, American biologist, born 4 Dec; with M.C. Chase showed DNA to be the carrier of genetic information in virus reproduction, 1952, *JGP* **36**:39. Shared Nobel Prize (Physiology or Medicine), 1969, with Max Delbrück, for work on replication mechanisms and genetic structure of viruses, *NPL*. *256*

1908:55 Ogden Carr **Bruton**, American paediatrician, born; first reported agammaglobulinaemia, 1952, *Ped* **9**:722. *2578.9*

1908:56 Alexander John Balmanno **Squire** died; introduced chrysarobin in dermatology; in his *On the treatment of psoriasis by an ointment of chrysophanic acid*, 1878. *4075.1*

1908: Nicholas **Senn** died, **born** 1844. *intestinal perforation, rectal insufflation, pancreas removal*

1908: Oscar **Liebreich** died, **born** 1839. *chloral hydrate*

1908: Johann Friedrich August von **Esmarch** died, **born** 1823. *first-aid bandage*

1908: Henry Robert **Silvester** died, **born** 1828. *artificial respiration*

1908: Harold Leslie **Barnard** died, **born** 1866. *sphygmomanometer*

1908: Antoine Henri **Becquerel** died, **born** 1852. *radioactivity*

1908: Georg Eduard **Rindfleisch** died, **born** 1836. *pernicious anaemia*

1908: Thomas **Annandale** died, **born** 1838. *intestinal obstruction, gastrotomy*

1908: Friedrich **Bezold** died, **born** 1842. *mastoiditis*

1908: Joseph von **Mering** died, **born** 1849. *diabetes mellitus, pancreas, barbitone*

1908: George Michael **Edebohls** died, **born** 1853. *nephropexy, nephritis*

1908: Thomas **Annandale** died, **born** 1838. *knee-joint cartilage*

1908: Charles **Chamberland** died, **born** 1851. *anthrax immunization, rabies, bacterial filtration*

1908: Leonardo **Gigli** died, **born** 1863. *craniotomy, pubiotomy, Gigli saw*

1908: Victor **Galtier** died, **born** 1845. *rabies*

1908: George **Lawson** died, **born** 1831. *skin grafts*

1908: Henry Richard Lobb **Veale** died, **born** 1832. *rubella*

1908: Paul **Berger** died, **born** 1845. *surgery, face mask, interscapulothoracic amputation*

1908: Herman **Snellen** died, **born** 1834. *sight test types*

1908: Franz **Leydig** died, **born** 1821. *Leydig cells*

1908: Carl von **Voit** died, **born** 1831. *nutrition, metabolism*

**1909**
1909:1 **Nobel Prize** (Physiology or Medicine): Emil Theodor Kocher (1841–1917), for his pioneer work on **thyroidectomy**, *NPL. 3826*

1909:2 **University of Neuchâtel** founded

1909:3 **Society of Medical History, Chicago**

1909:4 **University College (National University of Ireland), Dublin**

1909:5 The experimental work of Samuel James Meltzer (1851–1920) and John Auer (1875–1948) on **intratracheal insufflation anaesthetization** led to modern **endotracheal anaesthesia**, *JEM* **11**:622. *5694*

1909:6 An extraperitoneal lower-segment **caesarean section** described by Wilhelm Latzko (1863–1945), *WKW* **22**:477. *6249*

1909:7 The operation of **sclero-corneal trephining** for **glaucoma** introduced by Robert Henry Elliot (1864–1927), *Oph* **7**:804. *5955*

1909:8 Treatment of **micrognathia** or **prognathism** by closed ramisection of the mandible introduced by Vilray Papin Blair (1871–1955), *JAMA* **53**:178. *5756.2*

1909:9 The **inclusion bodies** in **ophthalmia neonatorum** demonstrated by Karl Bruno Stargardt (1875–1927), *GAO* **69**:525. *5956*

1909:10 One of the first to observe *Bartonella bacilliformis*, causal organism of **bartonellosis** (**Oroya fever**, **verruga peruana**), was A.L. Barton, *CrM* **26:7**. *5533*

1909:11 The sanitation methods employed by William Crawford Gorgas (1854–1920) against **yellow fever** in Havana were so successful that in three months the disease was practically eradicated, *JAMA* **52**:1075. *5460*

1909:12 American mucocutaneous **leishmaniasis** first described by Adolpho Carlos Lindenberg (1872–1944), *BSPE* **2**:252. *5299.1*

1909:13 Treatment of **athetosis** by removal of precentral area of the brain demonstrated by Victor Alexander Haden Horsley (1857–1916), *BMJ* **2**:125. *4882*

1909:14 An operation for **tabes** devised by Fedor Krause (1857–1937) and Hermann Küttner (1870–1932), *BKC* **63**:245. *4881*

1909:15 Infantile **kala-azar** considered by Charles Jules Henri Nicolle (1866–1936) to be due to a distinct species of *Leishmania*, *L.infantum*, *AnIP* **23**:361, 441. *5300*

1909:16 A diagnostic reaction for **cerebrospinal** and **typhus fevers** described by William James Wilson (1879–1954), later developed as the **Weil-Felix reaction**, *JHyg* **9**:316. *5381, 5390*

1909:17 The causal organism of **Rocky Mountain spotted** fever described, in blood smears, by Howard Taylor Ricketts (1871–1910), *JAMA* **52**:379. *5379*

1909:18 It was shown by Friedrich Karl Kleine (1869–1950) that the African **trypanosome** undergoes a developmental cycle in the **tsetse fly**, *Glossina*, *DMW* **35**:469. *5283.1*

1909:19 The causal organism of American **trypanosomiasis** ('**Chagas's disease**') discovered by Carlos Ribeiro Justiniano Chagas (1879–1934) at the Instituto Oswaldo Cruz and named *Trypanosoma cruzi*, *MIOC* **1**:159. *5283*

1909:20 First transmission of **poliomyelitis** to monkeys by Karl Landsteiner (1868–1943) and Erwin Popper, *ZI* **2**,1:379. *4669*

1909:21 The **Kirschner wire**, for **skeletal traction** and **stabilization of bone fragments** or **joint immobilization**, introduced by Martin Kirschner (1879–1942), *BKC* **64**:266. *4378*

1909:22 **Orchiopexy** for the treatment of **undescended testis** introduced by Franz Torek (1861–1938), *NYMJ* **90**:948. *4196*

1909:23 The **Brown-Buerger cystoscope** introduced by Leo Buerger (1879–1943), *AnS* **49**:225. *4195.1*

1909:24 **Uveoparotid fever** ('**Heerfordt's disease**'), a form of **sarcoidosis**, described by Christian Frederik Heerfordt (1872–1953). *4145.1*

1909:25 A classic description of **inherited conditions** caused by a particular block in a **metabolic pathway** given by Archibald Edward Garrod (1857–1936); in his *Inborn errors of metabolism*. *244.1, 3921*

1909:26 Blunt dissection **tonsillectomy** introduced by George Ernest Waugh (1876–1940), *L* **1**:1314. *3317*

1909:27 Chronic **constipation** treated by William Arbuthnot Lane (1856–1943) by short-circuiting the intestine; in his *The operative treatment of chronic constipation*. *3531*

1909:28 William George MacCallum (1874–1944) and Carl Voegtlin (1879–1960) proved that **calcium metabolism** is controlled by the **parathyroid glands**, *JEM* **11**:118. *3859*

1909:29 **Syphilis: salvarsan ('606')**, specific in treatment of syphilis and **yaws,** introduced by Paul Ehrlich (1854–1915) and Sahachiro Hata (1873–1938), *Die experimentelle Chemotherapie der Spirillosen* ..., published 1910; in 1912 Ehrlich replaced this with neosalvarsan (neoarsphenamine). *2403*

1909:30 **Auricular fibrillation** established as a cause of **perpetual arrhythmia** by Thomas Lewis (1881–1945) and independently by Carl Julius Rothberger (b.1871) and Heinrich Winterberg (1867–1929), *BMJ* **2**:1528; *WKW* **22**:839. *2830, 2831*

1909:31 First definite clinical description of **subacute bacterial endocarditis** by William Osler (1849–1919), *QJM* **2**:219, in which he described '**Osler's nodes**', first seen by him in 1888. *2827*

1909:32 **Diathermy** introduced by Karl Franz Nagelschmidt (1875–1952), *MMW* **56**:2575. *2007*

1909:33 **Localization of cerebral function**, comprehensive account by Korbinian Brodmann in his *Vergleichende Lokalisationslehre der Grosshirnrinde*. *1435*

---

1909:34 Charles **Curnen**, American physician, born 5 Jan; with co-workers, isolated Coxsackie virus from patients with poliomyelitis, 1949, *JAMA* **141**:894. *5546*

1909:35 George Keble **Hirst**, American virologist born 2 Mar; discovered virus haemagglutination, 1941, *Science* **94**:22, independently of Laurella McClelland and Ronald Hare. *2577*

1909:36 Alan **Kekwick**, British physician, born 12 Apr; with Hugh Leslie Marriott, introduced the slow-drip method of blood transfusion, 1935, *L* **1**:977. Died 1974. *2023*

1909:37 Rita **Levi-Montalcini**, Italian/American neurobiologist, born 22 Apr; shared Nobel Prize (Physiology or Medicine), 1986, with Stanley Cohen, for discovery of growth factors, *NPL*.

1909:38 James Myrlin **McGuire**, American microbiologist, born 12 May; discovered erythromycin, 1952, *AC* **2**:281. *1946*

1909:39 Charles Herbert **Stuart-Harris**, British physician, born 12 Jul; with Wilson Smith, reported first successful passage of influenza from animal to man, 1936, *L* **2**:121. Died 1996. *5497*

1909:40 Vittorio **Erspamer**, Italian pharmacologist, born 30 Jul; with Maffo Vialli, isolated 5-hydroxytryptamine, 1933, *ZZ* **19**:743, named serotonin by M. Rapport et al. (1948). *1924.2*

1909:41 Rose Marise **Payne**, American haematologist/immunologist, born 5 Aug; introduced leucocyte typing, 1957, *ArIM* **99**:587. *2578.23*

1909:42 Charles Stuart **Welch**, American surgeon, born 4 Oct; carried out auxiliary whole liver transplantation in dogs, 1955, *TrB* **6**:103. *3666.1*

1909:43 Edward Lawrie **Tatum**, American biochemist, born 14 Dec; shared the Nobel Prize (Physiology or Medicine), 1958, with Joshua Lederberg and George Wells Beadle, for his research on the mechanism by which the chromosomes in the cell nucleus transmit inherited characters, 1941, *PNAS* **27**:499; 1946, *Nature* **158**:558, *NPL*. Died 1975. *254.3, 255.4*

1909:44 Edwin Bennett **Astwood**, American physician, born 29 Dec; treated hyperthyroidism with thiourea and thiouracil, 1943, *JAMA* **122**:78, and with thiobarbital, 1945, *JCE* **5**:345. Died 1976. *3854, 3855*

---

1909:45 Robert Louis **Judet**, French orthopaedic surgeon, born; with Jean Udet, introduced the use of acrylic prostheses for hip arthroplasty, 1950, *JBJS* **32B**:166. *4405*

1909:46 Hans **Franke**, German physician, born; with J. Fuchs, introduced carbutamide, the first sulphonylurea, in the treatment of diabetes mellitus, 1955, *DMW* **80**:1449. Died 1955. *3978.1*

1909:47 John Arthur **Evans**, American radiologist, introduced nephrotomography, 1954, *AmJR* **71**:213. *4256.2*

1909:48 Iwao **Yasuda** born; first demonstrated electrically-induced osteogenesis, 1953, *JKMS* **4**:395. *4435.4*

1909:49 Colin Munro **Macleod**, American bacteriologist, born; with Oswald Theodor Avery and Maclyn McCarty, demonstrated that deoxyribonucleic acid (DNA) is the basic material responsible for genetic transformation, 1944, *JEM* **79**:137. *255.3*

---

1909:  Ivan Romanovich **Tarchanoff** died, **born** 1848. *psychogalvanic reflex*

1909:  Louis Charles **Malassez** died, **born** 1842. *haemocytometer*

1909:  Hermann Johann **Pfannenstiel** died, **born** 1862. *gynaecology, icterus gravis neonatorum*

1909:  Ernest **Besnier** died, **born** 1831. *prurigo, sarcoidosis*

1909:  Douglas Moray Cooper Lamb **Argyll** died, **born** 1837. *Argyll Robertson pupil, loaiasis*

1909:  Désiré Magloire **Bourneville** died, **born** 1840. *tuberose sclerosis*

1909:  Stephen **Mackenzie** died, **born** 1844. *Mackenzie's syndrome*

1909:  Otto **Bollinger** died, **born** 1843. *actinomycosis*

1909:  Edwin Theodor **Saemisch** died, **born** 1833. *ophthalmology, corneal ulcer, conjunctivitis*

1909:  Ludwig **Laqueur** died, **born** 1839. *glaucoma, physostigmine*

1909:  Thomas **Smith** died, **born** 1865. *craniohypophyseal xanthomatosis*

1909:  Johann Hermann **Baas** died, **born** 1838. *history of medicine*

1909:  Cesare **Lombroso** died, **born** 1836. *pellagra, criminal type*

## 1910
1910:1 **Nobel Prize** (Physiology or Medicine): Karl Martin Leonhard Albrecht Kossel (1853–1927), for work on the chemistry of the **cell** and **cell nucleus**, *NPL*. *702*

1910:2 **Statens Seruminstitut, Copenhagen**, founded

1910:3 [**Austrian Society for Investigation and Prevention of Cancer**] founded

1910:4 **National Committee for Preventing Blindness, US**, organized

1910:5 **Association Internationale des Médecins Scolaires** founded

1910:6 **Institut Pasteur, Algiers** founded

1910:7 An operation for the correction of protruding **ears** developed by William Henry Luckett (1872–1929), *SGO* **10**:635. *5756.4*

1910:8 The **anaphylactic** theory of the pathogenesis of **sympathetic ophthalmia** suggested by Anton Elschnig (1863–1939), *GAO* **75**:459. *5957*

1910:9 A small flap **sclerotomy** for **glaucoma** introduced by Herbert Herbert (1865–1942), *TOUK* **30**:199. *5958*

1910:10 William Blair Bell (1871–1936), who wrote *The principles of gynaecology*, was an outstanding figure in the history of British **gynaecology**. He was a founder of the Royal College of Obstetricians and Gynaecologists (1929). *6121*

1910:11 Meltzer and Auer's method of **intratracheal insufflation anaesthetization** (1909) introduced clinically by Charles Albert Elsberg (1871–1948), *BKW* **47**:957. *5695, 5694*

1910:12 **Roseola infantum (roseola subitum)** first described by John Zahorsky (b.1871), *Ped* **22**:60. *5506*

1910:13 A new species of **trypanosome**, *Trypanosoma rhodesiense*, discovered by John William Watson Stephens (1865–1946) and Harold Benjamin Fantham (1876–1937), *PRS* **83**:28. *5285*

1910:14 Demonstration of the transmission of **typhus** by the body **louse**, *Pediculus corporis*, and production of the disease in monkeys and guinea-pigs by the injection of infected blood, by Charles Jules Henri Nicolle (1866–1936), *AnIP* **24**:243; **25**:97; **26**:250, 332. *5384*

1910:15 A form of tick-borne **typhus** found in Tunisia first described as **fièvre boutonneuse** by Alfred Leon Joseph Conor (1870–1914) and A. Bruch, *BSPE* **3**:492. *5383*

1910:16 **Rocky Mountain spotted** fever differentiated from **typhus** by Howard Taylor Ricketts (1871–1910) and Russell Morse Wilder (1885–1952), *ArIM* **5**:361. *5380*

1910:17 'Brill's disease', recrudescent **typhus**, first described by Nathan Edwin Brill (1860–1925), *AmJMS* **139**:484. *5382*

1910:18 'Kienböck's disease', slowly progressive **osteonecrosis** of the lunate bone of the **wrist, carpal lunate malacia**, was first described by Robert Kienböck (1871–1953), *FGR* **16**:103. *4379*

1910:19 Demonstration of **antibodies** in convalescent serum in monkeys infected experimentally with **poliomyelitis** by Simon Flexner (1863–1946) and Paul A. Lewis (1879–1929), *JAMA* **54**:1780. *4670*

1910:20 The first accurate cell counts of the **cerebrospinal fluid** in **poliomyelitis** made by Frederick Parker Gay (1874–1939) and William Palmer Lucas (1880–1960), *ArIM* **6**:330. *4670.1*

1910:21 Arnold Netter (1855–1936) and Constantin Levaditi (1874–1953) discovered **antibodies** in human **poliomyelitis** convalescent serum, *CRSB* **68**:855. In the same year Levaditi and Karl Landsteiner (1868–1943) mixed serum from a monkey that had recovered from experimental **poliomyelitis** with a mixture containing active virus; it failed to produce paralytic disease when injected into fresh monkeys, *CRSB* **68**:311. *4670.2, 4670.3*

1910:22 Juvenile **osteochondritis deformans**, first mentioned by H. Waldenström in 1909, described independently by Arthur Thornton Legg (1874–1939), *BMSJ* **162**:202, Jacques Calvé (1875–1954), *RC* **42**:54, and by Georg Clemens Perthes (1869–1927), *DZC* **107**:111, and given the name 'Calvé-Legg-Perthes disease'. *4380, 4381, 4382*

1910:23 The **phenolsulphonephthalein kidney function test** introduced by Leonard George Rowntree (1883–1959) and John Timothy Geraghty (1876–1924), *JPET* **1**:579. *4236*

1910:24 **Urethrography** for the diagnosis of **urethral stricture** introduced by John Henry Cunningham (b.1877), *TAAGS* **5**:369. *4196.1*

1910:25 Method of **transurethral fulguration** of **bladder tumours** introduced by Edwin Beer (1876–1938), *JAMA* **54**:1768, led to the operation of **transurethral prostatectomy**. *4268*

1910:26 **Wohlgemuth's pancreatic function test** introduced by Julius Wohlgemuth (1874–1948), *BKW* **47**:92. *3646*

1910:27 Experimental demonstration that **hypophysectomy** causes **genital atrophy** by Samuel James Crowe (1883–1955), Harvey Williams Cushing (1869–1939) and John Homans (1877–1955), *JHB* **21**:127. *3894*

1910:28 Reverse guillotine **tonsillectomy** introduced by Samuel Short Whillis (1870–1953) and Frederick Charles Pybus (1882–1975), *L* **2**:875. *3318*

1910:29 Test for simulated unilateral **deafness** devised by Etienne Lombard (b.1869), *BAM* **64**:127. *3402.1*

1910:30 Knowledge concerning **duodenal ulcer** greatly advanced by Berkeley George Andrew Moynihan (1865–1936); in his *Duodenal ulcer*. *3535*

1910:31 Radical operation for **carcinoma** of the **rectum** introduced by William James Mayo (1861–1939), *AnS* **51**:854. *3534*

1910:32 Donald Church Balfour (1882–1963) introduced his method of resection of the **sigmoid colon**, *AnS* **51**:239. *3532*

1910:33 A method of **extrapleural pneumolysis** introduced by Theodore Tuffier (1857–1929), *BSCP* **36**:529. *3191*

1910:34 New **anti-pneumococcus** serum introduced by Fred Neufeld (1861–1945) and Ludwig Haendel (1869–1939), *AKG* **34**:293. *3190*

1910:35 **Thoracoscopy** made possible when Hans Christian Jacobaeus (1879–1937) adapted the **cystoscope** for the study of the interior of the body, *MMW* **57**:2090. *3189*

1910:36 **Sickle-cell anaemia** identified by James Bryan Herrick (1861–1954), *ArIM* **6**:517. *3133*

1910:37 Demonstration of the transmissibility to normal hens of chicken **sarcoma** by Francis Peyton **Rous** (1879–1970), *JEM* **12**:696; **13**:397. *2637*

1910:38 **Tumour** tissue grown *in vitro* by Alexis Carrel (1873–1944) and Montrose Thomas Burrows (1884–1947), *CRSB* **69**:332. *2636*

1910:39 *Streptococcus viridans* isolated in **bacterial endocarditis** by Hugo Schottmüller (1867–1936), *MMW* **57**:617, 697. *2836*

1910:40 **Auricular flutter** first described by William Adam Jolly (1878–1939) and William Thomas Ritchie (1873–1945), *Heart* **2**:177; it had been recognized by Ritchie in 1906. *2833*, *2821*

1910:41 **Coronary thrombosis** first comprehensively described, diagnosed before death and confirmed at necroscopy by Vasili Parmenovich Obraztsov (1849–1920) and Nikolai Dmitrievich Strazhesko (1876–1952), *ZKM* **71**:116. *2835*

1910:42 **Bundle-branch block** described by Hans Eppinger (1879–1946) and Oscar Stoerck (1870–1926), *ZKM* **71**:157. *2832*

1910:43 **Bronchial asthma** attributed to **anaphylaxis** by Samuel James Meltzer (1851–1920), *JAMA* **55**:1021. *2600.1*

1910:44 Test for **anaphylaxis** devised by William Henry Schultz (1873–1947), *JPET* **1**:549; similar work by Henry Hallett Dale, 1913, led to the term '**Schultz-Dale test**'. *2600.2*

1910:45 **Anaphylactic shock** described by John Auer (1875–1948) and Paul A. Lewis (1879–1929), *JEM* **12**:151. *2600*

1910:46 **Histamine** discovered in ergot extract by George Barger (1878–1939) and Henry Hallett Dale (1875–1968), *JP* **41**:19. *1898*

1910:47 **Blood classified into four groups** by William Lorenzo Moss (1876–1957), *JHB*, **21**:63. (This had already been done by Janský, but his work, published in a Czech journal, was not at that time known to Moss.) *900*

1910:48 **Monakow's bundle**, the rubrospinal tract, described by Constantin von Monakow (1853–1930), *AHI* **3**:51; **4**:103. *1375*

1910:49 Abraham Flexner (1866–1959) prepared a highly critical report, *Medical education in the United States and Canada*, which led to important reforms in North America. *1766.502*

---

1910:50 Hugh Roland **Butt**, American physician, born 8 Jan; with Albert Markley Snell, used vitamin K in the treatment of haemorrhagic disease, 1938, *PMC* **13**:74. *3097*

1910:51 Jacques Lucien **Monod**, French biochemist, born 9 Feb; shared the Nobel Prize (Physiology or Medicine), 1965, with François Jacob and André Michael Lwoff, for their discovery of the genetic control of enzyme and virus synthesis, 1961, *JMB* **3**:318, *NPL*. Died 1976. *256.9*

1910:52 Archer John Porter **Martin**, British chemist, born 1 Mar; shared Nobel Prize (Chemistry), 1952, with Richard Laurence Millington Synge, for their invention of partition chromatography, *NPL*.

1910:53 Nathan Kenneth **Jensen**, American surgeon, born 3 Mar; with co-workers, introduced the sulphonamide dressing of wounds, 1939, *Surgery* **6**:1. *5645*

1910:54 Lloyd Joseph **Florio**, American public health physician, born Batavia, 9 Mar; with co-workers, isolated the virus of Colorado tick fever from *Dermacentor andersoni*, 1950, *JI* **64**:257. *5546.1*

1910:55 Matthew Charles **Dodd**, American bacteriologist, born 24 Mar; with William Barlow Stillman, introduced nitrofuran (nitrofurazone) as a bacteriostatic, 1944, *JPET* **82**:11. *1928.2*

1910:56 Murray **Sanders**, American biologist, born 11 Apr; with Claus W. Jungeblut, isolated the encephalomyocarditis virus, 1940, *JEM* **72**:407. With R.C. Alexander, reported the isolation and identification of a filterable virus in epidemic keratoconjunctivitis, 1943, *JEM* **77**:71. Died 1987. *4661.1, 5990*

1910:57 Dorothy Mary Crowfoot **Hodgkin**, British chemist, born 12 May; awarded Nobel Prize (Chemistry), 1964, for determining, by x ray crystallography, the structure of complex, biologically important, organic molecules, including insulin, *NPL*. Died 1994.

1910:58 Eric George Lapthorne **Bywaters**, British physician, born 1 Jun; with Desmond Beall, gave an authoritative account of the 'crush syndrome', with impairment of renal function found in victims of London air-raids of 1940–41, 1941, *BMJ* **1**:427. *4252*

1910:59 Dwight Emary **Harken**, American surgeon, born 5 Jun; with co-workers, introduced valvuloplasty for mitral stenosis, 1948, *NEJM* **239**:801. *3046.1*

1910:60 Desiderius Emerick **Szilagyi**, Hungarian/American surgeon, born 20 Jun; with co-workers, introduced a Dacron arterial prosthesis, 1958, *ArSu* **77**:538. *3047.12*

1910:61 Heinz Ludwig **Fraenkel-Conrat**, German/American molecular biologist, born 29 Jul; with Robley Cook Williams reconstituted active tobacco mosaic virus, 1955, *PNAS* **41**:690. *2527*

1910:62 Lowell Orlando **Randall**, American pharmacologist, born 11 Sep; with co-workers, introduced the psychosedative, librium, 1960, *JPET* **129**:163. *1931.3*

1910:63 Mauricio **Rocha e Silva**, Brazilian pharmacologist, born 19 Sep; with co-workers, discovered bradykinin, the hypotensive and smooth-muscle-stimulating factor, 1949, *AmJPh* **156**:261. *1930*

1910:64 Ian **Donald**, British obstetrician, born 27 Dec; with co-workers, used ultrasound scanner to investigate the pregnant uterus, 1958, *L* **1**:1188. With T.G. Brown, first reported biparietal fetal cephalometry by ultrasound, 1961, *BJR* **34**:539. Died 1987. *2682, 6235.1*

1910:65 John Essary **Dees** born; with John Archibald Campbell Colston, used sulphanilamide in the treatment of gonorrhoea, 1937, *JAMA* **108**:1855. *5214*

1910: Florence **Nightingale** died, **born** 1820. *hospitals, nursing*

1910: Jean Henri **Dunant** died, **born** 1828. *Red Cross*

1910: Angelo **Mosso** died, **born** 1846. *sphygmomanometer*

1910: Eduard Heinrich **Henoch** died, **born** 1820. *purpura*

1910: Emanuel **Zaufal** died, **born** 1833. *mastoid operation*

1910: Hermann Hugo Rudolf **Schwartze** died, **born** 1837. *mastoid operation*

1910: Christian Archibald **Herter** died, **born** 1865. *chronic intestinal infection, infantilism*

1910: Etienne **Lancereaux** died, **born** 1829. *diabetes mellitus, pancreatic lesions*

1910: Walter Butler **Cheadle** died, **born** 1836. *scurvy, rickets*

1910: Vittorio **Mibelli** died, **born** 1860. *porokeratosis, angiokeratoma*

1910: Joseph **Grünfeld** died, **born** 1840. *ureter, catheterization, endoscopy*

1910: Franz **König** died, **born** 1832. *osteochondritis dissecans*

1910: Friedrich Daniel von **Recklinghausen** died, **born** 1833. *neurofibromatosis, osteitis fibrosa*

1910: Howard Taylor **Ricketts** died, **born** 1871. *Rocky Mountain spotted fever, typhus*

1910: Ernst von **Leyden** died, **born** 1832. *myotonia congenita, ataxia*

1910: William **Rose** died, **born** 1847. *trigeminal neuralgia*

1910: William **James** died, **born** 1842. *experimental psychology*

1910: Edouard van **Beneden** died, **born** 1846. *mammalian ovum, centrosome*

1910: Robert **Koch** died, **born** 1843. *typhoid prophylaxis, Bacillus anthracis, cholera vibrio, antisepsis, sterilization, conjunctivitis, bacterial infection, tuberculin, tuberculosis, bacterial culturing and staining*

1910: Eduard Friedrich Wilhelm **Pflüger** died. *physiology*

1910: Elizabeth **Blackwell** died, **born** 1821. *medical education*

**1911**

1911:1 **Nobel Prize** (Physiology or Medicine): Allvar Gullstrand (1862–1930), for his investigations of the dioptrics of the **eye**, *NPL. 1525.2*

1911:2 **Nobel Prize** (Chemistry): Marie Sklodowska Curie (1867–1934), for her discovery of **radium** and **polonium** (the first time a scientist had received a second prize), *NPL. 2003*

1911:3 **Universities of Lisbon and Oporto** founded in **Portugal**

1911:4 **Kyushu Imperial University, Fukuoka**, founded

1911:5 **University of Iceland** founded at **Reykjavik**

1911:6 **Biochemical Society, London**, founded

1911:7 **National Society for Industrial Safety**, US, organized

1911:8 **International Society for Individual Psychology, Vienna**

1911:9 [**Kaiser Wilhelm Society for Advancement of Science**] founded in **Berlin**

1911:10 **National Insurance Act**, UK

1911:11 **X rays** first used for the **diagnosis** of **pregnancy** by Lars Edling (b.1878), *FGR* **17**:345. *6216*

1911:12 The first exact description of the chemical constitution of the **cerebrospinal fluid** given by William Mestrezat (1883–1928); in his *Le liquide céphalo-rachidien. 4596*

1911:13 **Measles** transmitted to monkeys by John F. Anderson (1873–1958) and Joseph Goldberger (1874–1929), *USPHR* **26**:847, 887. *5448*

1911:14 The modern technique of **uretero-intestinal anastomosis** followed experimental work by Robert Calvin Coffey (1869–1938), *JAMA* **56**:397. *4196.2*

1911:15 **Syphilis**: *Treponema pallidum* cultured by Hideyo Noguchi (1876–1928), *JEM* **14**:99. *2404*

1911:16 Edward Bright Vedder (1878–1952) demonstrated the amoebicidal action of **emetine**, *BMMS* **3**:48; his work led to its general adoption in the treatment of **amoebiasis**. *5189*

1911:17 An intermittent gas-oxygen machine for administration of **nitrous oxide-oxygen anaesthesia** introduced by Elmer Isaac McKesson (1881–1935), *SGO* **13**:456. *5697*

1911:18 **Trichloroethylene** as an **anaesthetic** introduced by Karl Bernhard Lehmann (1858–1940), *ArHyg* **74**:1. *5696*

1911:19 Carl Gustav Jung (1875–1961), originally a supporter of Freud, he broke away and founded the school of analytical **psychology**, published his *Wandlungen*, which later appeared in English translation as *Psychology of the unconscious*, 1912. *4985.2*

1911:20 A vacuum method of **cataract** extraction devised by Vard Houghton Hulen (1865–1939), *JAMA* **57**:188. *5959*

1911:21 The **Binet-Simon intelligence tests** devised by Alfred Binet (1857–1911) and Théodore Simon (1873–1961); in their *La mésure du developpement de l'intelligence chez les jeunes enfants*. Binet had published a plan for studying intelligence as early as 1895. *4985*

1911:22 The mode of reproduction of the **trypanosome** of American **trypanosomiasis**, *Trypanosoma cruzi*, demonstrated by Gaspar Oliviera de Vianna (1885–1914), *MIOC* **3**:276. *5285.1*

1911:23 **Tularaemia** first recorded (in rodents) by George Walter McCoy (1876–1952), *USPHB* **43**:53. *5173*

1911:24 A thermoprecipitin reaction for the diagnosis of **anthrax** introduced by Alberto Ascoli (1877–1957), *CV* **34**:2. *5171*

1911:25 The concept of **schizophrenia** introduced by Paul Eugen Bleuler (1857–1939), who showed, in his *Dementia praecox oder die Gruppe der Schizophrenien*, that **dementia praecox** should include all the schizophrenias. *4957*

1911:26 Rupert Waterhouse (1873–1958) described suprarenal apoplexy, *L* **1**:577, named **Waterhouse-Friderichsen syndrome** following the later account by Carl Friderichsen (1918). *4685, 4686*

1911:27 **Spinal fusion** in the treatment of **scoliosis** introduced by Russell Aubra Hibbs (1869–1932), *NYMJ* **93**:1013. *4383.1*

1911:28 Fred Houdlett Albee (1876–1945), a pioneer of living **bone-graft** surgery, used bone grafts as splints; he transplanted part of a tibia into the spine for Pott's disease, *JAMA* **57**:885. *4384.1*

1911:29 **Erythroplasia of Queyrat**, a condition similar to the precancerous dermatosis described by J.T. Bowen in 1912 (now considered to be variant of an intra-epidermal basal-cell **epithelioma**) described by Auguste Queyrat (b.1872). *4146, 4148*

1911:30 The operation of total suprapubic **prostatectomy** modified by John Bentley Squier (1873–1948), *BMSJ* **164**:911. *4269*

1911:31 The chemical nature of the substance in rice which could cure **beriberi** determined by Casimir Funk (1884–1967), *JP* **43**:395. *3744*

1911:32 **Bárány's syndrome** – unilateral deafness, vertigo, and pain in the occipital region – recorded by Robert Bárány (1876–1936), *MK* **7**:1818. *3402*

1911:33 The **Billroth II operation** for **cancer** of the **pylorus** modified by Eugen Alexander Pólya (1876–?1944), *ZCh* **38**:892. *3537, 3483*

1911:34 A straight **gastroscope** designed by Hans Elsner (b.1874); in his *Die Gastroskopie*. *3535.1*

1911:35 Successful **femoral artery embolectomy** by G. Labey, *BuAM* **66**:358. *3013*

1911:36 The classic *Haemophilia* published by William Bulloch (1868–1941) and Paul Fildes (1882–1971), in which they claimed to have established the fact of immunity in females and confirmed the **Law of Nasse**. *3081, 3056*

1911:37 **Hay fever** treatment by **pollen** injections introduced by Leonard Noon (1878–1913) and John Freeman (1877–1962), *L* **1**:1572; **2**:814. *2600.3, 2600.4*

1911:38 **Histamine** isolated from animal tissues by George Barger (1878–1939) and Henry Hallett Dale (1875–1968), *JP* **41**:499. *1901.1*

1911:39 Discovery of the intracapsular mechanism of **accommodation** by Alvar Gullstrand (1862–1930); in his *Methoden der Dioptrik des Auges*. *1526*

1911:40 Functions of the **thalamus** described by Henry Head (1861–1940) and Gordon Morgan Holmes (1876–1965), *Brain* **34**:102. *1438.1*

---

1911:41 Reginald Irving **Hewitt**, American parasitologist, born 6 Feb; with co-workers, used diethylcarbamazine (hetrazan) experimentally in the treatment of filariasis, 1947, *JLCM* **32**:1314. *5351.3*

1911:42 Willem Johan **Kolff**, Dutch/American physician, born 14 Feb; introduced an artificial kidney (artificial renal dialyser), 1944, *AcM* **117**:1916; with B. Watschinger, introduced a disposable twin coil artificial kidney, 1956, *JLCM* **47**:969. *4255, 4257.1*

1911:43 Denis Parsons **Burkitt**, British physician, born 28 Feb; described 'Burkitt's tumour' (African lymphoma), 1958, *BJS* **46**:218 – already noted by Alfred Cook, the missionary. Died 1993. *2660.12*

1911:44 Bernard **Katz**, German/British physiologist, born 26 Mar; published *The release of neural transmitter substances*, 1969. Shared Nobel Prize (Physiology or Medicine), 1970, with Julius Axelrod and Ulf Svante von Euler, for his research into the nature of the processes of chemical neurotransmission; *NPL*. *1354.2*

1911:45 Feodor Felix Konrad **Lynen**, German biochemist, born 6 Apr; shared Nobel Prize (Physiology or Medicine), 1964, with Konrad Emil Bloch, for their contributions to understanding the mechanism and regulation of cholesterol and fatty acid metabolism, *NPL*.

1911:46 Saul **Krugman**, American physician, born 7 Apr; with co-workers, showed evidence for two distinctive types of infective hepatitis, 1967, *JAMA* **200**:265. *3666.5*

1911:47 Maclyn **McCarty**, American medical bacteriologist, born 9 Jun; with Oswald Theodor Avery and Colin Munro Macleod, demonstrated that deoxyribonucleic acid (DNA) is the basic material responsible for genetic transformation, 1944, *JEM* **79**:137; discovered streptodornase, 1948, *JEM* **88**:181. *255.3, 1929.2*

504

1911:48 Luis Walter **Alvarez**, American physicist, born 13 Jun; introduced linear ion accelerator, 1946, *PsR* **70**:799. Died 1988. *2659.5*

1911:49 Steven Otto **Schwartz**, Hungarian/American haematologist, born 6 Jul; with William Dameshek, first recognition of an auto-immune disease, acquired haemolytic anaemia, 1938, *AJMS. 3787.1*

1911:50 Paul Maurice **Zoll**, American cardiologist, born 15 Jul; introduced external cardiac pacemaker in treatment of ventricular standstill, 1952, *NEJM* **247**:768. *2883*

1911:51 William H. **Stein**, American biochemist, born 15 Jul; shared Nobel Prize (Chemistry), 1972, with Stanford Moore and Christian Boehmer Anfinsen, for his contribution to the understanding of the connection between chemical structure and catalytic activity of active centre of ribonuclease molecule, *NPL.*

1911:52 Chester B. **McVay**, American surgeon, born 1 Aug; introduced the McVay (or Cooper) ligament repair in hernia, 1948, *ArSuC* **57**:524. Died 1987. *3611.2*

1911:53 John Julian **Wild**, British/American physicist, born 11 Aug; with J.M. Reid, introduced ultrasonic investigation (tomogram) of soft tissue, 1957, Kelly, E.C. *Ultrasound*, p. 30. *2681*

1911:54 John **Charnley**, British surgeon, born 29 Aug; introduced total hip-joint replacement, the Charnley arthroplasty, 1961, *L* **1**:1129. Died 1982. *4405.1*

1911:55 John Samuel **LaDue**, American physician, born 6 Sep; with Felix Wroblewski, introduced diagnostic test for myocardial infarction, 1955, *Cir* **11**:871. Died 1980. *2883.1*

1911:56 Donald William **Kerst**, American physicist, born 1 Nov; introduced the betatron, 1940, *PsR* **58**:841; **60**:47. *2659.1, 2010.2*

1911:57 Niels Kaj **Jerne**, Danish immunologist, born 23 Dec; proposed a network theory of the immune system, 1974, *AnI* **125**C:373. Shared the Nobel Prize (Physiology or Medicine), 1984, with Georges Jean Franz Kohler and César Milstein, for his theories concerning the specificity in development and control of the immune system, *NPL.* Died 1994. *2578.42*

1911:58 Inge **Edler**, Swedish scientist, born; with Carl Hellmuth Hertz, introduced echo-cardiography, 1954, *Kongliga Fysiografiska Sällskapets i Lund Förhandlingar*, **24**:1. *2883.01*

1911:59 Juan Carlos **Fascioli**, Argentinian physician, born; with Bernardo Alberto Houssay, showed hypertension to be due to the action of a pressor substance, 1937, *RSAB* **13**:284. *2721*

1911:60 William Grey **Walter**, British neurophysiologist, born; used electro-encephalography in the location of cerebral tumours, 1936, *L* **2**:305. Died 1977. *4907*

1911: Theodor **Escherich** died, **born** 1857. *Escherichia*

1911: Francis **Galton** died, **born** 1822. *eugenics*

1911: Henry Pickering **Bowditch** died, **born** 1840. *indefatigability of nerve*

1911: Albert **Ladenburg** died, **born** 1842. *scopolamine*

1911: Vasiliy Isayevich **Isayev [Issayaeff]** died, **born** 1854. *immune bacteriolysis, cholera vibrio*

1911: Giuseppe **Profeta** died, **born** 1840. *syphilis*

1911: Etienne Louis Arthur **Fallot** died, **born** 1850. *congenital heart disease*

1911: Bernhard **Fraenkel** died, **born** 1836. *ozaena, mycotic pharyngitis, cancer of larynx*

1911: August **Lucae** died, **born** 1835. *otoscope, sound transmission through cranial bones*

1911: Samuel Jones **Gee** died, **born** 1839. *steatorrhoea, coeliac disease*

1911: Odilon Marc **Lannelongue** died, **born** 1840. *cretinism, thyroid transplantation*

1911: Frederick William **Pavy** died, **born** 1829. *albuminuria*

1911: John Hughlings **Jackson** died, **born** 1835. *paralysis, nervous diseases, ophthalmoscope, epilepsy, syringomyelia, aphasia*

1911: Alfred **Binet** died, **born** 1857. *intelligence tests*

1911: Walter Remsen **Brinckerhoff** died, **born** 1875. *smallpox*

1911: Jeffery Allen **Marston** died, **born** 1831. *leptospirosis, Weil's disease, brucellosis (Malta fever)*

1911: Hermann Jakob **Knapp** died, **born** 1831. *cornea*

1911: Gustav August **Braun** died, **born** 1829. *decapitation hook*

1911: Samuel **Wilks** died, **born** 1824. *bacterial endocarditis, lymphadenoma, linea atrophicae, verrucae necrogenicae, alcoholic paraplegia, osteitis deformans, myasthenia gravis*

## 1912

1912:1 **Nobel Prize** (Physiology or Medicine): Alexis Carrel (1873–1944), for **surgical** and **cell-culture** experiments, *NPL. 559, 560*

1912:2 **Canada Medical Act**

1912:3 **Naval Medical School** established at **Royal Naval College, Greenwich**, England

1912:4 **South African Institute for Medical Research, Johannesburg**, founded

1912:5 **Division of Industrial Hygiene (US Public Health Service)** organized

1912:6 **Institut de Radium (Curie Foundation), Paris**

1912:7 **Olivo-pontocerebellar atrophy** first described by Joseph Jules Dejerine (1849–1917) and André Thomas (1867–1963), *NIS* **25**:223. *4716.1*

1912:8 The classic description of **progressive familial hepatolenticular degeneration** ('**Kinnier Wilson's disease**') given by Samuel Alexander Kinnier Wilson (1874–1937), *Brain* **34**:295, although it had been previously described by Frerichs (1861). *4717, 4693*

1912:9 Filtration of the **trachoma** agent, *Chlamydia trachomatis*, carried out by Charles Jules Henri Nicolle (1866–1936) and co-workers, *CRAS* **155**:241. *5961*

1912:10 Traumatic **angiopathy** of the **retina** ('**Purtscher's disease**') first described by Otto Purtscher (1852–1927), *GAO* **82**:347. *5962*

1912:11 The first comprehensive text on **maxillofacial surgery** was *Surgery and diseases of the mouth and jaws*, by Vilray Papin Blair (1871–1955). *5756.7*

1912:12 Filtration of the virus of **inclusion conjunctivitis** carried out by Albert Botteri (1879–1955), *KMA* **50**i:653. *5960*

1912:13 The first description of **Krönig's operation** of transperitoneal lower-segment **caesarean section** appears in *Operative Gynäkologie*, 3rd edn, p. 879, by Albert Siegmund Döderlein (1860–1941) and Bernard Krönig (1863–1917). *6250*

1912:14 **Phenobarbitone** introduced in the treatment of **epilepsy** by Alfred Hauptmann (1881–1948), *MMW* **59**:1907. *4823*

1912:15 **Melioidosis** first described by Alfred Whitmore (1876–1946) and C.S. Krishnaswami, *IMG* **47**:262. *5159*

1912:16 Intractable **pain** relieved by **spinal cordotomy** by William Gibson Spiller (1863–1940) and Edward Martin (1859–1938), *JAMA* **58**:1489. *4883*

1912:17 The school of **individual psychology** founded by Alfred Adler (1870–1937), who seceded from Freud's psychoanalytical group; in his *Über die nervösen Charakter*. *4985.1*

1912:18 *Pasteurella tularensis*, causal organism of **tularaemia**, isolated by George Walter McCoy (1876–1952) and Charles Willard Chapin (b.1877), *JID* **10**:61. *5174*

1912:19 *Glossina morsitans* shown by Allan Kinghorn (1880–1955) and Warrington Yorke (1883–1943) to be the transmitting fly of *Trypanosoma rhodesiense*, *AnTM* **6**:1. *5285.2*

1912:20 The life cycle of *Trypanosoma cruzi* described by Alexandre Emile Brumpt (1877–1951), *BSPE* **5**:360. *5285.3*

1912:21 The **malaria** parasites, *Plasmodium vivax* and *P.falciparum*, cultivated *in vitro* by Charles Cassidy Bass (b.1875) and Foster Matthew Johns (b.1889), *JEM* **16**:567. *5255.1*

1912:22 **Boothby and Cotton's flowmeter**, for administration of **nitrous-oxide oxygen anaesthesia** introduced by Frederic Jay Cotton (1869–1938) and Walter Meredith Boothby (1880–1953), *SGO* **15**:281. *5698*

1912:23 **Cranio-facial dysostosis (hypertelorism)** first described by Octave Crouzon (1874–1938), *BSMH* **33**:545. *4385*

1912:24 **Encephalitis periaxialis diffusa** ('**Schilder's disease**') described by Paul Ferdinand Schilder (1886–1940), *ZGN* **10**:1. *4646*

1912:25 **Poliomyelitis virus** recovered from the intestinal tract by Carl Kling (1887–1967) and co-workers, disproving that it was exclusively neurotropic; in *Investigations on epidemic infantile paralysis … XVth International Congress on Hygiene and Demography. 4670.4*

1912:26 An operation for the treatment of congenital **pyloric stenosis** devised by Wilhelm Conrad Rammstedt (1867–1963), *MK* **8**:1702. *3539*

1912:27 Suspension **laryngoscopy** introduced by Gustav Killian (1860–1921), *ArL* **26**:277. *3338*

1912:28 **Cardiospasm** with **oesophageal dilatation** recorded by Henry Stanley Plummer (1874–1937), *JAMA* **58**:2013; after a report by Porter Paisley Vinson (1919) named '**Plummer-Vinson syndrome**'. *3320*

1912:29 Absence or incomplete development of **cervical vertebrae** ('**Klippel-Feil syndrome**') first reported by Maurice Klippel (1858–1942) and André Feil (b.1884), *NIS* **25**:223. *4386*

1912:30 **Paravertebral anaesthesia** introduced in **urology** by Max Kappis (1881–1938), *ZCh* **39**:249. *4197*

1912:31 **Bowen's disease**, a type of intra-epidermal basal-cell **epithelioma**, named after John Templeton Bowen (1857–1940) although described a year earlier by Queyrat. *4148, 4146*

1912:32 **Sporotrichosis** ('**de Beurmann-Gougerot disease**') first fully described by Charles Lucien de Beurmann (1851–1923) and Henri Gougerot (1881–1955); in their *Les sporotrichoses. 4147*

1912:33 Harvey Williams Cushing (1868–1939), who published *The pituitary body and its disorders*, the first clinical monograph on the subject, added much to the knowledge of the **pituitary** and its disorders. *3896*

1912:34 Alfred Erich Frank (1884–1957) was first definitely to connect the posterior **pituitary** with **diabetes insipidus**, *BKW* **49**:393. *3897*

1912:35 **Growth-stimulating vitamins** discovered by Frederick Gowland Hopkins (1861–1947), *JP* **44**:425. *1048*

1912:36 Anatomical distribution and development of lesions in **pulmonary tuberculosis** in children ('**Ghon's primary focus**') described by Anton Ghon (1866–1936); in his *Die primäre Lungenherd bei der Tuberkulose der Kinder*; he was preceded by J. Parrot (1876). *3233*

1912:37 Classic description of **cor pulmonale** by Francisco C. Arrilaga; in his *Cardiacos negros*, Thesis no. 2536. *2914*

1912:38 Experimental production of **cancer** by **tar** injection by Henry Peter George Bayon (1876–1952), *L* **2**:1579. *2639*

1912:39 **Syphilis: neoarsphenamine (neosalvarsan)** introduced in treatment by Paul Ehrlich (1854–1915), *CZ* **36**:637. *2405*

1912:40 Abraham Flexner (1866–1959) published the first systematic and thorough comparisons of the major systems of **medical education** in Europe, *Medical education in Europe. 1766.503*

---

1912:41 Konrad Emil **Bloch**, German/American biochemist, born 21 Jan; shared Nobel Prize (Physiology or Medicine), 1964, with Feodor Felix Konrad Lynen, for their contributions to understanding the mechanism and regulation of cholesterol and fatty acid metabolism, *NLP*

1912:42 Harry Fitch **Klinefelter**, American physician, born 20 Mar; with E.C. Reifenstein and Fuller Albright, first described the Klinefelter syndrome, an endocrine disorder, 1942, *JCE* **2**:615. *3804*

1912:43 Julius **Axelrod**, American biochemist, born 30 May; studied the pharmacology of central transmitter substances, for this work he shared the Nobel Prize (Physiology or Medicine), 1970, with Bernard Katz and Ulf Svante von Euler, *NPL. 1931.6*

1912:44 Lorrin Andrews **Riggs**, American psychologist, born 11 Jun; introduced retinography, 1941, *PSEB* **48**:204. *1533*

1912:45 Albert Hewett **Coons**, American immunologist, born 28 Jun; with Melvin H. Kaplan, introduced antigen location by fluorescent antibody technique, 1950, *JEM* **91**:1. Died 1978. *2578.8*

1912:46 Philip Gerald **Stansly**, American microbiologist, born 23 Jul; he was among several who simultaneously discovered polymyxins, 1947, *BJH* **81**:43. *1941*

1912:47 Salvador Edward **Luria**, Italian/American microbiologist, born 13 Aug; for his work on the genetics and replication of bacteria, 1949, *Gen* **34**:93, he shared the Nobel Prize (Physiology or Medicine), 1969, with Alfred Day Hershey and Max Delbrück, *NPL. 2526.1*

1912:48 Edward Lawrence **Rickes**, American nutritionist, born 31 Aug; isolated vitamin $B_{12}$ in crystalline form, 1948, *Science* **107**:396. *1091*

1912:49 William Richard Shaboe **Doll**, British epidemiologist, born 28 Oct; with Austin Bradford Hill, proved association of lung cancer with cigarette smoking (Müller, 1939; Wynder & Graham, 1950), 1950, *BMJ* **2**:139. *3215.2, 3213, 3215.1*

1912:50 George Emil **Palade**, Romanian cell biologist, born 19 Nov; shared Nobel Prize (Physiology or Medicine), 1974, with Albert Claude and Christian de Duve, for their discoveries concerning the structural and functional organization of the cell, *NPL.*

1912:51 Edward Heinrich **Robitzek**, American physician, born 12 Dec; with colleagues, introduced isoniazid in treatment of tuberculosis, 1952, *QSVH* **13**:27. Died 1984. *2353*

1912:52 Laurella **McClelland**, Canadian virologist, born 15 Dec; with Ronald Hare, discovered virus haemagglutination, 1941, *CPHJ* **32**:530, independently of George Keble Hirst. *2578*

1912:53 Joseph Holland **Burchenal**, American physician, born 21 Dec; introduced treatment of leukaemia with 6-mercaptopurine, 1953, *Blood* **8**:965. *3108.3*

1912:54 Auguste **Loubatières**, French pharmacologist, born 28 Dec; initiated work on hypoglycaemic sulphonamides, 1944, *CRSB* **138**:766. Died 1977. *3976.1*

1912:55 Frank Louis **Knotts** born; with Edgar Jacob Poth, introduced sulphasuxidine, 1941, *PSEB* **48**:129. *1957*

1912:56 John **Cade**, Australian psychiatrist, born; he was the first to try lithium salts in the treatment of psychosis, 1949, *MJA* **36**:349. *1930.1*

1912:57 Anders **Grönwall**, Swedish chemist, born; with B. Ingleman, used dextran as plasma substitute in blood transfusion, 1944, *AcPS* **7**:97. *2028*

1912: Robert **Fletcher** died, **born** 1823. *Index Medicus, Index-Catalogue of the Library of the Surgeon General's Office*

1912: Gerhard Henrik Armauer **Hansen** died, **born** 1841. *leprosy, Mycobacterium*

1912: Joseph **Lister** died, **born** 1827. *antisepsis, carbolic acid, antiseptic catgut ligature, inflammation, Bacterium lactis*

1912: Alexander Hugh **Ferguson** died, **born** 1853. *hernia*

1912: William Henry **Allchin** died, **born** 1846. *ulcerative colitis*

1912: Dittmar **Finkler** died, **born** 1852. *cholera, Vibrio proteus*

1912: Giulio **Vassale** died, **born** 1862. *parathyroid glands, tetany*

1912: Wilhelm **Ebstein** died, **born** 1836. *lymphadenoma*

1912: Heinrich **Unverricht** died, **born** 1853. *epilepsy*

1912: Adelchi **Negri** died, **born** 1876. *rabies*

1912: Jean Baptiste Nicolas Voltaire **Masius** died, **born** 1836. *haemolytic anaemia*

1912: Joaquin Maria **Albarran y Dominguez** died, **born** 1860. *nephrostomy, nephropexy*

1912: Henri Alexandre **Danlos** died, **born** 1844. *lupus erythematosus, radium*

1912: William **Murrell** died, **born** 1853. *angina pectoris, nitroglycerine*

1912: Alessandro **Codivilla** died, **born** 1861. *surgical lengthening of limbs*

1912: Sophia Louisa **Jex-Blake** died, **born** 1840. *medical education*

**1913**

1913:1 **Nobel Prize** (Physiology or Medicine): Charles Robert Richet (1850–1935), for work on **anaphylaxis**, *NPL. 2590*

1913:2 **Medical Research Committee**, UK, established (**Medical Research Council**, 1920). Formation of its **National Institute for Medical Research** agreed

1913:3 **International Medical Congress, London**

1913:4 **Wellcome Medical Museums, London**

1913:5 **Rockefeller Foundation (New York)** endowed by John D. **Rockefeller** (1839–1937)

1913:6 **International Health Board (Rockefeller Foundation)** organized

1913:7 **Institute for Cancer Research** opened in **New York**

1913:8 **[Institute for Cancer Research], Hamburg**

1913:9 **American Society of Experimental Pathology** founded

1913:10 **American College of Surgeons** founded

1913:11 **[Mycological Institute]** at **Hamburg**

1913:12 Joseph Barcroft's (1872–1947) *Respiratory function of the blood*, 1913 (2 edn, 2 vols, 1925–28) recorded studies of the **oxygen-carrying capacity of the blood**, particularly the elucidation of the oxygen dissociation curve. *964*

1913:13 One of the best single-volume **histories of medicine** is the *Introduction to the history of medicine* by Fielding Hudson Garrison (1870–1935). The 4th edition appeared in 1929. *6408*

1913:14 Thomas Burr Osborne (1859–1929), with L.B. Mendel, showed, like McCollum and Davis in the same year, the necessity in diet of a factor later to be named **vitamin A**, *JBC* **23**:181. *1050*

1913:15 *Estudios sobre la degeneración del sistema nervioso* (2 vols, 1913–14) by Santiago Ramón y Cajal (1852–1934) was the most complete work of its time on degeneration of the **nervous system** (English translation, 1928). *560.1*

1913:16 An **intratracheal ether anaesthesia** apparatus introduced by Robert Ernest Kelly (1879–1944), *BJS* **1**:90. *5699.2*

1913:17 George Washington Crile (1864–1943) advanced the kinetic theory of **shock** and the anoci-association concept in which **local and general anaesthesia** combined in sequence to eliminate **pre-operative fear and tension**, 1913, *L* 2:7. *5629*

1913:18 The first important account of **lymphogranuloma venereum** given by Joseph Durand (b.1876), Joseph Nicolas (1868–1960) and Maurice Favre (1876–1955), *BSMH* **35**:274. It is sometimes called '**Durand-Nicolas-Favre disease**'. *5217*

1913:19 **Anaesthesia** by rectal injection of liquid **ether** with olive oil dissolved in it (**synergistic anaesthesia**) produced by James Tayloe Gwathmey (1865–1944), *NYMJ* **98**:1101; especially successful in **midwifery**. *5699*

1913:20 Ernest Linwood Walker (1870–1952) and Andrew Watson Sellards (1884–1941) determined the incubation period in **amoebiasis** and demonstrated that *Entamoeba tetragena* and *E.minuta* are identical with *E.histolytica*, *PhJS B* **8**:253. *5191*

1913:21 Successful removal of a **pineal tumour** reported by Hermann Oppenheim (1858–1919) and Fedor Krause (1856–1937), *BKW* **50**:2316. *4884.1*

1913:22 **Thymectomy** for **myasthenia gravis** performed by Ernst Ferdinand Sauerbruch (1875–1951), *MGMC* **25**:746. *4764*

1913:23 A pure culture of *Treponema pallidum* obtained by Hideyo Noguchi (1876–1928) and Joseph Waldron Moore (b.1879), from a patient with **dementia paralytica**, *JEM* **17**:232. *4805*

1913:24 William Henry Luckett (1872–1929) found air in the cerebral ventricles following skull fracture; this gave Dandy (1919) the idea for **ventriculography**, *SGO* **17**:37. *4884, 4602*

1913:25 Toxin-antitoxin for **diphtheria** immunization introduced by Emil Adolph von Behring (1854–1917), *DMW* **39**:873; **40**:1139. *5067*

1913:26 Bela Schick (1877–1967) developed his diphtheria susceptibility test for use as an indication as to whether or not prophylactic injections are necessary in children already exposed to **diphtheria**, *MMW* **60**:2608. *5066*

1913:27 **Punch prostatectomy** operation introduced by Hugh Hampton Young (1870–1945), *JAMA* **60**:253. *4270*

1913:28 The term **lipoid nephrosis** introduced by Fritz Munk (b.1879), who found that urine in such cases contained anisotropic lipoid droplets, *ZKM* **78**:1. *4237*

1913:29 The description of postpartum **pituitary necrosis, panhypopituitarism**, by Leon Konrad Gliński (1870–1918), *PrzL* **4**:13, preceded the case of **pituitary cachexia** ('**Simmonds' disease**') described by Morris Simmonds (1914). *3900*

1913:30 The **van den Bergh test** for **bilirubin** in serum introduced by Albert Abraham Hijmans van den Bergh (1869–1943) and J. Snapper, *DAKM* **110**:540. *3647*

1913:31 A classic account of **pituitary infantilism** given by Achille Alexandre Souques (1860–1944) and Stephen Chauvet (1885–1950), *NIS* **26**:69. *3899*

1913:32 The modern operation of fenestration for **otosclerosis** suggested by George John Jenkins (1874–1939), *IMC* **16**:609. *3403*

1913:33 **Carcinoma** of the **oesophagus** first successfully treated by resection of the thoracic portion by Franz Torek (1861–1938), *SGO* **16**:614. *3540*

1913:34 First successful **abdominal aorta embolectomy** by Fritz Bauer, *ZcH* **40**:1945. *3014.1*

1913:35 **Monocytic leukaemia** first reported by H. Reschad and V. Schilling-Torgau, *MMW* **60**:1981. *3082.1*

1913:36 **Phrenicotomy** in the treatment of **pulmonary tuberculosis** introduced by Ferdinand Sauerbruch (1875–1951), *MMW* **60**:625. *3234*

1913:37 Classical clinical description of **pulmonary artery** fat **embolism** by Aldred Scott Warthin (1866–1931), *IC* 24 ser., 4:171. *3015*

1913:38 Four types of **pneumococci** differentiated by Alphonse Raymond Dochez (1882–1964) and Louis John Gillespie (b.1886), *JAMA* **61**:727. *3192.1*

1913:39 '**Dumping syndrome**', an after-effect of **gastroenterostomy** first described by Arthur Frederick Hertz [Hurst] (1879–1944), *PRSM* 6 Surg:155. *3538*

1913:40 **Achlorhydric anaemia** described by Knud Helge Faber (1862–1956), *BKW* **50**:958. *3134*

1913:41 **Instantaneous heart radiography** reported by L. Huismans, *VDK* **30**:266. *2842*

1913:42 **Coolidge high-vacuum x ray tube** invented by William David Coolidge (1873–1975), *AmJR* **3**:115. *2692*

1913:43 **Bucky diaphragm** introduced in **radiology** by Gustav Bucky (1880–1963), *ArRR* **18**:6, later modified (**Potter-Bucky grid**) by Hollis Elmer Potter (1916), *AmJR* **3**:142. *2691, 2692.1*

1913:44 **Burns; keritherapy** (treatment with paraffin-resin solution, **ambrine**) introduced by Edmond Barthe de Sandfort, *JMI* **17**:211. *2251*

1913:45 **Syphilis; Lange's colloidal gold test** for cerebrospinal syphilis introduced by Karl Friedrich August Lange (b.1883), *ZChem* **1**:44. *2406*

1913:46 **Vitamin A** discovered by Elmer Verney McCollum (1879–1967) and Marguerite Davis, *JBC* **15**:167. *1049*

1913:47 Work on **anaphylaxis** by Henry Hallett Dale (1875–1968), *JPET* **4**:167, on lines similar to that of William Henry Schultz, 1910, led to the term 'Schultz-Dale test'. *2600.5*

1913:48 Johannes Andreas Grib Fibiger (1867–1928) was awarded Nobel Prize (Physiology or Medicine), 1926, for discovery of *Spiroptera* (a **nematode**) **carcinoma** (1913, *ZKr* **13**:217, 1914; **14**:295), *NPL*. This particular work was not confirmed and his results are no longer accepted. Died 1928. *2640*

---

1913:49 William Wallace **Scott**, American urologist, born 27 Jan; with Charles Brenton Huggins, introduced adrenalectomy for prostatic carcinoma, 1945, *AnS* **122**:1031. *4276.1*

1913:50 Frederick Mitchum **Owens**, American surgeon, born 21 Feb; with Lester Reynold Dragstedt, treated peptic ulcer by vagotomy, 1943, *PSEBM* **53**:152. *3557*

1913:51 Robert Henry **Barter**, American obstetrician and gynaecologist, born 15 Mar; with Cecil Bryant Jacobson, gave the first detailed report of amniocentesis for diagnosis *in utero* of genetic disorders, 1967, *AmJOG* **99**:796. *6235.2*

1913:52 Robert Walter **Schlesinger**, German/American microbiologist, born 27 Mar; with Albert Bruce Sabin, successfully propagated dengue in mice and produced a vaccine, 1945, *Science* **101**:604. *5475.1*

1913:53 Patrick Christopher **Steptoe**, British gynaecologist and obstetrician, born 9 Jun; *in vitro* fertilization of human oocytes with B.D. Bavister and Robert Geoffrey Edwards, 1969, *Nature* **221**:632. With Edwards, reported first successful human birth after re-implantation of human embryo, 1978, *L* **2**:366. Died 1988. *532.4, 532.5*

1913:54 Edward Penley **Abraham**, British biochemist, born 10 Jun; in collaboration with Ernst Boris Chain, produced penicillinase, a penicillin-inhibiting enzyme, 1940, *Nature* **146**:837. With Howard Walter Florey, Chain et al., first reported the chemotherapeutic action of penicillin on humans, 1940, *Lancet* **2**:226. With H.S. Burton, isolated cephalosporins, 1951, *BJ* **50**:168. *1933.3, 1934, 1945.2*

1913:55 Frank Milan **Berger**, Czechoslovak/American pharmacologist, born 25 Jun; introduced meprobamate, 1954, *JPET* **112**:413, later used in the treatment of anxiety. *4962.4*

1913:56 Forrest **Fulton**, British bacteriologist, born 13 Aug; with L. Joyner, introduced a vaccine against scrub typhus, 1945, *L* **2**:729. *5399*

1913:57 Francis Daniels **Moore**, American surgeon, born 17 Aug; with co-workers, carried out liver transplantation in dogs following total hepatectomy, 1959, *TrB* **6**:103. *3666.2*

1913:58 Roger Wolcott **Sperry**, American psychobiologist, born 20 Aug; shared Nobel Prize (Physiology or Medicine), 1981, with David Hunter Hubel and Torsten Nils Wiesel, for his discoveries concerning the functional specialization of the cerebral hemispheres, *NPL*.

1913:59 Choh Hao **Li**, Chinese/American endocrinologist, born 21 Aug; with co-workers isolated the interstitial-cell-stimulating hormone, 1940, *En* **27**:303, and pure adrenocorticotrophic hormone (ACTH), 1943, *JBC* **149**:413. *1173.1, 1174*

1913:60 Stanford **Moore**, American biochemist, born 4 Sep; shared Nobel Prize (Chemistry), 1972, with William H. Stein and Christian Boehmer Anfinsen, for his contribution to the understanding of the connection between chemical structure and catalytic activity of active centre of ribonuclease molecule, *NPL*.

---

1913:61 James Porter **Baker**, American physician, born; with Soma Weiss, first described carotid sinus syndrome, 1933, *Medicine* **12**:297. *2921*

1913:62 Jean Pierre **Soulier**, French haematologist, born; with Jean Gueguen, introduced phenindione (phenylindanedione) as an anticoagulant, 1947, *CRSB* **141**:1007. *3107*

1913:63 Edwin W. **Shearburn**, American surgeon, born; with Richard N. Myers, introduced the Canadian or Shouldice repair for inguinal hernia, 1969, *Surgery* **66**:450. *3611.3*

1913:64 Robert Andrew **Hingson** born; with Waldo Berry Edwards, first reported continuous caudal anaesthesia during labour and delivery, 1942, *CRA* **21**:301. *6232.1*

---

1913: John Shaw **Billings** died, **born** 1838. *Library of the Surgeon General's Office, Index Medicus, Index-Catalogue of the Library of the Surgeon General's Office*

1913: Ira Van **Gieson** died, **born** 1866. *acid fuchsin and picric acid stains*

1913: Francis **Gotch** died, **born** 1853. *electroretinogram*

1913: Leonard **Noon** died, **born** 1878. *hay fever, pollen*

1913: Theodor Albrecht Edwin **Klebs** died, **born** 1834. *diphtheria, Corynebacterium diphtheriae, typhoid, Salmonella typhi, glomerulonephritis, syphilis, tuberculosis*

1913: Arnold **Heller** died, **born** 1840. *syphilis, aortic aneurysm*

1913: Karel **Maydl** died, **born** 1853. *colostomy*

1913: Rudolph **Frank** died, **born** 1862. *gastrostomy*

1913: Charles **McBurney** died, **born** 1845. *appendicitis*

1913: Mathieu **Jaboulay** died, **born** 1860. *gastroduodenoscopy, vascular disease, sympathectomy, interilio-abdominal amputation*

1913: Jonathan **Hutchinson** died, **born** 1828. *intussuception, syphilis, progeria, cheiropompholyx, sarcoidosis, hydradenitis destruens suppurativa, varicella gangrenosa*

1913: Norman William **Kingsley** died, **born** 1829. *teeth deformities*

1913: Louis Adolphus **Duhring** died, **born** 1845. *dermatitis herpetiformis*

1913: Edward **Nettleship** died, **born** 1845. *urticaria pigmentosa*

1913: Karel **Maydl** died, **born** 1853. *uretero-ureteral anastomosis*

1913: Antonin **Poncet** died, **born** 1849. *tuberculous rheumatism*

1913: Frank **Hartley** died, **born** 1856. *facial neuralgia, neurectomy*

1913: Erwin **Baelz** died, **born** 1849. *scrub typhus, tsutsugamushi disease*

1913: Emil **Ponfick** died, **born** 1844. *actinomycosis*

1913: Alfred Russel **Wallace** died, **born** 1823. *natural selection*

1913: Just Marcellin **Lucas-Championnière** died, **born** 1843. *antisepsis*

**1914**

1914:1 **Nobel Prize** (Physiology or Medicine): Robert Bárány (1876–1036), for work on the **vestibular apparatus**, *NPL. 3400, 3401, 3402*

1914:2 **Mayo Clinic** opened in **Rochester**, Minn. The Mayo Family were well-established in Rochester and moved into a purpose-built clinic

1914:3 **[Royal Hungarian University]** at **Debrecen** founded

1914:4 **[Prussian State University]** at **Frankfurt a.M.** founded

1914:5 **Brady Urological Institute, Johns Hopkins University**

1914:6 **Hydrocephalus** produced experimentally by Walter Edward Dandy (1886–1946) and Kenneth Daniel Blackfan (1883–1941), *AmJDC* **8**:406; **14**:43. *4597*

1914:7 The first full description of **acrodynia** ('**pink disease**', '**Swift's disease**') given by Harry Swift (1858–1937), *TAMC* **10**:547. *6348*

1914:8 Aldo Castellani (1877–1971) first to suspect that **toxoplasmosis** could affect humans, *JTM* **17**:113. *5535.1, 5544.1*

1914:9 A nitrous oxide-oxygen **ether** apparatus described by James Tayloe Gwathmey (1865–1944), one of the first specialists in **anaesthesiology** in the US; in his *Anesthesia*, p. 334. *5669.1*

1914:10 The inhibitory action of **acetylcholine** on the **heart** demonstrated, and its possible role in the chemical mediation of **nervous impulses** postulated by Henry Hallett Dale (1875–1968), *JPET* **6**:147. *1340*

1914:11 Experimental proof that **rubella** is caused by a virus, provided by Alfred Fabian Hess (1875–1933), *ArIM* **13**:913. *5506.1*

1914:12 **Salpingography**, to determine the patency of the **Fallopian tubes**, performed by William Hollenback Cary (b.1883), *AmJOD* **69**:462, independently of Isador Clinton Rubin (1883–1958), *SGO* **20**:435. *6122, 6123*

1914:13 **Snails** confirmed as the intermediate hosts of *Schistosoma japonicum* by Keinosuke Miyairi (1865–1946) and M. Suzuki, *MMFK* **1**:187. *5350.2*

1914:14 A **streptobacillus**, *Streptobacillus muris ratti*, isolated from a case of streptobacillary **rat-bite fever** by Hugo Schöttmüller (1867–1936), *DeW* **58** Suppl., 77. *5325*

1914:15 **Tartar emetic** introduced in the treatment of South American **leishmaniasis** by Gaspar Oliveira de Vianna (1885–1914), *AnPa* **2**:167. *5301*

1914:16 *Pasteurella tularensis*, causal organism of **tularaemia**, first isolated from lesions in humans by William Buchanan Wherry (1875–1936) and Benjamin Harrison Lamb (b.1889), *JID* **15**:331. *5175*

1914:17 The mechanism of transmission of **plague** bacillus from rat to man by the rat **flea** demonstrated by Arthur William Bacot (1866–1922) and Charles James Martin (1866–1955), *JHyg* Plague Suppl. 3:423. *5129.1*

1914:18 **Anosognosia** (unconcern for, or denial of, striking **neurological disorders**) described and named by Joseph François Félix Babinski (1857–1932), *ReN* **22**:845. *4596.2*

1914:19 The first full description of **pure nephrosis** given by Franz Volhard (1872–1950) and Karl Theodor Fahr (1877–1945); in their *Die Brightsche Nierenkrankheit. 4238*

1914:20 The origin of **bile pigment** demonstrated by John William McNee (1887–1984), *JPB* **18**:325. *3648*

1914:21 The rare, genetically-determined **Niemann-Pick disease**, first described by Albert Niemann (1880–1921), *JaK* **79**:1; later by Ludwig Pick, 1926. *3784, 3785*

1914:22 First successful experimental surgical treatment for chronic **valvular** disease by Théodore Tuffier (1857–1929), *BuAM* **71**:293. *3029*

1914:23 Important account of **heart arrhythmias**, reporting the value of **quinine** in **paroxysmal fibrillation**, by Karel Frederik Wenckebach (1864–1940); in his *Die unregelmässige Herztätigkeit und ihre klinische Bedeutung. 2844*

1914:24 *Geriatrics; the diseases of old age and their treatment* ..., the first modern treatise on **geriatrics**, published by Ignatz Leo Nascher (1863–1944). *1641.1*

1914:25 **Blood transfusion** with citrated blood carried out by Luis Agote (1868–1954), *AnIMod* **1**:24. *2020*

1914:26 **Acetylcholine** isolated in ergot by Arthur James Ewins (1882–1957), *BJ* **8**:44. *1341*

1914:27 **Localization of cerebral function** mapped by Constantin von Monakow (1853–1930) in his classical work, *Die Lokalisation im Grosshirn. 1438.2*

1914:28 Morris Simmonds (1855–1925) described **pituitary cachexia**, ('**Simmonds' disease**'), *DMW* **40:322;** *VA* **217**:226. *3901*

---

1914:29 Alan Lloyd **Hodgkin**, British biophysicist, born 5 Feb. With Andrew Fielding Huxley, recorded action potentials from inside a nerve fibre, 1939, *Nature* **144**:710. They shared the Nobel Prize (Physiology or Medicine), 1963, with John Carew Eccles, for their discoveries concerning the ionic mechanisms involved in the excitation and inhibition in the peripheral and central portions of the nerve cell membrane, *NPL. 1310.1*

1914:30 Renato **Dulbecco**, Italian/American tumour virologist, born 22 Feb; independently of both David Baltimore and Howard Martin Temin, discovered the interaction between tumour viruses and genetic material of the cell, *NCIM* **17**; *Nature* **226**:1209, 1211; shared Nobel Prize, 1975, with them, *NPL. 2660.20, 2660.22, 2660.23, 2660.27*

1914:31 Robert Joseph **Huebner**, American virologist, born 23 Feb; with W.L. Jellison and C. Pomerantz, described rickettsialpox and isolated the aetiological agent, *Rickettsia akari*, 1946, *USPHR* **61**:1677. *5400*

1914:32 Mark Arnold **Stahmann**, American biochemist, born 30 Mar; with C. Huebner and K.P. Link, isolated dicoumarol (bis-hydroxycoumarin), an anticoagulant, 1941, *JBC* **138**:513. *3102*

1914:33 James Fred **Denton**, American microbiologist, born 16 May; with co-workers, isolated *Blastomyces dermatitidis* from soil, 1961, *Science* **133**:1126. *4154.7*

1914:34 Max Ferdinand **Perutz**, Austrian/British molecular biologist, born 19 May; shared Nobel Prize (Chemistry), 1962, with John Cowdery Kendrew, for his work on globular proteins, particularly haemoglobin, *NPL.*

1914:35 Elvin Abraham **Kabat**, American immunochemist, born 1 Sep; with Arne Wilhelm Tiselius, showed antibodies to be gamma globulins, 1939, *JEM* **69**:119. *2576.8*

1914:36 Carlos **Galli Mainini**, Argentinian obstetrician, born 7 Oct; introduced the male toad test for the diagnosis of pregnancy, 1947, *SMB* **1**:337. Died 1961. *6234*

1914:37 Richard Laurence Millington **Synge**, British chemist, born 28 Oct; shared Nobel Prize (Chemistry), 1952, with Archer John Porter Martin, for their invention of partition chromatography, *NPL*. Died 1994.

1914:38 Jonas **Salk**, American virologist, born 28 Oct; with co-workers, carried out immunization against poliomyelitis with a killed-virus vaccine, 1953, *JAMA* **151**:1081. Died 1995, *4672.2*

1914:39 Charles Carter **Shepard**, American leprologist, born 18 Dec; successfully transmitted leprosy to animals (mice), 1960, *AmJH* **71**:147. Died 1985. *2442.4*

1914:40 Frank John **Fenner**, Australian physician, born 21 Dec; with Frank Macfarlane Burnet, explained acquired immunological tolerance; in *The production of antibodies*, 1949. *2578.7*

---

1914:41 Örjan Thomas Gunnersson **Ouchterlony**, Swedish immunologist, born; introduced agar gel immunodiffusion method, 1948, *AcPMS* **25**:186. *2578.6*

1914:42 Charles **Dubost**, French surgeon, born; with co-workers, successfully resected an abdominal aortic aneurysm and inserted a homologous graft, 1951, *MAC* **77**:381. *2993.1*

1914:43 Denis John **Bauer** born; with Frederic Ogden MacCallum, proved the nature of infective hepatitis, 1944, *L* **1**:622. *3664.3*

1914:44 Knud **Hallas-Møller** born; with co-workers, initiated clinical trials of slow-acting insulin zinc suspensions, 1951, *UL* **113**:1767. *3978*

1914:45 Theodor Behn **Steinhausen**, American radiologist, born; with co-workers, introduced pantopaque for the myelographic diagnosis of cerebral tumours, 1944, *Rad* **43**:230. *4615*

1914:46 Charles William **Ordman**, American immunologist, born; with C.G. Jenning and C.A. Janeway, used gamma globulin for passive immunization against measles, 1944, *JCI* **23**:541. *5449.1*

---

1914: Alphonse **Bertillon** died, **born** 1853. *anthropomorphic measurement*

518

1914: Rudolph **Emmerich** died, **born** 1852. *pyocyanase*

1914: Mstislav **Novinsky** died, **born** 1841. *tumours, transplantation*

1914: Daniel Elmer **Salmon** died, **born** 1850. *Salmonella cholerae-suis*

1914: Charles Barrett **Lockwood** died, **born** 1856. *femoral hernia*

1914: Constant **Vanlair** died, **born** 1839. *haemolytic anaemia*

1914: Karel **Pawlik** died, **born** 1849. *cystectomy*

1914: Silas Weir **Mitchell** died, **born** 1829. *nervous diseases, chorea, pain, neuralgia, erythromelalgia, neuritis*

1914: Jean Alfred **Fournier** died, **born** 1832. *parasyphilis, tabes dorsalis*

1914: Otto Ivar **Wickman** died, **born** 1872. *poliomyelitis*

1914: Albert Freeman Africanus **King** died, **born** 1914. *malaria, mosquito*

1914: Angelo **Celli** died, **born** 1857. *malaria, Plasmodium malariae*

1914: David Douglas **Cunningham** died, **born** 1843. *leishmaniasis, Delhi boil*

1914: Alfred Leon Joseph **Conor** died, **born** 1870. *typhus*

1914: Gaspar Oliviera de **Vianna** died, **born** 1885. *trypanosomiasis, Trypanosoma cruzi, leishmaniasis, tartar emetic*

1914: Paul **Reclus** died, **born** 1847. *cystic mastitis*

1914: Robert Charles **Moon** died, **born** 1844. *retinitis pigmentosa*

1914: August Friedrich Leopold **Weismann** died, **born** 1834. *germ plasm*

1914: Carl **Breus** died, **born** 1852. *tuberous mole, pelvic deformities*

1914: Walter Holbrook **Gaskell** died, **born** 1847. *neurophysiology*

**1915**
1915:1 **Nobel Prize**: no awards

1915:2 **American College of Physicians** founded

1915:3 **Mayo Foundation for Medical Education and Research** organized at **Rochester**, Minn.

1915:4 **Institute of Medicine** organized at **Chicago**

1915:5 Artur Schüller (1874–1958) described two cases of the condition later termed the **Hand-Schüller-Christian syndrome**, *FGR* **23**:12. *6359–6363*

1915:6 William Edward Fothergill (1865–1926) modified A. Donald's operation for **prolapse** of the **uterus**, *JOG* **27**:146. *6124, 6119*

1915:7 The first to employ living **bone grafts** as internal splints was Fred Houdlett Albee (1876–1945); he wrote *Bone graft surgery*. *5757*

1915:8 A method of extraction of **cataract** with forceps introduced by Arnold Hermann Knapp (1869–1956), *ArOp* **50**:426. *5964*

1915:9 **Dakin's solution**, a solution of sodium hypochlorite and boric acid, introduced by Henry Drysdale Dakin (1880–1952) as an antiseptic, *BMJ* **2**:318. Used by Alexis Carrel (1873–1944) for the continuous **irrigation of wounds (Carrel-Dakin treatment)**, *BuAM* **74**:361. *1903.1, 5643, 5642*

1915:10 The snail responsible for the transmission of *Schistosoma mansoni* and *S.haematobium* identified by Robert Thomson Leiper (1881–1969), *JRAMC* **25**:1, 147, 253; **27**:171; **30**:235. *5350.4*

1915:11 **Trench fever**, a louse-borne infection, first described by John Henry Porteus Graham (?1869–1957), *L* **2**:703 and so named by George Herbert Hunt (1884–1926) and Allan Coats Rankin (1877–1959), *L* **2**:1133. *5385, 5386*

1915:12 A pure culture of **vaccinia** virus obtained by Hideyo Noguchi (1876–1928), *JMR* **21**:539. *5430.1*

1915:13 Stanislaus Joseph Matthias von Prowazek (1875–1915), like Ricketts and Wilder, demonstrated the specific causal agent in **typhus**, *BKI* **4**:5. *5384.1, 5379, 5380.1*

1915:14 A test for the diagnosis of **smallpox** introduced by Gustav Paul (1859–1933), *ZPB* I Abt.**75**:518. *5431*

1915:15 Attention drawn to a causal organism in bacillary **dysentery** by Carl Olaf Sonne (1882–1948) and later named *Shigella sonnei*, *ZBP* I **75**:408. *5094*

1915:16 **Osteopoikilosis**, a structural anomaly of the skeleton, first definitely described by Heinrich Ernst Albers-Schönberg (1865–1921), *FGR* **23**:174. *4386.1*

1915:17 A dietetic treatment of **peptic ulcer** ('**Sippy diet**') introduced by Bertram Welton Sippy (1866–1924), *JAMA* **64**:1625. *3541*

1915:18 *The mechanism of Mendelian heredity*, recording epoch-making work on **heredity**, published by Thomas Hunt Morgan (1866–1945), Alfred Henry Sturtevant (1891–1970), Hermann Joseph Muller (1890–1967) and Colin Blackman Bridges (1889–1938). *246*

1915:19 **Aortic genesis** of **angina pectoris** suggested by Clifford Allbutt (1836–1925); in his *Diseases of the arteries, including angina pectoris*. *2894*

1915:20 **Essential thrombopenia** reported by Alfred Erich Frank (1884–1957), *BKW* **52**:454, 490. *3083*

1915:21 *Clostridium oedematiens* isolated by Michel Weinberg (1868–1940) and P. Seguin, *CRSB* **78**:274. *2520*

1915:22 **Antibody response** suppression by **x rays** demonstrated by Ludvig Hektoen (1863–1951), *JID* **17**:415. *2569*

1915:23 **Blood transfusion** with citrated blood carried out by Richard Lewisohn (1875–1962), *MR* **87**:141. *2021*

1915:24 **Bacteriophage**, so named by Félix Hubert d' Herelle who independently discovered it in 1917, the agent involved in the transmissible lysis of **bacteria** by **viruses (Twort-d'Herelle phenomenon)** first pointed out by Frederick William Twort (1877–1950), *L* **2**:1241. *2571, 2572*

1915:25 **Thyroxine** isolated by Edward Calvin Kendall (1886–1972), *JAMA* **64**:2042. *1133*

1915:26 Peter Brian **Medawar**, British zoologist and immunologist, born 28 Feb; with Thomas Gibson, explained transplantation rejection mechanism in skin homografts, 1943, *JA* **77**:299, **78**:176. With Rupert Everett Billingham, Leslie Brent and E.M. Sparrow, provided proof of Burnet-Fenner theory (1949) of acquired immunological tolerance, 1953, *Nature* **172**:603. Demonstrated the homograft (delayed sensitivity) reaction, 1958, *PRSB* **149**:145. Shared the Nobel Prize (Physiology or Medicine), 1960, with Frank Macfarlane Burnet, for their discovery of acquired immunological tolerance, *NPL*. Died 1987. *2578.4, 2578.11, 2578.24*

1915:27 James Van Gundia **Neel**, American geneticist, born 22 Mar; provided genetic evidence that sickle-cell anaemia is inherited in a simple Mendelian manner, 1949, *Science* **110**:64. *3154.2*

1915:28 Thomas Huckle **Weller**, American physician, born 15 Jun; with John Francis Enders and F.C. Robbins, grew poliomyelitis virus in cultures of various tissues, removing obstacles to vaccine production, 1949, *Science* **109**:85. First isolated the varicella-herpes virus, 1953, *PSEB* **83**:340. With Franklin Allen Neva, isolated the rubella virus, 1962, *PSEB* **111**:215, simultaneously with Parkman and co-workers. *4671.1, 5440.1, 5509.1, 5509.2*

1915:29 Eleanor **Zaimis**, Greek pharmacologist, born 16 Jun; with William Drummond MacDonald Paton, discovered the curare-like anaesthetic action of methonium compounds, 1948, *Nature* **161**:718. Died 1982. *1929.3, 5726*

1915:30 Earl Wilbur **Sutherland**, American biochemist, born; with G.A. Robson and R.W. Butcher, elucidated the role of cyclic AMP, the second messenger mediating actions in a wide range of hormonal effects, 1968, *AnRB* **37**:149. For this work he received the Nobel Prize (Physiology or Medicine), 1971, *NPL*. Died 1974. *7527*

1915:31 Thomas **Gibson** born; with Peter Brian Medawar, explained transplantation rejection mechanism in skin homografts, 1943, *JA* **77**:299; **78**:176. *2578.4*

1915: Austin **Flint** Jr died, **born** 1836. *coprosterol*

1915: George **Oliver** died, **born** 1841. *adrenaline*

1915: Paul **Ehrlich** died, **born** 1854. *trypanosomiasis, salvarsan, chemotherapy, malaria, methylene blue, diphtheria antitoxin, biological standardization, antibodies, syphilis, leukaemia, aplastic anaemia, reticulocyte*

1915: Friedrich Albert Johann **Loeffler** died, **born** 1852. *foot-and-mouth disease virus, Salmonella typhi-murium, glanders, Pfeifferella mallei*

1915: George Miller **Sternberg** died, **born** 1838. *pneumococcus*

1915: Adolf Fredrik **Lindstedt** died, **born** 1847. *volvulus*

1915: Theodor **Langhans** died, **born** 1839. *lymphadenoma*

1915: Kanehiro **Takaki** died, **born** 1849. *beriberi*

1915: Arthur Cecil Hamel **Rothera** died, **born** 1880. *acetone bodies in urine*

1915: Eduard **Jacobi** died, **born** 1862. *poikiloderma vascularis atrophicans*

1915: Otto Gerhard Karl **Sprengel** died, **born** 1852. *congenital elevation of scapula, upward displacement of scapula*

1915: Julius **Arnold** died, **born** 1835. *Arnold-Chiari malformation*

1915: Martin **Bernhardt** died, **born** 1844. *meralgia paraesthetica*

1915: Alexander Hughes **Bennett** died, **born** 1848. *brain tumour*

1915: Henry Charlton **Bastian** died, **born** 1837. *Bastian's law, aphasia, knee-jerk, Dracunculus medinensis*

1915: Thomas Smith **Clouston** died, **born** 1840. *general paresis, syphilis*

1915: Carl **Fraenkel** died, **born** 1861. *diphtheria, Corynebacterium diphtheriae*

1915: Alois **Alzheimer** died, **born** 1864. *presenile dementia*

1915: John Brown **Buist** died, **born** 1846. *vaccinia*

1915: Eugène **Koeberlé** died, **born** 1828. *ovariotomy*

1915: Robert von **Olshausen** died, **born** 1835. *excision of vagina, retroversion of uterus*

1915: Stanislaus Joseph Matthias von **Prowazek** died, **born** 1875. *trachoma, typhus*

1915: George **Coats** died, **born** 1876. *retinitis circinata*

1915: Carlos Juan **Finlay** died, **born** 1833. *yellow fever, mosquito*

1915: Theodor **Boveri** died, **born** 1862. *chromosomes, development*

1915: William Richard **Gowers** died, **born** 1845. *epilepsy, spinocerebellar tract, spinal cord tumour, progressive muscular dystrophy, panatrophy*

**1916**
1916:1 **Nobel Prize**: no awards

1916:2 **Royal College of Nursing (London)** founded (Royal Charter, 1963)

1916:3 **American Radium Society (St Louis)** founded

1916:4 **National Research Council (Washington, DC)** organized

1916:5 **[National Bacteriological Institute] Buenos Aires**

1916:6 **Bucky diaphragm** introduced in **radiology** by Gustav Bucky (1913), *ArRR* **18**:6, and modified by Hollis Elmer Potter (1880–1964), *AmJR* **3**:142, **Potter-Bucky grid**. *2692.1, 2691*

1916:7 **Heparin** extracted from dog liver by Jay McLean (1890–1957), *AmJPh* **41**:250. *904*

1916:8 **Histocompatibility antigens** studied by Clarence Cook Little (1888–1971) and Ernest Edward Tyzzer (1875–1966), *JMR* **33**:393. *2570*

1916:9 *Clostridium histolyticum* isolated by Michel Weinberg (1868–1940) and P. Seguin, *CRAS* **163**:449. *2521*

1916:10 Concept of **atopy** originated from work by Robert Anderson Cooke (1880–1960) and Albert Vander Veer (b.1879), *JI* **1**:201. *2600.6*

1916:11 **Lutembacher's syndrome, mitral stenosis** with interatrial septal defect, described by René Lutembacher (b.1884), *ArMC* **9**:237. *2846*

1916:12 **Kymography** introduced in clinical **cardiology** by Augustus Warren Crane (1868–1937), *AmJR* **3**:513. *2845*

1916:13 Experimental production of **cancer** by painting with a **tar** product by Katsusaburo Yamagiwa (1863–1930) and Koichi Ichikawa (1888–1948), *VJPJ* **6**:169; **7**:191. *2643*

1916:14 Injection treatment of **varicose veins** introduced by Paul Linser (1871–1963), *MK* **12**:897. *3000*

1916:15 **'Reiter's syndrome'**, characterized by initial diarrhoea, urethritis, conjunctivitis and arthritis occurring in males, first described by Noel Fiessinger (1881–1946) and Edgar Leroy, *BSMH* **40**:2030; was so named after the description by Hans Conrad Julius Reiter (1881–1969), *DMW* **42**:1535. *6370, 6371*

1916:16 The **'Stevens-Johnson syndrome'** first described by Robert Rendu (b.1886), *JPr* **30**:351. *6365*

1916:17 The **Kielland (obstetric) forceps** introduced by Christian Kielland (1871–1941), *MonG* **43**:48. *6219*

1916:18 A tubed pedicle flap used in **plastic surgery** as early as September 1916 by Vladimir Petrovich Filatov (1875–1956), *VO* **34**, 4–5:149. *5757.1*

1916:19 Attention first drawn to discoloration of the skin about the **umbilicus** as a sign of ruptured **ectopic pregnancy** ('**Cullen's sign**') by Thomas Stephen Cullen (1868–1953); in his *Embryology, anatomy, and diseases of the umbilicus. 6124.1*

1916:20 *Torula histolytica*, later found to be identical with *Cryptococcus neoformans*, causal organism in **cryptococcosis**, first isolated by James Leavitt Stoddard (b.1889) and Elliott Carr Cutler (1888–1947), *RIM* 6. *5537*

1916:21 An apparatus for the administration of warm **anaesthetic** vapours (**Shipway apparatus**) introduced by Francis Edward Shipway (1875–1968), *L* 1:70. *5699.3*

1916:22 '**Bipp**' (an **antiseptic paste**) introduced in the treatment of **wounds** by James Rutherford Morison (1853–1939), *L* 2:268. *5644*

1916:23 A spirillum, *Spirillum morsus muris*, found in the lymphatics and blood stream in cases of **rat-bite fever** by Kenzo Futaki (1873–1966) and co-workers, *JEM* **23**:249; **25**:33. *5326*

1916:24 *Spirillum (Leptospira) icterohaemorrhagiae* proved to be causal organism in **Weil's disease** by Ryukichi Inada (1874–1950) and co-workers, *JEM* **23**:377. *5334*

1916:25 A form of **trench fever** encountered by Wilhelm His Jr (1863–1934) in Volhynia, Russia, named by him **Volhynia fever**, *BKW* **53**:322. *5387*

1916:26 The **Weil-Felix reaction** for the diagnosis of **typhus** developed by Edmund Weil (1880–1922) and Arthur Felix (1887–1956), *WKW* **29**:33. *5390, 5381*

1916:27 The causal organism of **typhus** first isolated by Henrique de Rocha Lima (1879–1956), who named it *Rickettsia prowazeki* after Ricketts and Prowazek, both of whom had died of typhus, *BKW* **53**:567. *5388, 5379, 5394.1*

1916:28 *Rickettsia quintana* isolated from lice found on patients with **trench fever** by Hans Willi Töpfer (b.1876), *MMW* **63**:1495. *5389*

1916:29 The modern method of **trephining** and draining **inflammatory processes of the brain** initiated by Harris Peyton Mosher (b.1867), *SGO* **23**:740. *4886*

1916:30 **Causalgia** treated with **periarterial sympathectomy** by René Leriche (1879–1955), *PrM* **24**:178. *4885*

1916:31 The posterior **retroparotid space syndrome** ('**Villaret's syndrome**') described by Maurice Villaret (1877–1946), *ReN* **23**, I:188. *4719*

1916:32 **Acute infective polyneuritis (Guillain-Barré syndrome)** described by Georges Guillain (1876–1961), Jean Alexandre Barré (b.1880) and A. Strohl, *BSMH* **40**:1462. *4647*

1916:33 A test for determining the patency of the spinal **subarachnoid space** ('**Queckenstedt's test**') introduced by Hans Heinrich Georg Queckenstedt (1876–1918), *DZN* **55**:325. *4600*

1916:34 Method of **tendon transplantation** described by Leo Mayer (1884–1972), *SGO* **22**:182. *4386.3*

1916:35 **Pituitary dwarfism** termed **nanosomia pituitaria** by Jakob Erdheim (1874–1937) during his studies of pituitary pathology, *BPA* **62**:302. *3902*

1916:36 The *Involuntary nervous system*, by Walter Holbrook Gaskell (1847–1914) published. *1331*

---

1916:37 Sune **Bergström**, Swedish biochemist, born 10 Jan; with co-workers he isolated *nor*-adrenaline, 1949, *AcCS* **3**:305; *AcPS* 1950 **20**:101. With co-workers, elucidated the chemical structure of prostaglandins, 1962, *AcCS* **16**:501. Shared the Nobel Prize (Physiology or Medicine), 1982, with Bengt Ingemar Samuelsson and John Robert Vane, for this work, *NPL 1155, 1931.4*

1916:38 Clarence Chancelum **Lushbaugh**, American pathologist, born 15 Mar; with Paul Eby Steiner, first described amniotic fluid embolism, 1941, *JAMA* **117**:1245,1340. *6232*

1916:39 Christian Boehmer **Anfinsen**, American biochemist, born 26 Mar; shared Nobel Prize (Chemistry), 1972, with Stanford Moore and William H. Stein, for his work on ribonuclease, especially the connection between the amino acid sequence and the biologically active configuration, *NPL*. Died 1995.

1916:40 John Bernard **Kinmonth**, British surgeon, born 9 May; introduced lymphangiography, 1952, *CS* **11**:13. Died 1982. *2700.1*

1916:41 Francis Harry Compton **Crick**, British biologist, born 8 Jun; with James Dewey Watson determined molecular structure of DNA, 1953, *Nature* **171**:737; for this work they shared the Nobel Prize (Physiology or Medicine), 1962, with Maurice Hugh Frederick Wilkins, *NPL*. *256.3*

1916:42 Manfred Martin **Mayer**, German/American immunologist, born 15 Jun; with Robert Armstrong Nelson, introduced Nelson treponemal immobilization test for syphilis diagnosis, 1949, *JEM* **89**:369, With Lawrence Levine, introduced complement fixation technique, 1954, *JI* **72**:511. Died 1984. *2419, 2578.14*

1916:43 Robert **Guthrie**, American microbiologist, born 28 Jun; with Ada Susi, devised a bacterial inhibition test for phenylketonuria, 1963, *Ped* **32**:338. *3924.4*

1916:44 Charles Anthony **Hufnagel**, American cardiovascular surgeon, born 15 Aug; designed and inserted first workable prosthetic heart valve in man, 1951, *BGUMC* **4**:128. Died 1989. *3047.2*

1916:45 Frederick Chapman **Robbins**, American microbiologist, born 25 Aug. With John Franklin Enders and Thomas Huckle Weller, successfully transferred poliomyelitis in cultures of different tissues, 1949, *Science* **109**:85. Their method of growing the virus in this way removed the final obstacle to vaccine production and earned them the Nobel Prize (Physiology or Medicine), 1954, *NPL*. *4671.1*

1916:46 Henry George **Kunkel**, American physician, born 9 Sep; with co-workers, discovered idiotypy of isolated antibodies, 1963, *Science* **140**:405. Died 1963. *2578.35*

1916:47 Frederick Stanley **Philips**, American pharmacologist, born 25 Sep; with Albert Gilman, introduced nitrogen mustard in the treatment of Hodgkin's disease, 1946, *Science* **103**:409. *3788*

1916:48 Jean Baptiste **Dausset**, French haematologist, born 19 Oct; with A. Nenna, discovered leuco-agglutinins, 1952, *CRSB* **146**:1539. Discovered first histocompatibility antigen, 1958, *AcHa* **20**:156; for this work he shared the Nobel Prize (Physiology or Medicine), 1980, with Baruj Benacerraf and George Davis Snell, *NPL. 2578.10, 2578.26*

1916:49 Marvin Joseph **Weinstein**, American microbiologist, born 20 Oct; with co-workers isolated the antibiotic, gentamycin, 1963, *JMC* **6**:463. *1947.5*

1916:50 Hilary **Koprowski**, Polish/American microbiologist, born 5 Dec; with co-workers, achieved successful immunization against poliomyelitis with a living attenuated virus, 1952, *AmJH* **55**:108. *4672.1*

1916:51 Martin Hugh Frederick **Wilkins**, New Zealand biophysicist, born 15 Dec; with colleagues, discovered the helical structure of DNA, 1953, *Nature* **172**:759. Shared the Nobel Prize (Physiology or Medicine), 1962, with Francis Harry Compton Crick and James Dewey Watson, *NPL. 256.4*

---

1916:52 Robert Rocco **De Nicola** born; implantated a permanent artificial (silicone) urethra, 1950, *JU* **63**:168. *4203*

1916:53 A Bernard **Pasternack**, American physician, born; with Lee Foshay, used streptomycin in treatment of tularaemia, 1946, *JAMA* **130**:393. *5180.*

1916:54 Alberto Francis **Inclan**, Cuban orthopaedic surgeon, born; his work forms the basis of the modern use of bone preserved by refrigeration, 1941, *JBJS* **24**:81. *5764*

---

1916: Elie **Metchnikoff** died, **born** 1845. *phagocytosis, inflammation, immunity*

1916: Thomas Lauder **Brunton** died, **born** 1844. *angina pectoris, amyl nitrite*

1916: Wharton Peter **Hood** died, **born** 1835. *joint manipulation*

1916: Wilhelm **Türk** died, **born** 1871. *agranulocytosis*

1916: William **Cayley** died, **born** 1836. *haemoptysis, pneumothorax*

1916: Georg **Avellis** died, **born** 1864. *palate*

1916: John Benjamin **Murphy** died, **born** 1857. *gastric and intestinal anastomosis, suture of femoral artery*

1916: Harald **Hirschsprung** died, **born** 1830. *megacolon, pyloric stenosis*

1916: Ludwig **Heusner** died, **born** 1846. *gastric ulcer*

1916: Frederic Samuel **Eve** died, **born** 1853. *intersigmoid hernia*

1916: Charles **Girard** died, **born** 1850. *hind-quarter amputation*

1916: Paul **Bruns** died, **born** 1846. *neurofibroma*

1916: Hans **Chiari** died, **born** 1851. *Arnold-Chiari malformation, chorionepithelioma*

1916: Victor Alexander Haden **Horsley** died, **born** 1857. *spinal cord tumour, stereotactic surgery, athetosis, localization of cerebral function, stereotactic apparatus*

1916: Alfred Ludwig Siegmund **Neisser** died, **born** 1855. *syphilis, gonorrhoea, gonococcus, Neisseria gonorrhoeae, leprosy, Mycobacterium, aniline*

1916: Adolf **Weil** died, **born** 1848. *leptospirosis icterohaemorrhagica*

1916: Léon **Labbe** died, **born** 1832. *pre-anaesthetic medication*

1916: Frederic William **Hewitt** died, **born** 1857. *anaesthesia, ether, nitrous oxide/oxygen*

1916: Hans **Eppinger** died, **born** 1846. *nocardiosis, Nocardia asteroides*

1916: Vincenz **Czerny** died, **born** 1842. *uterine fibroids, hysterectomy*

1916: Andrew Woods **Smyth** died, **born** 1832. *innominate artery ligation*

1916: Walter Stanborough **Sutton** died, **born** 1877. *chromosomal basis of Mendelism*

1916: Antonio **Placido da Costa** died, **born** 1849. *keratoscope*

1916: Bernhard Moritz Carl Ludwig **Riedel** died, **born** 1846. *Riedel's lobe of the liver, Riedel's thyroiditis*

1916: George **Huntington** died, **born** 1850. *chorea*

**1917**
1917:1 **Nobel Prize**: no awards

1917:2 **School of Hygiene, Johns Hopkins University**, established

1917:3 **[Institute for Experimental Biology], Moscow**, organized

1917:4 **[State Pharmaceutical Institute], Warsaw**

1917:5 **Municipal Contagious Diseases Hospital, Chicago**, opened

1917:6 **Blindenstudienanstalt** established at **Marburg**

1917:7 **[Netherlands Society for Psychoanalysis]** established at **The Hague**

1917:8 **Lipochondrodystrophy** and **gargoylism** occurring in two brothers (**Hurler syndrome**) first described by Charles Hunter (1872–1955), *PRSM* **10** Dis.Child.:104. *6371, 6371.2*

1917:9 Tests for **colour-blindness** devised by Shinobu Ishihara (1879–1963); in his *Tests for colour-blindness. 5966*

1917:10 A tubed pedicle flap introduced by Harold Delf Gillies (1882–1960); in his *Plastic surgery of the face*, 1920. *5758*

1917:11 The Stockholm method of **radium** treatment of **cancer** of the **uterus**, as carried out at the Radiumhemmet, Stockholm, follows the technique devised by Carl Gustav Abrahamsson Forssell (1876–1950), *Hos* **10**:273. *6125*

1917:12 A continuous-flow **anaesthetic** machine introduced by Henry Edmund Gaskin Boyle (1875–1941), *PRSM* **11**: Anaes. 30. *5700*

1917:13 Rats shown by Yutako Ido (1881–1919) and co-workers to be the carriers of *Spirillum (Leptospira) icterohaemorrhagiae*, causal organism in **Weil's disease**, *JEM* **26**:341. *5334.1*

1917:14 *Shigella schmitzi*, a cause of bacillary **dysentery**, isolated by Karl Eitel Friedrich Schmitz (b.1889), *ZHyg* **84**:449. *5095*

1917:15 The **Binet-Simon** scale for measurement of **intelligence** revised by Lewis Madison Terman (1877–1957) and co-workers; in *The Stanford revision and extension of the Binet-Simon scale for measuring intelligence. 4986*

1917:16 The bacillus of **melioidosis**, *(Pfeifferella whitmori)* identified by Ambrose Thomas Stanton (1875–1938), *SIMR* **14**. He reproduced the disease in animals by feeding and inoculation of cultures. *5159.1*

1917:17 A classic account of **epidemic encephalitis (encephalitis lethargica, 'von Economo's disease')** given by Constantin von Economo (1876–1931), *WKW* **30**:381. *4650*

1917:18 While investigating **Murray Valley encephalitis (Australian X disease)**, an acute **polioencephalomyelitis**, John Burton Cleland (1878–1971) and Alfred Walter Campbell (1868–1937) isolated a virus from cerebral tissue, *RDNSW* p.150. *4648*

1917:19 Jean René Cruchet (1875–1959) and co-workers reported 40 cases of **epidemic encephalitis**, *BSMH* **41**:614, 13 days before the classic description given by von Economo. *4649, 4650*

1917:20 Jörgen Nilsen Schaumann (1879–1953) established the systemic nature of **sarcoidosis** ('**Besnier-Boeck-Schaumann disease**'), *AnD* **6**:357. *4095, 4128, 4149*

1917:21 The **Stevens-Johnson syndrome**, a generalized eruption with fever and conjunctivitis, described by Albert Mason Stevens (1884–1945) and Frank Chambliss Johnson (1894–1934). *4150*

1917:22 Arthur Robertson Cushny's (1866–1926) theory of **urinary secretion**, in his *The secretion of the urine*, followed and modified that of Carl Ludwig. *1237*

1917:23 The first clear account of **galactosaemia** published by Friedrich Göppert (1870–1927), *BKW* **54**:473. *3921.1*

1917:24 **Electrocardiographic changes** during an attack of **angina pectoris** recorded by Guy William John Bousfield (1893–1974), *L* **2**:457. *2894.1*

1917:25 **Effort syndrome** described by Thomas Lewis (1881–1945); previously noted by A.B.R. Myers (1870) and J.M. Da Costa (1871), *MRC* **8**. *2847*

1917:26 Experimental use of **lipiodol** in **bronchoscopy** introduced by Charles Alexander Waters (b.1885), S. Bayne-Jones, and Leonard George Rowntree (1883–1959), *ArIM* **19**:538. *3194.1*

1917:27 Ignacio Barraquer (1884–1965) invented a machine with which he extracted **cataract** by suction, *CO* **22**:328. *5965*

1917:28 **Bronchospirochaetosis** ('**Castellani's bronchitis**') described by Aldo Castellani (1877–1971), *PrM* **25**:377. *3193*

1917:29 **Endothelioma** of the **bronchus** removed by peroral **bronchoscopy** by Chevalier Jackson (1865–1958), *AmJMS* **153**:371. *3194*

1917:30 **Syphilis: Meinicke diagnostic reaction** introduced by Ernst Meinicke (1878–1945), *BKW* **66**:613. *2407*

1917:31 The **bacteriophage**, the agent involved in the transmissible lysis of **bacteria** by **viruses – Twort-d'Herelle phenomenon** – (originally noted by Frederick William Twort in 1915), so named by Félix Hubert d'Herelle (1873–1949) who discovered it independently, *CRAS* **165**:373. *2571, 2572*

1917:32 **Acriflavine** introduced by Carl Hamilton Browning (1881–1972) and co-workers, *BMJ* **1**:73. *1905*

1917:33 **Blood transfusion** with stored red cells carried out by Oswald Hope Robertson (1886–1966), *MB* **1**:436. *2021.1*

1917:34 **Decompression sickness** in aviators discussed by Yandell Henderson (1873–1944), *AvAeE* **2**:145. *2137.3*

1917:35 **Oxygen therapy** introduced by John Scott Haldane (1860–1936), *BMJ* **1**:161. *1977*

1917:36 Carlton Everett **Schwerdt**, American virologist, born 2 Jan; with Frederick Leland Schaffer crystallized poliomyelitis virus particles, 1955, *PNAS* **41**:1020. *2527.1*

1917:37 Gustav William **Rapp**, German/American biochemist, born 3 Jan; with Garwood Colvin Richardson, introduced a saliva test for prenatal sex determination, 1952, *Science* **115**:265. *6235*

1917:38 John Putnam **Merrill**, American physician, born 10 Mar; with co-workers, reported successful kidney transplant, between identical twins, 1956, *JAMA* **160**:277. Died 1986. *4257*

1917:39 John Cowdery **Kendrew**, British molecular biologist, born 24 Mar; shared Nobel Prize (Chemistry), 1962, with Max Ferdinand Perutz, for his studies on globular proteins, particularly myoglobin, *NPL*

1917:40 Robert Bruce **Angier**, American chemist, born 24 Mar; with co-workers, reported the isolation, structural determination and final synthesis of folic acid, 1946, *Science* **103**:667. *3151*

1917:41 Robert Burns **Woodward**, American chemist, born 10 Apr; with co-workers, synthesized cortisone, 1952, *JACS* **74**:4423; awarded the Nobel Prize (Chemistry), 1965, *NPL*. Died 1979. *1155.2*

1917:42 William Drummond MacDonald **Paton**, British pharmacologist, born 5 May; with Eleanor Zaimis, discovered the curare-like anaesthetic action of methonium compounds, 1948, *Nature* **161**:718; introduced hexamethonium bromide, an anaesthetic, 1949, *BJP* **4**:381. Died 1993. *1929.3, 5726*

1917:43 Richard John William **Rees**, British leprologist, born 11 Aug; introduced rifampicin in treatment of leprosy, 1970, *BMJ* **1**:89. *2442.5*

1917:44 John Warcup **Cornforth**, Australian/British chemist, born 7 Sep; shared Nobel Prize (Chemistry), 1975, with Vladimir Prelog, for his contribution to the stereochemistry of enzyme-catalyzed reactions, *NPL*

1917:45 Christian de **Duve**, Belgian cell biologist, born 2 Oct; shared Nobel Prize (Physiology or Medicine), 1974, with Albert Claude and George Emil Palade, for his discoveries concerning the structural and functional organization of the cell, *NPL*.

1917:46 Rodney Robert **Porter**, British immunologist, born 8 Oct; separated and isolated antibodies by partition chromatography, 1955, *BJ* **59**:405. Shared the Nobel Prize (Physiology or Medicine), 1972, with Gerald Maurice Edelman, for their studies concerning the chemical structure of antibodies, *NPL*. Died 1985. *2578.16*

1917:47 Andrew Fielding **Huxley**, British physiologist, born 22 Nov; with A.L. Hodgkin, recorded action potentials form inside a nerve fibre, 1939, *Nature* **144**:710. With R. Niedergerke published fundamental research on the physiology of muscle contraction, 1954, *Nature* **173**:971; 1958, *JP* **144**:403. He shared the Nobel Prize (Physiology or Medicine), 1963, with John Carew Eccles and Alan Lloyd Hodgkin, for their discoveries concerning the ionic mechanisms involved in the excitation and inhibition in the peripheral and central portions of the nerve cell membrane, *NPL*. *1310.1*

---

1917:48 Anne **Goetsch**, American physician, born; treated hypochromic anaemia with iron administered intravenously, 1946, *Blood* **1**:129. *3152*

---

1917: Theodor **Leber** died, **born** 1840. *optic atrophy, diabetes mellitus, eye disorders*

1917: Anton **Wölfler** died, **born** 1850. *gastroenterostomy, thyroid tumours, adenoma*

1917: Caesar Peter Moeller **Boeck** died, **born** 1845. *benign sarcoid*

1917: Emil Theodor **Kocher** died, **born** 1841. *carcinoma of tongue, goitre, myxoedema, thyroidectomy, cachexia strumipriva, subluxation of shoulder-joint, hernia, silk sutures*

1917: Friedrich Georg Rudolph **Wegner** died, **born** 1843. *syphilis*

1917: Joseph Jules **Dejerine** died, **born** 1849. *progressive muscular atrophy, olivo-ponto-cerebellar atrophy, neuritis, peripheral neuritis, tabetic muscular atrophies*

1917: Vladimir Mikhailovich **Kernig** died, **born** 1840. *cerebral meningitis*

1917: Friedrich **Pelizaeus** died, **born** 1850. *centrolobar sclerosis*

1917: Emil Adolf von **Behring** died, **born** 1854. *diphtheria and tetanus antitoxins and immunization*

1917: Louis Théophile Joseph **Landouzy** died, **born** 1845. *herpes zoster, leptospirosis icterohaemorrhagica, progressive muscular atrophy*

1917: Jean Baptiste Auguste **Chauveau** died, **born** 1827. *smallpox*

1917: Leo **Leistikow** died, **born** 1847. *gonococcus*

1917: Tomas **Salazar** died, **born** 1830. *bartonellosis*

1917: Alfred **Einhorn** died, **born** 1856. *local anaesthesia, procaine*

1917: Richard **Liebreich** died, **born** 1830. *fundus oculi, eye*

1917: Arthur von **Hippel** died, **born** 1841. *keratoplasty*

1917: Bernard **Krönig** died, **born** 1863. *caesarean section*

**1918**
1918:1 **Nobel Prize**: no awards

1918:2 **Hokkaido Imperial University** established at **Sapporo**

1918:3 Chair of **Industrial Hygiene** established at **Harvard University**

1918:4 **Deutsche Forschungsinstitut für Psychiatrie** established at **Munich** by Emil **Kraepelin** (1856–1926)

1918:5 **Industrial Fatigue Research Board** established in **London**

1918:6 **[Institute for Experimental Endocrinology]** at **Moscow**

1918:7 **British Orthopaedic Association** founded

1918:8 The most widespread pandemic of **influenza**, affecting people in all inhabited areas of the world and resulting in the death of 20 million persons, occurred in 1918–19. It is comprehensively recorded in *Report on the pandemic of influenza 1918–19, Reports on Public Health and Medical Subjects*, No. 4, London, 1920. *5492*

1918:9 The **Schultz-Charlton reaction** for the diagnosis of **scarlet fever** introduced by Werner Schultz (1878–1944) and Willy Charlton (b.1889), *ZK* **17**:328. *5081*

1918:10 Extirpation of the choroid plexus of the lateral ventricles in communicating **hydrocephalus** introduced by Walter Edward Dandy (1886–1946), *AnS* **68**:569. *4888*

1918:11 Resection of the trigeminal nerve, with conservation of the motor root, used for the treatment of **trigeminal neuralgia** by Max Minor Peet (1885–1949), *JMSMA* **17**:91. *4889*

1918:12 **Tartar emetic (antimony)** introduced in the treatment of **bilharziasis** by John Brian Christopherson (1868–1955), *L* **2**:325. *5350.6*

1918:13 Otto Meyerhof's (1884–1951) work on the chemistry of **muscle** laid the basis for the elucidation of the chemical pathway in the intracellular breakdown of **glucose** to provide energy for biological processes, *HSZ* **101**:165. *959*

1918:14 Mice shown by Yutako Ido (1881–1919) and co-workers to be the carriers of *Leptospira hebdomadis*, causal organism in **seven-day fever**, *JEM* **28**:435. *5334.2*

1918:15 Carl Friderichsen (b.1886) gave an account of the **Waterhouse-Friderichsen syndrome**, *JaK* **87**:109. *4686, 4685*

1918:16 Julius Wagner von Jauregg (1857–1940) inoculated **paretics** with **malaria** to induce **pyrexia**, *PNW* **20**:132, 251; he first used this form of treatment in 1887, to study the effect of **fevers** upon **psychotic conditions**. *4806, 4946*

1918:17 **Cerebral ventriculography** introduced by Walter Edward Dandy (1886–1946), *AnS* **68**:5. *4602*

1918:18 **Kineplastic surgery** (suggested by Vanghetti in 1898) was developed and improved by Vittorio Putti (1880–1940), *BMJ* **1**:635. *4477, 4474*

1918:19 **Cholangiograms** first obtained by Adolph Reich (b.1864), *JAMA* **71**:1555. *3650*

1918:20 The first convincing evidence that **rickets** is a deficiency disease submitted by Edward Mellanby (1884–1955), *JP* **52**: xi, liii; *L* **1**:407. *3733, 3734*

1918:21 *Shigella alkalescens*, an organism causing bacillary **dysentery**, discovered by Frederick William Andrewes (1859–1932), *L* **1**:560. *3542*

1918:22 The **Billroth II gastro-enterostomy** was further modified by Hans Finsterer (1877–1955), *ZCh* **45**:434, and named the **Hofmeister-Finsterer gastro-enterostomy**. *3543, 3529*

1918:23 **Quinidine** shown to be the most effective **cinchona** alkaloid in treatment of **auricular fibrillation** by Walter Frey (b.1884), *BKW* **55**:450. *2848*

1918:24 Vasomotor action of **histamine** studied by Henry Hallett Dale (1875–1968) and Alfred Newton Richards (1876–1966), *JP* **52**:110. *792*

1918:25 **Starling's 'law of the heart'**; Ernest Henry Starling (1866–1927); in his *Linacre Lecture on the law of the heart. 12 853*

---

1918:26 Gertrude Belle **Elion**, American biochemist and pharmacologist, born 23 Jan; shared Nobel Prize (Physiology or Medicine), 1988, with James W. Black and George H. Hitchings, for their discoveries of important principles for drug therapy, *NPL*.

1918:27 Arthur **Kornberg**, American biochemist, born 3 Mar; synthesized DNA, 1956, *BBA* **21**:197. Shared the Nobel Prize (Physiology or Medicine), 1959, with Severo Ochoa, *NPL*. *752.4*

1918:28 Solomon Aaron **Berson**, American physician, born 22 Apr; with Rosalyn Sussman Yalow, carried out first radioimmunoassay of a hormone (insulin), 1960, *JCI* **39**:1157. Yalow shared Nobel Prize (Physiology or Medicine), 1977, for this work, *NPL*. Died 1972. *2578.28*

1918:29 James Daniel **Hardy**, American surgeon, born 14 May; with seven other authors gave an account of an unsuccessful heart transplant from chimpanzee to man, 1964, *JAMA* **188**:1132. *3047.19*

1918:30 Edward B. **Lewis**, American geneticist, born 20 May; shared Nobel Prize (Physiology or Medicine), 1995, with Christiane Nüsslein-Volhard and Eric F. Wieschaus, for their discoveries concerning the genetic control of early embryonic development, *NPL*

1918:31 Edwin Gerhard **Krebs**, American biochemist, born 6 Jun; shared Nobel Prize (Physiology or Medicine), 1992, with Edmond Henri Fischer, for discoveries concerning reversible protein phosphorylation as a biological regulatory mechanism, *NPL*.

1918:32 Frederick **Sanger**, British biochemist, born 13 Aug. For his work on the structure of insulin, 1955, *BJ* **60**:541, he was awarded the Nobel Prize (Chemistry), 1958, *NPL*; for his work on sequencing of DNA he shared the Nobel Prize (Chemistry), 1980, with Paul Berg and Walter Gilbert, *NPL. 1207*

1918:33 Edwin Homer **Ellison**, American surgeon, born 4 Sep; with Robert Milton Zollinger, described the Zollinger-Ellison syndrome, 1955, *AnS* **142**:709. *3558.2*

1918:34 Harold Horace **Hopkins**, British physician, born 6 Dec; with N.S. Kapany, introduced a flexible fibrescope, using static scanning, 1954, *Nature* **173**:39. *3558.1*

---

1918:35 William Edward R. **Greer**, American physician, born; with Chester Scott Keefer, first described cat-scratch fever, 1951, *NEJM* **244**:545. *5546.2*

---

1918: Karl Edwin Konstantin **Hering** died, **born** 1834. *vision*

1918: Korbinian **Brodmann** died, **born** 1868. *Brodmann's area, localization of cerebral function*

1918: Philippe Charles Ernest **Gaucher** died, **born** 1854. *splenic anaemia*

1918: Ernst **Neumann** died, **born** 1834. *leukaemia*

1918: Carlo **Forlanini** died, **born** 1847. *pulmonary tuberculosis, pneumothorax*

1918: Ephraim Fletcher **Ingals** died, **born** 1848. *nasal septum*

1918: Mikolaj **Reichmann** died, **born** 1851. *gastrosuccorrhoea*

1918: George Walter **Caldwell** died, **born** 1834. *maxillary sinus abscess*

1918: Ludwig **Stacke** died, **born** 1859. *excision of auditory ossicles, mastoidectomy*

1918: Leon Konrad **Gliński** died, **born** 1870. *pituitary necrosis, panhypopituitarism*

1918: Max **Wilms** died, **born** 1867. *kidney embryoma*

1918: Hermann David **Weber** died, **born** 1823. *hemiplegia*

1918: Frederick Eustace **Batten** died, **born** 1865. *spinal cord degeneration*

1918: Hans Heinrich Georg **Queckenstedt** died, **born** 1876. *subarachnoid space*

1918: Charles Karsner **Mills** died, **born** 1845. *paralysis*

1918: Georg **Gaffky** died, **born** 1850. *typhoid, Salmonella typhi*

1918: Alexander **Kolisko** died, **born** 1847. *pelvic deformities*

## 1919
1919:1 **Nobel Prize** (Physiology or Medicine): Jean Jules Baptiste Vincent Bordet (1870–1961), for work in **immunology**, *NPL. 2547, 2551, 2552*

1919:2 **Ministry of Health, England**, established to supersede **Local Government Board**

1919:3 **University of Brno (Masaryk University)** established

1919:4 **University of Cologne** founded

1919:5 **University of Hamburg** founded

1919:6 **University of Ljubljana** founded

1919:7 **University of Riga** founded

1919:8 **University of Posen** founded

1919:9 **University of Pressburg** (1914) becomes **University of Bratislava**

1919:10 **School of Hygiene and Public Health, Johns Hopkins University**, opened at **Baltimore**

1919:11 **General Nursing Council**, UK, established

1919:12 **League of Red Cross Societies** founded

1919:13 **Purkyne Neurological Society** founded at **Prague**

1919:14 [**Moscow Medical Institute**] founded

1919:15 **International Bureau of Labour (Geneva)**

1919:16 **Mercurochrome** introduced for the treatment of urinary tract infections by Hugh Hampton Young (1870–1945) and colleagues, *JAMA* **73**:1483. *1908*

1919:17 Experimental transmission of **epidemic encephalitis** carried out by Leo Loewe (b.1876) and Israel Strauss (b.1873), *JAMA* **73**:1056. *4651*

1919:18 **Metropathia haemorrhagica** first described by Robert Schroeder (1884–1959), *ArGy* **110**:633. *6126*

1919:19 The **Hurler syndrome (lipochondrodystrophy and gargoylism)** so named after the description by Gertrud Hurler, *ZK* **24**:220, although she was preceded in this by C. Hunter. *6371.2, 6371.1*

1919:20 A low cervical **caesarean section** operation (**laparotrachelotomy**) described by Joseph Bolivar DeLee (1869–1942), *JAMA* **73**:91. *6251*

1919:21 A description of what later became known as the **Hand-Schüller-Christian syndrome**, given by Henry Asbury Christian (1876–1951); in his paper in *Contributions to medical and biological research dedicated to Sir William Osler*, **1**, 390. *6359–6363*

1919:22 Important studies on **Rocky Mountain spotted fever** carried out by Simeon Burt Wolbach (1880–1954); he mentioned the causal agent, ***Dermacentroxenus rickettsii*** (later named ***Rickettsia rickettsii***), *JMR* **41**:1. *5391*

1919:23 Causal organism of **typhus** demonstrated by Howard Taylor Ricketts (1871–1910), *JAMA* **54**:1373. *5380.1*

1919:24 The principal exponent of **behaviourist psychology** was John Broadus Watson (1878–1958); *Psychology from the standpoint of a behaviorist*. *4987*

1919:25 **Pneumoencephalography** introduced by Walter Edward Dandy (1886–1946), *AnS* **70**:397. *4603*

1919:26 **Rickets** cured with **ultraviolet irradiation** by Kurt Huldschinsky (1883–1941), *DMW* **45**:712. *3732*

1919:27 The **Folin-Wu test** for **blood sugar** devised by Otto Knut Olof Folin (1867–1934) and Hsien Wu (1895–1959), *JBC* **38**:81. *3922*

1919:28 Thomas Peel Dunhill (1876–1957), a pioneer in **thyroid surgery**, devised a new technique for the removal of **exophthalmic goitre**, *BJS* **7**:195. *3849.1*

1919:29 Serge Voronoff (1866–1951) reported his experimental **rejuvenation operation (testicular transplantation)**; in his *Greffes testiculaires*, 1923. *3797*

1919:30 Classical work on surgery of **temporal bone**, *Essays on the surgery of the temporal bone*, published by Charles Alfred Ballance (1856–1926) and Charles David Green (1862–1937). *3403.1, 4889.1*

1919:31 Modification of the standard operative procedures for the cure of **femoral** and **inguinal hernia** by G. Paul Laroque (1876–1934), *SGO* **29**:507. *3608.2*

1919:32 **Cardiospasm** with **oesophageal dilatation** reported by Porter Paisley Vinson (1890–1959), *MCNA* **3**:623; a condition already noted by Henry Stanley Plummer (1912) and named '**Plummer-Vinson syndrome**'. *3321*

1919:33 A classic account of severe **anaemias of pregnancy**, with a classification, given by William Osler (1849–1919), *BMJ* **1**:1. *3136*

1919:34 **Syphilis: Sachs-Georgi diagnostic reaction** introduced by Hans Sachs (1877–1945) and Walter Georgi (1889–1920), *MMW* **66**:440. *2408*

1919:35 **Mitsuda (lepromin) reaction** introduced by Kensuke Mitsuda (b.1876) for diagnosis of **leprosy**, *Hinyoka Zasshi* **19**:697 [*IJL* (1953) **21**:347, English translation by Mitsuda]. *2440*

1919:36 **Tryparsamide** introduced in treatment of trypanosome infections by Walter Abraham Jacobs (1883–1967) and Michael Heidelberger (1888–1991), *JEM* **30**:411. *1907*

1919:37 First textbook on **aviation medicine**, *Medical and surgical aspects of aviation*, published by H. Graeme Anderson. *2137.5*

1919:38 Isolation of **heparin** by William Henry Howell (1860–1945) and Luther Emmett Holt (1855–1924), *AmJPh* **47**:328. *905*

1919:39 Experimental **shock** produced by **histamine**, reported by Henry Hallett Dale (1875–1968) and Patrick Playfair Laidlaw (1881–1940) and shown to be similar to traumatic and surgical shock, *JP* **52**:355. *5630*

1919:40 Joe-Hin **Tjio**, Indonesian/American biologist, born 11 Feb; with J.A. Levan (b.1905), showed the chromosome number in man to be 46, 1956, *Her* **42**:1. *256.5*

1919:41 Hunter Hall **Comly**, American physician, born 31 Jul; reported methaemoglobinaemia, 1945, *JAMA* **129**:112. *3103*

1919:42 Godfrey Newbold **Hounsfield**, British electrical engineer, born 28 Aug; introduced computer-assisted tomography (CAT), or computed tomography (CT), 1973, *BJR* **46**:1016. For this work he shared the Nobel Prize (Physiology or Medicine), 1979, with Alan Macleod Cormack, *NPL*. *2700.4*

1919:43 Joseph E. **Murray**, American surgeon, born; shared Nobel Prize (Physiology or Medicine), 1990, with Edward Donnall Thomas, for their discoveries concerning organ and cell transplantation in the treatment of human diseases, *NPL*. *4257*

1919:44 Wyndham **Cottle** died; first described angiokeratoma, 1879, *SGHR* **9**:753; called 'Mibelli's disease' after the description by the latter in 1891. *4071, 4105*

1919: Franz **Nissl** died, **born** 1860. *Nissl's stain, Nissl's granules*

1919: Emil **Fischer** died, **born** 1852. *barbitone*

1919: Thomas Richard **Fraser** died, **born** 1841. *physostigmine (eserine), Strophanthus*

1919: Vincenzo **Cervello** died, **born** 1854. *paraldehyde*

1919: Pieter Klazes **Pel** died, **born** 1852. *lymphadenoma*

1919: François Henri **Hallopeau** died, **born** 1842. *pemphigus vegetans*

1919: Wilhelm Heinrich **Erb** died, **born** 1840. *brachial plexus paralysis*

1919: William Allen **Sturge** died, **born** 1850. *naevus*

1919: Edward **Liveing** died, **born** 1832. *migraine*

1919: Johann **Hoffmann** died, **born** 1857. *progressive muscular atrophy*

1919: James Ewing **Mears** died, **born** 1838. *trigeminal neuralgia*

1919: William **Alexander** died, **born** 1844. *epilepsy, retroversion of uterus*

1919: Leonardo **Bianchi** died, **born** 1848. *frontal lobes and character changes*

1919: André **Chantemesse** died, **born** 1851. *bacillary dysentery, Shigella, anti-typhoid inoculation*

1919: Hermann **Oppenheim** died, **born** 1858. *amyotonia congenita, pineal tumour*

1919: Masanori **Ogata** died, **born** 1852. *plague, flea*

1919: Yutako **Ido** died, **born** 1881. *leptospirosis icterohaemorrhagica, seven-day fever*

1919: Franz **Kuhn** died, **born** 1866. *anaesthesia, intratracheal insufflation*

1919: Thomas Addis **Emmet** died, **born** 1828. *vesico-vaginal fistula, perineorrhaphy, cystitis, vaginal cystotomy*

1919: Hippolyte **Morestin** died, **born** 1869. *mammaplasty*

1919: Abraham **Jacobi** died, **born** 1830. *paediatrics*

1919: Luigi Maria **Bossi** died, **born** 1859. *induction of premature labour*

1919: Ernst Heinrich Philipp August **Haeckel** died, **born** 1834. *Darwinism*

1919: William **Osler** died, **born** 1849. *medical textbook, telangiectasis, bacterial endocarditis, polycythaemia, erythraemia, pernicious anaemia, anaemias of pregnancy*

**1920**

1920:1 **Nobel Prize** (Physiology or Medicine): Schack August Steenberg Krogh (1874–1949), for work on the **physiology of capillaries**, *NPL. 793*

1920:2 **Medical Research Committee (UK)** renamed **Medical Research Council**

1920:3 **Association for Research in Nervous and Mental Diseases (New York)** founded

1920:4 **Union Internationale Contre la Tuberculose (Paris)** organized

1920:5 **National Health Council (US)** organized

1920:6 **[Society of Czechoslovak Physicians]** founded

1920:7 **Deutsche Pharmakologische Gesellschaft** founded

1920:8 **Société Internationale d'Histoire de la Médecine** founded, **Paris**

1920:9 **Institut International d'Anthropologie (Paris)** founded

1920:10 **Institut Pasteur Hellenique** opened at **Athens**

1920:11 A tubal insufflation method for diagnosis and treatment of **sterility** due to occlusion of the **Fallopian tubes** introduced by Isador Clinton Rubin (1883–1958), *JAMA* **74**:1017; **75**:661. *6127*

1920:12 Studies on the production of heat in **muscle** published by Archibald Vivian Hill (1886–1977), *JP* **54**:84. *659*

1920:13 **Herpangina** first described by John Zahorsky (b.1871), *SMJ* **13**:871. *5538*

1920:14 Demonstration that bilateral destruction of the **frontal lobes** caused **character changes** by Leonardo Bianchi (1848–1919); in his *La mecanica del cervello e la funzione dei lobe frontale. 4891*

1920:15 **Suramin (Bayer 205)** introduced in the treatment of **trypanosomiasis** by Ludwig Haendel (1869–1939) and Karl Wilhelm Joetten (b.1886), *BKW* **57**:821. *5286*

1920:16 In their classic account of the condition, Thomas Peck Sprunt (b.1884) and Frank Alexander Evans (b.1889) introduced the term '**infectious mononucleosis**', *BJH* **31**:410. *5486.1*

1920:17 **Splanchnic anaesthesia** introduced by Max Kappis (1881–1938), *ZCh* **47**:98. *5701*

1920:18 **Cisternal puncture** introduced by James Bourne Ayer (1882–1963), *ArNP* **4**:529. *4890*

1920:19 **Spastic pseudosclerosis ('Creutzfeldt-Jakob disease')** described by Hans Gerhard Creutzfeldt (1885–1964), *ZGN* **57**:1. Jakob also described it (1921). *4719.1, 4722*

1920:20 The treatment of **tetany** with **ultraviolet light** introduced by Kurt Huldschinsky (1883–1941), *ZK* **26**:207. *4836*

1920:21 Disease of the **corpora striata** (**status dysmyelinatus syndrome, 'Vogt syndrome'**) described by Cécile Vogt (1875–1962) and Oskar Vogt (1870–1959), *JPN*, Ergänz. iii:627. *4720*

1920:22 Demonstration of the experimental production of **pellagra** and its prevention by proper diet by Joseph Goldberger (1874–1929), *USPHL* **120**:7. *3757*

1920:23 Eugen Steinach (1861–1944) introduced his **rejuvenation** operation (ligation of the **vas deferens**); in his *Verjüngung durch experimentelle Neubelebung der alternden Pubertätsdrüse*. *3796*

1920:24 **Vesiculography** first demonstrated by Hugh Hampton Young (1870–1945) and Charles Alexander Waters (b.1885), *AmJR* **7**:16. *4198*

1920:25 George Lenthal Cheatle (1865–1951) was first to adopt the preperitoneal approach in the repair of **hernia**, *BMJ* **2**:68. *3608.3*

1920:26 Classification of **tumours** introduced by Albert Compton Broders (1885–1964), as an index of malignancy, *JAMA* **74**:656. *2645*

1920:27 **Angina pectoris** treated by cervical sympathectomy by Thomas Jonnesco (1860–1926), *BuAM* **84**:93. *2895*

1920:28 **Vectorcardiography** initiated by Hubert Mann (1891–1975), *ArIM* **25**:283. *2853.1*

1920:29 Emil Abderhalden (1877–1950) contributed notably to the technique and methodology of **physiology** and **biochemistry**, especially through his editorship of the *Handbuch der biologischen Arbeitsmethoden*, 107 vols, 1920–1939. *136*

---

1920:30 Albert **Schatz**, American microbiologist, born 2 Feb; with E. Bugie and Selman Abraham Waksman, discovered streptomycin, 1944, *PSEB* **55**:66. *1935*

1920:31 Edward Donnall **Thomas**, American physician and oncologist, born 15 Mar; shared Nobel Prize (Physiology or Medicine), 1990, with Joseph E. Murray, for their discoveries concerning organ and cell transplantation in the treatment of human disease, *NPL*.

1920:32 Edmond Henri **Fischer**, American biochemist, born 6 Apr; shared Nobel Prize (Physiology or Medicine), 1992, with Edwin Gerhard Krebs, for discoveries concerning reversible protein phosphorylation as a biological regulatory mechanism, *NPL*.

1920:33 François **Jacob**, French geneticist, born 17 Jun; shared the Nobel Prize (Physiology or Medicine), 1965, with Jacques Lucien Monod and André Michael Lwoff, for their work on the genetic control of enzyme and virus synthesis, 1961, *JMB* **3**:318, *NPL*. *256.9*

1920:34 Denton Arthur **Cooley**, American cardiovascular surgeon, born 22 Aug; with D.E. Mahaffey and M.E. DeBakey, excised the aortic arch for aortic aneurysm and replaced it with a prosthesis, 1955, *SGO* **101**:667. With co-workers, treated ventricular aneurysm by excision and cardiopulmonary bypass, 1959, *AnS* **150**:595. *2993.2, 3047.13*

1920:35 Peter Denis **Mitchell**, British biochemist, born 30 Sep; awarded Nobel Prize (Chemistry), 1978, for his contribution to the understanding of biological energy transfer through the formulation of the chemiosmotic theory, *NPL*. Died 1992.

1920:36 Carl Hellmuth **Hertz**, German physicist, born 15 Oct; with Inge Edler, introduced echocardiography, 1954, *Kongliga Fysiografiska Sällskapets i Lund Förhandlingar*, **24**:1. *2883.01*

1920:37 Baruj **Benacerraf**, Venezuelan/American immunologist, born 29 Oct; with Hugh O'Neill McDevitt, showed that immune response was genetically determined, 1972, *Science* **175**:273. Shared Nobel Prize (Physiology or Medicine), 1980, with Jean Baptiste Gabriel Joachim Dausset and George Davis Snell, for his work on histocompatibility-linked immune response genes, *NPL. 2578.29*

1920:38 Melvin H. **Kaplan**, American immunologist, born 23 Dec; with Albert Hewett, introduced antigen location by fluorescent antibody technique, 1950, *JEM* **91**:1. *2578.8*

1920:39 Charles **Heidelberger**, American oncologist, born 23 Dec; with co-workers, synthesized 5-fluorouracil, a tumour-inhibiting compound, 1957, *Nature* **179**:663. *2660.9*

---

1920: Dmitri Iosifovich **Ivanovski** died, **born** 1864. *tobacco mosaic disease virus*

1920: Walter **Georgi** died, **born** 1889. *syphilis*

1920: Nicolai Sergeievich **Korotkov** died, **born** 1874. *blood pressure, stethoscope*

1920: Vasili Parmenovich **Obraztsov** died, **born** 1849. *coronary thrombosis*

1920: Moritz Wilhelm Hugo **Ribbert** died, **born** 1855. *embryonal theory of cancer*

1920: Adam **Politzer** died, **born** 1835. *eustachian tube, membrana tympani, otosclerosis, acumeter, otology*

1920: Dagobert **Schwabach** died, **born** 1846. *hearing test*

1920: Ludwik **Rydygier** died, **born** 1850. *carcinomatous pylorus*

1920: William James **Morton** died, **born** 1845. *dental radiography*

1920: Benjamin Robinson **Schenck** died, **born** 1872. *sporotrichosis*

1920: Henri **Triboulet** died, **born** 1864. *rheumatism, streptococci*

1920: Rocco **Gritti** died, **born** 1826. *amputation of thigh*

1920: Moritz **Benedikt** died, **born** 1835. *oculomotor nerve paralysis*

1920: Anton **Weichselbaum** died, **born** 1845. *cerebral meningitis, Neisseria meningitidis*

1920: Stephanos **Kartulis** died, **born** 1852. *amoebiasis*

1920: Wilhelm Max **Wundt** died, **born** 1832. *experimental psychology, sensory perception*

1920: William Crawford **Gorgas** died, **born** 1854. *yellow fever*

1920: Samuel James **Meltzer** died, **born** 1851. *anaesthesia, intratracheal insufflation, asthma, anaphylaxis*

1920: Ernst **Wertheim** died, **born** 1864. *gonorrhoeal infection of uterus, gonococcal cystitis, cancer of uterus*

**1921**
1921:1 **Nobel Prize** (Physiology or Medicine): No award

1921:2 **Harvard School of Public Health, Boston**, founded

1921:3 **National Institute for Industrial Psychology, London**, founded

1921:4 **Dental Board of the United Kingdom** established

1921:5 **American Birth Control League** founded by Margaret **Sanger** (1883–1966)

1921:6 **Schweizerisches Gesellschaft für Geschichte der Medizin** founded in **Zürich**

1921:7 **[State Microbiological Institute]**, **Moscow**, founded

1921:8 **Australian National Research Council (Sydney)** organized

1921:9 **Gorgas Memorial Institute of Tropical and Preventive Medicine (Chicago)** founded

1921:10 **[Society of History of Science and Medicine]**, **Munich**, founded

1921:11 **International Conference on Standardization of Diphtheria Antitoxin, London**, which marked the beginning of international **biological standardization**, the major centres being the National Institute for Medical Research, London [Henry Hallett Dale] and the Statens Serum Institut, Copenhagen [Thorvald Madsen]

1921:12 A new operation for the repair of **cleft palate** introduced by Harold Delf Gillies (1882–1960) and William Kelsey Fry (1889–1963), *BMJ* **1**:335. *5759*

1921:13 The true nature of **endometrioma** of the **ovary** explained by John Albertson Sampson (1873–1946), *ArSuC* **3**:245. *6128*

1921:14 The **carbon tetrachloride** treatment of **ankylostomiasis** introduced by Maurice Crowther Hall (1881–1938), *JAMA* **77**:1641. *5368*

1921:15 **Peridural anaesthesia** introduced by Fidel Pagés Miravé (d.1924), *RSM* **11**:351, 389. *5702*

1921:16 *Rickettsia prowazeki*, causal agent in **typhus**, first isolated from blood by Leo Loewe (b.1896) and co-workers, *JAMA* **77**:1967. *5392*

1921:17 **Tryparsamide** introduced in the treatment of **trypanosomiasis** by Louise Pearce (1885–1959), *JEM* **34** Suppl. 1. *5287*

1921:18 The method of **myelography** by air injection into the **spinal subarachnoid space** introduced by Sofus Wideröe (b.1880), *ZCh* **48**:394. *4605.1*

1921:19 Positive contrast **myelography** with iodized oil (**lipiodol**) introduced by Jean Athanase Sicard (1872–1929) and Jacques Forestier (b.1890), *ReN* **28**:1264. *2693, 4605*

1921:20 A test ('**inkblot**') to determine **personality traits** devised by Hermann Rorschach (1884–1922); in his *Psychodiagnostik. 4988.1*

1921:21 **Kyphosis** due to **epiphyseal necrosis in vertebrae** ('**Scheuermann's disease**') noted by Holger Werfel Scheuermann (1877–1960), *ZOC* **41**:305. *4389*

1921:22 A rare form of **bone sarcoma** ('**Ewing's sarcoma**'), diffuse endothelioma of bone, described by James Ewing (1866–1943), *PNYP* **21**:17. *4388*

1921:23 First report of the use of the **laparoscope** for **arthroscopy** by Eugen Bircher, *ZCh* **48**:460. *4388.2*

1921:24 The importance of **encephalitis** as a cause of **parkinsonism** recognized by Achille Alexandre Souques (1860–1944), *ReN* **28**:534. *4723*

1921:25 Charles Foix (1882–1927) showed that the specific lesion in **Parkinson's disease** is located in the substantia nigra of the midbrain, *ReN* **28**:593. *4721*

1921:26 Alfons Maria Jakob (1884–1931) described **spastic pseudosclerosis**, already recorded by Creutzfeldt (1920), *ZGN* **64**:147; it is also named '**Creutzfeldt-Jakob disease**'. *4722, 4719.1*

1921:27 **Ryle's tube** for obtaining specimens of **gastric juice** devised by John Alfred Ryle (1889–1950), *GHR* **71**:42. *3544*

1921:28 The **Achard-Thiers syndrome**, the combination of hirsutism with **diabetes**, established by Emile Charles Achard (1860–1944) and Joseph Thiers, *BuAM* **86**:51. *3870*

1921:29 Nicolas Constantin Paulescu (1869–1931) isolated **insulin** before Frederick Grant Banting and Charles Herbert Best; he named it '**pancréine**', *ArIPh* **17**:**85**. *3965*

1921:30 First successful ligation of **abdominal aorta** by George Tully Vaughan (1859–1948), *AnS* **74**:308. *2970*

1921:31 First **pericardiectomy** for constrictive **pericarditis** by Paul Hallopeau (1876–1924), *BSCP* **47**:1120. *3030*

1921:32 **Erythrocyte sedimentation rate** measurement, **Westergren's method**, introduced by Alf Vilhelm Westergren (b.1891), *AcM* **54**:247. *3085*

1921:33 Antispasmodic action of **theophylline** on **bronchial smooth muscle** demonstrated by David Israel Macht (1882–1961) and Gui-ching Ting, leading to its use in management of **asthma**, *JPET* **18**:373. *3197.1*

1921:34 **Carcinoma** of **pharynx** treated with **radiotherapy** by Henri Coutard (1876–1950), ('**Coutard method**'), *BAFC* **10**:160. *3196*

1921:35 **Syphilis: bismuth** treatment introduced by Robert Sazerac (b.1875) and Constantin Levaditi (1874–1953), *CRAS* **173**:338. *2411*

1921:36 '**Prausnitz-Küstner reaction**', the presence of **antibodies** in the serum of persons suffering from atopic diseases, demonstrated by Otto Carl Willy Prausnitz (1876–1963) and Heinz Küstner (1897–1931), *ZBP* **I 86**:160. *2601.1*

1921:37 The history of the **British medical services in the First World War** (1914–1918) recorded in *History of the Great War. Medical Services*, 12 vols, 1921–29. *2178*

1921:38 The history of the **US Army medical services in the First World War** recorded in *The Medical Department of the U.S. Army in the World War*, 15 vols, 1921–29. *2179*

1921:39 Isolation of **glutathione** by Frederick Gowland Hopkins (1861–1947), *BJ* **15**:286. *745*

1921:40 **Growth hormone** of the anterior pituitary discovered by Herbert McLean Evans (1882–1971) and Joseph Abraham Long (b.1879), *AR* **21**:62. *1163*

1921:41 **Insulin** isolated by Frederick Grant Banting (1891–1941) and Charles Herbert Best (1899–1978), *JLCM* **7**:251, *AmJPh* 1922, **59**:479. *1205*

1921:42 **Blood grouping, medicolegal applications**, pioneer work by Reuben Ottenberg (b.1882), *JAMA* **77**:682, **78**:873, **79**:2137. *1756*

1921:43 **Ergotamine** isolated by Karl Spiro (1867–1932) and Arthur Stoll (1887–1971), *SMW* **2**:525. *1910*

1921:44 **Involuntary nervous system** mapped out by John Newport Langley (1852–1925); in his *The autonomic nervous system*. *1332*

1921:45 Research on the chemical mediation of **nervous impulses** reported by Otto Loewi (1873–1961), 1921–24, *HSZ* **189**:239; **193**:201; **203**:408; **204**:361,629. *1343*

---

1921:46 Robin Royston Amos **Coombs**, British immunologist, born 9 Jan; with co-workers, devised test for Rhesus sensitization, ('Coombs' test'), 1945, *L* **2**:15; *BJEP* **26**:255. *3104*

1921:47 Michael Anthony **Epstein**, British pathologist, born 18 May; with Y.M. Barr, discovered Epstein-Barr virus, a human herpesvirus implicated in Burkitt's lymphoma, 1964, *L* **1**;252, 272. *2660.17, 2660.18*

1921:48 Frederick Leland **Schaffer**, American biochemist and microbiologist, born 5 Jul; with Carlton Everett Schwerdt, crystallized poliomyelitis virus particles, 1955, *PNAS* **41**:1020. *2527.1*

1921:49 Alick **Isaacs**, British virologist, born 17 Jul; with Jean Lindenmann, discovered interferon, 1957, *PRSB* **147**:258. Died 1967. *2578.22*

1921:50 Rosalyn Sussman **Yalow**, American immunologist and endocrinologist, born 19 Jul; with Solomon A. Berson, carried out first radioimmunoassay of a hormone (insulin), 1960, *JCI* **39**:1157. She shared Nobel Prize (Physiology or Medicine), 1977, with Roger Charles Louis Guillemin and Andrew Victor Schally, for her development of radioimmunoassays of peptide hormones, *NPL*. *2578.28*

1921:51 Felix **Wroblewski**, American physician, born 8 Aug; with John Samuel LaDue, introduced diagnostic test for myocardial infarction, 1955, *Cir* **11**:871. *2883.1*

1921:52 Rupert Everett **Billingham**, British zoologist and immunologist, born 15 Oct; with Peter Brian Medawar, Leslie Brent and E.M. Sparrow, provided proof of Burnet-Fenner theory (1949) of acquired immunological tolerance, 1953, *Nature* **172**:603. *2578.11*

1921:53 Frederick Reuben **Hanson**, American microbiologist, born; with Thomas Eugene Eble, isolated fumagillin, an amoebicidal antibiotic, 1949, *JB* **58**:527, *Science* **113**:202. *1945*

1921:54 Thomas C. **Peebles**, American physician, born; with John Franklin Enders, isolated measles virus, 1954, *PSEB* **86**:277. *5449.2*

1921: Felix **Semon** died, **born** 1849. *thyroid, myxoedema, cachexia strumipriva, cretinism*

1921: Jan **Janský** died, **born** 1873. *blood classification*

1921: Johann Ernst Oswald **Schmiedeberg** died, **born** 1838. *digitoxin*

1921: Richard Julius **Petri** died, **born** 1852. *Petri dish*

1921: Heinrich Wilhelm Gottfried **Waldeyer-Hartz** died, **born** 1836. *cancer, epithelial cells*

1921: John Wickham **Legg** died, **born** 1843. *telangiectasis*

1921: Arthur Bowen Richards **Myers** died, **born** 1838. *effort syndrome*

1921: Carl Ludwig **Fiedler** died, **born** 1835. *myocarditis*

1921: Charles-Emile **François-Franck** died, **born** 1849. *cardiac valvulotomy*

1921: Gustav **Killian** died, **born** 1860. *bronchoscopy, laryngoscopy*

1921: Albert **Niemann** died, **born** 1880. *Niemann-Pick disease*

1921: Heinrich Ernst **Albers-Schönberg** died, **born** 1865. *osteopetrosis fragilis, osteopoikilosis, radiography*

1921: Wilhelm Heinrich **Erb** died, **born** 1840. *nervous disorders, paralysis, muscular dystrophies, syphilitic spinal paralysis, tabes dorsalis, knee-jerk, myasthenia pseudoparalytica, tetany*

1921: André Louis François Justin **Martin** died, **born** 1853. *diphtheria antitoxin*

1921: Dmitriy Leonidovich **Romanovsky** died, **born** 1861. *malaria stain*

1921: Emil **Pfeiffer** died, **born** 1846. *infectious mononucleosis*

1921: Ernesto **Odriozola** died, **born** 1862. *bartonellosis, Carrión's disease*

**1922**
1922:1 **Nobel Prize** (Physiology or Medicine): Archibald Vivian Hill (1886–1977), for his discoveries relating to the production of **heat** in **muscles**, *NPL. 659*; Otto Fritz Meyerhof (1884–1951), for research on consumption of **oxygen** and metabolism of **lactic acid** in man, *NPL. 959*

1922:2 **Finnish University, Tartu**, opened

1922:3 **University of Kaunas, Lithuania**, founded

1922:4 **[German Society of Industrial Hygiene]** founded

1922:5 **[Institute for the History of Science], Heidelberg**

1922:6 **[State Radium Institute], Leningrad**

1922:7 **Institut Pasteur** at **Brazzaville**

1922:8 **American Society of Clinical Pathologists, Denver**, founded

1922:9 **[Biological Institute], Guadalajara, Mexico**

1922:10 **Army Medical Library, Washington** (formerly Library of the Surgeon General's Office) established

1922:11 ***Premature and congenitally diseased infants***, by Julius H. Hess (1876–1955) was the first book dealing solely with the subject. *6348.1*

1922:12 The regulation of the motor mechanism of **capillaries** discovered by Schack August Sternberg Krogh (1874–1949); in his *The anatomy and physiology of the capillaries. 793*

1922:13 Cases of what was later named the **Laurence-Moon-Biedl syndrome, retinitis pigmentosa** with familial developmental imperfections, reported by Artur Biedl (1869–1933), *DMW* **48**:1630. *6369, 6368*

1922:14 Overlapping of the fetal skull bones as a sign of **fetal death** *in utero* ('**Spalding's sign**'), first described by Alfred Baker Spalding (1874–1942), *SGO* **35**:754. *6221.1*

1922:15 *Rickettsia prowazeki* confirmed as causal agent in **typhus** by Simeon Burt Wolbach (1880–1954) and co-workers; in his *The etiology and pathology of typhus. 5393*

1922:16 An association of a port-wine **naevus** with a vascular abnormality of the **meninges** on the same side described by Frederick Parkes Weber (1863–1962), *JNP* **3**:134, already recorded by Sturge (1879) – ('**Sturge-Weber syndrome**'). *4605.2, 4560.1*

1922:17 A syndrome affecting the **extrapyramidal system** ('**Hallervorden-Spatz syndrome**') described by Julius Hallervorden (1882–1965) and Hugo Spatz (1888–1969), *ZGN* **79**:254. *4724*

1922:18 *Lactobacillus odontolyticus*, suspected of causing **dental caries** isolated in them by James McIntosh and co-workers, *BJEP* **3**:138; **5**:175. *3691*

1922:19 The **chromaffin cell tumour** of the **adrenal medulla** first fully described by Ernest Marcel Labbe (1870–1939) and co-workers, *BSMH* **46**:982. *3871*

1922:20 A **pancreatic extract** isolated by Frederick Grant Banting (1891–1941), Charles Herbert Best (1899–1978) and John James Rickard Macleod (1876–1935) was named **insulin**, *AmJPh* **66**:479; *JLCM* **7**:251. *3966, 3967*

1922:21 The first clinical application of **insulin** in the treatment of **diabetes mellitus** made by Frederick Grant Banting and co-workers, *CMAJ* **12**:141. *3968*

1922:22 **Sickle-cell anaemia** so named by Vern Rheem Mason (b.1889), *JAMA* **79**:1318. *3136.1*

1922:23 **Agranulocytic angina** ('**Schultz's syndrome**') first described by Werner Schultz (1878–1944), *DMW* **48**:1195. *3086*

1922:24 Value of **theophylline** in the management of **asthma** established by Samson Hirsch, *KW* **1**:615. *3197.2*

1922:25 **Angina pectoris** treated by paravertebral injection of **novocaine** by Arthur Laewen (1876–1958), *ZCh* **49**:1510. *2896*

1922:26 **Lysozyme**, a bacteriolytic secretion, isolated by Alexander Fleming (1881–1955), *PRSB* **93**:306. *1910.1*

1922:27 **Syphilis: Kahn precipitation test** introduced by Reuben Leon Kahn (b.1887), *ArDS* **5**:570. *2412*

1922:28 **Syphilis: Kolmer complement-fixation test** introduced by John Albert Kolmer (1886–1962), *AmJSy* **6**:82. *2413*

1922:29 **Vitamin E** discovered by Herbert McLean Evans (1882–1971) and Katharine Scott Bishop (1888–1976), *Science* **56**:650. *1055*

1922:30 **Vitamin D** discovered by Elmer Verney McCollum (1879–1967) and co-workers, *JBC* **53**:297. *1054.1*

1922:31 **Gastroscopy** developed by Rudolph Schindler (1888–1968), *ArV* **69**:535. *3545*

1922:32 *Plasmodium ovale*, a **malaria** parasite, first described by John William Watson Stephens (1865–1946), *AnTM* **16**:383. *5255.2*

1922:33 The photometric **spectacle lens** introduced by Marius Hans Erik Tscherning (1851–1939), *AnO* **159**:625. *5967*

_____

1922:34 Har Gobind **Khorana**, Indian/American chemist, born 9 Jan; reported chemical synthesis of deoxyribonucleotides, 1958, *JACS* **80**:1580; shared Nobel Prize (Physiology or Medicine), 1968, with Robert William Holley and Marshall Warren Nirenberg, for his establishment of techniques for the synthesis of polynucleotides, *NPL*. *752.6*

1922:35 Robert William **Holley**, American biochemist, born 28 Jan; reported complete sequence of alanine transfer RNA, 1965, *Science* **147**:1462; shared Nobel Prize (Physiology or Medicine), 1968, with Marshall Warren Nirenberg and Har Gobind Khorana, for his work on RNA, *NPL*. *257.2*

1922:36 George Eugene **Moore**, American physician, born 22 Feb; introduced radioactive isotopes (fluorescein) in neuroradiology, 1947, *Science* **106**:130. *4615.1*

1922:37 Ernest Ludwig **Wynder**, German/American physician, born 30 Apr; with Evarts Ambrose Graham, proved association of lung cancer with cigarette smoking by case-control study, 1950), *JAMA* **143**:329. *3215.1*

1922:38 Harold James Charles **Swan**, Irish/American cardiologist, born 1 Jun; with co-workers, used flow-guided balloon-tipped catheter in cardiac catheterization, 1970, *NEJM* **283**:447. *2883.9*

1922:39 Robert Armstrong **Nelson**, American microbiologist, born 2 Oct; with Manfred Martin Mayer, introduced Nelson treponemal immobilization test for syphilis diagnosis, 1949, *JEM* **89**:369. *2419*

1922:40 Donald Nixon **Ross**, British cardiac surgeon, born 4 Oct; replaced aortic valve with a homograft placed below the coronary orifice, 1964, *L* **2**:487. *3047.17*

1922:41 Christiaan Neethling **Barnard**, S. African surgeon, born 8 Nov; performed the first human heart transplant on 3 Dec. 1967, *SAMJ* **41**:1271; the patient died on 21 Dec. *3047.20*

1922:42 Stanley **Cohen**, American biochemist, born 17 Nov; shared Nobel Prize (Physiology or Medicine), 1986, with Rita Levi-Montalcini, for their discovery of growth factors, *NPL*.

_____

1922:43 Franklin Allen **Neva**, American physician born; with Thomas Huckle Weller, isolated the rubella virus, 1962, *PSEB* **111**:215, simultaneously with Parkman and co-workers. *5509.1, 5509.2*

_____

1922: Augustus Désiré **Waller** died, **born** 1856. *electrocardiography*

1922: Sydney **Ringer** died, **born** 1834. *Ringer's solution*

1922: Jokichi **Takamine** died, **born** 1854. *adrenaline*

1922: William Williams **Keen** died, **born** 1837. *x rays*

1922: Alfred **Kirstein** died, **born** 1863. *laryngoscopy*

1922: Arthur William **Bacot** died, **born** 1866. *plague, flea*

1922: Heinrich Irenaeus **Quincke** died, **born** 1842. *hepatic artery aneurysm, angioneurotic oedema, lumbar puncture, Entamoeba histolytica, Escherichia coli*

1922: Gustav **Fütterer** died, **born** 1854. *typhoid, Salmonella typhi*

1922: Hermann **Rorschach** died, **born** 1884. *personality, inkblot test*

1922: Patrick **Manson** died, **born** 1844. *tropical disease, mosquito-malaria transmission hypothesis, filarial elephantiasis, Wuchereria bancrofti, paragonimiasis, Paragonimus rigeri*

1922: Arthur **Felix** died, **born** 1887. *typhus*

1922: Charles Louis Alphonse **Laveran** died, **born** 1845. *malaria, Toxoplasma*

1922: Carl Ludwig **Schleich** died, **born** 1859. *local infiltration anaesthesia*

1922: William Stewart **Halsted** died, **born** 1852. *surgery, rubber gloves, subclavian artery ligation, inguinal hernia, local infiltration anaesthesia, mastectomy*

1922: Edmund **Weil** died, **born** 1880. *typhus*

1922: Otto **Busse** died, **born** 1867. *blastomycosis, cryptococcosis*

1922: Nikolai Evgenievich **Vvedensky** died, **born** 1852. *reaction of living tissue to stimulants, indefatigability of nerve*

1922: Ernst Gottlob **Orthmann** died, **born** 1858. *ovarian tumour*

1922: Wilhelm August Oscar **Hertwig** died, **born** 1849. *fertilization, embryology, cytology*

## 1923
1923:1 **Nobel Prize** (Physiology or Medicine): Frederick Grant Banting (1891–1941) and John James Richard Macleod (1876–1935), for their work on isolation of **insulin** and its clinical application in the treatment of **diabetes mellitus**, *NPL. 3966, 3967, 3968*

1923:2 **University of Milan** founded

1923:3 **Health Organization of the League of Nations, Geneva**

1923:4 **Cancer Research Campaign (UK)** founded

1923:5 **Ross Institute and Hospital for Tropical Diseases** opened in London

1923:6 **[Epidemiological Institute]** opened at **Zagreb**

1923:7 **[Scientific Institute for Microbiological Investigation], Moscow**

1923:8 [**Alfonso XIII Institute for Cancer Research**], **Madrid**

1923:9 [**Cancer Institute**], **Buenos Aires**, opened

1923:10 **Maudsley Hospital for Nervous Diseases** established in **London**

1923:11 A plastic operation for the treatment of atrophied and enlarged **breasts** devised by Hans Kraske, *MMW* **70**:672. *5760*

1923:12 **Ethylene** introduced as an **anaesthetic** by Arno Benedict Luckhardt (1885–1957) and Jay Bailey Carter (b.1889), *JAMA* **80**:765. *5705*

1923:13 The use of **sodium amytal** as an **anaesthetic** first described by Irvine Heinly Page (b.1901), *JLCM* **9**:194. *5706*

1923:14 The **McCarthy foroblique panendoscope** for **cysto-urethroscopy** introduced by Joseph Francis McCarthy (1874–1965), *JU* **10**:519. *4198.1*

1923:15 **Sodium iodide** introduced as a contrast medium in **uretero-pyelography** by Earl Dorland Osborne (1895–1960) and co-workers, *JAMA* **80**:368. *4199*

1923:16 Experimental use of **peritoneal dialysis** in **uraemia** first carried out by G. Ganter, *MMW* **70**:1478. *4242*

1923:17 The '**crush syndrome**', with its effect on the **kidney**, first reported by S. Minami, *VA* **245**:247. *4243*

1923:18 Fascial suture used in the repair of **inguinal hernia** by William Edward Gallie (1882–1959) and Arthur Baker LeMesurier (b.1889), *CMAJ* **13**:469. *3609*

1923:19 **Holmgren's fenestration operation** for **otosclerosis** devised by Gunnar Holmgren (1875–1954), *AcOL* **5**:460. *3404*

1923:20 First complete **pericardiectomy** for constrictive **pericarditis** by Franz Volhard (1872–1950) and Victor Schmieden (1874–1945), *KW* **2**:5. *3031*

1923:21 **Mitral valve** section for relief of **mitral stenosis** successfully carried out by Elliott Carr Cutler (1888–1947) and Samuel Albert Levine (1891–1966), *BMSJ*, **188**:1023. *3030.1*

1923:22 **Bone marrow biopsy** by **sternal puncture** introduced by Carl Pauly Seyfarth (b.1890), *DMW* **49**:180. *3087*

1923:23 First **angiogram** of a living patient by Josef Berberich (b.1897) and S. Hirsch, *KW* **2**:2226. *2916*

1923:24 Pioneer English work on **birth control** published by Marie Stopes (1880–1958), *Contraception (birth control). 1641.2*

1923:25 **Oestrin**, the ovarian hormone, isolated by Edgar Allen (1892–1943) and Edward Adelbert Doisy (1893–1986), *JAMA* **81**:819. *1183*

1923:26 Norman E. **Shumway**, American cardiac surgeon, born 9 Feb; with Richard Rowland Lower, carried out heart transplantation in dogs, ('Shumway technique'), 1960, *SF* **11**:18. *3047.14*

1923:27 Rose Ruth **Ellison**, American oncologist, born 5 Jun; with co-workers, introduced cytosine arabinoside in the treatment of acute leukaemia, 1968, *Blood* **32**:507. *3108.9*

1923:28 Daniel Carleton **Gajdusek**, American paediatrician, born 9 Sep; with V. Zigas, first described Kuru, a disease occurring in natives of New Guinea, 1957, *NEJM* **257**:974; with Clarence J. Gibbs, transmitted kuru and Creutzfeldt-Jakob disease to primates, 1971, *Nature* **230**:588. Shared Nobel Prize (Physiology or Medicine), 1976, with Baruch Samuel Blumberg, for their discoveries concerning new mechanisms for the origin and dissemination of infectious diseases, *NPL. 4729.1, 4729.2*

1923:29 Thomas Eugene **Eble** born 15 Sep; with Frederick Reuben Hanson, isolated fumagillin, an amoebicidal antibiotic, 1949, *JB* **58**:527, *Science* **113**:202. *1945*

---

1923: Aleksandr Yakovlevich **Danilevsky** died, **born** 1838. *trypsin*

1923: Robert Adolf Armand **Tigerstedt** died, **born** 1853. *renin*

1923: Otto **Josue** died, **born** 1869. *arteriosclerosis*

1923: Wilhelm Conrad **Röntgen** died, **born** 1845. *x rays*

1923: Johannes **Orth** died, **born** 1847. *kernicterus*

1923: Frederick **Treves** died, **born** 1853. *haemophilia*

1923: Marie Ernest **Gellé** died, **born** 1834. *stapes fixation test, deafness*

1923: Ernst Leopold **Salkowski** died, **born** 1844. *pentosuria*

1923: William Augustus **Hardaway** died, **born** 1850. *prurigo nodularis*

1923: Charles Lucien de **Beurmann** died, **born** 1851. *sporotrichosis*

1923: Johann Karl **Proksch** died, **born** 1840. *venereal disease*

1923: Arthur **Looss** died, **born** 1861. *Ankylostoma duodenale*

1923: Max **Wolff** died, **born** 1844. *Actinomyces bovis*

1923: James Leonard **Corning** died, **born** 1855. *spinal anaesthesia*

1923: David Tod **Gilliam** died, **born** 1844. *prolapse of uterus*

1923: Fritz **Frank** died, **born** 1856. *caesarean section*

1923: Anton Julius Friedrich **Rosenbach** died, **born** 1842. *Streptococcus, Staphylococcus*

**1924**

1924:1 **Nobel Prize** (Physiology or Medicine): Willem Einthoven (1860–1927), for his development of **electrocardiography**, *NPL. 842*

1924:2 **International Society of Medical Officers of Health, Geneva,** founded

1924:3 **[Russian Society of Endocrinology]** founded

1924:4 **American Society of Parasitologists, Baltimore,** founded

1924:5 **[Werner Siemens Institute for Röntgenology]** at **Berlin**

1924:6 **History of Science Society** founded at **Boston**

1924:7 **London School of Hygiene and Tropical Medicine** founded; formerly London School of Tropical Medicine, 1899.

1924:8 Mathematical theory of **natural and artificial selection** proposed by John Burdon Sanderson Haldane (1892–1964), (Part I) *TCPS* **23**:19; (Parts II–IX) *PCPS* **1**:23, 26, 27, 28; (Part X) *Gen*, 1934, **19**:412. *254*

1924:9 The **Portes operation** – the classic **caesarean section** followed by temporary exteriorization of the uterus – described by Louis Portes (1891–1950), *BSOG* **13**:171. *6252*

1924:10 The **insulin-fattening** method of treatment of **malnutrition in infants** introduced by Williams McKim Marriott (1885–1936), *JAMA* **83**:600. *6350*

1924:11 **Letterer-Siwe disease** first described by Erich Letterer (1895–1982), *FZP* **30**:377. *6272, 6373*

1924:12 Demonstration that *Leishmania donovani* is capable of reproduction in the **sandfly**, *Phlebotomus argentipes* by Robert Knowles (1883–1936) and co-workers, *IMG* **59**:593. *5301.1*

1924:13 The 'scratch test', a cutaneous reaction for determination of susceptibility to **diphtheria** introduced by Karl Erhard Kassowitz (b.1886), *KW* **3**:1317. *5069*

1924:14 The **Dick test** for determination of susceptibility to **scarlet fever** devised by George Frederick Dick (1881–1967) and Gladys Rowena Dick (1881–1963), *JAMA* **82**:265. *5082*

1924:15 Proof that the **streptococcus** is the cause of **scarlet fever** given by George Frederick Dick (1881–1967) and Gladys Rowena Dick (1881–1963), *JAMA* **82**:301. *5082.1*

1924:16 **Sympathetic ramisection** for the treatment of **spastic paralysis** introduced by Norman Dawson Royle (d.1944), *MJA* **1**:77. *4894*

1924:17 The first planned operation for **intracranial aneurysm** diagnosed pre-operatively performed by Wilfred Trotter (1872–1939); reported by J.L. Birley (1928), *Brain* **51**:184. *3004.1, 4897.2*

1924:18 The **stretch reflex** investigated by Charles Scott Sherrington (1857–1952), with E.G.T. Liddell, 1924, *PRSB* **96**:212; 1925, *PRSB* **97**:267. *3004.1, 1443*

1924:19 The mechanism that makes it possible to control the direction in which a part of the **embryo** will develop ('**the organizer**') discovered by Hans Spemann (1869–1941), *Roux* **100**:599. *530*

1924:20 A syndrome of **finger agnosia**, right-left disorientation and **acalculia** ('**Gerstmann's syndrome**') due to **cerebral lesion** described by Josef Gerstmann (b.1887), *WKKW* **37**:1010. *4605.3*

1924:21 The use of a **cathode ray oscillograph** for transmission of impulses through single **nerve fibres** devised by Joseph Erlanger (1874–1965) and Herbert Spencer Gasser (1888–1963), *AmJPh* **70**:624. *1305*

1924:22 **Hypertelorism** as a separate entity first described by David Middleton Greig (1864–1936), *EMJ* **31**:560. *4392*

1924:23 The combination of **rheumatoid arthritis** with **splenomegaly** and **leucopenia** ('**Felty's syndrome**') described by Augustus Roy Felty (b.1895), *JHB* **35**:16. *4506*

1924:24 The **diazo-colour test** of **kidney function** introduced by Christopher Howard Andrewes (1896–1988), *L* **1**:590. *4244*

1924:25 The **bromsulphthalein test** for **liver function** devised by Sanford Morris Rosenthal (b.1897) and Edwin Clay White (b.1888), *JPET* **24**:265. *3653*

1924:26 **Cholecystography** introduced by Evarts Ambrose Graham (1883–1957) and Warren Henry Cole (b.1898), *JAMA* **82**:613. *3652*

1924:27 Intratracheal **lipiodol** introduced into **bronchography** by Jean Athanase Sicard (1872–1929) and Jacques Forestier (b.1890), *JMF* **13**:*33199*

1924:28 First successful treatment ('**Trendelenburg's operation**') for **pulmonary artery embolism** by Martin Kirschner (1879–1942), *ArKC* **133**:312. *3016*

1924:29 **Libman-Sacks disease, endocarditis** with **lupus erythematosus disseminatus** described by Emanuel Libman (1872–1946) and Benjamin Sacks (b.1896), *ArIM* **33**:701. *2855*

1924:30 Scraped-incision slit-skin method introduced by Herbert Windsor Wade (1886–1968) for diagnosis of **leprosy**, *JPMA* **4**:132. *2440.1*

1924:31 **Antigenic structure** of **pneumococcus** elucidated by Michael Heidelberger (1888–1991) and Oswald Theodore Avery (1877–1955), *JEM* **38**:73. *2573.2, 3198*

1924:32 **Tuberculosis; BCG (Bacille Calmette-Guérin)** prophylactic vaccine introduced by Léon Charles Albert Calmette (1863–1935), C. Guérin and B. Weill-Hallé, *BuAM* **91**:787. *2343*

1924:33 **Homograft reaction** in tissue **transplantation** shown by Clarence Cook Little (1888–1971) to be due to genetic differences between donor and recipient, *JCR* **8**:75. *2573.1*

---

1924:34 Roger Charles Louis **Guillemin**, French/American neuroendocrinologist, born 11 Jan; shared Nobel Prize (Physiology or Medicine), 1977, with Andrew Victor Schally and Rosalyn Yalow, for his discoveries concerning peptide hormone production in the brain, *NPL*.

1924:35 Brian Gerald **Barratt-Boyes**, New Zealand cardio-thoracic surgeon, born 13 Jan; replaced aortic valve with a subcoronary homograft for aortic incompetence and stenosis, 1964, *Thorax* **19**:131. *3047.18*

1924:36 Allan MacLeod **Cormack**, South African/American physicist, born 23 Feb; shared Nobel Prize (Physiology or Medicine), 1979, with Godfrey Newbold Hounsfield, for his contribution to the development of computer-assisted tomography, *NPL*.

1924:37 Torsten Nils **Wiesel**, Swedish/American neurobiologist, born 3 Jun; shared Nobel Prize (Physiology or Medicine), 1981, with Roger Wolcott Sperry and David Hunter Hubel, for discoveries concerning information processing in the visual system, *NPL*.

1924:38 James Learmonth **Gowans**, British immunologist, born 7 May; showed lymphocyte to be the immunologically competent cell, 1962, *Nature* **196**:651. *2578.33*

1924:39 James Whyte **Black**, British pharmacologist, born 14 Jun; with co-workers, introduced propranolol, 1964, *L* **1**:1080. Shared Nobel Prize (Physiology or Medicine), 1988, with Gertrude Belle Elion and George H. Hitchings, for their discoveries of important principles for drug treatment, *NPL. 1931.5*

1924:40 Lawrence **Levine**, American biochemist, born 18 Jul; with Manfred Martin Mayer, introduced complement fixation technique, 1954, *JI* **72**:511. *2578.14*

1924:41 John Harold **Edgcomb**, American pathologist, born 15 Aug; with co-workers, introduced primaquine (diaprim) in the treatment of malaria, 1950, *JNMS* **9**:285. *5262.3*

1924:42 John Joseph **Shea**, American otolaryngologist, born 4 Sep; introduced the operation of stapedectomy, 1958, *AnOt* **67**:932. *3412.7*

---

1924:43 Jean **Lindenmann**, Swiss virologist, born; with Alick Isaacs, discovered interferon, 1957, *PRSB* **147**:258. *2578.22*

1924:44 Earl K. **Shirley** born; with Frank Mason Sones, performed coronary arteriography, 1962, *MCCD* **31**:735. *2924.3*

---

1924:45 Francis **Paxton** died; first description of trichorrhexis nodosa, 1869, *JCuM* **3**:133. *4058*

1924:46 Fidel Pagés **Miravé** died; introduced peridural anaesthesia, 1921, *RSM* **11**:351, 389. *5702*

1924: Luther Emmett **Holt** died, **born** 1855. *heparin*

1924: William Maddock **Bayliss** died, **born** 1860. *hormones*

1924: Arnold **Pick** died, **born** 1851. *Pick's bundle, Pick's disease*

1924: Friedrich **Fehleisen** died, **born** 1854. *Streptococcus pyogenes*

1924: Paul **Hallopeau** died, **born** 1876. *pericardiectomy*

1924: Friedrich **Trendelenburg** died, **born** 1844. *congenital dislocation of hip-joint, varicose veins, saphenous vein ligation, hydronephrosis, endotracheal anaesthesia*

1924: Henry Orlando **Marcy** died, **born** 1837. *hernia*

1924: Edoardo **Bassini** died, **born** 1844. *femoral and inguinal hernia, nephropexy*

1924: Bertram Welton **Sippy** died, **born** 1866. *peptic ulcer*

1924: Andrew Rose **Robinson** died, **born** 1845. *hydrocystoma*

1924: John Timothy **Geraghty** died, **born** 1876. *kidney function test*

1924: William **Macewen** died, **born** 1848. *allograft transplantation of bone, pulmonary tuberculosis, endotracheal anaesthesia, inguinal hernia, brain surgery*

1924: Simon **Duplay** died, **born** 1836. *frozen shoulder syndrome*

1924: Jaroslav **Hlava** died, **born** 1855. *amoebiasis*

1924: Jacques **Loeb** died, **born** 1859. *tropisms, psychology, fertilization*

1924: Wilhelm **Roux** died, **born** 1850. *embryology*

## 1925
1925:1 **Nobel Prize** (Physiology or Medicine): No award

1925:2 **Hebrew University of Jerusalem** opened

1925:3 **University of Bari, Italy,** founded

1925:4 **Radiologic Institute (Foundation Bergonié), at Paris**

1925:5 **British Social Hygiene Council** (founded 1914) organized

1925:6 An intradermal pigment test used by Alan Churchill Woods (1889–1963) in the diagnosis and treatment of **sympathetic ophthalmia,** *TOUK* **45**:208. *5969*

1925:7 A **gonioscope** introduced by Manuel Uribe Troncoso (b.1867), *AmJOp* **8**:433. *5968*

1925:8 The first media upon which **amoebae** could be cultivated for indefinite periods were evolved by William Charles Boeck (b.1894) and Jaroslav Drbohlav (1893–1946), *AmJH* **5**:371. *5194*

1925:9. Transmission of **tularaemia** from man to rodents through insects demonstrated by Edward Francis (1872–1957), *JAMA* **84**:1243; he named the disease from Tulare County, California, where it was discovered. *5176*

1925: 10 Intracranial section of the **trigeminal nerve** used for the treatment of **glossopharyngeal neuralgia** by Walter Edward Dandy (1886–1946), *BJH* **36**:105. *4896*

1925: 11 **Presacral neurectomy** introduced by Gaston Cotte (1879–1951), *PrM* **33**:98. *4895*

1925: 12 The infectivity of **herpes zoster** first demonstrated by Karl Kundratitz, *MonK* **29**:516. *4652*

1925: 13 **Non-suppurative nodular panniculitis** ('**Weber-Christian disease**') reported by Frederic Parkes Weber (1863–1962) and later, in 1928, by Henry Asbury Christian. *4151, 4152*

1925: 14 Removal of a tumour of the **adrenal cortex** (by P. Sargent), with subsequent disappearance of the accompanying virilism, was recorded by Gordon Morgan Holmes (1876–1965), *QJM* **18**:143; thus establishing the relationship between **sexual abnormality** and **adrenal tumours**. *3872*

1925: 15 Felix Mandl (1892–1957) successfullly treated **osteitis fibrosa generalisata** by removal of a **parathyroid tumour**, *WKW* **38**:1343. *3863*

1925: 16 **Cytochrome** discovered by David Keilin (1887–1963), *PRSB* **98**:312. *968*

1925: 17 Research on the role of the anterior **pituitary** in **carbohydrate** metabolism published by Bernardo Alberto Houssay (1887–1971), *CRSB* **92**:822; 1929, **101**:940.

1925: 18 'Bite-wing' **dental radiograph** described by Howard Riley Raper, *IJO* **11**:275, 370, 470. *3692*

1925: 19 The **Takata-Ara reaction** for the diagnosis of **liver disease** devised by Mari Takata (b.1892) and Kiyoshi Ara (b.1894), *Far 6*, 1:667. *3654*

1925: 20 James Bertram Collip (1892–1965) extracted a **parathyroid hormone** ('**parathormone**'), *JBC* **63**:395, and, with Douglas Burrows Leitch (b.1888) used it in the treatment of **tetany**, *CMAJ* **15**:59. *3861, 3862, 4837*

1925: 21 **Follicular lymphadenopathy** described by Nathan Edwin Brill (1860–1925) and co-workers, *JAMA* **84**:668; later described by Douglas Symmers, 1927, and named '**Brill-Symmers disease**'. *3786, 3787*

1925: 22 First successful **mitral valvulotomy** for **mitral stenosis** by Henry Sessions Souttar (1875–1964), *BMJ* **2**:603. *3032*

1925: 23 **Thalassaemia** ('**Cooley's erythroblastic anaemia**') described by Thomas Benton Cooley (1871–1945) and co-workers, *AmJDC* **34**:347. *3141*

1925: 24 **Lederer's anaemia**, a form of acute haemolytic anaemia, described by Max Lederer (1885–1952), *AmJMS* **170**:500. *3138*

555

1925:25 Beneficial effect of raw **liver** in the treatment of **anaemia** demonstrated by Frieda Saur Robscheit-Robbins (b.1893) and George Hoyt Whipple (1878–1976), *AmJPH* **72**:408, paving the way for the establishment of this treatment by Minot and Murphy (1926). *3139, 3140*

1925:26 Arthur Robertson Cushny (1866–1926) reported important studies in *The action and uses in medicine of digitalis. 1912*

1925:27 Successful **exchange blood transfusion** for **icterus gravis neonatorum** by Alfred Purvis Hart (1887–1954), *CMAJ* **15**:1088. *3087.1*

1925:28 Theory of **viral origin of cancer** advanced by William Ewart Gye (1884–1952) supported photomicrographically by Joseph Edwin Barnard (1870–1949), *L* **2**:109, 117. *2647, 2468*

1925:29 **Sanocrysin** introduced in treatment of **tuberculosis** by Holger Møllgaard (b.1885), *TB* **20**:1. *2344*

1925:30 **Tannic acid** treatment of **burns** introduced by Edward Clark Davidson (1894–1933), *SGO* **41**:202. *2254*

1925:31 The **Frei skin test** for the diagnosis of **lymphogranuloma venereum** introduced by Wilhelm Siegmund Frei (1885–1943), *KW* **4**:2148. *5218*

1925:32 The first successful **embolectomy** in Britain was carried out by Geoffrey Jefferson (1886–1961), *BMJ* **2**:965. *3017*

1925:33 Joshua **Lederberg**, American geneticist, born 23 May; his work with Edward Lawrie Tatum on gene recombination in *Escherichia coli*, 1946, *Nature* **158**:558, resulted in his sharing of the Nobel Prize (Physiology or Medicine), 1958, with Tatum and George Wells Beadle, *NPL. 255.4*

1925:34 Irving Stanley **Johnson**, American experimental biologist, born 30 Jun; with co-workers, introduced vinblastine in the treatment of Hodgkin's disease (and other lymphomas) and vincristine in acute leukaemia of childhood, 1963, *CR* **23**:1390. *2660.16, 3788.2*

1925:35 Leslie **Brent**, British immunologist, born 5 Jul; with Rupert Everett Billingham, Peter Brian Medawar and E.M. Sparrow, provided proof of Burnet-Fenner theory (1949) of acquired immunological tolerance, 1953, *Nature* **172**:603. *2578.11*

1925:36 Baruch Samuel **Blumberg**, American medical anthropologist and immunologist, born 28 Jul; with H.J. Alter and S. Visnich, discovered the hepatitis B antigen (Australia antigen), 1965, *JAMA* **191**:541. Shared Nobel Prize (Physiology or Medicine), 1976, with Daniel Carleton Gajdusek, for their discoveries concerning new mechanisms for the origin and dissemination of infectious diseases, *NPL. 3666.4*

1925:37 Robert Geoffrey **Edwards**, British reproductive biologist, born 27 Sep; *in vitro* fertilization of human oocytes with B.D. Bavister and Patrick Christopher Steptoe, 1969, *Nature* **221**:632. With Steptoe, reported first successful human birth after re-implantation of human embryo, 1978, *L* **2**:366. *532.4, 532.5*

1925:38 Martin **Rodbell**, American biochemist, born 1 Dec; shared Nobel Prize (Physiology or Medicine), 1994, with Alfred G. Gilman, for discovery of G-proteins and their role in transduction in cells, *NPL*.

———————

1925: Heinrich **Dreser** died, **born** 1860. *acetylsalicylic acid (aspirin)*

1925: William Joseph **Dibdin** died, **born** 1850. *sewers*

1925: Karl Wilhelm Arthur **Heffter** died, **born** 1859. *mescaline*

1925: Carle **Gessard** died, **born** 1850. *Pseudomonas aeruginosa*

1925: Johann Georg **Mönckeberg** died, **born** 1877. *medial sclerosis of blood vessels*

1925: Thomas Clifford **Allbutt** died, **born** 1836. *clinical thermometer, angina pectoris*

1925: James **Mackenzie** died, **born** 1853. *digitalis, auricular fibrillation, pulse*

1925: Franz **Nowotny** died, **born** 1872. *asthma, bronchoscopy*

1925: Henri **Luc** died, **born** 1855. *maxillary sinus abscess*

1925: Nathan Edwin **Brill** died, **born** 1860. *typhus, follicular lymphadenopathy*

1925: Guido **Banti** died, **born** 1852. *splenomegalic anaemia*

1925: Morris **Simmonds** died, **born** 1855. *pituitary cachexia*

1925: Viktor **Janovsky** died, **born** 1847. *acanthosis nigricans*

1925: John **Cleland** died, **born** 1835. *Arnold-Chiari malformation*

1925: Rickman John **Godlee** died, **born** 1849. *brain tumour*

1925: August von **Wassermann** died, **born** 1866. *syphilis, general paresis*

1925: Ernst Adolf Gustav Gottfried **Strümpell** died, **born** 1853. *polioencephalomyelitis, brain pseudosclerosis, spastic spinal paralysis, ankylosing spondylitis*

1925: Hugo Karl **Liepmann** died, **born** 1863. *apraxia*

1925: Howard Henry **Tooth** died, **born** 1856. *peroneal muscular atrophy*

1925: Josef **Breuer** died, **born** 1842. *psychoanalysis*

1925: Edward Emanuel **Klein** died, **born** 1844. *scarlet fever, streptococcus*

1925: Eugen **Fraenkel** died, **born** 1853. *vulvovaginitis, gonococcus*

1925: Giovanni Battista **Grassi** died, **born** 1854. *malaria, ankylostomiasis*

1925: Samuel Taylor **Darling** died, **born** 1872. *histoplasmosis, Histoplasma capsulatum*

1925: Henry Rose **Carter** died, **born** 1852. *yellow fever*

1925: Alwin Karl **Mackenrodt** died, **born** 1859. *plastic reconstruction of vagina*

1925: Julius **Hirschberg** died, **born** 1843. *ophthalmology, electromagnet*

1925: John Newport **Langley** died, **born** 1852. *autonomic nervous system*

1925: Maximilian **Oberst** died, **born** 1849. *conduction anaesthesia, anaesthetic block*

## 1926
1926:1 **Nobel Prize** (Physiology or Medicine): Johannes Andreas Grib Fibiger (1867–1928), for demonstration in rodents of the effect of **nematodes (Spiroptera)** in the development of **carcinoma**, *NPL*. His results are no longer accepted. *2640*

1926:2 **School of Hygiene, Johns Hopkins University** (1916) officially opened

1926:3 **School of Tropical Medicine, University of Puerto Rico**, opened at San Juan

1926:4 **University of Agra, India**, founded

1926:5 An important histological study of **haemangiomatosis retinae** ('**Lindau's disease**') made by Arvid Vilhelm Lindau (b.1892), *AcPMS* Sup. 1. *5971*

1926:6 **Haverhill fever**, a streptobacillary form of **rat-bite fever**, first reported by Edwin Hemphill Place (b.1880) and co-workers, who isolated an organism later found to be identical with *Streptothrix muris ratti* and *Streptobacillus moniliformis*, *BMSJ* 194:285. *5328*

1926:7 **Pamaquin (plasmoquine)** introduced in the treatment of **malaria** by Wilhelm Roehl (d.1929), *ArST* **30** Beihefte 311. *5256*

1926:8 Murine (flea-borne) **typhus** described by Kenneth Fuller Maxcy (1889–1966), *USPHR* **41**:1213, 2967. *5396*

1926:9 A test for the diagnosis of **smallpox** introduced by John Charles Grant Ledingham (1875–1944), *JSM* **34**:125. *5433*

1926:10 *Aphasia and kindred disorders of speech*, by Henry Head (1861–1940), is considered the most important work on the subject in English. His theory of **aphasia** conceived it as being a disorder of symbolic formulation and expression. *4633*

1926:11 An important classification of **glioma group tumours** published by Percival Bailey (1892–1973) and Harvey Williams Cushing (1869–1939); in their *A classification of the tumours of the glioma group on a histogenetic basis. 4608*

1926:12 The first modern account of **kwashiorkor** was probably that given by L. Normet, *BSPE* **19**:207. *3759*

1926:13 Ludwig Pick's (1868–1935) account of a rare genetically-determined disorder, *EIM* **29**:519, also described by Albert Niemann (1914), led to the term '**Niemann-Pick disease**'. *3785, 3784*

1926:14 **Pemphigus erythematodes** ('**Senear-Usher syndrome**') first noted by Francis Eugene Senear (b.1889) and Barney David Usher (b.1899). *4151.2*

1926:15 The response of single **sensory end-organs** to natural stimuli (adaptation of **receptors**) observed by Edgar Douglas Adrian (1889–1977) and Y. Zotterman, *JP* **61**:151; see also Adrian's *The basis of sensation. The action of the sense organs*, 1928. *1307, 1308*

1926:16 The first isolation of an **enzyme**, crystalline **urease**, by James Batcheller Sumner (1887–1955), *JBC* **69**:435.

1926:17 A **resectoscope** for use in **prostatic surgery** introduced by Maximilian Stern (b.1877), *IJMS* **39**:72. *4273*

1926:18 Isolation of an **anti-pellagra** factor related to **vitamin B** by Joseph Goldberger (1874–1929) and co-workers, *USPHR* **41**:297. *3578*

1926:19 **Insulin** crystallized by John Jacob Abel (1857–1938), *PNAS* **12**:132. *1206, 3971*

1926:20 Isolation of **vitamin B₁ (aneurine, thiamine)**, lack of which causes **beriberi**, by Barend Coenraad Petrus Jansen (1884–1962) and Willem Frederik Donath (1889–1957), *CW* **23**:201,1387. *1058, 3746*

1926:21 Introduction of the raw **liver** diet in the treatment of **pernicious anaemia** by George Richards Minot (1885–1950) and William Parry Murphy (b.1892), *JAMA* **87**:470, as suggested by Robscheit-Robbins and Whipple (1925). *3140,3139*

1926:22 Displacement treatment of **nasal sinusitis** introduced by Arthur Walter Proetz (1888–1966), *ArOt(C)* **4**:1. *3325*

1926:23 **Pseudohaemophilia type B (von Willebrand's disease)** first reported by Erik Adolf von Willebrand (1870–1949), *FLH* **68**:87. *3087.2*

1926:24 Bendien test for **diagnosis of cancer** introduced by S.G.T. Bendien (d.1942) and co-workers, *NTG* **70, i:2856.** *2650*

1926:25 *Listeria monocytogenes* isolated by Everitt George Dunne Murray (1890–1964) et al., *JPB* **29**:407. *2522.1*

1926:26 *Aviation medicine*; important text published by Louis Hopewell Bauer (1888–1964). *2137.6*

1926:27 Metabolism of **tumours** studied by Otto Heinrich Warburg (1883–1970), who observed that malignant cells can grow without oxygen and utilize glucose by **glycolysis**; in his *Ueber die Stoffwechsel der Tumoren. 2651*

1926:28 **Vitamin B₂ (riboflavine)** discovered by Joseph Goldberger (1874–1929) et al., *USPHR* **41**:297. *1057*

1926:29 Wallace Prescott **Rowe**, American virologist, born 20 Feb; with co-workers discovered adenoviruses, 1953, *PSEB* **84**:570. *2526.2*

1926:30 David Hunter **Hubel**, Canadian/American neurobiologist, born 27 Feb; shared Nobel Prize (Physiology or Medicine), 1981, with Roger Wolcott Sperry and Torsten Nils Wiesel, for discoveries concerning information processes in the visual system, *NPL.*

1926:31 Thomas Earl **Starzl**, American surgeon, born 11 Mar; with co-workers, carried out the first liver transplant in humans, 1963, *SGO* **117**:659. *3666.3*

1926:32 Hubert Arthur **Lechevalier**, French/American microbiologist, born 12 May; with Selman Abraham Waksman, discovered neomycin, 1949, *Science* **113**:305. *1944*

1926:33 Ian McIntosh **Rollo**, British/Canadian pharmacologist, born 28 May; first used pyrimethamine (daraprim) in the treatment of proguanil-resistant malaria, 1951, *Nature* **168**:332. *5262.5*

1926:34 Albert **Starr**, American thoracic surgeon, born 1 Jun; with M. Lowell Edwards, introduced shielded ball valve prosthesis for mitral valve replacement, 1960, *JTCS* **42**:673; the first mitral valve replacement in a human. *3047.16*

1926:35 Jérôme **Lejeune**, French human geneticist, born 13 Jun; with co-workers, discovered trisomy-21, the cause of Down's syndrome, 1959, *CRAS* **248**:1721. *4962.5*

1926:36 Paul **Berg**, American biochemist, born 30 Jun; shared Nobel Prize (Chemistry), 1980, with Walter Gilbert and Frederick Sanger, for his fundamental studies of the biochemistry of nucleic acids, with particular regard to recombinant DNA, *NPL.*

1926:37 Aaron **Klug**, British molecular biologist, born 11 Aug; awarded Nobel Prize (Chemistry), 1982, for his development of crystallographic electron microscopy and his structural elucidation of biologically important nucleic acid – protein complexes, *NPL.*

1926:38 Andrew Victor **Schally**, Polish/American endocrinologist, born 30 Nov; shared Nobel Prize (Physiology or Medicine), 1977, with Roger Charles Louis Guillemin and Rosalyn Yalow, for his discoveries concerning peptide hormone production in the brain, *NPL.*

1926:39 Richard A. **DeWall**, American thoracic surgeon, born 16 Dec; with co-workers, introduced bubble oxygenator in heart surgery, 1956, *SCNA* **36**:1025. *3047.9*

---

1926: Robert Henry **Clarke** died, **born** 1850. *stereotactic surgery, stereotactic apparatus*

1926: Richard von **Krafft-Ebing** died, **born** 1840. *sexual psychopathology, forensic psychopathology, psychiatry*

1926: Franz **Ziehl** died, **born** 1857. *tuberculosis, Mycobacterium*

1926: Oscar **Stoerck** died, **born** 1870. *bundle-branch block*

1926: Friedel **Pick** died, **born** 1867. *constrictive pericarditis*

1926: Thomas **Jonnesco** died, **born** 1860. *angina pectoris*

1926: Adolf **Passow** died, **born** 1859. *otosclerosis, fenestration*

1926: Oscar Thorvald **Bloch** died, **born** 1847. *colon cancer*

1926: Giuseppe **Gradenigo** died, **born** 1859. *otitis media, abductor paralysis, tone decay in hearing*

1926: Luigi **Lucatello** died, **born** 1863. *liver puncture*

1926: Henry **Morris** died, **born** 1844. *nephrolithotomy*

1926: Otto Wilhelm **Madelung** died, **born** 1846. *wrist joint deformity*

1926: Johann Otto Leonhard **Heubner** died, **born** 1843. *meningococcus, paediatrics, infant feeding*

1926: Victor **Babès** died, **born** 1854. *glanders*

1926: William Boog **Leishman** died, **born** 1865. *malaria parasite stain, leishmaniasis, trypanosome*

1926: Camillo **Golgi** died, **born** 1843. *Golgi cells, malaria*

1926: George Herbert **Hunt** died, **born** 1884. *trench fever*

1926: James **Israel** died, **born** 1848. *actinomycosis, Actinomyces bovis, rhinoplasty, bone grafts*

1926: William Edward **Fothergill** died, **born** 1865. *prolapse of uterus*

1926: Carl Joseph **Eberth** died, **born** 1835. *typhoid, Salmonella typhi*

1926: William **Bateson** died, **born** 1861. *genetics*

1926: Franz von **Soxhlet** died, **born** 1848. *milk, lactodensimeter*

1926: Arthur Robertson **Cushny** died, **born** 1866. *auricular fibrillation, digitalis, urinary secretion*

1926: Fritz **Hitschmann** died, **born** 1870. *cyclic changes in endometrium*

**1927**
1927:1 **Nobel Prize** (Physiology or Medicine): Julius Wagner von Jauregg (1857–1948), for the use of **malaria fever therapy** in **general paralysis**, *NPL. 4806*

1927:2 **School of Hygiene, University of Toronto**, opened

1927:3 **Royal Australian College of Surgeons** founded

1927:4 **Ceylon Medical Association** founded

1927:5 Artificial transmutation of the **gene** by **irradiation** by Herman Joseph Muller (1890–1967), *Science* **66**:84. *251.1*

1927:6 **Ignipuncture** for the treatment of **detached retina** introduced by Jules Gonin (1870–1935), *AnO* **164**:817. *5972*

1927:7 Buttonhole **iridectomy** employed by Frederick Herman Verhoeff (b.1874) for the removal of **cataract** within the capsule, *TAOS* **25**:54. *5974*

1927:8 The successful **radium** treatment of **cancer** of the **breast** by Geoffrey Langdon Keynes (1887–1982), *BJS* **19**:415, established this conservative method. *5786*

1927:9 **Avertin (tribromethanol)** first used experimentally as an **anaesthetic** by Fritz Eichholtz (b.1889), *DMW* **53**:710. It was used clinically by O. Butzengeiger, *DMW* **53**:712, in the same year. *5708, 5709*

1927:10 *Bact. granulosis* isolated by Hideyo Noguchi (1876–1928) who believed it to be the causal organism in **trachoma**, *JAMA* **89**:739. *5973*

1927:11 The causal agent in **tsutsugamushi disease** (scrub **typhus**) isolated by Norio Ogata (b.1883); in reporting it in 1931, *ZBP* I Abt.122:249, he named it *Rickettsia tsutsugamushi*. *5396.3*

1927:12 The infective agent in **lymphogranuloma venereum** first seen by José Antonio Gay Prieto (1905–1979), *ACDS* **20**:122. *5219*

1927:13 The **vector** of **onchocerciasis** shown by Donald Breadalbane Blacklock (1879–1955) to be *Simulium damnosum*, *BMJ* **1**:129. *5350.8*

1927:14 **Child psychology** was a field given special study by Anna Freud (1895–1982), daughter of Sigmund Freud; in her *Einführung in die Technik der Kinderanalyse*. *4990.1*

1927:15 **Encephalitis periaxialis concentrica** ('Baló's disease') described by Jószef Baló (b.1896), *MOA* **28**:108. *4653*

1927:16 **Cerebral arteriography** and **carotid arteriography** introduced by Antonio Caetano de Abreu Freire Egas Moniz (1874–1955), *ReN* **34**ii, 72; *PrM* **35**:969. *4610, 4610.1*

1927:17 Activity of **gonads** maintained by anterior **pituitary** shown experimentally by Philip Edward Smith (1884–1970), *AmJPh* **80**:114; *AmJA* **40**:159. *1166, 1167*

1927:18 Experimental evidence that **bladder calculus** could follow a diet deficient in **vitamin A**, provided by Robert McCarrison (1878–1960), *IJMR* **14**:895, **15**:197, 485, 801. *4296*

1927:19 **Harris's operation** of suprapubic **prostatectomy** with closure described by Samuel Henry Harris (1881–1936), *MJA* **1**:460; *AuNZ* **4**:226. *4275*

1927:20 **Follicular lymphadenopathy** described by Douglas Symmers (1879–1952), *ArPa* **3**:816; previously described by Nathan Edwin Brill and co-workers, 1925, and named '**Brill-Symmers disease**'. *3787, 3786*

1927:21 A **bilirubin excretion test** of **liver function** devised by Wilhelm Eilbott (b.1900), *ZKM* **106**:529. *3655*

1927:22 **Fanconi's syndrome**, a metabolic disorder, described by Guido Fanconi (1892–1979), *JaK* **117**:257. *3142*

1927:23 **Bone marrow biopsy** by **needle puncture** introduced by Mikhail Arinkin (1876–1948), *VK* **30**:57. *3088*

1927:24 **Syphilis: bismarsen (bismuth arsphenamine sulphate)** treatment introduced by John Hinchman Stokes (b.1885) and Stanley Owen Chambers (b.1897), *JAMA* **89**:1500. *2414*

1927:25 **Burns**; a classification introduced by David Goldblatt (b.1894), *AnS* **85**:490. *2255*

1927:26 **Mescaline** poisoning described comprehensively by Kurt Beringer (1893–1949); in his *Der Meskalinrausch. 2086.1*

1927:27 **X ray dose fractionation** introduced by Claude Regaud (1870–1940) and R. Ferroux, *CRSB* **97**:431. *2008*

1927:28 **Gonadotrophic hormone** isolated by Bernhard Zondek (1891–1966) and Selmar Aschheim (1878–1965), *KW* **6**:348, **7**:831. *1168*

1927:29 Synthesis of **thyroxine** by Charles Robert Harington (1897–1972) and George Barger (1878–1939), *BJ* **21**:169. *1138*

1927:30 **Blood groups** M, N and P discovered by Karl Landsteiner (1868–1943) and Philip Levine (1900–1987), *PSEB* **24**:600, 941. *910*

---

1927:31 John Robert **Vane**, British pharmacologist, born 29 Mar; shared Nobel Prize (Physiology or Medicine), 1982, with Sune Bergström and Bengt Ingemar Samuelsson, for discoveries concerning the prostaglandins and related biologically active substances, *NPL.*

1927:32 Marshall Warren **Nirenberg**, American biochemist, born 10 Apr; reported DNAase-sensitive protein synthesis, 1961, *PNAS* **47**:1580; shared Nobel Prize (Physiology or Medicine), 1968, with Robert W. Holley and Har Gobind Khorana, for his work on DNA, *NPL. 256.11*

1927:33 Samuel Lawrence **Katz**, American virologist, born 29 May; with M. Milovanovič and John Franklin Enders, propagated the measles virus in cultures of chick embryo cells, 1958, *PSEB* **97**:23; with Enders, Milovanovič and A. Holloway, produced a live virus vaccine, 1960, *NEJM* **263**:153. *5449.3, 5449.4*

1927:34 Ivan Maurice **Roitt**, British immunologist, born 30 Sep; with co-workers, demonstrated autoantibodies, 1956, *L* **2**:820. *2578.19*

1927:35 César **Milstein**, Argentinian molecular biologist, born 8 Oct; with Georges F. Köhler, produced monoclonal antibodies, 1975, *Nature* **256**:495. Shared Nobel Prize (Physiology or Medicine), 1984, with Köhler and Niels Kaj Jerne, for the discovery of the principle of production of monoclonal antibodies, *NPL. 2578.43*

1927:36 Noel Richard **Rose**, American immunologist, born 3 Dec; with Ernest Witebsky, produced autoimmune thyroiditis experimentally, 1956, *JI* **76**:408. *3855.3*

_____

1927: Ernest Henry **Starling** died, **born** 1866. *hormonal control of heart, law of the heart*

1927: Willem **Einthoven** died, **born** 1860. *string galvanometer, electrocardiography, phonocardiography*

1927: Wilhelm **Filehne** died, **born** 1844. *antipyrene, pyramidon*

1927: Charles **Creighton** died, **born** 1847. *epidemiology*

1927: Georg Clemens **Perthes** died, **born** 1869. *carcinoma, x rays, osteochondritis deformans*

1927: Jacob da Silva **Solis-Cohen** died, **born** 1838. *cancer of larynx, otorhinolaryngology*

1927: Friedrich **Göppert** died, **born** 1870. *galactosaemia*

1927: Vladimir Michailovich **Bechterev** died, **born** 1857. *ankylosing spondylitis*

1927: Charles **Foix** died, **born** 1882. *Parkinson's disease*

1927: Waren **Tay** died, **born** 1843. *amaurotic familial idiocy*

1927: Oskar **Medin** died, **born** 1847. *poliomyelitis*

1927: Augusta **Dejerine-Klumpke** died, **born** 1859. *paralysis of hand muscles*

1927: Antonio **Carle** died, **born** 1854. *tetanus*

1927: Max **Gruber** died, **born** 1853. *typhoid, bacterial agglutination*

1927: Henry **Koplik** died, **born** 1858. *measles*

1927: Thomas Caspar **Gilchrist** died, **born** 1862. *blastomycosis*

1927: Karl Bruno **Stargardt** died, **born** 1875. *ophthalmia neonatorum*

1927: Robert Henry **Elliot** died, **born** 1864. *glaucoma*

1927: Adrian **Stokes** died, **born** 1887. *yellow fever*

1927: Robert Fulton **Weir** died, **born** 1839. *rhinoplasty*

1927: Wilhelm Ludvig **Johannsen** died, **born** 1857. *gene, genotype, phenotype*

1927: Karl Martin Leonhard Albrecht **Kossel** died, **born** 1853. *cell, cell nucleus*

1927: Otto **Purtscher** died, **born** 1852. *angiopathy of the retina*

**1928**

1928:1 **Nobel Prize** (Physiology or Medicine): Charles Jules Henri Nicolle (1866–1936), for his experimental proof of the role of **lice** in the transmission of exanthematous **typhus**, *NPL. 5384*

1928:2 **Nobel Prize** (Chemistry): Heinrich Otto Wieland (1877–1957), for investigations of the constitution of the **bile acids** and related substances, *NPL.*

1928:3 **New Presbyterian Hospital (New York Medical Center)** opened

1928:4 **Vasopressin** and **oxytocin** isolated by Oliver Kamm (1888–1965) and colleagues, *JACS* **50**:573. *1168.1*

1928:5 The anti-**beriberi** factor, **vitamin B₁**, discovered and synthesized by Robert Runnels Williams (1886–1965), *JBC* **78**:311. *1060, 1073*

1928:6 **Vitamin C (ascorbic acid)** isolated by Albert Szent-Györgyi (1893–1986), *BJ* **20**:537. *1059*

1928:7 **Shwartzman phenomenon**, local skin reactivity to *Bacillus typhosus* filtrate, observed by Gregory Shwartzman (1896–1965), *JEM* **48**:247. *2576*

1928:8 Humphry Davy Rolleston (1862–1944) published several contributions to the history of medicine, notably *Cardiovascular disease since Harvey's discovery. 3156*

1928:9 Important investigations in **conditioned reflexes** were published by I.P. Pavlov (1849–1936) under the title *Lectures on conditioned reflexes*, 1928–1941. *1445*

1928:10 **Heredity** of **cancer** studied by Maud Slye (1879–1954), *AnIM* **1**:951. *2652*

1928:11 **Dandy's** operation for treatment of **Menière's disease** devised by Walter Edward Dandy (1886–1946), *ArSuC* **16**:1127. *3406*

1928:12 Theory of dissociation of **bone growth** published by Murk Jansen (1863–1935); in the *Robert Jones Birthday Volume*, p. 43. *4395*

1928:13 **Japanese encephalitis** distinguished from **epidemic encephalitis** ('**encephalitis lethargica**') by Renjiro Kaneko (b.1886) and Y. Aoki, *EIM* **34**:342. *4654*

1928:14 The **diphtheria** toxin was so modified by Gaston Léon Ramon (1886–1963) that it lost its toxic properties while retaining its antigenic virtues, *AnIP* **42**:959. This **anatoxin** (**toxoid**) superseded toxin-antitoxin as an immunizing agent. *5070*

1928:15 **Electrocoagulation in neurosurgery** introduced by Harvey Williams Cushing (1869–1939), *SGO* **47**:751. *4897.1*

1928:16 Murine **typhus** differentiated from epidemic typhus by Hermann Mooser (1891–1971); the causal organism later named *Rickettsia mooseri*, *JID* **43**:241. *5396.1*

1928:17 A classic account of the life-cycle of *Entamoeba histolytica* given by Clifford Dobell (1886–1949), *Para* **20**:357. *5194.1*

1928:18 'Maitland's medium' introduced by Hugh Bethune Maitland (1895–1972) and Mary Cowan Maitland (d.1972) for the cultivation of vaccinia virus, *L* 2:596. *5434.1*

1928:19 A diagnostic test for smallpox introduced by Neil E. McKinnon (b.1894) and Robert Davies Defries (b.1889), *AmJH* 8:93. *5434*

1928:20 Yellow fever virus successfully transmitted to the *Macacus rhesus* monkey by Adrian Stokes (1887–1927) and co-workers, *AmJTM* 8:103; Stokes died of the disease during his investigations. *5462*

1928:21 The first vaccine for immunization against yellow fever introduced by Edward Hindle (1886–1973), *BMJ* 1:976. *5461*

1928:22 Modern mammectomy, with transplantation of nipple and areola, developed by Louis Dartigues (1869–1940), *BCChnP* 20:739. *5783*

1928:23 An operation for the repair of cleft palate devised by William Edward Mandell Wardill (1894–1960), *BJS* 16:127. *5761*

1928:24 The Aschheim-Zondek test for the diagnosis of pregnancy introduced by Selmar Aschheim (1878–1965) and Bernhard Zondek (1891–1966), *KW* 7:8, 1404, 1453. *6222*

1928:25 Fundamental work on transformation of pneumococcal types by Frederick Griffith (1879–1941), *JHyg* 27:113, which led to the work of Avery, MacLeod and McCarty demonstrating the role of DNA in genetics. *251.2, 255.3*

1928:26 Febrile nodular non-suppurative panniculitis ('Weber-Christian disease') reported by Henry Asbury Christian (1876–1951), *ArIM* 42:338; earlier reported (1925) by Frederic Parkes Weber. *6359–6363*

---

1928:27 Nicholas Avrion Mitchison, British zoologist and immunologist, born 5 Mar; carried out passive transfer of immunity, 1954, *PRSB* 142:72. *2578.15*

1928:28 James Dewey Watson, American biologist, born 6 Apr; with Francis Harry Compton Crick determined molecular structure of DNA, 1953, *Nature* 171:737. They shared the Nobel Prize (Physiology or Medicine), 1962, with Maurice Hugh Frederick Wilkins, *NPL*. *256.3*

1928:29 Daniel Nathans, American microbial geneticist, born 30 Oct; shared Nobel Prize (Physiology or Medicine), 1978, with Werner Arber and Hamilton Othanel Smith, for discovery of restriction enzymes and their application to problems of molecular genetics, *NPL*.

1928:30 Harry Martin Meyer, American virologist, born 25 Nov; with Paul Douglas Parkman and T.C. Panos, produced an experimental live-virus rubella vaccine, 1966, *NEJM* 275:575. *5509.2*

1928:31 John H. Menkes, Austrian/American paediatrician, born 28 Dec; with co-workers, first to describe maple syrup urine disease, an inherited metabolic disorder, 1954, *Ped* 14:462. *3924.3*

---

1928: Hubert Sattler died, born 1844. *Sattler's layer*

566

1928: Paul **Frosch** died, **born** 1860. *foot-and-mouth disease virus*

1928: John **MacIntyre** died, **born** 1859. *x ray cinematography*

1928: Karl Gottfried Paul **Döhle** died, **born** 1855. *syphilis, aortic aneurysm*

1928: Edmund **Jelinek** died, **born** 1852. *laryngology, anaesthetics, cocaine*

1928: Hugo Karl **Plaut** died, **born** 1858. *Plaut's angina*

1928: Felix Jacob von **Marchand** died, **born** 1846. *carotid body tumours, chorionepithelioma*

1928: Louis Anne Jean **Brocq** died, **born** 1856. *parasporosis*

1928: Amand **Coyon** died, **born** 1871. *rheumatism, streptococcus*

1928: Hideyo **Noguchi** died, **born** 1876. *Treponema, syphilis, dementia paralytica, vaccinia, bartonellosis, Phlebotomus, trachoma, Bact.granulosis*

1928: Ludwig **Lichtheim** died, **born** 1845. *aphasia*

1928: Robert **Abbe** died, **born** 1851. *rhizotomy, cleft lip*

1928: Greenfield **Sluder** died, **born** 1865. *sphenopalatine-ganglion neuralgia*

1928: Jean Albert **Pitres** died, **born** 1848. *agraphia, paraphrasia*

1928: William **Mestrezat** died, **born** 1883. *cerebrospinal fluid*

1928: Eugen **Bostroem** died, **born** 1850. *actinomycosis, Actinomyces graminis*

1928: David **Ferrier** died, **born** 1843. *brain function, cortical localization*

1928: Pierre Félix **Lagrange** died, **born** 1857. *glaucoma, sclerectomy*

1928: Johannes Andreas Grib **Fibiger** died, **born** 1867. *cancer*

**1929**
1929:1 **Nobel Prize** (Physiology or Medicine): Frederick Gowland Hopkins (1861–1947) and Christiaan Eijkman (1858–1930), for their work on **vitamins**, *NPL. 1048, 3741*

1929:2 **Royal College of Obstetricians and Gynaecologists, London** founded

1929:3 Work on the **sinus-aorta** mechanism in **respiration** published by Cornèille Jean François Heymans (1892–1968); *Le sinus carotidien et la zone homologue cardio-aortique. 967*

1929:4 **Electroencephalogram** described by Johannes [Hans] Berger (1873–1941), *ArPN* **87**:527. *1446*

1929:5 The nature and function of the **respiratory ferment** (Atmungsferment) discovered by Otto Heinrich Warburg (1883–1970), 1929, *BcZ* **214**:64; 1932, *BcZ* **254**:438. *969, 970*

1929:6 **Androsterone** isolated by Carl Richard Moore (1892–1955) and associates, *En* **13**:367; it was obtained in crystalline form by Adolf Friedrich Johann Butenandt (b.1903) in 1931, *ZAngC* **44**:905. *1191, 1195*

1929:7 **Progesterone**, the corpus luteum hormone, discovered by George Washington Corner (1889–1981) and Willard Myron Allen (b.1904), *AmJPh* **88**:326. *1188*

1929:8 **Vitamin K**, the dietary anti-haemorrhagic factor, discovered by Carl Pieter Henrik Dam (1895–1976), *BcZ* **215**:475. In 1939 he isolated vitamin K₁ from alfalfa. *1062*

1929:9 **Thyroid-stimulating hormone** of the anterior pituitary isolated by Max Aron (1892–1974) and by Leo Loeb (1869–1959) and R.B. Bassett, *PSEB* **26**:860; *CRSB* **102**:682. *1138.01, 1138.02*

1929:10 **Prolactin**, the pituitary lactogenic hormone, demonstrated by P. Stricker and P. Grueter, *CRSB* **99**:1978. *1168.2*

1929:11 **Pregnanediol** isolated by Guy Frederic Marrian (1904–1981), *BJ* **23**:1090. *1190*

1929:12 Discovery of the growth-inhibiting action of a **penicillin** on certain bacteria by Alexander Fleming (1881–1955), *BJEP* **10**:226. *1933*

1929:13 The **quantitative precipitin reaction** introduced by Michael Heidelberger (1888–1991) and Forrest E. Kendall (1898–1975), *JEM* **50**:809. *2576.01*

1929:14 **Drinker respirator** ('**iron lung**') introduced by Philip Drinker (1894–1972) and C.F. McKhann, *JAMA* **92**:1658. *1978*

1929:15 **Aortography** carried out by Reynaldo dos Santos (b.1880) and co-workers, *MCon* **47**:93. *2859*

1929:16 **Heart catheterization** performed, on himself, by Werner Theodor Otto Forssmann (1904–1979), *KW* **8**:2085. *2858*

1929:17 **Thorotrast (thorium dioxide)** first used in **radiological** diagnosis by Mitsumoto Oka, *FGR* **40**:497. *2695*

1929:18 Keith-Wagener-Barker classification of **essential hypertension** devised by Norman Macdonnell Keith (1885–1976), Henry Patrick Wagener (1890–1961), and N.W. Barker, *AmJMS* **197**:332, *Medicine*, 1939, **18**:317. *2716, 2723*

1929:19 One-stage **lung lobectomy** introduced by Harold Brunn (1874–1950), *ArSuC* **18**:490. *3202*

1929:20 Type I lobar **pneumonia** treated by monovalent antiserum by Rufus Ivory Cole (1872–1966), *JAMA* **93**:741. *3202.2*

1929:21 **Pernicious anaemia** shown by William Bosworth Castle (b.1897) to be due to absence from the gastric juice of **haemopoietin (Castle's instrinsic factor)**, necessary for the absorption of **vitamin B$_{12}$**, *AmJMS* **178**:748. *3143*

1929:22 Bronchial **asthma** first treated with **adrenaline** by the respiratory route by Percy William Leopold Camps (1877–1956), *GHR* **79**:496. *3202.1*

1929:23 Tubo-valvular **gastrostomy** introduced by Julius Leo Spivack (1889–1956), *BKC* **147**:308. *3549*

1929:24 **Gastrophotography** introduced by Otto Porges (b.1879), *WKW* **42**:89. *3548*

1929:25 An extensive study of **idiopathic steatorrhoea** (nontropical **sprue, coeliac disease**) by Thorald Einar Hess Thaysen (1883–1936), *L* **1**:1086, previously described by Samuel Jones Gee, 1888, led to the eponym '**Gee-Thaysen disease**'. *3550, 3491*

1929:26 Alfred Fabian Hess (1875–1933) showed that **rickets** and **scurvy** could be prevented by the **ultraviolet irradiation** of oils and foodstuffs; in his *Rickets, including osteomalacia and tetany*. *3735*

1929:27 **Addison's disease** first treated with **adrenal cortical extract** by Julius Moses Rogoff (1884–1966) and George Neil Stewart (1860–1930), *JAMA* **92**:1569. *3873*

1929:28 The **glycogen storage disease** known as '**von Gierke's disease**' described by Edgar Otto Konrad von Gierke (1877–1945), *BPA* **82**:497. *3656*

1929:29 The **blood urea clearance test** introduced by Eggert Hugo Heiberg Möller and co-workers, *JCI* **6**:427. *4246*

1929:30 **Uroselectan** introduced as a contrast medium in **excretion urography** by Moses Swick (b.1900) and Alexander von Lichtenberg (1880–1949), *KW* **8**:2087. *4200*

1929:31 New methods and apparatus for the management of **fractures** introduced by Lorenz Böhler (1885–1973); see his *Technik der Knochenbruchbehandlung*. *4433*

1929:32 **Gold therapy** introduced in chronic **rheumatism** by Jacques Forestier (b.1890), *BSMH* p. 323. *4506.1*

1929:33 A form of **osteochondrodystrophy** described by Luis Morquio (1867–1935), *ArME* **32**:129, *BSPP* **27**:145, and was named '**Morquio's disease**'. James Frederick Brailsford (1888–1961) also described it in the same year, *AmJMS* **7**:404, leading to the term '**Morquio-Brailsford disease**'. *4397, 4397.1*

1929:34 The theory of **gestalt psychology** advanced by Wolfgang Köhler (1887–1967); in his *Gestalt psychology*. *4991*

1929:35 **Avertin** first used intravenously by Martin Kirschner (1879–1942), *Ch* **1**:673. *5710*

1929:36 **Sodium amytal**, first described by Page (1923), first used as an intravenous **anaesthetic** by Leon Grotius Zerfas (b.1897) and co-workers, *PSEB* **26**:399. *5712*

1929:37 The vector of **bartonellosis (Oroya fever, Carrión's disease)** shown by Hideyo Noguchi (1876–1928) and co-workers to be *Phlebotomus*, *JEM* **49**:993. *5538.2*

1929:38 **Cyclopropane** introduced as an **anaesthetic** by George Herbert William Lucas (b.1894) and Velyien Ewart Henderson (1877–1945), *CMAJ* **21**:173. *5711*

1929:39 **Split-skin grafts** for covering large areas of granulating surfaces introduced by Vilray Papin Blair (1871–1955) and James Barrett Brown (1899–1971), *SGO* **49**:82. *5761.1*

1929:40 Gerald Maurice **Edelman**, American biochemist, born 1 Jul; shared Nobel Prize (Physiology or Medicine), 1972, with Gerald Maurice Edelman, for studies concerning the chemical nature of antibodies, *NPL. 2578.39*

1929:41 Werner **Arber**, American microbial geneticist, born 30 Oct; shared Nobel Prize (Physiology or Medicine), 1978, with Daniel Nathans and Hamilton Othanel Smith, for discovery of restriction enzymes and their application to problems of molecular genetics, *NPL.*

1929:42 Richard Rowland **Lower**, American thoracic surgeon, born 15 Aug; with Norman E. Shumway, carried out heart transplantation in dogs, ('Shumway technique'), 1960, *SF* **11**:18. *3047.14*

1929:43 Richard N. **Myers**, American surgeon, born; with Edwin W. Shearburn, introduced the Canadian or Shouldice repair for inguinal hernia, 1969, *Surgery* **66**:450. *3611.3*

1929:44 Wilhelm **Roehl** died; introduced pamaquin (plasmoquine) in the treatment of malaria, 1926, *ArST* **30** Beihefte 311. *5256*

1929: Joseph **Goldberger** died, **born** 1874. *measles, vitamins, pellagra, vitamin D*

1929: Samuel **Rideal** died, **born** 1863. *test for disinfectants*

1929: Georges Fernand Isidor **Widal** died, **born** 1862. *bacterial agglutination, haemolytic anaemia, bacillary dysentery, Shigella, typhoid*

1929: Clemens Peter **Pirquet von Cesenatico** died, **born** 1874. *allergy, serum sickness, tuberculosis*

1929: Alexander **Ogston** died, **born** 1844. *Staphyloccus aureus*

1929: Felix **Balzer** died, **born** 1849. *syphilis, bismuth*

1929: Jean Athanase **Sicard** died, **born** 1872. *radiography, bronchography, myelography, lipiodol*

1929: Heinrich **Winterberg** died, **born** 1867. *heart arrhythmia, auricular fibrillation*

1929: Théodore **Tuffier** died, **born** 1857. *urinary tract, radiography, pulmonary tuberculosis, valvular disease, extrapleural pneumolysis*

1929: Thomas Rushmore **French** died, **born** 1849. *larynx*

1929: Jacques-Louis **Reverdin** died, **born** 1842. *myoedema, thyroidectomy, skin grafts*

1929: Edmond **Delorme** died, **born** 1847. *empyema, lung decortication*

1929: Charles **Sajous** died, **born** 1852. *endocrinology*

1929: Paul Gerson **Unna** died, **born** 1850. *eczema, ichthammol, resorcinol, dermatology, acne bacillus*

1929: Domenico **Majocchi** died, **born** 1849. *purpura annularis telangiectodes*

1929: Paul A. **Lewis** died, **born** 1879. *anaphylactic shock, poliomyelitis*

1929: Amico **Bignami** died, **born** 1862. *malaria, alcoholism*

1929: Nagajosi **Nagai** died, **born** 1844. *ephedrine*

1929: Philip Hedgeland **Ross** died, **born** 1876. *relapsing fever, Ornithodorus moubata*

1929: Thomas Burr **Osborne** died, **born** 1859. *vitamin A*

1929: William Henry **Luckett** died, **born** 1872. *protruding ear surgery, ventriculography*

**1930**
1930:1 **Nobel Prize** (Physiology or Medicine): Karl Landsteiner (1868–1943), for his work on **blood groups**, *NPL. 889, 910*

1930:2 **Nobel Prize** (Chemistry): Hans Fischer (1881–1945), for researches into the chemical constitution of **haemin** and **chlorophyll** and synthesis of haemin, *NPL.*

1930:3 **US Hygienic Laboratory** becomes **National Institute(s) of Health**

1930:4 **Bethlem Royal Hospital** removed from **London** to **Beckenham**, Kent

1930:5 The foundations for **biometric genetics** laid by Ronald Aylmer Fisher (1890–1962), in his *The genetical theory of natural selection. 253*

1930:6 **Oestriol** isolated in crystalline form by Guy Frederic Marrian (1904–1981), *BJ* **24**:435. *1194*

1930:7 **Pepsin** crystallized by John Howard Northrop (b.1891), *JGP* **13**:739. *1038.1*

1930:8 **Digoxin** isolated by Sydney Smith, *JCS* 508. *1920*

1930:9 **Short-wave diathermy** introduced by Erwin Schliephake (b.1894), *KW* **9**:2333. *2009*

1930:10 Template or instruction theory of **antibody formation** proposed by Friedrich Breinl (b.1888) and Felix Haurowitz, *HSZ* **192**:45. *2576.1*

1930:11 **Temporal arteritis** first described by Max Schmidt (b.1898), *Brain* **53**:489. *2919*

1930:12 **Wolff-Parkinson-White syndrome** described by Louis Wolff (b.1898), John Parkinson (1885–1976) and Paul Dudley White (1886–1973), *AmHJ* **5**:685. *2860*

1930:13 The **hypoglycaemic** effect of certain **sulphonamides** discovered by Celestino L. Ruiz (b.1904) and co-workers, *RSAB* **6**:134. *3973*

1930:14 **Osteomalacia** shown to be due to lack of **vitamin D** by John Preston Maxwell (1871–1961), *PRSM* **23**:639. *4396*

1930:15 **Osteomalacia** with pseudofractures due to lack of **calcium** described by Louis Arthur Milkman (1895–1951), *AmJR* **24**:29, and named '**Milkman's syndrome**'. *4398*

1930:16 **Haemolytic streptococcal infection** shown as a cause of acute **rheumatism** in children by Bernard Schlesinger (1896–1984), *ArDiC* **5**:411. *4507*

1930:17 Alum-precipitated toxoid for active immunization against **diphtheria** introduced by Alexander Thomas Glenny (1882–1965), *BMJ* **2**:244. *5071*

1930:18 **Electric convulsion therapy** in **psychosis** introduced by Ugo Cerletti (1877–1963) and Lucio Bini (1908–1964), *BAMR* **64**:136. *4962*

1930:19 **Surgical shock** shown by Alfred Blalock (1899–1964) to be due to a decrease in circulating blood volume, *ArSuC* **20**:959. *5630.3*

1930:20 **Pentobarbitone sodium** first used as an intravenous **anaesthetic** by Richard Homer Fitch (b.1903) and co-workers, *AmJSu* **9**:110. *5712.1*

1930:21 The first full description of epidemic **myositis** ('**Bornholm disease**') made by Ejnar Oluf Sorenson Sylvest (1880–1931), *UL* **92**:798. *5540*

1930:22 The causal agent of **psittacosis** found by Claude Walter Levinthal (1886–1963) to be *Chlamydia psittaci*, *KW* **9**:654. The same discovery was made simultaneously by A.C. Coles (*Lancet*, **1**, 1011) and R.D. Lillie (*Publ. Hlth. Rep., Wash.*, **45**, 773). *5539*

1930:23 The intracerebral protection test in mice, for the diagnosis of **yellow fever** and for the determination of its past existence in the community, introduced by Max Theiler (1899–1972), *AnTM* **24**:249. *5463*

1930:24 **Colorado tick fever** first described as a separate entity by Frederick Edward Becker (b.1888), who suggested that it was transmitted by the tick, *Dermacentor andersoni*, *CoM* **27**:36. *5538.3, 5546.1*

1930:25 The **anaesthetic** properties of **divinyl ether** first demonstrated by Chauncey Depew Leake (1896–1978) and Mei-Yu Chen, *PSEB* **28**:151. *5713*

1930:26 The method of **corneal grafting (keratoplasty)** introduced by von Hippel developed with good results by Anton Elschnig (1863–1939), *ArOp* **4**:165. *5975*

1930:27 Important experimental work on **corneal transplantation** carried out by James William Tudor Thomas (1893–1976), *TOUK* **50**:127. *5979*

1930:28 The manufacture of modern **contact lenses** made possible by the work of Leopold Heine (b.1870), *MMW* **77**:6,271. *5976*

1930:29 Mirault's technique for the repair of **cleft palate** modified by Vilray Papin Blair (1871–1955) and James Barrett Brown (1899–1971), *SGO* **51**:81. *5762*

1930:30 **Amniography** introduced by Thomas Orville Menees (1890–1937), J.D. Miller and L.E. Holly, *AmJR* **24**:363. *6223*

------------

1930:31 Charles Freemont **McKhann**, American surgeon, born 29 Jan; with Ronald A. Malt, first successfully reattached a completely severed human limb, 1964, *JAMA* **189**:716. *4405.3*

1930:32 John R. **David**, British/American immunologist, born 15 Feb; discovered lymphokines, 1966, *PNAS* **56**:72; also discovered independently by B.R. Bloom and B. Bennett. *2578.36*

------------

1930: Alvar **Gullstrand** died, **born** 1862. *vision, ophthalomology, monochromatic aberrations*

1930: Constantin von **Monakow** died, **born** 1853. *rubrospinal tract, localization of cerebral function*

1930: Christine **Ladd-Franklin** died, **born** 1847. *vision*

1930: Salomon Eberhard **Henschen** died, **born** 1847. *visual centre*

1930: J.T. Ainslie **Walker** died, **born** 1868. *test for disinfectants*

1930: Katsusaburo **Yamagiwa** died, **born** 1863. *cancer, tar*

1930: Ernst Georg Ferdinand von **Küster** died, **born** 1839. *empyema, thoracotomy, mastoidectomy, hydronephrosis*

1930: Paul **Kraske** died, **born** 1851. *carcinoma of rectum*

1930: Louis **Bard** died, **born** 1857. *carcinoma of pancreas*

1930: Edward Hartley **Angle** died, **born** 1855. *orthodontics*

1930: George Neil **Stewart** died, **born** 1860. *Addison's disease*

1930: Ludwig **Rehn** died, **born** 1849. *heart suture, exophthalmic goitre, thyroidectomy*

1930: Christiaan **Eijkman** died, **born** 1858. *vitamins, beriberi*

1930: Karl **Leiner** died, **born** 1871. *desquamative erythroderma*

1930: Achille **Sclavo** died, **born** 1861. *anthrax immunization*

1930: Waldemar Mordecai Wolff **Haffkine** died, **born** 1860. *cholera vaccine, plague vaccine*

1930: Paul **Fürbringer** died, **born** 1849. *spinal puncture*

1930: Karl Theodor Paul Polykarpos **Axenfeld** died, **born** 1867. *metastatic ophthalmia, conjunctivitis*

1930: Ernst **Fuchs** died, **born** 1851. *keratoconjunctivitis, optic nerve atrophy*

**1931**
1931:1 **Nobel Prize** (Physiology or Medicine): Otto Heinrich Warburg (1883–1970), for his discovery of the nature and function of **iron oxygenase**, the **respiratory ferment**, *NPL. 969, 970*

1931:2 **Calciferol** isolated from irradiated ergosterol by Robert Benedict Bourdillon (1889–1971) and colleagues; *The quantitative estimation of vitamin D by radiography. 1065*

1931:3 **Androsterone** isolated by Adolf Friedrich Johann Butenandt (1903–1995), *ZAngC* **44**:905. *1195*

1931:4 Treatment of **hay fever** by **zinc** ionization introduced by Philip Franklin (1880–1951), *BMJ* **1**:1115. *2604*

1931:5 **Roentgenkymography** introduced by Pleikart Stumpf (b.1888), *FGR*, Erg. 41 . *2696*

1931:6 A quantitative theory of the effect of mutation, migration, selection and population size on changes in **gene frequencies in populations** advanced by Sewall Wright (1889–1988), *Genetics* **16**:97. *253.1*

1931:7 Introduction of **thorotrast** in **arteriography** by Reynaldo dos Santos (b.1880) and J. Caldas, *MCon* **49**:234. *2920*

1931:8 First successful surgical intervention for **cardiac aneurysm** by Ernst Ferdinand Sauerbruch (1875–1951), *ArKC* **167**:586. *2990*

1931:9 Successful complete removal of **bronchiectatic lung** by Rudolph Nissen (b.1896), *ZCh* **58**:3003. *3203*

1931:10 **Folic acid** shown by Lucy Wills (1888–1964) to have a haemopoietic effect in **anaemia**, *BMJ* **1**:1059. *3146*

1931:11 **Benedict's test** for **blood sugar** introduced by Stanley Rossiter Benedict (1884–1936), *JBC* **92**:141. *3923*

1931:12 '**Fanconi syndrome**', multiple defects in **renal tubular function**, described by Guido Fanconi (1892–1979), *JaK* **133**:257. *4248*

1931:13 The **Smith-Petersen nail**, a three-flanged nail which prevented rotation of the femoral head during treatment of **fractures of the neck of the femur** introduced by Marius Nygaard Smith-Petersen (1886–1953), *ArSuC* **23**:719 *4434*

1931:14 **Osteomyelitis** treatment with maggots inaugurated by William Stevenson Baer (1872–1931), *JBJS* **13**:438, ('**Baer therapy**'). *4399*

1931:15 The **arthroscopic appearance of joints** other than the knee first described by M.S. Burman, *JBJS* **13**:669. *4400.1*

1931:16 '**Adie's syndrome**', a condition in which a pupil that is usually larger than its fellow and reacts poorly to light ('**Adie's pupil**') is associated with absent tendon reflexes described by William John Adie (1886–1935), *BMJ* **1**:928. *4611*

1931:17 **High altitude physiology** studied by Joseph Barcroft (1872–1947), *ArSB* **16**:609. *2137.7*

1931:18 Precise **radiography** of the **skull** made possible by the **Lysholm-Schönander skull table** introduced by Erik Lysholm (1891–1947), *AcR* Sup.12. *4611.1*

1931:19 Immunological differences between strains of **poliomyelitis virus** demonstrated by Frank Macfarlane Burnet (1899–1985) and Jean Macnamara, *BJEP* **12**:57. *4670.5*

1931:20 The *gravis, mitis,* and intermediate types of *Corynebacterium diphtheriae* distinguished by James Stirling Anderson (1891–1976) and co-workers, *JPB* **34**:667. *5072*

1931:21 **Reserpine** introduced in the treatment of **psychoses** by G. Sen and K.C. Bose, *IMW* **2**:194. *4959*

1931:22 **Subarachnoid injection of alcohol** for the relief of **pain** introduced by Achile Mario Dogliotti (1897–1966), *PrM* **39**:1249. *4898*

1931:23 The **Kauffmann-White classification** of *Salmonella*, based on antigenic structure, described by Fritz Kauffmann, *ZGH* **25**:273. *5044.1*

1931:24 **Lymphogranuloma venereum** transmitted to animals and attributed to a virus by Sven Curt Alfred Hellerström (b.1901) and Erik Wassén, *CRDS* 1930, p. 1147. *5220*

1931:25 Murine **typhus** shown by Rolla Eugene Dyer (b.1886) to be caused by an organism, later named *Rickettsia mooseri, USPHR* **46**:334. *5396.2*

1931:26 The intraperitoneal test for immunity against **yellow fever** introduced by Wilbur Augustus Sawyer (1879–1931) and Wray Devere Marr Lloyd (1902–1936), *JEM* **54**:533. *5464*

1931:27 *Aëdes albopictus* shown to be a vector of **dengue** by James Stevens Simmons (1890–1954) and co-workers, *PhJS* **41**:215. *5475*

1931:28 **Rift Valley fever** described by Robert Daubney (b.1891) and John Richard Hudson, *JPB* **34**:545. *5541*

1931:29 An epidemiological and historical study of **yellow fever** compiled by Henry Rose Carter (1852–1925); *Yellow fever: an epidemiological and historical study of its place of origin*, edited after his death by L.A. Carter and W.H. Frost. *5468*

1931:30 The first to employ **ovarian hormone** systematically in the treatment of chronic **mastitis** was Max Cutler (1899–1984), *JAMA* **96**:1201. *5785*

1931:31 Victor Veau's (1871–1949) operation for **cleft palate** is described in his *Division palatine*. *5763*

1931:32 The **Friedman test** for the **diagnosis of pregnancy** introduced by Maurice Harold Friedman (b.1903) and Maxwell Edward Lapham (1899–1983), *AmJOG* **21**:405. *6224*

1931:33 Chemical **embryology** published by Joseph Needham (1900–1995). *531*

1931:34 **Substance P**, the first **peptide neurotransmitter**, isolated by John Henry Gaddum (1900–1965) and Ulf Svante von Euler (1905–1983), *JP* **72**:74.

1931:35 Jacques Albert Pierre **Miller**, French/Australian immunologist, born 2 Apr; demonstrated the immunological function of the thymus, 1961, *L* **2**:748. *2578.32*

1931:36 Hamilton Othanel **Smith**, American microbial geneticist, born 23 Aug; shared Nobel Prize (Physiology or Medicine), 1978, with Werner Arber and Daniel Nathans, for their discovery of restriction enzymes and their application to problems of molecular genetics, *NPL*.

1931:37 Ronald A. **Malt**, American surgeon, born 12 Nov; with Charles Freemont McKhann, first successfullly reattached a completely severed human limb, 1964, *JAMA* **189**:716. *4405.3*

1931:38 Philip Alfred **Brunel** born; with co-workers, first used zoster immune globulin for the prevention of varicella, 1969, *NEJM* **280**:1191. *5440.2*

1931: Auguste Henri **Forel** died, **born** 1848. *neuron theory*

1931: Edward R. **Henry** died, **born** 1931. *fingerprints*

1931: Emile Pierre Marie van **Ermengem** died, **born** 1851. *Clostridium botulinum, food poisoning*

1931: Harry de Riemer **Morgan** died, **born** 1863. *Proteus morgani*

1931: Felix von **Winiwater** died, **born** 1852. *thrombo-angiitis obliterans*

1931: Martin William **Flack** died, **born** 1882. *physiology, sino-auricular node (pacemaker of the heart)*

1931: Guido **Holzknecht** died, **born** 1872. *radiotherapy*

1931: Aldred Scott **Warthin** died, **born** 1866. *pulmonary fat embolism*

1931: Arthur **Hartmann** died, **born** 1849. *audiometer*

1931: Oscar **Minkowski** died, **born** 1858. *diabetes mellitus, oxybutyric acid, haemolytic jaundice, acromegaly, pituitary*

1931: Francis Xavier **Dercum** died, **born** 1856. *adiposis dolorosa*

1931: Nicolas Constantin **Paulescu** died, **born** 1869. *insulin*

1931: Axel **Holst** died, **born** 1861. *scurvy*

1931: William Stevenson **Baer** died, **born** 1872. *osteomyelitis*

1931: Charles Karsner **Mills** died, **born** 1845. *nervous system, paralysis*

1931: Alfons Maria **Jakob** died, **born** 1884. *spastic pseudosclerosis*

1931: William Henry **Bennett** died, **born** 1852. *rhizotomy*

1931: Constantin von **Economo** died, **born** 1876. *encephalitis*

1931: Shibasaburo **Kitasato** died, **born** 1852. *diphtheria and tetanus antitoxins, tetanus bacillus, Clostridium tetani*

1931: David **Bruce** died, **born** 1855. *brucellosis (Malta fever), Brucella melitensis, trypanosomiasis, tsetse fly, nagana, Trypanosoma brucei*

1931: Ludwig **Haendel** died, **born** 1869. *trypanosomiasis, suramin*

1931: Aristide **Agramonte y Simoni** died, **born** 1868. *yellow fever, mosquito*

1931: Ejnar Oluf Sorenson **Sylvest** died, **born** 1880. *myositis*

1931: Wilbur Augustus **Sawyer** died, **born** 1879. *yellow fever*

1931: Eugen von **Hippel** died, **born** 1869. *angiomatosis of retina*

1931: John Whitridge **Williams** died, **born** 1866. *obstetrics*

1931: Heinz **Küstner** died, **born** 1897. *antibodies, Prausnitz-Küstner reaction*

**1932**
1932:1 **Nobel Prize** (Physiology or Medicine): Charles Scott Sherrington (1857–1952) and Edgar Douglas Adrian (1889–1977), for their researches in **neuromuscular coordination** and function of **neurons**, *NPL. 1308, 1432*

1932:2 First **electron microscope** produced by Max Knoll (1879–1969) and Ernst Ruska (1906–1988), *AnPh* **12**:607. *269.3*

1932:3 **Mepacrine (atebrine, quinacrine)**, an anti-**malarial**, introduced by Walter Kikuth (1896–1968), *DMW* **58**:530. *5257*

1932:4 **Hypothalamus** shown to be the heat-regulating mechanism by Allen Dudley Keller (b.1901) and William Kendrick Hare (b.1908), *PSEB* **29**:1069. *1446.2*

1932:5 The role of the **sympathetic-adrenal mechanism** discussed by Walter Bradford Cannon (1871–1945); in his *The wisdom of the body. 664*

1932:6 **Artificial respiration**; 'arm-lift' method introduced by Holger Nielsen (1866–1955), *UL* **94**:1201. *2028.60*

1932:7 A new rocking method of **artificial respiration** described by Frank Cecil Eve (1871–1952); it became associated with his name, *L* 2:995. *1979*

1932:8 **Syphilis: Eagle flocculation test** introduced by Harry Eagle (b.1905), *JLCM* **17**:787. *2414.1*

1932:9 **Roentgen cinematography** introduced by Cesare Gianturco (b.1905) and Walter Clement Alvarez (b.1884), *PMC* **7**:669. *2697*

1932:10 A benign infectious **tumour** of viral origin, **Shope papilloma**, described by Richard Edwin Shope (1901–1966), *JEM* **56**:793. *2656*

1932:11 **Carcinogenic** properties of **dibenzanthracene** compounds discovered by James Wilfred Cook (1900–1975) with I. Hieger, Ernest Lawrence Kennaway (1881–1958) and W.V. Mayneord, *PRSB* **111**:455. *2654*

1932:12 **Hilar tourniquet** introduced in **lung** surgery by Norman Strahan Shenstone (b.1881) and Robert Meredith Janes (b.1894), *CMAJ* **27**:138. *3203.2*

1932:13 **Decompression apparatus** for the treatment of acute **intestinal obstruction** introduced by Owen Harding Wangensteen (1898–1981), *WJS* **40**:1. *3554*

1932:14 Burrill Bernard Crohn (1884–1983), L. Ginzburg and G.D. Oppenheimer described the clinical and pathological features of regional **ileitis** ('**Crohn's disease**'), *JAMA* **99**:1323. *3551*

1932:15 Flexible **gastroscope** introduced by Rudolph Schindler (1888–1968), *MMW* **79**:1268. *3553*

1932:16 Attention to **tyrosinosis**, an error of **tyrosine metabolism**, was drawn by Grace Medes (1886–1967), *BJ* **26**:917. *3923.1*

1932:17 An **adrenal cortical hormone** ('**eschatin**') prepared by Wilbur Willis Swingle (b.1891) and Joseph John Pfiffner (1903–1975) and used effectively in the treatment of **Addison's disease**, *Medicine* **11**:371. *3874*

1932:18 Harvey Williams Cushing (1869–1939) described '**Cushing's syndrome**', now known to be due to **adrenal disease**, *BJH* **50**:137; advanced the theory that the **hypothalamus** is responsible for the development of **peptic ulcer**, in his *Papers relating to the pituitary body, hypothalamus*, etc., p. 175; his operating technique enabled a dramatic reduction of mortality rate in **intracranial surgery**, shown in his *Intracranial tumours*. *3904, 3552, 4900*

1932:19 The use of **neostigmine** in the treatment of **myasthenia gravis** introduced by Lazar Remen (b.1907), *DZN* **128**:66. *4767*

1932:20 A skin test for the diagnosis of **tularaemia** introduced by Lee Foshay (1896–1960), *JID* **51**:286. *5178*

1932:21 **Lumbar encephalography** introduced by Leo Max Davidoff (1898–1975) and C.G. Dyke, *BNI* **2**:75. *4611.3*

1932:22 An intradermal test for the diagnosis of **trichinosis** introduced by Donald Leslie Augustine (b.1895) and Hans Theiler (b.1894), *Para* **24**:60. *5351.1*

1932:23 The '**Paul-Bunnell test**' for the diagnosis of **infectious mononucleosis** introduced by John Rodman Paul (1893–1971) and Walls Willard Bunnell (b.1902), *AmJMS* **183**:90. *5487*

1932:24 An immune serum for prophylactic inoculation against **yellow fever** devised by Wilbur Augustus Sawyer (1879–1931), S.F. Kitchen and Wray Devere Marr Lloyd (1902–1936), *JEM* **55**:945. *5465*

1932:25 **Yellow fever** virus grown in culture by Eugen Haagen and Max Theiler (1899–1972), *ZBP* Abt.I **125**:145. *5465.1*

1932:26 **Evipan** (**hexobarbitone**) introduced as an **anaesthetic** by Helmut Weese (1897–1954) and Walther Scharpff, *DMW* **58**:1205. *5714*

1932:27 Conclusive proof that the causal agent in **psittacosis** is *Chlamydia psittaci* given by Samuel Philips Bedson (1886–1969) and J.O.W. Bland, *BJEP* **13**:461. *5541.1*

1932:28 Intracapsular extraction of **cataract** by **diathermy** with the **electrodiaphake** carried out by Julio Lopez Lacarrere, *ArOH* **32**:293. *5983*

1932:29 A new method of **keratoplasty** (**corneal grafting**) introduced by Ramon Castroviejo (1904–1987), *AmJOp* **15**:825, 905. *5981*

1932:30 The **carcinogenic** effect of **ovarian hormone** demonstrated by Antoine Marcellin Lacassagne (1884–1971), *CRAS* **195**:30. *5787*

1932:31 The *Biographisches Lexikon der hervorragenden Ärzte der letzen fünfzig Jahre*, 1 vol. [in 2], 1932–33, compiled by Isidor Fischer (1868–1943); it is a supplement to the great source for **medical biography** to 1880, *Biographisches Lexikon*, 6 vols, 1884–1888, of A. Hirsch. *6732*

---

1932:32 Walter **Gilbert**, American biochemist, born 21 Mar; shared Nobel Prize (Chemistry), 1980, with Paul Berg and Frederick Sanger, for his contribution concerning the determination of base sequences in nucleic acids, *NPL*.

1932:33 Michael **Smith**, British biochemist, born 26 Apr; shared Nobel Prize (Chemistry), 1993, with Kary B. Mullis, for his fundamental contribution to the establishment of oligonucleotide-based, site-directed mutagenesis and its development for protein studies, *NPL*.

1932:34 Paul Douglas **Parkman**, American paediatrician and virologist, born 29 May; with co-workers isolated the rubella virus, 1962, *PSEB* **111**:225; with Harry Martin Meyer and T.C. Panos, produced an experimental live-virus rubella vaccine, 1966, *NEJM* **275**:575. *5509.2, 5509.3*

---

1932:35 Richard K. **Gerson** born; with K. Kondo, discovered suppressor T cells, 1970, *I* **18**:723. Died 1983. *2578.41*

---

1932:36 Arthur Dawson **Milne** died; with Philip Hedgeland Ross, discovered that African relapsing fever (tick fever) is conveyed by *Ornithodorus moubata*, 1904, *BMJ* **2**:453. *5317*

1932: Frederick William **Andrewes** died, **born** 1859. *dysentery, Shigella alkalescens*

1932: Karl **Spiro** died, **born** 1867. *ergotamine*

1932: Maurice **Nicolle** died, **born** 1862. *anaphylaxis*

1932: Rudolf **Kraus** died, **born** 1868. *antigens, antibodies, precipitin reaction*

1932: Georg **Klemperer** died, **born** 1865. *pneumococcus*

1932: Anatole Marie Emile **Chauffard** died, **born** 1855. *haemolytic jaundice, pseudoxanthoma elasticum*

1932: Alfred Leftwich **Gray** died, **born** 1873. *bladder carcinoma, radiotherapy*

1932: Paul Albert **Grawitz** died, **born** 1850. *hypernephroma*

1932: Fritz **Steinmann** died, **born** 1872. *fractures*

1932: Russell Aubra **Hibbs** died, **born** 1869. *scoliosis, spinal fusion*

1932: Joseph François Félix **Babinski** died, **born** 1857. *Frölich's syndrome, pyramidal-tract disease, syndrome of Babinski-Nageotte, anosognosia of neurological disorders*

1932: Samuel Vulvovich **Goldflam** died, **born** 1852. *myasthenia pseudoparalytica*

1932: Hermann **Küttner** died, **born** 1870. *tabes*

1932: Bernhard Laurits Frederik **Bang** died, **born** 1848. *brucellosis, Brucella abortus*

1932: William Williams **Keen** died, **born** 1837. *craniotomy, spasmodic torticollis*

1932: Petr Fokich **Borovskii** died, **born** 1863. *leishmaniasis, Leishmania tropica*

1932: Ronald **Ross** died, **born** 1857. *mosquito transmission of malaria*

1932: Max **Rubner** died, **born** 1854. *dynamic effect of foodstuffs, conservation of energy*

1932: Gustav Adolf **Neuber** died, **born** 1850. *asepsis*

## 1933

1933:1 **Nobel Prize** (Physiology or Medicine): Thomas Hunt Morgan (1866–1945), for establishing the **chromosome** theory of **heredity**, *NPL. 246*

1933:2 Experiments on **hearing** by Georg von Békésy (1899–1972) first appeared in *PhZ* **34**:577. *1570.1*

1933:3 *Leptospira canicola* first isolated from dog urine by Arie Klarenbeek (b.1888) and Wilhelm August Paul Schüffner (1867–1949), *NTG* **77**:4271. *5335*

1933:4 **Prolactin** prepared, identified and assayed by Oscar Riddle (1877–1968) and co-workers, *AmJPh* **105**:191. *1171*

1933:5 Synthesis of **vitamin** C by Tadeus Reichstein (1897–1996) and co-workers, *HCA* **16**;1019. *1068*

1933:6 **Burns**; gentian violet treatment introduced by Robert Henry Aldrich (b.1902), *NEJM* **208**:299. *2258*

1933:7 **Streptokinase**, a fibrinolysin, discovered by William Smith Tillett (1892–1974) and Raymond Loraine Garner (b.1906), *JEM* **58**:485. *1924.1*

1933:8 **5-Hydroxytryptamine** isolated by Maffo Vialli and Vittorio Erspamer (b.1909), *ZZ* **19**:743, named **serotonin** by M. Rapport et al., 1948. *1924.2*

1933:9 **Haemolytic streptococcus**; differentiation of types by Rebecca Craighill Lancefield (1895–1981), *JEM* **57**:571. *2524.2*

1933:10 Fundamental research on **antigen-antibody** reactions by Karl Landsteiner (1868–1943); *Die Specifizität der serologischen Reaktionen*. *2576.2*

1933:11 **Carotid sinus syndrome** described by Soma Weiss (1898–1942) and James Porter Baker (b.1913), *Medicine* **12**:297. *2921*

1933:12 **Angina pectoris** and **congestive heart failure** treated by **thyroidectomy** by Herman Ludwig Blumgart (b.1895), Samuel Albert Levine (1891–1966) and D.D. Berlin, *ArIM* **51**:866. *2899, 3033*

1933:13 **Chest leads** introduced in the **electrocardiographic** diagnosis of **coronary occlusion** by Christian Wolferth (1887–1965) and Francis Clark Wood (b.1901), *AmJMS* **183**:30. *2863*

1933:14 **Tomography** introduced into **radiography** by D.L. Bartelink, *FGR* **47**:399. *2698*

1933:15 **Bronchiectasis** associated with **sinusitis** and **situs inversus** ('**Kartagener's syndrome**') reported by Manes Kartagener (b.1897), *BKT* **83**:489. *3206*

1933:16 **Hyperventilation** syndrome reported by Charles Koran Maytum (b.1895), *PMC* **8**:282. *3207*

1933:17 Total **pneumonectomy** for **carcinoma** of **bronchus** by Evarts Ambrose Graham (1885–1957) and Jacob Jesse Singer (1882–1954), *JAMA* **101**:1371. *3205*

1933:18 Total **pneumonectomy** for **sarcoma** in a **tuberculous** patient performed by Howard Lilienthal (1861–1946), *JTS* **2**:600. *3207*

1933:19 Treatment of bilateral **pulmonary tuberculosis** by artificial **pneumoperitoneum** introduced by Ludwig Vajda, *ZTb* **67**:371. *3236*

1933:20 **Quick's liver function test** introduced by Armand James Quick (1894–1977), *AmJMS* **185**:630. *3659*

1933:21 Infantile **scurvy** first treated by administration of **ascorbic acid** by Leonard Gregory Parsons (1879–1950), *PRSM* **26**:1533. *3725*

1933:22 **Chaoul therapy (radiotherapy)** in the treatment of malignant **tumours** introduced by Henri Chaoul (b.1887) and Albert Adam, *Str* **48**:31. *4007*

1933:23 **Hippuran (sodium ortho-hippurate)** introduced by Moses Swick (b.1900), *SGO* **56**:62. *4201*

1933:24 **Epiphysiodesis** to inhibit the **bone growth** of a longer leg introduced by Dallas B. Phemister (1882–1951), *JBJS* **15**:1. *4400.3*

1933:25 **St Louis encephalitis virus** isolated by Ralph S. Muckenfuss and co-workers, *USPHR* **48**:1341. *4656*

1933:26 The *Culex* **mosquito** reported as vector of **St Louis encephalitis virus** by Leslie Leon Lumsden (1875–1946), *USPHR* **73**:340 [published in 1958]. *4661.2*

1933:27 **A.T. 10 (dihydrotachysterol)** introduced in the treatment of **tetany** by Friedrich Holtz, *ArKC* **177**:32. *4838*

1933:28 **Tetanus** toxoid first employed in the immunization of humans by Gaston Léon Ramon (1886–1963) and Christian Zoeller (1888–1934), *CRSB* **112**:347. *5151*

1933:29 **Lumbar sympathectomy** carried out by the antero-lateral extraperitoneal approach by René Leriche (1879–1955) and R. Fontaine, *PrM* **41**:1819. *4902*

1933:30 Prophylactic **vaccination** against **leptospirosis** introduced by H. Wani, *ZI* **79**:1. *5335.1*

1933:31 **Influenza A** virus recovered from throat washings of influenza patients by Wilson Smith (1897–1965), Christopher Howard Andrewes (1896–1988) and Patrick Playfair Laidlaw (1881–1940), *L* **2**:66. *5494*

1933:32 **Divinyl ether** first put to clinical use by Samuel Gelfan (b.1903) and I.R. Bell, *JPET* **47**:1. *5715*

1933:33 A serum for the treatment of **tularaemia** devised by Lee Foshay (1896–1960), *JAMA* **98**:552, **101**:1047. *5179*

1933:34 Cultivation of *Histoplasma capsulatum* by George Henry Hansmann (b.1890) and John Rudolph Schenken (b.1905), *Science* **77** (No. 2002), Supplement, p. 8, 1934, *AmJPa* **10**:731. Almost simultaneously it was cultivated by DeMonbreun. *5541.2, 5542*

1933:35 The first description of **plasma-cell mastitis** given by Frank Earl Adair (b.1887), *ArSuC* **26**:735. *5788*

1933:36 **Contact lenses** introduced by Josef Dallos (1905–1979), *KMA* **91**:640. *5985*

1933:37 The modern classification of the female **pelvis** is based on the work of William Edgar Caldwell (1880–1943) and Howard Carman Moloy (1903–1953), *AmJOG* **26**:479. *6266*

1933:38 **Amenorrhoea** first treated with **oestrogenic hormone** by Carl Kaufmann, *KW* **12**:1557. *6130*

1933:39 Grantly Dick-Read (1890–1959) advocated **natural childbirth** and demonstrated that prenatal education in methods of relaxation in many cases makes **labour** almost painless. He wrote *Natural childbirth*. *6225*

1933:40 The Paris method of **radium** treatment for **cancer** of the **uterus** devised by Claude Regaud (1870–1940), *RR* **3**:155. *6131*

1933:41 Sture August Siwe (b.1897) published his account of **Letterer-Siwe disease**, *ZK* **55**:212. *6373, 6372*

1933:42 A test for early diagnosis of **carcinoma** of the **cervix uteri** introduced by Walter Schiller (1887–1960), *SGO* **56**:210. *6132*

---

1933:43 Heinrich **Rohrer**, Swiss physicist, born 1933; shared Nobel Prize (Physics), 1986, with Gerd Binnig and Ernst Ruska, for the design of the scanning tunnelling microscope, *NPL*.

1933:44 Frank H. **Gunston** born; carried out an arthroplasty replacement of the knee-joint, 1971, *JBJS* **53b**:272. *4405.5*

---

1933: Walter Morley **Fletcher** died, **born** 1873. *Medical Research Committee (Council), lactic acid, muscular contraction*

1933: Weller **Van Hook** died, **born** 1862. *ureteral repair*

1933: Edward Clark **Davidson** died, **born** 1894. *burns*

1933: Léon Charles Albert **Calmette** died, **born** 1863. *tuberculosis, plague bacillus, inoculation*

1933: Robert **Jones** died, **born** 1858. *x rays*

1933: Viktor von **Hacker** died, **born** 1852. *resection of pylorus, gastrostomy*

1933: Hermann **Sahli** died, **born** 1856. *functional activity of stomach*

1933: Georges **Hayem** died, **born** 1841. *blood platelets, haemolytic anaemia, hepatitis, chlorosis*

1933: Alfred Fabian **Hess** died, **born** 1875. *rickets, scurvy, ultraviolet irradiation, rubella*

1933: Robert Calvin **Coffey** died, **born** 1869. *uretero-intestinal anastomosis*

1933: William Thomas **Councilman** died, **born** 1854. *amoebic dysentery*

1933: Pierre Paul Émile **Roux** died, **born** 1853. *diphtheria, Corynebacterium diphtheriae, antitoxin, rabies, anthrax immunization*

1933: Gustav **Paul** died, **born** 1859. *smallpox*

1933: Thomas Lane **Bancroft** died, **born** 1860. *dengue, mosquito*

1933: Joseph Léon Marcel **Lignières** died, **born** 1868. *actinobacillus*

1933: George Thomas **Beatson** died, **born** 1848. *oöphorectomy*

1933: George Howard **Monks** died, **born** 1853. *rhinophyma*

1933: Artur **Biedl** died, **born** 1869. *retinitis pigmentosa*

1933: Noel **Fiessinger** died, **born** 1881. *Reiter's syndrome*

1933: Carl Franz Joseph Erich **Correns** died, **born** 1864. *genetics*

1933: Alfred **Dührssen** died, **born** 1862. *caesarean section*

## 1934

1934:1 **Nobel Prize** (Physiology or Medicine): George Richards Minot (1885–1950), William Parry Murphy (1892–1987) and George Hoyt Whipple (1878–1976), for their treatment of pernicious **anaemia** with raw **liver** diet, *NPL. 3139, 3140*

1934:2 Isolation of **herpesvirus (B virus) simiae** by Albert Bruce Sabin (b.1906) and Arthur M. Wright, 1934, *JEM* **59**:115. *4658*

1934:3 **Vitamin F (linolenic acid)** isolated by Herbert McLean Evans (1882–1971) and co-workers, *JBC* **106**:431. *1070*

1934:4 **Androsterone** synthesized (first complete synthesis of a sex hormone) by Leopold Ruzicka (1887–1976) and co-workers, *HCA* **17**:1395. *1201*

1934:5 **Progesterone** isolated in crystalline form by Adolf Friedrich Johann Butenandt (1903–1995), *WKW* **47**:897,934. *1200*

1934:6 Action of **acetylcholine** in transmission of nerve impulses determined by Wilhelm Feldberg (1900–1993) and John Henry Gaddum (1900–1965), *JP* **81**:305. *1352*

1934:7 Crystalline **secretin** prepared by Gunnar Ågren (b.1907), *SkAP* **70**:10. *1039*

1934:8 **Prostaglandins** extracted from seminal fluid by Ulf Svante von Euler (1905–1983), *ArEP* **175**:78. *1924.3*

1934:9 **Serological classification of Streptococcus** by Frederick Griffith (?1879–1941), *JHyg* **34**:542. *2524.3*

1934:10 Atopic **dermatitis** shown to be due to inhaled **allergens** by Marion B. Sulzberger (1895–1983), *JAI* **5**:554. *2605.1*

1934:11 **Syphilis: mapharsen** used experimentally in treatment by Arthur Lawrie Tatum (1884–1955) and Garrett Arthur Cooper (b.1904), *JPET* **50**:198. (Its clinical use was initiated by Otto Foerster et al. in 1935.) *2415*

1934:12 **Unipolar leads** introduced into **electrocardiography** by Frank Norman Wilson (1890–1952) and co-workers, *AmHJ* **9**:447. *2864*

1934:13 Important studies on **experimental hypertension** carried out by Harry Goldblatt (1891–1977) and co-workers, *JEM* **59**:347. *2719*

1934:14 **Haemophilia** treatment by **snake venom** introduced by Robert Gwyn Macfarlane (1907–1987) and Burgess Barnett, *L* **2**:985. *3093*

1934:15 **Meulengracht diet** for treatment of **haematemesis** and **melaena** introduced by Einar Meulengracht (b.1887), *AcM* Sup. 59:375. *3555*

1934:16 **Phenylketonuria**, the first hereditary **metabolic disorder** shown to be responsible for **mental retardation**, first described by Ivar Asbjorn Følling (1888–1973), *NoMT* **8**:1054. *3924*

1934:17 Karel Frederik Wenckebach (1864–1940) wrote *Das Beriberi-Herz*, an important account of the **heart** in **beriberi**. *3747*

1934:18 The causal role of **intravertebral disk herniation** in **sciatica** demonstrated by William Jason Mixter (1880–1958) and Joseph Seton Barr (1901–1963), *NEJM* **211**:210. *4435*

1934:19 Benign **lymphocytic choriomeningitis virus** isolated by Charles Armstrong (1886–1967) and Ralph Dougall Lillie (b.1896), *USPHR* **49**:1019. *4688*

1934:20 The experimental transmission of **Japanese B encephalitis** accomplished by Michotomo Hayashi, *PIAJ* **10**:41. *4657*

1934:21 **Hydrocephalus** treated by endoscopic coagulation of the choroid plexus by Tracy Jackson Putnam (b.1894), *NEJM* **210**:1373. *4903*

1934:22 **Insulin shock therapy** introduced in the treatment of **schizophrenia** by Manfred Joshua Sakel (1900–1957), *WMW* **84**:1211. *4960*

1934:23 **Vi antigen**, the antigen of the **typhoid** bacillus, first described by Arthur Felix (1887–1956) and R.M. Pitt, *Lancet* **2**:186. *5045*

1934:24 Hans Zinsser (1878–1940) advanced the theory that **Brill's disease** is a recrudescence of epidemic **typhus**, *AmJH* **20**:513; the condition was subsequently named '**Brill-Zinsser disease**'. *5396.4, 5382*

1934:25 **Leptospirosis** due to infection with *Leptospira canicola* first reported in humans by C.M. Dhont, Arie Klarenbeek (b.1888) and Wilhelm August Paul Schüffner (1867–1949), *NTG* **78**:5297. *5336*

1934:26 **Cyclopropane anaesthesia** first used clinically by John Alden Stiles (b.1905) and co-workers, *CRA* **13**:56. *5717*

1934:27 The closed-circuit method of using **cyclopropane anaesthesia** introduced by Ralph Milton Waters (b.1883) and Erwin Rudolph Schmidt (b.1890), *JAMA* **103**:975. *5718*

1934:28 *Histoplasma capsulatum* cultivated by William Andrew DeMonbreun (b.1899), *AmJTM* **14**:93, almost simultaneously with Hansmann and Schenken. *5542, 5541.2*

1934:29 The **mumps** virus isolated by Claud D. Johnson and Ernest William Goodpasture (1886–1960), *JEM* **59**:1. *5543*

1934:30 **Trichloroethylene**, introduced by Lehmann (1911), first used experimentally as an **anaesthetic** by Dennis Emerson Jackson (b.1878), *CRA* **13**:198. *5716*

1934:31 **Fibroma** of the **ovary** with pleural effusion ('**Meigs' syndrome**') described by Joe Vincent Meigs (b.1892); in his *Tumors of the female pelvic organs*, p. 262.; described earlier by Lawson Tait, 1892. *6132.01, 6093.1*

1934:32 An apparatus for the self-administration of gas-air **analgesia** in **labour** (the '**Minnitt apparatus**') introduced by Robert James Minnitt (1889–1974), *L* **1**:1278. *6228*

1934:33 A test for the **diagnosis of pregnancy** introduced by Regine Kapeller-Adler, *KW* **13**:21. *6227*

1934:34 The *Xenopus* **toad test** for the **diagnosis of pregnancy** introduced by Charles William Bellerby, following the demonstration that *Xenopus* responds by ovulation to the **gonadotrophic hormone**, *Nature* **133**:494. *6226*

1934:35 Direct **radiography** of the **placenta** achieved by William Snow (b.1898) and Clilian Bethany Powell (b.1894), *AmJR* **31**:37. *6229*

---

1934:36 Bengt Ingemar **Samuelsson**, Swedish biochemist, born 21 May; shared Nobel Prize (Physiology or Medicine), 1982, with Sune Bergström and John Robert Vane, for their discoveries concerning the prostaglandins and related biologically active substances, *NPL*.

1934:37 Howard Martin **Temin**, American virologist, born 10 Dec; independently of both Renato Dulbecco and David Baltimore, discovered the interaction between tumour viruses and genetic material of the cell, 1964, *NCIM* **17**; 1970, *Nature* **226**:1211; *Nature* **226**:1209; shared Nobel Prize (Physiology or Medicine), 1975, with them, *NPL*. Died 1994. *2660.20, 2660.22, 2660.23, 2660.27*

---

1934: Marie Sklodowska **Curie** died, **born** 1867. *radium*

1934: William Henry **Welch** died, **born** 1850. *Clostridium perfringens, gas gangrene, Staphylococcus epidermidis albus, wound infection*

1934: Theobald **Smith** died, **born** 1859. *Salmonella cholerae-suis, tuberculosis, Mycobacterium, viral immunity, Babesia bigemina, Boophilus annulatus, Texas cattle fever*

1934: August **Gaertner** died, **born** 1848. *Salmonella enteritidis*

1934: Friedrich **Schultze** died, **born** 1848. *acroparaesthesia*

1934: G. Paul **Laroque** died, **born** 1876. *femoral and inguinal hernia*

1934: Otto Knut Olof **Folin** died, **born** 1867. *blood sugar test*

1934: Jay Frank **Schamberg** died, **born** 1870. *progressive pigmentary dermatosis*

1934: Frank Chambliss **Johnson** died, **born** 1894. *Stevens-Johnson syndrome*

1934: Carl **Schlatter** died, **born** 1864. *gastroscope, gastrectomy, tibial tuberosity lesions*

1934: Marmaduke Stephen **Mayou** died, **born** 1876. *amaurotic familial idiocy*

1934: Christian **Zoeller** died, **born** 1888. *tetanus toxoid, immunization*

1934: Edward Ernest **Maxey** died, **born** 1867. *Rocky Mountain spotted fever*

1934: Carlos Ribeiro Justiniano **Chagas** died, **born** 1879. *trypanosomiasis, Trypanosoma cruzi*

1934: Vasili Iakovlevich **Danilevski** died, **born** 1852. *malaria, Plasmodium*

1934: Wilhelm **His** Jr died, **born** 1863. *atrioventricular bundle, trench fever*

1934: Santiago **Ramón y Cajal** died, **born** 1852. *histology, degeneration and regeneration of nervous system*

1934: Heinrich Friedrich Wilhelm **Braun** died, **born** 1862. *anaesthesia, procaine*

**1935**
1935:1 **Nobel Prize** (Physiology or Medicine): Hans Spemann (1869–1941), for his discovery of the 'organizer' in **embryonic development**, *NPL. 530*

1935:2 Isolation of a **virus**, in crystalline form, later shown to be a **nucleoprotein**, by Wendell Meredith Stanley (1904–1971), *Science* **81**:644. *2524.5*

1935:3 Therapeutic value of **sulphanilamide** discovered by Daniel Bovet (b.1907), the Tréfouëls and other co-workers, *CRSB* **120**:756. *1950*

1935:4 **Testosterone** isolated from the testis by K. David and co-workers, *HSZ* **233**:281. *1201.1*

1935:5 **Burns**; **tannic acid-silver nitrate** method of treatment introduced by Adalbert Goodman Bettman (b.1883), *NM* **34**:46. *2259*

1935:6 **Prontosil**, the first drug containing a **sulphonamide**, introduced by Gerhard Domagk (1895–1964), *DMW* **61**:250. *1949*

1935:7 **Blood transfusion**, slow-drip method, introduced by Hugh Leslie Marriott (1900–1963) and Alan Kekwick (1909–1974), *L* **1**:977. *2023*

1935:8 **Syphilis: mapharsen** used in treatment by Otto Foerster (1876–1965) and co-workers, *ArDS* **32**:868. *2416*

1935:9 **Pleuropneumonia-like organisms (mycoplasma)** isolated from *Streptobacillus moniliformis* by Emmy Klieneberger (1892–1985), *JPB* **40**:93. *2524.4*

1935:10 Collateral **blood supply** to the **heart** provided by pericardial **implantation** of **pectoral muscle** by Claude Schaeffer Beck (1894–1971), *AnS* **102**:801. *3034*

1935:11 Collateral **blood supply** to the **heart** provided by **cardio-omentopexy** by Claude Schaeffer Beck (1894–1971) and Vladimir Leslie Tichy (1899–1967), *AmHJ* **10**:849. *3035*

1935:12 First planned lobectomy in **pulmonary tuberculosis** by Samuel Oscar Freedlander (b.1893), *JTS* **5**:132. *3238*

1935:13 **Prothrombin clotting time** estimation ('**Quick's method**') introduced by Armand James Quick (1894–1977), *JBC* **109**:lxxiii. *3095*

1935:14 **Wintrobe's method** for determination of **erythrocyte sedimentation rate** introduced by Maxwell Myer Wintrobe (1901–1986) and J. Walter Landsberg (b.1907), *AmJMS* **189**:102. *3096*

1935:15 Surgical treatment for **hypertension** ('**Peet's operation**') introduced by Max Minor Peet (1885–1949), *PCAM* **5**:58. *3036*

1935:16 **Achrestic anaemia** first described by John Frederick Wilkinson (b.1897) and Martin Cyril Gordon Israëls, *BMJ* **1**:139,194. *3148*

1935:17 **Thoracoplasty** with extrafacial **apicolysis** ('**Semb's operation**') in **pulmonary tuberculosis** carried out by Carl Boye Semb (1895–1972), *AcC* Suppl. 37ii:1. *3239*

1935:18 **Pancreaticoduodenectomy** for **cancer** of the **pancreas** ('**Whipple's operation**') introduced by Allen Oldfather Whipple (1881–1963), *AnS* **102**:763. *3659.1*

1935:19 Cicely Delphine Williams (1893–1992) gave the first accurate description of **kwashiorkor**, *L* **2**:1151. *3759*

1935:20 **Mandelic acid** first used in the treatment of **urinary infections** by Max Leonard Rosenheim (1908–1972), *L* **1**:1032. *4202*

1935:21 A one-stage **interinnomino-abdominal (hind-quarter) amputation** introduced by Gordon Gordon-Taylor (1878–1960) and Philip Wiles (1899–1967), *BJS* **22**:671. *4478*

1935:22 **Cardiazol (metrazol, pentylenetetrazol) convulsion therapy** introduced in the treatment of **schizophrenia** by Ladislaus Joseph Meduna (1896–1965), *ZGN* **152**:235. *4961*

1935:23 *d*-**Tubocurarine chloride** isolated from **curare** by Harold King (1887–1956), *Nature* **135**:469. *5719*

1935:24 **Phase contrast microscopy** developed by Frits Zernike (1888–1966), *PhZ* **36**:848. *269.5*

588

1935:25 **Thiopentone sodium** introduced as an **anaesthetic** by John Silas Lundy (b.1894), *PMC* **10**:536. *5720*

1935:26 Human **anaesthetization** with **trichloroethylene** first reported by Cecil Striker (b.1897) and co-workers, *CRA* **14**:68. *5721*

1935:27 **Influenza A** virus successfully cultivated by Frank Macfarlane Burnet (1899–1985), *MJA* **2**:687. *5496*

1935:28 Earlier work on **corneal transplantation** by Vladimir Petrovich Filatov (1875–1956), published in Russian journals, summarized, *ArOp* **13**:321. *5986*

1935:29 **Ergometrine** isolated by Harold Ward Dudley (1887–1935) and John Chassar Moir (1900–1977), *BMJ* **1**:520. *6230*

1935:30 The first report of the use of an antimicrobial agent (**prontosil**) in the treatment of **puerperal fever** made by Eugen Anselm, *DMW* **61**:264. *6280.1*

1935:31 **Amenorrhoea** associated with bilateral **polycystic ovaries** described by Irving Freiler Stein (b.1887) and Michael Leo Leventhal (b.1901) was named the **Stein-Leventhal syndrome**, *AmJOG* **29**:181. *6132.1*

1935: Carl **Sternberg** died, **born** 1872. *lymphogranulomatosis*

1935: Edward Albert **Sharpey-Schafer** died, **born** 1850. *adrenaline, artificial respiration*

1935: Charles Robert **Richet** died, **born** 1850. *anaphylaxis*

1935: Gustav **Hauser** died, **born** 1856. *Proteus vulgaris*

1935: Michael Idvorsky **Pupin** died, **born** 1858. *radiography*

1935: Joseph Colt **Bloodgood** died, **born** 1867. *inguinal hernia*

1935: Pierre Eugène **Menetrier** died, **born** 1859. *giant hypertrophic gastritis*

1935: Ludwig **Pick** died, **born** 1868. *Niemann-Pick disease*

1935: John James Rickard **Macleod** died, **born** 1876. *insulin*

1935: Carl **Sternberg** died, **born** 1872. *lymphadenoma, aleukaemic anaemia*

1935: Max Leonard **Rosenheim** died, **born** 1908. *urinary infections, mandelic acid*

1935: Luis **Morquio** died, **born** 1867. *osteochondrodystrophy*

1935: Murk **Jansen** died, **born** 1863. *bone growth*

1935: William John **Adie** died, **born** 1886. *Adie's syndrome*

1935: Wilhelm **Kolle** died, **born** 1868. *cholera vaccine*

1935: Charles **Norris** died, **born** 1867. *relapsing fever, spirochaete*

1935: Griffith **Evans** died, **born** 1835. *surra, trypanosome*

1935: Achille **Breda** died, **born** 1850. *yaws, framboesia*

1935: Ettore **Marchiafava** died, **born** 1847. *malaria, Plasmodium, alcoholism*

1935: Elmer Isaac **McKesson** died, **born** 1881. *anaesthesia, nitrous-oxide-oxygen*

1935: Jules **Gonin** died, **born** 1870. *detached retina*

1935: Victor **Morax** died, **born** 1866. *conjunctivitis*

1935: Camille Louis Antoine **Champetier de Ribes** died, **born** 1848. *cervix dilatation, Champetier de Ribes bag*

1935: Gustav Adolf **Walcher** died, **born** 1856. *gynaecology, 'Walcher position'*

1935: Harold Ward **Dudley** died, **born** 1887. *ergometrine*

1935: Hugo Marie de **Vries** died, **born** 1848. *genetics*

1935: Fielding Hudson **Garrison** died, **born** 1870. *history of medicine*

## 1936

1936:1 **Nobel Prize** (Physiology or Medicine): Henry Hallett Dale (1875–1968) and Otto Loewi (1873–1961), for their work on the chemical mediation of the **nervous impulse**, *NPL*. *1340, 1343*

1936:2 **Wellcome Trust** created, on the death of Henry Solomon Wellcome (1853–1936), to support **medical research** and the study of the **history of medicine**

1936:3 **Irish Medical Association** founded

1936:4 A **milk factor** in **cancer** transmission in mice isolated by John Joseph Bittner (1904–1961), *Science* **84**:162. *2658*

1936:5 **Poliomyelitis virus** isolated and propagated in pure culture by Albert Bruce Sabin (b.1906) and Peter Kosciusko Olitsky (1886–1964), *PSEB* **34**:357. *4670.6*

1936:6 Robert Bews Kerr (b.1908) and co-workers combined zinc with insulin, and later also with protamine, to form **protamine zinc insulin**, to delay the absorption rate, *CMAJ* **34**:400. *3975*

1936:7 **Vitamin E** isolated by Herbert McLean Evans (1882–1971), *JBC* **113**:319. *1071*

1936:8 **Oestradiol** isolated by Donald William McCorquodale (b.1898) and co-workers, *JBC* **115**:435. *1202*

1936:9 *The endocrine organs in health and disease* published by Humphry Davy Rolleston (1862–1944). *3909*

1936:10 **Cortisone** isolated by Edward Calvin Kendall (1886–1972) and associates, *JBC* **114**:lvii, 613; **116**:267. It was also isolated by Osker Paul Wintersteiner (1898–1971) and Joseph Pfiffner (1903–1975), *JBC* **111**:599; **116**:291, and by Tadeus Reichstein (1897–1996), *HCA* **19**:1107, in the same year. *1151, 1152, 1153*

1936:11 **Blood transfusion**, using heparin introduced by Per Johannes Hedenius (b.1906), *AcM* **89**:263. *2024*

1936:12 **Thiocyanate** treatment of **hypertension** developed by Marion Herbert Barker (1899–1947), *JAMA* **106**:762. *2720*

1936:13 *Atlas of congenital cardiac disease* compiled by Maude Elizabeth Seymour Abbott (1869–1940). *2865*

1936:14 **Vectorcardiogram** introduced by Fritz Schellong, *VDIM* **48**:288. *2865.1*

1936:15 **Thalassaemia** shown by J. Caminopetros to be genetically determined, *AnM* **43**:104. *3148.2*

1936:16 Mass **chest radiography** introduced by Manoel de Abreu (1892–1962), *RAPM* **9**:313. *3209.1*

1936:17 Operation for **femoral hernia**, using a midline extraperitoneal approach, devised by Arnold Kirkpatrick Henry (1886–1962), *L* **1**:531. *3611*

1936:18 **Cystic fibrosis (mucoviscidosis)** first described by Guido Fanconi (1892–1979) and co-workers, *WMW* **86**:753. *3659.2*

1936:19 **Insulin** combined with **protamine**, to delay its absorption rate, introduced by Hans Christian Hagedorn (1888–1971) and co-workers, *JAMA* **106**:177. *3974*

1936:20 '**Kimmelstiel-Wilson syndrome**', nodular **intercapillary glomerulosclerosis**, first described by Paul Kimmelstiel (1900–1970) and Clifford Wilson (b.1906), *AmJPa* **12**:83. *4250*

1936:21 A **virus** aetiology for **Japanese B encephalitis** established by Tenji Taniguchi (1896–1961) and co-workers, *JJEM* **14**:185. *4659*

1936:22 **Prefrontal lobotomy** used in treatment of certain **psychotic conditions** by Walter Freeman (1895–1972) and James Winston Watts (b.1904), *MADC* **5**:326. *4906*

1936:23 **Prefrontal lobotomy** used in treatment of **psychotic conditions** by Antonio Caetano de Abreu Freire Egas Moniz (1874–1955), *BuAM* **115**:385. *4905*

1936:24 The location of **cerebral tumours** by **electro-encephalography** determined by William Grey Walter (1911–1977), *L* **2**:305. *4907*

1936:25 **Facial palsy** treated by nerve grafts into the Fallopian canal and by other intratemporal methods by Charles Alfred Ballance (1856–1936) and Arthur Baldwin Duel (1870–1936), *ArOt(C)* **15**:1. *4899*

1936:26 Laurence O'Shaughnessy (1900–1940) attached a pedicled **graft** to the surface of the **heart** (**cardio-omentopexy**) – first carried out experimentally by Beck and Tichy (1935) – thus providing a collateral circulation to that organ and an advance in the treatment of **angina** and **cardiac ischaemia**, *BJS* **23**:665. *3037, 3034, 3035*

1936:27 Successful passage of **influenza** from animal to man first reported by Wilson Smith (1897–1965) and Charles Herbert Stuart-Harris (1909–1996), *L* **2**:121. *5497*

1936:28 The **rabies** virus grown in tissue culture and the culture virus used as anti-rabies vaccine by Leslie Tillotson Webster (1894–1943) and Anna D. Clow, *Science* **84**:487. *5484.2*

1936:29 The virus of **phlebotomus fever** cultivated by Henry Edward Shortt (1887–1987) and co-workers, *IJMR* **23**:865. *5480*

1936:30 The *Histoire générale de la médecine, de la pharmacie, de l'art dentaire et de l'art vétérinaire*, 3 vols, 1936–1949, a well-produced and fully illustrated **history of medicine**, written by experts, under the general editorship of Maxime Paul Marie Laignel-Lavastine (1875–1953). *6430*

1936:31 An experimental study of the use of **prontosil** in the treatment of **puerperal fever** made by Leonard Colebrook (1883–1967) and Méave Kenny, *L* **1**:1279. *6281*

---

1936:32 J. Michael **Bishop**, American microbiologist, born 22 Feb; with Harold E. Varmus (and co-workers) discovered the first oncogene, 1976, *Nature* **260**:170. Shared Nobel Prize (Physiology or Medicine), 1989, with Varmus, for their discovery of cellular origin of retroviral oncogenes, *NPL*. *2660.28*

---

1936:33 Cecil Bryant **Jacobson** born; with Robert Henry Barter, gave the first detailed report of amniocentesis for diagnosis *in utero* of genetic disorders, 1967, *AmJOG* **99**:796. *6235.2*

---

1936: Williams McKim **Marriott** died, **born** 1885. *infant malnutrition, insulin-fattening*

1936: Henry Solomon **Wellcome** died, **born** 1853. *Wellcome Trust*

1936: Ivan Petrovich **Pavlov** died, **born** 1849. *digestion, conditioned reflexes*

1936: Friedrich **Stolz** died, **born** 1860. *adrenaline*

1936: John Scott **Haldane** died, **born** 1860. *respiratory gas analysis, oxygen therapy, high altitude physiology*

1936: Stewart Rankin **Douglas** died, **born** 1871. *opsonins, immune serum*

1936: Francis Henry **Williams** died, **born** 1852. *fluoroscope, heart fluoroscopy, x rays*

1936: Louis Henri **Vaquez** died, **born** 1860. *polycythaemia, erythraemia*

1936: Anton **Ghon** died, **born** 1866. *pulmonary tuberculosis*

1936: Thorald Einar Hess **Thaysen** died, **born** 1883. *steatorrhoea, sprue, coeliac disease*

1936: Robert **Bárány** died, **born** 1876. *labyrinthine function, cerebellar lesions, Bárány's syndrome*

1936: Berkeley George Andrew **Moynihan** died, **born** 1865. *duodenal ulcer*

1936: William Henry **Battle** died, **born** 1855. *femoral hernia*

1936: Stanley Rossiter **Benedict** died, **born** 1884. *blood sugar test*

1936: Archibald Edward **Garrod** died, **born** 1857. *inborn metabolic errors*

1936: Josef **Jadassohn** died, **born** 1863. *maculopapular erythroderma*

1936: Samuel Henry **Harris** died, **born** 1881. *prostatectomy*

1936: David Middleton **Greig** died, **born** 1864. *hypertelorism*

1936: Arnold **Netter** died, **born** 1855. *poliomyelitis*

1936: Charles Alfred **Ballance** died, **born** 1856. *temporal bone, subdural haematoma and hydroma, brain abscess, brain tumours, facial palsy*

1936: William Buchanan **Wherry** died, **born** 1875. *tularaemia, Pasteurella tularensis*

1936: Charles Harrison **Frazier** died, **born** 1870. *intracranial trigeminal neurotomy*

1936: Arthur Baldwin **Duel** died, **born** 1870. *facial palsy*

1936: Charles Jules Henri **Nicolle** died, **born** 1866. *kala-azar, Leishmania infantum, typhus, trachoma, Chlamydia trachomatis*

1936: Hugo **Schöttmüller** died, **born** 1867. *rat-bite fever, Streptobacillus muris ratti, bacterial endocarditis, Streptococcus viridans*

1936: Robert **Knowles** died, **born** 1883. *Leishmania donovani, Phlebotomus*

1936: Enrique **Paschen** died, **born** 1860. *vaccinia*

1936: Wray Devere Marr **Lloyd** died, **born** 1902. *yellow fever*

1936: William Blair **Bell** died, **born** 1871. *gynaecology*

1936: James Fairchild **Baldwin** died, **born** 1850. *artificial vagina*

## 1937

1937:1 **Nobel Prize** (Physiology or Medicine): Albert von Szent-Györgyi (1893–1986), for discoveries concerning the biological combustion processes with special reference to **vitamin C** and the catalysis of **fumaric acid**, *NPL. 1059*

1937:2 **Nobel Prize** (Chemistry): Paul Karrer (1889–1971), for research into the constitution of **carotenoids**, **flavonoids**, and **vitamins A and B**, *NPL. 1079* Walter Norman Haworth (1883–1950), for research into constitution of **carbohydrates** and **vitamin C**, *NPL.*

1937:3 The **citric acid cycle** of **carbohydrate metabolism** discovered by Hans Adolf Krebs (1900–1981), *Enz* **4**:148. *751.1*

1937:4 **Sulphanilamide** used in the treatment of **gonorrhoea** by John Essary Dees (b.1910) and John Archibald Campbell Colston (b.1886), *JAMA* **108**:1855. *5214*

1937:5 A syndrome characterized by **osteitis fibrosa cystica** with other abnormalities ('**Albright's syndrome**') described by Fuller Albright (1900–1969) and co-workers, *NEJM* **216**:727. *4401*

1937:6 **Corticosterone** isolated from the adrenal cortex by P. de Fremery et al., *Nature* **139**:26 *1154*

1937:7 Frank George Young (1908–1988) produced permanent experimental **diabetes** by anterior **pituitary** injections (**anterior pituitary diabetogenic hormone**), *L* **2**:372. *3976*

1937:8 **Antihistamine** described by Daniel Bovet (1907–1992) and Anne-Marie Staub, *CRSB* **124**:547. *1925*

1937:9 **Blood transfusion**; establishment of a blood bank reported by Bernard Fantus (1874–1940), *JAMA* **129**:108. *2026*

1937:10 **Antigen II** discovered and **transplantation immunology** laws established by Peter Alfred Gorer (1907–1961), *JPB* **44**:691, **47**:231. *2576.5*

1937:11 **Leucotaxine**, factor responsible for increased capillary permeability, isolated by Valy Menkin (b.1901), *PSEB* **36**:164. *2312*

1937:12 **Tuberculosis; tuberculin patch test** introduced by Hermann Vollmer (1896–1955) and Esther White Goldberger (b.1905), *AmJDC* **54**:1019. *2348*

1937:13 **Hypertension** shown to be due to the action of a pressor substance by Bernardo Alberto Houssay (1887–1971) and Juan Carlos Fascioli (b.1911), *RSAB* **13**:284. *2721*

1937:14 **Arteriectomy** for relief of **arterial thrombosis** introduced by René Leriche (1879–1955), R. Fontaine and M. Dupertuis, *SGO* **64**:149. *3038*

1937:15 **Antihaemophilic globulin (Factor VIII)** isolated by Arthur Jackson Patek (b.1904) and Francis Henry Laskey Taylor (1900–1959), *JCI* **16**:113. *3096.1*

1937:16 First clinical use of **heparin** as **anticoagulant** by Donald Walter Gordon Murray (1894–1976) and co-workers, *Surgery* **2**:163. *3019*

1937:17 Isolation of **pleuropneumonia-like organism** from man by Louis Dienes and Geoffrey Edsall, *PSEB* **36**:740. *3215*

1937:18 **Hearing** restoration by **fenestration** in **otosclerosis** achieved by Maurice Sourdille (1885–1961), *BNYA* **13**:673. *3408*

1937:19 **Foreign bodies** in air and food passages and their removal was the subject of a comprehensive treatise, *Diseases of the air and food passages of foreign body origin*, by Chevalier Jackson (1865–1958) and his son Chevalier L. Jackson (1900–1961). *3338.1*

1937:20 **Pancreatoduodenectomy** introduced by Alexander Brunschwig (1901–1969), *SGO* **65**:681. *3660*

1937:21 'Sheehan's disease' – **hypopituitarism** due to postpartum **pituitary necrosis** – described by Harold Leeming Sheehan (1900–1988), *JPB* **45**:189. *3907.1*

1937:22 Plastic operation for the relief of **hydronephrosis** introduced by Frederic Eugene Basil Foley (1891–1966), *JU* **38**:643. *4250.1*

1937:23 **Vitallium** introduced experimentally in **bone replacement** by Charles Scott Venable (b.1877) and co-workers, *AnS* **105**:917. *4402*

1937:24 **Vitallium cup arthroplasty** of the **hip-joint** introduced by Marius Nygaard Smith-Petersen (1886–1953) and co-workers, *JBJS* **21**:269. *4403*

1937:25 In her *Infantile paralysis and cerebral diplegia*, the nurse Elizabeth Kenny (1886–1952) described the methods she used for the restoration of function in patients suffering from these conditions. 4671

1937:26 Changes in the **electroencephalogram** in **epilepsy** demonstrated by Frederick Lucian Golla (1878–1968) and co-workers, *JMS* **83**:137. *4824*

1937:27 **Trigeminal tractotomy** introduced in the treatment of **trigeminal neuralgia** by Carl Olof Sjöqvist (b.1901), *ZN* **2**:274. *4908*

1937:28 Constantin Levaditi (1874–1953) and A. Vaisman showed that **sulphanilamide** protected against experimental **gonococcal infection**, *PrM* **45**:1371. *5213.1*

1937:29 The **rickettsial** infection, Q (query) **fever** first described by Edward Holbrook Derrick (1898–1976), *MJA* **2**:281. *5397*

1937:30 The causal agent in Q (query) **fever**, *Rickettsia burneti*, discovered by Frank Macfarlane Burnet (1899–1976) and Mavis Freeman, *MJA* **2**:299. *5398*

1937:31 **Toxoplasmosis** definitely recognized in humans by Abner Wolf (b.1902) and David Cowen (b.1907), *BNI* **6**:306. *5544.1*

1937:32 The method of immunization against **yellow fever** without the use of immune serum devised by Max Theiler (1899–1972) and Hugh Hollingsworth Smith (b.1902), *JEM* **65**:787. *5467*

1937:33 **Cyclodiathermy** for **glaucoma** introduced by Alfred Vogt (1879–1943), *KMA* **99**:9. *5988*

1937:34 **Behçet's syndrome**, named after the description by Hulüsi Behçet (1889–1948), *DeW* **105**:1152, had already been described by H. Planner and F. Remenovsky (1922). *6374*

1937:35 **ß-tocopherol, vitamin E**, isolated by Alexander Robertus Todd (b.1907), *BJ* **31**:2257. *1075*

---

1937:36 Barry R. **Bloom**, American immunologist, born 13 Apr; with B. Bennett, discovered lymphokines, 1966, *Science* **153**:80; also discovered independently by John R. David. *2578.36*

---

1937: John Davidson **Rockefeller** died, **born** 1839. *Rockefeller Foundation, Rockefeller Institute for Medical Research*

1937: Samuel Alexander Kinnier **Wilson** died, born 1874. *Wilson's disease (lenticular degeneration with liver cirrhosis), neurology*

1937: George Henry Falkiner **Nuttall** died, **born** 1862. *bactericidal action of blood, Clostridium perfringens, gas gangrene*

1937: Augustus Warren **Crane** died, **born** 1868. *kymography, cardiology*

1937: Hans Christian **Jacobaeus** died, **born** 1879. *thoracoscopy, cystoscope*

1937: Werner **Körte** died, **born** 1853. *bronchiectasis, lobectomy*

1937: Charles David **Green** died, **born** 1862. *temporal bone*

1937: Henry Stanley **Plummer** died, **born** 1874. *cardiospasm, oesophageal dilatation*

1937: Jakob **Erdheim** died, **born** 1874. *pituitary dwarfism*

1937: Hermann **Schloffer** died, **born** 1868. *pituitary tumour*

1937: Sigmund **Pollitzer** died, **born** 1859. *acanthosis nigricans*

1937: Edvard **Ehlers** died, **born** 1863. *cutis laxa*

1937: Henri Alexandre **Danlos** died, **born** 1844. *cutis laxa*

1937: Emerich **Ullmann** died, **born** 1861. *kidney autotransplantation*

1937: Erich **Lexer** died, **born** 1867. *osteoarticular joint transplant*

1937: Hermann **Kümmell** died, **born** 1852. *spondylitis*

1937: Samuel Alexander Kinnier **Wilson** died, **born** 1874. *hepatolenticular degeneration*

1937: Alfred Walter **Campbell** died, **born** 1868. *Murray Valley encephalitis*

1937: Fedor **Krause** died, **born** 1857. *facial neuralgia, neurectomy, neurosurgery, tabes, pineal tumour, skin grafts*

1937: Alfred **Adler** died, **born** 1870. *inferiority complex, individual psychology*

1937: Janos **Bokay** died, **born** 1858. *varicella, herpes zoster*

1937: Harold Benjamin **Fantham** died, **born** 1876. *Trypanosoma rhodesiense*

1937: Sören **Holth** died, **born** 1863. *glaucoma, iridencleisis*

1937: Archibald **Donald** died, **born** 1860. *prolapse of uterus*

1937: Harry **Swift** died, **born** 1858. *acrodynia*

1937: Scipione **Riva-Rocci** died, **born** 1863. *sphygmomanometer*

1937: Thomas Orville **Menees** died, **born** 1890. *amniography*

1937: Karl Wilhelm Theodor Richard von **Hertwig** died, **born** 1850. *embryology, protozoology, cytology*

**1938**
1938:1 **Nobel Prize** (Physiology or Medicine): Corneille Jean François Heymans (1892–1968), for his work on the **sinus and aortic mechanisms** in regulation of **respiration**, *NPL. 967*

1938:2 **Nobel Prize** (Chemistry): Richard Kuhn (1900–1967), for his work on **carotenoids** and **vitamins**, *NPL.*

1938:3 **Australian College of Physicians** founded

1938:4 Fundamental discoveries on the **electrical conductance** of living **cell membranes** published by Kenneth Stewart Cole (1900–1984) and H.J. Curtis, *Nature* **142**:209; *JGP* **22**:37,649.

1938:5 Research on the **electrical discharges** of the **optic nerve** carried out by Haldan Keffer Hartline (1903–1983), *AmJPh* **121**:400. *1532*

1938:6 Synthesis of **vitamin E (α-tocopherol)** by Paul Karrer (1889–1971) et al., *HCA* **21**:520 *1079*

1938:7 Isolation of **nicotinic acid** by Conrad Arnold Elvehjem (1901–1962) et al., *JBC* **123**:137. *1077*

1938:8 **Sulphapyridine (M & B 693)** shown experimentally by Lionel Whitby (1895–1956) to be effective in pneumococcal and staphylococcal infections, *L* **1**:1210. *1951*

1938:9 **Pneumonia** treated with **M & B 693 (sulphapyridine)** by Gladys Mary Evans and Wilfrid Fletcher Gaisford (1902–1988), *L* **2**:14. *3210*

1938:10 **BLB (Boothby-Lovelace-Bulbulian) oxygen inhalation apparatus** devised by William Randolph Lovelace (1907–1965) and Arthur H. Bulbulian (b.1900), *PMC* **13**:646, 654. *1981, 1982*

1938:11 **Praecordial leads** introduced in **electrocardiography**, *BMJ* **1**:187. *2868*

1938:12 **Angiocardiography** introduced by George Porter Robb (b.1898) and Israel Steinberg (b.1902), *JCI* **17**:507. *2869*

1938:13 **Vitamin K** used in the treatment of **haemorrhagic disease** by Hugh Roland Butt (b.1910) and Albert Markley Snell (1896–1960), *PMC* **13**:74. *3097*

1938:14 The histological changes in **Menière's syndrome** described by Charles Skinner Hallpike (1900–1979) and Hugh William Bell Cairns (1896–1952), *PRSM* **31**:1317. *3409*

1938:15 Atypical **pneumonia** described by Hobart Ansteth Reimann (b.1897), *JAMA* **111**:2377. *3211*

1938:16 One-step **fenestration** operation (**Lempert's operation**) for **otosclerosis** devised by Julius Lempert (b.1891), *ArOt(C)* **28**:42. *3410*

1938:17 **Riboflavin (vitamin B complex) deficiency, ariboflavinosis**, subject of a report by William Henry Sebrell (b.1901) and Roy Edwin Butler (b.1902), *USPHR* **53**:2284. *3707*

1938:18 **Cephalin-cholesterol liver-function test** introduced by Franklin McCue Hanger (1894–1971), *TAAP* **53**:148. *3662*

1938:19 '**Turner's syndrome**' (infantilism, congenital webbed neck, and cubitus valgus) noted by Henry Hubert Turner (1892–1970), *En* **23**:566. *3801.1*

1938:20 **Hexoestrol** isolated by N.E. Campbell and co-workers, *Nature* **142**:1121. *3801*

1938:21 **Dienoestrol** introduced by Edward Charles Dodds (1899–1975) and co-workers, *Nature* **142**:34. *3800*

1938:22 **Wang's test** for **vitamin deficiency (avitaminosis)** developed by Y.L. Wang and Leslie Julius Harris (1898–1973), *BJ* **33**:1356. *3708*

1938:23 **Stilboestrol**, the first synthetic **oestrogen**, introduced by Edward Charles Dodds (1899–1975) and co-workers, *Nature* **141**:247. *3799*

1938:24 **Quick's** intravenous **hippuric acid liver-function test** introduced by Armand James Quick (1894–1977), H.N. Ottenstein and H. Weltchek, *PSEB* **38**:77. *3663*

1938:25 **Nicotinic acid**, a constituent of the **vitamin B** complex, was isolated as the **pellagra-**preventing factor by Conrad Arnold Elvehjem (1901–1962) and co-workers, *JBC* **123**:137. *3760*

1938:26 First recognition of an **auto-immune disease, acquired haemolytic anaemia**, by William Dameshek (1900–1969) and Steven Otto Schwartz (b.1911), *AJMS* **196**:769. *3787.1*

598

1938:27 During the Spanish Civil War Josep Trueta (1897–1977) developed the **closed plaster treatment** of wounds and **compound fractures**, after packing the excised wound with sterile vaselined gauze, which he termed the biological treatment of wounds; in his *El tratamiento de la fractura de guerra. 4435.1, 5632*

1938:28 **Eastern equine encephalitis virus** isolated from man by LeRoy Dryden Fothergill (1901–1967) and co-workers, *NEJM* **219**:411. *4659.1*

1938:29 **Western equine encephalitis virus** recovered from man by Beatrice Fay Howitt (b.1891), *Science* **88**:455. *4660*

1938:30 The **meningiomas** classified by Harvey Williams Cushing (1869–1939) and Louise Charlotte Eisenhardt (1891–1967); in their *Meningiomas. Their classification,* etc. *4612, 4909.01*

1938:31 **Diphenylhydantoin** introduced in the treatment of **convulsive disorders** by Hyram Houston Merritt (1902–1979) and Tracy J. Putnam (b. 1894), *JAMA* **111**:1068. *4824.1*

1938:32 Surgical section of the **lemniscus lateralis** first employed for the relief of severe intractable **pain** by Achile Mario Dogliotti (1897–1966), *CRA* **17**:143. *4909*

1938:33 **Typhoid** antiserum first prepared by Arthur Felix (1887–1956) and George Ford Petrie (1863–1955), *JHyg* **38**:673. *5045.1*

1938:34 The significance of maternal age in the aetiology of **Down's syndrome** pointed out by Lionel Sharples Penrose (1898–1972); in *A clinical and genetic study of 1,280 cases of mental defect* (Spec. Rep. Ser., MRC, No. 229). *4962.1*

1938:35 **Measles** virus cultivated by Harry Plotz (1890–1947), *BuAM* **119**:598. *5449*

1938:36 **Pinta** shown by Braulio Saenz to be caused by *Treponema carateum, ArMI* **4**:112. *5308.1*

1938:37 An operation for the construction of an **artificial vagina** devised by Archibald Hector McIndoe (1900–1960) and John Bright Banister (1880–1938), *JOG* **45**:490. *6133*

1938:38 David **Baltimore**, American virologist, born 7 Mar; independently of both Renato Dulbecco and Howard Martin Temin, discovered the interaction between tumour viruses and genetic material of the cell, 1970, *Nature* **226**:1209; 1964, *NCIM* **17**; 1970, *Nature* **226**:1211; shared Nobel Prize, 1975, with them, *NPL. 2660.20, 2660.22, 2660.23, 2660.27*

1938: Arthur Henry **Downes** died, **born** 1851. *bacterial action of sunlight*

1938: Hans Christian Joachim **Gram** died, **born** 1853. *bacterial stain*

1938: Sahachiro **Hata** died, **born** 1873. *salvarsan, syphilis*

1938: Colin Blackman **Bridges** died, **born** 1889. *heredity*

1938: Friedrich **Moritz** died, **born** 1861. *heart orthodiagraphy*

1938: Franz **Torek** died, **born** 1861. *undescended testis, orchiopexy, carcinoma of oesophagus*

1938: Ismar Isidor **Boas** died, **born** 1858. *duodenal aspiration*

1938: John Jacob **Abel** died, **born** 1857. *insulin*

1938: Jean **Darier** died, **born** 1856. *acanthosis nigricans, keratosis follicularis, tuberculides*

1938: Raymond Jacques Adrien **Sabouraud** died, **born** 1864. *fungous skin diseases, ringworm, radiotherapy, acne bacillus, Trichophyton*

1938: Edwin **Beer** died, **born** 1876. *bladder tumours, prostatectomy*

1938: Octave **Crouzon** died, **born** 1874. *craniofacial dysostosis*

1938: Ambrose Thomas **Stanton** died, **born** 1875. *melioidosis, Pfeifferella whitmori*

1938: Edward **Martin** died, **born** 1859. *pain, spinal cordotomy*

1938: Maurice Crowther **Hall** died, **born** 1881. *ankylostomiasis, carbon tetrachloride*

1938: George Burgess **Magrath** died, **born** 1870. *smallpox*

1938: Max **Kappis** died, **born** 1881. *urology, paravertebral anaesthesia, splanchnic anaesthesia*

1938: Frederic Jay **Cotton** died, **born** 1969. *anaesthesia, nitrous oxide/oxygen*

1938: Karl Friedrich Jakob **Sudhoff** died, **born** 1853. *medical history*

1938: John Bright **Banister** died, **born** 1880. *artificial vagina*

## 1939
1939:1 **Nobel Prize** (Physiology or Medicine): Gerhard Domagk (1895–1964), for the introduction into medicine of **prontosil**, the first **sulphonamide**-containing **antibacterial** drug, *NPL. 1949*

1939:2 **Nobel Prize** (Chemistry): Alfred Friedrich Johann Butenandt (1903–1995), for isolation in crystalline form of the male **sex hormone, androsterone**, and Leonard Stephen Ruzicka (1887–1976), for its synthesis, *NPL. 1195, 1201*

1939:3 **Nuffield Provincial Hospitals Trust** founded by Sir William **Morris**, Lord **Nuffield** (1877–1963)

1939:4 **Emergency Public Health Laboratory Service (England and Wales)** established, administered by the **Medical Research Council**

1939:5 **Blood groups** shown by William Clouser Boyd (1903–1983) to be inherited and not changed by environment, *Tab* **17**:113. *912*

1939:6 **Action potentials** recorded from inside a **nerve** by Andrew Fielding Huxley (b.1917) and A.L. Hodgkin (b.1914), 1939, *Nature* **144**:710. *1310.1*

1939:7 **Vitamin K**$_1$ isolated from alfalfa by Carl Pieter Henrik Dam (1895–1976) et al., *HCA* **22**:310. Died 1976. *1080*

1939:8 **Pethidine (meperidine)** synthesized by O. Eisler and O. Schaumann, *DMW* **65**:967. *1927*

1939:9 **Gramicidin** isolated by René Jules Dubos (1901–1982), *PSEB* **40**:311. *1933.1*

1939:10 **Ultrasonics** first used therapeutically by R. Pohlmann, R. Richter and E. Parow, *DMW* **65**:251. *2010.1*

1939:11 **Antibodies** shown to be **gamma globulins** by Arne Wilhelm Tiselius (1902–1971) and Elvin Abraham Kabat (b.1914), *JEM* **69**:119. *2576.8*

1939:12 **Ballistocardiogram** introduced by Isaac Starr (b.1895) and co-workers, *AmJPh* **127**:1. *2870*

1939:13 Successful surgical repair of a **patent ductus arteriosus** in **congenital heart disease** by Robert Edward Gross (1905–1988) and John Perry Hubbard (b.1903), *JAMA* **112**:729. *3039*

1939:14 **Heart-lung machine** first successfully used on an animal by John Heysham Gibbon (1903–1973), *JLCM* **24**:1192. *3038.1*

1939:15 **Lung cancer** associated with **cigarette smoking** by Franz Hermann Müller, *ZKr* **49**:57. *3213*

1939:16 **Leukaemia** treated with **radiophosphorus** by John Hundale Lawrence (b.1904) and co-workers, *NIC* **3**:33; *Rad* **35**:51. *3098, 3099*

1939:17 **Deoxycorticosterone acetate** introduced in the treatment of **adrenal insufficiency** by George Widmer Thorn (b.1906) and co-workers, *BJH* **64**:155. *3877*

1939:18 Aspiration **liver biopsy** technique introduced by Poul Iverson (b.1889) and Kaj Roholm, *AcM* **102**:1. *3664*

1939:19 **Triphenylchloroethylene**, a synthetic **oestrogen**, introduced into clinical use by Archibald Ian Macpherson and Edward Moody Robertson (b.1902), *L* **2**:1362. *3803*

1939:20 **Radiotherapy** in **Hodgkin's disease** first used with effect by René Gilbert, *AJR* **41**:198. *3787.2*

1939:21 A method of treating congenital **club-foot (talipes)**, using a series of **plaster casts** and **wedgings** introduced by Joseph Hiram Kite (b.1891), *JBJS* **21**:595. *4403.1*

1939:22 **Spring-summer (Russian Far East) encephalitis virus** isolated by L.A. Zil'ber, *ArBN* **56** No.2:9. *4660.1*

1939:23 Immunization against **whooping cough** made possible by the **pertussis** vaccine of Pearl L. Kendrick (b.1890) and Grace Eldering, *AmJH* **29B**:138. *5087.2*

1939:24 **Ventriculocisternostomy** for the relief of obstructive **hydrocephalus** introduced by Arne Torkildsen, *AcC* **82**:117. *4909.1*

1939:25 The **sulphonamide** dressing of **wounds** introduced by Nathan Kenneth Jensen (b.1910) and co-workers, *Surgery* **6**:1. *5645*

1939:26 The **Padgett dermatome**, for cutting calibrated **skin grafts**, introduced by Earl Calvin Padgett (1893–1946), *SGO* **69**:779. *5763.1*

1939:27 **Hormone treatment** in **pregnancy** first reported by Priscilla White (b.1900) and co-workers, *AmJMS* **198**:482. *6231*

1939:28 Alfred Blalock (1899–1964) treated **myasthenia gravis** by **thymectomy**, *AnS* **110**:544. *4771*

---

1939:29 Sidney **Altman**, American molecular biologist, born 7 May; shared Nobel Prize (Chemistry), 1989, with Thomas Robert Cech, for their discovery of catalytic RNA, *NPL*.

1939:30 Susumu **Tonegawa**, Japanese molecular biologist and immunologist, born 6 Sep; awarded Nobel Prize (Physiology or Medicine), 1987, for his discovery of the genetic principle for generation of antibody diversity, *NPL*.

1939:31 Harold E. **Varmus**, American virologist, born 18 Dec; with J. Michael Bishop (and co-workers) discovered the first oncogene, 1976, *Nature* **260**:170. Shared Nobel Prize (Physiology or Medicine), 1989, with Bishop, for their discovery of the cellular origin of retroviral oncogenes, *NPL*. *2660.28*

---

1939: Harvey Williams **Cushing** died, **born** 1869. *hypothalamus, peptic ulcer, Cushing's syndrome, glioma, meningioma, trigeminal neuralgia, electrocoagulation in neurosurgery, pneumatic tourniquet for craniotomy, intracranial haemorrhage of newborn, cerebral hernia in brain tumour surgery, local infiltration anaesthesia, hypophysectomy, genital atrophy*

1939: Sigmund **Freud** died, **born** 1856. *aphasia, agnosia, cerebral palsy, psychoanalysis, dreams*

1939: George **Barger** died, **born** 1878. *thyroxine, ergotoxine, histamine*

1939: Stephane Armand Nicolas **Leduc** died, **born** 1853. *electric convulsion therapy, ionic medication*

1939: Oscar Heinrich **Hinsberg** died, **born** 1857. *phenacetin*

1939: William Adam **Jolly** died, **born** 1878. *auricular flutter*

1939: Efim Semenovic **London** died, **born** 1869. *cancer, x rays*

1939: Tage Anton Ultimus **Sjögren** died, **born** 1859. *cancer, x rays*

1939: Ludwig **Haendel** died, **born** 1869. *pneumococcus*

1939: William James **Mayo** died, **born** 1861. *partial gastrectomy, umbilical hernia, carcinoma of rectum*

1939: Anton von **Eiselsberg** died, **born** 1860. *thyroidectomy, tetanus*

1939: George John **Jenkins** died, **born** 1874. *otosclerosis, fenestration*

1939: Ernest Marcel **Labbe** died, **born** 1870. *adrenal medulla, chromaffin cell tumour*

1939: Arthur Thornton **Legg** died, **born** 1874. *osteochondritis deformans*

1939: James Samuel Risien **Russell** died, **born** 1863. *spinal cord degeneration*

1939: Frederick Parker **Gay** died, **born** 1874. *poliomyelitis*

1939: Wilfred **Trotter** died, **born** 1872. *intracranial aneurysm*

1939: Paul Eugen **Bleuler** died, **born** 1857. *schizophrenia, dementia praecox*

1939: Henry Havelock **Ellis** died, **born** 1859. *psychology of sex*

1939: Henri Amadée **Lafleur** died, **born** 1863. *amoebic dysentery*

1939: Pietro **Canalis** died, **born** 1856. *malaria, Plasmodium spp.*

1939: James Rutherford **Morison** died, **born** 1853. *antiseptic paste*

1939: Anton **Elschnig** died, **born** 1863. *corneal transplantation, sympathetic ophthalmia*

1939: Vard Houghton **Hulen** died, **born** 1865. *cataract*

1939: Marius Hans Erik **Tscherning** died, **born** 1851. *spectacle lens*

1939: Edmund Beecher **Wilson** died, **born** 1856. *cytology, development, heredity*

## 1940
1940: 1 **Nobel Prize**: no awards

1940: 2 **Burns**; **Bunyan bag** method of treatment introduced by John Bunyan (1907–1983), *PRSM* **34**:65. *2260*

1940: 3 **Rh antigen** recognized by Karl Landsteiner (1868–1943) and Alexander Solomon Wiener (1907–1976), *PSEB* **43**:223. *912.2*

1940: 4 **Interstitial-cell-stimulating (luteinizing) hormone** isolated by Choh Hao Li (b.1913) and co-workers, *En* **27**:303. *1173.1*

1940: 5 **Folic acid (vitamin $B_c$)** isolated by Albert Garland Hogan (1884–1961) and Ernest Milford Parrott (b.1903), *JBC* **132**:507. *1086*

1940:6 **Sulphaguanidine** introduced by Eli Kennerly Marshall (1889–1966) and colleagues, *BJH* **67**:163. *1954*

1940:7 Chemotherapeutic action of **penicillin** proved by Ernst Boris Chain (1906–1979), Howard Walter Florey (1898–1968), Edward Penley Abraham (b.1913) et al, *Lancet* **2**:226. *1934*

1940:8 **Penicillinase** isolated by Edward Penley Abraham (b.1913) and Ernst Boris Chain (1906–1979), *Nature* **146**:837. *1933.3*

1940:9 Synthesis of **sulphamerazine** by Richard Owen Roblin (b.1907) et al., *JACS* **62**:2002. *1955*

1940:10 **Promin (sodium glucosulphone)** used in treatment of **tuberculosis** by William Hugh Feldman (1892–1974) et al., *PMC* **15**:295 *2349*

1940:11 **Angiotensin** isolated by Eduardo Braun-Menendez (b.1903) and co-workers, *JP* **98**:283; and independently by Irving Heinly Page (b.1901) and O.M. Helmer, *JEM* **71**:29. *2724.1, 2724.2*

1940:12 **Betatron** introduced by Donald William Kerst (b.1911), *PsR* **58**:841. *2010.2, 2659.1*

1940:13 Surgical obliteration of the **abdominal aorta** by René Leriche (1879–1955, *PrM* **48**:601. *3040*

1940:14 The **inulin clearance test** for the measurement of the **glomerular filtration rate** introduced by Alf Sven Alving (b.1902) and Benjamin Frank Miller (b.1907), *ArIM* **66**:306. *4251*

1940:15 Paul Durand (1895–1961) isolated a virus (**D virus**) from his own blood. The infection was named '**Durand's disease**', *ArIP* **29**:179. *4661*

1940:16 The **encephalomyocarditis virus** isolated by Claus W. Jungeblut (b.1897) and Murray Sanders (b.1910), *JEM* **72**:407. *4661.1*

1940:17 A **typhus** vaccine introduced by Herald Rea Cox (b.1907) and E.J. Bell, *USPHR* **55**:110. *5398.1*

1940:18 A complement-fixation test for the diagnosis of **lymphogranuloma venereum** introduced by C.M. McKee, G.W. Rake and M.F. Shaffer, *PSEB* **44**:410. *5224*

1940:19 Scrub **typhus** and **tsutsugamushi disease** shown to be identical by Raymond Lewthwaite (1894–1972) and S.R. Savoor (1900–1980), *L* **1**:255, 304. *5398.2*

1940:20 **Influenza B** virus recovered by Thomas Pleines Magill (b.1903), *PSEB* **45**:162, independently of Thomas Francis (1900–1969), *Science* **92**:405. *5498, 5499*

1940:21 Continuous **spinal analgesia** introduced by William Thomas Lemmon (b.1896), *AnS* **111**:141. *5722*

604

1940:22 **Splanchnic resection** in the treatment of **essential hypertension**, the '**Smithwick operation**', devised by Reginald Hammerick Smithwick (1899–1987), *Surgery* 7:1. *3041*

1940:23 *Neurology*, the monumental work by Samuel Alexander Kinnier Wilson (1874–1937) published posthumously. *4614*

---

1940:24 Joseph L. **Goldstein**, American physician, born 18 Apr; shared Nobel Prize (Physiology or Medicine), 1985, with Michael S. Brown, for their discoveries concerning the regulation of cholesterol metabolism, *NPL.*

---

1940: Max **Bielschowsky** died, **born** 1869. *Bielschowsky's stain, nerve fibre staining*

1940: Henry **Head** died, **born** 1861. *thalamus, hyperalgesia, herpes zoster, aphasia*

1940: John Sydney **Edkins** died, **born** 1863. *gastrin*

1940: Bernard **Fantus** died, **born** 1874. *blood bank*

1940: Jacques Arsène **d'Arsonval** died, **born** 1851. *electrotherapy*

1940: John Templeton **Bowen** died, **born** 1857. *epithelioma*

1940: Alexander **Besredka** died, **born** 1870. *anti-anaphylaxis*

1940: Guy Henry **Faget** died, **born** 1891. *leprosy, promin*

1940: Michel **Weinberg** died, **born** 1868. *Clostridium oedematiens, Clostridium histolyticum*

1940: Karel Frederik **Wenckebach** died, **born** 1864. *heart arrhythmia, quinine, beriberi*

1940: Oliver **Lodge** died, **born** 1851. *x rays*

1940: Maude Elizabeth Seymour **Abbott** died, **born** 1869. *congenital cardiac disease*

1940: George Ernest **Waugh** died, **born** 1876. *tonsillectomy*

1940: Max **Askanazy** died, **born** 1865. *parathyroid tumours, osteitis fibrosa cystica*

1940: Francis Randall **Hagner** died, **born** 1873. *epididymitis*

1940: Giuliano **Vanghetti** died, **born** 1861. *kinematization of amputation stump*

1940: Vittorio **Putti** died, **born** 1880. *kineplastic surgery*

1940: Paul Ferdinand **Schilder** died, **born** 1886. *encephalitis periaxialis diffusa*

1940: Alfred Walter **Campbell** died, **born** 1868. *herpes zoster*

1940: Pierre **Marie** died, **born** 1853. *cerebellar ataxia, peroneal muscular atrophy, aphasia, acromegaly, ankylosing spondylitis*

1940: Julius **Wagner von Jauregg** died, **born** 1857. *psychoses, fevers, malaria*

1940: William Gibson **Spiller** died, **born** 1863. *pain, spinal cordotomy, intracranial trigeminal neurotomy*

1940: Alexander **Rennie** died, **born** 1859. *plague bacillus*

1940: Laurence **O'Shaughnessy** died, **born** 1900. *cardio-omentopexy*

1940: Hans **Zinsser** died, **born** 1878. *typhus, Brill's disease*

1940: Augusto **Ducrey** died, **born** 1860. *chancroid, Haemophilus ducreyi*

1940: Percy Moreau **Ashburn** died, **born** 1872. *dengue*

1940: Karl Bernhard **Lehmann** died, **born** 1858. *anaesthesia, trichlorethylene*

1940: Patrick Playfair **Laidlaw** died, **born** 1881. *influenza, shock, histamine*

1940: Adolpho **Lutz** died, **born** 1855. *blastomycosis*

1940: Louis **Dartigues** died, **born** 1869. *mammectomy*

1940: Claude **Regaud** died, **born** 1870. *x ray dose fractionation, cancer of uterus, radium*

## 1941
1941:1 **Nobel Prize**: no awards

1941:2 **Mutations** induced with *Neurospora* by George Wells Beadle (1903–1989) and Edward Lawrie Tatum (1909–1975), *PNAS* **27**:499. This work laid the foundations of biochemical genetics. *254.3*

1941:3 **Electroretinography** introduced by Lorrin Andrews Riggs (b.1912), *PSEB* **48**:204. *1533*

1941:4 **Sulphasuxidine** introduced by Edgar Jacob Poth (b.1899) and Frank Louis Knotts (b.1912), *PSEB* **48**:129. *1957*

1941:5 **Sulphadiazine** introduced by Maxwell Finland (b.1902) et al., *JAMA* **116**:2641 *1956*

1941:6 **Virus haemagglutination** discovered by George Keble Hirst (b.1909) and independently by Laurella McClelland (b.1912) and Ronald Hare (1899–1986), *Science* **94**:22; *CPHJ* **32**:530. *2577, 2578*

1941:7 **Syphilis: cardiolipin antigen serodiagnosis** introduced by Mary Candace Pangborn (b.1907), *PSEB* **48**:484. *2417*

1941:8 **Cardiac catheterization** first used in clinical investigation by André Frédéric Cournand (1895–1988) and Hilmert Albert Ranges (1906–1969), *PSEB* **46**:462. *2871*

606

1941:9 **Dicoumarol (bis-hydroxycoumarin)**, an **anticoagulant**, isolated by Mark Arnold Stahmann (b.1914), C. Huebner and K.P. Link, *JBC* **138**:513. *3102*

1941:10 **Erythroblastosis foetalis** due to **rhesus incompatibility** between mother and child reported by Philip Levine (1900–1987) and co-workers, *AmJOG* **42**:925. *3100*

1941:11 The treatment of **prostatic carcinoma** with **stilboestrol** introduced by Charles Brenton Huggins (b.1901) and Clarence Vernard Hodges, *CR* **1**:293. *4276*

1941:12 The **Kveim test** for **sarcoidosis** introduced by Morten Ansgar Kveim (b.1892), *NoM* **9**:169. *4153*

1941:13 An authoritative account of the '**crush syndrome**', with impairment of **renal function** found in victims of London air-raids of 1940–41 given by Eric George Lapthorne Bywaters (b.1910) and Desmond Beall, *BMJ* **1**:427. *4252*

1941:14 A classification of **nephritis** published by Arthur William Mickle Ellis (1883–1966), *L* **1**:1,34,72. *4254*

1941:15 The fact that **chondrodystrophy** may be inherited established by Ernst Trier Morch (b.1908); in his *Chondrodystrophic dwarfism in Denmark*. *4404*

1941:16 The accuracy and reliability of **encephalography** improved by Edward Graeme Robertson (b.1903); in his *Encephalography*. *4614.1*

1941:17 **Sulphaguanidine** introduced in the treatment of bacillary **dysentery** by Eli Kennerley Marshall (1889–1966) and co-workers, *JHB* **68**:94. *5096*

1941:18 Proof of the transmission of *Leishmania tropica*, causal organism of cutaneous **leishmaniasis**, by the bite of *Phlebotomus papatasii* given by Saul Adler (1895–1966) and Mordehai Ber (d.1952), *IJMR* **29**:803. *5301.2*

1941:19 Norman McAlister Gregg (1892–1966) pointed out that **rubella** in early pregnancy could result in congenital defects in the infant, *TOSA* **3**:35. *5507*

1941:20 The **Oxford vaporisers** 1 and 2, for **anaesthesia**, introduced by Hans Georg Epstein, *L* **2**:62. *5723*

1941:21 The work of Alberto Francis Inclan (b.1916) forms the basis of the modern use of **bone preserved** by **refrigeration**, *JBJS* **24**:81. *5764*

1941:22 **Amniotic fluid embolism** first described by Paul Eby Steiner (b.1902) and Clarence Chancelum Lushbaugh (b.1916), *JAMA* **117**:1245, 1340. *6232*

1941:23 The diagnostic value of **cervical smears** in **carcinoma** of the **cervix** pointed out by George Nicholas Papanicolaou (1883–1962) and Herbert Frederick Traut (b.1894), *AmJOG* **42**:193. *6135*

---

1941:24 Michael S. **Brown**, American physician, born 13 Apr; shared Nobel Prize (Physiology or Medicine), 1985, with Joseph L. Goldstein, for their discoveries concerning the regulation of cholesterol metabolism, *NPL*.

1941:25 Alfred G. **Gilman**, American biochemist, born 1 Jul; shared Nobel Prize (Physiology or Medicine), 1994, with Martin Rodbell, for their discovery of G-proteins and their role in signal transduction in cells, *NPL*.

---

1941: Johannes [Hans] **Berger** died, **born** 1873. *electroencephalogram*

1941: Frederick **Griffith** died, **born** 1879. *transformation of pneumococcal types, serological classification of Streptococcus*

1941: Graham **Steell** died, **born** 1851. *pulmonary diastolic murmur*

1941: William **Bulloch** died, **born** 1868. *haemophilia, adrenogenital syndrome*

1941: Frank Thomas **Paul** died, **born** 1851. *intestinal drainage, colon resection*

1941: Kurt **Huldschinsky** died, **born** 1883. *rickets, ultraviolet irradiation*

1941: Hastings **Gilford** died, **born** 1861. *progeria*

1941: Frederick Grant **Banting** died, **born** 1891. *insulin*

1941: George Frederic **Still** died, **born** 1868. *paediatrics, diseases of children, rheumatism*

1941: Kurt **Huldschinsky** died, **born** 1883. *tetany, ultraviolet light*

1941: Kenneth Daniel **Blackfan** died, **born** 1883. *hydrocephalus*

1941: Otfrid **Foerster** died, **born** 1873. *spastic paralysis, rhizotomy*

1941: Charles Wardell **Stiles** died, **born** 1867. *Necator americanus*

1941: Andrew Watson **Sellards** died, **born** 1884. *amoebiasis, Entamoeba spp., hookworm*

1941: Henry Edmund Gaskin **Boyle** died, **born** 1875. *anaesthesia*

1941: Albert Siegmund Gustav **Döderlein** died, **born** 1860. *puerperal fever, lactobacillus*

1941: Emile Charles **Achard** died, **born** 1860. *paratyphoid, Salmonella paratyphi B*

1941: Hans **Spemann** died, **born** 1869. *embryology*

1941: Christian **Kielland** died, **born** 1871. *obstetric forceps*

## 1942
1942: 1 **Nobel Prize**: no awards

1942: 2 **Tanner slide operation** for **inguinal** and **femoral hernia** introduced by Norman Cecil Tanner (1906–1982), *BJS* **29**:285. *3611.1*

1942: 3 Diffuse **collagen disease** described by Paul Klemperer (1887–1964) and co-workers, *JAMA* **119**:331. *2237*

608

1942:4 Imhoff system of **sewage** purification devised by Karl Imhoff (b.1876); in his *Fortschritte der Abwasserreinigung. 1642*

1942:5 **Freund's adjuvant**, for use with **antigens**, introduced by Jules Thomas Freund (1890–1960) and Katherine McDermott, *PSEB* **49**:548. *2578.1*

1942:6 **Radioisotopic bone-scanning** introduced by Anne G. Treadwell and co-workers, *AmJMS* **204**:521. *2700.01*

1942:7 First successful excision of **arteriovenous aneurysm** of the **lung** by John Hepburn (b.1888) and James Arnold Dauphinee (b.1903), *AmJMS* **204**:681. *2992*

1942:8 The **Klinefelter syndrome**, an endocrine disorder, first described by Harry Fitch Klinefelter (b.1912), E.C. Reifenstein and Fuller Albright (1900–1969), *JCE* **2**:615. *3804*

1942:9 Transmission of the agent of **infective hepatitis** by H. Voegt, *MMW* **89**:76. *3664.1*

1942:10 **Exophthalmic goitre** treated with **radioactive iodine** by Saul Hertz (b.1905) and A. Roberts, *JCI* **21**:624. *3853*

1942:11 **Kala-azar** (visceral **leishmaniasis**) successfully transmitted to man through the bite of *Phlebotomus argentipes* by C.S. Swaminath and co-workers, who thus showed it to be the vector of *Leishmania, IJMR* **30**:473. *5302*

1942:12 **Curare** introduced into general **anaesthesia** by Harold Randall Griffith (b.1894) and G. Enid Johnson, *Ane* **3**:418. *5724*

1942:13 Continuous **caudal anaesthesia** during **labour** and **delivery** first reported by Robert Andrew Hingson (b.1913) and Waldo Berry Edwards (b.1905), *CRA* **21**:301. *6232.1*

1942:14 **Retrolental fibroplasia** first described by Theodor Lasater Terry (1899–1946), *AmJOp* **25**:203. *5989*

1942:15 Passive cell transfer of **delayed hypersensitivity** discovered by Karl Landsteiner (1868–1943) and Merrill Wallace Chase (b.1905), *PSEB* **49**:688. *2578.3*

1942:16 *Biochemistry and morphogenesis* published by Joseph Needham (1900–1995).

1942:17 Bert **Sakmann**, German physiologist, born 12 Jun; shared Nobel Prize (Physiology or Medicine), 1991, with Erwin Neher, for their discoveries concerning the function of single ion channels in cells, *NPL*.

1942:18 Christiane **Nüsslein-Volhard**, German geneticist, born; shared Nobel Prize (Physiology or Medicine), 1995, with Edward B. Lewis and and Eric F. Wieschaus, for their discoveries concerning the genetic control of early embryonic development, *NPL*.

1942: S.G.T. **Bendien** died. *cancer diagnosis*

1942: Herbert **Herbert** died, **born** 1865. *glaucoma*

1942: Ludwig **Aschoff** died, **born** 1866. *rheumatic myocarditis*

1942: Martin **Kirschner** died, **born** 1879. *anaesthesia, avertin, pulmonary embolism, skeletal traction and stabilization*

1942: James Emmons **Briggs** died, **born** 1869. *prostatectomy*

1942: Francis Sedgwick **Watson** died, **born** 1853. *prostatectomy*

1942: Bernard Jean Antonin **Marfan** died, **born** 1858. *Marfan's syndrome*

1942: Maurice **Klippel** died, **born** 1858. *cervical vertebrae abnormalities, angio-osteohypertrophy*

1942: Arthur **Nicolaier** died, **born** 1862. *tetanus bacillus, Clostridium tetani*

1942: Joseph Bolivar **DeLee** died, **born** 1869. *caesarean section, laparotrachelotomy*

1942: Alfred Baker **Spalding** died, **born** 1874. *fetal death*

## 1943

1943:1 **Nobel Prize** (Physiology or Medicine): Carl Peter Henrik Dam (1895–1976), for the discovery of **vitamin K**, the **anti-haemorrhagic** factor, *NPL. 1062*; Edward Adlebert Doisy (1893–1986), for the discovery of the chemical structure of **vitamin K**, *NPL.*

1943:2 Pure **adrenocorticotrophic hormone** isolated by Choh Hao Li and co-workers, 1943, *JBC* **149**:413. *1174*

1943:3 **Lysergic acid-diethylamide** synthesized by Arthur Stoll (1887–1971) and Albert Hofmann (b.1906), *HCA* **26**:944. *1928.1*

1943:4 **Sulphetrone (solapsone)** used in treatment of **leprosy** by Arthur Herbert Harkness and G. Brownlee, *PRSM* **41**:309. *2442.1*

1943:5 **Promin (sodium glucosulphone)** treatment of **leprosy** introduced by Guy Henry Faget (1891–1940) et al., *USPHR* **58**:1729. *2441*

1943:6 **Transplantation rejection mechanism** in **skin homografts** explained by Peter Brian Medawar (1915–1987) and Thomas Gibson (b.1915), *JA* **77**:299, **78**:176. *2578.4*

1943:7 **Syphilis: penicillin treatment** introduced by John Friend Mahoney (1889–1957) et al., *VDI* **24**:355, *AmJPu* **33**:1387 *2418*

1943:8 **Vagotomy** used in treatment of **peptic ulcer** by Lester Reynold Dragstedt (1893–1975) and Frederick Mitchum Owens (b.1913), *PSEB* **53**:152. *3557*

1943:9 **Hyperthyroidism** treated with **thiourea** and **thiouracil** by Edwin Bennett Astwood (1909–1976), *JAMA* **122**:78. *3854*

1943:10 **Calciferol** introduced in the treatment of **lupus vulgaris** by Jacques Charpy (b.1900), *AnD* 8 Ser. **3**:331; it was introduced independently by Geoffrey Barrow Dowling (1891–1976) and Ebenezer William Prosser Thomas in 1945. *4010, 4011*

1943:11 A classification of **nerve injuries** published by Herbert John Seddon (1903–1977), *Brain* **66**:237. *4911*

1943:12 Plasma clot **nerve suture** introduced by Isador Max Tarlov (b.1905) and Bernard Benjamin (b.1903), *SGO* **76**;366. *4912*

1943:13 Following the observations of Gregg (1941), Charles Spencer Swan and co-workers showed that **rubella** in the first or second month of pregnancy always results in an abnormal infant, *MJA* **2**:201. *5509*

1943:14 The isolation and identification of a filterable virus in epidemic **keratoconjunctivitis** reported by Murray Joseph Sanders (1910–1987) and R.C. Alexander, *JEM* **77**:71. *5990*

1943:15 The first use of **fibrin glue** for **skin grafting** was by Machteld Elisabeth Sano (b.1903), *AmJS* **61**:105. *5765*

---

1943:16 Richard J. **Roberts**, British molecular biologist, born 6 Sep; shared Nobel Prize (Physiology or Medicine), 1993, with Phillip Allen Sharp, for their discovery of split genes, *NPL*.

---

1943:17 Eric F. **Wieschaus**, American geneticist, born; shared Nobel Prize (Physiology or Medicine), 1995, with Edward B. Lewis and Christiane Nüsslein-Volhard, for their discoveries concerning the genetic control of early embryonic development, *NPL*.

---

1943: Karl **Landsteiner** died, **born** 1868. *poliomyelitis, Rh antigen, antigen-antibody reactions, auto-antibody*

1943: Leo **Buerger** died, **born** 1879. *thrombo-angiitis obliterans, cystoscope*

1943: William **Pasteur** died, **born** 1856. *massive lung collapse*

1943: William Arbuthnot **Lane** died, **born** 1856. *mastoidectomy, antrectomy, constipation, fractures*

1943: Albert Abraham **Hijmans van den Bergh** died, **born** 1869. *bilirubin test*

1943: Arthur Dean **Bevan** died, **born** 1861. *undescended testicle, inguinal hernia*

1943: Howard Atwood **Kelly** died, **born** 1858. *ureters, bladder, uretero-ureteral anastomosis, renal and ureteral calculi, catheter, gynaecology*

1943: Abraham **Buschke** died, **born** 1868. *scleroderma adultorum syndrome, blastomycosis, cryptococcosis*

1943: James **Ewing** died, **born** 1886. *bone sarcoma*

1943: Frederick John **Poynton** died, **born** 1869. *rheumatism, diplococcus*

1943: Alexandre Emile Jean **Yersin** died, **born** 1863. *plague, Pasteurella pestis, diphtheria, Corynebacterium diphtheriae*

1943: Warrington **Yorke** died, **born** 1883. *Trypanosome rhodesiense, tsetse fly*

1943: Wilhelm Siegmund **Frei** died, **born** 1885. *lymphogranuloma venereum*

1943: George Washington **Crile** died, **born** 1864. *anaesthetic blocking of nerve trunks, surgical shock, anaesthesia*

1943: Emile **Marchoux** died, **born** 1862. *yellow fever*

1943: Leslie Tillotson **Webster** died, **born** 1894. *rabies*

1943: William Edgar **Caldwell** died, **born** 1880. *pelvis*

1943: Alfred **Vogt** died, **born** 1879. *glaucoma, cyclodiathermy*

1943: Edgar **Allen** died, **born** 1892. *oestrin, oestradiol*

1943: Isidor **Fischer** died, **born** 1868. *medical biography*

1943: Russell Henry **Chittenden** died, **born** 1856. *nutrition, digestion*

## 1944

1944:1 **Nobel Prize** (Physiology or Medicine): Joseph Erlanger (1874–1965) and Herbert Spencer Gasser (1888–1963), for their demonstration that **nervous impulse velocity** is directly proportional to fibre diameter. *NPL. 1305*

1944:2 **Para-aminobenzoic acid** introduced in the treatment of **scrub typhus** by Andrew Yeomans (b.1907) and co-workers, *JAMA* **126**:349. *5398.3*

1944:3 **Blood transfusion** with **dextran** as plasma substitute introduced by Anders Grönwall (b.1912) and B. Ingleman, *AcPS* **7**:97. *2028*

1944:4 **Streptomycin** discovered by Albert Schatz (b.1920), E. Bugie, and Selman Abraham Waksman (1888–1974), *PSEB* **55**:66. *1935*

1944:5 **Dichlorodiphenyltrichloroethane** (DDT) introduced as an **insecticide** by Paul Hermann Müller (1899–1965), *HCA* **27**:892. *1928.3*

1944:6 **Nitrofuran (nitrofurazone)** introduced as a bacteriostatic by Matthew Charles Dodd (b.1910) and William Barlow Stillman (b.1904), *JPET* **82**:11. *1928.2*

1944:7 Demonstration that **deoxyribonucleic acid** (DNA) is the basic material responsible for **genetic transformation** by Oswald Theodor Avery (1877–1955), Colin Munro MacLeod (1909–1972) and Maclyn McCarty (b.1911), *JEM* **79**:137. *255.3*

1944:8 **Diasone** treatment of **leprosy** introduced by Ernest Muir (1880–1974), *IJL* **12**:1. *2442*

1944:9 Regression of **mammary cancer** with **oestrogen** administration achieved by Alexander Haddow (1907–1976) and co-workers, *BMJ* **2**:393. *2659.3*

612

1944:10 **Folic acid** concentrate used to inhibit **tumour** growth by Cecile Leuchtenberger (b.1906) and co-workers, *PSEB* **59**:204. *2659.2*

1944:11 Isolation of **Eaton agent** in patients with primary atypical **pneumonia** by Monroe Davies Eaton (b.1904) and co-workers, *JEM* **79**:649. *3213.1*

1944:12 **Hearing tests** for children devised by Irene Rosetta Ewing (1883–1959) and Alexander William Gordon Ewing (1896–1980), *JLO* **59**:309. *3412.1*

1944:13 **Waldenström's macroglobulinaemia** described by Jan Gösta Waldenström (b.1906), *AcM* **117**:216. *3924.1*

1944:14 The **serum colloidal gold reaction** and the **thymol turbidity test** used by Noel Francis Maclagen (b.1904) as **liver function tests**, *BJEP* **25**:15, 234. *3665, 3666*

1944:15 Work on **hypoglycaemic sulphonamides** initiated by Auguste Loubatières (1912–1977), *CRSB* **138**:766. *3976.1*

1944:16 The nature of **infective hepatitis** proved by Frederic Ogden MacCallum and Denis John Bauer (b.1914), *L* **1**:622. *3664.3*

1944:17 The nature of **serum hepatitis** proved by Frederic Ogden MacCallum and W.H. Bradley, *L* **2**:228. *3664.2*

1944:18 An **artificial kidney (artificial renal dialyser)** introduced by Willem Johan Kolff (b.1911), *AcM* **117**:1916. *4255*

1944:19 **Pantopaque** introduced for the **myelographic** diagnosis of **cerebral tumours** by Theodore Behn Steinhausen (b.1914) and co-workers, *Rad* **43**:230. *4615*

1944:20 **Gamma globulin** used by Charles William Ordman (b.1914) and co-workers for passive immunization against **measles**, *JCI* **23**:541. *5449.1*

---

1944:21 Erwin **Neher**, German biophysical chemist, born 20 Mar; shared Nobel Prize (Physiology or Medicine), 1991, with Bert Sakmann, for their discoveries concerning the function of single ion channels in cells, *NPL*.

1944:22 Phillip Allen **Sharp**, American molecular biologist, born 6 Jun; shared Nobel Prize (Physiology or Medicine), 1993, with Richard John Roberts, for the discovery of split genes, *NPL*.

1944:23 George Lewis **Stewart**, American parasitologist, born 30 Oct; with co-workers, introduced a **rubella virus haemagglutination-inhibition test**, 1967, *NEJM* **276**:554. *5509.4*

---

1944:24 Kary B. **Mullis**, American biochemist, born; shared Nobel Prize (Chemistry), 1993, for the invention of the polymerase chain reaction (PCR) method, *NPL*.

---

1944:25 Norman Dawson **Royle** died; introduced sympathetic ramisection for the treatment of spastic paralysis, 1924, *MJA* **1**:77. *4894*

---

1944: Alexis **Carrel** died, **born** 1873. *wound irrigation, kidney transplantation, heart transplantation, blood vessel transplantation, arterial suture, tumour growth in vitro*

1944: Bartolomeo **Gosio** died, **born** 1863. *penicillin*

1944: Yandell **Henderson** died, **born** 1873. *aviation medicine, decompression sickness*

1944: Leopold **Freund** died, **born** 1868. *deep radiation therapy*

1944: Ignatz Leo **Nascher** died, **born** 1863. *geriatrics*

1944: Karl **Herxheimer** died, **born** 1861. *syphilis*

1944: Werner **Schultz** died, **born** 1878. *agranulocytic angina, scarlet fever*

1944: Arthur Frederick **Hertz [Hurst]** died, **born** 1879. *dumping syndrome, gastroenterostomy*

1944: (?) Eugen Alexander **Pólya** died, **born** 1876. *cancer of pylorus*

1944: Emile Charles **Achard** died, **born** 1860. *Achard-Thiers syndrome*

1944: Achille Alexandre **Souques** died, **born** 1860. *parkinsonism, encephalitis, pituitary infantilism*

1944: Eugen **Steinbach** died, **born** 1861. *rejuvenation*

1944: Sandor **Korány** died, **born** 1866. *kidney function test*

1944: Bernard **Sachs** died, **born** 1858. *amaurotic familial idiocy*

1944: William George **MacCallum** died, **born** 1874. *parathyroid glands, calcium metabolism, malaria*

1944: Frederick Percival **Mackie** died, **born** 1875. *relapsing fever, Pediculus corporis*

1944: John Charles Grant **Ledingham** died, **born** 1875. *smallpox*

1944: Adolpho Carlos **Lindenberg** died, **born** 1872. *leishmaniasis*

1944: James Tayloe **Gwathmey** died, **born** 1865. *anaesthesia, midwifery*

1944: Carl **Koller** died, **born** 1857. *ophthalmology, cocaine anaesthesia*

1944: Robert Ernest **Kelly** died, **born** 1879. *intratracheal ether anaesthesia*

1944: Eduard Konrad **Zirm** died, **born** 1863. *corneal transplantation*

## 1945
1945:1 **Nobel Prize** (Physiology or Medicine): Alexander Fleming (1881–1955), for the discovery of **penicillin**, *NPL. 1933*; Howard Walter Florey (1898–1968) and Ernst Boris Chain (1906–1979), for its development as an **antibacterial antibiotic** for use in man, *NPL. 1934*

614

1945:2 **Dimercaprol, British anti-lewisite** (BAL), a heavy metal antagonist, developed by Rudolph Albert Peters (1889–1982) and co-workers, *Nature* **156**:616. *1929*

1945:3 **Bacitracin** introduced by Balbina A. Johnson, *Science* **102**:376. *1936*

1945:4 **Streptomycin** used in treatment of **tuberculosis** by Horton Corwin Hinshaw (b.1902) and William Hugh Feldman (1892–1974), *PMC* **20**:313. *2350*

1945:5 **Angina pectoris** treated with **thiouracil** by Wilhelm Raab (1895–1969), *JAMA* **128**:249. *2900*

1945:6 **Rhesus sensitization**, ('Coombs' test'), devised by Robin Royston Amos Coombs (b.1921) and co-workers, *L* **2**:15; *BJEP* **26**:255. *3104*

1945:7 **Conglutination** test for **rhesus sensitization** devised by Alexander Solomon Wiener (1907–1976), *JLCM* **30**:662. *3105*

1945:8 Surgical treatment of **coarctation of aorta** pioneered by Clarence Crafoord (1899–1984) and Karl Gustav Vilhelm Nylin (1892–1961), *JTS* **14**:347, and Robert Edward Gross (1905–1988), *Surgery* **18**:673. *3044, 3044.1*

1945:9 Operation for congenital defects of the **pulmonary artery** ('Blalock-Taussig operation') devised by Alfred Blalock (1899–1964) and Helen Brooke Taussig (1898–1986), *JAMA* **128**:189. *3043*

1945:10 The **Roth-Kvale histamine test** for the diagnosis of **phaeochromocytoma** introduced by Grace M. Roth and Walter Frederick Kvale (b.1907), *AmJMS* **210**:653. *3869*

1945:11 **Methaemoglobinaemia** reported by Hunter Hall Comly (b.1919), *JAMA* **129**:112. *3103*

1945:12 **Hyperthyroidism** treated with **thiobarbital** by Edwin Bennett Astwood (1909–1976), *JCE* **5**:345. *3855*

1945:13 **Adrenalectomy** for **prostatic carcinoma** introduced by Charles Brenton Huggins (b.1901) and William Wallace Scott (b.1913), *AnS* **122**:1031. *4276.1*

1945:14 A new extravesical technique for retropubic **prostatectomy** introduced by Terence John Millin (1903–1980), *L* **2**:693. *4277*

1945:15 **Calciferol** introduced in the treatment of **lupus vulgaris** by Geoffrey Barrow Dowling (1891–1976) and Ebenezer William Prosser Thomas, *PRSM* **39**:96. It was also used by Jacques Charpy in 1943, at that time isolated by the war in France. *4010, 4011*

1945:16 A vaccine against scrub **typhus** introduced by Forrest Fulton (b.1913) and L. Joyner, *L* **2**:729. *5399*

1945:17 **Proguanil (paludrine)** first used in the treatment of human **malaria** by Alfred Robert Davies Adams and co-workers, *AnTM* **39**:225. *5261*

1945:18 **Dengue** successfully propagated in mice and vaccine produced by Albert Bruce Sabin (b.1906) and Robert Walter Schlesinger (b.1913), *Science* **101**:604. *5475.1*

1945:19 A method of replacement of the **inverted uterus** by intravaginal hydraulic pressure introduced by James Vincent O'Sullivan, *BMJ* **2**:282. *6233*

---

1945: William Henry **Howell** died, **born** 1860. *heparin*

1945: Hugh Hampton **Young** died, **born** 1870. *vesiculography, mercurochrome, prostatectomy*

1945: Nicolas Maurice **Arthus** died, **born** 1862. *anaphylaxis*

1945: Fred **Neufeld** died, **born** 1861. *bacteriotropins, pneumococcus*

1945: Herbert Edward **Durham** died, **born** 1866. *typhoid, bacterial agglutination, Salmonella aertrycke, food poisoning*

1945: Hans **Sachs** died, **born** 1877. *syphilis*

1945: Richard Friedrich Johannes **Pfeiffer** died, **born** 1858. *bacterial influenza, immune bacteriolysis, cholera vibrio*

1945: Ernst **Meinicke** died, **born** 1878. *syphilis*

1945: Thomas Hunt **Morgan** died, **born** 1866. *heredity*

1945: William Thomas **Ritchie** died, **born** 1873. *auricular flutter*

1945: Thomas **Lewis** died, **born** 1881. *effort syndrome, heart arrhythmia, auricular fibrillation*

1945: Victor **Schmieden** died, **born** 1874. *pericardiectomy*

1945: Thomas Benton **Cooley** died, **born** 1871. *thalassaemia*

1945: Walter Bradford **Cannon** died, **born** 1871. *digestive tract, radiology, bismuth, sympathetic-adrenal mechanism*

1945: Edgar Otto Konrad von **Gierke** died, **born** 1877. *glycogen storage disease*

1945: Pierre **Abrami** died, **born** 1879. *haemolytic anaemia*

1945: Thomas **Barlow** died, **born** 1845. *scurvy*

1945: Karl Theodor **Fahr** died, **born** 1877. *nephrosis*

1945: Fred Houdlett **Albee** died, **born** 1876. *bone grafts*

1945: Walter Essex **Wynter** died, **born** 1866. *lumbar puncture*

1945: Alois **Pick** died, **born** 1859. *Phlebotomus fever*

1945: Albert Mason **Stevens** died, **born** 1884. *Stevens-Johnson syndrome*

1945: Velyien Ewart **Henderson** died, **born** 1877. *anaesthesia, cyclopropane*

1945: Wilhelm **Latzko** died, **born** 1863. *caesarean section*

1945: Hans **Fischer** died, **born** 1881. *chlorophyll, haemin*

**1946**
1946: 1 **Nobel Prize** (Physiology or Medicine): Hermann Joseph Muller (1890–1967), for the induction of **genetic mutation** by exposing *Drosophila* to **x rays**, *NPL. 251.1*

1946: 2 **Nobel Prize** (Chemistry): John Howard Northrop (1891–1987) and Wendell Meredith Stanley (1904–1971), for the preparation of **enzymes** and **viruses** in pure form, *NPL. 1038.1, 2524.5*; James Batcheller Sumner (1881–1955) for the discovery that **enzymes** can be **crystallized**, *NPL*

1946: 3 **National Insurance Act (UK)**

1946: 4 **National Health Service Act (UK)**

1946: 5 **Nitrogen mustard therapy** (methyl-bis amine hydrochloride and methyl-tris amine hydrochloride) for **Hodgkin's disease, lymphosarcoma**, etc. introduced by Louis Sanford Goodman (b.1906) and co-workers, *JAMA* **105**:475. *2659.6*

1946: 6 **Nitrogen mustard** introduced in the treatment of **Hodgkin's disease** by Albert Gilman (b.1908) and Frederick Stanley Philips (b.1916), *Science* **103**:409. *3788*

1946: 7 **Noradrenaline** shown to be predominant transmitter of the effects of sympathetic nerve impulses by Ulf Svante von Euler (1905–1983), *AcPS* **12**:73. *1354.1*

1946: 8 **Genetic recombination** in **bacteriophage** induced by Max Delbrück (1906–1981) and W.T. Bailey, *CSHS* **11**:33. *2578.5*

1946: 9 **Genetic recombination** in *Escherichia coli* reported by Joshua Lederberg (b.1925) and Edward Lawrie Tatum (1909–1975), *Nature* **158**:558. *255.4*

1946: 10 **Thiosemicarbazone** was introduced in the treatment of **tuberculosis** by Gerhard Domagk (1895–1964) and co-workers, *NW* **33**:315. *2351*

1946: 11 **Linear ion accelerator** introduced by Luis Walter Alvarez (1911–1988), *PsR* **70**:799. *2659.5*

1946: 12 **Folic acid** – isolation, structural determination and final synthesis carried out by Robert Bruce Angier (b.1917) and co-workers, *Science* **103**:667. *3151*

1946: 13 **Leukaemia** treated with **urethane** by Edith Paterson and co-workers, *L* **1**:677. *3106*

1946: 14 Introduction of *p*-**aminosalicylic acid**, first specific anti-tuberculosis drug, in the treatment of **pulmonary tuberculosis** by Jörgen Lehmann (b.1898), *L* **1**:15. *3241*

1946:15 **Hypochromic anaemia** treated with **iron** administered intravenously by Anne Goetsch (b.1917), *Blood* **1**:129. *3152*

1946:16 **Acoustic impedance hearing test** developed by Otto Metz (b.1905), *AcOL*, Suppl. 63. *3412.2*

1946:17 **'Refsum's syndrome'**, an inherited disorder of **lipid metabolism**, first described by Sigvald Refsum (1907–1991), *AcPsS* suppl. 38. *3924.2*

1946:18 **Streptomycin** used in the treatment of **tularaemia** by Lee Foshay (1896–1960) and A. Bernard Pasternack (b.1916), *JAMA* **130**:393. *5180*

1946:19 **Rickettsialpox** first described by several writers in 1946–7. Robert Joseph Huebner (b.1914), W.L. Jellison and C. Pomerantz described it and isolated the aetiological agent, *Rickettsia akari*, *USPHR* **61**:1677. *5400*

1946:20 Clinical trials of **chloroquine** in the treatment of **malaria** were first undertaken by Harry Most (b.1907) and co-workers, *JAMA* **131**:963. *5261.1*

1946:21 **Gallamine triethiodide (flaxedil)** introduced into **anaesthesia** by Daniel Bovet (1907–1992) and co-workers, *CRAS* **223**:597. *5725*

1946:22 **Mumps** vaccine introduced by Joseph Stokes (1896–1972) and co-workers, *JEM* **84**:407. *5544.2*

1946:23 **Lucanthone hydrochloride (Miracil D)** introduced for the treatment of **bilharziasis** by Walter Kikuth (1896–1968) and co-workers, *NW* **33**:253. *5351.2*

---

1946:24 Georges Jean Franz **Köhler**, German immunologist, born 17 Apr; with César Milstein, produced monoclonal antibodies, 1975, *Nature* **256**:495; shared Nobel Prize (Physiology or Medicine), 1984, with Niels Kaj Jerne and César Milstein, for the discovery of the principle of production of monoclonal antibodies, *NPL*. Died 1995. *2578.43*

---

1946: Hans **Eppinger** died, **born** 1879. *bundle-branch block*

1946: Emanuel **Libman** died, **born** 1872. *endocarditis, lupus erythematosus disseminatus*

1946: Felix **Klemperer** died, **born** 1866. *pneumococcus*

1946: Howard **Lilienthal** died, **born** 1861. *sarcoma, pneumonectony*

1946: Adolf **Lorenz** died, **born** 1854. *congenital hip dislocation*

1946: Maurice **Villaret** died, **born** 1877. *retroparotid space syndrome*

1946: Walter Edward **Dandy** died, **born** 1886. *Menière's disease, cerebral ventriculography, pneumoencephalography, hydrocephalus, glossopharyngeal neuralgia*

1946: Simon **Flexner** died, **born** 1863. *poliomyelitis, bacillary dysentery, Shigella flexneri, cerebrospinal meningitis*

1946: Alfred **Whitmore** died, **born** 1876. *melioidosis*

1946: Keinosuke **Miyairi** died, **born** 1865. *Schistosoma japonicum, snail*

1946: John William Watson **Stephens** died, **born** 1865. *malaria, Plasmodium ovale, Trypanosoma rhodesiense*

1946: Fujiro **Katsurada** died, **born** 1868. *schistosomiasis, Schistosoma japonicum*

1946: Jaroslav **Drbohlav** died, **born** 1893. *amoebae*

1946: Theodor Lasater **Terry** died, **born** 1899. *retrolental fibroplasia*

1946: Earl Calvin **Padgett** died, **born** 1893. *skin grafts, dermatome*

1946: John Albertson **Sampson** died, **born** 1873. *endometrioma of ovary*

1946: Alfred **Eddowes** died, **born** 1850. *osteogenesis imperfecta*

1946: Leslie Leon **Lumsden** died, **born** 1875. *St Louis encephalitis*

1946: Friedrich Ernst **Krukenberg** died, **born** 1870. *Krukenberg's tumour, ovary tumours*

**1947**
1947:1 **Nobel Prize** (Physiology or Medicine): Carl Ferdinand Cori (1896–1984) and Gerty Theresa Cori (1896–1957), for the first synthesis of **glycogen** *in vitro, NPL. 751.4*; Bernardo Alberto Houssay (1887–1971), for his work on the role of the anterior **pituitary** in **carbohydrate** metabolism, *NPL.*

1947:2 **Nobel Prize** (Chemistry): Robert Robinson (1886–1975) for research on products of biological importance, including **alkaloids**, **sterols**, **sex hormones**, and **penicillin**, *NPL.*

1947:3 **World Medical Association** founded

1947:4 **Women medical students** accepted in all **United Kingdom medical schools**

1947:5 *Sensory mechanisms of the retina*, published by Ragnar Arthur Granit (1900–1991). *1534*

1947:6 Factors determining the release of **antidiuretic hormone** elucidated by Ernest Basil Verney (1894–1967), *PRS* **135**:26. *1244.2*

1947:7 **Chloramphenicol (chloromycetin)** produced by John Ehrlich (b.1907) et al., *Science* **106**:417. *1938*

1947:8 **Polymyxin (aerosporin)** discovered by Geoffrey Clough Ainsworth (b.1905) and others, *Nature* **160**:263. Other polymyxins were discovered simultaneously by R.G. Benedict and A.F. Langlykke and by P.G. Stansly et al., *BJH* **81**:43. *1937, 1941*

1947:9 **Electrokymograph** for recording movements of the **heart** introduced by George Christian Henny (b.1899) and co-workers, *AmJR* **57**:409. *2876*

1947:10 Treatment of **ventricular fibrillation** by direct application of **electric shock** introduced by Claude Schaefer Beck (1894–1971) and co-workers, *JAMA* **135**:985. *2878.1*

1947:11 Successful division of the **pulmonary valve (valvulotomy)** for the treatment of **pulmonary stenosis** by Thomas Holmes Sellors (1902–1987), *L* **1**:988. *3046.2*

1947:12 First **thromboendarterectomy** for **arterial thrombosis** performed by Jean Cid dos Santos (d.1970), *MAC* **73**:409. *3019.1*

1947:13 **Phenindione (phenylindanedione)** introduced as an **anticoagulant** by Jean Pierre Soulier (b.1913) and Jean Gueguen, *CRSB* **141**:1007. *3107*

1947:14 **Atresia** of the **ileum** successfully treated by **enterostomy** alone by James R. Judd, *JPe* **30**:679. *3558*

1947:15 **Békésy** (semiautomatic) **audiometer** introduced by Georg von Békésy (1899–1972), *AcOL* **35**:411. *3412.3*

1947:16 **Radioactive isotopes (fluorescein)** introduced in **neuroradiology** by George Eugene Moore (b.1922), *Science* **106**:130. *4615.1*

1947:17 **Stereotactic surgery** first performed on the human brain by Ernest Adolf Spiegel and co-workers, *Science* **106**:349. *4912.1*

1947:18 **Revascularization of the brain** by the establishment of a cervical arteriovenous fistula carried out by Claude Schaeffer Beck (1894–1971) and co-workers, *JPe* **35**:317. *4914*

1947:19 **Chloramphenicol** introduced in the treatment of **typhus** by Joseph Edwin Smadel (1907–1963) and Elizabeth B. Jackson, *Science* **106**:418. *5402*

1947:20 **Diethylcarbamazine (hetrazan)** used experimentally in the treatment of **filariasis** by Reginald Irving Hewitt (b.1911) and co-workers, *JLCM* **32**:1314. *5351.3*

1947:21 **Suramin** introduced for the treatment of **onchocerciasis** by L. van Hoof and co-workers, *ASBMT* **27**:173. *5351.4*

1947:22 The **male toad test** for the **diagnosis of pregnancy** introduced by Carlos Galli Mainini (1914–1961), *SMB* **1**:337. *6234*

---

1947:23 Thomas Robert **Cech**, American biochemist, born 8 Dec; shared Nobel Prize (Chemistry), 1989, with Sidney Altman, for their discovery of catalytic DNA, *NPL*.

---

1947:24 Gerd **Binnig**, German physicist, born; shared Nobel Prize (Physics), 1986, with Heinrich Rohrer and Ernst Ruska, for design of the scanning tunnelling microscope, *NPL*.

---

1947: Frederick Gowland **Hopkins** died, **born** 1861. *vitamins, tryptophan, glutathione, lactic acid and muscular contraction*

1947: Joseph **Barcroft** died, **born** 1872. *physiology, respiratory function of blood*

1947: William Henry **Schultz** died, **born** 1873. *anaphylaxis, Schultz-Dale test*

1947: Charles **Mantoux** died, **born** 1877. *tuberculosis, tuberculin*

1947: Montrose Thomas **Burrows** died, **born** 1884. *tumour growth in vitro*

1947: Marion Herbert **Barker** died, **born** 1899. *hypertension, thiocyanate*

1947: Rudolph von **Jaksch** died, **born** 1855. *infantile pseudoleukaemic anaemia*

1947: William Ernest **Miles** died, **born** 1869. *abdominoperineal resection*

1947: Felix **Pinkus** died, **born** 1868. *lichen nitidus*

1947: Erik **Lysholm** died, **born** 1891. *radiography, skull table*

1947: Pierre Marie Félix **Janet** died, **born** 1859. *psychasthenia*

1947: Almroth Edward **Wright** died, **born** 1861. *opsonins, immune serum, typhoid inoculation, brucellosis*

1947: Harry **Plotz** died, **born** 1890. *measles*

1947: Elliott Carr **Cutler** died, **born** 1888. *cryptococcosis, mitral valve section*

**1948**
1948:1 **Nobel Prize** (Physiology or Medicine): Paul Hermann Müller (1899–1965), for his discovery of the high efficiency of **DDT** as an **insecticide**, *NPL. 1928.3*

1948:2 **Nobel Prize** (Chemistry): Arne Wilhelm Kaurin Tiselius (1902–1971), for his research on **electrophoresis** and **adsorption analysis**, especially for his discoveries concerning the complex nature of the **serum proteins**, *NPL. 2576.8*

1948:3 **National Health Service (NHS)** comes into operation in **UK**

1948:4 **World Health Organization** established by United Nations Organization, assuming the functions of the **League of Nations Organisation** (1920) and the **Office d'Hygiène Publique** (1907)

1948:5 **Vitamin B$_{12}$** isolated in crystalline form independently by Edward Lawrence Rickes (b.1912) et al., *Science* **107**:396, and by Ernest Lester Smith (1904–1992), *Nature* **162**:144. *1091, 1092*

1948:6 **Vitamin B$_{12}$** shown to be effective in treatment of **pernicious anaemia** by Randolph West (b.1890), *Science* **107**:398. *3154*

1948:7 Walter Rudolf Hess (1881–1973) published his researches on the functional organization of the **interbrain** as a coordinator of the activities of the internal organs, *Die funktionelle Organisation des vegetativen Nervensystems. 1451.1*

1948:8 Discovery of **chlortetracycline (aureomycin)** reported. *ANYAS* **51**:175. *1942*

1948:9 **Aureomycin** isolated and introduced by Bernard Minge Duggar (1872–1956), *ANYAS* **51**:175. *1942*

1948:10 **Agar gel immunodiffusion** method introduced by Örjan Thomas Gunnersson Ouchterlony (b.1914), *AcPMS* **25**:186. *2578.6*

1948:11 '**Antabuse**' (tetraethylthiuramdisulphide) introduced for the treatment of **alcoholism** by Jens Hald and co-workers, *AcPha* **4**:285. *2091*

1948:12 **Streptodornase** discovered by Maclyn McCarty (b.1911), *JEM* **88**:181. *1929.2*

1948:13 First successful **pulmonary-azygos shunt** for **mitral stenosis** performed by Edward Franklin Bland (b.1901) and Richard Harwood Sweet (b.1901), *AmPr* **2**:756. *3047*

1948:14 **Pulmonary valvulotomy** in the treatment of **congenital stenosis** introduced by Russell Claude Brock (1903–1980), *BMJ* **1**:1121. *3046*

1948:15 **Valvuloplasty** for **mitral stenosis** introduced by Dwight Emary Harken (b.1910) and co-workers, *NEJM* **239**:801. *3046.1*

1948:16 Exchange **blood transfusion** used in the treatment of **erythroblastosis foetalis** by Louis Klein Diamond (b.1902), *Ped* **2**:520. *3107.1*

1948:17 **McVay** (or **Cooper**) **ligament repair** in **hernia** introduced by Chester B. McVay (1911–1987), *ArSuC* **57**:524. *3611.2*

1948:18 Francis Curtis Dohan (b.1907) and Francis Dring Wetherill Lukens (b.1899) produced experimental **diabetes** by artificially-induced **hyperglycaemia**, *En* **42**:244. *3977*

1948:19 The science of **cybernetics** founded by Norbert Wiener (1894–1966); he wrote *Cybernetics: or control and communication in the animal and the machine. 4991.1*

1948:20 The pre-erythrocytic stage of **malaria** demonstrated by Henry Edward Shortt (1887–1987) and co-workers, *BMJ* **1**:192, 547; 1949, **2**:1006. *5262*

1948:21 **Melarsen** introduced in the treatment of **trypanosomiasis** by E.A.H. Friedheim, *AnTM* **42**:357

1948:22 **Pentaquine** was the subject of clinical trials in **malaria** by Alf Sven Alving (b.1902) and co-workers, *JCI* **27**, 3II:25. *5261.2*

1948:23 The **curare**-like **anaesthetic** action of **methonium** compounds discovered by William Drummond MacDonald Paton (1917–1993) and Eleanor Zaimis (1915–1982), *Nature* **161**:718. *19129.2, 5726*

1948:24 The **coxsackie** virus isolated by Gilbert Julius Dalldorf (b.1900) and Grace Mary Sickles (1898–1959) from children with paralysis, *Science* **108**:61. *5545*

---

1948: Alfred **Wolff-Eisner** died, **born** 1877. *tberculosis, tuberculin*

1948: Koichi **Ichikawa** died, **born** 1888. *cancer, tar*

1948: Mikhail **Arinkin** died, **born** 1876. *bone marrow biopsy*

1948: George Tully **Vaughan** died, **born** 1859. *abdominal artery ligation*

1948: Julius **Wohlgemuth** died, **born** 1874. *pancreatic function test*

1948: James Harry **Sequeira** died, **born** 1865. *adrenogenital syndrome*

1948: John Bentley **Squier** died, **born** 1873. *prostatectomy*

1948: Jean **Nageotte** died, **born** 1866. *syndrome of Babinski-Nageotte*

1948: Alfred **Hauptmann** died, **born** 1881. *epilepsy, phenobarbitone*

1948: Carl Olaf **Sonne** died, **born** 1882. *bacillary dysentery, Shigella sonnei*

1948: Charles Albert **Elsberg** died, **born** 1871. *anaesthesia, intratracheal insufflation*

1948: Richard Pearson **Strong** died, **born** 1872. *Histoplasma capsulatum*

1948: John **Auer** died, **born** 1875. *anaphylactic shock, anaesthesia, intratracheal insufflation*

1948: Henry **Smith** died, **born** 1862. *cataract*

1948: Hulüsi **Behçet** died, **born** 1889. *Behçet's syndrome*

**1949**
1949:1 **Nobel Prize** (Physiology or Medicine): Walter Rudolph Hess (1881–1973), for his discovery of the functional organization of the **interbrain** as a coordinator of the activities of the internal organs, *NPL. 1451.1*; Antonio Caetano de Abreu Freire Egas Moniz (1874–1955), for his discovery of frontal **leucotomy** as a treatment for certain **psychoses**, *NPL. 4905*

1949:2 **Wellcome Institute for the History of Medicine Library**, **London**, opened to public

1949:3 **School of Pharmacy**, **London**, becomes part of **University of London**

1949:4 Work on the **genetics** and replication of **bacteria** published by Salvador Edward Luria (b.1912), *Gen* **34**:93. *2526.1*

1949:5 **Poliomyelitis virus** grown in cultures of various tissues by John Francis Enders (1897–1985), Thomas Huckle Weller (b.1915) and F.C. Robbins, removing obstacles to **vaccine** production, *Science* **109**:85. *4671.1*

1949:6 **Pernicious anaemia** treated by parenteral **vitamin B$_{12}$** by Charles Cady Ungley, *BMJ* **2**:1370. *3155*

1949:7 Isolation of *nor*-**adrenaline** by Sune Bergström (b.1916) and co-workers, *AcCS* **3**:305; *AcPS* 1950 **20**:101. *1155*

1949:8 Clinical trials of **lithium** by John Cade (b.1912), *MJA* **36**:349. *1930.1*

1949: 9 **Microwave radiation therapy** introduced by Georges Wakim (b.1907) et al., *JAMA* **139**:989. *2010.5*

1949: 10 **Neomycin** discovered by Selman Abraham Waksman (1888–1973) and Hubert Arthur Lechevalier (b.1926), *Science* **113**:305. *1944*

1949: 11 **Bradykinin**, a hypotensive and smooth-muscle-stimulating factor, discovered by Mauricio Rocha e Silva (b.1910) et al., *AmJPh* **156**:261 *1930*

1949: 12 Isolation of **fumagillin**, an amoebicidal antibiotic, by Frederick Reuben Hanson (b.1921) and Thomas Eugene Eble (b.1923), *JB* **58**:527; *Science* **113**:202. *1945*

1949: 13 **Syphilis: Nelson treponemal immobilization test** introduced by Robert Armstrong Nelson (b.1922) and Manfred Martin Mayer (b.1916), *JEM* **89**:369. *2419*

1949: 14 **Acquired immunological tolerance** explained by Frank Macfarlane Burnet (1899–1985) and Frank John Fenner (b.1914); in *The production of antibodies. 2578.7*

1949: 15 **Sickle-cell anaemia** shown to be due to a structural **haemoglobin** variant (the first recognition of a haemoglobin variant) by Linus Pauling (1901–1994) and co-workers, *Science* **110**:543. *3154.1*

1949: 16 **Sickle-cell anaemia** shown to be inherited in a simple Mendelian manner by James Van Gundia Neel (b.1915), *Science* **110**:64. *3154.2*

1949: 17 **Tympanoplasty** operation for treatment of chronic suppurative **otitis media** introduced by William Ingledew Daggett (1900–1980), *JLO* **63**:635. *3412.4*

1949: 18 **Methimazole (mercazole)**, a potent **anti-thyroid** drug, synthesized by Reuben G. Jones and co-workers, *JACS* **71**:4000. *3855.1*

1949: 19 **Cortisone** and **adrenocorticotrophic hormone** (ACTH) introduced in the treatment of **rheumatoid arthritis** by Philip Showalter Hench (1896–1965) and co-workers, *PMC* **24**:181. *4508*

1949: 20 The use of **epiphyseal stapling (Blount staple)** to control **bone growth** introduced by Walter P. Blount (b.1900) and G.R. Clarke, *JBJS* **31**A:464. *4404.2*

1949: 21 '**Rush pins**', made of specially hardened stainless steel, introduced by Leslie V. Rush (b.1905) and H. Lowry Rush (1897–1965) for the fixation of **fractures** of long bones, *AmJSu* **78**:324. *4435.2*

1949: 22 **Artane** introduced in the treatment of **Parkinson's disease** by Kendall Brooks Corbin (b.1907), *JAMA* **141**:377. *4729*

1949: 23 The diagnosis of **lymphogranuloma venereum** by a skin-test antigen introduced by Samuel Phillips Bedson (1886–1969) and co-workers, *JCP* **2**:241. *5225*

1949: 24 **Influenza** C virus recovered by Richard Moreland Taylor (b.1887), *AmJPuH* **39**:171. *5500*

1949:25 **Succinylcholine chloride**, a muscle relaxant used in **anaesthesia**, introduced by Daniel Bovet (1907–1992) and co-workers, *RISS* **12**:106. *5728*

1949:26 **Hexamethonium bromide**, an **anaesthetic**, introduced by William Drummond MacDonald Paton (1917–1993), *BJP* **4**:381. *5727*

1949:27 **Coxsackie** virus isolated from patients with **poliomyelitis** by Edward Charles Curnen (b.1909) and co-workers, *JAMA* **141**:894. *5546*

1949:28 **Corneal graft** fixation by minute direct interrupted stitches carried out by José Ignacio Barraquer Moner, *ArSOH* **9**:912. *5990.1*

---

1949: Kurt **Beringer** died, **born** 1893. *mescaline*

1949: Félix Hubert **d'Herelle** died, **born** 1873. *bacteriophage*

1949: Joseph Edwin **Barnard** died, **born** 1870. *cancer, viruses*

1949: Erik Adolf von **Willebrand** died, **born** 1870. *pseudohaemophilia*

1949: Max Minor **Peet** died, **born** 1885. *hypertension, trigeminal neuralgia*

1949: Georg Ludwig **Zuelzer** died, **born** 1870. *insulin*

1949: Alexander von **Lichtenburg** died, **born** 1880. *pyelography, cystogram, excretion urography, uroselectan*

1949: Moritz **Oppenheim** died, **born** 1876. *gonorrhoea*

1949: Clifford **Dobell** died, **born** 1886. *Entamoeba histolytica*

1949: Charles Albert **Bentley** died, **born** 1873. *Ankylostoma duodenale*

1949: John Lancelot **Todd** died, **born** 1876. *relapsing fever, Ornithodorus moubata*

1949: Wilhelm August Paul **Schüffner** died, **born** 1867. *leptospirosis, Leptospira canicola, ankylostomiasis*

1949: August Karl Gustav **Bier** died, **born** 1861. *spinal anaesthesia, cocaine, hyperaemia in surgery*

1949: Ernest **Fourneau** died, **born** 1872. *anaesthesia, stovaine*

1949: John Elmer **Weeks** died, **born** 1853. *conjunctivitis*

1949: Victor **Veau** died, **born** 1871. *cleft palate*

1949: Schack August Steenberg **Krogh** died, **born** 1874. *regulation of motor mechanism of capillaries*

1949: Alfred **Hand** died, **born** 1868. *Hand-Schüller-Christian syndrome*

**1950**

1950:1 **Nobel Prize** (Physiology or Medicine): Edward Calvin Kendall (1886–1972), Philip Showalter Hench (1896–1955), and Tadeus Reichstein (1897–1996), for the isolation of **cortisone** and the use of cortisone and **ACTH** in the treatment of **rheumatoid arthritis**, *NPL. 1150, 1153, 4508*

1950:2 **Skin homografts** to prove the relationship of identical twins carried out by Archibald McIndoe (1900–1960) and Adolphe Franceschetti (b.1896), *BJPS* **2**:283. *1757*

1950:3 **DNA** research was revolutionized by the chemical studies of Erwin Chargaff (b.1905), *Ex* **6**:201. *255.6*

1950:4 **Oxytetracycline (terramycin)** discovered by Alexander Carpenter Finlay (b.1906) et al., *Science* **111**:85. *1945.1*

1950:5 '**General adaptation syndrome**' reaction to **stress** or injury advanced by Hans Selye (1907–1982); *The physiology and pathology of exposure to stress. 2238*

1950:6 **Antigen** location by **fluorescent antibody** technique introduced by Albert Hewett Coons (1912–1978) and Melvin H. Kaplan (b.1920), *JEM* **91**:1. *2578.8*

1950:7 Use of **scintillation counters** in the location of **tumours** introduced by Benedict Cassen (b.1902) and co-workers, *Nuc* **6**:78. *2660.2*

1950:8 Association of **lung cancer** with **cigarette smoking** proved by case-control study by Ernest Ludwig Wynder (b.1922) and Evarts Ambrose Graham (1883–1957), *JAMA* **143**:329. *3215.1*

1950:9 Association of **lung cancer** with **cigarette smoking** (Müller, 1939; Wynder & Graham, 1950) confirmed by William Richard Shaboe Doll (b.1912) and Austin Bradford Hill (1897–1991), *BMJ* **2**:139. *3215.2, 3213, 3215.1*

1950:10 **Triethylene melamine (TEM)** introduced in the treatment of **Hodgkin's disease** by Cornelius Packard Rhoads (1898–1959) and co-workers, *TAAP* **63**:136. *3788.1*

1950:11 **Fluoridation** of water supplies as a preventive against **dental caries** studied by Henry Trendley Dean (d.1962) and co-workers, *USPHR* **65**:1403. *3692.1*

1950:12 The first human **kidney transplant** in which the patient survived, carried out by Richard H. Lawler (1895–1982) and co-workers, *JAMA* **144**:844. *4256.1*

1950:13 Implantation of a permanent artificial (silicone) **urethra** by Robert Rocco De Nicola (b.1916), *JU* **63**:168. *4203*

1950:14 The use of an acrylic **prosthesis** for **hip arthroplasty** introduced by Jean Judet (b.1905) and Robert Louis Judet (b.1909), *JBJS* **32B**:166. *4405*

1950:15 **Primaquine (diaprim)** introduced in the treatment of **malaria** by John Harold Edgcomb (b.1924) and co-workers, *JNMS* **9**:285. *5262.3*

626

1950:16 The virus of **Colorado tick fever** isolated from *Dermacentor andersoni* by Lloyd Joseph Florio (b.1910) and co-workers, *JI* **64**:257. *5546.1*

1950: Frederick William **Twort** died, **born** 1877. *bacteriophage*

1950: Emil **Abderhalden** died, **born** 1877. *physiology, biochemistry*

1950: Julius **Donath** died, **born** 1870. *auto-antibody*

1950: Henri **Coutard** died, **born** 1876. *carcinoma of pharynx, radiotherapy*

1950: George Richards **Minot** died, **born** 1885. *liver treatment in anaemia*

1950: John Alfred **Ryle** died, **born** 1889. *gastric juice*

1950: Leonard Gregory **Parsons** died, **born** 1879. *scurvy, ascorbic acid*

1950: Emil **Abderhalden** died, **born** 1877. *cystinosis*

1950: Stephen **Chauvet** died, **born** 1885. *pituitary infantilism*

1950: Jean Hyacinthe **Vincent** died, **born** 1862. *ulcerative stomatitis, mycetoma*

1950: Franz **Volhard** died, **born** 1872. *nephrosis, pericardiectomy*

1950: Antonio **Garcia Tapia** died, **born** 1875. *palato-pharyngo-laryngeal hemiplegia*

1950: Friedrich Karl **Kleine** died, **born** 1869. *trypanosome, tsetse fly*

1950: Ryukichi **Inada** died, **born** 1874. *leptospirosis icterohaemorrhagica*

1950: Charles Franklin **Craig** died, **born** 1872. *dengue, malaria*

1950: Carl Gustav Abrahamsson **Forssell** died, **born** 1876. *cancer of uterus, radium*

1950: Louis **Portes** died, **born** 1891. *caesarean section*

1950: Harold **Brunn** died, **born** 1874. *lung lobectomy*

1950: Walter Norman **Haworth** died, **born** 1883. *carbohydrates, vitamin C*

**1951**
1951:1 **Nobel Prize** (Physiology or Medicine): Max Theiler (1899–1972), for diagnosis of, and prophylaxis against, **yellow fever**, *NPL. 5463*

1951:2 **Heaf multipuncture tuberculin test** for **tuberculosis** introduced by Frederick Roland George Heaf (1894–1973), *L* **2**:151. *2352.1*

1951:3 **Cytosine arabinoside** used in therapy of acute **myeloblastic leukaemia** by Werner Bergmann and Robert J. Feeney, *JOC* **16**:981. *2660.3*

1951:4 Successful resection of an **abdominal aortic aneurysm** and insertion of a homologous graft by Charles Dubost (b.1914) and co-workers, *MAC* **77**:381. *2993.1*

1951:5 **Aortic arterial homograft** performed for **thrombosis** by Jacques Oudot, *PrM* **59**:234. *3020.1*

1951:6 First workable **prosthetic heart valve** designed and inserted in man by Charles Anthony Hufnagel (1916–1989), *BGUMC* **4**:128. *3047.2*

1951:7 **Carbimazole**, an anti-**thyroid** drug, synthesized by Alexander Lawson and co-workers, *L* **2**:619. *3855.2*

1951:8 Clinical trials of slow-acting **insulin zinc** suspensions initiated by Knud Hallas-Møller (b.1914) and co-workers, *UL* **113**:1767. *3978*

1951:9 Artificial **bladder** constructed by Roger Couvelaire (1903–1986), *JUMC* **57**:408. *4203.1*

1951:10 An important account of the pathogenesis of acute **kidney failure** published by Jean Oliver (1889–1976) and co-workers, *JCI* **30**:1305. *4256.11*

1951:11 **Waardenburg's syndrome**, combining developmental anomalies of the eyelids and nose root with pigmentary defects of the iris and head hair and congenital deafness reported by Petrus Johannes Waardenburg (1886–1979), *AmJHG* **3**:195. *4154.4*

1951:12 The gradual development of excision of the **cerebral cortex** in the treatment of medically refractory focal **epilepsy** made by Wilder Graves Penfield (1891–1976); in his *Epilepsy and cerebral localization. 4910.1*

1951:13 **Pyrimethamine (daraprim)** first used in the treatment of **proguanil**-resistant **malaria** by Ian McIntosh Rollo (b.1926), *Nature* **168**:332. *5262.5*

1951:14 **Cat-scratch fever** first described by William Edward R. Greer (b.1918) and Chester Scott Keefer (1897–1972), *NEJM* **244**:545. *5546.2*

1951:15 **Succinylcholine chloride** first clinically used as a muscle relaxant in **anaesthesia** by H. Brücke and co-workers, *WKW* **63**:464. *5729*

1951:16 The first intra-ocular acrylic **lens** implanted by Nicholas Harold Lloyd Ridley (b.1906), *TOUK* **71**:617. *5991*

1951:17 **Cephalosporins** isolated by Edward Penley Abraham (b.1913) amd H.S. Burton, *BJ* **50**:168. *1945.2*

---

1951: Ludvig **Hektoen** died, **born** 1863. *liver cirrhosis, antibody response, x rays*

1951: Philip **Franklin** died, **born** 1880. *hay fever, zinc*

1951: Ernst **Moro** died, **born** 1874. *tuberculosis, tuberculin, serum sickness, Lactobacillus acidophilus*

1951: Walter **Broadbent** died, **born** 1868. *adherent pericardium*

1951: Ludolph **Brauer** died, **born** 1865. *pneumothorax, pulmonary tuberculosis,*

1951: Ernst Ferdinand **Sauerbruch** died, **born** 1875. *pneumothorax, cardiac aneurysm, pulmonary tuberculosis, myasthenia gravis, phrenicotomy*

1951: George Lenthal **Cheatle** died, **born** 1865. *hernia*

1951: Serge **Voronoff** died, **born** 1866. *rejuvenation*

1951: Dallas B. **Phemister** died, **born** 1882. *epiphysiodesis to inhibit bone growth*

1951: Louis Arthur **Milkman** died, **born** 1895. *osteomalacia, calcium*

1951: Gaston **Cotte** died, **born** 1879. *presacral neurectomy*

1951: Charles **Donovan** died, **born** 1863. *leishmaniasis, Leishmania donovani*

1951: Alexandre Emile **Brumpt** died, **born** 1877. *Trypanosoma cruzi*

1951: Otto Fritz **Meyerhof** died, **born** 1884. *muscle chemistry, glucose*

1951: Henry Asbury **Christian** died, **born** 1876. *Hand-Schüller-Christian syndrome*

**1952**
1952:1 **Nobel Prize** (Physiology or Medicine). Selman Abraham Waksman (1888–1973), for the isolation of **streptomycin** and its use in the treatment of **tuberculosis**, *NPL. 1935*

1952:2 **Nobel Prize** (Chemistry): Archer John Porter Martin (b.1910) and Richard Laurence Millington Synge (1914–1994), for the invention of **partition chromatography**, *NPL.*

1952:3 Army Medical Library, Washington (formerly Library of the Surgeon General's Office), renamed **Armed Forces Medical Library**; later (1956) National Library of Medicine

1952:4 **Aldosterone** isolated by Hilary M. Grundy and colleagues, *Nature* **169**:795. *1155.1*

1952:5 **DNA** shown to be the carrier of **genetic** information in **virus** reproduction by Alfred Day Hershey (b.1908) and M.C. Chase, *JGP* **36**:39. *256*

1952:6 **Heart bypass apparatus** devised by Forest Dewey Dodrill (b.1902) and co-workers, *JTS* **24**:134. *859.1*

1952:7 **Cortisone** synthesized by Robert Burns Woodward (1917–1979) and co-workers, *JACS* **74**:4423. *1155.2*

1952:8 *The Medical Department of the United States Army in World War II*, commenced publication. *2180.1*

1952:9 **British medical services in the Second World War** recorded in *History of the Second World War. Medical series*, 13 vols, 1952–62. *2180*

1952:10 **Erythromycin** discovered by James Myrlin McGuire (b.1909), *AC* **2**:281. *1946*

1952:11 **Isoniazid** introduced in treatment of **tuberculosis** by Edward Heinrich Robitzek (1912–1984) and colleagues, *QSVH* **13**:27. *2353*

1952:12 **Agammaglobulinaemia** first reported by Ogden Carr Bruton (b.1908), *Ped* **9**:722. *2578.9*

1952:13 **Leuco-agglutinins** discovered by Jean Dausset (b.1916) and André Nenna, *CRSB* **146**:1539. *2578.10*

1952:14 **Reserpine** isolated by J.M. Müller, *Ex* **8**:338. *1931*

1952:15 External **cardiac pacemaker** in treatment of **ventricular standstill** introduced by Paul Maurice Zoll (b.1911), *NEJM* **247**:768. *2883*

1952:16 **Lymphangiography** introduced by John Bernard Kinmonth (1916–1982), *CS* **11**:13. *2700.1*

1952:17 **Haemophilia B (Christmas disease)**, due to lack of **Factor IX**, reported by Rosemary Peyton Biggs and co-workers, *BMJ* **2**:1378. *3108.1*

1952:18 Trials of prophylaxis of **poliomyelitis** by **gamma globulin** carried out by William McDowell Hammon (b.1904) and co-workers, *JAMA* **150**:739. *4672*

1952:19 Successful **immunization** against **poliomyelitis** with a living attenuated virus achieved by Hilary Koprowski (b.1916) and co-workers, *AmJH* **55**:108. *4672.1*

1952:20 **Chlorpromazine** introduced in the treatment of **psychosis** by Jean Delay (b.1907) and Pierre Deniker; in *C.R. Congr. Alien. et Neurol. de Langue Franç. 4962.3*

1952:21 A **saliva test** for prenatal **sex determination** introduced by Gustav William Rapp (b.1917) and Garwood Colvin Richardson (b.1897), *Science* **115**:265. *6235*

1952:22 6- **Mercaptopurine** synthesized by Gertrude Belle Elion (b.1918), George H. Hitchings (b.1905), and E. Burgi, *JACS* **74**:411.

---

1952:23 Mordehai **Ber** died; with Saul Adler, proved that *Leishmania tropica*, causal organism of cutaneous leishmaniasis, is transmitted by the bite of *Phlebotomus papatasii*, 1941, *IJMR* **29**:803. *5301.2*

1952: Sydney William **Cole** died, **born** 1877. *tryptophan*

1952: Charles Scott **Sherrington** died, **born** 1857. *nervous system, muscle innervation, proprioceptive system, stretch reflex*

1952: Karl Franz **Nagelschmidt** died, **born** 1875. *diathermy*

1952: Henry Drysdale **Dakin** died, **born** 1880. *wound irrigation, chloramine-T*

1952: Richard **Otto** died, **born** 1872. *anaphylaxis*

1952: Leonard Erskine **Hill** died, **born** 1866. *sphygmomanometer*

1952: William Ewart **Gye** died, **born** 1884. *cancer, viruses*

1952: Frank Norman **Wilson** died, **born** 1890. *electrocardiography*

1952: Nikolai Dmitrievich **Strazhesko** died, **born** 1876. *coronary thrombosis*

1952: Henry Peter George **Bayon** died, **born** 1876. *cancer, tar*

1952: Max **Lederer** died, **born** 1885. *haemolytic anaemia*

1952: Douglas **Symmers** died, **born** 1879. *follicular lymphadenopathy*

1952: Elizabeth **Kenny** died, **born** 1886. *infantile paralysis, cerebral diplegia*

1952: Norman Beechey **Gwyn** died, **born** 1875. *Salmonella paratyphi A*

1952: George Walter **McCoy** died, **born** 1876. *tularaemia, Pasteurella tularensis*

1952: Ernest Linwood **Walker** died, **born** 1870. *amoebiasis, Entamoeba*

1952: George Carmichael **Low** died, **born** 1872. *transmission of filarial infection*

1952: Russell Morse **Wilder** died, **born** 1885. *Rocky Mountain spotted fever, typhus*

1952: Edward Bright **Vedder** died, **born** 1878. *amoebiasis, emetine*

1952: Robert **Doerr** died, **born** 1871. *Phlebotomus fever*

1952: Hugh William Bell **Cairns** died, **born** 1896. *Menière's syndrome*

1952: Frank Cecil **Eve** died, **born** 1871. *artificial respiration*

1952: Maria **Montessori** died, **born** 1870. *education system*

## 1953

1953:1 **Nobel Prize** (Physiology or Medicine): Hans Adolf Krebs (1900–1981), for his discovery of the **citric acid cycle** of aerobic **carbohydrate metabolism**, *NPL. 751.1*; Fritz Albert Lipmann (1899–1986), for the discovery of **co-enzyme A**, *NPL. 751.3*

1953:2 **Nobel Prize** (Physics): Frits Zernike (1888–1966), for his invention of **phase contrast microscopy**, *NPL. 269.5*

1953:3 **DNA molecular structure** determined by James Dewey Watson (b.1928) and Francis Harry Compton Crick (b.1916), *Nature* **171**:737. *256.3*

1953:4 The helical structure of DNA discovered by Maurice Hugh Frederick Wilkins (b.1916) and co-workers, *Nature* **172**:759. *256.4*

1953:5 **Oxytocin** synthesized by Vincent du Vigneaud (1901–1978) et al., *JACS* **75**:4879. *1175.3*

1953:6 **Adenoviruses** discovered by Wallace Prescott Rowe (b.1926) et al., *PSEB* **84**:570 *2526.2*

1953:7 **Immunoelectrophoresis** introduced by Pierre Grabar (1898–1986) and Curtis A. Williams, *BBA* **10**:193. *2578.13*

1953:8 **Acquired immunological tolerance**; proof of Burnet-Fenner theory (1949) by Rupert Everett Billingham (b.1921), Peter Brian Medawar (1915–1987), Leslie Brent (b.1925) and E.M. Sparrow, *Nature* **172**:603. *2578.11*

1953:9 **Chlorpromazine** introduced by S. Courvoisier and co-workers, *ArPha* **92**:305. *1931.1*

1953:10 **Nitrogen mustard (chlorambucil)** used in chemotherapy of **cancer** by James Lionel Everett and co-workers, *JCS* 2386. *2660.4*

1953:11 **TEPA (triethylenephosphoramide)** used in the treatment of **cancer** by Sidney Farber (1903–1973) and co-workers, *Cancer* **6**:135. *2660.5*

1953:12 Experimental oral **contraception**, using **progesterone** and related compounds, demonstrated by Gregory Goodwin Pincus (1903–1967) and Min Chueh Chang (b.1908), *AcPL* **3**:177. *1931.2*

1953:13 **Percutaneous arterial catheterization** introduced by Sven Ivar Seldinger, *AcR* **39**:368. *2924.2*

1953:14 Treatment of **leukaemia** with **6-mercaptopurine** introduced by Joseph Holland Burchenal (b.1912), *Blood* **8**:965. *3108.3*

1953:15 Treatment of chronic **myeloid leukaemia** with **myleran** introduced by Alexander Haddow (1907–1976) and Geoffrey Milward Timmis, *L* **1**:207. *3108.4*

1953:16 Electrically-induced **osteogenesis** first demonstrated by Iwao Yasuda (b.1909), *JKMS* **4**:395. *4435.4*

1953:17 **Immunization** against **poliomyelitis** with a killed-virus **vaccine** carried out by Jonas Salk (1914–1995) and co-workers, *JAMA* **151**:1081. *4672.2*

1953:18 The **varicella-herpes** virus first isolated by Thomas Huckle Weller (b.1915), *PSEB* **83**:340. *5440.1*

1953:19 **Fluroxene**, the first fluorine-containing **anaesthetic**, introduced by John Christian Krantz (b.1899) and co-workers, *JPET* **108**:488. *5729.1*

---

1953: Max **Einhorn** died, **born** 1862. *achylia gastrica, gastrodiaphany*

1953: Samuel Short **Whillis** died, **born** 1870. *tonsillectomy*

1953: Jörgen Nilsen **Schaumann** died, **born** 1879. *sarcoidosis*

1953: Christian Frederik **Heerfordt** died, **born** 1872. *sarcoidosis*

1953: Marius Nygaard **Smith-Petersen** died, **born** 1886. *hip-joint, vitallium cup arthroplasty, fractures of femur*

1953: Robert **Kienböck** died, **born** 1871. *progressive osteonecrosis, spinal cord cavity formation, bone atrophy*

1953: Constantin **Levaditi** died, **born** 1874. *poliomyelitis, gonococcal infection, sulphanilamide, syphilis, bismuth*

1953: Walter Meredith **Boothby** died, **born** 1880. *anaesthesia, nitrous oxide/oxygen, oxygen inhalation mask*

1953: Frederick **Edridge-Green** died, **born** 1863. *colour-blindness*

1953: Thomas Stephen **Cullen** died, **born** 1868 *ectopic pregnancy, hyperplasia of endometrium*

1953: Howard Carman **Moloy** died, **born** 1903. *pelvis*

1953: Maxime Paul Marie **Laignel-Lavastine** died, **born** 1875. *history of medicine*

1953: Alfred **Fröhlich** died, **born** 1871. *Fröhlich's syndrome*

**1954**
1954:1 **Nobel Prize** (Physiology or Medicine): John Franklin Enders (1897–1985), Frederick Chapman Robbins (b.1916), and Thomas Huckle Weller (b.1915), for evolving a method of growing the **poliomyelitis** virus that removed the final obstacle to **vaccine** production, *NPL. 4671.1*

1954:2 **Nobel Prize** (Chemistry): Linus Carl Pauling (1901–1994), for research on the **chemical bond** and its application to the elucidation of the structure of complex substances, *NPL. 3154.1*

1954:3 **Vasopressin** synthesized by Vincent du Vigneaud (1901–1978) et al., *JACS* 76:4751. *1175.4*

1954:4 **Passive transfer of immunity** carried out by Nicholas Avrion Mitchison (b.1928), *PRSB* 142:72. *2578.15*

1954:5 **Complement fixation** technique introduced by Manfred Martin Mayer (1916–1984) and Lawrence Levine (b.1924), *JI* 72:511. *2578.14*

1954:6 **Echocardiography** introduced by Inge Edler (b.1911) and Carl Hellmuth Hertz (b.1920), *Kongliga Fysiografiska Sällskapets i Lun Förhandlingar,* 24:1. *2883.01*

1954:7 **Synchrotron** introduced by Edwin Mattison McMillan (b.1907), *PsR* 68:143. *2659.4*

1954:8 **Nitrogen mustard (melphalan)** introduced by Franz Bergel (b.1900) and J.A. Stock, *JCS* 2409; it was later used in the chemotherapy of **cancer**. *2660.7*

1954:9 First use on humans of mechanical **heart-lung machine (pump-oxygenator)** by John Heysham Gibbon (1903–1973), *MinnM* 37:171, 185. *3047.5*

1954: 10 A flexible **fibrescope**, using static scanning, introduced by Harold Horace Hopkins (b.1918) and N.S. Kapany, *Nature* **173**:39. *3558.1*

1954: 11 **Maple syrup urine disease**, an inherited metabolic disorder, described by John H. Menkes (b.1928) and co-workers, *Ped* **14**:462. *3924.3*

1954: 12 **Nephrotomography** introduced by John Arthur Evans (b.1909) and co-workers, *AmJR* **71**:213. *4256.2*

1954: 13 **Meprobamate** introduced by Frank Milan Berger (b.1913), *JPET* **112**:413, and later used in the treatment of **anxiety**. *4962.4*

1954: 14 **Measles** virus isolated by John Franklin Enders (1897–1985) and Thomas C. Peebles. (b.1921), *PSEB* **86**:277. *5449.2*

1954: 15 Fundamental research on physiology of **muscular contraction** reported by Andrew Fielding Huxley (b.1917) and R. Niedergerke, *Nature* **173**:971; 1958, *JP* **144**:403.

---

1954: Luis **Agote** died, **born** 1868. *blood transfusion*

1954: Franz **Hamburger** died, **born** 1874. *serum sickness*

1954: Auguste **Rollier** died, **born** 1874. *heliotherapy, tuberculosis*

1954: Maud **Slye** died, **born** 1879. *cancer, heredity*

1954: Jacob Jesse **Singer** died, **born** 1885. *pneumonectomy, carcinoma of bronchus*

1954: Alfred Purvis **Hart** died, **born** 1887. *icterus gravis neonatorum*

1954: James Bryan **Herrick** died, **born** 1861. *sickle-cell anaemia*

1954: Gunnar **Holmgren** died, **born** 1875. *otosclerosis, fenestration*

1954: Jacques **Calvé** died, **born** 1875. *osteochondritis deformans*

1954: Simeon Burt **Wolbach** died, **born** 1880. *typhus, Rickettsia rickettsii*

1954: William James **Wilson** died, **born** 1879. *cerebrospinal fever, typhus fever*

1954: James Stevens **Simmons** died, **born** 1890. *dengue, mosquito*

1954: Helmut **Weese** died, **born** 1897. *anaesthesia, hexobarbitone*

## 1955

1955: 1 **Nobel Prize** (Physiology or Medicine): Axel Hugo Teodor Theorell (1903–1982), for his discoveries relating to the nature and mode of action of **oxidising enzymes**, *NPL.* *752.5*

1955: 2 **Nobel Prize** (Chemistry): Vincent du Vigneaud (1901–1978), for his work in the synthesis of **oxytocin** and other posterior **pituitary hormones**, *NPL.* *1175.3*

634

1955:3 Synthesis of **nucleic acids** by Marianne Grunberg-Manago and Severo Ochoa (b.1905), *JACS* **77**:3165. *752.3*

1955:4 A live attenuated **poliomyelitis virus vaccine** produced by Albert Bruce Sabin (b.1906), *ANYAS* **61**:924. *4672.3*

1955:5 **Amphotericins A and B** isolated from a streptomycete by W. Gold et al., *AA*: 579 *1947.2*

1955:6 Molecular separation of **antibodies** by Rodney Robert Porter (1917–1985), *BJ* **59**:405. *2578.16*

1955:7 **Tobacco mosaic virus** reconstituted by Heinz Ludwig Fraenkel-Conrat (b.1910) and Robley Cook Williams (b.1908), *PNAS* **41**:690. *2527*

1955:8 First crystallization of an animal **virus**, **poliomyelitis**, by Frederick Leland Schaffer (b.1921) and Carlton Everett Schwerdt (b.1917), *PNAS* **41**:1020. *2527.1*

1955:9 Diagnostic test for **myocardial infarction** introduced by John Samuel LaDue (1911–1980) and Felix Wroblewski (b.1921), *Cir* **11**:871. *2883.1*

1955:10 Resection of an **aortic** arch for **aneurysm** and replacement by a polyvinyl sponge prosthesis by Denton Arthur Cooley (b.1920), D.E. Mahaffey and M.E. DeBakey, *SGO* **101**:667. *2993.2*

1955:11 Chronic **lymphatic leukaemia** treated with **chlorambucil** by David Abraham Goiten Galton, *L* **2**:1172. *3108.6*

1955:12 The **Zollinger-Ellison syndrome** described by Robert Milton Zollinger (b.1903) and Edwin Homer Ellison (b.1918), *AnS* **142**:709. *3558.2*

1955:13 Primary **aldosteronism** ('**Conn's syndrome**') first recorded by Jerome W. Conn (b.1907), *JLCM* **45**:661. *3877.1*

1955:14 **Carbutamide**, the first **sulphonylurea**, introduced in the treatment of **diabetes mellitus** by Hans Franke (1909–1955) and J. Fuchs, *DMW* **80**:1449. *3978.1*

1955:15 Auxiliary whole **liver transplantation** in dogs carried out by Charles Stuart Welch (b.1909), *TrB* **6**:103. *3666.1*

1955: Per Gustav **Bergman** died, **born** 1874. *renin*

1955: Carl Richard **Moore** died, **born** 1892. *androsterone*

1955: Holger **Nielsen** died, **born** 1866. *artificial respiration*

1955: Alexander **Fleming** died, **born** 1881. *penicillin, lysozyme*

1955: Arthur Lawrie **Tatum** died, **born** 1884. *mapharsen, syphilis*

1955: Oswald Theodore **Avery** died, **born** 1877. *antigenic structure of pneumococcus, deoxyribonucleic acid (DNA) and genetic transformation*

1955: Hermann **Vollmer** died, **born** 1896. *tuberculosis, tuberculin*

1955: Wolfgang **Pauli** died, **born** 1869. *hypertension, thiocyanates*

1955: Hans **Finsterer** died, **born** 1877. *gastro-enterostomy*

1955: Samuel James **Crowe** died, **born** 1883. *hypophysectomy, genital atrophy*

1955: Edward **Mellanby** died, **born** 1884. *rickets*

1955: Hans **Franke** died, **born** 1909. *diabetes mellitus, carbutamide*

1955: Henri **Gougerot** died, **born** 1881. *sporotrichosis*

1955: Friedrich **Voelcker** died, **born** 1872. *cystogram, pyelography, kidney function test*

1955: Charles James **Martin** died, **born** 1866. *plague, flea*

1955: George Ford **Petrie** died, **born** 1938. *typhoid antiserum*

1955: René **Leriche** died, **born** 1879. *abdominal aorta, arterial thrombosis, arteriectomy, lumbar sympathectomy, causalgia*

1955: Antonio Caetano de Abreu Freire **Egas Moniz** died, **born** 1874. *cerebral and carotid arteriography, prefrontal lobotomy, psychoses*

1955: Maurice **Favre** died, **born** 1876. *lymphogranuloma venereum*

1955: John Brian **Christopherson** died, **born** 1868. *schistosomiasis, tartar emetic*

1955: John **Homans** died, **born** 1877. *hypophysectomy, genital atrophy*

1955: Allan **Kinghorn** died, **born** 1880. *Trypanosoma rhodesiense, tsetse fly*

1955: Vilray Papin **Blair** died, **born** 1871. *skin grafts, maxillofacial surgery, micrognathia, prognathism*

1955: Albert **Botteri** died, **born** 1879. *conjunctivitis*

1955: Charles **Hunter** died, **born** 1872. *lipochondrodystrophy, gargoylism*

1955: James Batcheller **Sumner** died, **born** 1887. *enzymes, urease*

1955: Donald Breadalbane **Blacklock** died, **born** 1879. *onchocerciasis, Simulium damnosum*

1955: Arthur **Keith** died, **born** 1866. *sino-auricular node (pacemaker of the heart)*

**1956**

1956:1 **Nobel Prize** (Physiology or Medicine): Werner Theodor Otto Forssmann (1904–1979), for his work on **cardiac catheterization**, *NPL. 2858*; André Frédéric Cournand (1895–1988) and Dickinson W. Richards (1895–1973), for investigations with the **cardiac catheter** as a clinical method of investigation, *NPL. 2871*

1956:2 **National Library of Medicine**, Bethesda, Maryland, founded; formerly Library of the Surgeon General's Office (1836), Army Medical Library (1922), Armed Forces Medical Library (1952)

1956:3 Enzymatic synthesis of **DNA** by Arthur Kornberg (b.1918) and co-workers, *BBA* **21**:197. *752.4*

1956:4 **Chromosome** number in man shown by J.H. Tjio (b.1919) and Albert Johan Levan (b.1905) to be 46, *Her* **42**:1. *256.5*

1956:5 **Mitomycin** C isolated by Toju Hata et al., *JAnt* **A9**:141. *1947.3*

1956:6 **Cytomegalovirus** isolated from salivary gland virus disease by Margaret G. Smith, *PSEB* **92**:424. *2527.2*

1956:7 **Autoantibodies** demonstrated by Ivan Maurice Roitt (b.1927) and co-workers, *L* **2**:820. *2578.19*

1956:8 **Diphenylthiourea (thiambutosine)** introduced in treatment of **leprosy** by Thomas Frank Davey (1907–1983) and G. Currie, *LR* **27**:94. *2442.2*

1956:9 Introduction of **bubble oxygenator** in **heart surgery** by Richard A. DeWall (b.1926) and co-workers, *SCNA* **36**:1025. *3047.9*

1956:10 First successful **aortic valve homograft** by Donald Walter Gordon Murray (1894–1974), *Angiology* **7**:466. *3047.8*

1956:11 **Autoimmune thyroiditis** produced experimentally by Ernest Witebsky (1901–1969) and Noel Richard Rose (b.1927), *JI* **76**:408. *3855.3*

1956:12 A disposable twin coil **artificial kidney** introduced by Willem Johan Kolff (b.1911) and B. Watschinger, *JLCM* **47**:969. *4257.1*

1956:13 Successful **kidney transplant**, between identical twins, reported by John Putnam Merrill (1917–1986) and co-workers, *JAMA* **160**:277. *4257*

1956:14 **Halothane (fluothane)**, an **anaesthetic**, synthesized by J. Raventós. *BJP* **11**:394, and first used clinically by Michael William Johnstone, *BJA* **28**:392. *5729.3, 5729.2*

---

1956: Ervin Sidney **Ferry** died, **born** 1868. *Ferry-Porter law*

1956: Lionel Ernest Howard **Whitby** died, **born** 1895. *sulphapyridine*

1956: Knud Helge **Faber** died, **born** 1862. *achlorhydric anaemia*

1956: Percy William Leopold **Camps** died, **born** 1877. *asthma, adrenaline*

1956: Julius Leo **Spivack** died, **born** 1889. *gastrostomy*

1956: Robert Bayley **Osgood** died, **born** 1873. *tibial tuberosity lesions*

1956: Arthur **Felix** died, **born** 1887. *typhoid bacillus, Vi antigen, typhoid antiserum*

1956: Henrique de **Rocha Lima** died, **born** 1879. *typhus, Rickettsia prowazeki*

1956: Harold **King** died, **born** 1887. *anaesthesia, tubocurarine*

1956: Arnold Hermann **Knapp** died, **born** 1869. *cataract*

1956: Bernard Minge **Duggar** died, **born** 1872. *aureomycin*

1956: Vladimir Petrovich **Filatov** died, **born** 1875. *tubed pedicle flap in surgery, corneal transplantation*

**1957**
1957:1 **Nobel Prize** (Physiology or Medicine): Daniel Bovet (1907–1992), for the discovery of the antibacterial properties of **sulphanilamide**, *NPL. 1950*

1957:2 **Nobel Prize** (Chemistry): Alexander Robertus Todd (b.1907), for his work on **nucleotides** and **nucleotide co-enzymes**, *NPL.*

1957:3 **Catheterization** of the right **heart** investigated by Dickinson Woodruff Richards (1895–1973), *AmHJ* **54**:161. *2883.2*

1957:4 **Kanamycin** isolated by Hamao Umezawa et al., *JAnt* **A10**:181. *1947.4*

1957:5 **Clonal selection** theory of **acquired immunity** proposed by Frank Macfarlane Burnet (1899–1985); in his *Clonal selection theory of acquired immunity. 2578.31*

1957:6 **Interferon** discovered by Alick Isaacs (1921–1967) and Jean Lindenmann (b.1924), *PRSB* **147**:258. *2578.22*

1957:7 **Syphilis: fluorescent treponemal antibody test** introduced by William Eugene Deacon (b.1907) et al., *PSEB* **96**:477. *2419.2*

1957:8 **Leucocyte typing** introduced by Rose Marise Payne (b.1909), *ArIM* **99**:587. *2578.23*

1957:9 **Ultrasonic** investigation (**tomogram**) of soft tissue by John Julian Wild (b.1911) and J.M. Reid, Kelly, E.C. *Ultrasound*, p. 30. *2681*

1957:10 **Papovavirus** isolated by Sarah Elizabeth Stewart (b.1906) and co-workers, *Vir* **3**:380. *2660.10*

1957:11 **5-fluorouracil**, a **tumour**-inhibiting compound, synthesized by Charles Heidelberger (b.1920) and co-workers, *Nature* **179**:663. *2660.9*

638

1957:12 **Follicular mucinosis, alopecia mucinosa**, recorded by Hermann Pinkus (b.1905), *ArDS* **76**:419. *4154.5*

1957:13 **Phenformin, a hyperglycaemic biguanide**, introduced into the treatment of **diabetes** by Georges Ungar (b.1906) and co-workers, *PSEB* **95**:190. *3978.3*

1957:14 **Kuru**, a disease occurring in natives of New Guinea, first described by Daniel Carleton Gajdusek (b.1923) and V. Zigas, *NEJM* **257**:974. In 1971, with Gibbs, he transmitted kuru and **Creutzfeldt-Jakob disease** to primates. *4729.1, 4729.2*

1957:15 The **trachoma** agent, *Chlamydia trachomatis*, isolated by Fei Fan Chang and co-workers, *ChMJ* **75**:429. *5991.1*

1957: Gerty Theresa **Cori** died, born 1896. *glycogens*

1957: Arthur James **Ewins** died, **born** 1882. *acetylcholine*

1957: Jay **McLean** died, **born** 1890. *heparin*

1957: William Lorenzo **Moss** died, **born** 1876. *blood classification*

1957: John Friend **Mahoney** died, **born** 1889. *penicillin, syphilis*

1957: Evarts Ambrose **Graham** died, **born** 1883. *pneumonectomy, carcinoma of bronchus, cholecystography, lung cancer, smoking*

1957: Rudolph **Matas** died, **born** 1860. *aneurysmorrhaphy*

1957: Alfred Erich **Frank** died, **born** 1884. *pituitary, diabetes insipidus, thrombopenia*

1957: Felix **Mandl** died, **born** 1892. *parathyroid tumors, osteitis fibrosa generalisata*

1957: Thomas Peel **Dunhill** died, **born** 1876. *exophthalmic goitre, thyroid surgery*

1957: Willem Frederik **Donath** died, **born** 1889. *beriberi, vitamin B1*

1957: Lewis Madison **Terman** died, **born** 1877. *intelligence tests*

1957: Edward **Francis** died, **born** 1872. *tularaemia*

1957: Manfred Joshua **Sakel** died, **born** 1900. *schizophrenia, insulin shock therapy*

1957: Octave **Gengou** died, **born** 1875. *whooping cough, Bordetella pertussis, complement-fixation reaction*

1957: Kiyoshi **Shiga** died, **born** 1870. *bacillary dysentery, Shigella dysenteriae*

1957: Alberto **Ascoli** died, **born** 1877. *anthrax*

1957: John Henry Porteus **Graham** died, **born** ?1869. *trench fever*

1957: Frederick George **Novy** died, **born** 1864. *relapsing fever, spirochaete*

1957: Arno Benedict **Luckhardt** died, **born** 1885. *anaesthesia, ethylene*

1957: Carl Joseph **Gauss** died, **born** 1875. *labour pains, twilight sleep*

1957: Paul Theodor **Uhlenhuth** died, **born** 1870. *Salmonella paratyphi C, organ-specific antigens*

1957: Heinrich Otto **Wieland** died, **born** 1877. *bile acids*

## 1958

1958:1 **Nobel Prize** (Physiology or Medicine): George Wells Beadle (1903–1989), Joshua Lederberg (b.1925), and Edward Lawrie Tatum (1909–1975), for their researches on the mechanism by which the **chromosomes** in the **cell nucleus** transmit **inherited characters**, *NPL. 254.3, 255.4*

1958:2 **Nobel Prize** (Chemistry): Frederick Sanger (b.1918) for work on the structure of **proteins**, especially **insulin**, *NPL. 1207*

1958:3 **Histocompatibility genes** (genes governing transplantation) so named by George Davis Snell (1903–1996), *JNCI* 20:787. *2578.30*

1958:4 **Homograft reaction** in **transplantation** (delayed sensitivity reaction) demonstrated by Peter Brian Medawar (1915–1987), *PRSB* 149:145. *2578.24*

1958:5 **Histocompatibility antigen** discovered by Jean Dausset (b.1916), *AcHa* 20:156. *2578.26*

1958:6 **Ultrasonic** investigation of **pregnant uterus** by Ian Donald (1910–1987) and co-workers, *L* 1:1188. *2682*

1958:7 '**Burkitt's tumour**' (African **lymphoma**) described by Denis Parsons Burkitt (1911–1993), *BJS* 46:218. *2660.12*

1958:8 **Cyclophosphamide** introduced in the chemotherapy of **cancer** by Herbert Arnold and co-workers, *Nw* 45:64. *2660.11*

1958:9 Dacron **arterial prosthesis** introduced by Desiderius Emerick Szilagyi (b.1910) and co-workers, *ArSu* 77:538. *3047.12*

1958:10 **Stapedectomy** introduced by John Joseph Shea (b.1924), *AnOt* 67:932. *3412.7*

1958:11 A new **fibrescope** introduced by Basil I. Hirschcowitz, *Gast* 35:50. *3558.3*

1958:12 **Griseofulvin** introduced in the treatment of **tinea (ringworm)** by James Clark Gentles, *Nature* 182:476. *4011.1*

1958:13 The *Culex* **mosquito** reported as vector of **St Louis encephalitis virus** by Leslie Leon Lumsden (1875–1946), *USPHR* 73:340 [original unpublished report was in 1933]. *4661.2*

1958:14 **Measles** virus propagated in cultures of chick embryo cells by Samuel Lawrence Katz (b.1927), M. Milovanovič and John Franklin Enders (1897–1985), *PSEB* **97**:23. *5449.3*

1958:15 *System of ophthalmology*, 19 vols, 1958–1976, edited by William Stewart Duke-Elder (1898–1978).

1958:16 Chemical **synthesis** of **deoxyribonucleotides** reported by Har Gobind Khorana (b.1922), *JACS* **80**:6212. *752.6*

1958: Albert Frank Stanley **Kent** died, **born** 1863. *atrioventricular bundle*

1958: Marie **Stopes** died, **born** 1880. *birth control*

1958: Arthur **Laewen** died, **born** 1876. *angina pectoris, novocaine*

1958: Ernest Lawrence **Kennaway** died, **born** 1881. *carcinogens, dibenzanthracene*

1958: Chevalier **Jackson** died, **born** 1865. *endothelioma of bronchus, bronchoscopy*

1958: Paul **Sainton** died, **born** 1868. *cleidocranial dysostosis*

1958: William Jason **Mixter** died, **born** 1880. *sciatica*

1958: Rupert **Waterhouse** died, **born** 1873. *adrenal apoplexy*

1958: John Broadus **Watson** died, **born** 1878. *behaviourist psychology*

1958: John F. **Anderson** died, **born** 1873. *measles*

1958: Isador Clinton **Rubin** died, **born** 1883. *salpingography, sterility*

1958: Artur **Schüller** died, **born** 1874. *Hand-Schüller-Christian syndrome*

1958: Ludwig **Adler** died, **born** 1876. *cyclic changes in endometrium*

**1959**
1959:1 **Nobel Prize** (Physiology or Medicine): Severo Ochoa (b.1905) and Arthur Kornberg (b.1918) for their artificial synthesis of **nucleic acids** by means of **enzymes**, *NPL. 752.3, 752.4*

1959:2 **Ditophal (Etisul)** introduced in treatment of **leprosy** by Thomas Frank Davey (1907–1983) and L. Hogerzeil, *LR* **30**:61. *2442.3*

1959:3 **Ethionamide** introduced in treatment of **tuberculosis** by Noel Rist and co-workers, *AMRT* **79**:1. *2353.2*

1959:4 **Ventricular aneurysm** treated by **excision** and **cardiopulmonary bypass** by Denton Arthur Cooley (b.1920) and co-workers, *AnS* **150**:595. *3047.13*

1959:5 **Liver transplantation** in dogs following total hepatectomy carried out by Francis Daniels Moore (b.1913) and co-workers, *TrB* **6**:103. *3666.2*

1959: 6 **Trisomy-21**, the cause of **Down's syndrome**, discovered by Jerome Lejeune (b.1926) and co-workers, *CRAS* **248**:1721. *4962.5*

---

1959: Abraham **Flexner** died, **born** 1866. *medical education*

1959: Leo **Loeb** died, **born** 1869. *thyroid-stimulating hormone*

1959: Oskar **Vogt** died, **born** 1870. *corpora striata disease*

1959: Adolf Otto Reinhold **Windaus** died, **born** 1876. *histamine, sterols, vitamins*

1959: Erich **Hoffmann** died, **born** 1868. *syphilis, Treponema pallidum*

1959: Francis Henry Laskey **Taylor** died, **born** 1900. *antihaemophilic globulin (Factor VIII)*

1959: Porter Paisley **Vinson** died, **born** 1890. *cardiospasm, oesophageal dilatation*

1959: William Edward **Gallie** died, **born** 1882. *inguinal hernia*

1959: Irene Rosetta **Ewing** died, **born** 1883. *hearing tests*

1959: Hsien **Wu** died, **born** 1895. *blood sugar test*

1959: Cornelius Packard **Rhoads** died, **born** 1898. *Hodgkin's disease, triethylene melamine*

1959: Leonard George **Rowntree** died, **born** 1883. *kidney function test, bronchoscopy, lipiodol*

1959: Jean René **Cruchet** died, **born** 1875. *encephalitis*

1959: Allan Coats **Rankin** died, **born** 1877. *trench fever*

1959: Louise **Pearce** died, **born** 1885. *trypanosomiasis, tryparsamide*

1959: Grace Mary **Sickles** died, **born** 1898. *Coxsackie virus*

1959: Grantly **Dick-Read** died, **born** 1890. *natural childbirth*

1959: Robert **Schroeder** died, **born** 1884. *metropathia haemorrhagica*

## 1960

1960: 1 **Nobel Prize** (Physiology or Medicine): Frank Macfarlane Burnet (1899–1985) and Peter Brian Medawar (1915–1987), for their discovery of acquired **immunological tolerance**, *NPL. 2578.7, 2578.11, 2578.12*

1960: 2 **Salk Institute for Biological Studies** opened in **California**

1960: 3 **Radioimmunoassay** of a **hormone (insulin)** carried out by Rosalyn Sussman Yalow (b.1921) and Solomon A. Berson (1918–1972), *JCI* **39**:1157. *2578.28*

1960: 4 **Leprosy** transmitted experimentally to animals by Charles Carter Shepard (1914–1985), *AmJH* **71**:147. *2442.4*

1960:5 Psychosedative, **librium**, introduced by Lowell Orlando Randall (b.1910) and co-workers, *JPET* **129**:163. *1931.3*

1960:6 First fully-implantable **pacemaker** for **heart block** introduced by William M. Chardack, *Surgery* **48**:643. *3047.15*

1960:7 Shielded ball-valve prosthesis for **mitral valve replacement** introduced by Albert Starr (b.1926) and M. Lowell Edwards, *JTCS* **42**:673; the first mitral valve replacement in a human. *3047.16*

1960:8 **Heart transplantation** in dogs, ('**Shumway technique**'), carried out by Richard Rowland Lower (b.1929) and Norman E. Shumway (b.1923), *SF* **11**:18. *3047.14*

1960:9 An important improvement in **haemodialysis** made by W.E. Quinton and co-workers by the development of indwelling Teflon-Silastic **arteriovenous shunts**, *TASAO* **6**:104. *4257.2*

1960:10 A live virus vaccine against **measles** prepared by John Franklin Enders (1897–1985), Samuel Lawrence Katz (b.1927), M. Milovanovič and A. Holloway, *NEJM* **263**:153. *5449.4*

1960:11 First report of **amniocentesis** for the diagnosis *in utero* of **genetic disorders** by Poul Riis and Fritz Fuchs, *L* **2**:180. *6235.2*

---

1960: Robert **Hutchison** died, **born** 1871. *thyroglobulin, adrenal sarcoma*

1960: Robert Anderson **Cooke** died, **born** 1880. *atopy*

1960: Jules Thomas **Freund** died, **born** 1890. *adjuvants, antigens*

1960: Albert Markley **Snell** died, **born** 1896. *haemorrhagic disease, vitamin K*

1960: Carl **Voegtlin** died, **born** 1870. *parathyroid glands, calcium metabolism*

1960: Earl Dorland **Osborne** died, **born** 1895. *ureteropyelography, sodium iodide*

1960: Holger Werfel **Scheuermann** died, **born** 1877. *kyphosis, epiphyseal necrosis*

1960: Gordon **Gordon-Taylor** died, **born** 1878. *hind-quarter amputation*

1960: Robert **McCarrison** died, **born** 1878. *bladder calculi, vitamin A*

1960: William Palmer **Lucas** died, **born** 1880. *poliomyelitis*

1960: Lee **Foshay** died, **born** 1896. *tularaemia, streptomycin*

1960: Joseph **Nicolas** died, **born** 1868. *lymphogranuloma venereum*

1960: Frederick Creighton **Wellman** died, **born** 1871. *yaws, Treponema pertenue*

1960: Ernest William **Goodpasture** died, **born** 1886. *Histoplasma capsulatum*

1960: Harold Delf **Gillies** died, **born** 1882. *plastic surgery, tubed pedicle flap in surgery, cleft palate*

1960: William Edward Mandell **Wardill** died, **born** 1894. *cleft palate*

1960: Archibald Hector **McIndoe** died, **born** 1900. *skin homografts, artificial vagina*

1960: Walter **Schiller** died, **born** 1887. *carcinoma of cervix uteri*

## 1961

1961:1 **Nobel Prize** (Physiology or Medicine): Georg von Békésy (1899–1972), for his discoveries concerning the physical mechanism of stimulation within the **cochlea**, *NPL. 1570.1*

1961:2 **(Royal) College of General Practitioners, London,** founded (chartered 1972)

1961:3 **Public Health Laboratory Service (England and Wales)** established; originally set up in 1939 as the Emergency Public Health Laboratory Service (administered by the Medical Research Council)

1961:4 **Immunological** function of the **thymus** demonstrated by Jacques Albert Pierre Miller (b.1931), *L* 2:748. *2578.32*

1961:5 **Ethambutol** tried in treatment of **tuberculosis** by J.P. Thomas et al., *AmRRD* **83**:891. *2353.3*

1961:6 ***Blastomyces dermatitidis*** isolated from soil by James Fred Denton (b.1914) and co-workers, *Science* **133**:1126. *4154.7*

1961:7 Total **hip-joint replacement**, the **Charnley arthroplasty**, introduced by John Charnley (1911–1982), *L* **1**:1129. *4405.1*

1961:8 Biparietal **fetal cephalometry** by **ultrasound** first reported by Ian Donald (1910–1987) and T.G. Brown, *BJR* **34**:539. *6235.1*

1961:9 **DNAase**-sensitive **protein synthesis** reported by Marshall Warren Nirenberg (b.1927), *PNAS* **47**:1580. *256.11*

1961:10 **Genetic** mechanisms in **protein synthesis** reported by François Jacob (b.1920) and Jacques Lucien Monod (1910–1976), *JMB* **3**:318. *256.9*

---

1961: John Joseph **Bittner** died, **born** 1904. *milk factor in cancer transmission*

1961: Albert Garland **Hogan** died, **born** 1884. *folic acid*

1961: Thomas Renton **Elliott** died, **born** 1877. *chemical mediation of nerve impulses, adrenaline*

1961: Paul **Gelmo** died, **born** 1879. *sulphanilamide*

1961: Peter Alfred **Gorer** died, **born** 1907. *antigen II, transplantation immunology*

1961: Henry Patrick **Wagener** died, **born** 1890. *hypertension*

1961: Carl Gustav Vilhelm **Nylin** died, **born** 1892. *coarctation of aorta*

1961: David Israel **Macht** died, **born** 1882. *asthma, theophylline*

1961: Maurice **Sourdille** died, **born** 1885. *otosclerosis, fenestration*

1961: Chevalier L. **Jackson** died, **born** 1900. *foreign bodies in air and food passages*

1961: Otto **Loewi** died, **born** 1873. *chemical mediation of nerve impulses, pancreatic function test*

1961: John Preston **Maxwell** died, **born** 1871. *osteomalacia. vitamin D*

1961: James Frederick **Brailsford** died, **born** 1888. *osteochondrodystrophy*

1961: Tenji **Taniguchi** died, **born** 1896. *Japanese B encephalitis*

1961: Georges **Guillain** died, **born** 1876. *polyneuritis*

1961: Paul **Durand** died, **born** 1895. *Durand's disease*

1961: Théodore **Simon** died, **born** 1873. *intelligence tests*

1961: Jules Jean Baptiste Vincent **Bordet** died, **born** 1870. *whooping cough, Bordetella pertussis, complement-fixation reaction, antibody, complement, bacteriolysis, immune haemolysis*

1961: Carl Gustav **Jung** died, **born** 1875. *psychology*

1961: Carlos **Galli Mainini** died, **born** 1914. *pregnancy diagnosis*

1961: Geoffrey **Jefferson** died, **born** 1886. *embolectomy*

**1962**
1962:1 **Nobel Prize** (Physiology or Medicine): Maurice Hugh Frederick Wilkins (b.1916), Francis Harry Compton Crick (b.1916), and James Dewey Watson (b.1928), for their discovery of the structure of **DNA**, *NPL. 256.3, 256.4*

1962:2 **Nobel Prize** (Chemistry): Max Ferdinand Perutz (b.1914) and John Cowdery Kendrew (b.1917), for their studies on **globular proteins, haemoglobin, myoglobin**, *NPL.*

1962:3 **Royal College of Physicians and Surgeons of Glasgow** (formerly Faculty, 1599)

1962:4 **Lymphocyte** shown to be the **immunologically** competent cell by James Learmonth Gowans (b.1924), *Nature* 196:651. *2578.33*

1962:5 Chemical structure of **prostaglandins** elucidated by Sune Bergström (b.1916) and co-workers, *AcCS* **16**:501. *1931.4*

1962:6 **Coronary arteriography** performed by Frank Mason Sones and Earl K. Shirley (b.1924), *MCCD* **31**:735. *2924.3*

1962:7 The **rubella** virus isolated by Paul Douglas Parkman (b.1932) and co-workers, *PSEB* **111**:225, simultaneously with Thomas Huckle Weller (b.1915) and Franklin Allen Neva (b.1922). *PSEB* **111**:215. *5509.2, 5509.1*

---

1962: Ronald Aylmer **Fisher** died, **born** 1890. *biometric genetics*

1962: Barend Coenraad Petrus **Jansen** died, **born** 1884. *vitamins, beriberi*

1962: Richard **Lewisohn** died, **born** 1875. *blood transfusion*

1962: John Albert **Kolmer** died, **born** 1886. *syphilis*

1962: Paul **Portier** died, **born** 1866. *anaphylaxis*

1962: John **Freeman** died, **born** 1877. *hay fever, pollen*

1962: Manoel de **Abreu** died, **born** 1892. *chest radiography*

1962: Arnold Kirkpatrick **Henry** died, **born** 1886. *femoral hernia*

1962: Conrad Arnold **Elvehjem** died, **born** 1901. *pellagra, nicotinic acid*

1962: Frederick Parkes **Weber** died, **born** 1863. *telangiectasis, erythrokeratoma, naevus*

1962: Leonard **Rogers** died, **born** 1868. *leishmaniasis, kala-azar*

1962: William Sampson **Handley** died, **born** 1872. *breast cancer*

1962: George Nicholas **Papanicolaou** died, **born** 1883. *carcinoma of cervix, cervical smears*

1962: Erich **Tschermak von Seysenegg** died, **born** 1871. *genetics*

1962: Cécile **Vogt** died, **born** 1875. *corpora striata disease*

# 1963
1963:1 **Nobel Prize** (Physiology or Medicine): John Carew Eccles (b.1903), Alan Lloyd Hodgkin (b.1914), and Andrew Fielding Huxley (b.1917), for their discoveries concerning the ionic mechanisms involved in the excitation and inhibition in the peripheral and central portions of the **nerve cell membrane**, *NPL. 1310.1, 1310.2*

1963:2 **Gentamycin** isolated by Marvin Joseph Weinstein (b.1916), *JMC* **6**:463. *1947.5*

1963:3 **Idiotypy** of isolated **antibodies** discovered by Henry George Kunkel (1916–1963) and co-workers, *Science* **140**:405. *2578.35*

1963:4 Introduction of **balloon catheter embolectomy** by Thomas J. Fogarty and co-workers, *SGO* **116**:241. *3020.2*

1963:5 **Intrauterine blood transfusion** for **haemolytic disease** by Albert William Liley, *L* **2**:1107. *3108.7*

1963:6 Introduction of **vinblastine** in the treatment of **Hodgkin's disease** (and other **lymphomas**) and **vincristine** in **acute leukaemia of childhood** by Irving Stanley Johnson (b.1925) and co-workers, *CR* **23**:1390. *2660.16, 3788.2*

1963:7 A bacterial inhibition test for **phenylketonuria** devised by Robert Guthrie (b.1916) and Ada Susi, *Ped* **32**:338. *3924.4*

1963:8 The first **liver transplantation** in humans carried out by Thomas Earl Starzl (b.1926) and co-workers, *SGO* **117**:659. *3666.3*

1963:9 Henry Trendley **Dean** died; with co-workers, studied fluoridation of water supplies as a preventive against dental caries, 1950, *USPHR* **65**:1403. *3692.1*

1963: Otto Carl Willy **Prausnitz** died, **born** 1876. *antibodies, Prausnitz-Küstner reaction*

1963: Henry George **Kunkel** died, **born** 1916. *idiotypy of antibodies*

1963: Gustav **Bucky** died, **born** 1880. *radiography*

1963: Paul **Linser** died, **born** 1871. *varicose veins*

1963: Charles Claude **Guthrie** died, **born** 1880. *heart transplantation*

1963: Donald Church **Balfour** died, **born** 1882. *resection of sigmoid colon*

1963: Wilhelm Conrad **Rammstedt** died, **born** 1867. *pyloric stenosis*

1963: Allen Oldfather **Whipple** died, **born** 1881. *pancreatic cancer, pancreaticoduodenectomy*

1963: Joseph Seton **Barr** died, **born** 1901. *sciatica*

1963: André **Thomas** died, **born** 1867. *olivo-ponto-cerebellar atrophy*

1963: Gladys Rowena **Dick** died, **born** 1881. *scarlet fever. streptococcus*

1963: James Bourne **Ayer** died, **born** 1882. *cisternal puncture*

1963: Ugo **Cerletti** died, **born** 1877. *psychoses, electric convulsion therapy*

1963: Gaston Léon **Ramon** died, **born** 1886. *tetanus toxoid, immunization, diphtheria toxoid*

1963: Joseph Edwin **Smadel** died, **born** 1907. *typhus, chloramphenicol*

1963: Claude Walter **Levinthal** died, **born** 1886. *psittacosis, Chlamydia psittaci*

1963: William Kelsey **Fry** died, **born** 1889. *cleft palate*

1963: Alan Churchill **Woods** died, **born** 1889. *sympathetic ophthalmia*

1963: Hugh Leslie **Marriott** died, **born** 1900. *blood transfusion*

1963: David **Keilin** died, **born** 1887. *cytochrome*

1963: Herbert Spencer **Gasser** died, **born** 1888. *nerve impulse transmission and velocity*

1963: Shinobu **Ishihara** died, **born** 1879. *colour-blindness*

1963: Claude Gordon **Douglas** died, **born** 1882. *high altitude physiology*

### 1964

1964:1 **Nobel Prize** (Physiology or Medicine): Konrad Bloch (b.1912) and Feodor Lynen (b.1911), for researches on the mechanism and control of **cholesterol** and **fatty acid** metabolism, *NPL*.

1964:2 **Nobel Prize** (Chemistry): Dorothy Mary Crowfoot Hodgkin (1901–1994), for determining, by **x ray crystallography**, the structure of complex, biologically-important, organic molecules, including **insulin**, *NPL*.

1964:3 **Syphilis: absorbed fluorescent treponemal antibody (FTA-ABs) test** introduced by Elizabeth F. Hunter et al., *USPHR* **79**:410. *2419.3*

1964:4 **Epstein-Barr virus**, a human **herpesvirus** implicated in Burkitt's **lymphoma**, discovered by Michael Anthony Epstein (b.1921) and Y.M. Barr, *L* **1**:252, 272. *2660.17, 2660.18*

1964:5 **Propranolol** introduced by James Whyte Black (b.1924) and co-workers, *L* **1**:1080. *1931.5*

1964:6 **Percutaneous transluminal coronary arteriography** performed by C.T. Dotter and M.P. Judkins, *Cir* **30**:654. *2924.4*

1964:7 **Homograft** replacement of **aortic valve** by Donald Nixon Ross (b.1922), *L* **2**:487. *3047.17*

1964:8 Replacement of **aortic valve** with a subcoronary **homograft** for aortic incompetence and **stenosis** by Brian Gerald Barratt-Boyes (b.1924), *Thorax* **19**:131. *3047.18*

1964:9 Unsuccessful **heart transplant** from chimpanzee to man by James Daniel Hardy (b.1918) and co-workers, *JAMA* **188**:1132. *3047.19*

1964:10 The first successful reattachment of a **completely severed human limb** achieved by Ronald A. Malt (b.1931) and Charles Freemont McKhann (b.1930), *JAMA* **189**:716. *4405.3*

1964:11 **Niridazole (Ambilhar)** introduced in the treatment of **bilharziasis** by C.R. Lambert, *AnTM* **58**:292. *5351.6*

---

1964: John Burdon Sanderson **Haldane** died, **born** 1892. *genetics*

1964: Gerhard **Domagk** died, **born** 1895. *prontosil, sulphonamide, thiosemicarbazone, tuberculosis*

648

1964: Louis Hopewell **Bauer** died, **born** 1888. *aviation medicine*

1964: Paul **Klemperer** died, **born** 1887. *collagen disease*

1964: Everitt George Dunne **Murray** died, **born** 1890. *Listeria monocytogenes*

1964: Albert Compton **Broders** died, **born** 1885. *tumour classification*

1964: Lucy **Wills** died, **born** 1888. *anaemia, folic acid*

1964: José **Goyanes Capdevila** died, **born** 1876. *arterial blood flow, vein grafts*

1964: Alphonse Raymond **Dochez** died, **born** 1882. *pneumococcus*

1964: Henry Sessions **Souttar** died, **born** 1875. *mitral valvulotomy*

1964: Alfred **Blalock** died, **born** 1899. *pulmonary artery defects, shock, myasthenia gravis*

1964: Hans Gerhard **Creutzfeldt** died, **born** 1885. *spastic pseudosclerosis*

1964: Lucio **Bini** died, **born** 1908. *psychoses, electric convulsion therapy*

1964: Hollis Elmer **Potter** died, **born** 1888. *radiology*

1964: Peter Kosciusko **Olitsky** died, **born** 1886. *poliomyelitis virus*

**1965**
1965:1 **Nobel Prize** (Physiology or Medicine): François Jacob (b.1920), André Michael Lwoff (1902–1994), and Jacques Lucien Monod (1910–1976), for their work on the **genetic** control of **enzyme** and **virus** synthesis, *NPL. 256.9*

1965:2 **Nobel Prize** (Chemistry): Robert Burns Woodward (1917–1979), for contributions to the art of organic synthesis, including the synthesis of **cortisone**, *NPL. 1155.2*

1965:3 **Francis A. Countway Library** formed by amalgamation of Boston Medical Library (1875) and Harvard Medical Library (1783)

1965:4 **Hepatitis B antigen (Australia antigen)** discovered by Baruch Samuel Blumberg (b.1925), H.J. Alter and S. Visnich, *JAMA* 191:541. *3666.4*

1965:5 Sex-linked recessive **ichthyosis** shown to be an important entity by Robert Stuart Wells and Charles Baldwin Kerr, *ArDS* 92:1. *4154.8*

1965:6 **Stereotactic tractotomy** in the treatment of **mental illness** carried out by Geoffrey Cureton Knight (b.1906), *JNNP* 28:304. *4914.3*

1965:7 Complete sequence of **alanine transfer** RNA reported by Robert William Holley (b.1922), *Science* 147:1462. *257.2*

---

1965: Ladislaus Joseph **Meduna** died, **born** 1896. *schizophrenia, cardiazol convulsion therapy*

1965: Oliver **Kamm** died, **born** 1888. *oxytocin*

1965: Selmar **Aschheim** died, **born** 1878. *pregnancy diagnosis, growth hormone*

1965: John Henry **Gaddum** died, **born** 1900. *acetylcholine, substance P, neurotransmission*

1965: William Randolph **Lovelace** died, **born** 1907. *oxygen inhalation apparatus*

1965: Paul Hermann **Müller** died, **born** 1899. *dichlorodiphenyltrichloroethane (DDT)*

1965: Otto **Foerster** died, **born** 1876. *mapharsen, syphilis*

1965: Gregory **Shwartzman** died, **born** 1896. *Schwartzman phenomenon, Bacillus typhosus*

1965: Christian **Wolferth** died, **born** 1887. *coronary occlusion, electrocardiography*

1965: Gordon Morgan **Holmes** died, **born** 1876. *thalamus, adrenal cortex tumour*

1965: Joseph Francis **McCarthy** died, **born** 1874. *cysto-urethroscopy*

1965: Philip Showalter **Hench** died, **born** 1896. *rheumatoid arthritis, cortisone, adrenocorticotrophic hormone*

1965: H. Lowry **Rush** died, **born** 1897. *fractures*

1965: James Bertram **Collip** died, **born** 1892. *tetany, parathyroid hormone*

1965: Julius **Hallervorden** died, **born** 1882. *Hallervorden-Spatz syndrome*

1965: Alexander Thomas **Glenny** died, **born** 1882. *diphtheria toxoid*

1965: Ernest Edward **Tyzzer** died, **born** 1875. *varicella, histocompatibility antigens*

1965: Wilson **Smith** died, **born** 1965. *influenza*

1965: Robert Runnels **Williams** died, **born** 1886. *vitamin $B_1$*

1965: Joseph **Erlanger** died, **born** 1874. *nerve impulse transmission and velocity*

1965: Ignacio **Barraquer** died, **born** 1884. *cataract*

1965: Albert **Schweitzer** died, **born** 1875. *medical missionary*

## 1966
1966:1 **Nobel Prize** (Physiology or Medicine): Charles Brenton Huggins (b.1901), for work on the **hormonal** treatment of **cancer**, *NPL. 4276*; Francis Peyton Rous (1879–1970), for work on **hormone-dependent tumours**, *NPL. 2637*

1966:2 An experimental live-virus **rubella** vaccine produced by Harry Martin Meyer (b.1928), Paul Douglas Parkman (b.1932) and T.C. Panos, *NEJM* **275**:575. *5509.3*

1966:3 A flexible silicone rubber **finger-joint prosthesis** introduced by A.B. Swanson, *NYUPG* 6:16. *4405.4*

1966:4 **Lymphokines** discovered by John R. David (b.1930), *PNAS* **56**:72, and independently by B.R. Bloom (b.1937) and B. Bennett, *Science* **153**:80. *2578.36*

1966: Alfred Newton **Richards** died, **born** 1876. *histamine*

1966: Eli Kennerley **Marshall** died, **born** 1889. *bacillary dysentery, sulphaguanidine*

1966: Oswald Hope **Robertson** died, **born** 1886. *blood transfusion*

1966: Richard Edwin **Shope** died, **born** 1901. *tumours, papilloma, viruses*

1966: Samuel Albert **Levine** died, **born** 1891. *angina pectoris, heart failure, thyroidectomy, mitral valve section*

1966: Rufus Ivory **Cole** died, **born** 1872. *pneumonia*

1966: Arthur Walter **Proetz** died, **born** 1888. *nasal sinusitis*

1966: Julius Moses **Rogoff** died, **born** 1884. *Addison's disease*

1966: Frederic Eugen Basil **Foley** died, **born** 1891. *hydronephrosis*

1966: Arthur William Mickle **Ellis** died, **born** 1883. *nephritis*

1966: Achile Mario **Dogliotti** died, **born** 1897. *pain, section of lemniscus lateralis*

1966: Norbert **Wiener** died, **born** 1894. *cybernetics*

1966: Kenneth Fuller **Maxcy** died, **born** 1889. *typhus*

1966: Kenzo **Futaki** died, **born** 1873. *rat-bite fever, Spirillum morsus muris*

1966: Norman McAlister **Gregg** died, **born** 1892. *rubella*

1966: Frits **Zernike** died, **born** 1888. *phase contrast microscopy*

1966: Bernhard **Zondek** died, **born** 1891. *pregnancy diagnosis, growth hormone*

1966: Saul **Adler** died, **born** 1895. *leishmaniasis, Leishmania tropica, Phlebotomus*

### 1967

1967:1 **Nobel Prize** (Physiology or Medicine): Haldan Keffer Hartline (1903–1983), for work on **visual mechanisms**, *NPL. 1532*; George Wald (b.1906), for work on the photosensitive pigments of the **visual receptor** apparatus, *NPL. 1535*; Ragnar Arthur Granit (1900–1991), for elucidation of the mechanism of the **visual process**, *NPL. 1534*

1967:2 First detailed report of **amniocentesis** for diagnosis *in utero* of **genetic disorders** by Cecil Bryant Jacobson (b.1936) and Robert Henry Barter (b.1913), *AmJOG* **99**:796. *6235.2*

1967:3 A **rubella** virus haemagglutination-inhibition test introduced by George Louis Stewart (b.1936) and co-workers, *NEJM* **276**:*554. 5509.4*

1967:4 Evidence for two distinctive types of **infective hepatitis** shown by Saul Krugman (b.1911) and co-workers, *JAMA* **200**:*265. 3666.5*

1967:5 First human **heart transplant** reported by Christiaan Neethling Barnard (b.1922), *SAMJ* **41**:1271; the operation took place on 3 Dec and the patient died on 21 Dec. *3047.20*

1967:6 **Syphilis: treponemal haemagglutination test** introduced by Tara Rathlev, *BJVD* **43**:181. *2419.4*

----

1967: Ernest Basil **Verney** died, **born** 1894. *antidiuretic hormone*

1967: Elmer Verney **McCollum** died, **born** 1879. *vitamins*

1967: Walter Abraham **Jacobs** died, **born** 1883. *tryparsamide*

1967: Alick **Isaacs** died, **born** 1921. *interferon*

1967: Hermann Joseph **Muller** died, **born** 1890. *heredity, artificial transmutation of gene*

1967: Gregory Goodwin **Pincus** died, **born** 1903. *contraception, progesterone*

1967: Vladmir Leslie **Tichy** died, **born** 1899. *cardio-omentopexy*

1967: Casimir **Funk** died, **born** 1884. *beriberi*

1967: Grace **Medes** died, **born** 1886. *tyrosinosis*

1967: Philip **Wiles** died, **born** 1899. *hindquarter amputation*

1967: LeRoy Dryden **Fothergill** died, **born** 1901. *Eastern equine encephalitis*

1967: Carl **Kling** died, **born** 1887. *poliomyelitis*

1967; Charles **Armstrong** died, **born** 1886. *lymphocytic choriomeningitis*

1967: Louise Charlotte **Eisenhardt** died, **born** 1891. *meningiomas*

1967: Bela **Schick** died, **born** 1877. *diphtheria, serum sickness*

1967: George Frederick **Dick** died, **born** 1881. *scarlet fever, streptococcus*

1967: Wolfgang **Köhler** died, **born** 1887. *gestalt psychology*

1967: Leonard **Colebrook** died, **born** 1883. *puerperal fever, prontosil*

1967: Richard **Kuhn** died, **born** 1900. *carotenoids, vitamins*

**1968**

1968:1 **Nobel Prize** (Physiology or Medicine): Robert William Holley (b.1922), for his work on **transfer RNA**, *NPL. 257.2*; Marshall Warren Nirenberg (b.1927), for his work on DNA, *NPL. 256.11*; Har Gobind Khorana (b.1927), for the techniques he established for the **synthesis** of **polynucleotides**, *NPL. 752.6*

1968:2 The **Epstein-Barr virus** shown by Gertrude Henle and co-workers to be the causal agent in **infectious mononucleosis**, *PNAS* **59**:94. *5487.1*

1968:3 The role of **cyclic AMP**, the second messenger mediating actions in a wide range of **hormonal** effects, elucidated by Earl Wilber Sutherland (1915–1974), G.A. Robson, and R.W. Butcher, *AnRB* **37**:149. *752.7*

1968:4 **Leukaemia** treated with **cytosine arabinoside** by Rose Ruth Ellison (b.1923) and co-workers, *Blood* **32**:507. *3108.9*

1968:5 First report of **coronary artery autograft bypass** by R.G. Favaloro, *AnTS* **5**:354. *3047.21*

---

1968: Henry Hallett **Dale** died, **born** 1875. *histamine, anaphylactic shock, Schultz-Dale test, acetylcholine, chemical mediation of nerve impulses, biological standardization*

1968: Cornèille Jean François **Heymans** died, **born** 1892. *sinus-aorta mechanism in respiration*

1968: Oscar **Riddle** died, **born** 1877. *prolactin*

1968: Howard Walter **Florey** died, **born** 1898. *penicillinase, penicillin*

1968: Herbert Windsor **Wade** died, **born** 1896. *leprosy*

1968: Frederick Lucian **Golla** died, **born** 1878. *epilepsy, electroencephalography*

1968: Walter **Kikuth** died, **born** 1896. *malaria, mepacrine, schistosomiasis, lucanthone hydrochloride*

1968: Francis Edward **Shipway** died, **born** 1875. *anaesthesia*

**1969**

1969:1 **Nobel Prize** (Physiology or Medicine): Max Delbrück (1906–1981) and Salvador Edward Luria (1912–1991), for their work on **genetics** and replication of **bacteria**, *NPL. 2526.1, 2578.5*; Alfred Day Hershey (b.1908), for work on replication mechanisms and **genetic** structure of **viruses**, *NPL. 256*

1969:2 **Zoster immune globulin** first used for the prevention of **varicella** by Philip Alfred Brunel (b.1931) and co-workers, *NEJM* **280**:1191. *5440.2*

1969:3 Work on the nature of the processes of chemical **neurotransmission** published by Bernard Katz (b.1911); *The release of neural transmitter substances. 1354.2*

1969:4 **Oxamniquinine** introduced in the treatment of **bilharziasis** by Hugh Colin Richards and Raymond Foster, *Nature* **222**:581. *5351.7*

1969:5 The Canadian or Shouldice repair for **inguinal hernia** published by Edwin W. Shearburn (b.1913) and Richard N. Myers (b.1929), *Surgery* **66**:450. *3611.3*

1969:6 *In vitro* **fertilization of human oocytes** by Robert Geoffrey Edwards (b.1925), B.D. Bavister and Patrick Christopher Steptoe (1913–1988), *Nature* **221**:632. *532.4*

1969:7 **Immunoglobulin** molecule sequence reported by Gerald Maurice Edelman (b.1929), *PNAS* **63**:78. *2578.39*

---

1969: Hilmert Albert **Ranges** died, **born** 1906. *cardiac catheterization*

1969: Wilhelm **Raab** died, **born** 1895. *angina pectoris, thiouracil*

1969: Rudolph **Schindler** died, **born** 1888. *gastroscopy*

1969: Fuller **Albright** died, **born** 1900. *osteitis fibrosa cystica*

1969: Ernest **Witebsky** died, **born** 1901. *autoimmune thyroiditis*

1969: William **Dameshek** died, **born** 1900. *haemolytic anaemia, auto-immune disease*

1969: Alexander **Brunschwig** died, **born** 1901. *pancreatoduodenectomy*

1969: Hugo **Spatz** died, **born** 1888. *Hallervorden-Spatz syndrome*

1969: Samuel Phillips **Bedson** died, **born** 1886. *psittacosis, Chlamydia psittaci, lymphogranuloma venereum*

1969: Robert Thomson **Leiper** died, **born** 1881. *Schistosoma mansoni, S. haematobium, snail*

1969: Thomas **Francis** died, **born** 1900. *influenza*

1969: Hans Conrad Julius **Reiter** died, **born** 1881. *Reiter's syndrome*

1969: Max **Knoll** died, **born** 1879. *electron microscope*

## 1970

1970:1 **Nobel Prize** (Physiology or Medicine): Bernard Katz (b.1911) and Ulf Svante von Euler (1905–1983), for their research into the nature of the processes of **neurotransmission**, *NPL. 1354.1, 1354.2*; Julius Axelrod (b.1912), for his studies on the pharmacology of central **neurotransmitter** substances, *NPL. 1931.6*

1970:2 **Nobel Prize** (Chemistry): Luis Frederico Leloir (1906–1987), for discovery of **sugar nucleotides** and their role in the biosynthesis of **carbohydrates**, *NPL.*

1970:3 Flow-guided balloon-tipped catheter used in **cardiac catheterization** by Harold James Charles Swan (b.1922) and co-workers, *NEJM* **283**:447. *2883.9*

1970:4 **Epstein-Barr virus** shown to be a cause of **Burkitt's lymphoma** by Thomas Shope, *PNAS* **70**:2487. *2660.25*

1970:5 Interaction between **tumour viruses** and genetic material of the cell discovered by David Baltimore (b.1938), Renato Dulbecco (b.1914) and Howard Martin Temin (1934–1994), *Nature* **226**:1209, 1211. *2660.20, 2660.22, 2660.23, 2660.27*

1970:6 **Rifampicin** introduced in treatment of **leprosy** by Richard John William Rees (b.1917), *BMJ* **1**:89. *2442.5*

1970:7 Suppressor **T cells** noted by Richard K. Gerson (1932–1983) and K. Kondo, *I* **18**:723. *2578.41*

---

1970:8 Jean **Cid dos Santos** died; performed first thrombo-endarterectomy, 1947, *MAC* **73**:409. *3019.1*

1970: Otto **Warburg** died, **born** 1883. *tumours, metabolism, respiratory ferments*

1970: Alfred Henry **Sturtevant** died, **born** 1891. *heredity*

1970: Francis Peyton **Rous** died, **born** 1879. *sarcoma*

1970: Henry Hubert **Turner** died, **born** 1892. *Turner's syndrome*

1970: Philip Edward **Smith** died, **born** 1884. *gonads, anterior pituitary*

1970: Paul **Kimmelstiel** died, **born** 1900. *glomerulosclerosis*

## 1971

1971:1 **Nobel Prize** (Physiology or Medicine): Earl W. Sutherland (1915–1974), for his discoveries concerning the mechanisms of the action of **hormones**, *NPL.* **7527**

1971:2 **Royal Medico-Psychological Association, London**, becomes **Royal College of Psychiatrists**

1971:3 **Kuru** and **Creutzfeldt-Jakob disease** transmitted to primates by Daniel Carleton Gajdusek (b.1923) and Clarence J. Gibbs, *Nature* **230**:588. *4729.2*

1971:4 An **arthroplasty** replacement of the **knee-joint** carried out by Frank H. Gunston (b.1933), *JBJS* **53b**:272. *4405.5*

---

1971: Wendell Meredith **Stanley** died, **born** 1904. *virus, nucleoprotein, enzymes*

1971: Robert Benedict **Bourdillon** died, **born** 1889. *calciferol*

1971: Paul **Karrer** died, **born** 1889. *vitamins*

1971: Herbert McLean **Evans** died, **born** 1882. *vitamins, hormones*

1971: Osker Paul **Wintersteiner** died, **born** 1898. *cortisone*

1971: Arthur **Stoll** died, **born** 1887. *ergotamine, lysergic acid-diethylamide*

1971: Clarence Cook **Little** died, **born** 1888. *homograft reaction, transplantation, histocompatibility antigens*

1971: Arne Wilhelm **Tiselius** died, **born** 1902. *antibodies, gamma globulins, serum proteins, electrophoresis*

1971: Bernardo Alberto **Houssay** died, **born** 1887. *hypertension, carbohydrate metabolism, anterior pituitary*

1971: Claude Schaeffer **Beck** died, **born** 1894. *pericardial implantation of pectoral muscle, cardio-omentopexy, ventricular fibrillation, electric shock, revascularization of brain*

1971: Paul **Fildes** died, **born** 1882. *haemophilia*

1971: John Heysham **Gibbon** died, **born** 1903. *heart-lung machine*

1971: Aldo **Castellani** died, **born** 1877. *trypanosomiasis, Trypanosoma gambiense, toxoplasmosis, yaws, Treponema pertenue, bronchospirochaetosis*

1971: Eugene Lindsay **Opie** died, **born** 1873. *malaria, diabetes, islets of Langerhans*

1971: Franklin McCue **Hanger** died, **born** 1894. *liver-function test*

1971: Hans Christian **Hagedorn** died, **born** 1888. *protamine insulin*

1971: John Burton **Cleland** died, **born** 1878. *Murray Valley encephalitis*

1971: Hermann **Mooser** died, **born** 1891. *typhus, Rickettsia mooseri*

1971: John Rodman **Paul** died, **born** 1893. *infectious mononucleosis*

1971: Antoine Marcellin **Lacassagne** died, **born** 1884. *carcinogenesis, ovarian hormone*

1971: James Barrett **Brown** died, **born** 1899. *skin grafts*

## 1972

1972: 1 **Nobel Prize** (Physiology or Medicine): Gerald Maurice Edelman (b. 1929) and Rodney Robert Porter (1917–1985), for their studies concerning the chemical structure of **antibodies**, *NPL. 2578.25, 2578.39*

1972: 2 **Nobel Prize** (Chemistry): Christian Boehmer Anfinsen (1916–1995), for work on **ribonuclease**, especially connection between the **amino acid** sequence and the biologically active conformation, *NPL*; Stanford Moore (1913–1982) and William H. Stein (1911–1980), for contributions to understanding of the connection between chemical structure and catalytic activity of the active centre of the **ribonuclease** molecule, *NPL.*

1972: 3 **Mayo Medical School** (for undergraduates) founded at **Rochester**, Minn.

1972: 4 **Immune response** shown to be genetically determined, by Baruj Benacerraf (b. 1920) and Hugh O'Neill McDevitt, *Science* **175**:273. *2578.29*

1972:5 Mary Cowan **Maitland** died; with Hugh Bethune Maitland, introduced 'Maitland's medium' for the cultivation of vaccinia virus, 1928, *L* **2**:596. *5434.1*

1972: Hugh Bethune **Maitland** died, **born** 1895. *vaccinia virus*

1972: Georg von **Békésy** died, **born** 1899. *hearing, audiometer*

1972: Edward Calvin **Kendall** died, **born** 1886. *thyroxine, cortisone*

1972: Charles Robert **Harington** died, **born** 1897. *thyroxine*

1972: Philip **Drinker** died, **born** 1894. *Drinker respirator ('iron lung')*

1972: Carl Hamilton **Browning** died, **born** 1881. *acriflavine*

1972: Solomon A. **Berson** died, **born** 1918. *radioimmunoassay, insulin*

1972: Lester Reynold **Dragstedt** died, **born** 1893. *peptic ulcer, vagotomy*

1972: Leo **Mayer** died, **born** 1884. *tendon transplantation*

1972: Walter **Freeman** died, **born** 1895. *prefrontal lobotomy, psychoses*

1972: Lionel Sharples **Penrose** died, **born** 1898. *Down's syndrome*

1972: Raymond **Lewthwaite** died, **born** 1894. *scrub typhus, tsutsugamushi disease*

1972: Joseph **Stokes** died, **born** 1896. *mumps*

1972: Max **Theiler** died, **born** 1899. *yellow fever*

1972: Chester Scott **Keefer** died, **born** 1897. *cat-scratch fever*

1972: Carl Boye **Semb** died, **born** 1895. *thoracoplasty*

1972: Colin Munro **MacLeod** died, **born** 1909. *DNA, genetic transformation*

**1973**
1973:1 **Nobel Prize** (Physiology or Medicine): Karl von Frisch (1886–1982), Konrad Zacharias Lorenz (1903–1989), and Nikolaas Tinbergen (1907–1988), for their discoveries concerning organization and elicitation of **individual and social behaviour patterns**, *NPL.*

1973:2 A human diploid cell vaccine against **rabies** developed by T.J. Wiktor and co-workers, *JAMA* **224**:1170. *5484.4*

1973:3 **Computer-assisted tomography** (CAT), or computed tomography (CT) introduced by Godfrey Newbold Hounsfield (b.1919), *BJR* **46**:1016. *2700.4*

---

1973: Dickinson Woodruff **Richards** died, **born** 1895. *heart catheterization*

1973: Frederick Roland George **Heaf** died, **born** 1894. *tuberculosis, tuberculin*

1973: Sidney **Farber** died, **born** 1903. *cancer, triethylenephosphoramide*

1973: Paul Dudley **White** died, **born** 1886. *heart disease*

1973: John Heysham **Gibbon** died, **born** 1903. *heart-lung machine*

1973: Ivar Asbjorn **Følling** died, **born** 1888. *phenylketonuria*

1973: Leslie Julius **Harris** died, **born** 1898. *vitamin deficiency*

1973: Lorenz **Böhler** died, **born** 1885. *fractures*

1973: Arvid Johann **Wallgren** died, **born** 1889. *lymphocytic choriomeningitis*

1973: Percival **Bailey** died, **born** 1892. *glioma*

1973: Walter Rudolf **Hess** died, **born** 1881. *functional organization of interbrain*

1973: Edward **Hindle** died, **born** 1886. *yellow fever*

1973: Selman Abraham **Waksman** died, **born** 1888. *streptomycin, neomycin*

**1974**
1974:1 **Nobel Prize** (Physiology or Medicine): Albert Claude (1899–1983), Christian de Duve (b.1917), and George Emil Palade (b.1912), for their discoveries concerning the structural and functional organization of the **cell**, *NPL*.

1974:2 A network theory of the **immune system** proposed by Nils Kaj Jerne (1911–1994), *AnI* **125**C:373. *2578.42*

---

1974: Max **Aron** died, **born** 1892. *thyroid-stimulating hormone*

1974: Earl Wilbur **Sutherland** died, **born** 1915. *cyclic AMP, hormones*

1974: Alan **Kekwick** died, **born** 1909. *blood transfusion*

1974: William Smith **Tillett** died, **born** 1892. *streptokinase*

1974: William Hugh **Feldman** died, **born** 1892. *tuberculosis, promin, streptomycin*

1974: Ernest **Muir** died, **born** 1880. *leprosy, diasone*

1974: Guy William John **Bousfield** died, **born** 1893. *angina pectoris, electrocardiography*

1974: Alban **Köhler** died, **born** 1874. *heart teleradiography*

1974: Donald Walter Gordon **Murray** died, **born** 1894. *aortic valve homograft*

1974: Robert James **Minnitt** died, **born** 1889. *labour, analgesia*

**1975**

1975:1 **Nobel Prize** (Physiology or Medicine): David Baltimore (b.1938), Renato Dulbecco (b.1914), and Howard Martin Temin (1934–1994), for their discoveries concerning the interaction between **tumour viruses** and **genetic** material of the **cell**, *NPL. 2660.20, 2660.22, 2660.23, 2660.27*

1975:2 **Nobel Prize** (Chemistry): John Warcup Cornforth (b.1917), for contributions to the **stereochemistry** of **enzyme-catalyzed** reactions, *NPL;* Vladimir Prelog (b.1906), for contributions to **stereochemistry** of **organic molecules** and reactions, *NPL.*

1975:3 **Monoclonal antibodies** produced by César Milstein (b.1927) and Georges J. F. Köhler (1946–1995), *Nature* **256**:495; they received the Nobel Prize (Physiology or Medicine), 1984, for this work, *NPL. 2578.43*

1975: Joseph John **Pfiffner** died, **born** 1903. *Addison's disease, eschatin, cortisone*

1975: Edward Lawrie **Tatum** died, **born** 1909. *chromosomes*

1975: William David **Coolidge** died, **born** 1873. *x ray tube*

1975: James Wilfred **Cook** died, **born** 1900. *carcinogens, dibenzanthracene*

1975: Hubert **Mann** died, **born** 1891. *vectorcardiography*

1975: Frederick Charles **Pybus** died, **born** 1882. *tonsillectomy*

1975: Edward Charles **Dodds** died, **born** 1899. *stilboestrol, dienoestrol*

1975: Leo Max **Davidoff** died, **born** 1898. *lumbar encephalography*

1975: Forrest F. **Kendall** died, **born** 1898. *precipitin reaction*

1975: Robert **Robinson** died, **born** 1886, *alkaloids, sterols, sex hormones, penicillin*

**1976**

1976:1 **Nobel Prize** (Physiology or Medicine): Baruch Samuel Blumberg (b.1925) and Daniel Carleton Gajdusek (b.1923), for their discoveries concerning new mechanisms for the origin and dissemination of **infectious diseases**, *NPL. 3666.4, 4729.1, 4729.2*

1976:2 First **oncogene** discovered by Harold E. Varmus (b.1942) and J. Michael Bishop (b.1936) and co-workers, *Nature* **260**:170. *2660.28*

1976: Leopold **Ruzicka** died, **born** 1887. *androsterone*

1976: Jacques Lucien **Monod** died, **born** 1910. *genes, enzymes, viruses*

1976: Carl Pieter Henrik **Dam** died, **born** 1895. *vitamins*

1976: Katharine Scott **Bishop** died, born 1888. *vitamins*

1976: Alexander Solomon **Wiener** died, **born** 1907. *Rh antigen, rhesus sensitization*

1976: John **Parkinson** died, **born** 1885. *heart disease*

1976: Norman Macdonnell **Keith** died, **born** 1885. *hypertension*

1976: Alexander **Haddow** died, **born** 1907. *mammary cancer, oestrogen, myeloid leukaemia, myleran*

1976: George Hoyt **Whipple** died, **born** 1878. *liver treatment in anaemia, intestinal lipodystrophy*

1976: Donald Walter Gordon **Murray** died, **born** 1894. *anticoagulation, heparin*

1976: Edwin Bennett **Astwood** died, **born** 1909. *hyperthyroidism*

1976: Geoffrey Barrow **Dowling** died, **born** 1891. *lupus vulgaris, calciferol*

1976: Jean **Oliver** died, **born** 1889. *kidney failure*

1976: James Stirling **Anderson** died, **born** 1891. *Corynebacterium diphtheriae*

1976: Wilder Graves **Penfield** died, **born** 1891. *epilepsy*

1976: Edward Holbrook **Derrick** died, **born** 1898. *rickettsial Q fever*

1976: James William Tudor **Thomas** died, **born** 1893. *corneal transplantation*

**1977**
1977:1 **Nobel Prize** (Physiology or Medicine): Roger Charles Louis Guillemin (b.1924) and Andrew Victor Schally (b.1926), for their discoveries concerning the **peptide hormone** production of the **brain**, *NPL*; Rosalyn Sussman Yalow (b.1921), for the development of **radioimmunoassays** for **peptide hormones**, *NPL*.

1977:2 First major scientific account of **Legionnaires' disease** given by David William Fraser and co-workers, *NEJM* **297**:1189. *3215.7*

1977: Harry **Goldblatt** died, **born** 1891. *hypertension*

1977: Armand James **Quick** died, **born** 1894. *liver-function test, prothrombin clotting time*

1977: Auguste **Loubatières** died, **born** 1912. *hypoglycaemic sulphonamides*

1977: Josep **Trueta** died, **born** 1897. *closed plaster treatment of wounds and fractures*

1977: William Grey **Walter** died, **born** 1911. *cerebral tumours, electroencephalography*

1977: Archibald Vivian **Hill** died, **born** 1886. *heat production in muscle*

1977: Edgar Douglas **Adrian** died, **born** 1889. *sensory physiology*

1977: John Chassar **Moir** died, **born** 1900. *ergometrine*

660

1977: Henry John **Seddon** died, **born** 1903. *nerve injuries, classification*

**1978**
1978:1 **Nobel Prize** (Physiology or Medicine): Werner Arber (b.1929), Daniel Nathans (b.1928), and Hamilton Othanel Smith (b.1931), for the discovery of **restriction enzymes** and their application to problems of molecular **genetics**, *NPL.*

1978:2 **Nobel Prize** (Chemistry): Peter Denis Mitchell (1920–1992), for contributions to the understanding of **biological energy transfer** through the formulation of the **chemiosmotic theory**, *NPL.*

1978:3 **Medical Act (UK)** gives Education Committee of **General Medical Council** statutory responsibility for coordinating **medical education** and for promoting high standards of such education in the **UK**

1978:4 First successful **human birth** after **re-implantation of human embryo** reported by Patrick Steptoe (1913–1988) and Robert Geoffrey Edwards (b.1925), *L* 2:366. *532.5*

1978: Vincent du **Vigneaud** died, **born** 1901. *oxytocin, vasopressin*

1978: Albert Hewett **Coons** died, **born** 1912. *antigens, fluorescent antibodies*

1978: Charles Herbert **Best** died, **born** 1899. *insulin*

1978: Chauncey Depew **Leake** died, **born** 1896. *anaesthesia, divinyl ether*

1978: William Stewart **Duke-Elder** died, **born** 1898. *ophthalmology*

**1979**
1979:1 **Nobel Prize** (Physiology or Medicine): Allan MacLeod Cormack (b.1924) and Godfrey Newbold Hounsfield (b.1919), for the development of **computer assisted tomography**, *NPL.* *2700.4*

1979: Robert Burns **Woodward** died, **born** 1917. *cortisone*

1979: Ernst Boris **Chain** died, **born** 1906. *penicillinase, penicillin*

1979: Werner Theodor Otto **Forssmann** died, **born** 1904. *heart catheterization*

1979: Guido **Fanconi** died, **born** 1892. *Fanconi's syndrome, cystic fibrosis (mucoviscidosis), renal tubular function*

1979: Petrus Johannes **Waardenburg** died, **born** 1886. *Waardenburg's syndrome*

1979: Hyram Houston **Merritt** died, **born** 1902. *convulsive disorders, diphenylhydantoin*

1979: Josef **Dallos** died, **born** 1905. *contact lenses*

1979: José Antonio Gay **Prieto** died, **born** 1905. *lymphogranuloma venereum*

1979: Charles Skinner **Hallpike** died, **born** 1896. *Menière's syndrome*

## 1980

1980:1 **Nobel Prize** (Physiology or Medicine): George Davis Snell (1903–1996), for work on **transplantation genetics**, *NPL. 2578.30*; Jean Baptiste Dausset (b.1916), for the discovery of the first **histocompatibility antigen**, *NPL. 2578.26*; Baruj Benacerraf (b.1920), for work on **histocompatibility-linked immune response genes**, *NPL. 2578.29*

1980:2 **Nobel Prize** (Chemistry): Frederick Sanger (b.1918) and Walter Gilbert (b.1932), for contributions concerning the determination of base sequences of **nucleic acids**, *NPL*; Paul Berg (b.1926), for fundamental studies of the biochemistry of **nucleic acids**, with particular regard to **recombinant DNA**, *NPL*.

1980:3 The announcement that '**smallpox** eradication has been achieved throughout the world' made by the World Health Organization on 8 May; *The global eradication of smallpox. 5434.2*

---

1980: John Samuel **LaDue** died, **born** 1911. *myocardial infarction*

1980: Alexander William Gordon **Ewing** died, **born** 1896. *hearing tests*

1980: William Ingledew **Daggett** died, **born** 1900. *otitis media, tympanoplasty*

1980: Terence John **Millin** died, **born** 1903. *prostatectomy*

1980: S.R. **Savoor** died, **born** 1900. *scrub typhus, tsutsugamushi disease*

1980: Russell Claude **Brock** died, **born** 1903. *congenital stenosis, pulmonary valvulotomy*

1980: William H. **Stein** died, **born** 1911. *ribonuclease*

## 1981

1981:1 **Nobel Prize** (Physiology or Medicine): Roger Wolcott Sperry (1913–1994), for his discoveries concerning the functional specialization of the **cerebral hemispheres**, *NPL*; David Hunter Hubel (b.1926) and Torsten Nils Wiesel (b.1924), for their discoveries concerning information processing in the **visual system**, *NPL*.

1981:2 **Acquired immunodeficiency syndrome** (AIDS), a range of diseases associated with **human immunodeficiency virus** (HIV) infection, first recognized in male homosexuals in USA. It produces a slowly progressive weakening in the cellular immune system. In 1984 it was demonstrated that HIV (formerly lymphadenopathy-associated virus (LAV), isolated by workers at the Institut Pasteur, Paris, 1983) or human T-cell lymphotropic virus type III (HTLV III) was the probable cause. HTLV III was isolated by workers at US National Institute of Health, Bethesda, Md in 1984

---

1981: Hans Adolf **Krebs** died, **born** 1900. *citric acid cycle in carbohydrate metabolism*

1981: George Washington **Corner** died, **born** 1889. *progesterone*

1981: Guy Frederic **Marrian** died, **born** 1904. *pregnanediol, oestriol*

1981: Rebecca Craighill **Lancefield** died, **born** 1895. *haemolytic streptococci*

1981: Max **Delbrück** died, **born** 1906. *genetic recombination, bacteriophage*

1981: Owen Harding **Wangensteen** died, **born** 1898. *intestinal obstruction*

1981: Wilhelm Alexander **Freund** died, **born** 1833. *cancer, hysterectomy*

## 1982
1982:1 **Nobel Prize** (Physiology or Medicine): Sune Bergström (b.1916), Bengt Ingemar Samuelsson (b.1934), and John Robert Vane (b.1927), for their discoveries concerning the **prostaglandins** and related biologically active substances, *NPL.*

1982:2 **Nobel Prize** (Chemistry): Aaron Klug (b.1926), for his development of **crystallographic electron microscopy** and his structural elucidation of biologically important **nucleic acid – protein** complexes, *NPL.*

---

1982: Axel Hugo Teodor **Theorell** died, **born** 1903. *oxidizing enzymes*

1982: René Jules **Dubos** died, **born** 1901. *gramicidin*

1982: Hans **Selye** died, **born** 1907. *stress*

1982: Rudolph Albert **Peters** died, **born** 1889. *dimercaprol, British anti-lewisite (BAL)*

1982: John Bernard **Kinmonth** died, **born** 1916. *lymphangiography*

1982: Norman Cecil **Tanner** died, **born** 1906. *inguinal and femoral hernia*

1982: Richard H. **Lawler** died, **born** 1895. *kidney transplant*

1982: John **Charnley** died, **born** 1911. *hip-joint replacement*

1982: Anna **Freud** died, **born** 1895. *child psychology*

1982: Eleanor **Zaimis** died, **born** 1915. *anaesthesia, methonium compounds*

1982: Erich **Letterer** died, **born** 1895. *Letterer-Siwe disease*

1982: Karl von **Frisch** died, **born** 1886. *behaviour*

1982: Geoffrey Langdon **Keynes** died, **born** 1887. *breast cancer, radium*

1982: Stanford **Moore** died, **born** 1913. *ribonuclease*

## 1983
1983:1 **Nobel Prize** (Physiology or Medicine): Barbara McClintock (1902–1992), for her discovery of mobile **genetic elements**, *NPL.*

---

1983: William Clouser **Boyd** died, **born** 1903. *blood groups*

1983: Haldan Keffer **Hartline** died, **born** 1903. *optic nerve*

1983: John **Bunyan** died, **born** 1907. *burns*

1983: Ulf Svante von **Euler** died, **born** 1905. *noradrenaline, prostaglandin, Substance P, neurotransmission*

1983: Richard K. **Gerson** died, **born** 1932. *suppressor T cells*

1983: Thomas Frank **Davey** died, **born** 1907. *leprosy, diphenylthiourea, ditophal*

1983: Marion B. **Sulzberger** died, **born** 1895. *dermatitis, allergens*

1983: Maxwell Edward **Lapham** died, **born** 1899. *pregnancy diagnosis*

1983: Burrill Bernard **Crohn** died, **born** 1884. *ileitis*

1983: Albert **Claude** died, born 1899. *cytology*

## 1984
1984:1 **Nobel Prize** (Physiology or Medicine): Niels Kaj Jerne (1911–1994), Georges Jean Franz Köhler (1946–1995), and César Milstein (b.1927), for theories concerning the specificity in development and control of the **immune** system and the discovery of the principle of production of **monoclonal antibodies**, *NPL. 2578.42, 2578.43*

1984: Carl Ferdinand **Cori** died, **born** 1896. *glycogens*

1984: Kenneth Stewart **Cole** died, **born** 1900. *electrical conduction of living cell membranes*

1984: Manfred Martin **Mayer** died, **born** 1916. *complement fixation*

1984: Edward Heinrich **Robitzek** died, **born** 1912. *tuberculosis, isoniazid*

1984: Clarence **Crafoord** died, **born** 1899. *coarctation of aorta*

1984: John William **McNee** died, **born** 1887. *bile pigment*

1984: Bernard **Schlesinger** died, **born** 1896. *rheumatism, streptococci*

1984: Max **Cutler** died, **born** 1899. *mastitis*

## 1985
1985:1 **Nobel Prize** (Physiology or Medicine); Michael Stuart Brown (b.1941) and Joseph Leonard Goldstein (b.1940), for their discoveries concerning the regulation of **cholesterol** metabolism, *NPL*

1985:2 Epidemic of **bovine spongiform encephalopathy** (BSE) reported in beef cattle in Britain; later traced to cattle feed containing sheep carcasses infected with scrapie; in following year there were fears that beef consumption could possibly lead to **Creutzfeldt-Jakob disease** in humans. *4719.1, 4722*

1985: Frank Macfarlane **Burnet** died, **born** 1899. *clonal selection, acquired immunological tolerance, influenza, rickettsial Q fever, Rickettsia burneti, poliomyelitis*

1985: Rodney Robert **Porter** died, **born** 1917. *antibodies*

664

1985: Charles Carter **Shepard** died, **born** 1914. *leprosy*

1985: Emmy **Klieneberger** died, **born** 1892. *pleuropneumonia-like organisms, Streptococcus moniliformis*

1985: John Franklin **Enders** died, **born** 1897. *poliomyelitis, measles*

**1986**
1986:1 **Nobel Prize** (Physiology or Medicine): Stanley Cohen (b.1922) and Rita Levi-Montalcini (b.1909), for their discovery of **growth factors**, *NPL.*

1986:2 **Nobel Prize** (Physics): Ernst Ruska (1906–1988), for design of the first **electron microscope**, *NPL. 269.3*; Gerd Binnig (b.1947) and Heinrich Rohrer (b.1933), for design of the **scanning tunnelling microscope**, *NPL.*

---

1986: Fritz Albert **Lipmann** died, **born** 1899. *coenzyme A*

1986: Edward **Allen** died, **born** 1892. *oestrin*

1986: Ronald **Hare** died, **born** 1899. *virus haemagglutination*

1986: Pierre **Grabar** died, **born** 1898. *immunoelectrophoresis*

1986: Helen Brooke **Taussig** died, **born** 1898. *pulmonary artery defects*

1986: John Putnam **Merrill** died, **born** 1917. *kidney transplant*

1986: Maxwell Myer **Wintrobe** died, **born** 1901. *erythrocyte sedimentation rate*

1986: Roger **Couvelaire** died, **born** 1903. *artificial bladder*

1986: Edward Adelbert **Doisy** died. *oestradiol, vitamin K*

1986: Albert **Szent-Györgyi** died, **born** 1893. *vitamins*

**1987**
1987:1 **Nobel Prize** (Physiology or Medicine): Susumi Tonegawa (b.1939), for his discovery of the **genetic** principle for generation of **antibody** diversity, *NPL.*

---

1987: Peter Brian **Medawar** died, **born** 1915. *acquired immunological tolerance, transplant rejection mechanism, skin homografts*

1987: Ian **Donald** died, **born** 1910. *fetal cephalometry, ultrasonic scanning*

1987: Robert Gwyn **Macfarlane** died, **born** 1907. *haemophilia, snake venom*

1987: Philip **Levine** died, **born** 1900. *erythroblastosis fetalis, blood groups*

1987: Thomas Holmes **Sellors** died, **born** 1902. *pulmonary valvulotomy, pulmonary stenosis*

1987: Chester B. **McVay** died, **born** 1911. *hernia*

1987: Henry Edward **Shortt** died, **born** 1887. *malaria, Phlebotomus fever, Leishmania*

1987: Ramon **Castroviejo** died, **born** 1904. *corneal transplantation*

1987: Murray Joseph **Sanders** died, **born** 1910. *keratoconjunctivitis*

1987: Noel Francis **Maclagan** died, **born** 1904. *liver function test*

1987: Reginald Hammerick **Smithwick** died, **born** 1899. *Smithwick operation (splanchnic resection for essential hypertension)*

1987: John Howard **Northrop** died, **born** 1891. *pepsin, enzymes, proteins*

1987: Luis Frederico **Leloir** died, **born** 1906. *sugar nucleotides, carbohydrates*

## 1988
1988: 1 **Nobel Prize** (Physiology or Medicine): James Whyte Black (b.1924), Gertrude Belle Elion (b.1918), and George Herbert Hitchings (b.1905), for their discoveries of important principles for **drug treatment**, *NPL. 1931.5, 3108.2*

---

1988: André Frédéric **Cournand** died, **born** 1895. *cardiac catheterization*

1988: Frank George **Young** died, **born** 1908. *anterior pituitary diabetogenic hormone, diabetes*

1988: Patrick Christopher **Steptoe** died, **born** 1913. *in vitro fertilization of human oocytes*

1988: Luis Walter **Alvarez** died, **born** 1911. *linear ion accelerator*

1988: Robert Edward **Gross** died, **born** 1905. *coarctation of aorta, patent ductus arteriosus*

1988: Harold Leeming **Sheehan** died, **born** 1900. *hypopituitarism*

1988: Christopher Howard **Andrewes** died, **born** 1896. *influenza, kidney function test*

1988: Wilfred Fletcher **Gaisford** died, **born** 1902. *paediatrics, diabetes*

1988: Sewall **Wright** died, **born** 1889. *genetics*

1988: Nikolaas **Tinbergen** died, **born** 1907. *behaviour*

1988: Ernst **Ruska** died, **born** 1906. *electron microscope*

## 1989
1989: 1 **Nobel Prize** (Physiology or Medicine): Harold E. Varmus (b.1939) and J. Michael Bishop (b.1936), for their discovery of the cellular origin of **retroviral oncogenes**, *NPL. 2660.28*

1989: 2 **Nobel Prize** (Chemistry): Sidney Altman (b.1939) and Thomas Robert Cech (b.1947), for their discovery of catalytic **RNA**, *NPL.*

---

1989: Charles Anthony **Hufnagel** died, **born** 1916. *prosthetic heart valve*

1989: George Wells **Beadle** died, **born** 1903. *genetics*

1989: Konrad Zacharias **Lorenz** died, **born** 1903. *behaviour*

**1990**
1990:1 **Nobel Prize** (Physiology or Medicine): Joseph E. Murray (b.1919) and E. Donnall Thomas (b.1920), for their discoveries concerning **organ** and **cell transplantation** in the treatment of human disease, *NPL. 4257*

**1991**
1991:1 **Nobel Prize** (Physiology or Medicine): Erwin Neher (b.1944) and Bert Sakmann (b.1942), for their discoveries concerning the function of **single ion channels** in **cells**, *NPL.*

1991: Michael **Heidelberger** died, **born** 1888. *antigenic structure of pneumococcus, tryparsamide*

1991: Austin Bradford **Hill** died, **born** 1897. *lung cancer, smoking*

1991: Sigvald **Refsum** died, **born** 1907. *lipid metabolism disorders*

1991: Ragnar Arthur **Granit** died, **born** 1900. *retinal physiology*

**1992**
1992:1 **Nobel Prize** (Physiology or Medicine): Edmond Henri Fischer (b.1920) and Edwin Gerhard Krebs (b.1918), for their discoveries concerning reversible **protein phosphorylation** as a biological regulatory mechanism, *NPL.*

1992: Cicely Delphine **Williams** died, **born** 1893. *kwashiorkor*

1992: Daniel **Bovet** died, **born** 1907. *anaesthesia, gallamine triethiodide, succinylcholine chloride, antihistamine*

1992: Ernest Lester **Smith** died, **born** 1904. *vitamin $B_{12}$*

1992: Barbara **McLintock** died, **born** 1902. *genetics*

1992: Peter Denis **Mitchell** died, **born** 1920. *chemiosmotic theory*

**1993**
1993:1 **Nobel Prize** (Physiology or Medicine): Richard John Roberts (b.1943) and Phillip Allen Sharp (b.1944), for discovery of **split genes**, *NPL.*

1993:2 **Nobel Prize** (Chemistry): Kary B. Mullis (b.1944), for invention of the **polymerase chain reaction** (PCR) method for DNA-based chemistry, *NPL*; Michael J. Smith (b.1932), for contributions to the establishment of **oligonucleotide**-based, site-directed, **mutagenesis** and its development for **protein** studies, *NPL.*

1993: Wilhelm **Feldberg** died, **born** 1900. *acetylcholine*

1993: Denis Parsons **Burkitt** died, **born** 1911. *lymphoma*

1993: William Drummond MacDonald **Paton** died, **born** 1917. *anaesthesia, methonium compounds*

## 1994
1994: 1 **Nobel Prize** (Physiology or Medicine): Alfred G. Gilman (b.1941) and Martin Rodbell (b.1925), for discovery of **G-proteins** and their role in **signal transduction in cells**, *NPL*

---

1994: Linus **Pauling** died, **born** 1901. *chemical bond, sickle-cell anaemia, haemoglobin*

1994: Dorothy Crowfoot **Hodgkin** died, **born** 1910. *x ray crystallography, insulin*

1994: André Michael **Lwoff** died, **born** 1902. *genes, enzymes, viruses*

1994: Niels Kaj **Jerne** died, **born** 1911. *immune system*

1994: Howard Martin **Temin** died, **born** 1934. *genetics, tumour viruses*

1994: Richard Laurence Millington **Synge** died, **born** 1914. *partition chromatography*

## 1995
1995: 1 **Nobel Prize** (Physiology or Medicine): Edward B. Lewis (b.1918), Christiane Nüsslein-Volhard (b.1942), and Eric F. Wieschaus (b.1947), for their discoveries concerning the **genetic** control of early **embryonic development**, *NPL.*

---

1995: Georges Jean Franz **Köhler** died, **born** 1946. *monoclonal antibodies*

1995: Jonas **Salk** died, **born** 1914. *poliomyelitis vaccine*

1995: Joseph **Needham** died, **born** 1900. *embryology, morphogenesis, biochemistry*

1995: Adolf Friedrich Johann **Butenandt** died, **born** 1903. *androsterone, progesterone*

1995: Christian Boehmer **Anfinsen** died, **born** 1916. *amino acids, ribonuclease*

## 1996
1996: Charles **Stuart-Harris** died, **born** 1909. *influenza*

1996: George Davis **Snell** died, **born** 1903. *transplantation genes*

1996: Tadeus **Reichstein** died, **born** 1897. *vitamin C, cortisone*

# Index of personal names

References are to birth entries (in the very few cases where no birth date is known the reference is to the death entry, where known, or to event entries). Names containing umlauts (ä, ö, ü) are listed as if spelt out, i.e. ae, oe, ue. Mac and Mc are listed as Mac.

Bateman, T., 1778:13
Bateson, W., 1861:35
Batten, F.E., 1865:32
Battey, R., 1828:33
Battie, W., 1704:2
Battle, W.H., 1855:34
Baudelocque, J.L., 1746:8
Bauer, D.J., 1914:43
Bauer, F., 1913:34
Bauer, L., 1814:16
Bauer, L.H., 1888:51
Bauer, R., 1906:33
Baumann, E., 1846:36
Bayle, A.L.J., 1799:8
Bayle, G.L., 1774:11
Bayley, W., 1529:3
Bayliss, W.M., 1860:36
Bayne-Jones, S., 1917:26
Bayon, H.P.G., 1876:72
Bayrlant, O. von, 1400:1
Bazalgette, J.W., 1819:14
Bazin, P.E.A., 1807:8
Beadle, G.W., 1903:70
Beall, D., 1941:13
Beard, G.M., 1839:27
Beatson, G.T., 1848:25
Beaumont, W., 1785:14
Beauperthuy, L.D., 1807:16
Bechterev, V.M., 1857:21
Beck, C.S., 1894:48
Beck, T., 1791:9
Becker, F.E., 1888:67
Béclard, P.A., 1785:15
Becquerel, A.H., 1852:55
Bednař, A., 1816:22
Bedson, S.P., 1886:67
Beer, E., 1876:47
Beer, G.J., 1763:4
Beevor, C.E., 1854:40
Behçet, H., 1889:41
Behring, E.A. von, 1854:34
Békésy, G. von, 1899:39
Belgrand, M.F.E., 1810:9
Bell, B., 1749:2
Bell, C., 1774:7
Bell, E.J., 1940:17
Bell, I.R., 1933:32
Bell, J., 1763:2
Bell, W.B., 1871:35
Bellerby, C.W., 1934:34
Bellini, L., 1643:1
Benacerraf, B., 1920:37
Beneden, W. van, 1846:25
Benedict, R.G., 1947:8
Benedict, S.R., 1884:65
Benedikt, M., 1835:17
Benjamin, B., 1903:62

Bennet, J.H., 1816:21
Bennett, A.H., 1848:35
Bennett, B., 1966:4
Bennett, H.C., 1837:23
Bennett, J.H., 1812:16
Bennett, W.H., 1852:35
Bentley, C.A., 1873:25
Ber, M., 1952:23
Bérard, A., 1802:9
Berberich, J., 1897:45
Berdmore, T., 1740:9
Berengario da Carpi, G., 1460:2
Berenger-Féraud, E. von, 1832:27
Berg, P., 1926:36
Berg, T., 1806:10
Bergel, F., 1900:51
Berger, F.M., 1913:55
Berger, J. (Hans), 1873:26
Berger, P., 1845:43
Bergman, P.G., 1874:45
Bergmann, E. von, 1836:27
Bergmann, W., 1951:3
Bergström, S., 1916:37
Beringer, K., 1893:42
Berlin, D.D., 1933:12
Berlin, R., 1833:30
Bernard, C., 1813:11
Bernhardt, M., 1844:24
Berson, S.A., 1918:28
Bert, P., 1833:24
Berthold, A.A., 1803:6
Bertillon, A., 1853:21
Bertin, R.J.H., 1757:5
Besnier, E., 1831:22
Besredka, A., 1870:55
Best, C.H., 1899:36
Bettinger, J., 1802:6
Bettman, A.G., 1883:28
Beurmann, C.L. de, 1851:38
Bevan, A.D., 1861:36
Bezold, F., 1842:25
Bianchi, L., 1848:22
Bichat, M.F.X., 1771:11
Bidloo, G., 1649:3
Biedl, A., 1869:43
Bielschowsky, M., 1869:28
Bier, A.K.G., 1861:42
Biermer, A., 1827:19
Biett, L.T., 1781:6
Bigelow, H.J., 1818:17
Biggs, R.P., 1952:17
Bignami, A., 1862:30
Bilharz, T.M., 1825:13
Billard, 1800:13
Billingham, R.E., 1921:52
Billings, J.S., 1838:24
Billroth, T., 1829:22

Binet, A., 1857:35
Bini, L., 1900:63
Binnig, G., 1947:24
Bircher, E., 1921:23
Bishop, K.S., 1888:58
Bishop, M., 1936:32
Bittner, J.J., 1904:30
Bizzozero, G.C., 1846:26
Black, J.W., 1924:39
Blackfan, K.D., 1883:34
Blackley, C.H., 1820:22
Blacklock, D.B., 1879:29
Blackwell, E., 1821:24
Blaes, G., 1626:2
Blair, P., 1660:5
Blair, V.P., 1871:29
Blalock, A., 1899:37
Bland, E.F., 1901:39
Bland, J.O.W., 1932:27
Blane, G., 1749:4
Blasius, G., 1626:2
Blaud, P., 1774:12
Bleuler, P.E., 1857:29
Blickhahn, W.L., 1893:6
Bloch, K.E., 1912:41
Bloch, O.T., 1847:30
Blocq, P., 1860:59
Bloodgood, J.C., 1867:34
Bloom, B.R., 1937:36
Blount, W.P., 1900:78
Blumberg, B.S., 1925:36
Blumgart, H.L., 1895:45
Blundell, J., 1790:10
Blunt, T.P., 1877:25
Boas, I.I., 1858:33
Bobbs, J.S., 1809:14
Bodington, G., 1799:15
Boeck, C.P.M., 1845:33
Boeck, C.W., 1808:11
Boeck, W.C., 1894:37
Boerhaave, H., 1668:6
Böhler, L., 1885:33
Boghurst, W., 1631:2
Boivin, M.A.V., 1773:7
Bokay, J., 1858:31
Bollinger, O., 1843:25
Bollstadt, A. von, 1193:1
Bolton, J., 1812:13
Bonaventura, F., 1555:2
Bondt, J. de, 1592:1
Bonet, J.P., 1579:3
Bonet, T., 1620:3
Bonifacio, G., 1616:2
Bonomo, G.C., 1666:11
Bontius, 1592:1
Boorde, A., 1490:1
Boothby, W.M., 1880:43

Borde, A., 1490:1
Bordet, J.J.B.V., 1870:38
Borovskii, P.F., 1863:40
Bose, K.C., 1931:21
Bossi, L.M., 1859:44
Bostock, J., 1771:13
Bostroem, E., 1850:35
Botallo, L., 1519:4
Botteri, A., 1879:60
Bottini, E., 1837:29
Bouchard, A., 1833:28
Bouchut, E., 1818:18
Bouillaud, J.B., 1796:9
Bourdillon, R.B., 1889:53
Bourgeois, L., 1563:5
Bourneville, D.M., 1840:26
Bousfield, G.W.J., 1893:38
Boveri, T., 1862:41
Bovet, D., 1907:54
Bowditch, H.P., 1840:19
Bowen, J.T., 1857:45
Bowman, W., 1816:10
Boyd, W.C., 1903:60
Boyle, H.E.G., 1875:36
Boyle, R., 1627:2
Boylston, Z., 1679:6
Bozeman, N., 1825:14
Bozzini, P., 1773:8
Bradley, W.H., 1944:17
Bradwell, S., 1594:2
Braid, J., 1795:21
Braille, L., 1809:13
Brailsford, J.F., 1888:49
Brashear, W., 1776:9
Brauer, L., 1865:38
Braun, G.A., 1829:23
Braun, H.F.W., 1862:20
Braun-Menendez, E., 1903:82
Braunschweig, H., 1450:1
Bravais, L.F., 1842:36
Bravo, F., 1530:5
Breda, A., 1850:40
Breinl, A., 1905:14
Breinl, F., 1888:47
Breisky, A., 1832:25
Breithaupt, 1855:11
Brenner, F., 1877:62
Brent, L., 1925:35
Bretonneau, P.F., 1778:10
Breuer, J., 1842:23
Breus, C., 1852:37
Bricheteau, I., 1789:11
Bridges, C.B., 1889:40
Briggs, J.E., 1869:50
Briggs, W., 1642:5
Bright, R., 1789:13
Bright, T., 1551:5

Brill, N.E., 1860:27
Brinckerhoff, W.R., 1875:62
Brinton, W., 1823:24
Brisseau, M., 1676:4
Broadbent, W., 1868:42
Broca, P.P., 1824:15
Brock, R.C., 1903:71
Brocklesby, R., 1722:5
Brocq, L.A.J., 1856:21
Broders, A.C., 1885:42
Brodie, B., 1783:7
Brodmann, K., 1868:47
Brown, J., 1854:48
Brown, J.B., 1899:46
Brown, M.S., 1941:24
Brown, R., 1773:12
Brown, T.G., 1961:8
Brown, W., 1752:11
Brown-Séquard, C.É., 1817:15
Browne, J., 1642:4
Browne, T., 1605:1
Browning, C.H., 1881:43
Brownlee, G., 1943:4
Bruce, D., 1855:25
Bruch, A., 1910:15
Brücke, E.W. von, 1819:16
Brücke, H., 1951:15
Brumpt, A.E., 1877:31
Brunel, P.A., 1931:38
Brunn, H., 1874:47
Brunner, J.C. à, 1653:3
Bruns, P., 1846:31
Bruns, V. von, 1812:15
Brunschwig, A., 1901:49
Brunschwig, H., 1450:1
Brunton, J., 1836:31
Brunton, T.L., 1844:22
Bruton, O.C., 1908:55
Buchner, E., 1860:39
Buchner, H.E., 1850:41
Buck, G., 1807:9
Bucknill, J.C., 1817:23
Bucky, G., 1880:45
Budd, G., 1808:9
Budd, W., 1811:16
Bünger, C.H., 1782:8
Buerger, L., 1879:52
Bugie, E., 1944:4
Buist, J.B., 1846:27
Bulbulian, A.H., 1900:71
Bulloch, W., 1868:44
Bulwer, J., 1654:4
Bunnell, W.W., 1902:49
Bunon, R., 1702:3
Bunyan, J., 1907:73
Burchenal, J.H., 1912:53
Burckhardt, G., 1891:16

Burgauer, D., 1534:1
Burgi, E., 1952:22
Burkitt, D.P., 1911:43
Burman, M.S., 1931:15
Burnet, F.M., 1899:45
Burnham, W., 1808:7
Burns, A., 1781:4
Burrows, M.T., 1884:59
Burton, H., 1799:14
Burton, H.S., 1951:17
Burton, J., 1697:5
Burton, R., 1577:3
Buschke, A., 1868:54
Busk, G., 1807:12
Busquet, G.P., 1866:52
Buss, C.E., 1878:26
Busse, O., 1867:44
Butcher, R.W., 1968:3
Butenandt, A.F.J., 1903:61
Butler, R.E., 1902:47
Butt, H.R., 1910:50
Butzengeiger, O., 1927:9
Buxbaum, A., 1898:11
Bylon, D., 1780:7
Bywaters, E.G.L., 1910:58

Cade, J., 1912:56
Cadogan, W., 1711:3
Caelius Aurelianus, 500:1
Cagniard-Latour, C., 1777:9
Cahn, A., 1887:33
Cairns, H.W.B., 1896:69
Caius, J., 1510:1
Caldas, J., 1931:7
Calder, J., 1733:6
Caldwell, G.W., 1834:31
Caldwell, W.E., 1880:36
Callisen, A.C.P., 1787:12
Calmette, L.C.A., 1863:43
Calvé, J., 1875:56
Caminopetros, J., 1936:15
Campbell, A.W., 1868:31
Campbell, N.E., 1938:20
Camper, P., 1722:3
Camps, P.W.L., 1877:52
Canalis, P., 1856:36
Cannon, W.B., 1871:38
Canstatt, C.F., 1807:11
Capivaccio, G., 1523:2
Carabelli, G., 1787:9
Carcano Leone, G.B., 1536:3
Cardano, G., (Cardanus), 1501:2
Carey, M., 1760:4
Carle, A., 1854:37
Carnochan, J.M., 1817:17
Carpue, J.C., 1764:8
Carr, F.H., 1906:42

Carrel, A., 1873:29
Carrión, D.A., 1857:36
Carroll, J., 1854:39
Carter, H.R., 1852:45
Carter, H.V., 1831:15
Carter, J.B., 1889:72
Cary, W.H., 1883:45
Casal y Julian, G., 1679:7
Cassen, B., 1902:41
Castellani, A., 1877:43
Castle, W.B., 1897:40
Castro, R. de, 1541:1
Castroviejo, R., 1904:37
Cathelin, F., 1873:27
Catlin, G., 1796:8
Cavendish, H., 1731:4
Caventou, J.B., 1795:18
Cawley, T., 1788:5
Cayley, W., 1836:25
Cazenave, P.L.A., 1795:14
Cech, T.R., 1947:23
Celli, A., 1857:25
Celsus, 30:1
Cenci, F., 1907:22
Cerletti, U., 1877:44
Cervello, V., 1854:32
Cesalpino, A., 1519:3
Cestoni, G., 1637:3
Chabert, P., 1737:4
Chadwick, E., 1800:9
Chagas, C.R.J., 1879:38
Chain, E.B., 1906:55
Chamberland, C., 1851:22
Chamberlen family, 1631:3
Chambers, S.O., 1897:43
Champetier de Ribes, C.L.A., 1848:26
Champier, S., 1472:3
Chang, F.F., 1957:15
Chang, M.C., 1908:52
Channing, W., 1786:13
Chantemesse, A., 1851:35
Chaoul, H., 1887:55
Chapin, C.W., 1877:59
Chapuis, J., 1896:38
Charaka, 800 BC
Charcot, J.M., 1825:18
Chardack, W.M., 1960:6
Chargaff, E., 1905:40
Charlton, W., 1889:66
Charnley, J., 1911:54
Charpy, J., 1900:77
Chase, M.C., 1952:5
Chase, M.W., 1905:41
Chassaignac, P.M.E., 1804:15
Chatin, G.A., 1813:14
Chauffard, A.M.E., 1855:29
Chauliac, G. de, 1298:1

Chauveau, J.B.A., 1827:20
Chauvel, H., 1896:38
Chauvet, S., 1885:51
Cheadle, W.B., 1836:21
Cheatle, G.L., 1865:27
Cheevers, N., 1818:26
Cheselden, W., 1688:1
Chevreul, M.E., 1786:15
Cheyne, G., 1671:5
Cheyne, J., 1777:8
Chiari, H., 1851:21
Chiarugi, V., 1759:6
Chisholm, C., 1755:3
Chittenden, R.H., 1856:42
Chopart, F., 1743:7
Choulant, J.L., 1791:7
Christian, H.A., 1876:42
Christopherson, J.B., 1868:57
Chvostek, F., 1835:14
Cid dos Santos, J., 1970:8
Citois, F., 1572:4
Civiale, J., 1792:11
Clarke, G.R., 1949:20
Clarke, J., 1761:8
Clarke, J.A.L., 1817:24
Clarke, R.H., 1850:38
Claude, A., 1899:43
Clay, C., 1801:19
Cleland, A., 1744:2
Cleland, J., 1835:15
Cleland, J.B., 1878:34
Cloquet, J.H., 1787:7
Clouston, T.S., 1840:20
Clover, J.T., 1825:19
Clow, A.D., 1936:28
Clowes, W., 1540:3
Coats, G., 1876:67
Cock, E., 1805:7
Codivilla, A., 1861:26
Codronchi, G.B., 1547:3
Coffey, R.C., 1869:44
Cogswell, M.F., 1761:9
Cohen, S., 1922:42
Cohnheim, J., 1839:29
Coindet, J.F., 1774:6
Coiter, V., 1534:2
Cole, K.S., 1900:57
Cole, R.I., 1872:37
Cole, S.W., 1877:51
Cole, W.H., 1898:55
Colebrook, L., 1883:25
Coles, A.C., 1930:22
Colle, G., 1558:2
Colles, A., 1773:10
Collier, J.S., 1900:34
Collip, J.B., 1892:64
Colston, J.A.C., 1886:61

Daviel, J., 1693:5
Davis, J.B., 1780:16
Davis, M., 1913:46
Davy, H., 1778:12
Deacon, W.E., 1907:51
DeBakey, M.E., 1955:10
Dees, J.E., 1910:65
Defries, R.D., 1889:69
Deiters, O.F.C., 1834:28
Dejerine, J.J., 1849:28
Dejerine-Klumpke, A., 1859:48
Dekkers, F., 1648:4
Delabarre, C.F., 1777:13
Delamarre, G., 1866:18
Delay, J., 1907:78
Delbrück, M., 1906:61
Déléage, F., 1862:44
DeLee, J.B., 1869:45
Delorme, E., 1847:28
Delpech, J.M., 1777:12
Demarquay, J.N., 1814:11
DeMonbreun, W.A., 1899:41
De Nicola, R.R., 1916:52
Deniker, P., 1952:20
Denis, J., 1640:4
Denton, J.F., 1914:33
Denys, J., 1640:4
Dercum, F.X., 1856:31
Derosne, C.L., 1780:14
Derrick, E.H., 1898:56
Desault, P.J., 1744:5
Descartes, R., 1596:4
Descemet, J., 1732:5
Detmold, W., 1808:12
Deventer, H. van, 1651:3
Devergie, M.G.A., 1798:12
DeWall, A.V., 1926:39
Dewees, W.P., 1768:10
Dhanwantari, 500 BC
Diamond, L.K., 1902:36
Diaz, F., 1580:1
Diaz de Isla, R.R., 1462:1
Dibdin, W.J., 1850:43
Dick, G.F., 1881:47
Dick, G.R., 1881:55
Dick-Read, G., 1890:37
Dieffenbach, J.F., 1792:8
Diemerbroeck, Y. van, 1609:5
Dienes, L., 1937:17
Dietl, J., 1804:17
Dimsdale, T., 1712:3
Diocles *of Carystus*, 360 BC
Dioscorides, 54:1
Dobell, C., 1886:46
Dobson, M., 1731:6
Dochez, A.R., 1882:47
Dodd, M.C., 1910:55

Dodds, E.C., 1899:49
Dodrill, F.D., 1902:43
Döderlein, A.S.G., 1860:42
Döhle, K.G.P., 1855:27
Dörfler, J., 1899:22
Doerr, R., 1871:39
Dogliotti, A.M., 1897:39
Dohan, F.C., 1907:55
Doisy, E.A., 1893:39
Doll, W.R.S., 1912:49
Domagk, G., 1895:49
Donald, A., 1860:35
Donald, I., 1910:64
Donath, J., 1870:49
Donath, W.F., 1889:48
Donati, M., 1538:2
Donders, F.C., 1818:19
Donné, A., 1801:20
Donovan, C., 1863:51
Dorsey, J.S., 1783:11
Dotter, C.T., 1964:6
Double, F., 1776:10
Douglas, C.D., 1882:59
Douglas, J., 1675:2
Douglas, S.R., 1871:27
Douglass, W., 1691:4
Dover, T., 1662:7
Dowling, G.B., 1891:51
Downes, A.H., 1851:34
Dragstedt, L.R., 1893:37
Drbohlav, J., 1893:44
Dreschfeld, J., 1846:34
Dreser, H., 1860:55
Dressler, L.A., 1815:23
Drinker, P., 1894:51
Dubini, A., 1813:15
Du Bois, P.A., 1795:20
Dubois de Chemant, 1753:7
Du Bois Reymond, E., 1818:23
Dubos, R.J., 1901:40
Dubost, C., 1914:42
Duché, L.L., 1784:6
Duchenne de Boulogne, G.B.A., 1806:11
Ducrey, A., 1860:53
Dudley, B.W., 1785:8
Dudley, H.W., 1887:53
Düben, G.W.J., 1822:23
Dührssen, A., 1862:28
Duel, A.B., 1870:58
Duggar, B.M., 1872:46
Duhring, L.A., 1845:40
Duke-Elder, W.S., 1898:49
Du Laurens, A., 1558:3
Dulbecco, R., 1914:30
Dumas, J.B.A., 1800:14
Dunant, J.H., 1828:24
Duncan, J.M., 1826:17

Dunhill, T.P., 1876:63
Dupertuis, M., 1937:14
Duplay, S., 1836:35
Dupuytren, G., 1777:11
Durand, J., 1876:83
Durand, P., 1895:57
Duret, P., 1745:7
Durham, H.E., 1866:34
Durlacher, L., 1792:14
Duroziez, P.L., 1826:16
Dutton, J.E., 1874:36
Duve, C. de, 1917:45
Duverney, J.G., 1648:3
Du Vigneaud, V., 1901:45
Dyer, R.E., 1886:63
Dyke, C.G., 1932:21

Eagle, H., 1905:39
Eaton, M.D., 1904:41
Ebers, G., 1550 BC
Eberth, C.J., 1835:21
Eble, T.E., 1923:29
Ebstein, W., 1836:24
Eccles, J.C., 1903:59
Economo, C. von, 1876:57
Eddowes, A., 1850:39
Edebohls, G.M., 1853:22
Edelman, G.M., 1929:40
Edgcomb, J.H., 1924:41
Edkins, J.S., 1863:44
Edler, I., 1911:58
Edling, L., 1878:30
Edridge-Green, F., 1863:54
Edsall, G., 1937:17
Edwards, M.L., 1960:7
Edwards, R.G., 1925:37
Edwards, W.B., 1905:53
Egas Moniz, A.C. de A.F., 1874:40
Ehlers, E., 1863:59
Ehrenberg, C.G., 1795:13
Ehrlich, J., 1907:69
Ehrlich, P., 1854:33
Ehrmann, C.H., 1792:13
Eichholtz, F., 1889:71
Eichstedt, C.F., 1816:14
Eijkman, C., 1858:38
Eilbott, W., 1900:75
Einhorn, A., 1856:23
Einhorn, M., 1862:23
Einthoven, W., 1860:40
Eiselsberg, A. von, 1860:44
Eisenhardt, L.C., 1891:61
Eisenmenger, V., 1897:22
Eisler, O., 1939:8
Ekman, O.J., 1788:3
Eldering, G., 1939:23
Elion, G.B., 1918:26

Ellenbog, U., 1440:1
Elliot, R.H., 1864:30
Elliotson, J., 1791:6
Elliott, T.R., 1877:47
Ellis, A.W.M., 1883:32
Ellis, H.H., 1859:25
Ellison, E.H., 1918:33
Ellison, R.R., 1923:27
Eloy, N.F.J., 1714:7
Elsberg, C.A., 1871:32
Elschnig, A., 1863:48
Elsner, H., 1874:48
Elvehjem, C.A., 1901:46
Ely, E.T., 1850:47
Emmerich, R., 1852:46
Emmet, T.A., 1828:39
Enders, J.F., 1897:30
Eppinger, Hans (1846–1916), 1846:22
Eppinger, Hans (1879–1946), 1879:28
Epstein, H.G., 1941:20
Epstein, M.A., 1921:47
Erasistratus, 304 BC
Erb, W.H., 1840:28
Erdheim, J., 1874:30
Erichsen, J.E., 1818:22
Erlanger, J., 1874:21
Ermengem, E.P.M. van, 1851:32
Erspamer, V., 1909:40
Escherich, T., 1857:41
Esmarch, J.F.A. von, 1823:17
Esquirol, J.E., 1772:7
Eulenburg, M.M., 1811:13
Euler, U.S. von, 1905:33
Eustachi, B., 1510:2
Evans, F.A., 1889:45
Evans, G., 1835:20
Evans, G.M., 1938:9
Evans, H.M., 1882:52
Evans, J.A., 1909:47
Eve, F.C., 1871:26
Eve, F.S., 1853:41
Everett, J.L., 1953:10
Ewing, A.W.G., 1896:79
Ewing, I.R., 1883:39
Ewing, J., 1886:68
Ewins, A.J., 1882:55
Eysell, A., 1846:23

Fabbroni, A., 1787:2
Faber, K.H., 1862:38
Fabricius ab Aquapendente, 1533:3
Fabricius Hildanus, 1560:2
Fabrizio, G., 1533:3
Fabry, W., 1560:2
Faget, G.H., 1891:47
Fagge, C.H., 1838:26
Fahr, K.T., 1877:46

Faivre, J., 1856:19
Falloppio, G. (Fallopius), 1523:1
Fallot, E.L.A., 1850:34
Falret, J.P., 1794:21
Fanconi, G., 1892:71
Fantus, B., 1874:46
Farber, S., 1903:69
Farr, S., 1741:6
Farre, J.R., 1775:4
Fascioli, J.C., 1911:59
Fatham, H.B., 1876:73
Fauchard, P., 1678:3
Fauvel, S.A., 1813:17
Favaloro, R.G., 1968:5
Favre, M., 1876:75
Fechner, G.T., 1801:13
Fedchenko, A.P., 1844:44
Feeney, R.J., 1951:3
Fehleisen, F., 1854:46
Fehr, J.M., 1610:2
Feil, A., 1884:67
Feldberg, W., 1900:67
Feldman, W.H., 1892:65
Felix, A., 1887:44
Felty, A.R., 1895:56
Fenner, F.J., 1914:40
Ferguson, A.H., 1853:17
Fergusson, W., 1808:10
Fermi, C., 1862:21
Fernel, J., 1497:3
Ferrall, M., 1790:12
Ferrier, D., 1843:28
Ferry, E.S., 1868:41
Fibiger, J.A.G., 1867:27
Fiedler, C.L., 1835:19
Fiessinger, N., 1881:56
Filatov, N.F., 1847:38
Filatov, V.P., 1875:31
Fildes, P., 1882:44
Filehne, W., 1844:21
Fine, P., 1760:5
Finkler, D., 1852:44
Finland, M., 1902:32
Finlay, A.C., 1906:49
Finlay, C.J., 1833:27
Finsen, N.R., 1860:52
Finsterer, H., 1877:37
Fischer, E., 1864:14
Fischer, Emil (1852–1919), 1852:48
Fischer, E.H., 1920:32
Fischer, H., 1881:48
Fischer, I., 1868:59
Fisher, R.A., 1890:38
Fitch, R.H., 1903:80
Flack, M.W., 1882:43
Flajani, G., 1741:7
Fleischer, R., 1848:31

Fleming, A., 1881:49
Flemming, W., 1843:27
Fletcher, R., 1823:19
Fletcher, W.M., 1873:33
Flexner, A., 1866:48
Flexner, S., 1863:35
Flint, A., 1812:17
Flint, A. Jr, 1836:29
Florey, H.W., 1898:58
Florio, L.J., 1910:54
Flourens, M.J.P., 1794:14
Floyer, J., 1649:4
Foerster, Otfrid, 1873:37
Foerster, Otto, 1876:71
Fogarty, T.J., 1963:4
Foix, C., 1882:58
Foley, F.E.B., 1891:59
Folin, O.K.O., 1867:39
Følling, I.A., 1888:63
Fontaine, R., 1933:29, 1937:14
Fontana, F., 1730:8
Fonzi, G.A., 1768:14
Forel, A.H., 1848:29
Forestier, J., 1890:48
Forget, A., 1811:11
Forlanini, C., 1847:24
Forssell, C.G.A., 1876:44
Forssmann, W.T.O., 1904:38
Forster, J.C., 1823:23
Foshay, L., 1896:61
Foster, M., 1836:18
Foster, R., 1969:4
Fothergill, J., 1712:2
Fothergill, L.D., 1901:43
Fothergill, W.E., 1865:35
Fourneau, E., 1872:48
Fournier, J.A., 1832:28
Foville, A.L.F., 1799:16
Fowler, G.R., 1848:33
Fox, J., 1775:7
Fox, W.T., 1836:34
Fracastoro, G. (Fracastorius), 1478:2
Fraenkel, B., 1836:22
Fraenkel, C., 1861:29
Fraenkel, E., 1853:33
Fränkel, F., 1886:27
Fraenkel-Conrat, H.L., 1910:61
Franceschetti, A., 1896:75
Francis, E., 1872:34
Francis, T., 1900:58
Franco, P., 1500:3
François-Franck, C.-E., 1849:37
Frank, A.E., 1884:52
Frank, F., 1856:32
Frank, J.P., 1745:5
Frank, R., 1862:34
Franke, H., 1909:46

Franklin, P., 1880:35
Frapolli, F., 1773:13
Fraser, D.W., 1977:2
Fraser, T.R., 1841:15
Frazier, C.H., 1870:35
Freedlander, S.O., 1893:43
Freeman, J., 1877:40
Freeman, M., 1937:30
Freeman, W., 1895:50
Frei, W.S., 1885:45
Freind, J., 1675:3
Freke, J., 1688:2
Fremery, P., de 1937:6
French, T.R., 1849:38
Frerichs, F.T., 1819:13
Freud, A., 1895:51
Freud, S., 1856:26
Freund, A. von, 1835:18
Freund, J.T., 1890:42
Freund, L., 1868:36
Freund, W.A., 1833:22
Frey, W., 1884:46
Frick, G., 1793:21
Fricke, J.K.G., 1790:5
Friderichsen, C., 1886:73
Frieben, E., 1875:54
Friedheim, E.A.H., 1948:21
Friedländer, K., 1847:31
Friedman, H., 1903:84
Friedmann, M., 1906:25
Friedreich, N., 1826:18
Frisch, K. von, 1886:66
Fritsch, G.T., 1838:23
Fröhlich, A., 1871:31
Froin, G., 1874:50
Frosch, P., 1860:45
Fry, W.K., 1889:42
Fuchs, E., 1851:29
Fuchs, F., 1960:11
Fuchs, J., 1955:14
Fuchs, L., 1501:1
Fürbringer, P., 1849:29
Fütterer, G., 1854:49
Fuller, F., 1670:4
Fuller, H.W., 1820:23
Fulton, F., 1913:56
Funk, C., 1884:47
Funke, O., 1828:31
Futaki, K., 1873:45

Gaddum, J.H., 1900:53
Gaertner, A., 1848:23
Gaffky, G., 1850:22
Gaisford, W.F., 1902:33
Gajdusek, D.C., 1923:28
Gale, T., 1507:1
Galen, 129:1

Gall, F.J., 1758:3
Galli Mainini, C., 1914:36
Gallie, W.E., 1882:42
Galtier, V., 1845:36
Galton, D.A.G., 1955:11
Galton, F., 1822:14
Galvani, L., 1732:6
Ganter, G., 1923:16
Garcia, M., 1805:8
Garcia d'Orta, 1501:3
Garcia Tapia, A., 1875:59
Gardner, W., 1877:19
Garner, R.L., 1906:50
Garretson, J.E., 1828:30
Garrison, F.H., 1870:47
Garrod, A.B., 1819:15
Garrod, A.E., 1857:39
Gaskell, W.H., 1847:29
Gasser, H.S., 1888:48
Gasser, J.L., 1757:8
Gaucher, P.C.E., 1854:41
Gauss, C.J., 1875:46
Gay, F.P., 1874:34
Gay Prieto, J.A., 1905:50
Gayet, C.J.A., 1833:29
Gee, S.J., 1839:31
Gegenbaur, K., 1826:19
Geisböck, F., 1905:26
Gelfan, S., 1903:58
Gélineau, J.B.E., 1859:47
Gelmo, P., 1879:50
Generali, F., 1896:39
Gengou, O., 1875:33
Gentles, J.C., 1958:12
Georgi, W., 1889:46
Geraghty, J.T., 1876:78
Gerard, J., 1545:3
Gerbec, M. (Gerbezius), 1658:4
Gerhard, W.W., 1809:8
Gerland, H., 1852:28
Gersdorff, H. von, 1500:1
Gerson, R.K., 1932:35
Gerstmann, J., 1887:60
Gesner, C., 1516:1
Gessard, C., 1850:37
Ghedini, G., 1877:53
Ghon, A., 1866:51
Gianturco, C., 1905:34
Gibbon, J.H., 1903:68
Gibbs, C.J., 1971:3
Gibert, C.M., 1797:11
Gibson, T., 1915:31
Gibson, W., 1788:6
Gierke, E.O.K. von, 1877:29
Gigli, L., 1863:38
Gilbert, R., 1939:20
Gilbert, W., 1932:32

Hahnemann, C.F.S., 1755:5
Halberstaedter, L., 1876:64
Hald, J., 1948:11
Haldane, J.B.S., 1892:63
Haldane, J.S., 1860:37
Hales, S., 1677:2
Hall, M., 1790:6
Hall, M.C., 1881:46
Hall, R.J., 1856:41
Hallas-Møller, K., 1914:44
Haller, A. von, 1708:2
Hallervorden, J., 1882:57
Halley, E., 1656:4
Hallopeau, F.H., 1842:24
Hallopeau, P., 1876:74
Hallpike, C.S., 1900:59
Halsted, W.S., 1852:47
Haly Abbas, 930:1
Hamburger, G.E., 1697:4
Hamilton, F.H., 1813:13
Hamilton, R., 1721:5
Hammon, W.M., 1904:33
Hammond, W.A., 1828:29
Hammurabi, 1792 BC
Hanau, A.N., 1858:32
Hancock, H., 1809:9
Hand, A., 1868:34
Handley, W.S., 1872:36
Hanger, F.M., 1894:47
Hannover, A., 1814:10
Hanot, V.C., 1844:30
Hansen, G.H.A., 1841:17
Hansmann, G.H., 1890:53
Hanson, F.R., 1921:53
Hardaway, W.A., 1850:17
Hardy, J.D., 1918:29
Hare, R., 1899:44
Hare, W.K., 1908:46
Harington, C.R., 1897:38
Harington, J., 1560:4
Harken, D.E., 1910:59
Harkness, A.H., 1943:4
Harley, G., 1829:18
Harris, C.A., 1806:9
Harris, L.J., 1898:65
Harris, S.H., 1881:50
Harris, W., 1647:1
Harrison, F., 1896:36
Hart, A.P., 1887:58
Hartley, F., 1856:28
Hartline, H.K., 1903:76
Hartmann, A., 1849:19
Harvey, W., 1578:3
Hata, S., 1873:41
Hata, T., 1956:5
Haüy, V., 1745:8
Hauptmann, A., 1881:51

Haurowitz, F., 1930:10
Hauser, G., 1856:38
Havers, C., 1655:4
Hawkins, F.B., 1796:11
Haworth, W.N., 1883:26
Hayashi, M., 1934:20
Hayem, G., 1841:24
Haygarth, J., 1740:10
Head, H., 1861:34
Heaf, F.R.G., 1894:40
Heberden, W., Sr, 1710:7
Hebra, F. von, 1816:13
Hebra, H. von, 1847:23
Hedenius, P.J., 1906:65
Heerfordt, C.F., 1872:56
Heffter, K.W.A., 1859:33
Heidelberger, C., 1920:39
Heidelberger, M., 1888:45
Heine, J. von, 1799:17
Heine, L., 1870:53
Heister, L., 1683:6
Hektoen, L., 1863:42
Heller, A., 1840:21
Hellerström, S.C.A., 1901:57
Helmholtz, H.L.F. von, 1821:19
Helmont, J.B. van, 1579:2
Hench, P.S., 1896:63
Henderson, V.E., 1877:38
Henderson, W., 1810:7
Henderson, Y., 1873:23
Henke, P.J.W., 1834:23
Henle, F.G.J., 1809:7
Henle, G., 1968:2
Henny, G.C., 1899:35
Henoch, E.H., 1820:16
Henrotin, F., 1847:39
Henry, A.K., 1886:71
Henry, E.R., 1850:42
Henschen, S.E., 1847:22
Hepburn, J., 1888:62
Hepp, P., 1887:33
Herbert, H., 1865:23
d'Herelle, F.H., 1873:24
Hering, K.E.K., 1834:24
Hérisson, J., 1834:13
Herophilus, 350 BC
Herrick, J.B., 1861:38
Hershey, A.D., 1908:54
Herter, C.A., 1865:30
Hertwig, K.W.T.R., 1850:33
Hertwig, W.A.O., 1849:26
Hertz, A.F., 1879:39
Hertz, C.H., 1920:36
Hertz, S., 1905:47
Herxheimer, K., 1861:30
Hess, A.F., 1875:45
Hess, W.R., 1881:41

Hesselbach, F.K., 1759:5
Heubner, J.O.L., 1843:23
Heurteloup, C.L.S., 1793:11
Heusner, L., 1846:37
Hewitt, F.W., 1857:34
Hewitt, R.I., 1911:41
Hewson, W., 1739:4
Heyfelder, J.M., 1798:13
Heymans, C.J.F., 1892:56
Heysham, J., 1753:6
Hibbs, R.A., 1869:38
Hickman, H.H., 1800:12
Hicks, J.B., 1823:18
Hijmans van den Bergh, A.A., 1869:49
Hildenbrand, J.V. von, 1763:6
Hill, A.B., 1897:36
Hill, A.V., 1886:58
Hill, J., 1714:8
Hill, L.E., 1866:39
Hillier, T., 1831:24
Hilsmann, F.A., 1849:36
Hilton, J., 1804:11
Himly, C.G., 1772:9
Hindle, E., 1886:49
Hingson, R.A., 1913:64
Hinsberg, O.H., 1857:44
Hinshaw, H.C., 1902:45
Hippel, A. von, 1841:22
Hippel, E. von, 1869:36
Hippocrates, 460 BC
Hirsch, A., 1817:21
Hirsch, A.B.R., 1765:5
Hirsch, S., 1922:24, 1923:23
Hirschberg, J., 1843:26
Hirschcowitz, B.I., 1958:11
Hirschsprung, H., 1830:16
Hirst, G.K., 1909:35
His, W., Sr, 1831:17
His, W., Jr, 1863:55
Hitchings, G.H., 1905:36
Hitschmann, F., 1870:61
Hitzig, E., 1838:21
Hlava, J., 1855:35
Hobrecht, J., 1825:25
Hodge, H.L., 1796:7
Hodges, C.V., 1941:11
Hodgkin, A.L., 1914:29
Hodgkin, D.M.C., 1910:57
Hodgkin, T., 1798:10
Höck, H., 1893:19
Högyes, E., 1847:35
Hoffmann, E., 1868:37
Hoffmann, F., 1660:3
Hoffmann, J., 1857:46
Hofmann, A., 1906:46
Hogan, A.G., 1884:62
Hohenheim, T.P.A.B. von, 1493:2

Holder, W., 1616:6
Holley, R.W., 1922:35
Holloway, A., 1960:10
Holly, L.E., 1930:30
Holmes, G.M., 1876:43
Holmes, O.W., 1809:10
Holmgren, A.F., 1831:19
Holmgren, G., 1875:44
Holst, A., 1860:47
Holt, L.E., 1855:23
Holth, S., 1863:45
Holtz, F., 1933:27
Holzknecht, G., 1872:54
Homans, J., 1877:54
Home, E., 1756:4
Home, F., 1719:3
Homolle, A.E., 1808:13
Hood, W.P., 1835:24
Hoof, L. van, 1947:21
Hooke, R., 1635:2
Hope, J., 1801:12
Hopkins, F.G., 1861:32
Hopkins, H.H., 1918:34
Hoppe-Seyler, F., 1825:20
Horner, J.F., 1831:14
Horsley, V.A.H., 1857:28
Horst, G., 1688:3
Hounsfield, G.N., 1919:42
Houssay, B.A., 1887:47
Houston, R., 1678:2
Howard, J., 1726:3
Howell, W.H., 1860:30
Howitt, B.F., 1891:52
Huang-ti, 2700 BC
Hubbard, J.P., 1903:72
Hubel, D.H., 1926:30
Huddart, J., 1741:3
Hudson, J.R., 1931:28
Hübener, E.A., 1870:41
Huebner, C., 1941:9
Huebner, R.J., 1914:31
Hufnagel, C.A., 1916:44
Huggins, C.B., 1901:51
Huguier, P.C., 1804:18
Huismans, L., 1913:41
Huldschinsky, K., 1883:24
Hulen, V.H., 1865:40
Hunt, G.H., 1884:49
Hunter, C., 1872:32
Hunter, E.F., 1964:3
Hunter, J., 1728:2
Hunter, W., 1718:6
Huntington, G., 1850:24
Hurlock, J., 1742:5
Hurst, A.F., 1879:39
Hutchinson, John, 1811:9
Hutchinson, Jonathan, 1828:28

Kast, A., 1856:37
Kast, T., 1755:10
Katsurada, F., 1868:38
Katz, B., 1911:44
Katz, S.L., 1927:33
Kauffmann, F., 1931:23
Kaufmann, C., 1933:38
Keefer, C.S., 1897:32
Keen, W.W., 1837:20
Kehr, H., 1903:38
Keilin, D., 1887:42
Keith, A., 1866:30
Keith, N.M., 1885:40
Kekwick, A., 1909:36
Keller, A.D., 1901:44
Kelly, H.A., 1858:29
Kelly, R.E., 1879:34
Kendall, E.C., 1886:48
Kendall, F.E., 1898:60
Kendrew, J.C., 1917:39
Kendrick, P.L., 1890:45
Kennaway, E.L., 1881:44
Kenny, E., 1886:56
Kenny, M., 1936:31
Kent, A.F.S., 1863:36
Kerner, C.A.J., 1786:16
Kernig, V.M., 1840:30
Kerr, C.B., 1965:5
Kerr, R.B., 1908:51
Kerst, D.W., 1911:56
Keynes, G.L., 1887:43
Khorana, H.G., 1922:34
Kielland, C., 1871:46
Kienböck, R., 1871:23
Kikuth, W., 1896:80
Kilborne, F.L., 1858:43
Kilian, H.F., 1800:10
Killian, G., 1860:41
Kimball, G., 1804:14
Kimmelstiel, P., 1900:76
King, A.F.A., 1841:13
King, H., 1887:41
King, J., 1817:10, 1818:8
Kinghorn, A., 1880:55
Kinmonth, J.B., 1916:40
Kircher, A., 1602:3
Kirkes, W.S., 1823:28
Kirschner, M., 1879:45
Kirstein, A., 1863:41
Kitasato, S., 1852:53
Kite, J.H., 1891:54
Klarenbeek, A., 1888:66
Klebs, T.A.E., 1834:20
Klein, E.E., 1844:38
Kleine, F.K., 1869:32
Klemperer, F., 1866:44
Klemperer, G., 1865:25

Klemperer, P., 1887:50
Klencke, P.F.H., 1813:16
Klieneberger, E., 1892:55
Klinefelter, H.F., 1912:42
Kling, C., 1887:61
Klippel, M., 1858:34
Klug, A., 1926:37
Knapp, A.H., 1869:37
Knapp, J.H., 1832:24
Knapp, R.E., 1884:69
Kneisel, F.C., 1797:10
Knight, G.C., 1906:63
Knoll, M., 1879:61
Knotts, F.L., 1912:55
Knowles, R., 1883:43
Koch, R., 1843:32
Kocher, E.T., 1841:18
Koeberlé, E., 1828:26
Köhler, A., 1874:25
Köhler, G.J.F., 1946:24
Köhler, W., 1887:39
Kölliker, R.A. von, 1817:18
König, F., 1832:22
Körte, W., 1853:35
Kohn, M., 1837:31
Kolff, W.J., 1911:42
Kolisko, A., 1847:42
Kolle, W., 1868:46
Koller, K., 1857:42
Kolmer, J.A., 1886:53
Kondo, K., 1970:7
Koplik, H., 1858:41
Koprowski, H., 1916:50
Korány, S., 1866:51
Kornberg, A., 1918:27
Korotkov, N.S., 1874:24
Korsakoff, S.S., 1854:30
Kossel, K.M.L.A., 1853:31
Kraepelin, E., 1856:22
Krafft-Ebing, R. von, 1840:25
Krantz, J.C., 1899:48
Kraske, H., 1923:11
Kraske, P., 1851:26
Kraus, R., 1868:51
Krause, F., 1857:24
Krauss, J., 1841:27
Krebs, E.G., 1918:31
Krebs, H.A., 1900:62
Krishnaswami, C.S., 1912:15
Krönig, B., 1863:30
Krogh, S.A.S., 1874:39
Krugman, S., 1911:46
Krukenberg, F.E., 1870:60
Küchler, H., 1811:10
Kühne, W.F., 1837:22
Kümmell, H., 1852:57
Küster, E.G.F. von, 1839:34

Levaditi, C., 1874:35
Levan, J.A., 1905:35
Leventhal, M.L., 1901:58
Lever, J.C.W., 1811:17
Levi-Montalcini, R., 1909:37
Levine, L., 1924:40
Levine, P., 1900:73
Levine, S.A., 1891:42
Levinthal, C.W., 1886:75
Levret, A., 1703:3
Lewin, G.R., 1820:14
Lewis, E.B., 1918:30
Lewis, P.A., 1879:35
Lewis, T., 1881:57
Lewis, T.R., 1841:19
Lewisohn, R., 1875:53
Lewthwaite, R., 1894:49
Lexer, E., 1867:41
Leyden, E. von, 1832:26
Leydig, F., 1821:17
Li, C.H., 1913:59
Libman, E., 1872:45
Lichtenberg, A. von, 1880:33
Lichtheim, L., 1845:39
Liddell, E.G.T., 1924:18
Liébeault, A.A., 1823:21
Lieberkühn, J., 1711:2
Liebig, J. von, 1803:7
Liebreich, O., 1839:23
Liebreich, R., 1830:10
Liepmann, H.K., 1863:37
Lignières, J.L.M., 1868:58
Liley, A.W., 1963:5
Lilienthal, H., 1861:39
Lillie, R.D., 1896:70
Linacre, T., 1524:1
Lind, J., 1716:4
Lindau, A.V., 1892:73
Lindenberg, A.C., 1872:59
Lindenmann, J., 1924:43
Lindstedt, A.F., 1847:34
Ling, P.H., 1776:13
Link, K.P., 1941:9
Linnaeus, C., 1707:8
Linné, C. von, 1707:8
Linser, P., 1871:33
Lipmann, F.A., 1899:40
Lisfranc, J., 1790:7
Lister, J., 1827:16
Liston, R., 1794:16
Little, C.C., 1888:55
Little, W.J., 1810:13
Littré, A., 1658:3
Litzmann, C.C.T., 1815:19
Liveing, E., 1832:21
Livingstone, D., 1813:9
Lizars, J., 1794:22

Lloyd, W.D.M., 1902:50
Lobstein, J.G.C.F.M., 1777:14
Lockwood, C.B., 1856:40
Lodge, O., 1851:28
Loeb, J., 1859:29
Loeb, L., 1869:41
Loeffler, F.A.J., 1852:43
Lösch, F., 1840:31
Löw, O., 1844:41
Loewe, L., 1896:65
Loewenberg, B., 1836:30
Loewenhardt, S.E., 1796:12
Loewi, O., 1873:28
Lombard, E., 1869:51
Lombroso, C., 1836:23
London, E.S., 1869:48
Long, C.W., 1815:20
Long, J.A., 1879:32
Longmore, T., 1816:15
Looser, E., 1905:20
Looss, A., 1861:25
Lopez Lacarrere, J., 1932:28
Lorenz, A., 1854:43
Lorenz, K.Z., 1903:73
Loreta, P., 1831:23
Lorry, C. de, 1726:2
Lotheissen, G., 1868:53
Lotze, R.H., 1817:16
Loubatières, A., 1912:54
Louis, P.C.A., 1787:6
Lovelace, W.R., 1907:70
Low, G.C., 1872:49
Lowe, P., 1560:3
Lower, R., 1631:1
Lower, R.R., 1929:42
Lowson, D., 1850:44
Luc, H., 1855:19
Lucae, A., 1835:23
Lucas, G.H.W., 1894:45
Lucas, W.P., 1880:34
Lucas-Championnière, 1843:30
Lucatello, L., 1863:46
Luckett, W.H., 1872:60
Luckhardt, A.B., 1885:43
Ludwig, C., 1816:18
Ludwig, W.F., 1790:11
Lugol, J.G.A., 1786:14
Luke, J., 1798:11
Lukens, F.D.W., 1899:47
Lumsden, L.L., 1875:58
Lundy, J.S., 1894:41
Luria, S.E., 1912:47
Luschka, H. von, 1820:18
Lushbaugh, C.C., 1916:38
Lutembacher, R., 1884:58
Lutz, A., 1855:32
Lutz, H.C., 1860:15

Lwoff, A.M., 1902:35
Lynen, F.F.K., 1911:45
Lysholm, E., 1891:60

McBurney, C., 1845:21
MacCallum, F.O., 1944:16, 1944:17
MacCallum, W.G., 1874:28
McCarrison, R., 1878:31
McCarthy, J.F., 1874:31
McCarty, M., 1911:47
McClelland, L., 1912:52
McClintock, B., 1902:38
McCollum, E.V., 1879:31
MacCormac, W., 1836:17
McCorquodale, D.W., 1898:53
McCoy, G.W., 1876:54
McCreary, C., 1785:10
McDevitt, H.O., 1972:4
McDowell, E., 1771:10
Macewen, W., 1848:18
Macfarlane, R.G., 1907:59
McGill, A.F., 1846:38
Macgill, W.D., 1802:13
McGuire, J.M., 1909:38
Machin, J., 1751:4
Macht, D.I., 1882:45
McIndoe, A.H., 1900:54
McIntosh, J., 1922:18
Macintyre, J., 1859:41
Macintyre, W., 1850:8
McKee, C.M., 1940:18
Mackenrodt, A.K., 1859:42
Mackenzie, J., 1853:20
Mackenzie, M., 1837:27
Mackenzie, R.J., 1821:23
Mackenzie, S., 1844:37
Mackenzie, W., 1791:12
McKesson, E.I., 1881:61
McKhann, C.F., 1930:31
Mackie, F.P., 1875:32
McKinnon, N.E., 1894:36
Maclagan, N.F., 1904:42
Maclagan, T.J., 1838:31
McLean, J., 1890:44
Macleod, C.M., 1909:49
Macleod, J.J.R., 1876:59
Macleod, K., 1840:23
McMillan, B.M., 1907:64
Macnamara, J., 1931:19
McNee, J.W., 1887:56
Macpherson, A.I., 1939:19
McVay, C.B., 1911:52
Madelung, O.W., 1846:29
Maffucci, A., 1845:37
Magendie, F., 1783:10
Magill, T.P., 1903:64
Magnus, H.G., 1802:7

Magrath, G.B., 1870:44
Mahaffey, D.E., 1955:10
Mahoney, J.F., 1889:60
Maier, R., 1824:10
Maimon, M. ben, 1135:1
Maimonides, 1135:1
Maisonneuve, J.G.T., 1809:11
Maitland, H.B., 1895:59
Maitland, M.C., 1972:5
Maître-Jan, A., 1650:3
Majocchi, D., 1849:30
Major, J.D., 1634:2
Malassez, L.C., 1842:33
Malcarne, M.V.G., 1744:7
Malgaigne, J.F., 1806:7
Malmsten, P.H., 1811:15
Malpighi, M., 1628:3
Malt, R.A., 1931:37
Malthus, T.R., 1766:3
Mandl, F., 1892:69
Mann, H., 1891:53
Manson, P., 1844:35
Mantoux, C., 1877:34
Marcet, A.J.G., 1770:9
Marchand, F.J., 1846:40
Marchiafava, E., 1847:41
Marchoux, E., 1862:29
Marcy, H.O., 1837:25
Marey, E.J., 1830:7
Marfan, B.J.A., 1858:35
Marie, P., 1853:29
Marrian, G.F., 1904:31
Marriott, H.L., 1900:66
Marriott, W.M., 1885:36
Marsh, J., 1794:16
Marshall, E.K., 1889:47
Marston, J.A., 1831:25
Marten, B., 1720:3
Martin, A.J.P., 1910:52
Martin, A.L.F.J., 1853:43
Martin, C.J., 1866:27
Martin, E., 1859:38
Martine, G., 1702:4
Masius, J.B.N.V., 1836:32
Mason, V.R., 1889:50
Massa, N., 1489:3
Matas, R., 1860:49
Mathijsen, A., 1805:10
Mattioli, P.A., 1500:2
Mauriceau, F., 1637:4
Maury, F.F., 1840:24
Maxcy, K.F., 1889:49
Maxey, E.E., 1867:32
Maxwell, J.P., 1871:42
Maydl, K., 1853:18
Mayer, A., 1843:34
Mayer, L., 1884:68

Mayer, M.M., 1916:42
Mayo, C.H., 1900:1
Mayo, W.J., 1861:31
Mayo, W.W., 1900:1
Mayou, M.S., 1876:52
Mayow, J., 1641:2
Maytum, C.K., 1895:52
Mead, R., 1673:3
Mears, J.E., 1838:32
Meckel, J.F. *the elder*, 1724:4
Meckel, J.F. *the younger*, 1781:5
Meckel von Hemsbach, H., 1822:18
Medawar, P.B., 1915:26
Medes, G., 1886:64
Medin, O., 1847:36
Meduna, L.J., 1896:64
Meekeren, J.J. van 1, 611:3
Meibom, H., 1638:3
Meigs, J.V., 1892:62
Mein, 1831:9
Meinicke, E., 1878:39
Mélier, F., 1798:9
Mellanby, E., 1884:48
Meltzer, S.J., 1851:23
Mendel, G., 1822:20
Menees, T.O., 1890:52
Menetrier, P.E., 1859:43
Menière, P., 1799:9
Menkes, J.H., 1928:31
Menkin, V., 1901:41
Mercier, L.A., 1811:14
Merck, G.F., 1825:24
Mercuriali, G., 1530:4
Mercurio, G.S., 1550:1
Mering, J. von, 1849:34
Merrill, J.P., 1917:38
Merritt, H.H., 1902:30
Meryon, E., 1809:16
Merzbacher, L., 1875:30
Mesmer, F.A., 1734:2
Mestrezat, W., 1883:41
Metchnikoff, E., 1845:28
Mettauer, J.P., 1787:10
Metz, O., 1905:46
Meulengracht, E., 1887:45
Meyer, H.M., 1928:30
Meyer, H.W., 1825:21
Meyer, W., 1885:3
Meyerhof, O.F., 1884:50
Meynert, T.H., 1833:20
Mibelli, V., 1860:29
Michaelis, G.A., 1798:14
Middeldorpf, A.T., 1824:16
Middleton, P., 1781:7
Miescher, J.F., 1844:33
Mikulicz-Radecki, J., von 1850:25
Miles, W.E., 1869:26

Milkman, L.A., 1895:55
Millar, J., 1733:11
Miller, B.F., 1907:63
Miller, J.A.P., 1931:35
Miller, J.D., 1930:30
Miller, W.D., 1853:26
Millin, T.J., 1903:56
Mills, C.K., 1845:38
Milne, A.D., 1932:36
Milne, J., 1776:14
Milovanović, M., 1958:14, 1960:10
Milstein, C., 1927:35
Minami, S., 1923:17
Minkowski, O., 1858:28
Minnitt, R.J., 1889:55
Minot, G.R., 1885:48
Mirault, G., 1796:13
Miravé, F.P., 1924:46
Mitchell, J.K., 1793:14
Mitchell, P.D., 1920:35
Mitchell, S.W., 1829:19
Mitchison, N.A., 1928:27
Mitsuda, K., 1876:70
Mixter, W.J., 1880:53
Miyairi, K., 1865:26
Möbius, P.J., 1854:31
Möller, E.H.H., 1929:29
Möller, J.O.L., 1819:17
Mönckeberg, J.G., 1877:41
Mohr, B., 1809:15
Moir, J.C., 1900:81
Møllgaard, H., 1885:38
Moloy, H.C., 1903:83
Monakow, C. von, 1853:36
Monardes, N., 1493:3
Mondeville, H. de, 1260:1
Mondino de'Luzzi, 1275:1
Mongin, 1770:7
Monks, G.H., 1853:44
Monod, J.L., 1910:51
Monro, A., *Secundus*, 1733:8
Montessori, M., 1870:42
Montgomery, W.F., 1787:11
Moon, H., 1845:41
Moon, R.C., 1844:46
Moon, W., 1818:25
Moore, C.H., 1821:18
Moore, C.R., 1892:66
Moore, F.D., 1913:57
Moore, G.E., 1922:36
Moore, J.C., 1762:6
Moore, J.W., 1879:58
Moore, S., 1913:60
Mooser, H., 1891:46
Morand, S.-F., 1697:3
Morau, H., 1860:56
Morax, V., 1866:56

Morch, E.T., 1908:50
Moreau, J.-J., 1804:16
Morestin, H., 1869:53
Morgagni, G.B., 1682:1
Morgan, H. de R., 1863:58
Morgan, T.H., 1866:43
Morison, J.R., 1853:34
Moro, E., 1874:42
Morquio, L., 1867:40
Morris, H., 1844:20
Morton, R., 1637:2
Morton, T.G., 1835:26
Morton, W.J., 1845:30
Morton, W.T.G., 1819:19
Morvan, A.M., 1819:22
Mosetig-Moorhof, A. von, 1838:19
Mosher, H.P., 1867:33
Moss, W.L., 1876:58
Mosso, A., 1846:30
Most, H., 1907:65
Mott, V., 1785:13
Mouat, F.J., 1816:20
Mouton, C., 1786:18
Moynihan, B.G.A., 1865:33
Muckenfuss, R.S., 1933:25
Müller, H., 1820:21
Müller, J., 1801:16
Müller, J.M., 1952:14
Müller, O.F., 1730:9
Müller, P.H., 1899:31
Müller, R., 1877:60
Münchmeyer, E., 1846:39
Muir, E., 1880:50
Muller, H.J., 1890:47
Mullis, K.B., 1944:24
Mundinus, 1275:1
Munk, F., 1879:33
Murphy, J.B., 1857:43
Murphy, W.P., 1892:54
Murray, D.W.G., 1894:55
Murray, E.G.D., 1890:43
Murray, H.M., 1855:33
Murray, J.E., 1919:43
Murrell, W., 1853:39
Muybridge, E., 1830:8
Myers, A.B.R., 1838:30
Myers, R.N., 1929:43

Nabarro, D.N., 1903:24
Naegele, F.C., 1778:15
Naegele, H.F.J., 1810:8
Nagai, N., 1844:42
Nagelschmidt, K.F., 1875:52
Nageotte, J., 1866:31
Nascher, I.L., 1863:57
Nasmyth, A., 1848:37
Nasse, C.F., 1778:14

Nathans, D., 1928:29
Nau, P., 1904:27
Needham, J., 1900:74
Neel, J. van G., 1915:27
Neelsen, F., 1854:36
Negri, A., 1876:56
Neher, E., 1944:21
Neisser, A.L.S., 1855:21
Nélaton, A., 1807:10
Nelson, R.A., 1922:39
Nenna, A., 1952:13
Nepveu, G., 1841:23
Netter, A., 1855:31
Nettleship, E., 1845:22
Neuber, G.A., 1850:28
Neufeld, F., 1861:44
Neumann, E., 1834:19
Neumann, I. von, 1832:23
Neva, F.A., 1922:43
Nicholls, F., 1699:3
Nicolaier, A., 1862:25
Nicolas, J., 1868:43
Nicolle, C.J.H., 1866:42
Nicolle, M., 1862:43
Niedergerke, R., 1954:15
Nielsen, H., 1866:49
Niemann, Albert (1834–1861), 1834:30
Niemann, Albert (1880–1921), 1880:52
Nightingale, F., 1820:15
Nirenberg, M.W., 1927:32
Nisbet, W., 1759:8
Nissen, R., 1896:73
Nissl, F., 1860:48
Nitze, M., 1848:30
Nobele, J. de, 1865:28
Noble, G.H., 1860:60
Nocard, E.I.E., 1850:19
Noeggerath, E., 1827:18
Noguchi, H., 1876:62
Noon, L., 1878:42
Nordtmeyer, H., 1891:39
Normet, L., 1926:12
Normond, L.A., 1834:32
Norris, C., 1867:37
North, E., 1771:12
Northrop, J.H., 1891:49
Nothnagel, C.W.H., 1841:20
Nott, J.C., 1804:7
Novinsky, M., 1841:26
Novy, F.G., 1864:35
Nowotny, F., 1872:55
Noyes, H.D., 1832:32
Nüsslein-Volhard, C., 1942:18
Nuttall, G.H.F., 1862:36
Nylin, C.G.V., 1892:74

Obermeier, O.H.F., 1843:24

Oberst, M., 1849:32
Obraztsov, V.P., 1849:35
Ochoa, S., 1905:42
O'Connor, B., 1666:10
O'Connor, W., 1880:59
Odriozola, E., 1862:47
O'Dwyer, J.P., 1841:21
Ogata, M., 1852:59
Ogata, N., 1883:44
Ogston, A., 1844:26
Oka, M., 1929:17
Olitsky, P.K., 1886:70
Oliver, G., 1841:16
Oliver, J., 1889:51
Ollier, L.X.E.L., 1830:15
Olshausen, R. von, 1835:16
O'Neill, J., 1875:9
Opie, E.L., 1873:30
Oppenheim, H., 1858:26
Oppenheim, M., 1876:81
Oppenheimer, G.D., 1932:14
Ord, W.M., 1834:27
Ordman, C.W., 1914:46
Oré, P.C., 1828:38
Orth, J., 1847:21
Orthmann, E.G., 1858:44
Osborne, E.D., 1895:40
Osborne, T.B., 1859:37
Osgood, R.B., 1873:31
O'Shaughnessy, L., 1900:72
Osiander, F.B., 1759:10
Osler, W., 1849:27
O'Sullivan, J.V., 1945:19
Otis, F.N., 1825:15
Ottenberg, R., 1882:56
Ottenstein, H.N., 1938:24
Otto, J.C., 1774:5
Otto, R., 1872:51
Ouchterlony, Ö.T.G., 1914:41
Oudot, J., 1951:5
Ould, F., 1710:8
Owen, R., 1804:9
Owens, F.M., 1913:50

Pacini, F., 1812:12
Padgett, E.C., 1893:35
Page, I.H., 1901:38
Pagenstecher, A., 1828:22
Paget, J., 1814:8
Paine, A., 1900:37
Palade, G.E., 1912:50
Panaroli, D., 1657:4
Panas, P., 1832:20
Pancoast, J., 1805:11
Pangborn, M.C., 1907:62
Panos, T.C., 1966:2
Panum, P.L., 1820:12

Papanicolaou, G.N., 1883:33
Paquelin, C.A., 1836:28
Paracelsus, 1493:2
Paré, A., 1510:4
Paris, J.A., 1785:12
Park, H., 1744:6
Parker, W., 1800:16
Parkhill, C., 1860:34
Parkin, J., 1801:14
Parkinson, J.W.K., 1785:11
Parkinson, James (1755–1824), 1755:6
Parkinson, John (1567–1650), 1567:4
Parkinson, John (1885–1976), 1885:34
Parkman, P.D., 1932:34
Parow, E., 1939:10
Parrish, P.F., 1892:25
Parrot, J., 1829:28
Parrott, E.M., 1903:74
Parry, C.H., 1755:7
Parry, J.S., 1843:22
Parsons, L.G., 1879:49
Paschen, E., 1860:54
Passow, A., 1859:46
Pasternack, A.B., 1916:53
Pasteur, L., 1822:22
Pasteur, W., 1856:39
Patek, A.J., 1904:32
Paterson, E., 1946:13
Paterson, R., 1814:15
Paton, W.D.M., 1917:42
Paul *of Aegina*, 625:1
Paul, B.H., 1828:36
Paul, F.T., 1851:36
Paul, G., 1859:26
Paul, J.R., 1893:33
Paulescu, N.C., 1869:46
Pauli, W., 1869:39
Pauling, L.C., 1901:42
Pavlov, I.P., 1849:31
Pavy, F.W., 1829:24
Pawlik, K., 1849:22
Paxton, F., 1924:45
Payne, R.M., 1909:41
Peacock, T.B., 1812:18
Péan, J.E., 1830:14
Pearce, L., 1885:35
Peebles, T.C., 1921:54
Peet, M.M., 1885:46
Pel, P.K., 1852:33
Pelizaeus, F., 1850:46
Pelletier, P.J., 1788:7
Pellier de Quengsby, 1750:4
Penada, J., 1748:4
Penfield, W.G., 1891:44
Penrose, L.S., 1898:51
Percival, T., 1740:8
Perry, R., 1783:12

Perthes, G.C., 1869:40
Perutz, M.F., 1914:34
Peters, R.A., 1889:43
Petit, J.L., 1674:6
Petri, R.J., 1852:56
Petrie, G.F., 1863:62
Pettenkofer, M.J. von, 1818:24
Pfaff, P., 1716:5
Pfannenstiel, H.J., 1862:48
Pfeiffer, E., 1846:24
Pfeiffer, R.F.J., 1858:30
Pfiffner, J.J., 1903:77
Pflüger, E.F.W., 1829:25
Phaer (Phayer, Phayr), T., 1510:3
Phemister, D.B., 1882:49
Philips, F.S., 1916:47
Physick, P.S., 1768:11
Pic, A., 1862:39
Pick, Alois, 1859:40
Pick, Arnold, 1851:30
Pick, F., 1867:38
Pick, L., 1868:45
Pilarini, G., 1659:3
Pillore, H., 1776:3
Pincus, G.G., 1903:63
Pinel, P., 1745:6
Pinkus, F., 1868:55
Pinkus, H., 1905:43
Piorry, P.A., 1794:18
Piria, R., 1815:22
Pirogov, N.I., 1810:16
Pirquet von Cesenatico, C.P., 1874:29
Piso, W., 1611:2
Pitres, J.A., 1848:36
Pitt, R.M., 1934:23
Place, E.H., 1880:56
Place, F., 1771:14
Placido da Costa, A., 1849:41
Platner, Z., 1694:1
Platter, F., 1536:4
Plaut, H.K., 1858:40
Plenck, J.J. von, 1738:1
Plotz, H., 1890:39
Ploucquet, W.G., 1744:9
Plummer, H.S., 1874:26
Pohlmann, R., 1939:10
Poiseuille, J.L.M., 1797:8
Pol, B., 1854:26
Politzer, A., 1835:22
Pollender, F.A.A., 1800:11
Pollitzer, S., 1859:24
Pólya, E.A., 1876:51
Pomerantz, C., 1946:19
Poncet, A., 1849:40
Ponfick, E., 1844:40
Porges, O., 1879:51
Porro, E., 1842:30

Porter, R.R., 1917:46
Portes, L., 1891:63
Portier, P., 1866:38
Posadas, A., 1870:52
Post, P.W., 1766:4
Potain, P.C.É., 1825:16
Poth, E.J., 1899:33
Pott, P., 1714:5
Potter, H.E., 1880:48
Poupart, F., 1661:3
Pourfour du Petit, F., 1664:5
Powell, C.B., 1894:61
Poynton, F.J., 1869:34
Pratensis, J., 1486:1
Prausnitz, O.C.W., 1876:69
Pravaz, C.G., 1791:5
Praxagoras of Cos, 340 BC
Prelog, V., 1906:57
Prévost, J.L., 1790:9
Prichard, J.C., 1786:12
Priestley, J., 1733:9
Priestley, W.O., 1829:26
Pringle, J., 1707:7
Prior, J., 1884:30
Proetz, A.W., 1888:56
Profeta, G., 1840:22
Proksch, J.K., 1840:17
Prosser, T., 1769:3
Prowazek, S.J.M. von, 1875:47
Pupin, M.I., 1858:39
Purkyně, J.E., 1787:8
Purtscher, O., 1852:49
Puschmann, T., 1844:27
Putnam, T.J., 1894:39
Putti, V., 1880:37
Pybus, F.C., 1882:53
Pyl, T., 1742:3
Pylarini (Pilarini), G., 1659:3

Queckenstedt, H.H.G., 1876:80
Queyrat, A., 1872:57
Quick, A.J., 1894:42
Quincke, H.I., 1842:28
Quinquaud, C.E., 1841:25
Quinton, W.E., 1960:9
Quittenbaum, C.F., 1793:19

Raab, W., 1895:39
Rabanus Maurus, 776:1
Radcliffe, J., 1652:6
Rake, G.W., 1940:18
Ramazzini, B., 1633:2
Rammstedt, W.C., 1867:26
Ramon, G.L., 1886:59
Ramón y Cajal, S., 1852:40
Randall, L.O., 1910:62
Ranges, H.A., 1906:66

692

Rankin, A.C., 1877:61
Raper, H.R., 1925:18
Rapp, G.W., 1917:37
Rapport, M., 1933:8
Rathke, M.H., 1793:17
Rathlev, T., 1967:6
Rattone, G., 1884:21
Raventós, J., 1956:14
Ray, I., 1807:7
Rayer, P.F.O., 1793:12
Raynaud, M., 1834:25
Récamier, J.C.A., 1774:10
Recklinghausen, F.D. von, 1833:26
Reclus, P., 1847:40
Redi, F., 1626:1
Reed, D., 1902:21
Reed, W., 1851:33
Rees, G.O., 1813:18
Rees, R.J.W., 1917:43
Refsum, S., 1907:76
Regaud, C., 1870:54
Rehn, L.M., 1849:24
Reich, A., 1864:37
Reichmann, M., 1851:37
Reichstein, T., 1897:37
Reid, J.M., 1957:9
Reil, J.C., 1759:7
Reimann, H.A., 1897:42
Reissner, E., 1824:17
Reiter, H.C.J., 1881:58
Remak, R., 1815:17
Remen, L., 1907:77
Rendu, H.J.L., 1844:31
Rendu, R., 1886:77
Rennie, A., 1859:49
Renucci, S.F., 1835:8
Retzius, A.A., 1796:10
Reuter, K., 1906:38
Reverdin, J.-L., 1842:29
Reybard, J.F., 1790:4
Rhazes, 854:1
Rhoads, C.P., 1898:52
Ribbert, M.W.H., 1855:22
Richards, A.N., 1876:46
Richards, D.W., 1895:48
Richards, H.C., 1969:4
Richardson, G.C., 1897:51
Richet, C.R., 1850:31
Richter, A.G., 1742:8
Richter, R., 1939:10
Rickes, E.L., 1912:48
Ricketts, H.T., 1871:25
Ricord, P., 1800:17
Riddle, O., 1877:45
Rideal, S., 1863:56
Ridley, N.H.L., 1906:56
Riedel, B.M.C.L., 1846:33

Rieux, L., 1853:10
Riggs, J.M., 1811:18
Riggs, L.A., 1912:44
Riis, P., 1960:11
Rimpau, W., 1877:28
Rindfleisch, G.E., 1836:26
Ringer, S., 1834:29
Rinne, F.H., 1819:12
Ritchie, C., 1799:19
Ritchie, W.T., 1873:35
Ritgen, F.A.M.F., 1787:13
Ritter, J., 1879:9
Rittershain, G. von, 1820:24
Riva-Rocci, S., 1863:47
Riverius, 1589:1
Rivière, L., 1589:1
Robb, G.P., 1898:54
Robbins, F.C., 1916:45
Roberts, A., 1942:10
Roberts, R.J., 1943:16
Robertson, D.M.C.L.A., 1837:34
Robertson, E.G., 1903:79
Robertson, E.M., 1902:48
Robertson, O.H., 1886:54
Robinson, A.R., 1845:31
Robinson, J., 1813:19
Robinson, R., 1866:41
Robiquet, P.J., 1780:9
Robitzek, E.H., 1912:51
Roblin, R.O., 1907:68
Robscheit-Robbins, F.S., 1893:41
Robson, G.A., 1968:3
Rocha Lima, H. de, 1879:48
Rocha e Silva, M., 1910:63
Rockefeller, J.D., 1839:28
Rodbell, M., 1925:38
Rodgers, J.K., 1793:22
Rodrigues, J.C.B., 1511:2
Roehl, W., 1929:44
Röntgen, W.C., 1845:25
Rösslin, E., 1526:3
Roger, H., 1809:6
Rogers, L., 1868:32
Roget, P.M., 1779:10
Rogoff, J.M., 1884:61
Roholm, K., 1939:18
Rohrer, H., 1933:43
Roitt, I.M., 1927:34
Rokitansky, C., 1804:5
Rolfinck, G., 1599:2
Rolleston, H.D., 1862:35
Rollet, J.P., 1824:18
Rollier, A., 1874:38
Rollo, I.M., 1926:33
Romanovsky, D.L., 1861:41
Romberg, M.H., 1795:19
Romero, F., 1815:6

Roonhuyze, H. van, 1622:1
Roos, E., 1866:54
Rorschach, H., 1884:60
Rose, N.R., 1927:36
Rose, W., 1847:26
Rosén von Rosenstein, N., 1706:6
Rosenbach, A.J.F., 1842:32
Rosenheim, M.L., 1908:48
Rosenheim, T., 1896:35
Rosenthal, S.M., 1897:33
Ross, D.N., 1922:40
Ross, P.H., 1876:82
Ross, R., 1857:31
Roth, G.M., 1945:10
Rothberger, C.J., 1871:37
Rothera, A.C.H., 1880:41
Rothmund, A., 1830:11
Rous, F.P., 1879:43
Rousselot, 1772:10
Rousset, F., 1535:4
Roux, P.J., 1780:11
Roux, P.P.E., 1853:40
Roux, W., 1850:27
Rowe, W.P., 1926:29
Rowntree, L.G., 1883:29
Royle, N.D., 1944:25
Rubin, I.C., 1883:23
Rubner, M., 1854:38
Rueff, J., 1500:4
Ruete, C.G.T., 1810:10
Rufus *of Ephesus*, 100:1
Ruiz, C.L., 1904:43
Runge, F.F., 1795:12
Rush, B., 1746:7
Rush, H.L., 1897:47
Rush, L.V., 1905:48
Ruska, E., 1906:67
Russell, J., 1755:8
Russell, J.S.R., 1863:60
Rust, J.N., 1775:5
Rutherford, D., 1749:5
Rutty, J., 1698:3
Ruysch, F., 1638:4
Ruzicka, L., 1887:51
Rydygier, L., 1850:30
Ryff, W.H., 1548:1
Ryle, J.A., 1889:58
Rynd, F., 1801:21

Sabin, A.B., 1906:59
Sabouraud, R.J.A., 1864:34
Sachs, B., 1858:27
Sachs, H., 1877:36
Sacks, B., 1896:82
Saemisch, E.T., 1833:23
Sänger, M., 1853:19
Saenz, B., 1938:36

Sahli, H., 1856:27
Saint-Yves, C. de, 1667:7
Sainton, P., 1868:56
Sajous, C., 1852:52
Sakel, W., 1900:56
Sakmann, B., 1942:17
Salazar, T., 1830:17
Salicetti, G. da, 1210:1
Salimbeni, A.T., 1903:16
Salk, J., 1914:38
Salkowski, E.L., 1844:36
Salmon, D.E., 1850:29
Salter, H.H., 1823:22
Sampson, J.A., 1873:46
Samuelsson, B.I., 1934:36
Sanctorius, 1561:3
Sanders, M., 1910:56
Sandfort, E.B. de, 1913:44
Sandifort, E., 1742:9
Sandström, I.V., 1852:36
Sanger, F., 1918:32
Sano, M.E., 1903:81
Santo di Barletta, M., 1488:1
Santorio, S., 1561:3
Santos, R. dos, 1880:47
Saporta, A., 1573:2
Sassonia, E., 1551:4
Sattler, H., 1844:34
Saucerotte, N., 1741:5
Sauerbruch, E.F., 1875:40
Savoor, S.R., 1900:79
Sawyer, W.A., 1879:40
Sayre, L.A., 1820:13
Scarpa, A., 1752:9
Schaffer, F.L., 1921:48
Schally, A.V., 1926:38
Schamberg, J.F., 1870:48
Schatz, A., 1920:30
Schaudinn, F.R., 1871:34
Schaumann, J.N., 1879:57
Schaumann, O., 1939:8
Scheele, C.W., 1742:10
Schellong, F., 1936:14
Schenck, B.R., 1872:44
Schenken, J.R., 1905:32
Scheuermann, H.W., 1877:30
Schick, B., 1877:39
Schilder, P.F., 1886:44
Schiller, W., 1887:63
Schimmelbusch, C., 1860:51
Schindler, R., 1888:46
Schlatter, C., 1864:27
Schleich, C.L., 1859:35
Schleiden, M.J., 1804:8
Schlesinger, B., 1896:77
Schlesinger, R.W., 1913:52
Schliephake, E., 1894:53

694

Schloffer, H., 1868:39
Schmidt, E.R., 1890:51
Schmidt, M., 1898:62
Schmiedeberg, J.E.O., 1838:27
Schmieden, V., 1874:22
Schmitt, W.J., 1760:6
Schmitz, K.E.F., 1889:65
Schneider, C.V., 1614:8
Schönlein, J.L., 1793:20
Schoepff, J.D., 1752:8
Schottmüller, H., 1867:43
Schroeder, R., 1884:55
Schroeder van der Kolk, J.L.C., 1797:7
Schüffner, W.A.P., 1867:25
Schüller, A., 1874:43
Schütte, D., 1824:8
Schultz, W., 1878:36
Schultz, W.H., 1873:40
Schultze, F., 1848:28
Schwabach, D., 1846:28
Schwalbe, M.W., 1883:42
Schwann, T., 1810:17
Schwartz, S.O., 1911:49
Schwartze, H.H.R., 1837:28
Schweitzer, A., 1875:28
Schwerdt, C.E., 1917:36
Sclavo, A., 1861:27
Scott, W.W., 1913:49
Sebrell, W.H., 1901:50
Seddon, H.J., 1903:66
Sédillot, C.E., 1804:10
Seeber, G.R., 1900:39
Ségalas, P.S., 1792:12
Séguin, E., 1812:9
Seldinger, S.I., 1953:13
Sellards, A.W., 1884:70
Sellerbeck, H., 1842:35
Sellors, T.H., 1902:34
Selter, P., 1886:76
Selye, H., 1907:50
Semb, C.B., 1895:53
Semmelweis, I.P., 1818:21
Semon, F., 1849:33
Sen, G., 1931:21
Senear, F.E., 1889:64
Senn, N., 1844:39
Sennert, D., 1572:3
Sequeira, J.H., 1865:34
Sertürner, F.W.A., 1783:8
Sérullas, G.S., 1774:8
Servetus, M., 1511:1
Severino, M.A., 1580:2
Seyfarth, C.P., 1890:49
Shaffer, M.F., 1940:18
Sharp, A., 1944:22
Sharpey-Schafer, E.A., 1850:26
Shattuck, L., 1793:18

Shea, J.J., 1924:42
Shearburn, E.W., 1913:63
Sheehan, H.L., 1900:60
Shen Nung, 2700 BC
Shenstone, N.S., 1881:59
Shepard, C.C., 1914:39
Sherrington, C.S., 1857:40
Shiga, K., 1870:59
Shipway, F.E., 1875:50
Shirley, E.K., 1924:44
Shope, R.E., 1901:56
Shope, T., 1970:4
Shortt, H.E., 1887:48
Shrapnell, H.J., 1834:33
Shumway, N.E., 1923:26
Shwartzman, G., 1896:66
Sicard, J.A., 1872:39
Sichel, J., 1802:8
Sick, P.A., 1836:33
Sickles, G.M., 1898:46
Siebold, A.E. von, 1775:6
Silvester, H.R., 1828:35
Simmonds, M., 1855:20
Simmons, J.S., 1890:41
Simon Januensis, 1270:2
Simon, G., 1824:12
Simon, J., 1816:16
Simon, T., 1873:32
Simond, P.L., 1903:16
Simpson, J.Y., 1811:12
Sims, J.M., 1813:7
Singer, J.J., 1885:41
Sippy, B.W., 1866:47
Siwe, S.A., 1897:50
Sjögren, T.A.U., 1859:45
Sjöqvist, C.O., 1901:55
Skinner, R.C., 1834:34
Skoda, J., 1805:12
Slawyk, 1899:12
Sluder, G., 1865:29
Slye, M., 1879:30
Smadel, J.E., 1907:48
Smellie, W., 1697:6
Smith, E., 3000 BC
Smith, E.L., 1904:35
Smith, H., 1862:37
Smith, H.H., 1902:42
Smith, H.O., 1931:36
Smith, M., 1932:33
Smith, N., 1762:5
Smith, N.R., 1797:9
Smith, P.E., 1884:45
Smith, R.W., 1807:14
Smith, S., 1930:8
Smith, Theobald, 1859:36
Smith, Thomas, 1833:18
Smith, W., 1897:34

696

Sutton, T., 1767:9
Sutton, W.S., 1877:33
Swaminath, C.S., 1942:11
Swammerdam, J., 1637:1
Swan, C.S., 1943:13
Swan, H.J.C., 1922:38
Swanson, A.B., 1966:3
Sweet, R.H., 1901:47
Swick, M., 1900:82
Swift, H., 1858:37
Swingle, W.W., 1891:43
Sydenham, T., 1624:2
Sylvest, E.O.S., 1880:57
Syme, J., 1799:13
Symmers, D., 1879:41
Synge, R.L.M., 1914:37
Szent-Györgyi, A., 1893:36
Szilagyi, D.E., 1910:60

Tagliacozzi, G., 1546:4
Tait, R.L., 1845:27
Takaki, K., 1849:39
Takamine, J., 1854:45
Takata, M., 1892:70
Taliaferro, V.H., 1831:18
Taniguchi, T., 1896:83
Tanner, N.C., 1906:54
Tarchanoff, I.R., 1848:34
Tarlov, I.M., 1905:37
Tarnier, E.S., 1828:23
Tatum, A.L., 1884:64
Tatum, E.L., 1909:43
Taussig, H.B., 1898:50
Tay, W., 1843:36
Taylor, F.H.L., 1900:68
Taylor, R.M., 1887:52
Taylor, R.W., 1842:27
Temin, H.M., 1934:37
Terman, L.M., 1877:27
Terry, T.L., 1899:34
Thackrah, C.S., 1795:16
Thaysen, T.E.H., 1883:40
Theiler, H., 1894:58
Theiler, M., 1899:32
Theorell, A.H.T., 1903:65
Thiers, J., 1921:28
Thiersch, K., 1822:17
Thomas, A., 1867:42
Thomas, E.D., 1920:31
Thomas, E.W.P., 1945:15
Thomas, H.O., 1834:26
Thomas, H.W., 1905:14
Thomas, J.D., 1844:45
Thomas, J.P., 1961:5
Thomas, J.W.T., 1893:34
Thomas, T.G., 1831:21
Thompson, H., 1820:20

Thomsen, J.T., 1815:16
Thorn, G.W., 1906:47
Thudichum, J.L.W., 1829:27
Tichy, V.L., 1899:53
Tigerstedt, R.A.A., 1853:16
Tillett, W.S., 1892:59
Timmis, G.M., 1953:15
Timoni, E., 1718:7
Tinbergen, N., 1907:57
Tiselius, A.W.K., 1902:39
Tjio, J.-H., 1919:40
Todd, A.R., 1907:67
Todd, J.L., 1876:60
Töpfer, H.W., 1876:84
Tomes, J., 1815:13
Tonegawa, S., 1939:30
Tooth, H.H., 1856:24
Topham, W., 1842:6
Torek, F., 1861:28
Torkildsen, A., 1939:24
Torti, F., 1658:5
Toti, A., 1861:22
Toynbee, J., 1815:21
Traube, L., 1818:15
Traut, H.F., 1894:38
Treitz, W., 1819:21
Trenaunay, P., 1875:55
Trendelenburg, F., 1844:29
Treves, F., 1853:15
Triboulet, H., 1864:25
Trigt, A.C. van, 1825:26
Tröltsch, A.F. von, 1829:21
Trotter, T., 1760:7
Trotter, W., 1872:50
Trousseau, A., 1801:18
Trueta, J., 1897:41
Tschermak von Seysenegg, E., 1871:40
Tscherning, M.H.E., 1851:25
Türck, L., 1810:12
Türk, W., 1871:20
Tuffier, T., 1857:26
Tuke, D.H., 1827:17
Tuke, S., 1784:11
Tulp, N., 1593:3
Turner, D., 1667:8
Turner, G.A., 1845:42
Turner, H.H., 1892:61
Twitchell, A., 1781:3
Twort, F.W., 1877:49
Tyndall, J., 1820:19
Tyson, E., 1650:2
Tyzzer, E.E., 1875:42

Uhlenhuth, P.T., 1870:29
Ullmann, E., 1861:24
Umezawa, H., 1957:4
Underwood, M., 1737:6

Ungar, G., 1906: 52
Ungley, C.C., 1949: 6
Unna, P.G., 1850: 32
Unverricht, H., 1853: 32
Uribe Troncoso, 1867: 45
Usher, B.D., 1899: 55

Vaisman, A., 1937: 28
Vajda, L., 1933: 19
Valentin, G.G., 1810: 11
Vallambert, S. de, 1537: 1
Vander Veer, A., 1879: 54
Vane, J.R., 1927: 31
Van Gieson, I., 1866: 55
Vanghetti, G., 1861: 40
Van Hook, W., 1862: 45
Vanlair, C., 1839: 22
Vaquez, L.H., 1860: 46
Varmus, H.E., 1939: 31
Varoli, C., 1543: 5
Vassale, G., 1862: 33
Vaughan, G.T., 1859: 34
Vauquelin, L.N., 1763: 3
Veale, H.R.L., 1832: 33
Veau, V., 1871: 43
Vedder, E.B., 1878: 35
Velpeau, A.A.L.M., 1795: 15
Velse, C.H., 1742: 4
Venable, C.S., 1877: 57
Venel, J.A., 1740: 7
Verhoeff, F.H., 1874: 32
Verneuil, A.A.S., 1823: 25
Verney, E.B., 1894: 44
Vervoort, H., 1900: 25
Vesalius, A., 1514: 1
Vialli, M., 1933: 8
Vianna, G.O. de, 1885: 37
Vidal, J.B.E., 1825: 22
Vierordt, K., 1818: 20
Vieussens, R., 1641: 4
Vieusseux, G., 1746: 9
Villaret, M., 1877: 50
Villemin, J.A., 1827: 15
Vincent, J.H., 1862: 42
Vinci, Leonardo da, 1452: 2
Vinson, P.P., 1890: 36
Virchow, R.L.K., 1821: 21
Virgili, P., 1669: 4
Visnich, S., 1965: 4
Voegt, H., 1942: 9
Voelcker, F., 1872: 58
Vogt, A., 1879: 46
Vogt, C., 1875: 57
Vogt, H., 1875: 37
Vogt, K., 1880: 49
Vogt, O., 1870: 33
Voit, C. von, 1831: 20

Volhard, F., 1872: 38
Volkmann, R. von, 1830: 12
Vollgnad, H., 1634: 4
Vollmer, H., 1896: 81
Voltolini, F.E.R., 1819: 18
Voronoff, S., 1866: 40
Vries, H.M., de 1848: 21
Vulpian, E.F.A., 1826: 15
Vvedensky, N.E., 1852: 39

Waardenburg, P.J., 1886: 72
Wade, H.W., 1896: 76
Wagener, H.P., 1890: 40
Wagner, 1829: 8
Wagner, E.L., 1829: 20
Wagner, W., 1848: 17
Wagner von Jauregg, J., 1857: 23
Wakim, G., 1907: 58
Waksman, S.A., 1888: 52
Walcher, G.A., 1856: 34
Wald, G., 1906: 64
Waldenström, J.A., 1839: 32
Waldenström, J.G., 1906: 53
Waldeyer-Hartz, H.W.G., 1836: 20
Walker, E.L., 1870: 39
Walker, J.T.A., 1868: 50
Wallace, A.R., 1823: 16
Wallace, W., 1791: 8
Waller, A.D., 1856: 30
Waller, A.V., 1816: 17
Wallgren, A.J., 1889: 54
Wallis, J., 1616: 5
Walter, J.G., 1734: 3
Walter, W.G., 1911: 60
Walther, P.F. von, 1782: 5
Wang, Y.L., 1938: 22
Wangensteen, O.H., 1898: 57
Wani, H., 1933: 30
Warburg, O.H., 1883: 35
Ward, W.S., 1842: 6
Wardill, W.E.M., 1894: 60
Wardrop, J., 1782: 7
Warren, J., 1753: 5
Warren, J.C., 1778: 11
Warren, J.M., 1811: 21
Warthin, A.S., 1866: 46
Wassén, E., 1931: 24
Wassermann, A. von, 1866: 32
Watelle, T.J.J., 1854: 26
Waterhouse, B., 1754: 5
Waterhouse, R., 1873: 21
Waters, C.A., 1885: 52
Waters, R.M., 1883: 36
Waterton, C., 1782: 6
Watson, F.S., 1853: 42
Watson, J., 1807: 6
Watson, J.B., 1878: 29

Watson, J.D., 1928:28
Watson, W., 1715:2
Watts, J.W., 1904:29
Waugh, G.E., 1876:61
Weber, E.H., 1795:17
Weber, F.P., 1863:39
Weber, H.D., 1823:26
Webster, L.T., 1894:59
Weeks, J.E., 1853:27
Weese, H., 1897:48
Wegner, F.G.R., 1843:35
Weichselbaum, A., 1845:20
Weigert, C., 1845:23
Weil, A., 1848:20
Weil, E., 1880:39
Weill-Hallé, B., 1924:32
Weinberg, M., 1868:33
Weinstein, M.J., 1916:49
Weir, R.F., 1839:35
Weiss, S., 1898:48
Weissman, A.F.L., 1834:18
Welch, C.S., 1909:42
Welch, W.H., 1850:23
Wellcome, H.S., 1853:28
Weller, T.H., 1915:28
Wellman, F.C., 1871:45
Wells, H., 1815:11
Wells, R.S., 1965:5
Wells, T.S., 1818:16
Wells, W.C., 1757:6
Welsch, G.H., 1624:3
Weltchek, H., 1938:24
Wenckebach, K.F., 1864:28
Wenzel, C., 1769:9
Wepfer, J.J., 1620:5
Werdnig, G., 1862:46
Werlhof, P.G., 1699:2
Wernicke, C., 1848:24
Wernicke, R.J., 1873:47
Wertheim, E., 1864:26
West, C., 1816:11
West, R., 1890:50
Westergren, A.V., 1891:58
Westphal, C.F.O., 1833:17
Weyer, J., 1516:2
Wharton, T., 1614:6
Wherry, W.B., 1875:61
Whetstone, G., 1544:3
Whillis, S.S., 1870:57
Whipple, A.O., 1881:60
Whipple, G.H., 1878:38
Whitby, L.E.H., 1895:44
White, A., 1782:9
White, C., 1728:4
White, E.C., 1887:59
White, P., 1900:80
White, P.D., 1886:55

Whitmore, A., 1876:53
Whytt, R., 1714:6
Wichmann, J.E., 1740:6
Wickman, O.I., 1872:41
Widal, G.F.I., 1862:26
Wideröe, S., 1880:44
Wieland, H.O., 1877:35
Wiener, A.S., 1907:53
Wiener, N., 1894:50
Wier, J., 1516:2
Wieschaus, E.F., 1943:17
Wiesel, T.N., 1924:37
Wiktor, T.J., 1973:2
Wild, J.J., 1911:53
Wilde, W.R.W., 1815:14
Wilder, R.M., 1885:47
Wiles, P., 1899:42
Wilkins, M.H.F., 1916:51
Wilkinson, J.F., 1897:35
Wilks, S., 1824:13
Willan, R., 1757:7
Willcox, W., 1840:3
Willebrand, E.A. von, 1870:30
Williams, C.D., 1893:40
Williams, F.H., 1852:38
Williams, H.W., 1821:22
Williams, J.W., 1866:29
Williams, R.C., 1908:53
Williams, R.R., 1886:45
Willis, T., 1621:5
Wills, L., 1888:61
Wilmer, B., 1779:5
Wilms, M., 1867:35
Wilson, C., 1906:48
Wilson, E.B., 1856:35
Wilson, F.N., 1890:46
Wilson, S.A.K., 1874:41
Wilson, W.J., 1879:59
Wilson, W.J.E., 1809:12
Wilton, W., 1809:17
Windaus, A., 1876:66
Winge, E., 1827:21
Winiwater, F. von, 1852:34
Winterberg, H., 1867:28
Wintersteiner, O.P., 1898:59
Wintrobe, M.M., 1901:54
Witebsky, E., 1901:48
Withering, W., 1741:4
Wöhler, F., 1800:15
Wölfler, A., 1850:18
Wohlgemuth, J., 1874:27
Wolbach, S.B., 1880:42
Wolcott, E.B., 1804:13
Wolf, A., 1902:37
Wolfe, J.R., 1824:19
Wolferth, C., 1887:57
Wolff, C.F., 1733:10

Wolff, L., 1898:63
Wolff, M., 1844:28
Wolff-Eisner, A., 1877:42
Wollaston, W.H., 1766:7
Wood, A., 1817:22
Wood, F.C., 1901:52
Wood, W., 1774:13
Woodall, J., 1570:2
Woods, A.C., 1889:52
Woodward, J.J., 1833:25
Woodward, R.B., 1917:41
Worcester, N., 1812:14
Wreden, R.R., 1837:32
Wright, A.E., 1861:37
Wright, A.M., 1934:2
Wright, M.B., 1803:8
Wright, S., 1889:59
Wrisberg, H., 1739:3
Wroblewski, F., 1921:51
Wu, H., 1895:54
Wucherer, O.E.H., 1820:17
Würtz, F., 1518:4
Wunderlich, K., 1815:18
Wundt, W.M., 1832:29
Wynder, E.L., 1922:37
Wynter, W.E., 1860:38

Yalow, R.S., 1921:50
Yamagiwa, K., 1863:31

Yasuda, I., 1909:48
Yeomans, A., 1907:79
Yersin, A.E.J., 1863:53
Yonge, J., 1646:3
Yorke, W., 1883:30
Young, F.G., 1908:49
Young, H.H., 1870:43
Young, T., 1773:9

Zacchias, P., 1584:2
Zahorsky, J., 1871:36
Zaimis, E., 1915:29
Zambeccari, G., 1665:11
Zaufal, E., 1833:21
Zeis, E., 1807:13
Zenker, F.A., 1825:12
Zerbi, G., 1445:1
Zerfas, L.G., 1897:31
Zernike, F., 1888:50
Ziehl, F., 1857:27
Zigas, V., 1957:14
Zimmermann, J.G., 1728:3
Zinsser, H., 1878:41
Zirm, E.K., 1863:34
Zoeller, C., 1888:65
Zoll, P.M., 1911:50
Zollinger, R.M., 1903:67
Zondek, B., 1891:50
Zuelzer, G.L., 1870:34

# Subject index

Bilharziasis, 1852:15, 1904:11
treatment
– – lucanthone hydrochloride (miracil D),
  1946:23
– – niridazole (ambilhar), 1964:11
– – oxamniquinine, 1969:4
– – tartar emetic, 1918:12
– – *see also* Schistosoma
Biliary tract, calculi, radiography, 1896:38
Bilirubin
– excretion test, 1927:21
– van den Bergh test, 1913:30
Billroth I operation, 1881:27
Billroth II operation, 1885:23, 1911:33, 1918:22
Bills of Mortality, in England, 1532:2, 1629:1
Binet-Simon scale for measurement of
  intelligence, 1911:21, 1917:15
Biochemical Society, London, 1911:6
Biochemistry, Abderhalden's *Handbuch*, 1920:29
Biochemistry, foundation, 1648:1
*Biographisches Lexikon*, 1884:4, 1932:31
Biography, *see* Medicine, biography
Biological standardization, 1897:10, 1921:11
Biology, 384 BC, 1193:1
Biometric genetics, 1930:5
*Biometrika*, 1901:6
Bipp antiseptic, in wound treatment, 1916:22
Birmingham University, 1874:3
Birth control, 1822:13
– Stopes's treatise, 1923:24
– *see also* Contraception
Birth, human, after re-implantation of human
  embryo, 1978:4
Birth, premature, 1600:1
Births and Deaths Registration Act, England,
  1836:4
Births and Deaths Registration Acts, UK, 1871:2
Bismarsen, in syphilis, 1927:24
Bismuth
– in syphilis, 1889:34, 1921:35, 1927:24
– meal, 1898:37
Black death *see* Plague
Blackwater fever, 1874:13
Blackwell, Elizabeth, first woman to qualify in
  medicine, 1849:1
Bladder
– aeroscopic examination, 1893:15
– artificial, 1951:9
– calculus, 1535:2, 1625:1, 1797:5, 1927:18
– – lithotrity, 1829:10, 1833:6, 1878:7
– – *see also* Lithotomy
– carcinoma, radiotherapy, 1906:29
– caruncle, 1551:2
– cystectomy, total, 1891:41
– cystotomy, 1851:16
– diverticula, 1895:24
– epicystotomy, 1858:5

– examination, *see* Cystoscopy
– exstrophy, treatment, 1859:6
– extroversion, 1859:19
– gonococcal infection, 1896:10
– neck, diseases, 1834:12
– rupture, intraperitoneal, treatment, 1886:28
– tumour, 1884:26
– – excision, 1897:14
– – resection, 1875:19
– – transurethral fulguration, 1910:25
Blalock-Taussig operation, 1945:9
*Blastomyces dermatitidis*, 1961:6
Blastomycosis, 1895:12, 1896:19, 1908:14
Blaud's pill, 1832:11
BLB (Boothby-Lovelace-Bulbulian) oxygen
  inhalation apparatus, 1938:10
Blepharoplasty, 1818:9, 1829:3
Blind
– Braille system, 1837:8
– education, 1786:11, 1845:6, 1873:3
Blindness
– due to optic neuritis, 1860:14
– *see also* Colour-blindness
Blocq's disease, 1888:19
Blood, 1794:6
– analysis, 1684:3
– bactericidal action, 1888:40
– bank, 1937:9
– cells, 1771:9
– – red, *see* Erythrocytes
– circulation, 1210:2, 1553:2, 1571:2, 1615:1,
  1628:1
– classified, into three groups, 1900:10, 1927:30
– classified, into four groups, 1906:44, 1910:47
– coagulation, role of platelets, 1882:9
– corpuscles, 1693:2, 1843:15
– fibrinolysis, 1933:7
– flow, arterial, vein grafts for restoration,
  1906:37
– gases, quantitative analysis, 1837:15
– grouping, medicolegal applications, 1921:42
– groups, 1930:1
– – inheritance, 1939:5
– oxygen-carrying capacity, 1913:12
– platelets, 1842:19, 1878:28, 1882:9
– pressure, 1733:4
– – accurately estimated, 1856:19
– – examination, using stethoscope and
  sphygmomanometer, 1905:30
– – recording, 1834:13
– respiratory function, 1913:12
– sugar, tests, 1919:27, 1931:11
– transfusion, 1628:2, 1665:8, 1667:4
– – blood bank, 1937:9
– – human-to-human, 1819:11, 1828:10
– – in animals, 1821:14
– – in erythroblastosis foetalis, 1948:16

*Journal des Sçavans*, 1665:1
Junker's inhaler, 1867:7
Jurisprudence, medical, 1597:4, 1621:3, 1788:2
– – first notable American text, 1823:14

Kahn precipitation test, in syphilis, 1922:27
Kaiser-Wilhelms Akademie, Berlin, 1895:1
Kaiserliche Königliche Gesellschaft der Aertze,
    Vienna, founded, 1837:4
Kaiserliche Leopoldinische Akademie der
    Naturforscher, founded, 1677:1
Kala-azar, 1870:6, 1909:15
– Leishman-Donovan bodies, 1904:13
– transmission, through *Phlebotomus argentipes*,
    1941:11
– *see also* Leishmaniasis
Kanamycin, isolated, 1957:4
Kaposi's disease, 1882:18, 1886:29
Kaposi's sarcoma, 1872:25
Karolinska Institutet, Stockholm, 1810:1
Kartagener's syndrome, 1933:15
Keloid, 1816:9, 1854:20
Keratitis, 1808:5
Keratoconjunctivitis, 1889:5, 1943:14
Keratoconus, 1868:5
Keratoplasty, 1878:4, 1888:14, 1906:12,
    1930:26, 1930:27, 1932:29, 1935:28,
    1949:28
Keratoscope, 1882:8
Keratosis follicularis, 1860:15, 1899:27,
    1899:39
Keritherapy, in burns, 1913:44
Kernicterus, 1875:22
Kernig's sign, 1882:17
Khartoum, Wellcome Tropical Research
    Laboratories, 1903:6
Kidney, 1662:3
– artificial, 1944:18, 1956:12
– atrophy, arteriosclerotic, 1872:23
– calculus, 1880:18, 1896:31, 1901:17
– cancer, nephrectomy for, 1877:13
– in crush syndrome, 1923:17, 1941:13
– decortication, for chronic nephritis, 1901:22
– embryoma, 1899:18
– excretory ducts, 1662:3
– failure, pathogenesis, 1951:10
– function tests, 1903:33 1894:27, 1910:23,
    1924:24
– glomerular filtration rate, 1940:14
– Henle's loop, 1855:16
– hypernephroma, 1884:25
– mobile, 1881:23, 1882:22, 1893:17, 1906:31
– nephrotomography, 1954:12
– radiography, 1906:32
– secretion, 1843:21
– surgery, 1865:10
– transplantation, 1950:12, 1956:13

– – experimental, 1902:20, 1908:26
– tubule function, multiple defects, 1931:12
– tumour, treatment, 1861:16
– *see also* Glomerulonephritis
Kiel, University, 1665:4
Kielland (obstetric) forceps, 1916:17
Kienböck's atrophy, 1901:18
Kienböck's disease, 1902:17, 1910:18
Kiev, Bacteriological Institute, 1896:7
Kimmelstiel-Wilson syndrome, 1936:20
King Edward VII College of Medicine,
    Singapore, 1905:5
King's College, New York
– founded, 1754:2
– Medical Department, 1767:2
– becomes Columbia College, 1784:3
Kinnier Wilson's disease, 1861:11, 1912:8
Kirschner wire, 1909:21
Klebs' disease, 1879:18
Klebs-Loeffler bacillus, *see Corynebacterium
    diphtheriae*
*Klebsiella pneumoniae*, discovered, 1882:31
Klinefelter syndrome, 1942:8
*Klinische Wochenschrift*, 1864:7
Klippel-Feil syndrome, 1912:29
Klippel-Trenaunay syndrome, 1900:38
Klumpke's paralysis, 1885:15
Knee-jerk reflex
– term introduced, 1880:17
– in tabes dorsalis, 1875:11
Knee-joint
– ankylosis, treatment, 1845:11
– arthroplasty, 1971:4
– Baker's cysts, 1877:10
– internal derangement, relief, 1885:17
Knights Hospitallers, 1070:1
Koch's phenomenon, 1890:29
Koch's postulates, 1878:23
Koch-Weeks bacillus, 1883:6, 1886:7
Kolmer complement fixation test, in syphilis,
    1922:28
Kongelige Danske Videnskabernes Selskab,
    1742:2
Konglige Vetenskaps–Societeten i Uppsala,
    1710:4
Königliche Bayerische Akademie der
    Wissenschaften, Munich, 1759:1
Königliche Gesellschaft für Wissenschaften,
    Göttingen, 1751:1
Koninklijke Nederlandse Akademie van
    Wetenschappen, 1808:1, 1855:3
Koplik's spots, in measles, 1896:17
Korsakoff's psychosis (syndrome), 1887:37
Krakow
– Jagiellonian University, created, 1364:1
– Society of Physicians, founded, 1866:2
Kraurosis vulvae, 1885:4

734

Leprosy, 1847:18
– bacillus, 1873:17, 1879:25
– Council of Lyons interdicts migration of lepers, 583:1
– diagnosis, 1924:31
– – lepromin reaction, 1919:35
– hospitals
– – leprosarium at St Albans, 794:1
– – near Canterbury, 1080:1
– – at Ilford, near London, 1136:2
– – leprosarium at St Jürgen's Hospital, Bergen, 1411:2
– lazar houses, 1403:1, 1656:1
– lepers driven from London, 1346:1
– transmission, experimental, 1960:4
– treatment
– – chaulmoogra oil, 1854:25
– – diasone, 1944:8
– – diphenylthiourea (thiambutosine), 1956:8
– – ditophal (etisul), 1959:2
– – promin, 1943:5
– – rifampicin, 1970:6
– – sulphetrone, 1943:4
Leptospira canicola, 1933:3, 1934:25
Leptospira hebdomadis, 1918:14
Leptospira icterhaemorrhagiae, 1916:24, 1917:13
Leptospirosis, 1934:25
– vaccination, 1933:30
– icterohaemorrhagica, 1861:10, 1883:11, 1886:15
– – causal organism, 1916:24, 1917:13
Lethargy, 1672:3
Letterer-Siwe disease, 1924:11, 1933:41
Leuco-agglutinins, 1952:13
Leucocystosis, 1843:15
Leucocyte, typing, 1957:8
Leucopoiesis, 1868:28
Leucotaxine, 1937:11
Leucotomy, frontal, in psychoses, 1949:1
Leukaemia, 1844:16, 1845:16
– acute, 1857:16
– – of childhood, vincristine in, 1963:6
– diagnosis, 1846:14
– lymphatic and myelogenous, differentiated, 1891:34
– lymphatic, chronic, treatment, nitrogen mustard (chlorambucil), 1955:11
– monocytic, 1913:35
– myeloblastic, acute, therapy, cytosine arabinoside, 1951:3
– myelogenous, 1870:25
– myeloid, chronic, treatment, myleran, 1953:15
– treatment
– – cytosine arabinoside, 1968:4
– – 6-mercaptopurine, 1953:14
– – urethane, 1946:13

– – with radiophosphorus, 1939:16
Leyden's ataxia, 1891:21
Leydig cells of the testis, 1850:13
Libman-Sacks disease, 1924:29
Library of Congress, Washington, 1800:3
Librium, 1960:5
Lichen
– nitidus, 1901:21
– ruber moniliformis, 1886:29
– urticatus, 1813:6
Lichtheim's disease, 1885:2
Lieberkühn's glands, crypts, 1745:3
Liège, University, founded, 1816:3
Life-table for actuaries, 1771:1
Ligatures
– absorbable, 1816:6
– antiseptic, for hernia, 1878:20
– catgut, introduction, 1869:19
Light
– invisible, therapeutic value, 1896:57, 1903:1
– Newton's theory, 1672:1
– wave theory, 1802:1
Lille
– University, 1562:1
– Faculté de Médecine et Pharmacie, 1875:2
Lima, University, Medical Faculty, 1638:1
Limb
– human, severed, reattachment, 1964:10
– kinematization of amputation stump, 1898:26, 1918:18
– lengthening, surgical, 1905:19
– paralysis, unilateral, 1858:15
Lindau's disease, 1926:5
Lineae atrophicae, 1861:4
Linitis plastica, 1859:12
Linnaean classification, 1735:2
Linnean Society of London, 1788:1
Linolenic acid, see Vitamin F
Lip
– cleft, repair, 1844:5, 1845:9, 1884:7, 1898:15
– plastic surgery, 1868:7
Lipid, metabolism, disorder, 1946:17
Lipiodol
– in bronchoscopy, 1917:26
– intratracheal, in bronchography, 1924:27
– in myelography, 1921:19
Lipochondrodystrophy with gargoylism, 1917:8, 1919:19
Lipodystrophy, intestinal, 1907:27
Lisbon (by date)
– Academia das Sciencias, 1779:1
– Medical Society, 1834:6
– Instituto de Oftalmologia, 1891:4
– Instituto Bacteriológico de Câmara Pestana, 1892:2
– School of Tropical Medicine, 1903:3
Lisfranc's amputation, 1815:1

Meningitis (concluded)
– tuberculous, 1768:5, 1834:10
Meningococcus, 1887:13, 1896:28
Menstruation, pain, 1872:9
Mental diseases, classification, 1798:6
Mental defectives, classification, 1866:15
Mental retardation, 1934:16
Mepacrine, an antimalarial, 1932:3
Meperidine, *see* Pethidine
Meprobamate, in anxiety, 1954:13
Meralgia paraesthetica, 1878:14
Mercaptopurine
– synthesis, 1952:22
– in leukaemia treatment, 1953:14
Mercazole, antithyroid drug, synthesis, 1949:18
Mercuric chloride, as antiseptic, 1881:15
Mercurochrome, in urinary tract infections,
    1919:16
Mercury, in treatment of syphilis, 1533:2
Mercy Hospital, Chicago, chartered, 1852:6
Merida, hospital, 580:1
Mescaline, 1898:43, 1927:26
Mesmerism, 1779:9, 1842:9
– *see also* Hypnotism
Metabolism, 1881:5
– disorders, 1927:22
– inborn errors, 1909:25
– physiology, 1614:3
Metacarpus, Bennett's fracture, 1882:19
Metatarsalgia, anterior, 1845:10, 1876:26
Metatarsals, osteoperiostitis, 1855:11, 1897:16
Metatarsus varus, congenital, 1863:16
Methaemoglobinaemia, 1945:11
Methimazole, antithyroid drug, synthesis,
    1949:18
Methonium compounds, as anaesthetics, 1948:23
Methylene blue, 1881:34, 1891:13
Metrazol, *see* Cardiazol
Metropathia haemorrhagica, 1919:18
Meulengracht diet, 1934:15
Mexico
– first hospital erected in city by Cortes, 1524:2
– University, Chair of Medicine, 1578:1
Mibelli's disease, 1875:15, 1879:16, 1893:16,
    1896:34
Michigan, University, Ann Arbor, founded,
    1837:2
Microbes, pathogenic, 1835:12, 1840:11
Microfilariae, 1871:8
Micrognathia, 1909:8
Microscopy, 1658:1, 1665:7
– electron, 1932:2, 1982:2, 1986:2
– Galilean, 1610:1
– phase contrast, 1935:24, 1953:2
– scanning tunnelling, 1986:2
*Microsporon audouini*, 1843:16
Microtome, 1870:28

Microwave radiation therapy, 1949:9
Middlesex Hospital, London, 1834:8
Middlesex Infirmary (later Hospital), London,
    1745:2
Midwifery, 1631:3, 1742:6, 1751:3, 1752:7,
    1754:4, 1807:1, 1821:7
– chair founded at Edinburgh, 1739:1
– earliest textbook, 1513:1
– regulation, New York, 1716:1
– *see also* Obstetrics
Migraine, 1776:6, 1873:8, 1884:18
Mikulicz operation for colon cancer, 1892:33
Milan, Ospedale Maggiore, 1456:1
Military hospitals, 1764:4
Military medicine, 1752:5
Milk
– adulteration, laws, 1860:3
– factor, in cancer transmission in mice, 1936:4
– fat content, 1886:6
– lactodensimeter, 1886:6
– sterilization, 1886:6
Milkman's syndrome, 1930:15
Millar's asthma, 1769:2
Mills' disease, 1900:33
Miners' diseases, 1524:3, 1567:1
Ministry of Health, England, established, 1919:2
Minkowski-Chauffard disease, 1900:41, 1907:47
Minneapolis, University, founded, 1851:1
Minnitt apparatus, for self-administered analgesia
    in labour, 1934:32
Miracil D, in bilharziasis, 1946:23
*Miscellanea Curiosa Medico-Physica*, 1670:2
Missouri, University, Columbia, founded, 1839:2
Mitchell's disease, 1872:21
Mitomycin C, 1956:5
Mitral stenosis, 1674:4, 1695:1, 1916:11
– – congenital, 1877:20
– – mitral valve section in, 1923:21
– – mitral valvulotomy for, 1925:22
– – presystolic murmur in, 1843:20
– – treatment
– – – pulmonary-azygos shunt, 1948:13
– – – valvuloplasty, 1948:15
– – valve, prosthetic replacement, 1960:7
Mitsuda reaction, 1919:35
Mittelschmerz, 1872:9
Modena, University, 1678:1
Möbius's disease, 1884:18
Mönckenberg's sclerosis, 1903:42
Mole
– Breus, 1892:9
– hydatiform, 1827:2
– tuberous, 1892:9
Molluscum contagiosum, inclusion body, 1841:5
Monakow's bundle, 1910:48
Mongolism, 1866:15
Moniliasis, *see* Thrush

Oxygen
- in respiration, 1668:4, 1674:4
- inhalation apparatus, 1938:10
- isolation, 1772:4, 1775:3
- metabolism, 1922:1
- therapy, 1917:35
Oxygen-nitrous oxide, as anaesthetic, 1868:9
Oxytetracycline, 1950:4
Oxytocin
- isolation, 1928:4
- synthesis, 1953:5, 1955:2
Ozaena, 1876:33
- Friedländer group bacillus in, 1894:31

P-aminobenzoic acid, in scrub typhus, 1944:2
P-aminosalicylic acid, in pulmonary tuberculosis,
    1946:14
Pacemaker, heart, 1907:12, 1952:15, 1960:6
Pacini's corpuscles, 1840:13
Padgett dermatome, 1939:26
Padua
- University, formed, 1222:1
- anatomical theatre, 1549:1
- Botanic Garden, 1544:2
Paediatrics, 1565:3, 1748:3, 1764:6, 1767:8,
    1784:10, 1848:7
- first American textbook, 1825:5
- first French work, 1537:1
- first printed book, 1472:2
- first specialist in USA, 1887:6
- see also Children, diseases
Paget's disease of bone, 1877:11
Paget's disease of nipple, 1874:11
Pain
- abolition, in surgical operations, 1824:4
- intractable, relief, 1912:16, 1938:32
- relation to weather, 1877:12
- relief, subarachnoid alcohol injection for,
    1931:22
Palate
- aphthae, 1850:7
- cleft, repair, 1816:8, 1819:8, 1820:4, 1824:9,
    1825:6, 1843:9, 1862:6, 1921:12, 1928:23,
    1930:29, 1931:31
- paralysis, 1872:19, 1891:30
Palato-pharyngo-laryngeal hemiplegia, 1905:18
Palermo
- [Royal Academy of Medical Sciences],
    established, 1649:2
- University, 1778:2
Palsy, cerebral, 1897:12
Paludrine, see Proguanil
Pamaquin, in treatment of malaria, 1926:7
Pan-American Sanitary Bureau, established,
    1902:4
Panatrophy, 1886:19
Pancreas

- cancer, treatment, 1935:18
- carcinoma, 1888:27
- experimental studies, 1683:3
- function test, 1908:30, 1910:26
- in diabetes, 1788:5, 1877:16, 1890:25
- necrosis, 1882:30
- pancreatic juice, digestive action, 1857:20
- removal, partial, 1886:31
- see also Insulin
Pancreatoduodenectomy, 1935:18, 1937:20
Pancréine, 1921:29
Panniculitis, 1925:13, 1928:26
Pantopaque, for diagnosis of cerebral tumours,
    1944:19
Papaverine, isolation, 1848:12
Papilloma, Shope, 1932:10
Papovavirus, 1957:10
Pappataci fever, 1886:11
Papyrus, Ebers, 1550 BC
Papyrus, Edwin Smith, 3000 BC
Paquelin's cautery, 1877:26
Para-aminobenzoic acid, in scrub typhus, 1944:2
Para-aminosalicylic acid, in pulmonary
    tuberculosis, 1946:14
Paracusis, 1669:3
- of Willis, 1672:3
Paraffin, cancer due to, 1875:26
Paragonimiasis, 1880:8
*Paragonimus ringeri*, 1880:8
Paraldehyde, used as narcotic, 1884:41
Paralysis
- agitans, see Parkinson's disease
- ascending, unilateral, progressive, 1900:33
- bulbar, progressive, 1860:10
- descending, unilateral, 1906:26
- facial, 1797:4, 1821:11, 1936:25
- general, 1672:3, 1822:6
-- and congenital syphilis, 1877:8
-- diagnosis, 1906:24
-- malaria (fever) therapy, 1918:16, 1927:1
- oculomotor, unilateral, 1879:15
- spastic, treatment, 1908:19, 1924:16
Paramyoclonus multiplex, 1881:31
Paraphrasia, 1895:20
Paraplegia, alcoholic, 1868:16
Parasitology, 1700:6
Parasporosis, 1902:19
Parasyphilis, 1894:17
Parathyroid, 1880:32
- control of calcium metabolism, 1909:28
- extirpation and tetany, 1896:39
- hormone (parathormone), 1925:20
- tetany, 1830:3, 1831:6
- tumour, and osteitis, 1904:17, 1925:15
Paratyphoid, 1896:26, 1898:20
Paresis, see Paralysis, general

746

Paris (by date)
- Hôtel Dieu founded by St Landry, Bishop of Paris, 651:1
- University, founded, 1110:1
- anatomical theatre opened, 1551:1
- Jardin des Plantes, founded, 1597:2
- La Salpêtrière, founded, 1651:1, opened, 1657:2
- Académie des Sciences, Paris, 1666:1
- Hôpital des Enfants Malades, 1676:2
- Académie de Chirurgie, 1713:1
- Société Nationale de Chirurgie, 1731:1
- Académie Royale de Chirurgie, 1731:1
- Faculté de Médecine, Library, 1733:1
- Hôpital Necker, 1779:3
- Hôpital Cochin, 1780:3
- Hôpital Beaujon, 1785:1
- Hôpital St Antoine, 1795:4
- Société de Médecine de Paris, 1795:7
- Académie de Médecine, 1820:1
- Faculté de Médecine, 1823:3
- Société de Chirurgie, 1843:2
- Société de Biologie, 1848:1
- École de Médecine Militaire, Val-de-Grâce, 1852:5
- sewers, 1854:7, 1872:16
- Société Française d'Hygiène, 1876:5
- Institut Pasteur, 1888:1
- Société Française d'Ophthalmologie, 1888:6
- Association Française d'Urologie, organized, 1896:4
- Société de Pathologie Exotique, 1905:4
- Institut de Radium, 1912:6
Parkinson's disease, 1817:10
- encephalitis as cause of, 1921:24
- specific lesion, 1921:25
- treatment, artane, 1949:22
Parma, University, 1422:1
Parotid gland, 1662:4
- - removal, 1823:10, 1823:11
- - tumour, 1752:6, 1841:8
Parotitis, epidemic, see Mumps
Paschen elementary bodies, 1886:14, 1906:18
Pasteur Institut (by date)
- - Paris, founded, 1888:1
- - Saigon, established, 1890:4
- - Saigon, opened, 1891:5
- - Tunis, 1894:1
- - Annam, established, 1895:4
- - de la Loire-Inférieur, Nancy, 1896:5
- - Algiers, 1910:6
- - Hellenique, Athens, opened, 1920:10
- - Brazzaville, 1922:7
*Pasteurella pestis*, 1894:14, 1894:15
*Pasteurella tularensis*, 1912:18, 1914:16
Pasteurization, 1866:24

Pathological Society of Great Britain and Ireland, 1906:8
Pathological Society of London, 1846:4
Pathological Society of Philadelphia, founded, 1857:4
Pathology, 1761:2, 1793:3, 1797:4, 1799:6, 1802:2, 1842:15
- chair, at Strassburg, 1819:3
- first systematic treatise, 1554:1
- surgical, 1632:3, 1832:7
- Virchow's treatise, 1858:24
Paul's operation, 1895:27
Paul's tube, 1891:32
Paul-Bunnell test, 1932:23
Pavia, University, 1361:1
Pavy's disease, 1885:20
PCR, see Polymerase chain reaction
*Pediculus corporis*, 1907:11, 1910:14
Peet's operation, 1935:15
Peking Union Medical College, 1908:2
Pel-Ebstein disease, 1885:21, 1887:23
Pelizaeus-Merzbacher disease, 1885:18, 1908:21
Pellagra, 1735:4, 1771:4
- anti-pellagra factor, 1926:18
- experimental, 1920:22
- maize theory of origin, 1869:25
- nicotinic acid in prevention, 1938:25
Pelvimeter, 1781:1
Pelvis
- anomalies, 1753:4
- classification, 1861:7, 1933:37
- contracted, 1839:7
- deformities, 1851:7, 1852:9, 1854:10, 1861:7, 1871:4, 1900:12
- female, 1701:5
- haematocele, 1851:8
- rachitic, 1752:7, 1851:7
- spinosa, 1854:10
Pemphigus
- erythematodes, 1926:14
- foliaceus, 1844:10
- vegetans, 1886:30, 1889:21
Penicillin, 1896:55, 1929:12, 1940:7, 1943:7, 1945:1, 1947:2
Penicillinase, isolated, 1940:8
*Penicillium*, bacteria-inhibiting effect, 1876:35
*Penicillium glaucum*, 1896:55
Penis, 1743:4
Pennsylvania (by date)
- Quarantine Act, 1700:3
- University, founded (as College of Philadelphia), 1740:1
- Pennsylvania Hospital, Philadelphia, 1752:2
- Pennsylvania Hospital Library, Philadelphia, 1762:1
- University, Medical Department, 1765:1
- Quarantine Act, 1770:5

Pennsylvania (concluded)
- Western University of, 1786: 5
- *see also* Philadelphia
Pentaquine, in malaria, 1948: 22
Pentobarbitone sodium, as intravenous anaesthetic, 1930: 20
Pentosuria, 1895: 25
Pentylenetetrazol, *see* Cardiazol
Pepinière, Berlin, 1795: 8
Pepsin, 1836: 15
- crystallized, 1930: 7
Peptic ulcer, *see* Duodenum, ulcer; Stomach, ulcer
Peptide hormones
-- production, brain, 1977: 1
-- radioimmunoassay, 1977: 1
Percussion, 1828: 17, 1839: 20
Percussor, 1828: 17
Periarteritis nodosa, 1866: 23
Pericardiectomy, for constrictive pericarditis, 1923: 20
Pericardiocentesis, 1815: 6
Pericarditis
- constrictive, 1842: 20, 1896: 52, 1921: 31, 1923: 20
- suppurative, 1875: 24
Pericardium, adherent, Broadbent's sign, 1895: 34
Perineorrhaphy, 1883: 7
Perineum, female, suture, 1834: 9
Periodicals (by date)
- *Journal des Sçavans*, 1665: 1
- *Philosophical Transactions of the Royal Society of London*, 1665: 2
- *Miscellanea Curiosa Medico-Physica*, 1670: 2
- *Nouvelles Découvertes sur toutes les Parties de la Médecine*, 1679: 1
- *Medicina Curiosa*, 1684: 1
- *Vrachevnie Viedomosti*, 1792: 3
- *Archiv für die Physiologie*, 1795: 5
- *Journal der Practischen Arzneykunde*, 1795: 6
- *Medical Repository*, 1797: 1
- *Journal de Physiologie Expérimentale*, 1821: 6
- *New England Journal of Medicine and Surgery*, 1821: 1.1
- *Lancet*, 1823: 1
- *American Journal of the Medical Sciences*, 1827: 1
- *Boston Medical and Surgical Journal*, 1828: 4
- *Gazette des Hôpitaux*, 1828: 5
- *Lancette Française*, 1828: 5
- *Glasgow Medical Journal*, 1828: 6
- *Proceedings of the Royal Society of London*, 1831: 2
- *Archiv für Anatomie, Physiologie und Wissenschaftliche Medicin*, 1834: 5
- *Proceedings of the American Philosophical Society*, 1838: 1

- *Archiv für Pathologische Anatomie (Virchow's)*, 1847: 1
- *Annalen der Pharmacie*, 1832: 5
- *Wiener Medizinische Wochenschrift*, 1851: 5
- *Provincial Medical and Surgical Journal*, 1853: 2
- *Association Medical Journal*, 1853: 2
- *Aertzliches Intelligenz-Blatt*, 1854: 5
- *Münchener Medizinische Wochenschrift*, 1854: 5
- *Graefe's Archiv*, 1854: 6
- *Archiv für Ophthalmologie*, 1854: 6
- *British Medical Journal*, 1857: 1
- *Berliner Klinische Wochenschrift, (Klinische Wochenschrift, 1922)*, 1864: 7
- *Archiv für Mikroskopische Anatomie*, 1864: 8
- *Archiv für die Gesamte Physiologie (Pflüger's)*, 1868: 4
- *American Journal of Obstetrics*, 1869: 1
- *Deutsche Medizinische Wochenschrift*, 1875: 5
- *Journal of Physiology*, 1878: 1
- *Journal of the American Medical Association*, 1883: 1
- *Journal of Experimental Medicine*, 1896: 2
- *Journal of Hygiene*, 1901: 9
- *Biometrika*, 1901: 6
- *Archiv für Geschichte der Medizin (Sudhoff's Archiv)*, 1908: 10
Peritoneum, 1722: 3
- pouch of Douglas, 1730: 4
- processus vaginalis, 1722: 3
Peritonitis, 1785: 5, 1848: 14
Peroneal artery, *see* Artery, peroneal
Persecution mania, 1852: 18
Persian medicine, 854: 1, 930: 1, 980: 1, 1092: 1
Personality, traits, determination, 1921: 20
Pertussis, *see* Whooping cough
Perugia
- University, 1266: 1
- medical school established, 1321: 1
Peruvian bark, 1663: 3
Pethidine, synthesis, 1939: 8
Petit's hernia and triangle, 1774: 3
Petri dish, 1887: 29
Peyronie's disease, 1743: 4
Pfannenstiel's incision, 1900: 15
Pfeiffer's disease, 1889: 6
Pfeiffer phenomenon, 1894: 32
*Pfeifferella mallei*, 1882: 16
*Pfeifferella whitmori*, 1917: 16
*Pflüger's Archiv*, 1868: 4
Phaeochromocytoma, 1886: 27, 1945: 10
Phagocytosis, 1884: 34
Pharmacopoeia, 1546: 2
- *British Pharmacopoeia*, 1864: 23
- Florence, 1498: 1
- German, 1477: 3

Protozoa, 1693:2
– pathogenic, 1907:1
Provincial Medical and Surgical Association,
Worcester, England, 1832:1
*Provincial Medical and Surgical Journal*, 1853:2
Prurigo
– mitis, 1796:4
– nodularis, 1879:20
*Pseudomonas aeruginosa*, 1882:35
*Pseudomonas pyocyanea*, 1889:36
Pseudosclerosis, spastic, 1920:19, 1921:26
Pseudotuberculosis, 1891:11
Pseudoxanthoma elasticum, 1889:22
Psittacosis, 1879:9, 1930:22, 1932:27
Psoriasis, 1796:4, 1878:12
Psychasthenia, 1903:20
Psychiatry, 1567:2, 1621:4, 1758:2, 1793:6,
1801:7, 1803:5, 1838:3
– disorders, classification, 1798:6
– first American textbook, 1812:1
– forensic, 1838:5
Psychical process, reaction time, 1868:13
Psychoanalysis, 1893:7, 1895:16
Psychogalvanic reflex, 1890:34
Psychology
– analytical, 1911:19
– behaviourist, 1919:24
– child, 1927:14
– experimental, 1873:7, 1890:14
– gestalt, 1929:34
– individual, 1912:17
– medical, 1852:26, 1858:11
– of the unconscious, 1911:19
Psychoneuroses, application of hypnosis,
1872:18
Psychopathology, 1567:2
Psychophysics, 1860:9
Psychoses
– treatment
– – chlorpromazine, 1952:20
– – electric convulsion therapy in, 1830:18
– – frontal leucotomy, 1949:1
– – prefrontal lobotomy, 1936:22, 1936:23
– – reserpine in, 1931:21
– – sterotactic tractotomy in, 1965:6
Psychotherapy, 1666:5, 1866:13
Psychotic conditions
– effect of fevers on, 1887:15
– malaria (fever) therapy, 1918:16, 1927:1
Public health
– English, 1720:4
– in Britain, 1842:16, 1890:30
– measures against overcrowding in London,
1582:2
Public Health Act, Canada, 1882:3
Public Health Act, England, 1848:4, 1875:4

Public Health and Local Government Acts,
England, 1858:1
Public Health Laboratory Service, England and
Wales, established, 1939:4, 1961:3
Public hygiene, 1779:4
– – food regulations at Nuremberg, 1518:3
– – Royal Order against pollution of Thames,
1357:1
Puerperal
– convulsions, albuminous urine in, 1843:3
– fever, 1773:6, 1795:10, 1847:7, 1855:9,
1861:9, 1879:3, 1892:8
– – contagiousness, 1751:3, 1843:4
– – treatment, prontosil, 1935:30, 1936:31
Pulmonary artery, *see* Artery, pulmonary
Pulmonary valve, stenosis, treatment, 1947:11,
1948:14
Pulmonary-azygos shunt, for mitral stenosis,
1948:13
Pulse, 1902:25
– paradoxical, 1873:15
Pulse-clock, 1603:2, 1625:1
Pulse-watch, 1707:4
Pulsus alterans, 1872:29
Pump-oxygenator, 1954:9
Pupil
– Adie's syndrome, 1931:16
– Argyll Robertson, 1869:13
– artificial, 1729:2, 1811:2, 1852:13
– dilatation, with hyoscyamine, 1801:9
– response to light, 1751:2
Purgatives, Jalap, 1609:1
Purkyně cells, 1837:16
Purkyně fibres, 1839:21
Purpura, 1556:1
– anaphylactoid, 1837:11
– annularis telangiectoides, 1896:33
– fulminans, 1887:28
– haemorrhagica, 1735:3
– Schönlein-Henoch, 1868:21
Purtscher's disease, 1912:10
Putrefaction, biological process, 1837:18,
1863:26
Pyelitis, 1888:23, 1887:8
Pyelography, 1906:32
Pyknolepsy, 1906:25
Pyloroplasty, 1882:26
Pylorus
– cancer, Billroth II operation, 1911:33
– carcinoma, 1880:23, 1881:27
– resection, 1885:23
– stenosis, 1717:2, 1777:3, 1888:11, 1912:26
Pyocyanase, 1889:36
Pyorrhoea alveolaris, 1594:1, 1876:27
Pyramidal tract, 1890:32
– – disease, plantar response, 1896:27
Pyramidon, 1896:56

Skeleton, osteopoikilosis, 1915:16
Skin
– diseases, 1714:2, 1776:6, 1832:10
– – classification, 1845:12, 1856:10
– – colloid, 1865:19
– – first comprehensive American text, 1845:13
– – fungous, 1894:28
– – histopathology, 1894:23
– epithelia, 1837:5
– grafts, 1822:3, 1829:9, 1869:8, 1871:7
    1875:7, 1939:26
– – fibrin glue for, 1943:15
– – forensic use, 1950:2
– – full-thickness, 1804:4
– – in treatment of ulcers, 1854:15
– – intermediate-thickness grafts, 1872:11,
    1874:9
– – rejection mechanisms, 1943:6
– – split-skin, 1929:39
– – whole-thickness, 1893:4
– hyperalgesia, and visceral disease, 1893:10
– Schwartzman phenomenon, 1928:7
– see also Dermatology
Skull
– cleidocranial dysostosis, 1760:3, 1898:28
– linear craniotomy, 1891:14
– radiography, 1931:18
Sleeping sickness, see Trypanosomiasis
Slit-lamp, Gullstrand's, 1902:29
Sloane Maternity Hospital, New York, 1887:2
Sluder's neuralgia, 1901:16
Smallpox, 1685:4
– diagnostic test, 1915:14, 1926:9, 1928:19
– differentiated from:
– – measles, 854:1
– – syphilis, 1560:1
– – varicella, 1768:7
– Free Vaccination Act, England, 1840:1
– global eradication, 1980:3
– inoculation, 1671:3, 1701:1, 1714:4, 1715:1,
    1718:2, 1747:1, 1767:7, 1777:1
– – in America, 1721:3, 1726:1
– – in Wales, 1722:1
– – into monkey, 1904:14
– Prevention Act, Massachusetts, 1701:2
– vaccination, 1799:1
– – in USA, 1800:8
– – Jennerian, 1796:5, 1798:4
– – obligatory in Spain, 1903:7
– virus, 1868:10
Smell see Olfaction
Smellie manoeuvre, 1752:7
Smith-Petersen nail, 1931:13
Smithwick operation, 1940:21
Smoking, associated with lung cancer, 1939:15,
    1950:8, 1950:9
Snake venom, 1664:3, 1767:4, 1934:14

Snow's inhaler, 1847:11, 1848:9
Sociedad Cientifica Argentina, 1872:6
Società Italiana delle Scienze, 1782:3
Società Medico-Chirurgica, Bologna, 1823:4
Société de Biologie, Paris, 1848:1
Société de Chirurgie, Paris, 1843:2
Société Française d'Hygiène, Paris, 1876:5
Société Française d'Ophtalmologie, Paris,
    1888:6
Société de Médecine de Paris, 1795:7
Société Nationale de Chirurgie, 1731:1
Société de Pathologie Exotique, Paris, 1905:4
Society of Apothecaries, London, 1676:1
Sodium amytal, anaesthetic, 1923:13, 1929:36
Sodium glucosulphone, see Promin
Sodium iodide, contrast medium in
    ureteropyelography, 1923:15
Sodium ortho-huppurate, see Hippuran
Solapsone, in leprosy, 1943:4
Sorbonne, founded in Paris, 1257:1
South African Institute for Medical Research,
    Johannesburg, 1912:4
Spain, see Madrid; Seville; Valencia; Valladolid
Spalding's sign, 1922:14
Spectacles, 1270:1, 1623:2, 1922:33
Speculum, 1806:5
– duck-billed, 1866:10
– urethro-cystic, 1827:8
– vaginal, 1843:7, 1857:6
Speech
– cerebral localization, 1861:8
– disorders, 1864:15, 1877:9, 1887:16, 1898:25,
    1906:27, 1926:10
Spencer Wells' forceps, 1879:26
Spermatozoa, 1693:1, 1841:6
Sphygmograph, 1854:24, 1860:24
Sphygmomanometer, 1834:13, 1881:33,
    1889:35, 1895:33, 1896:48, 1897:23
Spielmayer-Vogt disease, 1905:16, 1907:25
Spinal cord, 1666:3
– – degeneration in tabes dorsalis, 1883:19
– – – subacute, combined, 1900:34
– – diseases, 1880:17
– – lesion, 1850:14, 1890:19
– – myelography, 1921:18
– – paralysis
– – – spastic, 1886:23
– – – syphilitic, 1892:24
– – posterior columns, disease, 1839:11
– – subacute combined degeneration, 1884:33
– – traumatic cavity formation, 1902:17
– – tumour, extramedullary, 1888:18
Spine
– deformities, 1769:4
– immobilization and fusion, 1891:24
– kyphosis, 1744:3, 1921:21
– neurotic, arthropathies, 1831:7

*Streptococcus*
– classification, serological, 1934: 9
– described, 1880: 29
– differentiation from Staphylococcus, 1881:35, 1884: 44
– haemolytic, 1879: 3
– – acute rheumatism in children due to, 1930: 16
– – type differentiation, 1933: 9
– in acute rheumatism, 1898: 29
– in scarlet fever, 1924: 15
*Streptococcus pyogenes*, discovered, 1882:36
*Streptococcus viridans*, isolated, in bacterial endocarditis, 1910:39
Streptodornase, 1948: 12
Streptokinase, 1933: 7
Streptomycin, 1944: 4
– in tuberculosis, 1945: 4, 1952: 1
– in tularaemia, 1946: 18
*Streptothrix muris ratti*, 1926: 6
Stress, general adaptation syndrome, 1950: 5
Stretch reflex, 1924: 18
*Strongyloides stercoralis*, 1876: 18
Strongyloidosis, 1876: 18
*Strophanthus hispidus*, 1890:31
Strümpell's disease, 1884: 21, 1885: 16, 1886:23
Strychnine, isolation, 1819: 10
Sturge-Weber syndrome, 1879: 14, 1922:16
Subarachnoid space, patency, 1916:33
Subclavian artery, *see* Artery, subclavian
Subconscious states, 1852: 26
Substance P, peptide neurotransmitter, 1931:34
Succinylcholine chloride, 1949: 25, 1951: 15
Sulphadiazine, 1941: 5
Suphaguanidine, 1940: 6
– in bacillary dysentery, 1941: 17
Sulphamerazine, synthesis, 1940: 9
Sulphanilamide, 1908: 43
– antibacterial, 1957: 1
– in treatment of gonorrhoea, 1937: 4
– protection by, in experimental gonococcal infections, 1937: 28
– therapeutic value, 1935: 3
Sulphapyridine, pneumococcal and staphylococcal infections, 1938: 8, 1938: 9
Sulphasuxidine, 1941: 4
Sulphetrone, in leprosy, 1943: 4
Sulphonal, 1884: 35, 1888: 10
Sulphonamide, 1935: 6, 1939: 1
– dressing, of wounds, 1939: 25
– hypoglycaemic effect, 1930: 13, 1944: 15
Sulphonylurea, 1955: 14
Sunlight, bactericidal action, 1877: 25
Sunstroke, 1665: 9
Suramin
– in onchocerciasis, 1947: 21
– in trypanosomiasis, 1920: 15

Surgeon General's Office Library, Washington, 1836: 2
Surgeons separated from barbers
– in England, 1745: 1
– in Austria, 1783: 2
Surgery, 1260: 1, 1307: 1, 1563:4, 1596:3, 1606: 1, 1718: 5
– Abernethy's treatise, 1809: 1
– antiseptic principle, 1867: 6
– bibliography, 1774: 1
– Billroth's treatise, 1863: 29
– Desault's treatise, 1798: 8
– diagnosis, x ray, 1896: 50
– Dorsey's treatise, 1813: 2
– experimental, 1838: 18
– first printed book, 1210: 1
– first printed treatise in German, 1497: 2
– French, 1290: 1, 1298: 1
– Gross's treatise, 1859: 22
– intracranial, 1932: 18
– kineplastic, 1898: 26, 1918: 18
– Liston's treatise, 1837: 19
– military, 1517: 1, 1812:8, 1829:7
– operative, 1807: 2, 1821: 9, 1832: 19, 1834: 17
– ophthalmic, 1823: 6, 1833: 7
– oral, *see* Mouth, surgery
– orthopaedic, 1822: 5, 1882: 20; *see also* Orthopaedics
– plastic, 1597: 5, 1822: 5, 1838: 8, 1847: 9, 1916: 18, 1917: 10
– – *see also* Cleft palate; Keratoplasty; Rhinoplasty; etc.
– reconstructive, 1876: 16
– rubber gloves, 1894: 12
– shock, 1899: 29
– *see also* Anaesthesia
Surra, 1881: 16
Susruta Samhita, 500 BC
Suture
– Lembert's, 1829: 11, 1836: 12
– silver, 1858: 25, 1888: 43
Sweat
– coloured, 1858: 16
– secretion, disorders, 1873: 10
Sweating sickness, 1529: 2, 1552: 2
Swift's disease, 1914: 7
Sycosis barbae, 1806: 2, 1842: 11
Sydenham Society, founded in London, 1843: 1
Sydenham's chorea, 1686: 1
Sydney, Botanic Garden, 1789: 2
Syme's amputation, 1843: 17
Sympathectomy
– for vascular disease, 1900: 45
– lumbar, 1933: 29
Sympathetic ramisection, in spastic paralysis, 1924: 16
Sympathetic-adrenal system, 1932: 5

Tumours (concluded)
– *see also* Cancer; *individual sites* Adrenals;
    Bladder; Brain; Breast; Kidney; Larynx;
    Oesophagus; Ovary; Parathyroid; Parotid;
    Pituitary; Spinal cord; Thyroid; Uterus
Tunis, Institut Pasteur, 1894:1
Turku, University, 1640:1
Turner's syndrome, 1938:19
Twilight sleep, 1902:6, 1906:10
Twort-d'Herelle phenomenon (bacteriophage),
    1915:24, 1917:31
Tympanic membrane, 1561:2, 1832:16, 1865:13
Tympanoplasty, in otitis media, 1949:17
Tyndallization, 1877:24
Typhoid, 1824:7, 1884:12
– aetiology, 1849:8
– agglutination reaction, 1896:24
– and typhus, differentiation, 1836:6, 1837:9,
    1840:4, 1847:16
– antiserum, 1938:33
– bacillus, 1880:10, 1881:17
– – Vi antigen, 1934:23
– epidemic, 1659:2
– fever, 1829:10, 1873:6
– identification, 1896:22
– inoculation, 1888:17, 1896:25
Typhus, 1536:2, 1546:3, 1810:3
– aetiology, 1849:8
– and famine, 1868:11
– at Cambridge Assizes, 1521:1
– at Oxford Assizes, 1577:2
– causal organism, 1915:13, 1916:27, 1919:23,
    1921:16, 1922:15
– diagnosis, 1916:26
– differentiated
– – from plague, 1666:4
– – from relapsing fever, 1844:6
– – from Rocky Mountain fever, 1910:16
– – from typhoid, 1836:6, 1837:9, 1840:4,
    1847:16
– epidemic, 1934:24
– exanthematous, transmission by lice, 1928:1
– fever, diagnostic reaction, 1909:16
– identical to 'hospital fever', 1750:3
– murine, 1926:8
– – aetiology, 1931:25
– – differentiated from epidemic typhus, 1928:16
– prophylaxis, 1905:18
– recrudescent, 1910:17
– *Rickettsia prowazeki* causal agent in, 1921:16,
    1922:15
– scrub, 1879:8
– – causal organism, 1927:11
– – identical to tsutsagamuchi disease, 1940:19
– – treatment, para-aminobenzoic acid, 1944:2
– – vaccine, 1945:16
– Spanish/Mexican (tabadillo), 1570:1

– transmission
– – by body louse, 1910:14
– – tick-born, 1910:15
– treatment, chloramphenicol, 1947:19
– vaccine, 1940:17
Tyrosinosis, 1932:16

Ulcers
– classification, 1778:8
– treatment by skin grafts, 1854:15
– *see also* Duodenum, ulcers; Stomach, ulcers
Ultraviolet irradiation
– – – of oils and foods, 1929:26
– – – rickets cured with, 1919:26
– – – tetany treatment with, 1920:20
– – – therapeutic value, 1896:57, 1903:1
– – – tuberculosis treatment, 1903:47
Ultrasonic investigation
– – cephalometry, 1961:8
– – in pregnancy, 1958:6
– – soft tissue, 1957:9
Ultrasonic therapy, 1939:10
Unconscious, psychology, 1852:26, 1911:19
Underwood's disease, 1784:10
Union Internationale Contre la Tuberculose,
    Paris, 1920:4
United Kingdom (by date)
– – Pharmacy Act, 1852:4
– – Medical Act, 1858:2
– – General Medical Council, established, 1858:3
– – Medical Register, first woman registered,
    1859:3
– – Births and Deaths Registration Acts, 1871:2
– – National Insurance Act, 1911:10
– – Medical Research Committee (later Council)
    established, 1913:2
– – Medical Research Council (formerly
    Committee) established, 1920:2
– – National Health Service (NHS) comes into
    operation, 1948:3
– – *see also* England; London; Cambridge;
    Oxford; Edinburgh etc.
United States (by date)
– – Marine Hospital Service, established, 1798:1
– – public health and hygiene, 1850:12
– – National Academy of Sciences, Washington,
    chartered, 1863:4
– – War of the Rebellion, 1870:27
– – National Board of Health, 1879:2
– – Public Health Service, Hygienic Laboratory,
    1901:8
– – Federal Food and Drugs Act, 1906:2
– – National Health Council, 1920:5
– – Hygienic Laboratory becomes National
    Institute(s) of Health, 1930:3
– – *see also* individual States and Cities
University College London, founded, 1826:3

Unna's eczema, 1887:21
Unverricht's disease, 1891:19
Uppsala
– – University, 1477:2
– – anatomical theatre, 1662:2
– – Konglige Vetenskaps-Societeten i Uppsala,
    1710:4
– – Nosocomium Academicum, established,
    1718:3
Uraemia, peritoneal dialysis, 1923:16
Urea, 1732:2
– blood, clearance test, 1929:29
– synthesis, 1828:19
Urease, isolation, in crystal form, 1926:16
Ureter
– calculus, radiographic demonstration, 1901:19
– catheterization, 1876:30, 1893:14, 1893:15,
    1901:17
– repair, 1893:18
Ureteral colic, 1864:19
Uretero-intestinal anastomosis, 1852:23,
    1894:26, 1911:14
Uretero-pyelography, sodium iodide contrast
    medium in, 1923:15
Uretero-ureteral anastomosis, 1894:25
Urethane, in leukaemia, 1946:13
Urethra
– artificial, 1950:13
– female, cancer, 1833:8
– stricture, diagnosis, 1910:24
Urethrography, 1910:24
Uric acid, discovery, 1776:8
Urinary
– catheter, 1845:14
– tract
– – diseases, 1791:4
– – fistula, 1870:15
– – infection
– – – mandelic acid in, 1935:20
– – – mercurochrome in, 1919:16
– – visualization, 1899:14
Urine
– acetone bodies in, Rothera's test, 1908:25
– cryoscopy, 1894:27
– dropsical, 1812:2
– in diagnosis, 1683:4
– secretion, 1917:22
Uriniferous tubules, 1666:7
Urinoscopy, 1350:1, 1529:1
Urography, excretion, 1929:30, 1933:23
Urology, 1588:2, 1791:4
– local anaesthesia first used, 1884:27
Uroselectan, as contrast medium, 1929:30
Urticaria pigmentosa, 1869:14
Uterine sound, 1843:5
Uterus
– cancer, 1824:3, 1858:7

– – radium treatment, 1917:11, 1933:40
– – surgery, 1902:7
– cervix, amputation, 1833:8, 1861:5
– – cancer diagnosis, 1933:42, 1941:2
– contractions, during pregnancy, 1872:10
– dilatation, 1888:12
– excision, 1863:6
– fibroids, 1853:6, 1881:11
– gonorrhoeal infection, 1896:14
– gravid, 1774:4, 1794:11
– inverted, replacement, 1945:18
– peritoneal folds, 1854:11
– pregnant, ultrasonic investigation, 1958:6
– prolapse, treatment, 1900:19, 1908:13, 1915:6
– retroposition, 1843:5
– retroversion, 1771:8
– – treatment, 1881:9, 1886:10
– tumours, 1845:7
– – removal, 1886:9
Utrecht, University, 1634:1
Uveo-parotid fever, 1909:24

Vaccinia, 1796:5, 1798:4
– virus, 1886:14
– – cultivation, 1928:18
– – Paschen elementary bodies in, 1906:18
– – pure culture, 1915:12
Vaccination, see Smallpox, Yellow fever, etc.
Vagina
– artificial, 1904:9, 1938:37
– atresia, 1900:16
– excision, 1895:7
– plastic reconstruction, 1896:16
Vagotomy, in duodenal ulcer, 1943:8
Valencia, School of Medicine established, 1345:2
Valladolid, hospital for insane, opened, 1489:1
Valsalva's manoeuvre, 1704:1
Valvuloplasty, in mitral stenosis, 1948:15
Valvulotomy, for pulmonary valve stenosis,
    1947:11, 1948:14
Van den Bergh test, for bilirubin, 1913:30
Van Gieson's stains for nervous tissue, 1889:38
Vaquez-Osler disease, 1892:43, 1903:37
Varicella, 1553:1
– and herpes zoster, aetiological relationship,
    1892:23
– differentiated from smallpox, 1768:7
– gangrenosa, 1882:14
– inclusion bodies, 1905:11
– prevention, zoster immune globulin, 1969:2
Varicella-herpes, virus, 1953:18
Varicose veins
– surgery, 1814:7
– treatment, 1890:27, 1916:14
Variolation, see Smallpox, inoculation

# Journal codes

| | |
|---|---|
| *AA* | Antibiotics Annual |
| *AbL* | Abhandlungen, Kgl. Sächs Gesellschaft der Wissenschaften, Math.-phys Kl. |
| *AC* | Antibiotics and Chemotherapy |
| *AcC* | Acta Chirurgica Scandinavica |
| *AcCS* | Acta Chemica Scandinavica |
| *AcDS* | Actas Dermo-Sifilográficas |
| *AcHa* | Acta Haematologica |
| *AcM* | Acta Medica Scandinavica |
| *ACMI* | Atti del Congresso della Associazione Medica Italiana |
| *AcOL* | Acta Oto-Laryngologica |
| *AcP* | Acta Paediatrica |
| *AcPha* | Acta Pharmacologica |
| *AcPL* | Acta Physiologica Latino-Americana |
| *AcPMS* | Acta Pathologica et Microbiologica Scandinavica |
| *AcPN* | Acta Psychiatrica et Neurologica |
| *AcPS* | Acta Physiologica Scandinavica |
| *AcPsS* | Acta Psychiatrica Scandinavica |
| *AcR* | Acta Radiologica |
| *ADGP* | Archiv der Deutschen Gesellschaft für Psychiatrie und Gerichtliche Psychologie |
| *AGPA* | Arbeiten auf dem Gebiete der Pathologischen Anatomie und Bacteriologie |
| *AHI* | Arbeiten aus dem Hirnanatomischen Institut in Zürich |
| *AIB* | Ärztliches Intelligenz-Blatt |
| *AKG* | Arbeiten aus dem Kaiserlichen Gesundheitsamte |
| *AMC* | Allgemeine Medizinische Central-Zeitung |
| *AMD* | Army Medical Dept., Statistical, Sanitary and Medical Reports |
| *AmHJ* | American Heart Journal |
| *AMHN* | Annales de Musée Nationale d'Histoire Naturelle de Paris |
| *AmJA* | American Journal of Anatomy |
| *AmJDC* | American Journal of Diseases of Children |
| *AmJH* | American Journal of Hygiene |
| *AmJHG* | American Journal of Human Genetics |
| *AmJMS* | American Journal of the Medical Sciences |
| *AmJOD* | American Journal of Obstetrics and Diseases of Women and Children |
| *AmJOG* | American Journal of Obstetrics and Gynecology |
| *AmJOp* | American Journal of Ophthalmology |
| *AmJOrS* | American Journal of Orthodontics and Oral Surgery |
| *AmJPa* | American Journal of Pathology |
| *AmJPh* | American Journal of Physiology |
| *AmJPm* | American Journal of Pharmacy |
| *AmJPuH* | American Journal of Public Health |
| *AmJR* | American Journal of Roentgenology |
| *AmJSc* | American Journal of Science (and the Arts) |
| *AmJSu* | American Journal of Surgery |
| *AmJSy* | American Journal of Syphilis, Gonorrhea, and Venereal Diseases |
| *AmJTM* | American Journal of Tropical Medicine |
| *AMKI* | Arbeiten, Medicinisch-Klinische Institute, Leipzig |

| | |
|---|---|
| *AmM* | American Medicine |
| *AmMG* | American Medical Gazette |
| *AmMM* | American Monthly Microscopical Journal |
| *AmMPR* | American Medical and Philosophical Register |
| *AmMR* | American Medical Recorder |
| *AmP* | American Practitioner (Louisville) |
| *AmPr* | American Practitioner (Philadelphia) |
| *AmQR* | American Quarterly of Roentgenology |
| *AmRRD* | American Review of Respiratory Diseases |
| *AmRT* | American Review of Tuberculosis |
| *Analyst* | Analyst |
| *AnBSG* | Annales et Bulletin de la Société Royale de Médecine de Gand |
| *AnC* | Annales de Chimie |
| *AnCK* | Annalen der Charité-Krankenhauses, Berlin |
| *AnCM* | Anales del Circulo Médico Argentino |
| *AnCP* | Annalen der Chemie und Pharmacie |
| *AnD* | Annales de Dermatologie et de Syphiligraphie |
| *Ane* | Anesthesiology |
| *AnG* | Annales de Gynécologie |
| *AnGH* | Annalen der Gesamte Heilkunde |
| *Angiology* | Angiology |
| *AnGO* | Annales de Gynécologie et d'Obstétrique |
| *AnH* | Annales d'Hygiène Publique |
| *AnI* | Annales d'Immunologie |
| *AnIM* | Annals of Internal Medicine |
| *AnIMod* | Anales del Instituto Modelo de Clinica Medica |
| *AnIP* | Annales de l'Institut Pasteur, Paris |
| *AnIS* | Annali d'Igiene Sperimentale |
| *AnM* | Annales de Médecine |
| *AnMP* | Annales des Maladies de la Peau et de la Syphilis |
| *AnMV* | Annales de Médecine Vétérinaire |
| *AnO* | Annales d'Oculistique |
| *AnOG* | Annali di Ostetricia e Ginecologia |
| *AnOt* | Annals of Otology, Rhinology, and Laryngology |
| *AnP* | Annalen der Pharmacie |
| *AnPa* | Annaes Paulistas de Medicina e Cirurgia |
| *AnPh* | Annalen der Physik und Chemie |
| *AnRA* | Anales de la Real Academia de Ciencias Medicas, Fisicas, y Naturales de Habana |
| *AnRB* | Annual Review of Biochemistry |
| *AnS* | Annals of Surgery |
| *AnSMP* | Annales de la Société de Médecine Pratique |
| *AnSR* | Annales de la Société Royale des Sciences Médicales et Naturelles de Bruxelles |
| *AnTM* | Annals of Tropical Medicine and Parasitology |
| *AnTS* | Annals of Thoracic Surgery |
| *AnU* | Annali Universali di Medicina |
| *ANYAS* | Annals of the New York Academy of Sciences |
| *APIH* | Arbeiten aus dem Pathologischen Institut, Universität, Helsingfors |
| *AR* | Anatomical Record |
| *ArAA* | Archiv für Anatomie, Physiologie, und Wissenschaftliche Medicin [Müller's] |

| | |
|---|---|
| *ArAP* | Archiv für Anatomie und Physiologie. Physiologische Abteilung |
| *ArBM* | Archivos Brasileiros de Medicina |
| *ArBN* | Arkhiv Biologicheskikh Nauk |
| *ArD* | Archiv für Dermatologie und Syphilis |
| *ArDiC* | Archives of Disease in Childhood |
| *ArDS* | Archives of Dermatology (and Syphilology) |
| *ArEP* | Archiv für Experimentelle Pathologie und Pharmakologie |
| *ArG* | Archiv für die Geburtshülfe |
| *ArGeM* | Archiv für die Gesamte Medizin |
| *ArGM* | Archives Générales de Médecine |
| *ArGy* | Archiv für Gynäkologie |
| *ArH* | Archiv der Heilkunde |
| *ArHyg* | Archiv für Hygiene |
| *ArIB* | Archives Italiennes de Biologie |
| *ArIL* | Archives International de Laryngologie, d'Otologie et de Rhinologie |
| *ArIM* | Archives of Internal Medicine |
| *ArIP* | Archives de l'Institut Pasteur de Tunis |
| *ArIPh* | Archives Internationales de Physiologie |
| *ArIPha* | Archives Internationales de Pharmacodynamie et de Therapie |
| *ArKC* | Archiv für Klinische Chirurgie |
| *ArL* | Archiv für Laryngologie und Rhinologie (Berlin) |
| *ArMA* | Archiv für Mikroskopische Anatomie |
| *ArMC* | Archives des Maladies du Coeur et des Vaisseaux |
| *ArME* | Archives de Médecine des Enfants |
| *ArMEA* | Archives de Médecine Experimentale et d'Anatomie Pathologique |
| *ArMEr* | Archiv für Medizinische Erfahrung |
| *ArMi* | Archivos de Medicina Interna |
| *ArN* | Archives de Neurologie |
| *ARNMD* | Association for Research in Nervous and Mental Disease, Research Publications |
| *ArNP* | Archives of Neurology and Psychiatry |
| *ArNS* | Archives Neerlandaises des Sciences Exactes et Naturelles |
| *ArO* | Archives d'Ophtalmologie |
| *ArOh* | Archiv für Ohrenheilkunde |
| *ArOH* | Archivos de Oftalmologia Hispano-Americanos |
| *ArOp* | Archives of Ophthalmology |
| *ArOt(C)* | Archives of Otolaryngology |
| *ArOt(NY)* | Archives of Otology |
| *ArP* | Archiv für Physiologie |
| *ArPa* | Archives of Pathology and Laboratory Medicine |
| *ArPC* | Archives Provinciales de Chirurgie |
| *ArPe* | Archives of Pediatrics |
| *ArPH* | Archiv für Physiologische Heilkunde |
| *ArPha* | Archives de Pharmacodynamie |
| *ArPhy* | Archives de Physiologie Normale et Pathologique |
| *ArPN* | Archiv für Psychiatrie und Nervenkrankheiten |
| *ArRR* | Archives of the Roentgen Ray |
| *ARSB* | Archivio di Scienze Biologiche |
| *ARSCI* | Annual Report, Sanitary Commission, India |
| *ArSk* | Archives of Skiagraphy |
| *ArSM* | Archivio per le Scienze Mediche |

| | |
|---|---|
| *ArSOH* | Archivos de la Sociedad Oftalmológica Hispano-Americana |
| *ArST* | Archiv für Schiffs- und Tropenhygiene |
| *ArSuC* | Archives of Surgery, Chicago |
| *ArV* | Archiv für Verdauungskrankheiten |
| *ASBMT* | Annales de la Société Belge de Médecine Tropicale |
| *ASMG* | Annales de la Société de Médecine, Gand |
| *ASML* | Annales de la Société de Médecine, Lyon |
| *AtMJ* | Atlanta Medical and Surgical Journal |
| *AuMG* | Australasian Medical Gazette |
| *AuNZ* | Australian and New Zealand Journal of Surgery |
| *AvAeE* | Aviation and Aeronautical Engineering |
| *AWMZ* | Allgemeine Wiener Medicinische Zeitung |
| *AZP* | Allgemeine Zeitschrift für Psychiatrie |
| | |
| *BAFC* | Bulletin de l'Association Française pour l'Etude du Cancer |
| *BAIS* | Bulletin de l'Académie Imperiale des Sciences St Petersburg |
| *BAMR* | Bolletino, R. Accademia Medica di Roma |
| *BARM* | Bulletin de l'Académie Royale de Médecine de Belgique |
| *BARS* | Bulletin de l'Académie Royale des Sciences, des Lettres, et des Beaux-Arts de Belgique |
| *BB* | Biological Bulletin |
| *BBA* | Biochimica et Biophysica Acta |
| *BcZ* | Biochemische Zeitschrift |
| *BDBG* | Berichte der Deutschen Botanischen Gesellschaft |
| *BDCG* | Berichte der Deutschen Chemischen Gesellschaft |
| *BEP* | Beiträge zur Experimentelle Pathologie |
| *BFM* | Bulletin de la Faculté de Médecine, Paris |
| *BFMCR* | British and Foreign Medico-Chirurgical Review |
| *BGJ* | British Gynaecological Journal |
| *BGT* | Bulletin Général de Thérapeutique Médicale |
| *BGUMC* | Bulletin of the Georgetown University Medical Center |
| *BHJ* | British Heart Journal |
| *BIP* | Bulletin de l'Institut Pasteur, Paris |
| *BJ* | Biochemical Journal |
| *BJA* | British Journal of Anaesthesia |
| *BJD* | British Journal of Dermatology (and Syphilis) |
| *BJEP* | British Journal of Experimental Pathology |
| *BJH* | Bulletin of the Johns Hopkins Hospital |
| *BJO* | British Journal of Ophthalmology |
| *BJP* | British Journal of Pharmacology and Chemotherapy |
| *BJPS* | British Journal of Plastic Surgery |
| *BJR* | British Journal of Radiology |
| *BJS* | British Journal of Surgery |
| *BJVD* | British Journal of Venereal Diseases |
| *BKC* | Beiträge zur Klinischen Chirurgie |
| *BKI* | Beiträge zur Klinik der Infektionskrankheiten und zur Immunitätsforschung |
| *BKl* | Berliner Klinik |
| *BKO* | Budapesti Kiralyi Orvosegyisulet |
| *BKT* | Beiträge zur Klinik der Tuberkulose |
| *BKW* | Berliner Klinische Wochenschrift |
| *Blood* | Blood |

| | |
|---|---|
| *BMCW* | Beobachtungen der K.K. Medicinisch-Chirurgischen Josephs-Academie zu Wien |
| *BMJ* | British Medical Journal |
| *BMMS* | Bulletin of the Manila Medical Society |
| *BMR* | Birmingham Medical Review |
| *BMSC* | Bulletin et Mémoires de la Société de Chirurgie de Paris |
| *BMSJ* | Boston Medical and Surgical Journal |
| *BNC* | Bulletin et Mémoires, Société Nationale de Chirurgie |
| *BNI* | Bulletin of the Neurological Institute of New York |
| *BNYA* | Bulletin of the New York Academy of Medicine |
| *BoAN* | Boletín de la Academia Nacional de Medicina de Buenos Aires |
| *BPA* | Beiträge zur Pathologischen Anatomie (und Physiologie) und zur Allgemeinen Pathologie |
| *BPJR* | Baltimore Philosophical Journal and Review |
| *Brain* | Brain |
| *BrM* | Brasil-Medico |
| *BSAnth* | Bulletins de la Sociéte d'Anthropologie de Paris |
| *BSAP* | Bulletin de la Société Anatomique de Paris |
| *BSCP* | Bulletins et Mémoires de la Société de Chirurgiens de Paris |
| *BSFD* | Bulletin de la Société Française de Dermatologie et de Syphiligraphie |
| *BSIC* | Bulletin de la Société Impériale de Chirurgie de Paris |
| *BSMH* | Bulletins et Mémoires de la Société Médicale des Hôpitaux de Paris |
| *BSMP* | Bolletino della Societa Medico-Chirurgica di Pavia |
| *BSOG* | Bulletin de la Société Obstetricale et Gynécologique de Paris |
| *BSP* | Bulletin de la Société de Pharmacologie |
| *BSPa* | Bulletin des Sciences Pharmacologiques |
| *BSPE* | Bulletin de la Société de Pathologie Exotique |
| *BSPP* | Bulletin de la Société de Pédiatrie de Paris |
| *BU* | Bibliothèque Universelle |
| *BuAIM* | Bulletin de l'Académie Imperiale de Médecine, Paris |
| *BuAM* | Bulletin de l'Académie de Médecine, Paris |
| *BuM* | Bulletin Médical |
| *BVDN* | Berichte über die Versammlung der Deutschen Naturforschungen und Aertze |
| *BVOG* | Berichte über die Versammlung der Deutschen Ophthalmologischen Gesellschaft |
| *BZ* | Biologisches Zentralblatt |
| | |
| *CA* | Charité-Annalen |
| *Cancer* | Cancer |
| *Ch* | Chirurg |
| *ChA* | Cholera-Archiv |
| *ChMJ* | Chinese Medical Journal |
| *Cir* | Circulation |
| *CLC* | Casopis Lékaru Ceskych |
| *CLLH* | Clinical Lectures and Reports, London Hospital |
| *CM* | Clinica Moderna |
| *CMAJ* | Canadian Medical Association Journal |
| *CMHD* | Clinique Médicale de l'Hôtel-Dieu |
| *CMI* | Clinica Medica Italiana |
| *CMSJ* | Canada Medical and Surgical Journal |
| *CO* | Clinique Ophtalmologique |

| | |
|---|---|
| *CoM* | Colorado Medicine |
| *CORC* | Collezione d'Osservazione e Riflessioni di Chirurgia |
| *CPHJ* | Canadian Public Health Journal |
| *CR* | Cancer Research |
| *CRA* | Current Researches in Anesthesia and Analgesia |
| *CRAFS* | Comptes-Rendus de l'Association Française pour l'Avancement des Sciences |
| *CRAS* | Comptes Rendus Hebdomadaires des Séances de l'Académie des Sciences |
| *CRCAN* | Comptes Rendus, Congrès Alien Neurologie de Langue Français, Paris |
| *CRDS* | Comptes Rendus, Congrès International de Dermatologie et de Syphiligraphie. |
| *CrM* | Cronica Medica |
| *CRSB* | Comptes Rendus Hebdomadaires des Séances et Mémoires de la Société de Biologie |
| *CS* | Clinical Science |
| *CSHS* | Cold Spring Harbor Symposia on Quantitative Biology |
| *CV* | Clinica Veterinaria |
| *CW* | Chemisch Weekblad |
| *CZ* | Chemiker-Zeitung |
| | |
| *DAKM* | Deutsches Archiv für Klinische Medizin |
| *DAP* | Deutsches Archiv für Physiologie |
| *DeC* | Dental Cosmos |
| *DeW* | Dermatologische Wochenschrift |
| *DeZ* | Dermatologische Zeitschrift |
| *DHR* | Dublin Hospital Reports |
| *DJMS* | Dublin Journal of Medical Science |
| *DK* | Deutsche Klinik |
| *DMP* | Dublin Medical Press |
| *DMPE* | Dublin Medical and Physical Essays |
| *DMW* | Deutsche Medizinische Wochenschrift |
| *DQMS* | Dublin Quarterly Journal of Medical Science |
| *DZC* | Deutsche Zeitschrift für Chirurgie |
| *DZN* | Deutsche Zeitschrift für Nervenheilkunde |
| | |
| *EaP* | Ergebnisse der Allgemeinen Pathologie und Pathologischen Anatomie |
| *EIM* | Ergebnisse der Inneren Medizin und Kinderheilkunde |
| *El* | Electricity |
| *EMJ* | Edinburgh Medical Journal |
| *EMSJ* | Edinburgh Medical and Surgical Journal |
| *En* | Endocrinology |
| *ENPJ* | Edinburgh New Philosophical Journal |
| *Enz* | Enzymologia |
| *ER* | Eclectic Repertory and Analytical Review |
| *Ex* | Experientia |
| | |
| *Far* | Far Eastern Association of Tropical Medicine, 6th Congress, 1925, Tokyo |
| *FGR* | Fortschritte auf dem Gebiete der Röntgenstrahlen |
| *FH* | Folia Haematologica |
| *FLH* | Finska Läkaresällskapets Handlingar |
| *FM* | Fortschritte der Medizin |
| *FSL* | Förhandlingar vid Svenska Läkaresällskapet Sammankomster |
| *FZP* | Frankfurter Zeitschrift für Pathologie |

| | |
|---|---|
| *Gal* | Galvani |
| *GAMT* | Giornale R. Accademia di Medicina di Torino |
| *GAO* | [Albrecht von Graefe's] Archiv für Ophthalmologie |
| *Gast* | Gastroenterology |
| *GBMO* | Great Britain, Privy Council, Report of Medical Officer |
| *Gen* | Genetics |
| *GH* | Gazette des Hôpitaux Civils et Militaires |
| *GHR* | Guy's Hospital Reports |
| *GIMV* | Giornale Italiano delle Malattie Veneree e della Pelle |
| *GiISM* | Giornale Internazionale delle Scienze Mediche |
| *GISM* | Gazzetta Internationale de Scienze Mediche |
| *GL* | Gazeta Lekarska |
| *GMB* | Gazeta Medica da Bahia |
| *GMC* | Gazette Hebdomadaire de Médecine et de Chirurgie |
| *GMI* | Gazzetta Medica Italiana Lombardo |
| *GMIFT* | Gazzetta Medica Italiana Fed.Tosc. |
| *GMJ* | Glasgow Medical Journal |
| *GML* | Gazette Médicale de Lyon |
| *GMLi* | Gaceta Médica de Lima |
| *GMP* | Gazette Médicale de Paris |
| *GMS* | Gazette Médicale de Strasbourg |
| *GMT* | Gazzetta Medica di Torino |
| *GOC* | Gazzetta degli Ospedali (et delle Cliniche) |
| *GOCu* | Gaceta Oficial de Cumana |
| *GSMB* | Gazette Hebdomadaire des Sciences Médicales de Bordeaux |
| *GTNI* | Geneeskundig Tijdschrift voor Nederlandsch-Indie |
| | |
| *HARS* | Histoire de l'Académie Royale des Sciences |
| *HCA* | Helvetica Chimica Acta |
| *Heart* | Heart |
| *Her* | Hereditas |
| *HKA* | Heidelberger Klinische Annalen |
| *Hos* | Hospitalstidende |
| *HSZ* | Hoppe-Seyler's Zeitschrift für Physiologische Chemie |
| *Hygiea* | Hygiea (Stockholm) |
| | |
| *I* | Immunology |
| *IAMS* | Indian Annals of Medical Science |
| *IC* | International Clinics |
| *ICH* | International Congress of Hygiene and Demography, 1912, Washington |
| *IJL* | International Journal of Leprosy |
| *IJMR* | Indian Journal of Medical Research |
| *IJMS* | International Journal of Medicine and Surgery |
| *IJO* | International Journal of Orthodontia |
| *IMC* | International Medical Congress |
| *IMG* | Indian Medical Gazette |
| *IMW* | Indian Medical World |
| *IOLE* | Izvestiia Imperial Obsch. Liub. Estes |
| *IRAFC* | Informations et Rapports, Association Française de Chirurgie |
| *IS* | Ijo Shinbun |
| *IVMA* | Izvestiia Imperial Voenno-Meditsinkaiia Akademia |

| | |
|---|---|
| *JA* | Journal of Anatomy |
| *JACS* | Journal of the American Chemical Society |
| *JaK* | Jahrbuch für Kinderheilkunde |
| *JAl* | Journal of Allergy |
| *JAMA* | Journal of the American Medical Association |
| *JAnt* | Journal of Antibiotics |
| *JANVB* | Jahresberichte Akademische-Naturwissenschaftliche Vereins Breslau |
| *JaP* | Jahrbücher für Psychiatrie |
| *JB* | Journal of Bacteriology |
| *JBC* | Journal of Biological Chemistry |
| *JBDA* | Journal of the British Dental Association |
| *JBJS* | Journal of Bone and Joint Surgery |
| *JC(M)* | Journal de Chirurgie (Malgaigne) |
| *JCA* | Journal für Chirurgie und Augenheilkunde |
| *JCBMA* | Journal of the Ceylon Branch, British Medical Association |
| *JCE* | Journal of Clinical Endocrinology and Metabolism |
| *JCGu* | Journal of Cutaneous and Genito-Urinary Diseases |
| *JCI* | Journal of Clinical Investigation |
| *JCMC* | Journal des Connaissances Médico-Chirurgicales |
| *JCMP* | Journal des Connaissances Médicales Pratiques et de Pharmacologie |
| *JCP* | Journal of Clinical Pathology |
| *JCR* | Journal of Cancer Research |
| *JCS* | Journal of the Chemical Society |
| *JCuM* | Journal of Cutaneous Medicine and Diseases of the Skin (London) |
| *JEM* | Journal of Experimental Medicine |
| *JEZ* | Journal of Experimental Zoology |
| *JGM* | Journal of General Microbiology |
| *JGMC* | Journal Générale de Médecine, de Chirurgie, et de Pharmacie |
| *JGP* | Journal of General Physiology |
| *JGSB* | Journal of the Gyn(a)ecological Society of Boston |
| *JHB* | Johns Hopkins Hospital Bulletin |
| *JHR* | Johns Hopkins Hospital Reports |
| *JHyg* | Journal of Hygiene |
| *JI* | Journal of Immunology |
| *JID* | Journal of Infectious Diseases |
| *JJEM* | Japanese Journal of Experimental Medicine |
| *JKMS* | Journal of Kyoto Medical Society |
| *JLCM* | Journal of Laboratory and Clinical Medicine |
| *JLO* | Journal of Laryngology (Rhinology) and Otology |
| *JMB* | Journal of Molecular Biology |
| *JMC* | Journal of Medicinal Chemistry |
| *JMCA* | K.K. Josephinische Medicinisch-Chirurgische Academie zu Wien |
| *JMCP* | Journal de Médecine, Chirurgie, Pharmacie, etc |
| *JMF* | Journal Médical Français |
| *JMI* | Journal de Médecine Interne |
| *JMR* | Journal of Medical Research |
| *JMS* | Journal of Mental Science |
| *JMSMA* | Journal of Michigan State Medical Association |
| *JN* | Journal of Neurosurgery |
| *JNCI* | Journal of the National Cancer Institute |
| *JNMD* | Journal of Nervous and Mental Disease |

| | |
|---|---|
| *JNMS* | Journal of the National Malaria Society |
| *JNNP* | Journal of Neurology, Neurosurgery and Psychiatry. |
| *JNP* | Journal of Neurology and Psychopathology |
| *JOC* | Journal of Organic Chemistry |
| *JOG* | Journal of Obstetrics and Gynaecology of the British Empire |
| *JP* | Journal of Physiology |
| *JPAA* | Journal der Pharmacie für Aertze und Apotheker |
| *JPB* | Journal of Pathology and Bacteriology |
| *JPC* | Journal de Pharmacie et de Chimie (Paris) |
| *JPe* | Journal of Pediatrics |
| *JPE* | Journal de Physiologie Expérimentale et Pathologique (Magendie) |
| *JPET* | Journal of Pharmacology and Experimental Therapeutics |
| *JPLSZ* | Journal (and Proceedings) of the Linnean Society, Zoology |
| *JPMA* | Journal of the Philippine Medical Association |
| *JPN* | Journal für Psychologie und Neurologie |
| *JPr* | Journal des Praticiens |
| *JPrC* | Journal für Praktische Chemie |
| *JPrH* | Journal der Practisen Heilkunde |
| *JRAMC* | Journal of the Royal Army Medical Corps |
| *JSI* | Journal of the Sanitary Institute of Great Britain |
| *JSM* | Journal of State Medicine |
| *JSP* | Journal des Sçavans |
| *JT(C)S* | Journal of Thoracic (and Cardiovascular) Surgery |
| *JTM* | Journal of Tropical Medicine |
| *JU* | Journal of Urology |
| *JUMC* | Journal d'Urologie Médicale et Chirurgicale |
| *JUSM* | Journal Universel des Sciences Médicales |
| *JZN* | Jenaische Zeitschrift für Naturwissenschaft |
| | |
| *KAAV* | Korrepondenz-Blätter des Allgemeinen Aerztlichen Vereins von Thüringen |
| *KAWS* | Koninklijke Akademie van Wetenschappen, Proc.Sect.Sci. |
| *KBSA* | Korrespondenz-Blatt (Correspondenz-Blatt) für Schweizer Ärzte |
| *KJ* | Klinisches Jahrbuch |
| *KMA* | Klinische Monatsblätter für Augenheilkunde |
| *KMJ* | Königsberger medicinische Jahrbucher |
| *KW* | Klinische Wochenschrift |
| | |
| *L* | Lancet |
| *LAGH* | Litterarische Annalen der Gesammten Heilkunde |
| *LCMI* | Lavori dei Congressi di Medicina Interna |
| *LEMJ* | London and Edinburgh Monthly Journal of Medical Science |
| *LM* | Lyon Médical |
| *LMG* | London Medical Gazette |
| *LMJ* | London Medical Journal |
| *LMSJ* | London Medical and Surgical Journal (Renshaw) |
| *LR* | Leprosy Review |
| *LV* | Landwirtschaftlichen Versuchswesen |
| | |
| *MAC* | Mémoires de l'Académie de Chirurgie |
| *MADC* | Medical Annals of the District of Columbia |
| *MAM* | Mémoires de l'Académie Impériale de Médécine |

| MANM | Mémoires de l'Académie Nationale de Médecine |
|---|---|
| MARC | Mémoires de l'Académie Royale de Chirurgie |
| MARM | Mémoires de l'Académie Royale de Médecine |
| MASB | Memorie della R. Accademia delle Scienze dell'Istituto di Bologna |
| MCCD | Modern Concepts of Cardiovascular Disease |
| MCE | Miscellanea Curiosa Ephemerides Naturae Curiosum |
| MCh | Medical Chronicle |
| MCMP | Miscellanea Curiosa Medico-Physica Academia Naturae Curiosorum |
| MCNA | Medical Clinics of North America |
| MCom | Medical Commentaries |
| MCon | Medicina Contemporanea |
| MCT | Medico-Chirurgical Transactions |
| MDGN | Mitteilungen der Deutschen Gesellschaft für Natur- und Völkerkunde Ostasiens |
| Medicine | Medicine |
| MEO | Medical Essays and Observations (Edinburgh) |
| MeS | Medical Sentinel |
| MEx | Medical Examiner and Record of Medical Science |
| MGH | Magazin für die Gesammte Heilkunde |
| MGMC | Mitteilungen aus dem Grenzgebieten der Medizin und Chirurgie |
| MhC | Monatshefte für Chemie |
| MHJ | Middlesex Hospital Journal |
| MinnM | Minnesota Medicine |
| MIOC | Memorias do Instituto Oswaldo Cruz |
| MJa | Medizinische Jahrbücher |
| MJA | Medical Journal of Australia |
| MJMS | Monthly Journal of Medical Science |
| MJOS | Medicinische Jahrbücher des K.K. Österreichischen Staates |
| MK | Medizinische Klinik |
| MKG | Mitteilungen aus dem Kaiserlichen Gesundheitsamte |
| MKW | Medizinisches Korrespondenzblatt für Württemburg |
| MM | Marseille-Médical |
| MMC | Movimento Medico-Chirurgico |
| MMFK | Mitteilungen aus der Medizinischen Fakultät der Universität Kyushu (Fukuoka) |
| MMSL | Memoirs of the Medical Society of London |
| MMW | Münchener Medizinische Wochenschrift |
| MN | Medical News |
| MOA | Magyar Orvosi Archivum |
| MOI | Medical Observations and Inquiries (London) |
| MoJ | Morphologisches Jahrbuch |
| MonG | Monatsschrift für Geburtshilfe und Gynäkologie |
| MonK | Monatsschrift für Kinderheilkunde |
| MonM | Monitor Médico |
| MonO | Monatsschrift für Ohrenheilkunde |
| MonP | Monatsschrift für Psychiatrie und Neurologie |
| MPD | Monatshefte für Praktische Dermatologie |
| MR | Medical Record |
| MRC | Great Britain, Medical Research Council, Special Report Series |
| MRecorder | Medical Recorder of Original Papers and Intelligence in Medicine and Surgery |
| MRep | Medical Repository |

| | |
|---|---|
| *MRpt* | Medical Reports, Imperial Maritime Customs, China |
| *MSMB* | Mémoires et Bulletins de la Société de Médecine et de Chirurgie de Bourdeaux |
| *MSMC* | Mémoires et Comptes-Rendus de la Société des Sciences Médicales de Lyon. |
| *MSR* | Medical and Surgical Register |
| *MSRep* | Medical and Surgical Reporter |
| *MSSPL* | Mémoires de la Société des Sciences Physicales de Lausanne |
| *MTG* | Medical Times and Gazette |
| *MTr* | Medical Transactions of College of Physicians in London |
| *MTR* | Medical Times and Register |
| *MV* | Meditsinskiy Vestnik |
| *MVMJ* | Maryland and Virginia Medical Journal |
| *MZ* | Medicinische Zeitung |
| | |
| *NAL* | Nelson's American Lancet |
| *NAMR* | North American Medico-Chirurgical Review |
| *Nat* | Naturwissenschaften |
| *Nature* | Nature |
| *NCASP* | Novi Commentariis Academiae Scientiarum Petropolitariae |
| *NCIM* | National Cancer Institute Monographs |
| *NEJM* | New England Journal of Medicine |
| *NEJMS* | New England Journal of Medicine and Surgery |
| *NEQJ* | New England Quarterly Journal of Medicine and Surgery |
| *NIC* | New International Clinics |
| *NIS* | Nouvelle Iconographie de la Salpêtrière |
| *NM* | Northwestern Medicine |
| *NML* | Norsk Magasin for Laegevidenskaben |
| *NNGN* | Neue Notizen aus dem Gebiete der Natur- und Heilkunde |
| *NoM* | Nordisk Medicin |
| *NoMA* | Nordiskt Medicinskt Arkiv |
| *NOMSJ* | New Orleans Medical and Surgical Journal |
| *NoMT* | Nordisk Medicinsk Tidskrift |
| *NPL* | Nobel Prize Lectures [Since 1901 the Nobel Foundation has published annually *Les Prix Nobel*, which includes the Lectures given by the laureates, together with biographies. The right to publish this material in English was given to Elsevier Publishing, who produced separate volumes covering Physiology or Medicine (4 vols), Chemistry (4 vols), Physics (4 vols), Literature (1 vol.), and Peace (3 vols), for the period 1901–1970. Later volumes (covering 10 year periods), are published by World Scientific Publishing.] |
| *NTG* | Nederlandsch Tijdschrift voor Geneeskunde |
| *NTT* | Nordisk Tidsskrift for Terapi |
| *Nuc* | Nucleonics |
| *NYJM* | New York Journal of Medicine |
| *NYMJ* | New York Medical Journal |
| *NYMM* | New York Medical Monatschrift |
| *NYMPJ* | New York Medical and Physical Journal |
| *NYUPG* | New York University Post-Graduate Medical School Inter-Clinic Information Bulletin |
| *NZ* | Neurologisches Zentralblatt |
| | |
| *OHP* | Ophthalmic Hospital Reports |
| *OJP* | Österreichisches Jahrbuch für Pädiatrik |

| Oph | Ophthalmoscope |
|---|---|
| OR | Ophthalmic Review Science |
| OrH | Orvosi Hetilap |
| Oss | Osservatore |
| OZPH | Österreichische Zeitschrift für Praktische Heilkunde |
| | |
| PAMC | Pan-American Medical Congress, Transactions |
| PANS | Proceedings of the Academy of Natural Sciences of Philadelphia |
| Para | Parasitology |
| PBSW | Proceedings of the Biological Society of Washington |
| PCAM | Proceedings of the California Academy of Medicine |
| PCPS | Proceedings of the Cambridge Philosophical Society |
| Ped | Pediatrics |
| PfA | Pflüger's Archiv für die Gesamte Physiologie |
| PGBMD | Proceedings of the Government of Bengal Medical Department |
| PhaZ | Pharmazeutische Zeitung |
| PhJ | Pharmaceutical Journal |
| PhJMS | Philadelphia Journal of the Medical and Physical Sciences |
| PhJS | Philippine Journal of Science |
| PhMeJ | Philadelphia Medical Journal |
| PhMoJ | Philadelphia Monthly Journal of Medicine and Surgery |
| PhMT | Philadelphia Medical Times |
| PhZ | Physikalische Zeitschrift |
| PIAJ | Proceedings of the Imperial Academy of Japan |
| PJDS | Pennsylvania Journal of Dental Science |
| PMC | Proceedings of the Staff Meetings of the Mayo Clinic |
| PMCP | Pester Medizinisch-Chirurgische Presse |
| PMW | Prager Medizinische Wochenschrift |
| PNAS | Proceedings of the National Academy of Sciences, USA |
| PNW | Psychiatrisch-Neurologische Wochenschrift |
| PNYP | Proceedings of the New York Pathological Society |
| PPSS | Proceedings of the Pathological Society of Philadelphia |
| Prac | Practitioner |
| PrM | Presse Médicale |
| PRMCS | Proceedings of the Royal Medical and Chirurgical Society of London |
| ProM | Progrès Médical |
| PRS | Proceedings of the Royal Society of London |
| PRSE | Proceedings of the Royal Society of Edinburgh |
| PRSM | Proceedings of the Royal Society of Medicine |
| Przl | Przeglad Lekarski |
| PsA | Psychologische Arbeiten |
| PSEB | Proceedings of the Society for Experimental Biology and Medicine |
| PSM | Popular Science Monthly |
| PsR | Physical Review |
| PT | Philosophical Transactions of the Royal Society of London |
| PVC | Procès Verbaux, Congrès (Association) Français de Chirurgie |
| | |
| QJM | Quarterly Journal of Medicine |
| QJMS | Quarterly Journal of Microscopical Science |
| QSGN | Quellen und Studien zur Geschichte der Naturwissenschaften und der Medizin |
| QSVH | Quarterly Bulletin, Sea View Hospital, New York |

| | |
|---|---|
| *Rad* | Radiology |
| *RAMA* | Revista de la Asociación Médica Argentina |
| *RAPM* | Revista da Associacão Paulista de Medicina |
| *RC* | Revue de Chirurgie |
| *RCB* | Rivista Clinica di Bologna |
| *RCP* | Rivista di Clinica Pediatrica |
| *RCSL* | Réunions Cliniques, Hôpital St Louis, Comptes Rendus |
| *RDNSW* | Report of the Director General of Public Health, New South Wales |
| *ReM* | Revue de Médecine |
| *ReMP* | Recueil Périodique de la Société de Médecine de Paris |
| *ReN* | Revue Neurologique |
| *ReO* | Recueil d'Ophtalmologie |
| *RGAP* | Répertoire Général d'Anatomie et de Physiologie Pathologique, et des Cliniques Chirurgicales |
| *RIER* | Revue Internationale d'Electrothérapie et de Radiothérapie |
| *RIL* | Rendiconti R. Istituto Lombardo di Scienze e Lettere |
| *RIM* | Rockefeller Institute for Medical Research, New York, Monographs on Medical and Allied Subjects |
| *RISP* | Rivista di Igiene e Sanità Pubblica |
| *RISS* | Rendiconti dell'Istituto Superiore di Sanità |
| *RMFE* | Revue Médicale Française et Étrangère |
| *RMSR* | Revue Médicale de la Suisse Romande |
| *Roux* | Wilhelm Roux' Archiv für Entwicklungsmechanik der Organismen |
| *RPH* | Reports on Public Health and Medical Subjects, Great Britain, Ministry of Health |
| *RPN* | Rivista di Patologia Nervosa e Mentale |
| *RR* | Radiophysiologie et Radiothérapie |
| *RSAB* | Revista de la Sociedad Argentina de Biologia |
| *RSI* | Report of the Smithsonian Institution |
| *RSM* | Revista de Sanidad Militar |
| | |
| *SAH* K | Svenska Vetenskapsakademien, Handlingar |
| *SAMJ* | South African Medical Journal |
| *SAW* | Sitzungsberichte, K. Akademie der Wissenschaften, Mathematisch-Naturwissenschaftliche Klasse |
| *SBHR* | St Bartholomew's Hospital Reports |
| *SBJH* | Studies, Biological Laboratory, Johns Hopkins University |
| *Science* | Science |
| *SCNA* | Surgical Clinics of North America |
| *SF* | Surgical Forum |
| *SGHR* | St George's Hospital Reports |
| *SGO* | Surgery, Gynecology, and Obstetrics |
| *SIMR* | Studies, Institute for Medical Research, Federated Malay States |
| *SK* | Sbornik Klinicky |
| *SKAP* | Skandinavisches Archiv für Physiologie |
| *SKU* | Schriften Kieler Universität |
| *SKV* | Sammlung Klinischer Vorträge |
| *SMB* | Semana Médica |
| *SMI* | Scientific Memoirs of Medical Officers of the Army of India |
| *SMJ* | Southern Medical Journal |
| *SMM* | Siglo Médico (Madrid) |

| | |
|---|---|
| *SMP* | Semaine Médical |
| *SMSJ* | Southern Medical and Surgical Journal |
| *SMW* | Schweizerische Medizinische Wochenschrift |
| *Spe* | Sperimentale |
| *SPKG* | Sitzungsberichte, Physikalisch-Medicinische Gesellschaft |
| *SPMW* | Saint Petersburger Medicinische Wochenschrift |
| *Str* | Strahlentherapie |
| *Surgery* | Surgery |
| *SVMG* | Stethoscope and Virginia Medical Gazette |
| | |
| *TAAG* | Transactions of the American Association of Genito-Urinary Surgeons |
| *TAAP* | Transactions of the Association of American Physicians |
| *Tab* | Tabulae Biologicae |
| *TADA* | Transactions of the American Dermatological Association |
| *TAGS* | Transactions of the American Gynecological Society |
| *TALA* | Transactions of the American Laryngological Association |
| *TAMA* | Transactions of the American Medical Association |
| *TAMC* | Transactions of the Australasian Medical Congress |
| *TAOrA* | Transactions of the American Orthopedic Association |
| *TAOS* | Transactions of the American Ophthalmological Society |
| *TASAO* | Transactions of the American Society for Artificial Internal Organs |
| *TB* | Tuberkulose-Bibliothek |
| *TCAP* | Transactions of the College of American Physicians and Surgeons |
| *TCPS* | Transactions of the Cambridge Philosophical Society |
| *TCSL* | Transactions of the Clinical Society of London |
| *TGe* | Therapie der Gegenwart |
| *THI* | Treasury of Human Inheritance |
| *Thorax* | Thorax |
| *TIMS* | Transactions of the Indiana State Medical Society |
| *TKMS* | Transactions of the Kentucky Medical Society |
| *TLS* | Transactions of the Linnean Society of London |
| *TM* | Therapeutische Monatshefte |
| *TMAG* | Transactions of Medical Association of Georgia |
| *TMCS* | Transactions of the Medico-Chirurgical Society of Edinburgh |
| *TMPB* | Transactions of the Medical and Physical Society of Bombay |
| *TNYM* | Transactions of the New York Medical Society |
| *TOSA* | Transactions of the Ophthalmological Society of Australia |
| *TOSG* | Transactions of the Odontological Society of Great Britain |
| *TOSL* | Transactions of the Obstetrical Society of London |
| *TOUK* | Transactions of the Ophthalmological Society of the United Kingdom |
| *TPNY* | Transactions of the Physico-Medical Society of New York |
| *TPS* | Transactions of the Pathological Society of London |
| *TrB* | Transplantation Bulletin |
| *TrJM* | Transylvania Journal of Medicine |
| *TRP* | Times and Register, Philadelphia |
| *TRSE* | Transactions of the Royal Society of Edinburgh |
| *TRSS* | Transactions of the Royal Society of South Africa |
| *TRST* | Transactions of the Royal Society of Tropical Medicine and Hygiene |
| *TSIK* | Transactions of Sei-I-Kwai |
| *TSIM* | Transactions of the Society for the Improvement of Medical and Chirurgical Knowledge |

| | |
|---|---|
| *TSSA* | Transactions of the Southern Surgical and Gynecological Association |
| *TYL* | Thompson Yates Laboratory Report, Liverpool University |
| *TZS* | Transactions of the Zoological Society of London |
| | |
| *UL* | Ugeskrift for Laeger |
| *ULF* | Uppsala Läkareforenings Forhandlingar |
| *UM* | Union Médicale |
| *UMM* | University Medical Magazine [Philadelphia] |
| *UPIH* | Untersuchungen der Physiologisches Institut, Universität Heidelberg |
| *UPMB* | University of Pennsylvania Medical Bulletin |
| *USPHB* | Public Health Bulletin, USA |
| *USPHL* | Public Health Service Laboratory Bulletin, USA |
| *USPHR* | Public Health Reports, USA |
| | |
| *VA* | Virchow's Archiv für Pathologische Anatomie und Physiologie |
| *VBG* | Verhandelingen, Bataavisch Genootschap van Kunsten en Wetenschappen |
| *VBMG* | Verhandlungen der Berliner Medizinischen Gesellschaft |
| *VDDG* | Verhandlungen der Deutschen Dermatologischen Gesellschaft |
| *VDGC* | Verhandlungen der Deutschen Gesellschaft für Chirurgie |
| *VDGG* | Verhandlungen der Deutschen Gesellschaft für Gynäkologie |
| *VDI* | Venereal Disease Information |
| *VDK* | Verhandlungen des (Deutschen) Kongresses für Innere Medizin |
| *VDOG* | Verhandlungen der Deutschen Otologischen Gesellschaft |
| *VDPG* | Verhandlungen der Deutschen Pathologischen Gesellschaft |
| *VDS* | Vierteljahrsschrift für Dermatologie und Syphilis |
| *VGDA* | Verhandlungen der Gesellschaft der Deutscher Naturforscher und Aerzte |
| *VGK* | Verhandlungen der Gesellschaft für Kinderheilkunde |
| *Vir* | Virology |
| *VJ* | Veterinary Journal and Annals of Comparative Pathology |
| *VJPG* | Verhandlungen der Japanischen Pathologischen Gesellschaft |
| *VK* | Vestnik Khirurgii i Pogranichnykh Oblastei |
| *VKP* | Vestnik Klinicheski Psichiatri |
| *VMZ* | Voenno-Meditsinskii Zhurnal |
| *VNMV* | Verhandlungen des Naturhistorisch-Medizinischen Vereins zu Heidelberg |
| *VNVB* | Verhandlungen des Naturforschenden Vereins in Brünn |
| *VO* | Vestnik Oftalmologiya |
| *VPH* | Vierteljahrsschrift für die Praktische Heilkunde |
| *VPMG* | Verhandlungen der Physikalisch-Medizinischen Gesellschaft zu Würzberg |
| *Vrach* | Vrach |
| | |
| *WGH* | Wochenschrift für die Gesammte Heilkunde |
| *WGS* | Western Journal of Surgery, Obstetrics, and Gynecology |
| *WKR* | Wiener Klinische Rundschau |
| *WKW* | Wiener Klinische Wochenschrift |
| *WMP* | Wiener Medizinische Presse |
| *WMW* | Wiener Medizinische Wochenschrift |
| | |
| *ZAngC* | Zeitschrift für Angewandte Chemie |
| *ZAP* | Zentralblatt für Allgemeine Pathologie und Pathologische Anatomie |
| *ZBP* | Zentralblatt für Bakteriologie und Parasitenkunde |
| *ZC* | Zentralblatt für Chirurgie |

784

| | |
|---|---|
| *ZChem* | Zeitschrift für Chemotherapie und Verwandte Gebiete |
| *ZenKM* | Zentralblatt für Klinische Medicin |
| *ZEP* | Zeitschrift für Experimentelle Pathologie und Therapie |
| *ZGA* | Zeitschrift der K.K. Gesellschaft der Ärzte zu Wien |
| *ZGG* | Zeitschrift für Geburtshülfe und Gynäkologie |
| *ZGH* | Zentralblatt für die Gesamte Hygiene |
| *ZGN* | Zeitschrift für die Gesamte Neurologie und Psychiatrie |
| *ZGy* | Zentralblatt für Gynäkologie |
| *ZHe* | Zeitschrift für Heilkunde |
| *ZHyg* | Zeitschrift für Hygiene und Infektionskrankheiten |
| *ZI* | Zeitschrift für Immunitätsforschung und Experimentelle Therapie |
| *ZK* | Zeitschrift für Kinderheilkunde (Berlin) |
| *ZKH* | Zentralblatt für die Medizinischen Wissenschaften |
| *ZKM* | Zeitschrift für Klinische Medizin |
| *ZKr* | Zeitschrift für Krebsforschung |
| *ZN* | Zentralblatt für Neurochirurgie |
| *ZOC* | Zeitschrift für Orthopädische Chirurgie |
| *ZOh* | Zeitschrift für Ohrenheilkunde |
| *ZPAu* | Zentralblatt für Praktische Augenheilkunde |
| *ZPPS* | Zeitschrift für Psychologie und Physiologie der Sinnesorgane |
| *ZRM* | Zeitschrift für Rationelle Medizin |
| *ZTb* | Zeitschrift für Tuberkulose |
| *ZTM* | Zeitschrift für Thiermedizin |
| *ZWZ* | Zeitschrift für Wissenschaftliche Zoologie |
| *ZZ* | Zeitschrift für Zellforschung und Mikroskopische Anatomie |